T0295020

THE REQUISITES

Thoracic Imaging

The Requisites Series

SERIES EDITOR

James H. Thrall, MD
Radiologist-in-Chief Emeritus
Massachusetts General Hospital
Distinguished Juan M. Taveras Professor of Radiology
Harvard Medical School
Boston, Massachusetts

TITLES IN THE SERIES

Breast Imaging
Cardiac Imaging
Emergency Imaging
Gastrointestinal Imaging
Genitourinary Imaging
Musculoskeletal Imaging
Neuroradiology Imaging
Nuclear Medicine
Pediatric Imaging
Radiology Noninterpretive Skills
Thoracic Imaging
Ultrasound
Vascular and Interventional Imaging

THE REQUISITES

Thoracic Imaging

THIRD EDITION

Edited by

Jo-Anne O. Shepard, MD
Professor of Radiology
Harvard Medical School;
Director, Thoracic Imaging and Intervention
Director, Cardiothoracic Imaging Fellowship
Massachusetts General Hospital
Department of Radiology
Boston, Massachusetts

Associate Editors

Gerald F. Abbott, MD
Associate Professor of Radiology
Harvard Medical School;
Radiologist, Thoracic Imaging and Intervention
Department of Radiology
Massachusetts General Hospital
Boston, Massachusetts

Jeanne B. Ackman, MD, FACR
Assistant Professor of Radiology
Harvard Medical School;
Radiologist, Thoracic Imaging and Intervention
Director, Thoracic MRI
Department of Radiology
Massachusetts General Hospital
Boston, Massachusetts

Subba R. Digumarthy, MBBS
Assistant Professor of Radiology
Radiologist, Thoracic Imaging and Intervention
Division Quality Director, Thoracic Imaging
Department of Radiology
Massachusetts General Hospital
Harvard Medical School
Boston, Massachusetts

Matthew D. Gilman, MD
Assistant Professor of Radiology
Harvard Medical School;
Associate Director, Thoracic Imaging and Intervention
Associate Director, Cardiothoracic Imaging Fellowship
Department of Radiology
Massachusetts General Hospital
Boston, Massachusetts

Anita Sharma, MD, MBBS
Assistant Professor of Radiology
Harvard Medical School;
Radiologist, Thoracic Imaging and Intervention Division
Department of Radiology
Massachusetts General Hospital
Boston, Massachusetts

Carol C. Wu, MD
Associate Professor of Diagnostic Radiology
University of Texas MD Anderson Cancer Center
Houston, Texas

ELSEVIER

ELSEVIER

1600 John F. Kennedy Blvd.
Ste 1800
Philadelphia, PA 19103-2899

THORACIC IMAGING : THE REQUISITES, 3rd edition ISBN: 978-0-323-44886-4

Notices

Knowledge and best practice in this field are constantly changing. As new research and experience broaden our understanding, changes in research methods, professional practices, or medical treatment may become necessary.

Practitioners and researchers must always rely on their own experience and knowledge in evaluating and using any information, methods, compounds, or experiments described herein. In using such information or methods they should be mindful of their own safety and the safety of others, including parties for whom they have a professional responsibility.

With respect to any drug or pharmaceutical products identified, readers are advised to check the most current information provided (i) on procedures featured or (ii) by the manufacturer of each product to be administered, to verify the recommended dose or formula, the method and duration of administration, and contraindications. It is the responsibility of practitioners, relying on their own experience and knowledge of their patients, to make diagnoses, to determine dosages and the best treatment for each individual patient, and to take all appropriate safety precautions.

To the fullest extent of the law, neither the Publisher nor the authors, contributors, or editors, assume any liability for any injury and/or damage to persons or property as a matter of products liability, negligence or otherwise, or from any use or operation of any methods, products, instructions, or ideas contained in the material herein.

Library of Congress Cataloging-in-Publication Data
Names: Shepard, Jo-Anne O., editor. | Preceded by (work): McLoud, Theresa C. Thoracic radiology.
Title: Thoracic imaging / edited by Jo-Anne O. Shepard; associate editors, Gerald F. Abbott, Jeanne B. Ackman, Subba Digumarthy, Matthew D. Gilman, Amita Sharma, Carol C. Wu.
Other titles: Thoracic imaging (Shepard) | Requisites series.
Description: Third edition. | Philadelphia, PA : Elsevier, [2019] | Series: Requisites series | Preceded by Thoracic radiology / Theresa McLoud, Phillip Boiselle. 2nd ed. c2010. | Includes bibliographical references and index.
Identifiers: LCCN 2017042687 | ISBN 9780323448864 (hardcover : alk. paper)
Subjects: | MESH: Thoracic Diseases–diagnostic imaging | Lung Diseases–diagnostic imaging | Radiography, Thoracic–methods
Classification: LCC RC941 | NLM WF 975 | DDC 617.5/407572-dc23 LC record available at https://lccn.loc.gov/2017042687

Content Strategist: Robin Carter
Content Development Specialist: Ann Anderson
Publishing Services Manager: Patricia Tannian
Project Manager: Ted Rodgers
Design Direction: Amy Buxton

Printed in the United States of America

Last digit is the print number: 9 8 7 6 5 4 3

To my husband Bill
and our children Sarah, John, and Bobby
with whose love and support all is possible

To my parents
Anne and John O'Malley
for their inspiration

Jo-Anne O'Malley Shepard, MD

In memory of our friends and colleagues
Henry J. Llewellyn, MD (1937-2009)
Beatrice Trotman-Dickenson, MBBS (1957-2015)
Joan Curran Dow (1949-2016)

Foreword

It is a pleasure to help introduce the Third Edition of *Thoracic Radiology: The Requisites*. Thoracic imaging is a cornerstone of radiology practice that touches more patients than any other area of sub-specialization in radiology. Many of the same technological innovations and advancements that have propelled other areas of radiology forward in the last several years have also substantially changed the landscape in thoracic imaging, making the publication of the Third Edition timely and important.

Dr. Jo-Anne O. Shepard is the editor of the new edition and has assembled a terrific team of co-editors and authors. In this regard, the Third Edition of *Thoracic Radiology: The Requisites* reflects an important trend in authorship. The original books were each written by a small number of people, many with only one or two authors. Over time, the breadth and complexity of each topic have increased to the point that a multi-author approach is now appropriate for the level of expertise required. Doctors Gerald F. Abbott, Jeanne B. Ackman, Subba R. Digmurthy, Mathew D. Gilman, Amita Sharma, and Carol C. Wu serve as Associate Editors for this edition. Additional contributing authors include Manudeep Kalra, Alexi Otraji, Melissa Price, Bojan Kovacina, Lan Qian (Lancia) Guo, Brett W. Carter, Mylene Truong, Christopher M. Walker, Susan Gutschow, Shaunagh McDermott, Efren J. Flores, Laura L. Avery, John W. Nance, Hristina Natcheva, Thomas Keimig, Jonathan Chung, Rydhwana Hossain, Victorine V. Muse, Milena Petranovic, Florian J. Fintelmann, Bradley S. Sabloff and Justin Stowell. It is difficult to imagine a stronger group of contributors. Dr. Shepard and her co-authors are to be congratulated on producing a high-quality book that will be both practical and manageable for the reader.

The format and layout of *Thoracic Radiology: The Requisites* remain largely intact with early chapters on technique and normal anatomy and chapters covering major diseases and conditions. However, several new chapters address advances in technology and provide for deeper coverage of increasingly specialized clinical applications. For example, in the interval since publication of the Second Edition of *Thoracic Radiology: The Requisites*, the National Lung Screening Trial (NLST) demonstrated that screening for lung cancer in a defined population saves lives. This was a major milestone in medical practice that has created important opportunities for thoracic radiologists but also challenges related to adopting best practices for screening and correct application of the lung cancer staging system. Correspondingly there are two chapters in this book that address these issues, one on screening and one on staging.

The digital transformation in radiology is now substantially complete. This transformation is fully incorporated into the Third Edition of *Thoracic Radiology: The Requisites*, including a chapter that covers PET/CT and PET/MR. While PET/CT is well established in thoracic imaging, especially for cancer diagnosis and follow-up, the potential for PET/MR is just becoming more widely available. Many of the chapters with familiar titles are now more richly illustrated with digital images with corresponding emphasis on high-resolution cross-sectional methods. The associated improvements in both image quality and diagnostic capabilities are highlighted.

The Requisites books are not intended to be exhaustive. There are "mega" reference texts that catalog rare and unusual cases and that present different sides of controversies. Rather, *The Requisites* books are intended to provide information on the conditions that radiologists see every day, the ones that are at the core of radiology practice. In fact, one of the requests to authors is to not look up anything unusual or obscure but to put in the book what they teach their own residents every day at the workstation. Since the authors are experienced experts in their respective areas, this is predictably the most important material.

The Requisites series is now well over 25 years old and has served thousands of radiologists. The books are familiar and trusted friends to many people. It is my hope and expectation that radiology trainees as well as practicing radiologists seeking to refresh their knowledge will find the Third Edition of *Thoracic Radiology: The Requisites* a useful text.

James H. Thrall, MD
Radiologist-in-Chief, Emeritus
Massachusetts General Hospital
Distinguished Taveras Professor of Radiology
Harvard Medical School

Preface

It is an honor and a privilege to be the Editor of the Third Edition of *Thoracic Imaging: The Requisites.* The prior editions, edited by Theresa McLoud and Philip Boiselle, have been embraced by students and practitioners of thoracic imaging throughout the world as a reliable source for the essentials of state-of-the-art thoracic imaging.

Much has changed since the earlier editions in 1998 and 2010. *Thoracic Requisites* has been rewritten to encompass a host of new imaging and interventional techniques, up-to-date disease classifications and staging, current approaches to diagnosis and management, and radiation dose reduction strategies. The content has been arranged into 25 focused chapters. An integrated approach to learning normal chest anatomy contains correlative radiographic and CT images. There is new material on acute and critical care imaging, including post-operative complications, trauma, ICU diagnosis, and implantable devices. There is extensive new information on thoracic MRI indications, protocols, and case material, as well as expanded content on interstitial lung disease, infections, and vascular diseases. Updated lung cancer coverage includes new tumor staging and diagnostic techniques, lung cancer screening, and updated pulmonary nodule management strategies. State-of-the-art interventional content includes diagnostic thoracic biopsy techniques, fiducial placement to aid VATS surgical resection of small pulmonary nodules, and ablative therapies for local control of thoracic tumors. More than 1000 new images encompass current digital radiographs, MDCT images including HRCT, and dual energy CT scanning, FDG-PET/CT, and PET/MRI. The content has been enhanced by many new diagrams and illustrations in full color. New tables and boxes contain concise differential diagnoses and diagnostic information.

In the tradition of the *Requisites* series, *Thoracic Imaging* is designed to provide a requisite curriculum in thoracic imaging for residents and fellows in radiology and allied specialties, as well as practicing radiologists and other healthcare providers. Thoracic imaging is growing as a specialty, and the demand for expertise is increasing within both hospital and community practices. *Thoracic Imaging: The Requisites* will be an invaluable educational resource for all involved in the diagnosis of thoracic disease.

Jo-Anne O. Shepard, MD

Contributors

Gerald F. Abbott, MD, FACR
Associate Professor of Radiology
Harvard Medical School;
Radiologist, Thoracic Imaging and Intervention
Department of Radiology
Massachusetts General Hospital
Boston, Massachusetts
Chapter 2, Normal Anatomy and Atelectasis
Chapter 16, Mycobacterial Infection
Chapter 17, Approach to Diffuse Lung Disease: Anatomic Basis and High-Resolution Computed Tomography

Jeanne B. Ackman, MD, FACR
Assistant Professor of Radiology
Harvard Medical School;
Radiologist, Thoracic Imaging and Intervention
Director, Thoracic MRI
Department of Radiology
Massachusetts General Hospital
Boston, Massachusetts
Chapter 3, Thoracic Magnetic Resonance Imaging: Technique and Approach to Diagnosis
Chapter 5, The Mediastinum
Chapter 7, The Pleura, Diaphragm, and Chest Wall
Chapter 13, Thoracic Trauma

Laura L. Avery, MD
Assistant Professor of Radiology
Harvard Medical School;
Associate Director, Emergency Radiology
Radiology Clerkship Director
Department of Radiology
Massachusetts General Hospital
Boston, Massachusetts
Chapter 13, Thoracic Trauma

Brett W. Carter, MD
Assistant Professor of Diagnostic Radiology
Quality Officer, Diagnostic Imaging
Director, CT and MRI
Clinical Co-Director, Quantitative Imaging Analysis Core
The University of Texas MD Anderson Cancer Center
Houston, Texas
Chapter 6, The Airways
Chapter 20, Obstructive Lung Diseases
Chapter 21, Pulmonary Tumors and Lymphoproliferative Disorders

Jonathan Chung, MD
Associate Professor of Radiology
Interim Chief of Quality
Section Chief, Thoracic Radiology
Department of Radiology
The University of Chicago Medicine
Chicago, Illinois
Chapter 18, Diffuse Lung Diseases

Subba R. Digumarthy, MD
Assistant Professor of Radiology
Radiologist, Thoracic Imaging and Intervention
Division Quality Director, Thoracic Imaging
Department of Radiology
Massachusetts General Hospital
Boston, Massachusetts
Chapter 1, Radiological Techniques and Dose Reduction Strategies in Chest Imaging
Chapter 4, PET-CT and PET-MRI: Technique, Pitfalls, and Findings
Chapter 12, The Postoperative Chest
Chapter 19, Pneumoconioses
Chapter 22, Incidental Pulmonary Nodule
Chapter 24, Lung Cancer Staging

Florian J. Fintelmann, MD
Assistant Professor of Radiology
Harvard Medical School;
Radiologist, Thoracic Imaging and Intervention
Department of Radiology
Massachusetts General Hospital
Boston, Massachusetts
Chapter 25, Interventional Techniques

Efren J. Flores, MD
Instructor of Radiology
Harvard Medical School;
Radiologist, Emergency Radiology
Director, Radiology Community Health Improvement
Department of Radiology
Massachusetts General Hospital
Boston, Massachusetts
Chapter 13, Thoracic Trauma

Matthew D. Gilman, MD
Assistant Professor of Radiology
Harvard Medical School;
Associate Director, Thoracic Imaging and Intervention
Associate Director, Cardiothoracic Imaging Fellowship
Department of Radiology
Massachusetts General Hospital
Boston, Massachusetts
Chapter 8, Congenital Thoracic Malformations
Chapter 9, Thoracic Lines and Tubes
Chapter 11, Pulmonary Embolus and Pulmonary Vascular Diseases

Lan Qian (Lancia) Guo, MD, FRCP(C)
Radiologist, Division of Cardiothoracic Imaging
Department of Medical Imaging
University of Toronto
Sunnybrook Health Sciences Centre
Toronto, Ontario, Canada
Chapter 5, The Mediastinum
Chapter 7, The Pleura, Diaphragm, and Chest Wall

Susan Gutschow, MD
Clinical Assistant Professor of Radiology
University of Missouri-Kansas City
Kansas City, Missouri
Chapter 10, Acute Thoracic Conditions in the Intensive Care Unit

Rydhwana Hossain, MD
Assistant Professor of Diagnostic Radiology and Nuclear Medicine
University of Maryland School of Medicine
Baltimore, Maryland
Chapter 19, Pneumoconioses

Mannudeep Kalra, MD, DNB
Associate Professor of Radiology
Harvard Medical School;
Radiologist, Thoracic and Cardiac Imaging
Director, Webster Center for Advanced Radiation Research and Education
Department of Radiology
Massachusetts General Hospital
Boston, Massachusetts
Chapter 1, Radiological Techniques and Dose Reduction Strategies in Chest Imaging

Thomas Keimig, MD
Radiologist
Henry Ford Hospital
Detroit, Michigan
Chapter 16, Mycobacterial Infection

Bojan Kovacina, MDCM
Assistant Professor of Radiology
McGill University;
Radiologist
Jewish General Hospital
Montreal, Quebec, Canada
Chapter 4, PET-CT and PET-MRI: Technique, Pitfalls, and Findings
Chapter 12, The Postoperative Chest
Chapter 24, Lung Cancer Staging

Suzanne Loomis, MS, FBCA
Production Supervisor
Radiology Education Media Services (REMS);
Department of Radiology
Massachusetts General Hospital
Boston, Massachusetts
Medical Illustrations

Shaunagh McDermott, MB, BCh, BAO, FFR, (RCSI)
Assistant Professor of Radiology
Harvard Medical School;
Radiologist, Thoracic Imaging and Intervention
Massachusetts General Hospital
Boston, Massachusetts
Chapter 11, Pulmonary Embolus and Pulmonary Vascular Diseases
Chapter 23, Lung Cancer Screening

Victorine V. Muse, MD
Assistant Professor of Radiology
Harvard Medical School;
Radiologist, Thoracic Imaging and Intervention
Department of Radiology
Massachusetts General Hospital
Boston, Massachusetts
Chapter 19, Pneumoconioses

John W. Nance, MD
Assistant Professor of Radiology
Director of Cardiovascular CT
Medical University of South Carolina
Charleston, South Carolina
Chapter 14, Community-Acquired Pneumonia

Hristina Natcheva, MD
Assistant Professor of Radiology
Boston University School of Medicine;
Radiologist, Department of Radiology
Boston Medical Center
Boston, Massachusetts
Chapter 15, Pulmonary Disease in the Immunocompromised Patient

Alexi Otrakji, MD
Research Fellow
Harvard Medical School;
Clinical Fellow in Radiology
Department of Radiology
Massachusetts General Hospital;
Research Fellow
Harvard Medical School
Boston, Massachusetts
Chapter 1, Radiological Techniques and Dose Reduction Strategies in Chest Imaging

Milena Petranovic, MD
Instructor of Radiology
Harvard Medical School
Radiologist, Thoracic Imaging and Intervention
Department of Radiology
Massachusetts General Hospital
Boston, Massachusetts
Chapter 22, Incidental Pulmonary Nodule

Melissa Price, MD
Instructor of Radiology
Harvard Medical School
Radiologist, Thoracic Imaging and Intervention
Department of Radiology
Massachusetts General Hospital
Boston, Massachusetts
Chapter 2, Normal Anatomy and Atelectasis

Amita Sharma, MD
Assistant Professor of Radiology
Harvard Medical School
Radiologist, Thoracic Imaging and Intervention
Department of Radiology
Massachusetts General Hospital
Boston, Massachusetts
Chapter 17, Approach to Diffuse Lung Disease: Anatomic Basis and High-Resolution Computed Tomography
Chapter 18, Diffuse Lung Diseases
Chapter 23, Lung Cancer Screening

Jo-Anne O. Shepard, MD
Professor of Radiology
Harvard Medical School;
Director, Thoracic Imaging and Intervention
Director, Cardiothoracic Imaging Fellowship
Massachusetts General Hospital
Department of Radiology
Boston, Massachusetts
Chapter 2, Normal Anatomy and Atelectasis
Chapter 6, The Airways
Chapter 16, Mycobacterial Infection
Chapter 20, Obstructive Lung Diseases
Chapter 23, Lung Cancer Screening
Chapter 25, Interventional Techniques

Bradley S. Sabloff, MD
Professor of Diagnostic Radiology
University of Texas MD Anderson Cancer Center
Houston, Texas
Chapter 21, Pulmonary Tumors and Lymphoproliferative Disorders

Justin Stowell, MD
Resident
Department of Radiology
University of Missouri-Kansas City
Kansas City, Missouri
Chapter 8, Congenital Thoracic Malformations

Mylene T. Truong, MD
Professor of Diagnostic Imaging
Section Chief of Thoracic Imaging
University of Texas MD Anderson Cancer Center
Houston, Texas
Chapter 6, The Airways
Chapter 21, Pulmonary Tumors and Lymphoproliferative Disorders

Christopher M. Walker, MD
Associate Professor of Radiology
University of Missouri-Kansas City;
Saint Luke's Hospital
Kansas City, Missouri
Chapter 8, Congenital Thoracic Malformations
Chapter 10, Acute Thoracic Conditions in the Intensive Care Unit

Carol C. Wu, MD
Associate Professor of Diagnostic Radiology
University of Texas MD Anderson Cancer Center
Houston, Texas
Chapter 6, The Airways
Chapter 20, Obstructive Lung Diseases
Chapter 21, Pulmonary Tumors and Lymphoproliferative Disorders

Contents

Acknowledgments

Massachusetts General Hospital has a long and venerable history of excellence in thoracic imaging. Many of the early icons in chest imaging were faculty at MGH, including Drs. Ross Golden, Aubrey Otis Hampton, and Felix Fleischner, whose radiographic signs we still acknowledge today and are referenced in this book. I was fortunate to have trained at MGH with Drs. Reginald Greene, Paul Stark, and Theresa McLoud, and as a fellow with Robert Pugatch, to whom I am most grateful for their outstanding teaching, mentoring, and leadership. In the MGH tradition of educational excellence, we have collectively trained hundreds of residents and fellows in thoracic imaging, many of whom are recognized today as leaders in the field both nationally and internationally.

This book would not have been possible without the help of my current and former colleagues in the Thoracic Division at MGH. The Associate Editors, Drs. Gerald Abbott, Jeanne Ackman, Subba Digumarthy, Matthew Gilman, Amita Sharma, and Carol Wu, have generously provided their expertise, creativity, and direction in producing this new, updated edition. I am thankful to all the contributing authors who have hailed from MGH as faculty, fellows, or trainees. A special thanks to Suzanne Loomis, a gifted medical illustrator, who has graced this edition with beautiful color illustrations, and to Dr. Gerald Abbott, who has artfully enhanced the images.

I am most grateful to Dr. Juan Taveras, who as Chairman of Radiology at Massachusetts General Hospital appointed me as faculty in the Thoracic Division at MGH, understanding the value of subspecialization in radiology. A special thanks to Dr. James Thrall, who as Chairman of the Department of Radiology at MGH provided me the opportunity to develop and lead the Thoracic Division that we enjoy today. Through his sage mentorship we have a robust and diverse division of incredibly talented faculty. I am so proud that the Cardiothoracic Fellowship Program, with the leadership of Dr. Matthew Gilman and all our faculty, produces so many wonderful thoracic radiologists. Thank you to our current Chairman, Dr. James Brink, for acknowledging the commitment and contributions of our group and for his continued strong support of our clinical, educational, and research missions.

Finally, this book would not have been possible without the support of so many others. Veronica Noah and Lisa Howell, Staff Assistants at MGH, have provided invaluable administrative assistants. I would also like to recognize the dedicated professionals at Elsevier whose advice, guidance, and support have made this publication possible.

Jo-Anne O. Shepard, MD

Chapter 1

Radiologic Techniques and Dose Reduction Strategies in Chest Imaging

Mannudeep K. Kalra, Alexi Otrakji, and Subba R. Digumarthy

INTRODUCTION

This chapter reviews various x-ray–based techniques used in thoracic imaging, including radiography, fluoroscopy, digital tomosynthesis, and computed tomography (CT).

CONVENTIONAL, COMPUTED, AND DIGITAL RADIOGRAPHY

Merely 1 year after discovery of x-rays by Wilhelm Konrad Roentgen, calcium tungstate was chosen as the material for the first screen cassettes based on Thomas Edison's assessment of about 5000 chemicals for their light-producing capabilities upon exposure to x-rays. For the next 75 years, conventional radiography remained confined to the radiographic films sandwiched between two calcium tungstate–based fluoroscopic screens. It was not until the mid-1970s that the first computer-based processing of radiographic images began to emerge with concomitant introduction of rare earth chemicals into intensifying screens, which had better x-ray absorption and lower radiation dose requirements.

The earlier versions of computed radiography (CR) used the cassettes with new fluorescent materials, which retained the information of x-ray exposure as a latent image. This information was retrieved by stimulation with a thin focused laser beam, which resulted in re-emission of light. This light was captured with light-sensitive diodes and converted to electrical signals stored and processed with computers. Although initial versions of CR required much higher radiation exposure, subsequent refinements in the detectors resulted in considerable decreases in radiation doses. The cassette-based CR systems also required specific readout stations, which have also decreased in size and cost. These systems are in common use because of their flexibility and lower costs.

Developments in CR technology finally led to direct digital radiography (DR), with electronic detectors. In the direct conversion type of DR system, the incident x-ray photons interact with photodiodes and generate electrons, which form digital images. In the indirect conversion type, x-ray photons interact with a scintillator to generate light photons, which then subsequently interact with photodiodes to release electrons to form digital images (Fig. 1.1).

The indirect conversion type of DR system is most commonly used in chest radiography, and commonly used scintillation detectors are cesium iodide and gadolinium oxysulfide. The direct type of DR systems is used in mammography units. Compared with CR, DR systems are faster, allow more efficient throughput, have better image quality, and have higher radiation dose efficiency. For these reasons, mobile and wireless DR systems have immense applications in critical care settings, emergency departments, and intraoperative imaging.

Digitization of radiographic images with CR and DR has also enabled benefits in the form of electronic image storage and display on the picture archiving and communication system (PACS) as well as image manipulations such as adjustment of brightness and contrast, edge enhancement, inverted image display, zooming, and subtraction capabilities.

Modern radiography units are more radiation dose efficient and use automatic exposure control techniques to terminate the radiographic exposure when the desired quality is reached. It is also important that the operators use appropriate guidelines (e.g., centering, breath-hold instruction, and coning) to minimize unnecessary repetition of radiographs.

As opposed to readout workstations for CR, which implied some readout time, with DR systems, radiographs could be ready for interpretation in as little as 5 seconds after their acquisition (Fig. 1.2).

CHEST RADIOGRAPHY: PROJECTIONS AND VIEWS

The plain chest radiograph is the most commonly performed imaging procedure in most radiology practices, constituting between 30% and 50% of studies. The standard routine chest radiograph consists of an erect radiograph made in the posteroanterior (PA) projection and a left lateral radiograph, both obtained at full inspiration. In the standard PA projection, the patient faces the cassette, and the x-ray tube is located 6 feet behind the patient. The arms are directed away from the chest with the hands resting on the waist. This technique prevents magnification of anterior structures such as the heart. The full inspiration allows complete expansion of the lungs and separation of pulmonary blood vessels to improve detection of pathology. In an ideally performed standard radiograph, the trachea is in midline projection over the spine and is equidistant from the heads of both clavicles. The lung apices, the lateral costophrenic (CP) angles of the lungs, and the diaphragm are completely visualized, and the diaphragm lies at or below the anterior sixth and posterior ninth ribs.

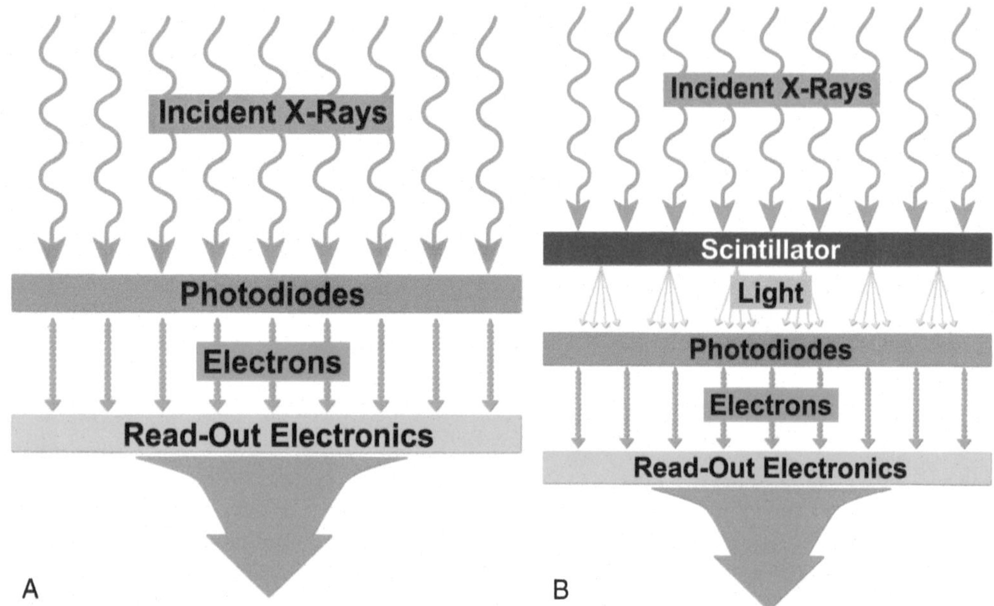

FIGURE 1.1 Digital radiography (DR). Schematic representation of direct conversion type of DR system **(A)** and indirect conversion type of DR system **(B)**.

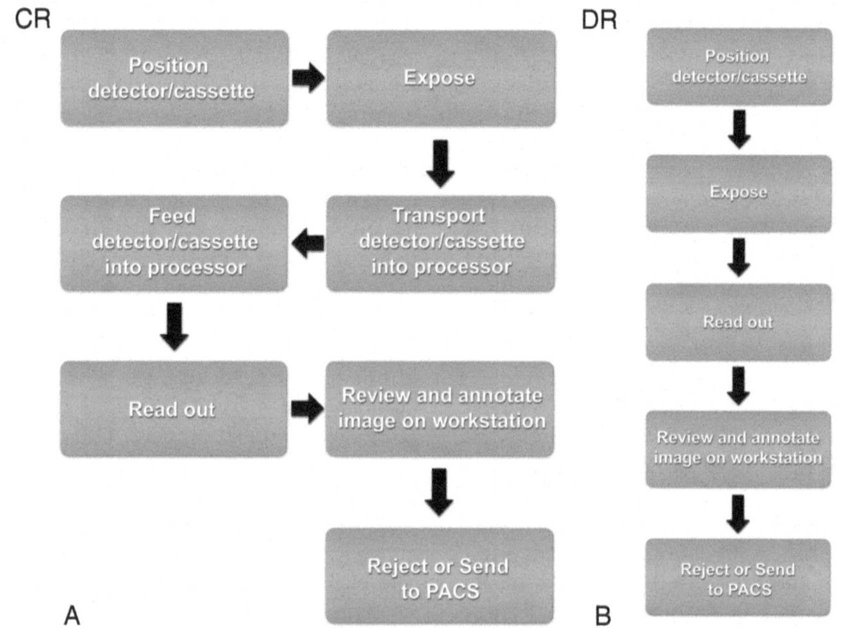

FIGURE 1.2 Workflow chart for computed radiography (CR) **(A)** and digital radiography (DR) **(B)** systems. *PACS*, Picture archiving and communication system.

Chest radiographs should be exposed using a high kilovoltage (kV) technique, usually in the range of 100 to 140 kV. With this technique, a grid or air gap is required to reduce scatter radiation. The main advantage of this technique is that the bony structures appear less dense, permitting better visualization of the underlying parenchyma and the mediastinum. The only drawbacks are the decreased detectability of calcified lesions and loss of bony detail.

With the emergence of CT, the use of additional projections and views in chest radiography has precipitously decreased because additional information in doubtful circumstances is typically resolved with cross-sectional imaging. Furthermore, emerging literature also demonstrates the use of digital tomosynthesis in these situations. Additional views of the chest may be required in special instances. Shallow oblique radiographs (15 degrees) may be useful in confirming the presence of a suspected nodule. Forty-five-degree oblique radiographs can be used for the detection of asbestos-related pleural plaques. Apical lordotic views project the clavicles above the chest, improving visualization of the apices and the middle lobe, particularly in cases of middle lobe atelectasis. Lateral decubitus radiographs (Fig. 1.3) can be used to determine the presence or mobility of pleural effusion and to detect small pneumothorax, particularly in patients who are confined to bed and unable to sit or stand erect. A PA radiograph done with nipple markers is useful

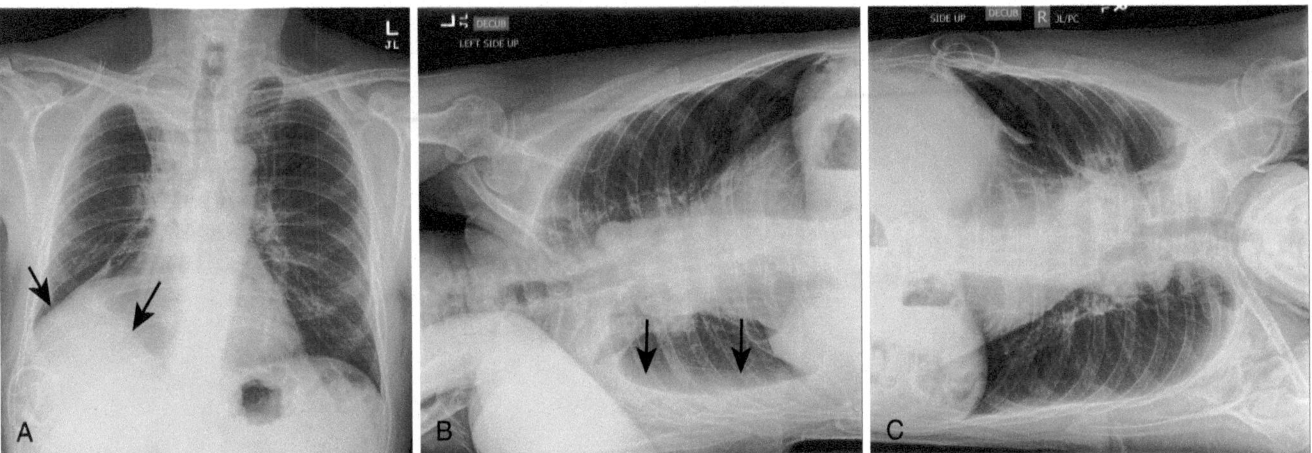

FIGURE 1.3 Decubitus views. Standard upright radiograph **(A)** demonstrates right subpulmonic pleural effusion *(arrows)*. In the right lateral decubitus position **(B)**, the pleural fluid is layering along the dependent right lateral chest wall *(arrows)*. In the left lateral decubitus position **(C)**, the fluid has moved away from chest wall, indicating freely flowing fluid. Note radiation therapy changes in the right perihilar lung related to treated lung cancer.

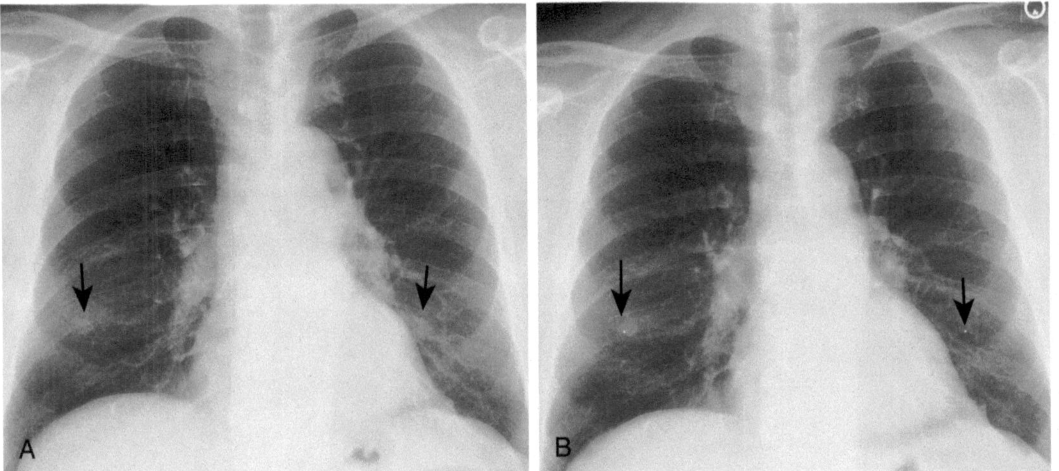

FIGURE 1.4 Nipple markers. A standard radiograph **(A)** demonstrates bilateral nodular opacities in the lower chest *(arrows)*. A radiograph with nipple markers **(B)** demonstrates that the nodules correspond to nipples.

in differentiating nipple shadows from true lung nodules (Fig. 1.4). Paired inspiratory and expiratory radiographs (Fig. 1.5) can improve the conspicuity of small pneumothorax in doubtful cases.

Bedside portable chest radiographs may account for up to 50% of chest radiographs in a hospital setting. Many critically ill patients, including patients in intensive care units (ICUs), must be radiographed at the bedside, resulting in radiographs with limited diagnostic information. The diagnostic quality of these images is often limited because of the increased exposure time needed, which results in respiratory motion. Because portable chest radiographs are acquired with reduced target film distance (<6 feet) and in anteroposterior projection, magnification occurs, particularly of the heart and anterior structures. In ICUs, often patients have lines and tubes overlying the chest; these must be moved to the side if possible. At the very least, coiling or bunching up of wires and electrodes over the chest should be avoided. Better quality radiographs can be obtained in large patients, with attention to centering, coning, and use of antiscatter grids to minimize scattering in large patients.

Digital Subtraction Techniques in Chest Radiography

With advances in DR and display systems, it is possible to apply subtraction techniques in chest radiography that include dual-energy subtraction and temporal subtraction. The former refers to removal of bone structures from the chest radiograph to improve the detectability of pulmonary findings, which can easily be missed (Fig. 1.6). There is a wide variation in the frequency of missed findings ranging from 10% to 50% as reported in different studies. To reduce the frequency of missed findings because of overlapping bones, dual-energy subtraction radiography has been explored in the chest. Such radiographs can be acquired with either single exposure of the patient using layered detectors (each detecting different energy spectra) or sequential exposure of the patient with high and low kV with minimum interval. Subtraction of bones from the soft tissue with dual-energy radiography helps improve visibility of pulmonary findings. Conversely, subtraction of soft tissues from bones can help assess the presence of calcifications in pulmonary nodules and pleural plaques. The visibility

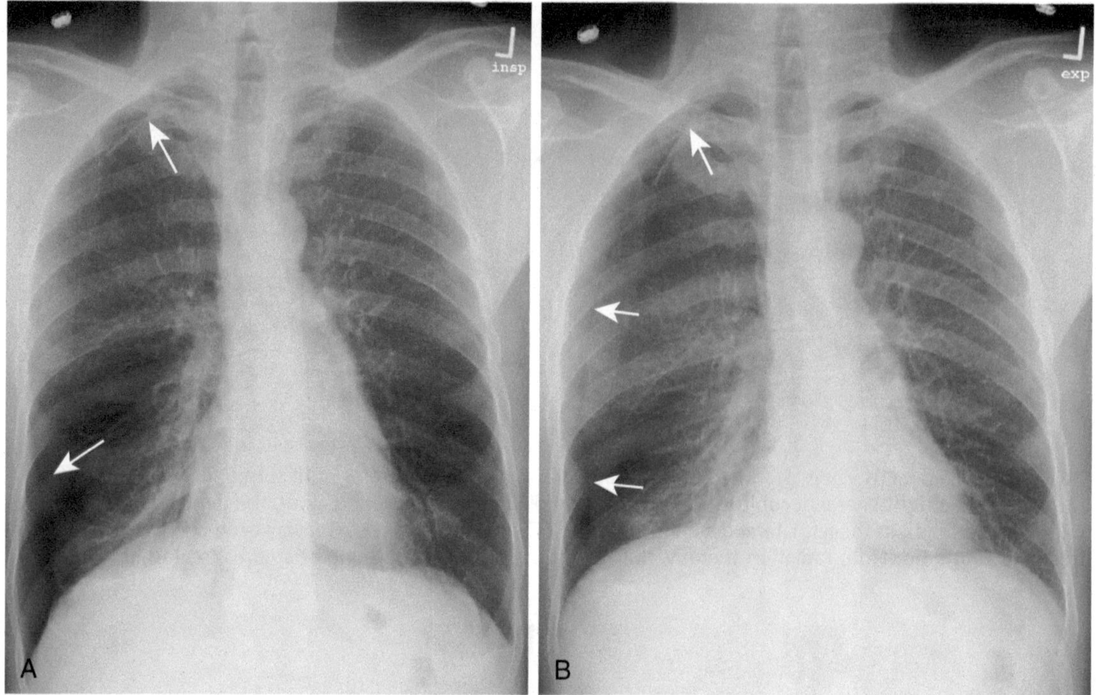

FIGURE 1.5 Inspiration and expiration radiographs. Right apical and lateral pneumothorax *(arrows)* on full inspiration **(A)** and in expiration **(B)** radiographs. Notice the increased conspicuity of the pneumothorax on expiration.

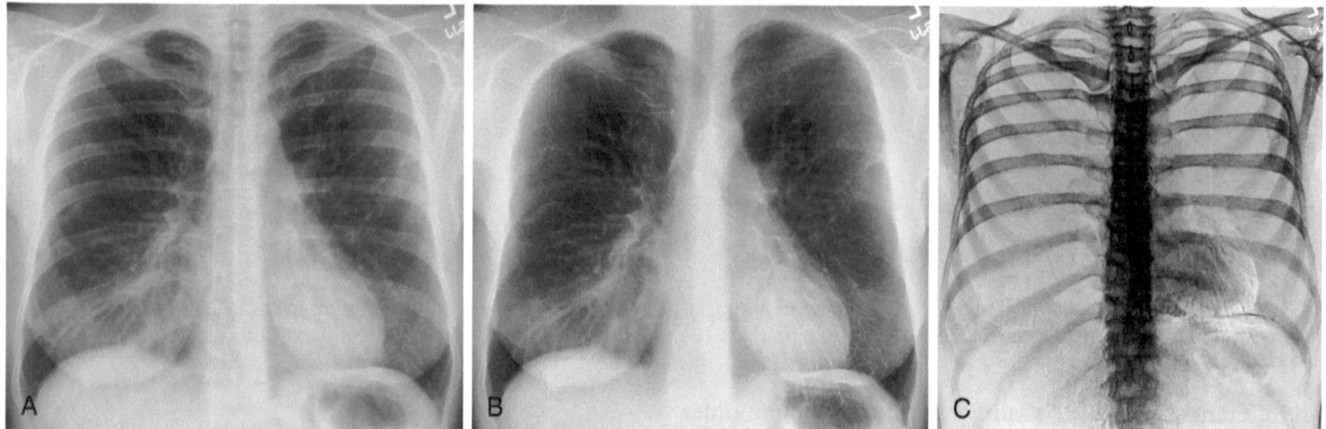

FIGURE 1.6 Subtraction using dual-energy double-exposure technique. Multiple bilateral pulmonary nodules and masses on the standard chest radiograph **(A)** are better seen on the bone-subtracted image **(B)**. Note the increased conspicuity of the ribs on the bone-subtraction image **(C)**. The bone-only image removes the lung findings and is helpful for the detection of bone findings.

of coronary and pericardial calcifications as well as chest implants is also improved with subtraction of soft tissues from the bones.

Temporal subtraction implies subtraction of chest radiograph at two different time points for the purpose of identifying changes in abnormalities over time. Studies have reported the effectiveness of this technique for the progression or regression of pulmonary findings as well as for the detection of new abnormalities. Although subtraction techniques have been around for several years, their clinical use in the United States remains low because of the cost of adopting these techniques, lack of reimbursement, and concerns over increases in interpretation time. Edge enhancement improves the conspicuity of pneumothorax and outlines of supporting devices and access lines (Fig. 1.7).

Chest Fluoroscopy

With the widespread application of CT, chest fluoroscopy is mainly restricted to the evaluation of diaphragmatic motion in patients with suspected diaphragmatic paralysis. Ideally, fluoroscopy for this purpose should be performed with the patient standing so that both hemidiaphragms can be visualized simultaneously. After the diaphragm is localized and centered, patients are instructed to perform a short quick inspiratory maneuver (e.g., a sniff). In patients with diaphragmatic paralysis, the affected hemidiaphragm moves up during a rapid inspiration instead of moving down.

When performing a fluoroscopic examination, it is important to limit the exposure duration to minimize the radiation dose to the patient and operator. Automatic brightness control should be used to allow adjustment of

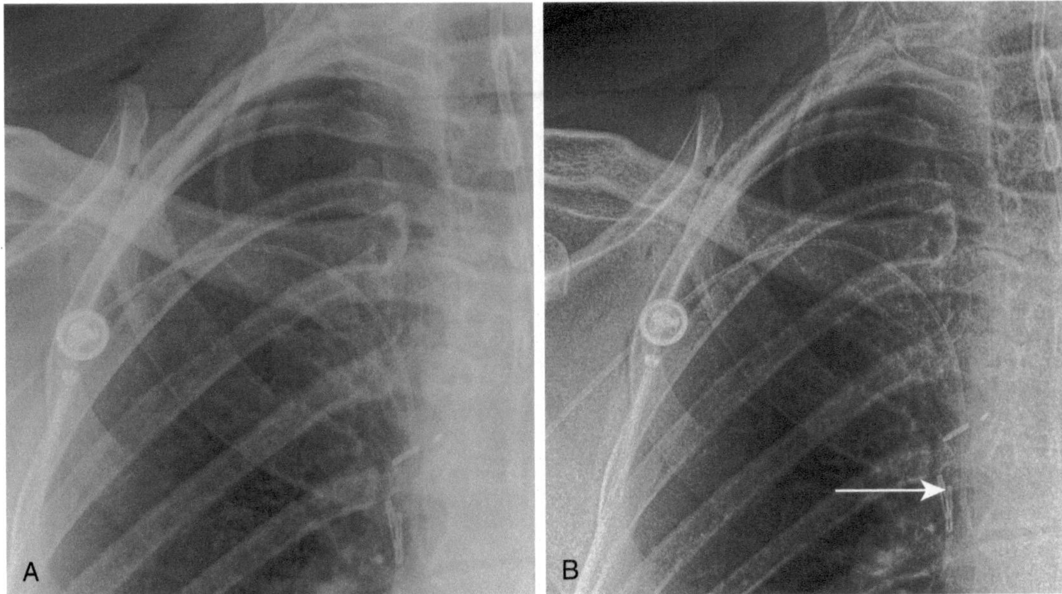

FIGURE 1.7 Edge enhancement technique. The tip of the right peripherally inserted central catheter (PICC) line is difficult to see on standard chest radiograph **(A)**. With edge enhancement technique **(B)**, the PICC line and its tip are better visualized *(arrow)*.

exposure to body habitus. Fluoroscopic time should be kept to the minimum, and the exposure factors should be recorded.

Digital Tomosynthesis in the Chest

In digital tomosynthesis, multiple projections (about 60) of very low-dose x-rays are obtained through the region of interest during a breath-hold of 10 seconds. The acquired data are then reconstructed into contiguous coronal images. At total estimated effective dose of about 0.12 mSv, the radiation dose from digital tomosynthesis is higher than typical PA chest radiographs (0.02 mSv) but significantly lower than most chest CT examinations (2–6 mSv). Compared with plain radiography, digital tomosynthesis provides superior lesion detectability from noise reduction, better depth assessment, and superior contrast resolution.

Although the driving application of chest digital tomosynthesis is improved detection of pulmonary nodules over conventional radiography, several other applications have been assessed as well—for example, suspected interstitial lung disease, cystic fibrosis, airway evaluation, and evaluation of thoracic skeleton fractures. Studies have shown that digital tomosynthesis can help detect more pulmonary nodules smaller than 9 mm in diameter compared with combined PA and lateral chest radiographs (Fig. 1.8).

COMPUTED TOMOGRAPHY

Similar to conventional radiography, CT also uses x-rays generated from an x-ray tube. Although x-rays in conventional radiography are projected from one direction only, the x-ray tube in CT revolves 360 degrees around the patient while continuously projecting x-rays so that cross-sectional images of the body can be generated. These x-rays traverse through the patient's body and reach the detector assembly, where they create a signal. This signal is represented by attenuation value or coefficient, which is a measure of attenuation of x-rays as it traverses through the material or body part being scanned.

The Hounsfield units (HU) or CT numbers are arbitrary units that represent the average of all attenuation values in a voxel of image. The voxel represents a three-dimensional (3D) volume element in the object consisting of each individual number in the image matrix. The Hounsfield value of water is considered "0." Fat, lung, and air have negative values (-50 to 100, -850 to -910, and -1000, respectively). Soft tissues, bone, and metals have positive values (45 to 65, 700 to 1500, and over 2000, respectively).

The earliest "step-and-shoot" CT scanners involved x-ray tube and detector assemblies with direct wire attachments, which meant that after each revolution, the wires had to "unwind" before rescanning. In the early 1990s, the x-ray tube and detector elements were mounted on a "slip ring" gantry system that was connected to the wires. This arrangement meant that both x-ray tube and detector elements could continuously revolve around the patient while the table moved in or out of the gantry aperture. Dubbed as spiral or helical CT, this enabled a much faster coverage compared with its predecessor step-and-shoot CT systems. Because there was only a single row of detectors along the patient length in the earlier helical scanners, only one image could be created per 360-degree gantry revolution.

Helical CT experienced a breakthrough in the 1990s, when multiple rows of finer detectors were introduced into the detector assembly along the patient length, enabling multiple images or slices per gantry revolution of the x-ray tube. These multidetector-row CT (MDCT) scanners began with a modest 2 to 16 rows, enabling two to four images per 360-degree revolution and led to slice wars among different CT vendors in the early 2000s. Modern MDCT scanners (Box 1.1) can now generate 64 to 640 overlapping images per gantry revolution, encompassing a length of up to 16 cm per gantry revolution!

In addition to wide area coverage, the finer detector rows in modern MDCT scanners can generate submillimeter images (up to 0.5 mm thickness) of the whole chest in under 1 second. Wide area coverage, fast gantry revolution times down to a quarter of a second, and high scanning

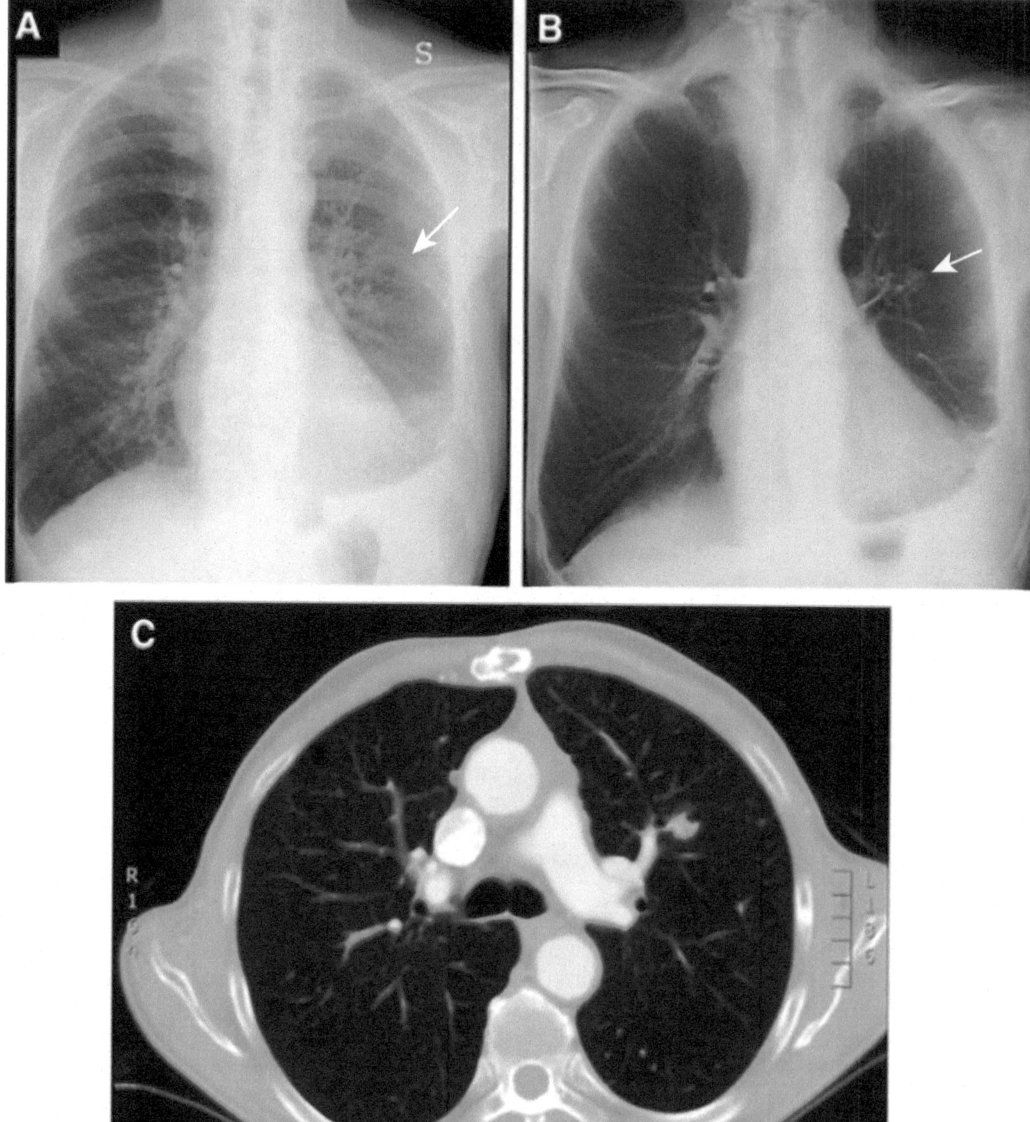

FIGURE 1.8 Digital tomosynthesis. A nodule in the left mid-lung zone on a standard radiograph *(arrow)* **(A)** is better seen on a radiograph obtained with the digital tomosynthesis technique **(B)**. Chest computed tomography demonstrates the lung nodule in the left upper lobe **(C)**. (From Terzi A, Bertolaccini L, Viti A, et al: Lung cancer detection with digital chest tomosynthesis: baseline results from the observational study SOS. J Thorac Oncol 2013;8(6):685-692.)

speeds have enabled users to substantially reduce or eliminate motion artifacts from CT images. In fact, some MDCT scanners can now enable free-breathing scanning of the entire chest in less than half a second.

X-ray tubes in newer MDCT scanners have also overcome tube heating issues for nonstop extended coverage examinations (e.g., multiple body part CT angiography) and for large patients. Simultaneous improvements in detector assemblies in certain MDCT scanners with better integration of electronics have helped improve scanner efficiency and have decreased image noise at low-dose levels as well as in very large patients.

Because of simultaneous improvements in computational capabilities, thanks to the video gaming industries and more accurate and efficient methods of image reconstruction, iterative reconstruction techniques have been introduced on most modern MDCT scanners. These techniques result in less image noise and fewer artifacts compared with the conventional filtered back projection methods, which in turn enables users to reduce radiation dose while maintaining or even enhancing image quality.

Applications of Computed Tomography of the Chest

Although chest CT is the imaging modality of choice for the evaluation of several clinical indications, chest radiography remains the most commonly performed test in the radiology department for assessment of the chest in both inpatient and outpatient settings. Compared with chest CT, chest radiography has a much lower cost and is associated with a substantially lower radiation dose.

BOX 1.1 Attributes and Advantages of Modern Multidetector-Row Computed Tomography Scanners

POWERFUL X-RAY TUBES

Heavy patients can be adequately scanned
Longer scan lengths without tube heating issues
Allows use of higher mA and lower kV to reduce contrast volume requirements

DETECTORS

Wide area detector assemblies enable faster scanning
Fine detector rows enable thinner images
Efficient detector assembly reduces image noise at low doses

FASTER GANTRY SPEED

Reduces motion artifacts
Enables better temporal resolution for cardiac and vascular CT
Reduces motion artifacts in patients unable to hold breath during CT

ITERATIVE RECONSTRUCTION TECHNIQUES

Enables image noise reduction at low radiation doses
Improves image quality without need for higher radiation doses
Reduces certain artifacts

CT, Computed tomography.

Some important clinical indications for chest CT are persistent cough, dyspnea, chest pain, abnormal chest radiograph findings, and cancer staging workup. Recently, low-dose CT for lung cancer screening has been approved for screening eligible patients at risk of developing lung cancer. A vast number of CTs are also performed for follow-up of indeterminate lung nodules seen on initial chest CT; these can be performed at low radiation dose levels in the absence of recent malignancy.

Chest CT angiography of pulmonary arteries is the imaging modality of choice for evaluation of patients with suspected or known pulmonary embolism (PE) and pulmonary arteriovenous malformations. A diffuse lung disease protocol (also referred to as high-resolution CT of the chest) is used for a host of clinical indications such as interstitial lung diseases, bronchiectasis, and post–lung transplantation evaluation. Abnormalities of the central airway and chest wall are also well assessed with CT. Indication-specific CT protocols can be designed to confine scan length to the area of interest and control the number of scan phases (inspiration, expiration, and prone images).

Dual-Energy Computed Tomography of the Chest

In CT, tissues interact with x-ray photons in two primary ways, Compton scattering and photoelectric absorption. The former is the most common interaction and results from transfer of x-ray energy to outer shell electrons with release of electrons and scattering of x-ray photons. The photoelectric interaction results from transfer of x-ray photon energy to an inner k-shell electron and its subsequent release from the k-shell. To fill the k-shell void, an outer shell electron jumps to the k-shell and releases a characteristic radiation. This type of interaction only occurs when the x-ray energy is close to the k-shell electron binding energy, which is referred to as the k-edge. Both these interactions (Compton and photoelectric) depend on the electron density of the substance, but the latter interaction also depends on the specific effective atomic number of the substance. Generally speaking, with single-energy CT at a higher x-ray energy level, Compton scattering predominates the photoelectric interaction that occurs at lower x-ray energy levels.

When scanning is performed in single-energy or single-kV settings, CT comprises information on x-ray attenuation coefficient values (HU) at that energy only. With dual energy, CT obtains information on two physical quantities (called density of two basis materials) because of changes in x-ray interactions and x-ray attenuation at two different energy levels. These differential interactions at dual x-ray energies result in the ability to decompose the images into a pair of basis materials such as iodine–water or iodine–calcium when their effective atomic numbers are substantially different. Thus, the body's soft tissues (mostly water component) can be decomposed from bones (high calcium content) or iodinated contrast media on contrast-enhanced CT. One can thus obtain material decomposition images from the dual-energy computed tomography (DECT) datasets, such as iodine density images (taking water from contrast-enhanced images) or water density images (taking out iodine-based contrast from water) (Fig. 1.9).

Dual-Energy Computed Tomography Techniques

There are different ways to acquire dual-energy images (Table 1.1). The initial method of scanning at high and then low kV (or vice versa) was used even in the non-MDCT era but was limited because the two sets were not acquired at the same time, which resulted in inaccuracies. This method of two separate x-ray rotations, though, is still used on some modern MDCT scanners (Toshiba), in which in one direction, the scanner uses one kV and in the reverse direction, the scanner uses another kV setting. This method is less than ideal because the datasets are not acquired at the same time.

The earliest simultaneous DECT technique used dual-source MDCT scanners, in which the two x-ray sources use different kV at the same time to generate two sets of high- and low-kV images. The latter are then blended to obtain DECT images. This method enables reconstruction of images at each kV while allowing use of automatic exposure control to optimize radiation dose. Because one of the detector arrays of dual source CT is smaller than the other, the field of view is limited (up to 35.5 cm) at the time of writing this manuscript.

The rapid kV switching technique was subsequently released as an alternative approach to DECT. This method uses only one x-ray source but changes the kV between high and low values (within 0.2 ms) to generate dual-energy images. Although near simultaneous dual-energy acquisition is possible with this technique over the entire 50-cm field of view, the automatic exposure control technique cannot be used, which may result in a higher radiation dose.

Some other vendors use the dual detector layers or sandwich detectors to absorb lower x-ray energies in the superficial layer and higher energies with the deeper detectors. Thus, any single kV dataset can be converted to DECT. To date, very little has been published on this technique since its commercial release.

Finally, instead of splitting the detectors into two layers, another vendor uses a twin-beam technique to obtain DECT from a single x-ray source and a single layer of detectors.

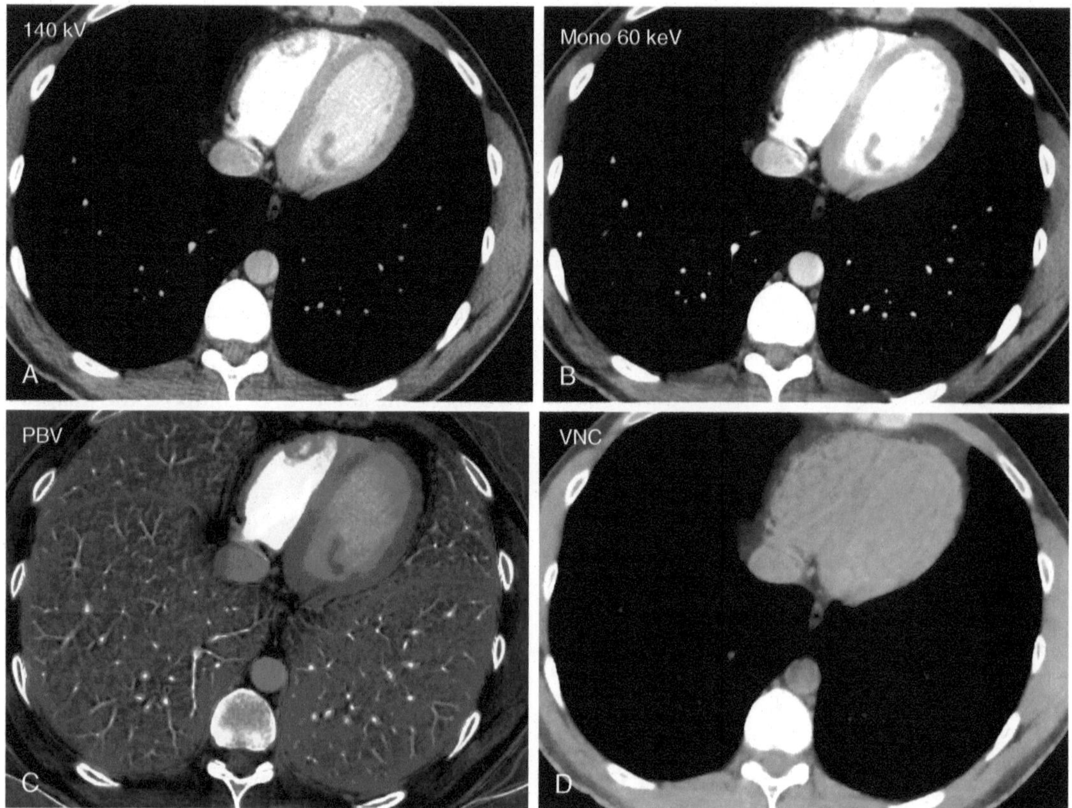

FIGURE 1.9 Normal dual-energy computed tomography. Standard 140-kV image **(A)** has low noise and low contrast. Mono 60-keV image **(B)** has increased contrast and increased image noise. Pulmonary blood volume (PBV) image **(C)** depicts iodine distribution, and virtual noncontrast (VNC) image **(D)** preferentially subtracts iodine density from the image.

TABLE 1.1 Different Techniques for Acquiring Dual-Energy Computed Tomography

Techniques	Description
Rapid kV switching (GE)	kV switches between high and low kV as x-ray tube moves around the patient.
Dual-layer detector (Philips)	Single kV is used. Inner detector layer picks up lower energy x-rays while other detects higher energy x-rays for DECT.
Dual-source CT (Siemens)	Two x-ray tubes and detector arrays are used. Each x-ray tube operates at a different kV (high and low kV) for DECT.
Twin-beam CT (Siemens)	Single kV x-ray beam is split into low- and high-energy x-rays by the gold and tin filters to generate DECT.
Twin rotations (Toshiba)	Wide area detector CT (16 cm) can acquire two rotations at two different kVs to generate DECT.

CT, Computed tomography; *DECT,* dual-energy computed tomography.

TABLE 1.2 Common Types of Images Generated From Dual-Energy Computed Tomography

Image Type	Description
Virtual monochromatic (keV)	Appear similar to conventional CT images Lower keV: better contrast enhancement Higher keV: lower noise and artifacts
Material decomposition	
Iodine or blood volume images	Assess pulmonary parenchymal enhancement
Water or virtual noncontrast images	Differentiate calcifications or blood from iodine
Blended images (Siemens)	Blend of low-kV and high-kV images with reduced image noise
High- and low-kV images (Siemens)	Dual-source CT allows users to view original high and low kV images
Quality Check images (GE)	Initial high-kV images generated from GE scanners

CT, Computed tomography.

In this technique, a special tin- and gold-based x-ray filter is used to split the x-ray beam into high (tin) and low (gold) energies.

Dual-Energy Computed Tomography Image Processing

Compared with single-energy CT protocols, DECT enables the generation of additional image series (Table 1.2). These series require a dedicated vendor-specific software program and depend on the technique of DECT used. For example, the rapid kV switching technique generates initial quality check images, which are generated using a 140-kV setting. The dual-source CT, on the other hand, generates both high- and low-kV image series in addition to a user-prescribed blended image series that combines the low- and high-kV images. The latter image series combines the high-contrast enhancement of low kV with lower image noise of the high-kV images.

Most DECT datasets can be used to generate additional virtual monoenergetic images (typically between 40 and 60 keV [kilo electron volts]) that have high-contrast enhancement because they are close to the k-edge of the iodine. To minimize contrast streak artifacts and image noise in larger patients, higher keV images (>70 keV) may be necessary. Iodine or pulmonary blood volume images represent material decomposition images (obtained from subtracting water from contrast-enhanced DECT images) that provide information on distribution of iodine in the lungs or remainder of the chest depending on the selected settings. The absolute iodine concentration expressed as milligrams per milliliter can be calculated from pulmonary blood volume images (Fig. 1.10). One can also generate water or virtual noncontrast images from contrast-enhanced DECT by subtracting iodine from the image datasets to differentiate calcium, hemorrhage, or high-protein content from iodinated contrast (Fig. 1.11). The DECT technique also allows generation of higher keV images, which can help reduce artifacts with metallic implants or prostheses (Fig. 1.12).

Radiation Doses With Dual-Energy Computed Tomography

Recent publications on dual-source DECT for chest applications have reported dose parity with single-energy CT protocols. With rapid kV switching DECT, the radiation dose can be higher than for single-energy CT. Given the importance of maintaining radiation dose levels at as low as reasonably achievable (ALARA principle), it is important

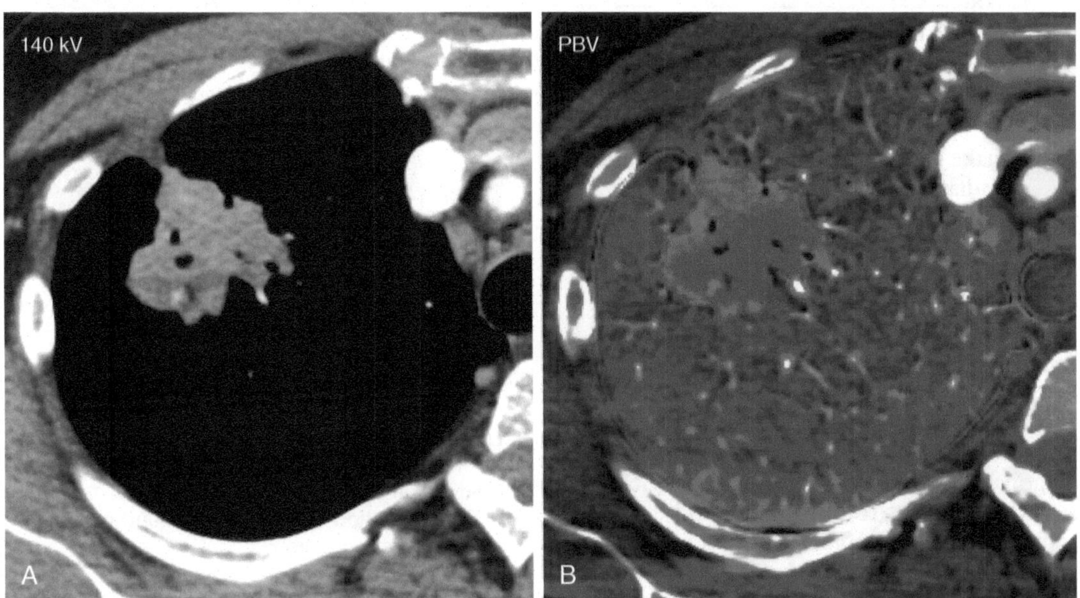

FIGURE 1.10 Estimation of iodine density in lung cancer. A standard computed tomography image **(A)** demonstrates an enhancing mass in the right upper lobe, particularly in the anterior aspect of the mass. The absolute iodine concentration expressed as milligrams per milliliter can be calculated from pulmonary blood volume (PBV) images **(B)**.

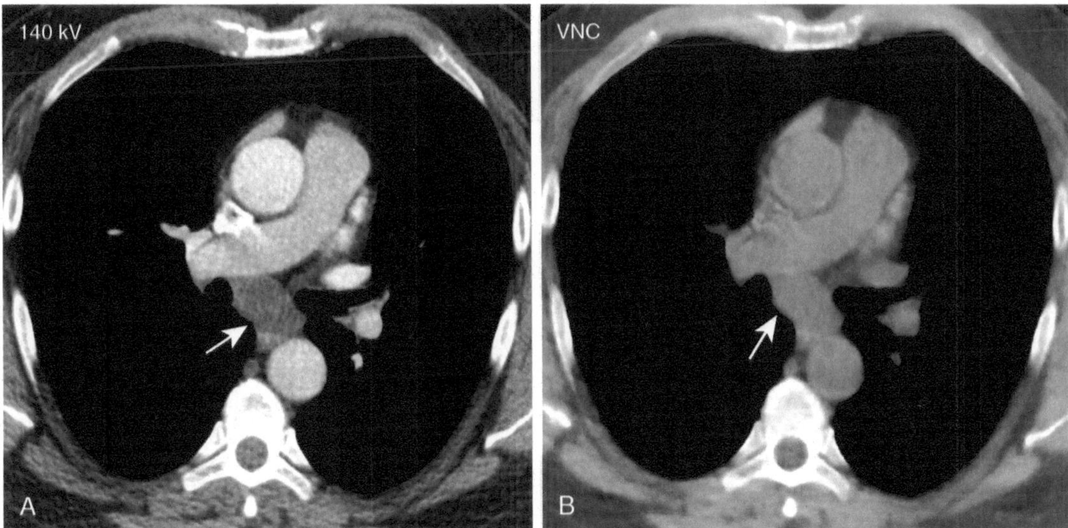

FIGURE 1.11 Virtual noncontrast image. A soft tissue density mass is seen in the subcarinal region on the 140-kV image **(A)**. On the virtual noncontrast (VNC) image **(B)**, after iodine substraction, there is no change in the density of the subcarinal mass, and therefore there is no evidence for enhancement. This mass is consistent with a nonenhancing bronchogenic cyst.

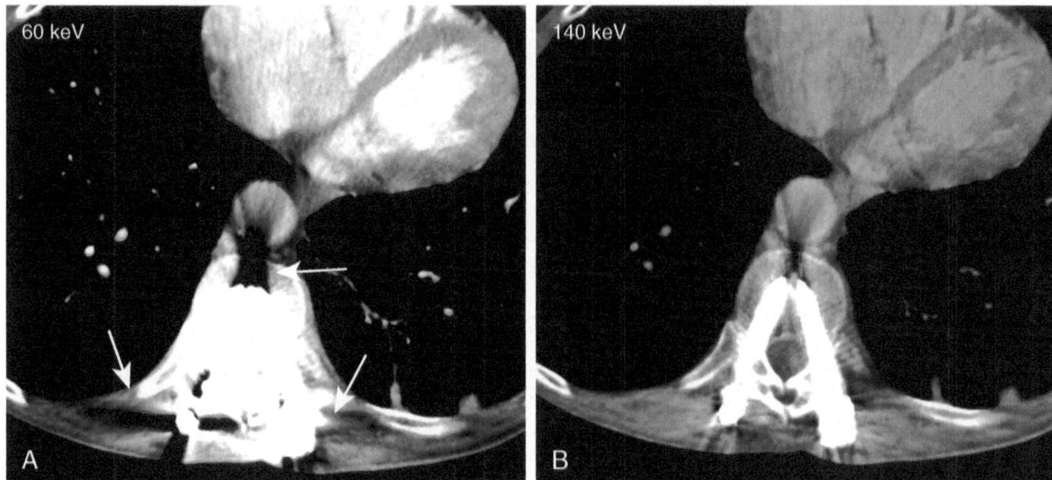

FIGURE 1.12 Metal artifact reduction. On the mono 60-keV computed tomography image **(A)**, there are dense streak artifacts from thoracic transpedicular screws that limit evaluation of the spinal canal *(arrows)*. With higher 140-keV images **(B)**, the artifacts are significantly reduced.

for the users to make sure that unless there is a compelling clinical reason, radiation doses should not increase with the use of DECT.

Clinical Applications of Dual-Energy Computed Tomography

Clinical applications of DECT in the chest are still evolving and are summarized in Box 1.2. The most often reported application of DECT in chest imaging is for evaluation of acute and chronic PE. DECT pulmonary angiograms have better contrast enhancement and enable evaluation of smaller pulmonary arteries compared with single-energy CT at higher kV settings (>100 kV). This can help reduce the number of cases with suboptimal contrast enhancement as well as potentially enable reduction of contrast volume in patients at risk of contrast-induced renal toxicity. Several studies have reported that DECT pulmonary angiography can be performed with a fraction of contrast volume compared with conventional CT pulmonary angiography (CTPA). In addition, the contrast injection rate can also be decreased with DECT, which helps make the procedure more comfortable for the patients.

In patients with PE, DECT images also provide information regarding contrast enhancement of the lung parenchyma. Published literature suggests that the presence of pulmonary enhancement defects (or perfusion defects) on iodine images is an independent predictor of the prognosis of patients with PE. These images also enable differentiation of pulmonary infarction from other causes of pulmonary opacities such as atelectasis or pneumonia (Fig. 1.13).

Another emerging pulmonary vascular application of DECT is in evaluation of patients with pulmonary hypertension. In chronic thromboembolic pulmonary hypertension, DECT datasets increased enhancement in the central pulmonary arteries with mismatch enhancement defects in the lung periphery on iodine images. Some software (e.g., SyngoVia, Siemens) also enables quantification of lung enhancement in the upper, mid, and lower thirds of the lungs similar to the quantitative perfusion nuclear scan.

Interpretation of enhancement defects on iodine or pulmonary blood volume images obtained from DECT must be performed cautiously and with the conventional attenuation-based images (virtual monoenergetic images) because enhancement defects in the lungs can also occur with other processes such as artifacts, emphysema, and air trapping. Although artifacts are easy to recognize because of their nonanatomic distribution, shape, and extent, emphysema and air trapping appear as areas of relative lucency in lung windows, but enhancement defects of vascular etiology show normal lung attenuation.

Applications of DECT in cancer imaging have been reported in small initial studies, but substantive evidence required for its general use or advantage over single-energy CT is lacking. For example, measurement of iodine content on iodine images has been used to differentiate benign from malignant lesions. Whereas malignant lesions demonstrate heterogeneous contrast enhancement and iodine content, benign lesions tend to show greater enhancement and iodine content on DECT. Likewise, good correlation has also been noted between iodine content in the lesion and F-18 fluorodeoxyglucose (FDG) uptake in non-small cell lung cancers. DECT has also been used to assess response to chemotherapy and radiofrequency ablation in separate studies.

Dual-energy CT with inhaled xenon is also used to perform qualitative and quantitative assessment of lung ventilation

BOX 1.2 Published Clinical Applications for Dual-Energy Computed Tomography of the Chest

- Pulmonary arteries
  - Acute pulmonary embolism
  - Chronic thromboembolic pulmonary hypertension
  - Pulmonary arteriovenous malformations
  - Low-contrast volume CTA
- Lung nodule characterization
  - Differentiation between benign and malignant causes
- Lung cancer
  - Treatment response to chemotherapy
- Mediastinal masses
  - Differentiation between benign and malignant causes
- Metal artifact reduction

CTA, Computed tomography angiography; *DECT*, dual-energy computed tomography.

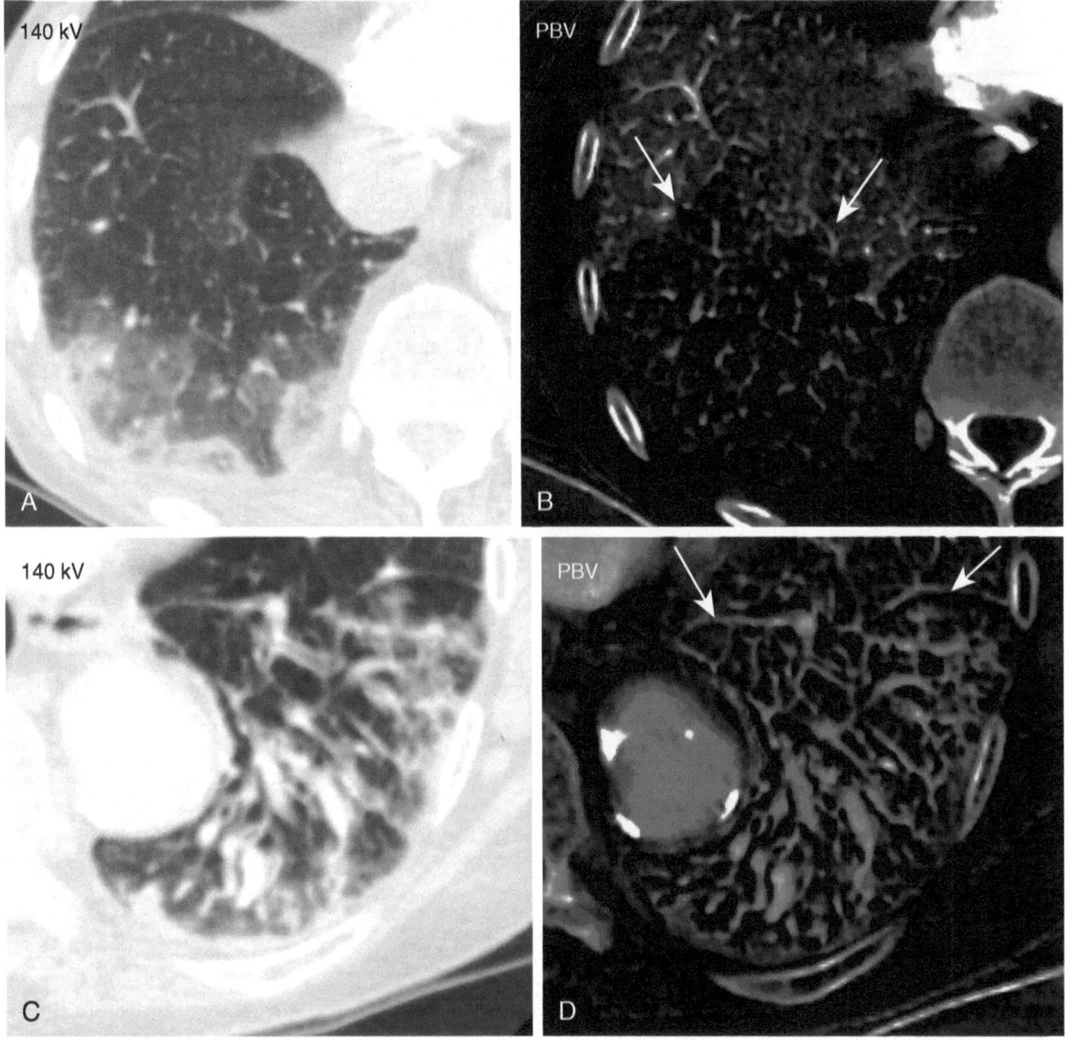

FIGURE 1.13 Iodine distribution on dual-energy computed tomography with pulmonary embolism and pneumonia. Acute pulmonary infarct on computed tomography in the lung window **(A)** and in pulmonary blood volume (PBV) image **(B)** demonstrates that the size of iodine distribution defect *(arrows)* is larger than the infarct seen in the lung window. In the case of pneumonia **(C)**, the alteration in iodine distribution in the PBV image **(D)** matches the size of the consolidation in the lung window.

with good correlation with pulmonary function tests and to demonstrate changes in airflow after bronchodilator administration. Unfortunately, use of xenon gas for CT is not approved by the Food and Drug Administration (FDA).

Computed Tomography Protocols and Radiation Dose

In the United States, more than 70 million CT examinations are performed each year. This increased use has resulted in attention on efforts to optimize and reduce radiation doses associated with CT scanning. To address these concerns, CT vendors have developed and introduced several technologies to enable radiation dose reduction. Examples of such technologies include automatic exposure control (also referred to as automatic tube current modulation), automatic tube potential selection, efficient detector assemblies, and iterative image reconstruction. Several clinical studies have described methods to enable radiation dose reduction based on clinical indications, patient weight, body mass index, and chest dimensions to tailor scan protocols. Several organizations and regulators (e.g., the FDA) have also proposed helpful guidelines, CT protocols, and recommendations regarding the use of CT. The American College of Radiology (ACR) appropriateness criteria help ensure justification of CT for different clinical indications. The ACR has also initiated a Dose Index Registry, a nationwide repository of CT radiation dose that enables institutions to monitor, track, and compare their CT doses with their peer institutions across the country. Recent guidelines from The Joint Commission recommend the use of the radiation dose registry for monitoring doses for various CT protocols.

On CT, the chest as an anatomic region has a high inherent tissue contrast, which means that there is a large difference between x-ray attenuation (and Hounsfield units) of air, blood vessels, and other soft tissues of the chest. The high inherent tissue contrast enables diagnostic interpretation at extremely low radiation doses compared with other body regions such as the abdomen and pelvis. Air-filled lungs have lower x-ray beam attenuation, which results in lower image noise and artifacts at lower radiation doses compared with other body regions as well. Likewise, as discussed in the subsequent sections, chest CT examinations are also amenable to effective clinical indication-based protocols and radiation dose reduction.

Optimization of radiation dose for CT begins with determining the appropriateness and justification of CT for a given clinical indication. When chest CT is likely to provide diagnostic and treatment-changing information, it should not be withheld for concerns of radiation dose regardless of patient age or gender. When CT is unlikely to provide meaningful diagnostic information, the lowest dose CT results from avoiding the CT altogether. Several resources are available for determining the appropriateness of chest CT for different clinical scenarios from several organizations such as the ACR, Royal College of Radiologists, and European Commission referral guidelines. In addition, online decision support programs are available to aid referring physicians in ordering the most appropriate imaging test for a given clinical indication. After the appropriateness is established, the next step in radiation dose optimization for CT involves modification of scan parameters based on clinical indication and patient size.

Scan Parameters

This section discusses the relationship of CT scan parameters with image quality and radiation dose. Box 1.3 provides a list of important scan parameters for chest CT.

Major parameters have profound effects on CT radiation dose. Other parameters have variable effects on radiation dose depending on the CT scanner and vendor.

Tube Current

Tube current (measured in milliamperes [mA]) is the most commonly adjusted scan parameter for adjusting image quality and radiation dose. This is because there is a direct linear relationship between the applied tube current and the radiation dose. Thus, a 50% increase in tube current increases the radiation dose by 50% if other scan parameters are not changed. Likewise, a 50% decrease in tube current decreases the radiation dose by half. CT scanners can operate with fixed tube current specified by the user. Different tube currents are needed for different clinical indications and patient sizes.

Most chest CT examinations on MDCT scanners must be performed with automatic exposure control (AEC) techniques, which automatically adjust tube current based on patient size as estimated from x-ray attenuation during acquisition of scout or planning radiographs. For a smaller or less dense body region, these AEC techniques automatically use less tube current when the x-ray tube revolves around the patient in the x-y plane (angular modulation), along the patient length or z-axis from one scan position to the next (longitudinal modulation), or in both planes (combined angular and longitudinal modulation). Conversely, these techniques increase the tube current for a larger or denser body region. Basically, AEC techniques help adjust the tube current automatically based on the image quality that users specify in the form of noise index (GE), quality reference mAs (Siemens), or standard deviation (Toshiba). The image quality settings should be specified based on clinical indications. When low-radiation-dose CT is desired (e.g., for lung nodule follow-up CT), a lower image quality is specified so that AEC uses a lower tube current. Conversely, when better image quality is needed (e.g., routine chest CT protocols), a relatively higher image quality is specified. Studies have shown that AEC techniques can enable substantial dose reduction (>50%) compared with fixed tube current-based CT protocols.

BOX 1.3 Scan Parameters

MAJOR PARAMETERS

Scan length (cm)
Number of phases (inspiration, expiration, prone)
Tube current (mA)
Tube potential (kV)
Gantry rotation time (seconds)
Detector configuration (mm)
Table speed (mm/rotation or mm/sec)

OTHER PARAMETERS

Beam pitch (no unit)
Reconstructed section thickness (mm)
Reconstruction method
- Filtered back projection (FBP)
- Iterative reconstruction techniques (IRT)

Tube Potential

Tube potential (measured in kilovoltage [kV]) has a more profound effect on radiation dose than tube current. In addition to radiation dose reduction, lower tube potential also increases the image contrast (brightness of intravenous [IV] contrast), an effect not seen with tube current. Traditionally, chest CT examinations were performed at 120 kV. Most nonobese patients should be scanned at 80 to 100 kV for chest CT. Most young children should be scanned at 80 kV to reduce radiation dose while obtaining sufficient contrast enhancement with lower contrast volume and rate of injection.

On most CT scanners, users still need to manually select an appropriate kV for scanning, although some modern MDCT now offer automatic kV selection techniques (KV Assist, GE; Care kV, Siemens) to enable automatic selection of the lowest tube potential while maintaining image quality. This selection is based on patient size (again coming from the initial scout or planning radiograph) and specified type of CT examination (noncontrast, postcontrast vs CT angiography). Lower tube potential (<120 kV) in adult patients undergoing chest CT has also increased with the availability of iterative reconstruction techniques, which help improve the quality of images acquired at lower tube potential or tube current. Some of the advanced MDCT scanners have powerful x-ray tubes to deliver higher tube current at lower tube potential so that advantages of lower tube potential in terms of radiation dose reduction and image contrast improvement can be extended to larger patients as well.

Gantry Rotation Time

This parameter alludes to the time it takes for the x-ray tube to complete one 360-degree rotation around the patient. If other scan parameters are kept constant, a faster gantry rotation time will imply a shorter scan duration and therefore less radiation dose. Most chest CT scans, particularly on MDCT scanners, regardless of clinical indications, should be performed at a gantry rotation time of less than or equal to 0.5 seconds to minimize motion artifacts and have shorter breath-hold time.

Detector Configuration or Beam Collimation

Beam collimation refers to the width of the x-ray beam used during CT scanning. It depends on the number of detector rows and width of each detector row in the CT scanner, a combination that is also referred to as detector configuration. On MDCT scanners, beam collimation can vary from submillimeter to 16 cm based on the CT vendor and scanner type. If all other CT parameters are kept the same, a wider beam collimation is more radiation dose efficient than a narrow one for most chest CT. However, on some legacy MDCT scanners, the widest beam collimation may not provide the thinnest images, so users have to make a compromise if thinner images are desired.

Table speed per gantry rotation (represented in millimeters per second or millimeters per gantry rotation) is also tied to the beam collimation and the pitch. A faster table speed is desirable for chest CT, especially for patients who cannot lie still or follow breathing instructions. For most chest CT protocols, including routine chest, PE, lung nodule follow-up, low-dose CT for lung cancer screening, and tracheal or airway protocols, a wider beam collimation is selected as long as desired slice thickness can be obtained.

Pitch

Pitch is an important scan parameter for multidetector helical CT that represents the ratio of table speed or travel and beam collimation (or detector configuration). It is a unitless entity. There is complex relationship of radiation dose with pitch based on the CT vendor. For Siemens and Philips scanners, a change in pitch (for a value of up to 1.5 : 1) does not result in a change in radiation dose because the tube current (mA) automatically changes to keep the radiation dose constant. For GE and Toshiba scanners, a decrease in pitch increases radiation dose, but an increase is associated with decrease in radiation dose because there is inadequate change in tube current with change in pitch. Most chest CT examinations are performed with a pitch close to 1 or higher.

A notable exception exists for dual-source CT scanners (Siemens Flash and Force) in which a pitch as high as 3.0 has been used to perform fast CT scanning of the entire chest in under 1 second and with substantially lower radiation dose. When available, this scanning mode can be used to reduce severity of motion artifacts in patients who cannot lie still or hold their breath during CT scanning. Most chest CT examinations are performed with a nonoverlapping pitch (>1.0 : 1).

Scan Length

Radiation dose is directly proportional to the length of the body scanned (scan length) during CT. Thus, efforts must be made to not overscan. Radiologists must clearly specify anatomic landmarks for different CT protocols. Whereas extending too high into the neck beyond lung apices increases the radiation dose to the radiosensitive thyroid gland, extending routine chest CT beyond the adrenal glands increases the radiation dose to patients. For some chest CT protocols, such as lung nodule follow-up CT, CTPA, airway evaluation, and low-dose CT for lung cancer screening, scan length must be limited to the chest only.

Another way to reduce the radiation dose to patients is by reducing the amount of overlapping radiation dose when contiguous body regions are imaged with separate scan runs. For example, when performing neck–chest or chest–abdomen CT, it is prudent to limit the extent of overlap of chest CT with neck and abdominal regions to reduce redundant radiation doses.

Number of Phases

The radiation dose increases with an increase in the number of phases or number of times CT is repeated over the same anatomic region. Therefore, acquisition of multiphase images (vascular or respiratory) should be limited to situations when it is absolutely necessary. As a rule of thumb, routine chest, CTPA, lung nodule follow-up CT, and low-dose CT for lung cancer screening must all be single-phase CT performed with inspiratory breath-hold. Routine acquisition of both noncontrast and contrast-enhanced images has little to no role in most chest CT and should be discouraged. The notable exception to this rule is CT angiography of the thoracic aorta.

Repetitive scanning of the chest is performed for evaluation of tracheobronchomalacia and diffuse lung diseases with CT in different phases of respiration. In such cases, the radiation dose for additional series must be kept in check.

Indication-Specific Chest Computed Tomography Protocols

Creation of indication-specific CT protocols not only helps in radiation dose optimization but also aids in ensuring that CT images can obtain the required clinical information. Each indication-based CT protocol should then have specifications for scan parameters to adapt radiation dose according to patient body habitus. The most commonly used chest CT protocols are summarized in Table 1.3. Each protocol must include specific sets of clinical indications for its use; phase(s) of breath-hold; scan coverage; and specific scan parameters such as field of view, section thickness, and reconstruction algorithms. Several studies have shown that radiation doses for certain chest CT protocols—notably, lung nodule follow-up and lung cancer screening—can be performed at less than a 1-mSv radiation dose. In fact, these CT protocols, with the help of iterative reconstruction techniques on certain CT scanners, can be performed at radiation doses (<0.1 mSv) approaching chest radiography.

Most chest CT protocols involve scanning at maximum inspiration breath-hold. Because motion artifacts and scanning in the wrong phase of respiration (in expiration or non–breath-hold phase) can negatively affect optimal assessment of chest findings, one should never underestimate the importance of breath-hold instructions. For contrast-enhanced chest CT, particularly CTPA protocols, appropriate breath-hold is crucial to avoid interruption of contrast bolus and suboptimal contrast enhancement in the pulmonary arteries.

By far, routine chest CT is the most commonly used CT protocol for a plethora of clinical indications such as abnormal chest radiographs, persistent cough, cancer staging and treatment response assessment, chest trauma, and mediastinal and pleural abnormalities. Routine chest CT may be performed with or without IV contrast media

TABLE 1.3 Creating Clinical Indication-Based Chest Computed Tomography Protocols

Protocol	Clinical Indications
Routine chest CT	Abnormal radiograph, lung cancer, metastatic workup, persistent cough, pleural effusion, chest trauma, hemoptysis
CTPA	Acute or chronic PE, AVM, pulmonary hypertension, pseudoaneurysm
Lung cancer screening low-dose CT	Lung cancer screening in eligible patients
Lung nodule follow-up CT	Follow-up CT for lung nodules
Diffuse lung disease protocol	Diffuse lung diseases
Airway or tracheal protocol CT	Tracheal abnormalities (tracheal stenosis, tumors, tracheomalacia)
Chest wall protocol CT	Chest wall abnormalities (thoracic skeleton and chest wall soft tissues)

AVM, Arteriovenous malformation; *CT*, computed tomography; *CTPA*, computed tomography pulmonary angiography; *PE*, pulmonary embolism.

administration. Routine acquisition of both noncontrast and postcontrast images should be strongly discouraged because it does not add information and increases the radiation dose associated with CT.

Multidector-row CT scanners use automatic exposure control or automatic kV selection techniques to help users adapt radiation dose according to patient size. However, adjustment of radiation dose and scan protocols according to indications require creation of clinical indication–based scan protocols to tailor the scan parameters, including these automatic techniques. The following section discusses practical aspects of individual clinical indication–based CT protocols (see Table 1.3).

Routine Chest Protocol

Routine chest CT is the most frequently used chest protocol and can be performed with or without IV contrast administration. Typically, the scan extends from the lung apices to the adrenal glands in inspiratory breath-hold, which requires good breath-hold instructions and patient compliance to minimize respiratory motion artifacts and scanning in expiration. CT images are reconstructed with skin-to-skin coverage with section thickness of about 1.0 to 1.5 mm or thinner for lung windows and 2.5 to 3.0 mm for the mediastinal windows. Coronal and sagittal reformat images are generated with multiplanar reformation. Maximum intensity projection (MIP) images with at least 5-mm section thickness are generated to aid in lung nodule detection. Minimum intensity projection (MinIP) is useful for the detection of emphysema (Fig. 1.14).

Pulmonary Embolism Protocol

Chest CT for the evaluation of PE requires careful attention to several details. First, patients must be given good breath-hold instructions because many PE protocol CTs are limited from respiratory motion. They should be instructed to avoid the Valsalva maneuver during breath-hold because it can lead to contrast bolus interruption with increased venous return from the lower half of the body. This maneuver can lead to suboptimal contrast enhancement. Second, to obtain sufficient contrast enhancement of PE, it is important to use a timing bolus or automatic bolus tracking technique to find the time when scanning should be started after the start of the contrast injection. An ideal contrast injection results in opacification of both pulmonary arteries and veins as well as at least some enhancement of the thoracic aorta. Third, CT techniques should be modified to maximize contrast opacification in pulmonary arteries, which can be accomplished with use of either lower tube potential (≤100 kV) with a single-energy scanning mode or a dual-energy scanning mode. Both techniques (low kV with single-energy CT and DECT) help improve the conspicuity of iodine in CT images and improve sensitivity of the examination to detect PE. Fourth, scan range for this protocol should be generally shorter than for routine chest CT, extending from the lung apices to the lung bases. Although some publications suggest coverage from the top of the aortic arch to the diaphragmatic domes to reduce radiation dose, in our practice, a sizeable number of patients have other pulmonary processes that can be missed with reduced coverage. Fifth, CT images must be reconstructed with finer (1.0–1.5 mm) overlapping section thickness using a soft tissue reconstruction algorithm to detect PE. Additional overlapping reformations in coronal and sagittal planes can help assess suspicious or subtler filling defects in the pulmonary arteries. Finally, lower extremity venous CT should not be performed routinely with PE CT to avoid additional radiation dose. Doppler ultrasonography is recommended for this purpose (Fig. 1.15).

Lung Nodule Follow-up Computed Tomography

A sizeable number of chest CT scans are performed for assessing changes in lung nodules from the initial examinations. Because lung nodules can be very well seen at a fraction of radiation doses compared with routine chest CT, special considerations should be given to this protocol. Recent studies have reported that lung nodule follow-up CT can be easily performed at less than 1-mSv radiation doses (one third of the annual individual radiation from the background), but others have reported doses as low as 0.1 mSv for lung nodule follow-up CT matching radiation doses from plain radiography. Iterative reconstruction techniques and efficient detector hardware make it possible to reduce radiation dose significantly compared with the more legacy scanners without these techniques.

Because low-dose and noncontrast images for this protocol usually do not enable optimal evaluation of abdomen structures, inferior scan coverage should extend to the lung bases and not include the adrenal glands. The remaining image reconstruction settings are similar to the routine chest CT protocol (Fig. 1.16).

Low-Dose Computed Tomography for Lung Cancer Screening

Similar to lung nodule follow-up CT, lung cancer screening should also be performed with a low radiation dose. Most principles applicable to lung nodule follow-up with low-radiation-dose CT are applicable to the lung cancer screening low-dose CT (LDCT) as well. The ACR discourages the use of four-slice or less MDCT for LDCT to avoid higher radiation dose and enable single short breath-hold scanning. According to the ACR recommendations, the radiation dose for LDCT for a standard size patient (typically 170 cm in height, 70 kg in weight, and body mass index of around 24 kg/m^2) must be 3.0 mGy or less, which implies that for a smaller subject, a lower radiation dose should be used, and higher radiation doses are necessary for a larger patient.

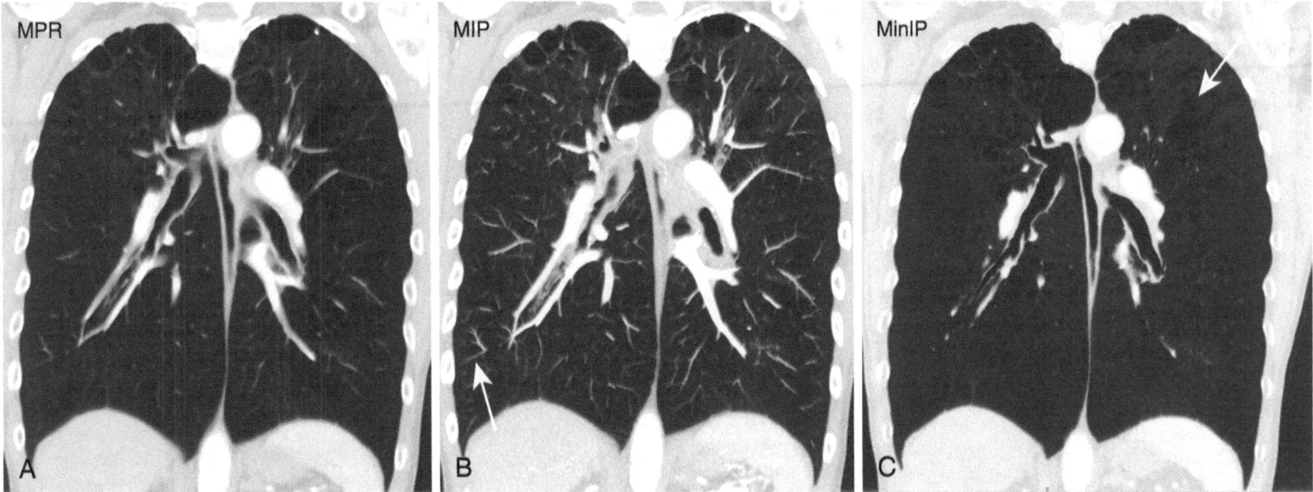

FIGURE 1.14 Intensity projection images. Coronal reformatted standard computed tomography image **(A)** shows emphysematous changes in the upper lungs and normal pulmonary blood vessels. In the maximum intensity projection **(B)**, high attenuation structures such as blood vessels are better seen *(arrows)*. In the minimum intensity projection) **(C)**, low-density structures and lesions such emphysema *(arrows)* are better depicted.

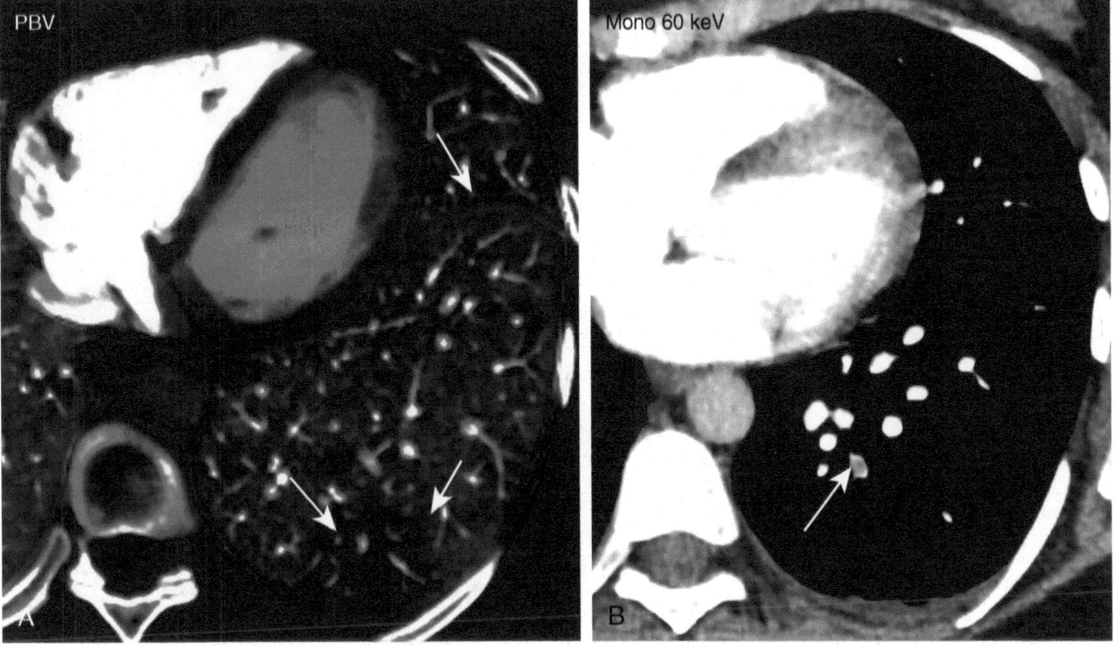

FIGURE 1.15 Iodine distribution defect in pulmonary infarct. A pulmonary blood volume image **(A)** from computed tomography pulmonary angiography done with dual-energy computed tomography demonstrates a peripheral iodine distribution defect *(arrows)* in the left lower lobe. The infarct is in the distribution of a nonocclusive subsegmental embolus *(arrow)* in the left lower lobe **(B)**.

Several publications have reported substantially lower radiation doses for LDCT, particularly with modern, more advanced MDCT using iterative reconstruction techniques. It is important to adhere to recommended standards for LDCT in lung cancer screening for reimbursement and regulatory purposes as well as to ensure that ALARA doses are delivered to an otherwise healthy screening population to reduce risk from the screening procedure itself (Fig. 1.17).

Tracheal or Airway Protocol Computed Tomography

This protocol is used for assessing the airways, with common indications being tracheal stenosis, tracheal neoplasms, and tracheobronchomalacia. Typically, images are acquired in inspiratory breath-hold, initially spanning both the neck and chest. Expiratory images are best acquired with scanning during dynamic forceful expiration to maximize the sensitivity of the examination to detect tracheal or bronchial collapsibility. Expiratory images are caudally restricted to just below the carina to encompass the mainstem bronchi. With wide area detector CT (16 cm), some studies have reported continuous scanning (4-D CT) during inspiration and expiration.

Because the intent of this examination is to assess the large airways, unless evaluation of other mediastinal soft tissues is necessary, both inspiration and expiration images should be performed at lower radiation doses than needed

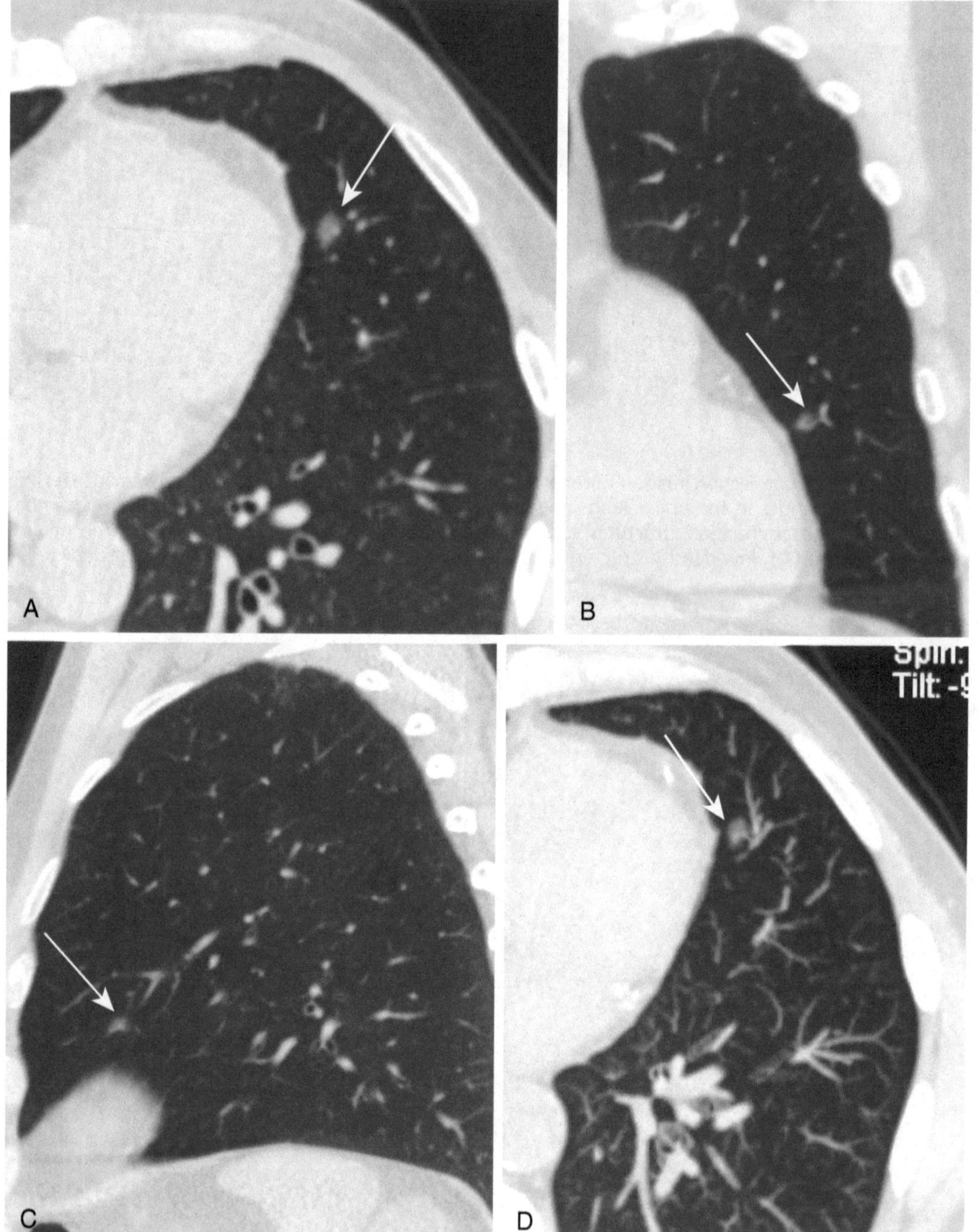

FIGURE 1.16 Nodule follow-up computed tomography (CT) protocol with low radiation dose. On this low-dose CT, there is a clear depiction of a 6-mm ground-glass nodule in axial **(A)**, coronal **(B)**, sagittal **(C)**, and maximum intensity projection **(D)** images. The radiation dose was 1.3 mSv.

for routine chest CT. For this protocol, additional coronal and sagittal reformats of the airways are generated along with virtual endoscopic (endoluminal views of the airway) and volume-rendered (external views of segmented trachea) 3D images to assess the craniocaudal extent of airway involvement and help the endoscopists and surgeons in treatment planning (Fig. 1.18).

High-Resolution Computed Tomography for Diffuse Lung Diseases

High-resolution CT (HRCT) in the chest is used to assess diffuse pulmonary parenchymal and small airway diseases. Modern MDCT can generate thin sections (≤1.25 mm) with high spatial frequency reconstruction algorithms (also known as sharp kernel) for routine chest CT without additional dose penalty. In addition to the thinner sections and sharper kernels, to maximize resolution, the HRCT protocol should also mandate use of a smaller scan field of view to include just rib-to-rib cage coverage instead of skin-to-skin coverage for a routine chest CT protocol. This is because the size of the image pixels is inversely related to the field of view when the image matrix is held constant. *Image matrix* refers to number of rows and columns of pixels that create the image. Modern CT scanners mostly use a 512 × 512 matrix although some newer scanners can enable a high-definition scanning mode with a 1024 × 1024 matrix (GE

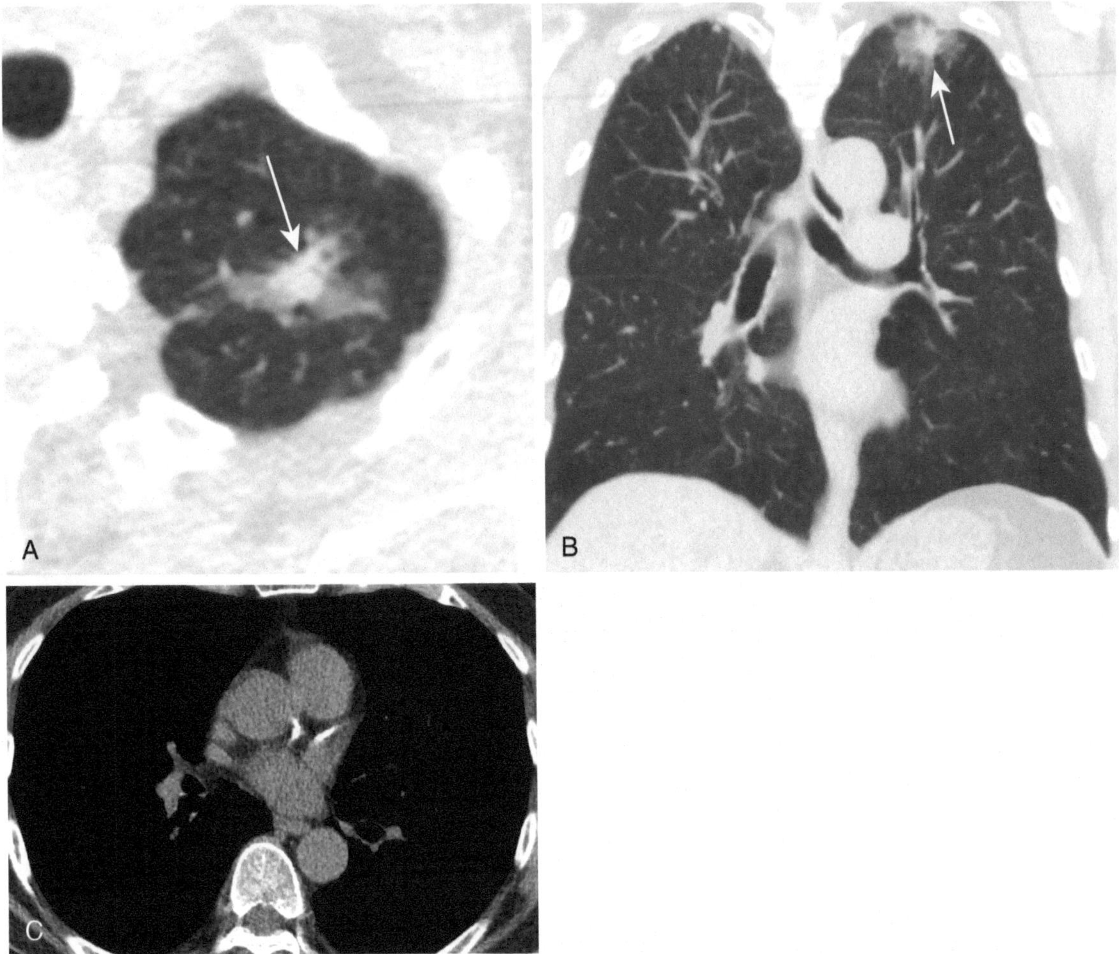

FIGURE 1.17 Lung cancer screening computed tomography (CT), adenocarcinoma, LungRADS 4X. CT images on lung window axial **(A)** and coronal image **(B)** demonstrate a subsolid nodule with spiculated borders. Moderate calcification of coronary arteries is seen on mediastinal window **(C)**. The radiation dose was 0.9 mSv.

revolution). The latter typically implies higher radiation dose compared with the traditional 512 × 512 matrix.

High-resolution CT also demands good patient instructions and cooperation in terms of breath-hold in full inspiration and then in expiration. Explaining and practicing breath-hold before scanning help with compliance. In our institution, inspiratory phase CT images are acquired in helical scanning mode, but expiration images can be acquired with a step-and-shoot (nonhelical) manner to reduce the dose by acquiring thin sections at 1- to 2-cm intervals. Some sites use the step-and-shoot scanning mode for both inspiration and expiration phases to reduce radiation dose. Others use helical scanning at reduced radiation doses for both the inspiratory and expiratory phases. Prone images are acquired to differentiate dependent densities from early subpleural reticulations and ground-glass opacities by eliminating dependent atelectasis. These images are typically acquired in step-and-shoot mode at 1- to 2-cm intervals through the lung bases only to keep the radiation dose low.

Contrast Usage in Chest Computed Tomography: Guidelines

Chest CT for lung nodule follow-up, lung cancer screening, airway evaluation, chest wall assessment, and interstitial lung diseases is typically performed without IV contrast. Routine chest CT may be performed with or without IV contrast medium. In general, routine chest CT can be performed with lower contrast volume compared with routine abdominal CT. Most adult patients can be scanned with 60 to 80 mL of contrast medium injected at 2.5 to 3.0 mL/sec on legacy CT systems. On the more modern MDCT scanners, with dual-energy or with lower kV single-energy scanning mode (≤100 kV), a much smaller contrast volume (as low as 25 mL) and lower injection rate can provide sufficient contrast enhancement for routine chest CT as well as CTPA.

A fixed time delay to trigger the start of scanning after the administration of contrast medium can provide variable contrast enhancement based on injected volume and rate, patient size, and cardiac output. Therefore, bolus tracking should be used to time the scan delay relative to the contrast injection for obtaining consistent contrast enhancement. In this method, a region of interest is drawn in the pulmonary trunk or aorta, and a threshold HU is set. When the threshold HU is exceeded, scanning begins automatically. Use of this technique requires acquiring additional images for tracking the contrast transit and accurate placement of the region of interest. At our institution, we have implemented a split-bolus contrast injection technique in

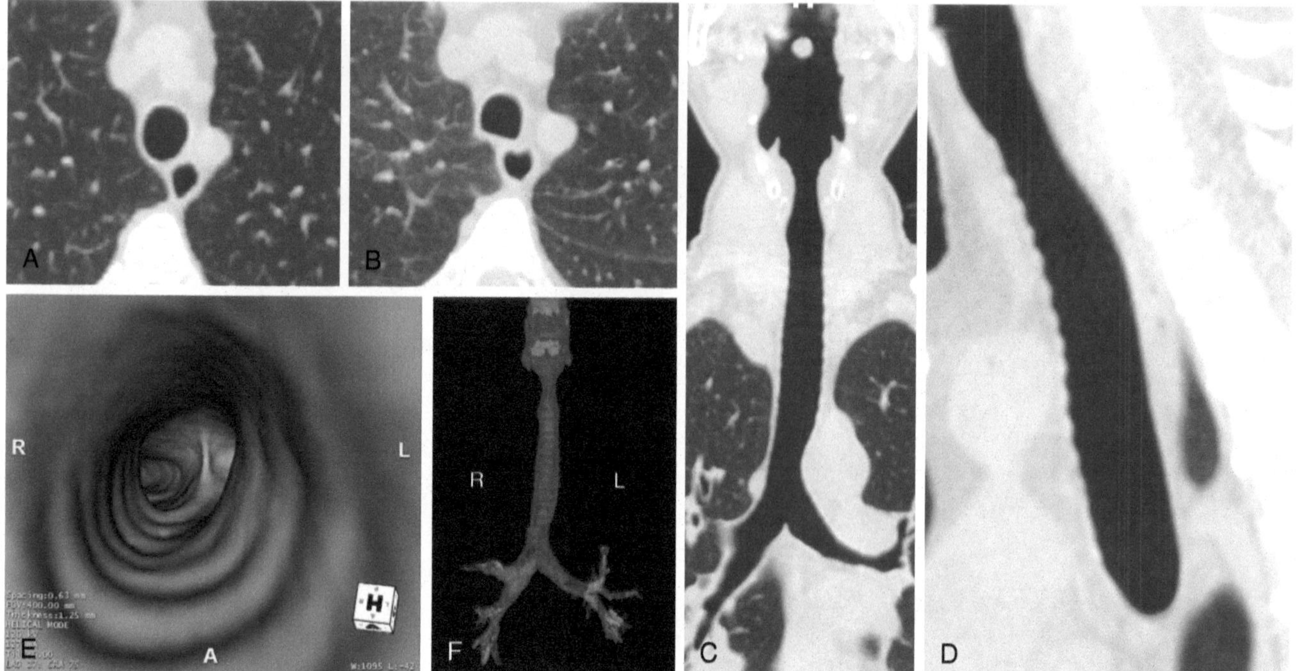

FIGURE 1.18 Tracheal protocol computed tomography. The standard tracheal protocol includes inspiratory **(A)** and expiratory **(B)** axial images and multiplanar reconstructed images in the coronal **(C)** and sagittal planes **(D)**. Images are also reconstructed with internal volume (virtual bronchoscopy) **(E)** and external volume-rendering techniques **(F)**. Note the normal flattening of the posterior wall of the trachea in expiratory images in **B**. The virtual bronchoscopic view **(E)** is at the level of the carina, showing both main bronchi.

which a initial slower rate of contrast injection (about 1 cc/sec for aortic and soft tissue enhancement) is followed by a relatively higher injection rate (about 2 cc/sec for pulmonary arterial enhancement). This method provides simultaneous pulmonary arterial, aortic, and soft tissue enhancement without the need for bolus tracking, which can only target one region of interest at a time.

The term *contrast-induced nephropathy* refers to deterioration of renal function caused by administration of intravascular iodinated contrast medium. According to the ACR's *Manual of Contrast Media Version 10.2* (2016), contrast-induced nephropathy is a rare but real entity that warrants further rigorous research. The ACR manual states that there is insufficient evidence of contrast-induced nephropathy in patients with estimated glomerular filtration rates (eGFR estimated from the formula of the Modification of Diet in Renal Disease) of 30 mL/min/1.73 m^2 or greater. Contrast medium can be administered in patients with lower eGFRs provided that there are substantial anticipated benefits of contrast enhancement that exceed the harm resulting from potential contrast nephrotoxicity and ensuring adequate pre- and postprocedural hydration.

CONCLUSIONS

In summary, radiographic and CT techniques should be modified according to the patient's body habitus and clinical indications for their use in the chest. Basic understanding of radiographic and CT scan parameters helps in key adjustments for achieving the desired image quality at reduced radiation doses.

SUGGESTED READINGS

ACR Manual of Contrast Media Version 10.2; 2016. Accessed at http://www.acr.org/Quality-Safety/Resources/Contrast-Manual on August 23, 2016.

ACR Practice guidelines for the performance of High Resolution Computed Tomography (HRCT) of the lungs in adults. Accessed at http://doseoptimization.jacr.org/Content/PDF/Lungs.pdf on August 23, 2016.

Kalra MK, Maher MM, Toth TL, et al. Strategies for CT radiation dose optimization. *Radiology*. 2004;230(3):619-628.

Kalra MK, Maher MM, Toth TL, et al. Techniques and applications of automatic tube current modulation for CT. *Radiology*. 2004;233(3):649-657.

Kazerooni EA, Austin JH, Black WC, et al; American College of Radiology; Society of Thoracic Radiology. ACR-STR practice parameter for the performance and reporting of lung cancer screening thoracic computed tomography (CT): 2014 (Resolution 4). *J Thorac Imaging*. 2014;29(5):310-316.

Machida H, Yuhara T, Tamura M, et al. Whole-body clinical applications of digital tomosynthesis. *Radiographics*. 2016;36(3):735-750.

MacMahon H, Li F, Engelmann R, et al. Dual energy subtraction and temporal subtraction chest radiography. *J Thorac Imaging*. 2008;23(2):77-85.

Murugan VA, Kalra MK, Rehani M, et al. Lung cancer screening: computed tomography radiation and protocols. *J Thorac Imaging*. 2015;30(5):283-289.

Otrakji A, Digumarthy SR, Lo Gullo R, et al. Dual-energy CT: spectrum of thoracic abnormalities. *Radiographics*. 2016;36(1):38-52.

Padole A, Ali Khawaja RD, Kalra MK, et al. CT radiation dose and iterative reconstruction techniques. *AJR Am J Roentgenol*. 2015;204(4):W384-W392.

Schaefer-Prokop CM, De Boo DW, Uffmann M, et al. DR and CR: recent advances in technology. *Eur J Radiol*. 2009;72(2):194-201.

Singh S, Kalra MK, Ali Khawaja RD, et al. Radiation dose optimization and thoracic computed tomography. *Radiol Clin North Am*. 2014;52(1):1-15.

Chapter 2

Normal Anatomy and Atelectasis

Melissa Price, Jo-Anne O. Shepard, and Gerald F. Abbott

NORMAL ANATOMY

Trachea and Main Bronchi

The trachea is a midline cartilaginous and fibromuscular tubular structure that extends from the inferior aspect of the cricoid cartilage to the carina. The intrathoracic length of the trachea normally ranges from 6 to 9 cm. The wall contains 16 to 22 horseshoe-shaped cartilage rings that are connected longitudinally by annular ligaments containing fibrous and connective tissue. The posterior wall of the trachea is membranous and contains transverse smooth muscle fibers of the trachealis muscle. Proximally, the trachea lies in close proximity to the skin surface but is posteriorly angulated as it descends inferiorly. The recurrent laryngeal and vagus nerves innervate the trachea, and sympathetic trunks provide sympathetic innervation. The left recurrent laryngeal nerve loops underneath the aortic arch and is located within or in close proximity to the tracheoesophageal groove. Arterial blood supply to the trachea derives from branches of the inferior thyroidal, intercostal, and bronchial arteries. The thoracic esophagus typically maintains a posterior location relative to the trachea; however, this varies, and the esophagus may be located laterally (Fig. 2.1, *A* and *B*).

At the carina, the trachea divides into the right and left main bronchi (Fig. 2.1, *C*). The angle of bifurcation can either be measured as the interbronchial angle, which represents the angle between the central axis of each main bronchus, or the subcarinal angle, defined as the angle between the inferior aspect of both the right and left main bronchi. The normal carinal angle can range from 45 to 90 degrees but is usually approximately 60 degrees. A variety of pathologies may result in widening of the carinal angle, including left atrial enlargement, subcarinal masses or lymphadenopathy, lobar collapse, and presence of a pericardial effusion.

The right main bronchus has a more vertical course than the left and a shorter length (see Fig. 2.1, *C*). The bronchial angle represents the angle created by the intersection of lines through the tracheal axis longitudinally and the origin of the bronchial axis. The steeper right bronchial angle and shorter length of the right main bronchus lead to a more accessible route for foreign bodies. However, in children up to 15 years of age, the right and left bronchial angles are relatively symmetric, with resultant near equal incidence of right- and left-sided aspiration in pediatric patients.

Lobar Bronchi and Bronchopulmonary Segments

Right Side

The right upper lobe bronchus arises from the lateral aspect of the right main bronchus, approximately 2 cm from the carina. The bronchus courses laterally and divides into three branches 1 to 2 cm from its origin, denoted anterior, posterior, and apical—each of which supplies a segment (see Fig. 2.1, *C* and *D*). This normal trifurcation pattern has been shown to vary considerably, and many individuals have a variable bifurcation pattern of segmental bronchi in the right upper lobe. The anterior segmental bronchus is typically located in the axial scan plane on computed tomography (CT) (see Fig. 2.1, *D*) and may appear as a rounded lucency on coronal CT images (Fig. 2.2). The angle of the posterior segmental bronchus is directly slightly cephalad after its take-off and can be seen typically on CT as it ascends cranially (see Fig. 2.1, *D*). The apical segmental bronchus can be identified on axial CT as a rounded lucency at the level of the carina (see Fig. 2.1, *C*).

The bronchus intermedius continues distally for 3 to 4 cm following the origin of the right upper lobe bronchus and bifurcates into the right middle and right lower lobe bronchi (Fig. 2.1, *E* and *F*). The posterior wall of the bronchus intermedius approximates the superior segment of the right lower lobe and should be less than 3 mm in thickness. The right middle lobe bronchus originates from the anterolateral wall of the bronchus intermedius, nearly opposite from the origin of the lower lobe superior segmental bronchus origin (see Fig. 2.1, *F*). It divides into the medial and lateral segmental bronchi approximately 1 to 2 cm beyond its origin, extending anteriorly and slightly inferiorly (Fig. 2.1, *G*).

The nondivided segment of the right lower lobe bronchus is short. The superior segmental bronchus of the right lower lobe arises from the posterior wall of the right lower lobe bronchus near its origin. The superior segmental bronchus courses posteriorly and laterally for approximately 1 cm (Fig. 2.3). After the superior segmental bronchus take-off, the right lower lobe bronchus continues caudally as the basal bronchial trunk or truncus basalis for 5 to 10 mm (see Fig. 2.1, *F*). There are four basal segments in the right lower lobe: anterior, lateral, posterior, and medial, which is the order from the lateral to medial aspect of the hemithorax on the standard PA radiograph (Fig. 2.1, *H*). The first branch of the basal trunk is typically the medial basal segmental bronchus, which has an anterior

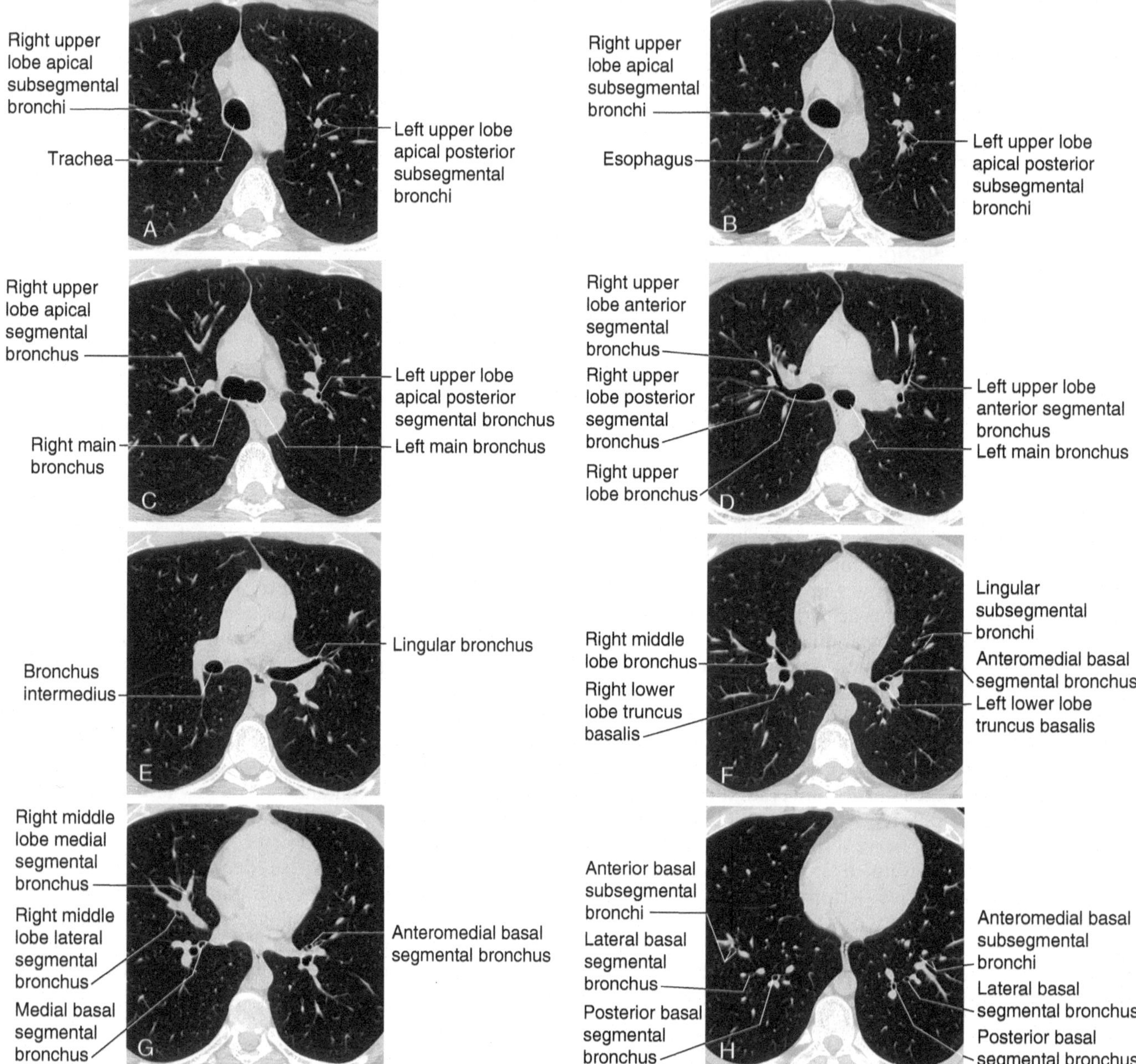

FIGURE 2.1 Airway anatomy. **A,** Axial computed tomography (CT) image at the level of the aortic arch shows the trachea and subsegmental branches of the apical bronchus in the right upper lobe and apical posterior subsegmental bronchi in the left upper lobe. **B,** Axial CT image slightly more inferiorly at the level of the aortopulmonary window show branches of the apical segmental bronchus in the right upper lobe and the apical posterior bronchus in the left upper lobe. **C,** Axial CT image at the level of the carina demonstrates the apical segmental bronchus in the right upper lobe. The apical posterior segmental bronchus is seen at the same level in the left upper lobe. **D,** Axial CT image shows the origin of the right upper lobe bronchus as it arises from the right main bronchus. The anterior and posterior segmental bronchi in the right upper lobe and the left upper lobe anterior segmental bronchus are seen at this level. **E,** Axial CT image demonstrates the bronchus intermedius and the lingular bronchus in the left upper lobe. **F,** Axial CT image shows the right middle lobe bronchus. In this patient, the right middle lobe bronchus originates below the superior segmental bronchi, and the basal bronchial trunks are seen in the right and left lower lobes at this level. **G,** Axial CT image demonstrates the medial and lateral segmental bronchi in the right middle lobe. The medial basal segmental bronchus is visible in the right lower lobe, and the left lower lobe anteromedial basal segmental bronchus is also seen. **H,** Axial CT image shows the segmental and subsegmental basal bronchi in the lower lobes. On the right, branches of the posterior, lateral, and anterior basal bronchi can be seen (from medial to lateral). In the left lower lobe, posterior, lateral, and anteromedial basal branches are visible (from medial to lateral).

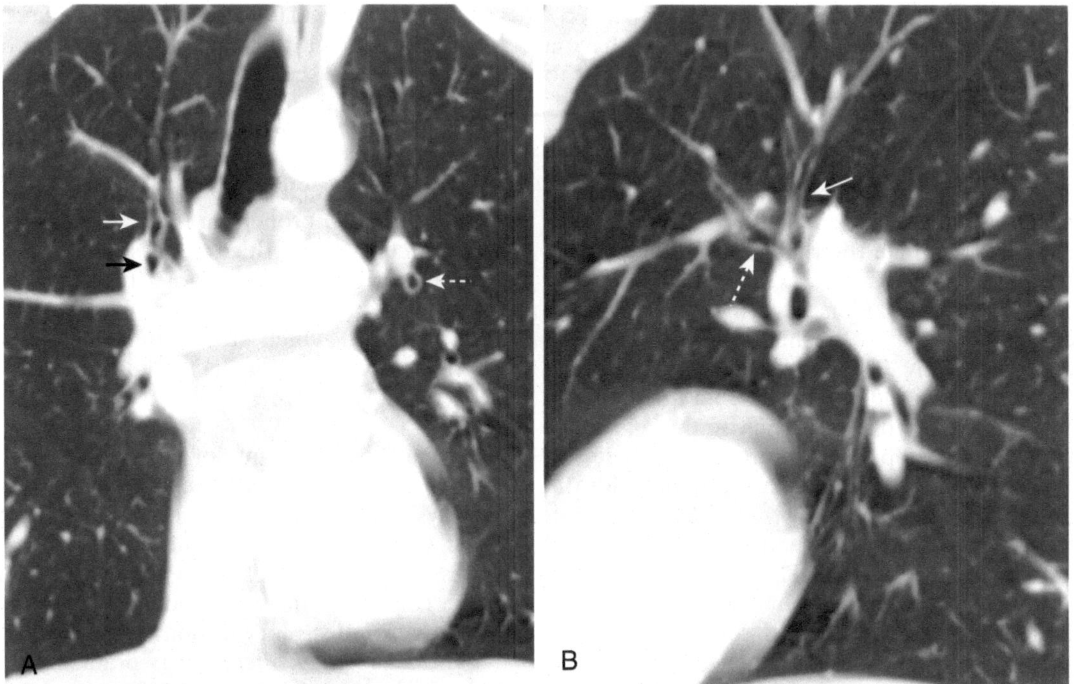

FIGURE 2.2 Upper lobe anterior segmental bronchi. **A,** Coronal computed tomography (CT) image shows the anterior segmental bronchi of the right and left upper lobes. The apical segmental bronchus in the right upper lobe is seen at the same level and ascends superiorly *(white arrow)*. The anterior segmental bronchus is located just lateral to the truncus anterior *(black arrow)*, and the left upper lobe anterior segmental bronchus is visible end-on *(dashed arrow)*. **B,** Sagittal CT image through the left lung shows that the apical posterior segmental bronchus extends superiorly in the left upper lobe *(arrow)*, while the anterior segmental bronchus courses anteriorly *(dashed arrow)*.

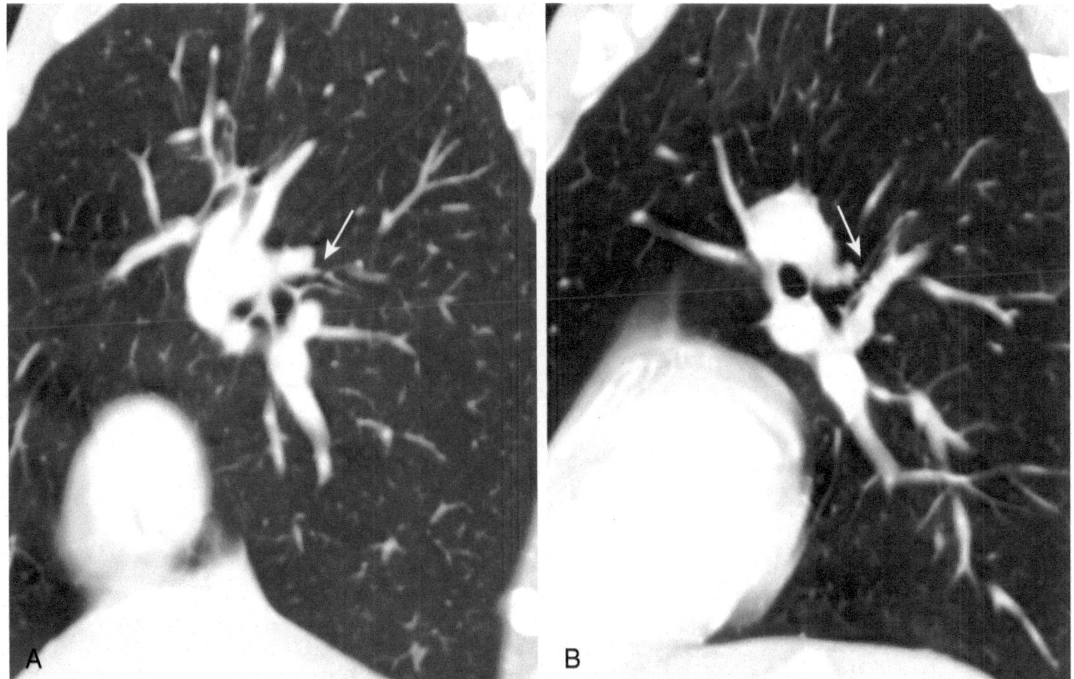

FIGURE 2.3 Lower lobe superior segmental bronchi. **A,** Sagittal image through the right lung shows the origin of the right lower lobe superior segmental bronchus *(arrow)*. **B,** Sagittal computed tomography image through the left lung shows the origin of the left lower lobe superior segmental bronchus *(arrow)*.

relationship to the right inferior pulmonary vein (Fig. 2.1, *G*). The anterior and lateral basilar bronchi tend to have a somewhat oblique course, which can make it difficult to identify them on axial CT.

Left Side

The left main bronchus is longer in length than the right and divides into the left upper and left lower lobe bronchi at a more caudal level than the right main bronchus (see Fig. 2.1, *D*).

The left upper lobe bronchus arises from the anterolateral aspect of the left main bronchus and is 2 to 3 cm in length. In approximately 75% of cases, the left upper lobe bronchus bifurcates into superior and inferior divisions, the latter of which is the lingular bronchus. In the remainder of individuals, the left upper lobe bronchus trifurcates in anterior, apical posterior, and lingular bronchi. With the most common branching pattern, the superior division divides almost immediately into the apical posterior and anterior segmental branches (see Figs. 2.1, *C* and *D*, and 2.2). The anterior segmental bronchus can be seen at the level of the left upper lobe bronchus coursing anteriorly (see Fig. 2.2). The apical posterior segmental bronchus has a vertical course and therefore is imaged in cross-section at axial CT, appearing as a circular lucency above the anterior segmental bronchus origin (see Figs. 2.1, *C*, and 2.2).

The lingular bronchus originates from the inferior aspect of the distal left upper lobe bronchus, approximately 1 to 2 cm inferior to the right middle lobe bronchus take-off (see Fig. 2.1, *E*). The lingular bronchus courses obliquely in the anterior inferior direction for 2 to 3 cm and then gives rise to the superior and inferior segmental branches (see Fig. 2.1, *F*). Because of the oblique cephalocaudad course of the lingular bronchus and its segmental branches, it may be difficult to clearly visualize them on axial CT.

The superior segmental bronchus of the left lower lobe originates within 1 cm of the origin of the left lower lobe bronchus and courses posteriorly and laterally (see Fig. 2.3). It arises from the left lower lobe bronchus at approximately the level of the lingular and right middle lobe bronchi. The basal segmental bronchi in the left lower lobe arise from the truncus basalis, which is visible inferior to the superior segment origin for a length of 1 to 2 cm. There are three basal segments in the left lower lobe: anteromedial, lateral, and posterior, which are situated from lateral to medial on the posteroanterior (PA) radiograph (see Fig. 2.1, *H*).

Variants

There are many variants of the normal tracheobronchial branching pattern, most frequently within the subsegmental airways but also among the lobar and segmental bronchi. Most variations have been found to occur in the upper lobes. Although bronchial segmental branching variations occur commonly, the bronchopulmonary segments maintain a relatively consistent location.

The *tracheal bronchus* was originally described as a bronchus to the right upper lobe arising from the trachea. More recently, the term *tracheal bronchus* has been used to refer to bronchial anomalies in which a bronchus supplying an upper lobe arises from either the trachea or a main bronchus. The majority of tracheal bronchi are located on the right and represent displaced rather than supernumerary bronchi. Tracheal bronchi to the right upper lobe typically arise from the right lateral tracheal wall within 2 cm of the carina and most frequently supply the apical segment (Fig. 2.4).

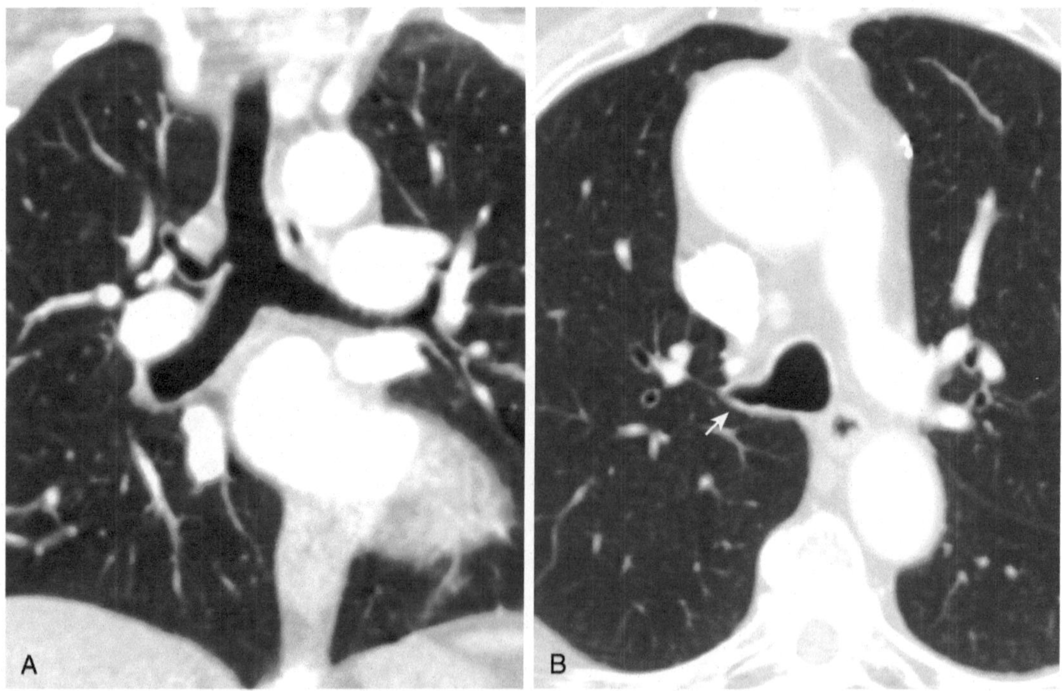

FIGURE 2.4 Tracheal bronchus. **A,** Coronal computed tomography (CT) image demonstrates the tracheal bronchus arising from the lateral wall of the trachea and supplying the apical segment of the right upper lobe. The tracheal bronchus is seen just below the azygous arch. **B,** Axial CT image from a different patient shows the tracheal bronchus origin from the right lateral aspect of the distal trachea *(arrow)*.

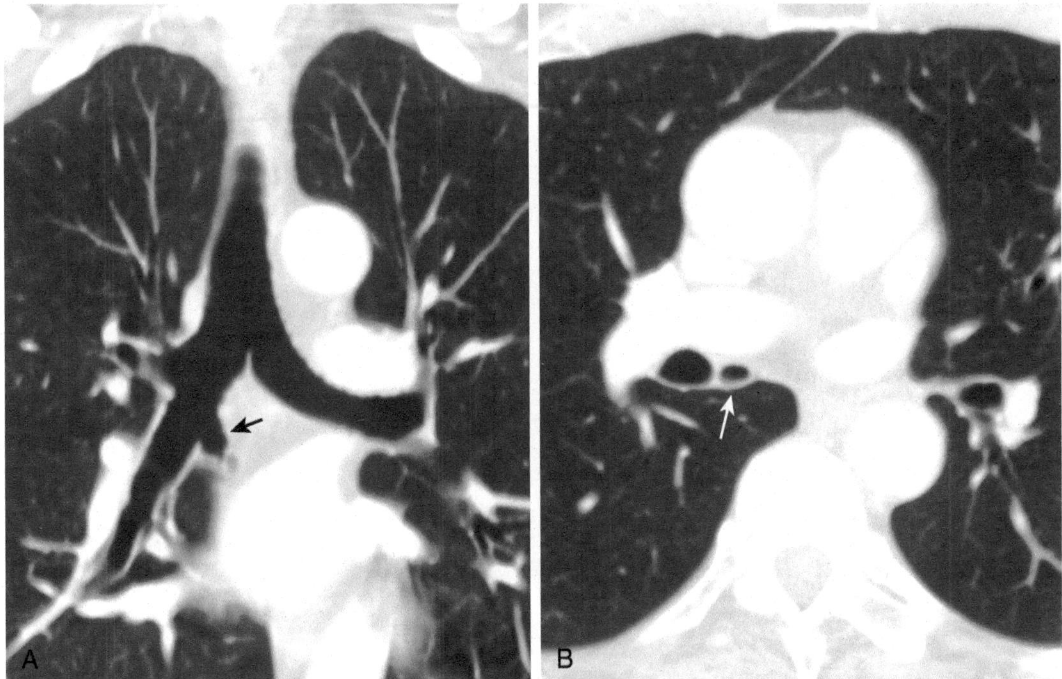

FIGURE 2.5 Accessory cardiac bronchus. **A,** Coronal computed tomography (CT) image demonstrates a blind-ending bronchial diverticulum arising from the medial wall of the bronchus intermedius *(arrow)*. There is no associated pulmonary parenchymal tissue in this patient. **B,** Axial CT image shows the accessory bronchus coursing inferiorly *(arrow)*, roughly parallel to the bronchus intermedius.

The *accessory cardiac bronchus* typically originates from the medial aspect of the bronchus intermedius or occasionally the right main bronchus and courses caudally, parallel to the bronchus intermedius, for 1 to 5 cm toward the heart or mediastinum (Fig. 2.5). The incidence is about 0.1%. The majority of accessory cardiac bronchi are blind ending, although some terminate in small bronchioles, which may be associated with vestigial bronchiolar parenchymal tissue located in the azygoesophageal recess.

Pulmonary Vessels

The main pulmonary artery arises from the pulmonic valve at the base of the right ventricle and passes superiorly, posteriorly, and to the left before bifurcating into the left and right pulmonary arteries (Figs. 2.6 and 2.7, *C*). The main, right, and left pulmonary arteries are located within the pericardium. The right pulmonary artery, which is longer than the left, courses to the right posterior to the ascending aorta before dividing in front of the right main bronchus into a right upper lobe branch, the *truncus anterior*, located anterior to the right upper lobe bronchus and the descending or interlobar pulmonary artery. The truncus anterior gives rise to segmental branches, which supply the right upper lobe. However, in many individuals, a separate branch originating from the interlobar artery supplies a portion of the right upper lobe posterior segment.

The right interlobar artery is located anterior and lateral to the bronchus intermedius and posterior to the right superior pulmonary vein (Fig. 2.7, *D*). The right middle lobe pulmonary artery arises from the interlobar artery and courses laterally, parallel to the right middle lobe bronchus. The right lower lobe pulmonary artery is directed perpendicular to the axial scan plane on CT at this level and can be seen as an ovoid structure at the level of the right middle lobe artery origin. The basilar segmental pulmonary arteries in the right lower lobe are located posterolateral to the associated basilar segmental bronchi.

The higher left pulmonary artery passes over the left main bronchus (see Fig. 2.6). It can give rise to a separate branch to the left upper lobe but more commonly continues directly into a vertical left interlobar or descending pulmonary artery, which directly gives to rise to segmental branches in the left upper and lower lobes. At the level of the lingular bronchus, the left interlobar artery is located lateral to the lower lobe bronchi and posterolateral to the lingular bronchus (see Fig. 2.7, *D*). The basilar segmental arteries in the left lower lobe are located posterolateral to the basilar bronchi, as in the right lower lobe.

Pericardial Recesses

The pericardial recesses appear as fluid attenuation structures on CT, which exhibit minimal or no mass effect on adjacent structures. The transverse sinus and oblique sinus are the two major pericardial sinuses, each of which gives rise to several recesses.

The transverse sinus is situated superior to the left atrium and posterior to the ascending aorta and pulmonary trunk. There are four recesses within the transverse sinus: the superior and inferior aortic recesses and the right and left pulmonic recesses.

The superior aortic recess is the most superior component of the transverse sinus, and it can extend along the right aspect of the ascending aorta. The anterior aspect of the recess insinuates between the ascending aorta and pulmonary trunk. The posterior division of the superior aortic recess, also denoted the superior pericardial recess, is

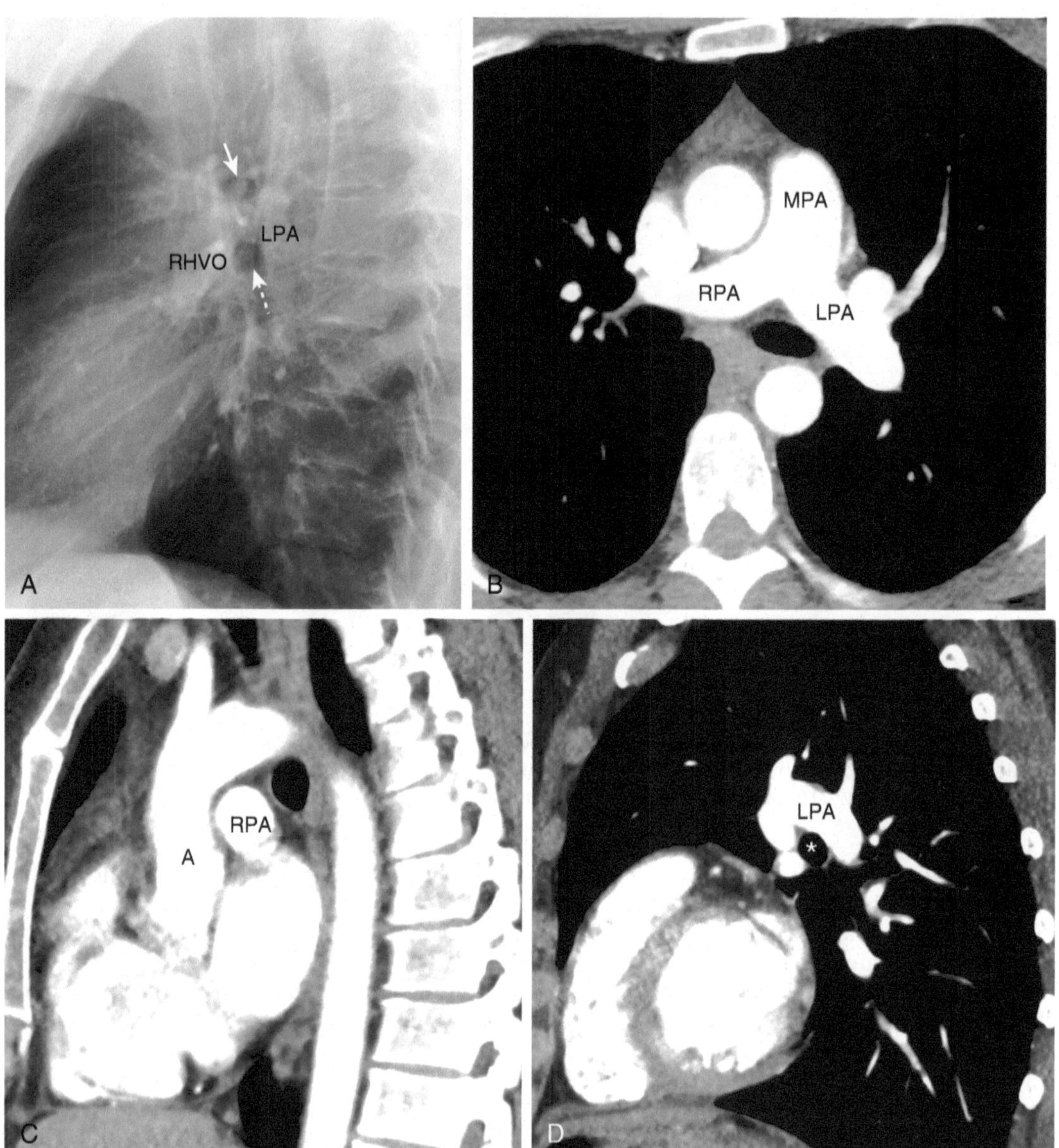

FIGURE 2.6 Hilar anatomy. **A,** Lateral chest radiograph shows the normal relationship between the hilar structures. The right upper lobe bronchus *(white arrow)* is seen as an ill-defined oval lucency anterior to the left pulmonary artery (LPA) and posterior to the aortic arch. The right hilar vascular opacity (RHVO) is an anterior round poorly marginated density. The left main–upper lobe continuum (LULC) *(dashed arrow)* is typically seen as a well-delineated round lucency inferior to the right upper lobe bronchus and anterior to the LPA. **B,** Axial computed tomography (CT) image shows the main pulmonary artery (MPA) and demonstrates the shorter mediastinal course of the left pulmonary artery compared with the right pulmonary artery (RPA). **C,** Sagittal CT image shows the right pulmonary artery (RPA) located posterior to the ascending aorta (A). **D,** Sagittal CT image shows the left pulmonary artery arching posteriorly and laterally over the LULC *(asterisk)*, which creates the comma-shaped opacity on the lateral radiograph.

typically visible as a crescentic fluid collection approximating the posterior aspect of the ascending aorta, just above the right pulmonary artery (Fig. 2.8). In some individuals, a "high-riding" superior pericardial recess may extend to the right paratracheal space and can be mistaken for lymphadenopathy or a cystic mediastinal lesion.

The left pulmonic recess is located inferior to the left pulmonary artery and is usually seen on CT as a crescentic or triangular fluid-attenuation structure paralleling the proximal right pulmonary artery (see Fig. 2.8). As with the superior aortic recess, the left pulmonic recess may have a round configuration and can be mistaken for lymphadenopathy.

The oblique pericardial sinus is posteriorly located within the pericardial space. It is situated anterior to the esophagus and posterior to the left atrium, approximating the subcarinal space. Fluid within the oblique sinus can mimic esophageal abnormalities or subcarinal lymphadenopathy.

The right and left pulmonary venous recesses and the postcaval recess originate from the pericardial cavity proper. The postcaval recess is located posterior to the superior vena cava (SVC). The right and left pulmonary venous recesses are situated between the superior and inferior pulmonary veins on their respective sides. Fluid distending the right pulmonary venous recess may have a

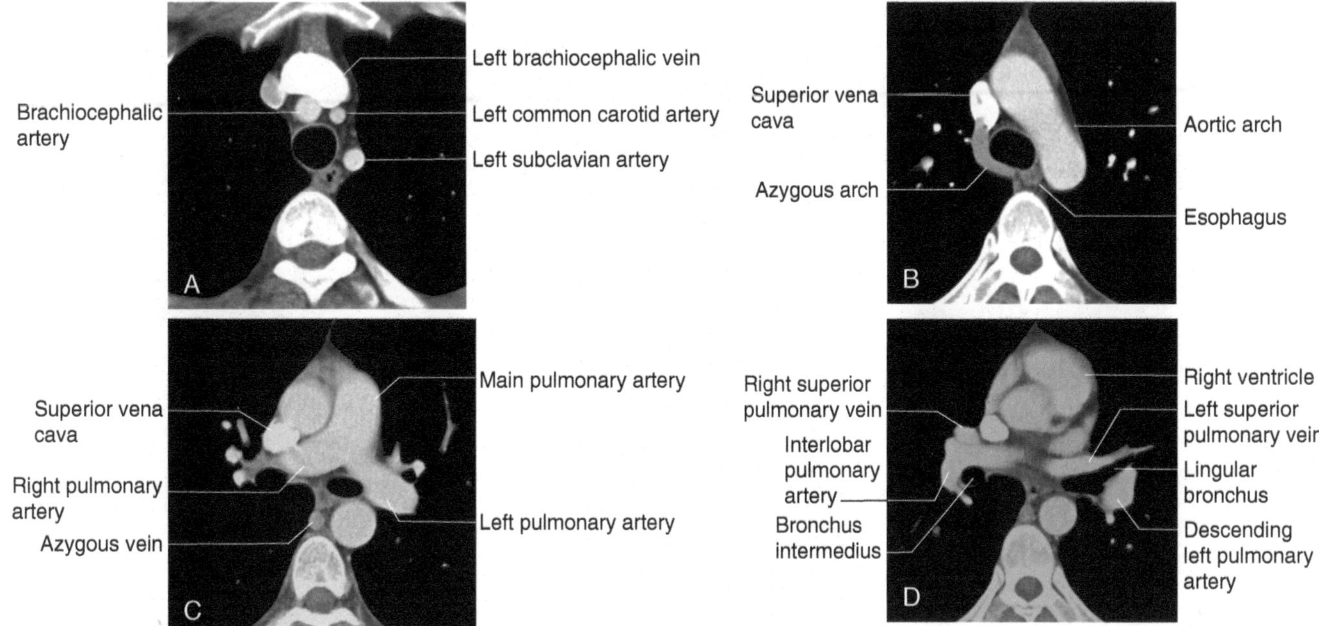

FIGURE 2.7 Pulmonary vessels. Sequential computed tomography images demonstrating normal mediastinal and hilar vascular anatomy. **A,** At the level of the left brachiocephalic vein, the three arterial branches arising from the aortic arch can be seen: the brachiocephalic artery, left common carotid artery, and left subclavian artery. **B,** At the level of the aortic arch, the azygous vein can be seen draining into the superior vena cava. **C,** The main pulmonary artery bifurcates into the right and left pulmonary arteries as shown. **D,** At the level of the superior pulmonary veins, the interlobar artery is seen lateral to the bronchus intermedius. The descending left pulmonary is located posterior and lateral to the lingular bronchus.

lobulated appearance and can also mimic lymphadenopathy (Fig. 2.9).

Fissures

The lobes of the lungs are separated by fissures, bounded by the visceral pleura. The majority of fissures are incomplete. On the lateral projection, the *major fissures* course from superior to inferior, from the fifth thoracic vertebra to the diaphragm, roughly paralleling the sixth rib. The entire length of the major fissures is not usually visible. Above the hila, the medial portions of the major fissures lie more anteriorly than the lateral portions, and below the hila, the lateral portions of the major fissures lie more anteriorly. The major fissure is usually not visible on the frontal projection. However, the superolateral major fissure can occasionally be seen when extrapleural fat enters the edge of the fissure where it contacts the posterior chest wall. It forms a curved line on the frontal radiograph that starts medially above the hilum and curves downward and laterally.

The *minor fissure* extends anteriorly and laterally from the right hilum to the lateral chest wall and separates the anterior segment of the right upper lobe from the middle lobe. It is seen in at least half of patients on the frontal view. The fissure terminates medially at the right interlobar artery. On the lateral radiograph, the posterior extent of the minor fissure can occasionally project posterior to the hilum and major fissure.

Accessory fissures can be found in up to 30% of patients and may occur between any segments. Such fissures are frequently incomplete and vary with the degree of development. The common accessory fissures include the azygous fissure, inferior accessory fissure, superior accessory fissure, and left minor fissure.

The azygous fissure is formed by the downward invagination of the azygous vein through the apical right upper lobe. It creates a curvilinear reflection composed of four pleural layers extending obliquely from the upper aspect of the right lung and terminating in a teardrop shadow, which is formed by the azygous vein above the right hilum (Fig. 2.10). The azygous lobe is the portion of the right lung located medial to the fissure.

The inferior accessory fissure separates the medial basal segment from the remaining lower lobe segments and may occur on the right or left. The fissure extends from the inner third of the hemidiaphragm superiorly and slightly medially (Fig. 2.11). It is visible in up to 16% of individuals on chest CT.

The superior accessory fissure divides the superior segment from the lower lobe basal segments. It is more frequent on the right and located in a horizontal plane similar to that of the right minor fissure (Fig. 2.12).

The left minor fissure divides the lingua from the superior division of the left upper lobe (Fig. 2.13). The left minor fissure is typically more superiorly located than the right.

The Diaphragm

The diaphragm is a muscular tendinous sheath that separates the thoracic and abdominal cavities. The right hemidiaphragm is usually found at about the right anterior sixth rib. In the majority of people, the right hemidiaphragm

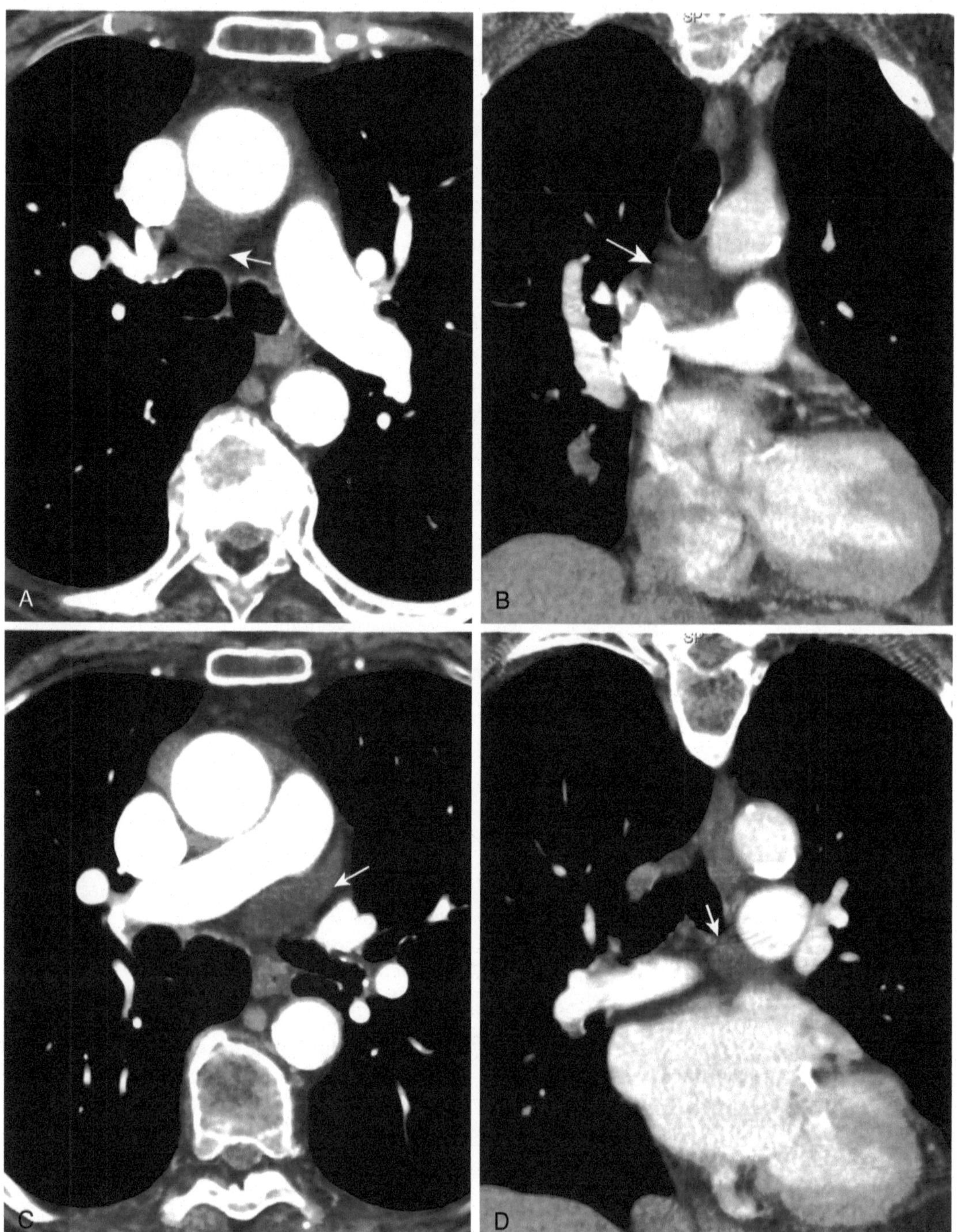

FIGURE 2.8 Pericardial recesses. **A,** Axial computed tomography (CT) image shows the superior aortic recess posterior to the aortic arch *(arrow)*. **B,** Coronal CT image shows the superior aortic recess *(arrow)*. **C,** Axial CT image at the level of the right pulmonary artery shows fluid left in the pulmonic recess *(arrow)*, which parallels the proximal right pulmonary artery. A thin fat plane posterior to the recess separates the adjacent esophagus. **D,** Coronal CT image shows the left pulmonic recess in the same patient *(arrow)*.

is higher than the left by 1.5 to 2.5 cm or approximately one half of an interspace on the standard PA radiograph.

There are three openings or hiatuses within the diaphragm, which allow passage of structures between the abdomen and thorax. At the T8 level, the inferior vena cava (IVC) hiatus contains the IVC and right phrenic nerve branches. The esophagus, vagus nerve, and sympathetic nerve branches traverse the esophageal hiatus at the T10 level. Most inferiorly at the level of T12, the retrocrural aortic hiatus contains the descending aorta, azygous and hemiazygous veins, and thoracic duct.

Several radiographic signs can be used to identify the right and left diaphragm on the lateral radiograph. The right ribs are magnified on lateral radiographs and appear larger and more posteriorly located. The presence of an air-filled gastric bubble localizes the left diaphragm.

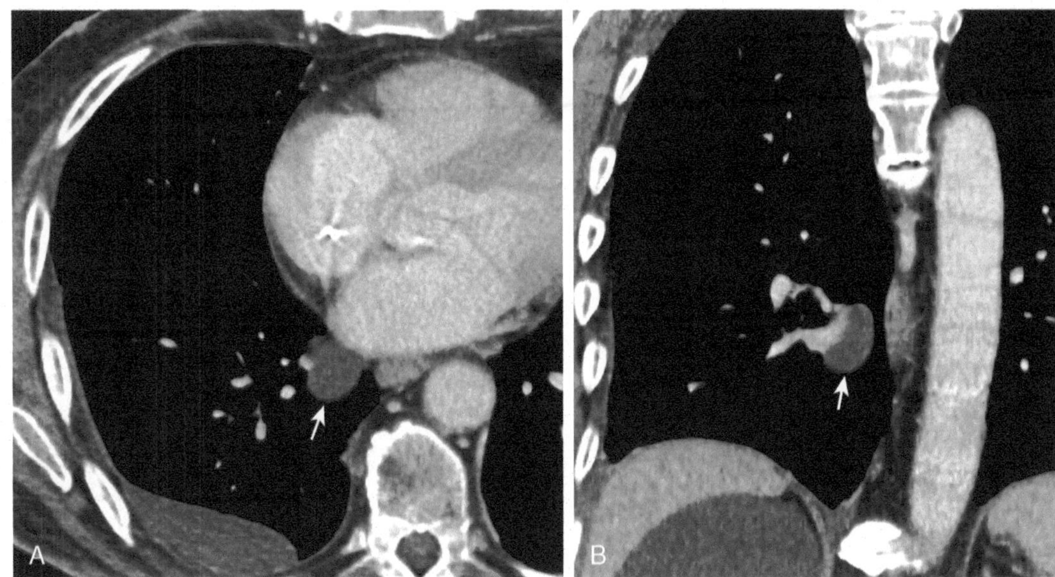

FIGURE 2.9 Right pulmonary venous recess. Axial **(A)** and coronal **(B)** computed tomography images show fluid in the right pulmonary venous recess *(arrows)* adjacent to the right inferior pulmonary vein. This is a common pseudolesion that may be mistaken for lymphadenopathy.

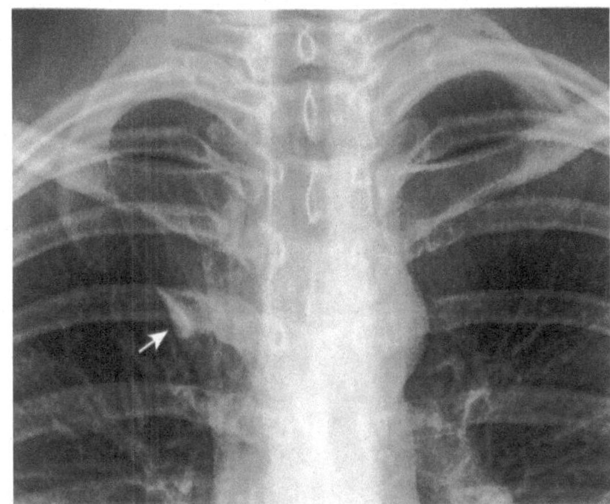

FIGURE 2.10 Accessory azygous fissure. Posteroanterior radiograph demonstrates the curvilinear accessory azygous fissure as it courses inferiorly to terminate above the right hilum. The teardrop-shaped opacity seen along the inferior aspect of the fissure represents the azygous vein *(arrow)*.

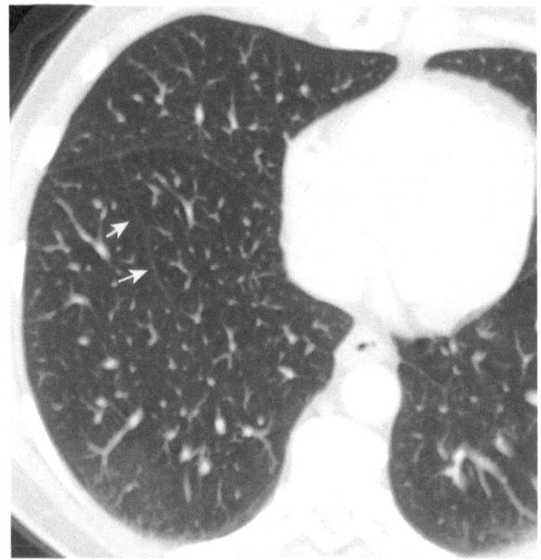

FIGURE 2.11 Right inferior accessory fissure. The right inferior accessory fissure demarcates the medial basal segment of the right lower lobe *(arrows)* as demonstrated on this axial computed tomography image.

Whereas the right diaphragm should be visible along its entire course on the lateral chest radiograph, the anterior left hemidiaphragm is frequently obscured by the cardiac silhouette (Fig. 2.14). Last, the left diaphragm is typically slightly lower than the right.

Normal Mediastinal Contours: The Frontal Projection

On the frontal projection chest radiograph, the right mediastinal border is composed of the right brachiocephalic vein, SVC, azygous vein, and right atrium from cephalad to caudad, where the right lung abuts these structures (Figs. 2.15 and 2.16). The left subclavian artery forms the left lateral margin of the superior mediastinum in the supraaortic region on the frontal radiograph (Figs. 2.17 to 2.19). The lateral aspect of the aortic arch forms the *aortic knob*.

The azygous vein arches anteriorly and inferiorly at approximately the level of the T4 to T5 vertebral bodies along the posterior trachea wall. The vein then courses laterally and anteriorly over the right main bronchus and drains into the SVC (see Fig. 2.7, *B*). On the PA radiograph, the *azygous arch* is seen as an ovoid density located along the inferior portion of the right paratracheal stripe at the right tracheobronchial angle. The azygous arch is bordered by air within the trachea medially and the aerated right upper lobe along its lateral border. The transverse diameter

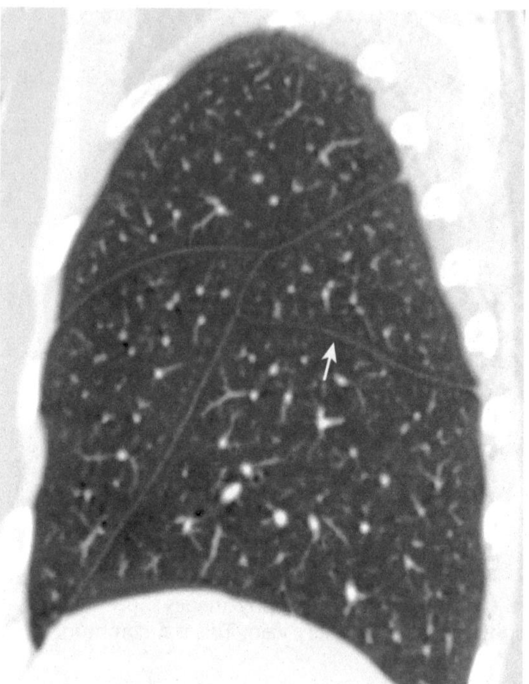

FIGURE 2.12 Superior accessory fissure. Sagittal computed tomography image shows the superior accessory fissure coursing in roughly the horizontal plane to separate the superior segment from the right lower lobe basal segments *(arrow)*.

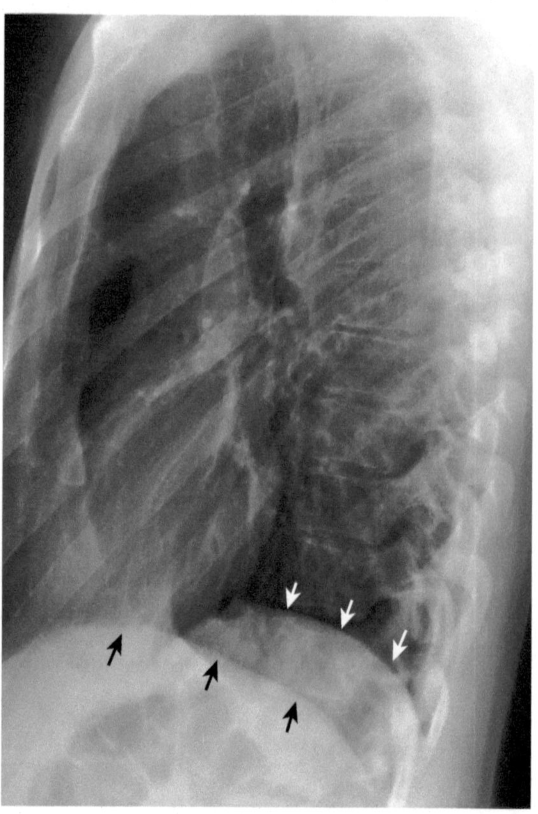

FIGURE 2.14 Diaphragm on the lateral radiograph. This lateral radiograph demonstrates that the left hemidiaphragm *(white arrows)* is not visible anterior to the cardiac silhouette. Although in most cases, the left hemidiaphragm is slightly lower than the right, in this patient, it is slightly superior. The right hemidiaphragm *(black arrows)* is typically visible along its entire anteroposterior course. The right ribs are slightly magnified and more posteriorly located than the left.

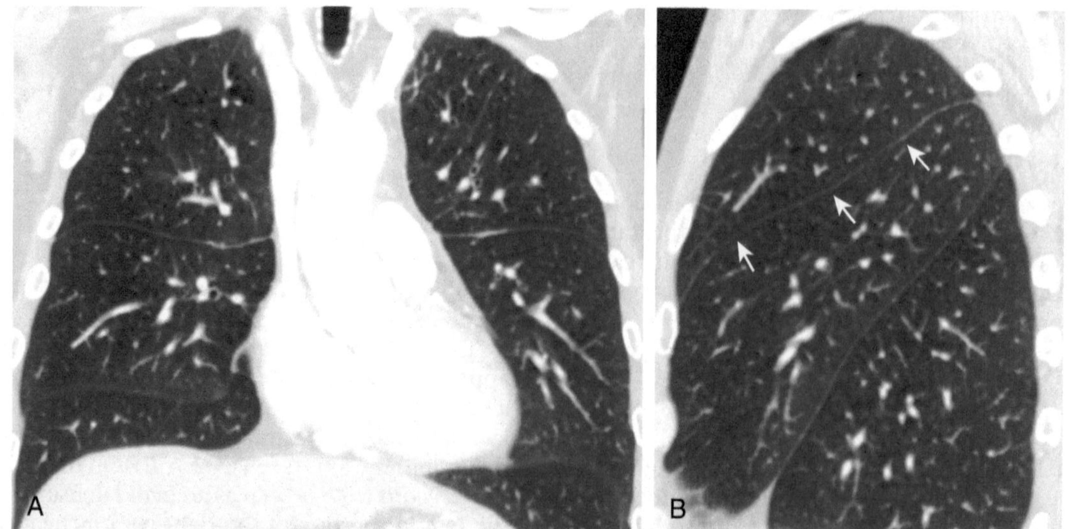

FIGURE 2.13 Left minor fissure. **A,** Coronal computed tomography (CT) image shows the left minor fissure at approximately the same level as the right minor fissure. **B,** Sagittal CT image shows the left minor fissure separating the lingula from the remainder of the left upper lobe *(arrows)*.

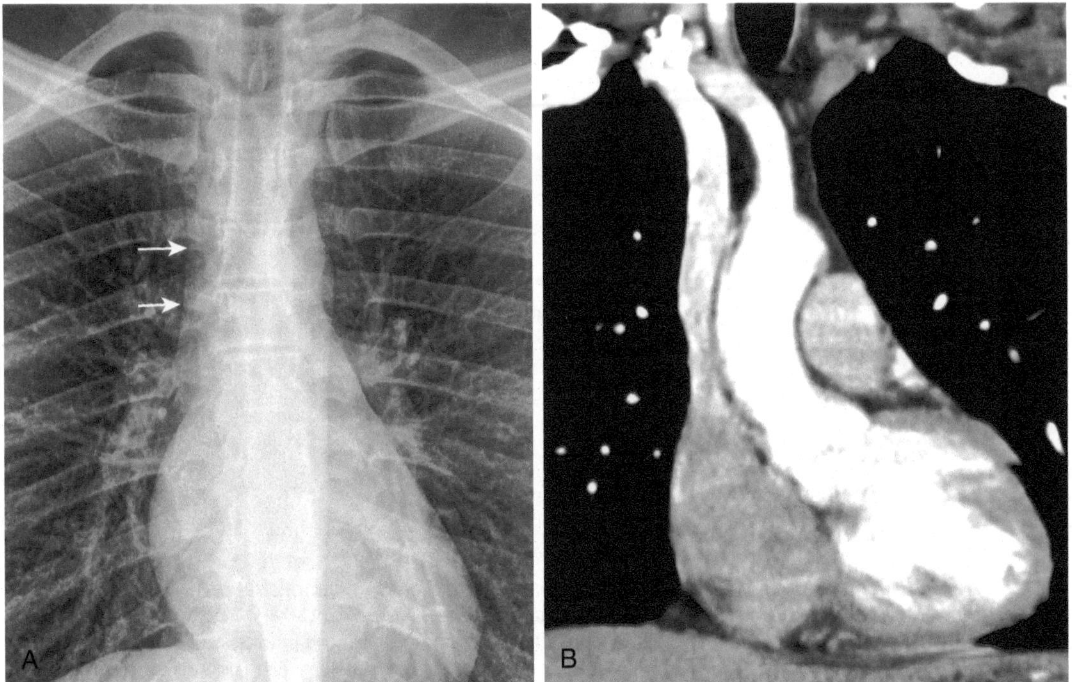

FIGURE 2.15 Normal mediastinal contours. **A,** Frontal radiograph shows the normal appearance of the superior vena cava (SVC) interface where the right lateral wall of the SVC interfaces with the right lung *(arrows)*. **B,** Coronal computed tomography image shows where the right lung abuts the superior vena cava, which may be minimally concave laterally as in this case.

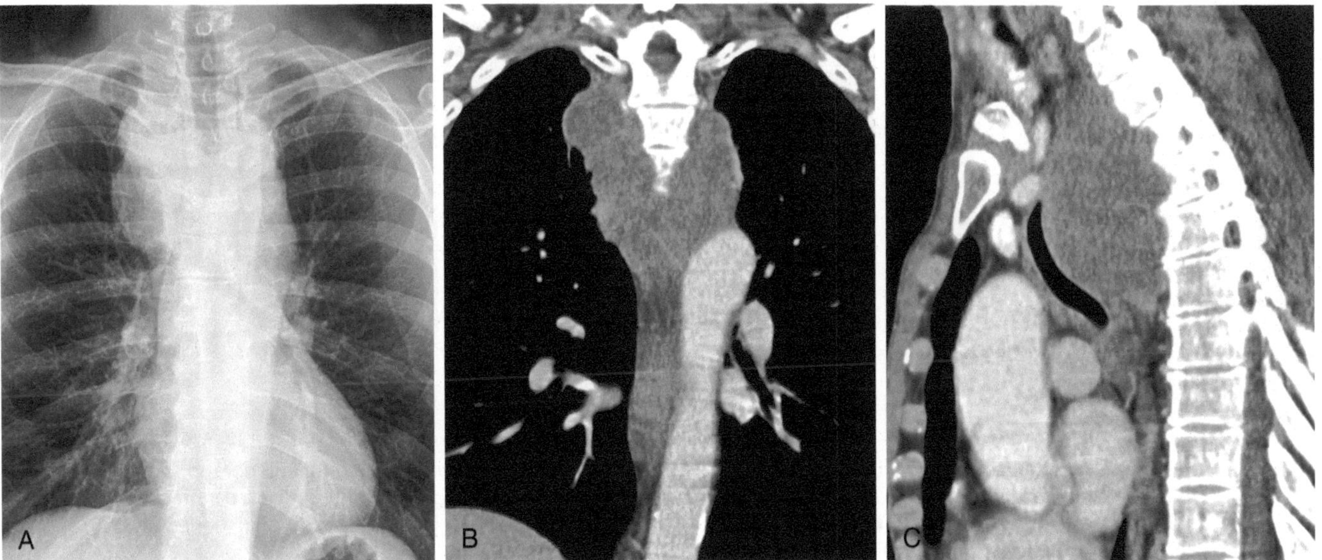

FIGURE 2.16 Abnormal superior mediastinal contour in a patient with poorly differentiated non–small cell lung cancer. **A,** Posteroanterior radiograph shows a mediastinal mass obscuring the adjacent vertebral bodies and normal contour of the superior vena cava and left subclavian artery interface. **B,** Coronal computed tomography (CT) image demonstrates a confluent mass involving the posterior and middle mediastinum. **C,** Sagittal CT image shows the mass displacing the trachea anteriorly and eroding the adjacent vertebral bodies.

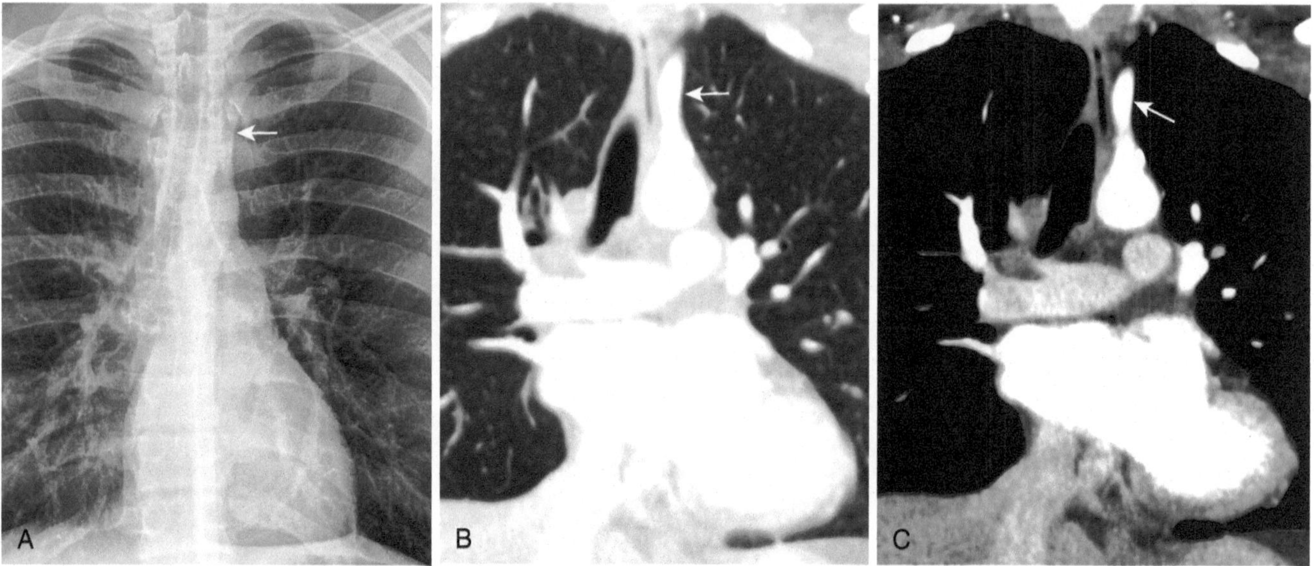

FIGURE 2.17 Left subclavian artery interface. **A,** Posteroanterior radiograph demonstrates the appearance of the left subclavian interface where the left upper lobe contacts the left subclavian artery. This interface is typically concave as shown here *(arrow)*. **B** and **C,** Coronal computed tomography images in lung and soft tissue windows show the normal course and contour of the left subclavian artery after it arises from the aortic arch *(arrows)*.

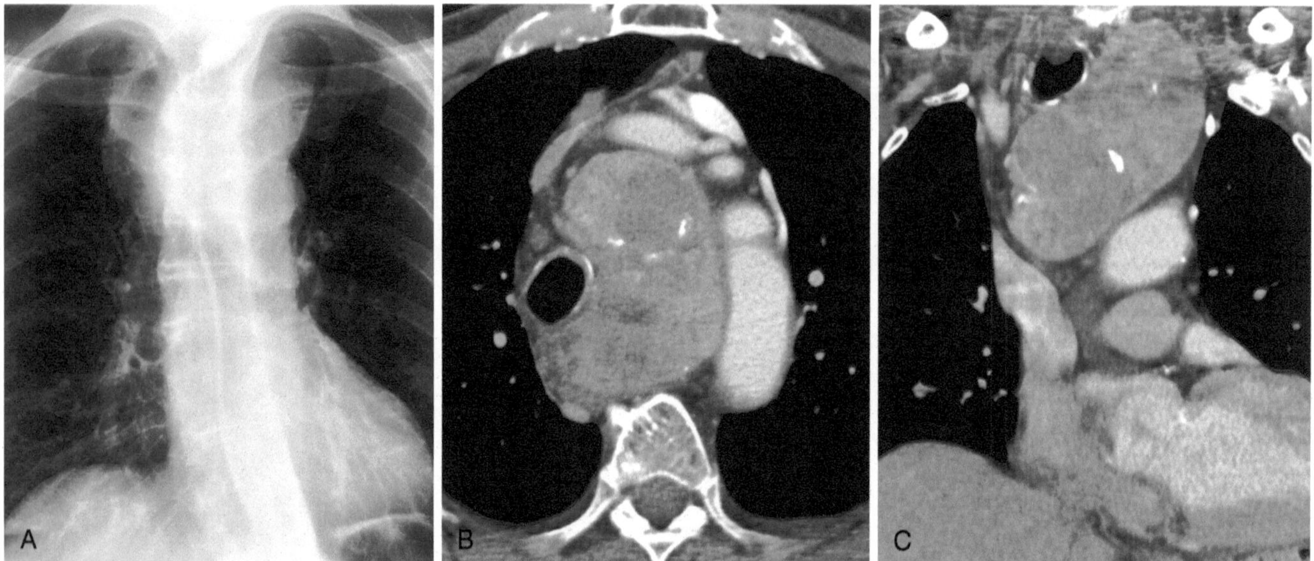

FIGURE 2.18 Abnormal left subclavian artery interface: intrathoracic thyroid goiter. **A,** Frontal radiograph shows rightward shift of the trachea and abnormal mediastinal widening with thickening of the right and left paratracheal stripes. Axial **(A)** and coronal **(B)** computed tomography images show an intrathoracic thyroid goiter that extends into the left paratracheal space.

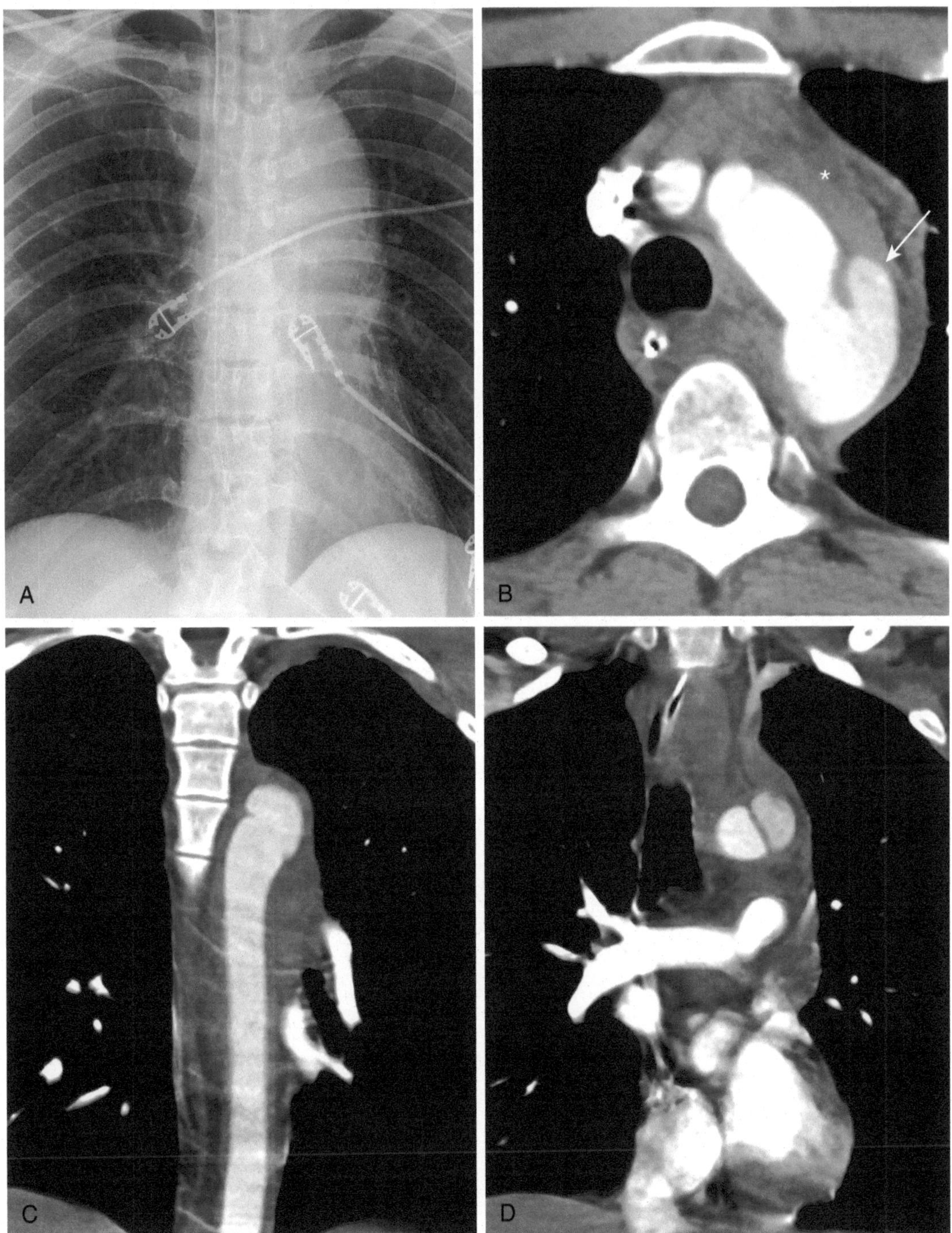

FIGURE 2.19 Abnormal left superior mediastinal contour in the setting of traumatic aortic transection. **A,** Frontal radiograph shows convex bulging of the normal left superior mediastinal interface. There is mass effect on the trachea, which is slightly deviated to the right. **B,** Axial computed tomography image shows aortic pseudoaneurysm formation *(arrow)* and adjacent mediastinal hematoma *(asterisk)*. **C** and **D,** Coronal images through the aortic arch show the traumatic aortic transection and surrounding mediastinal hematoma.

of the azygous arch on the frontal chest radiograph should be less than 10 mm (Fig. 2.20).

The *right paratracheal stripe* is seen through the right brachiocephalic vein and SVC as a smooth, vertically oriented soft tissue density line measuring no more than 4 mm in transverse diameter. The interface of the right lung in the supraazygous region with the right lateral tracheal wall creates the stripe that is composed of visceral and parietal pleura of the right upper lobe and a small amount of intervening mediastinal fat. The right paratracheal stripe extends from the level of the clavicles to the right tracheobronchial angle inferiorly at the level of the azygous arch (Fig. 2.21). Widening of the right paratracheal stripe can be seen in the setting of paratracheal lymphadenopathy, pleural disease, mediastinal infiltration, or malignancy arising from the trachea, thyroid gland, or parathyroid gland (Fig. 2.22).

The *left paratracheal stripe* is visible on the PA chest radiograph in a minority of individuals and is formed by the

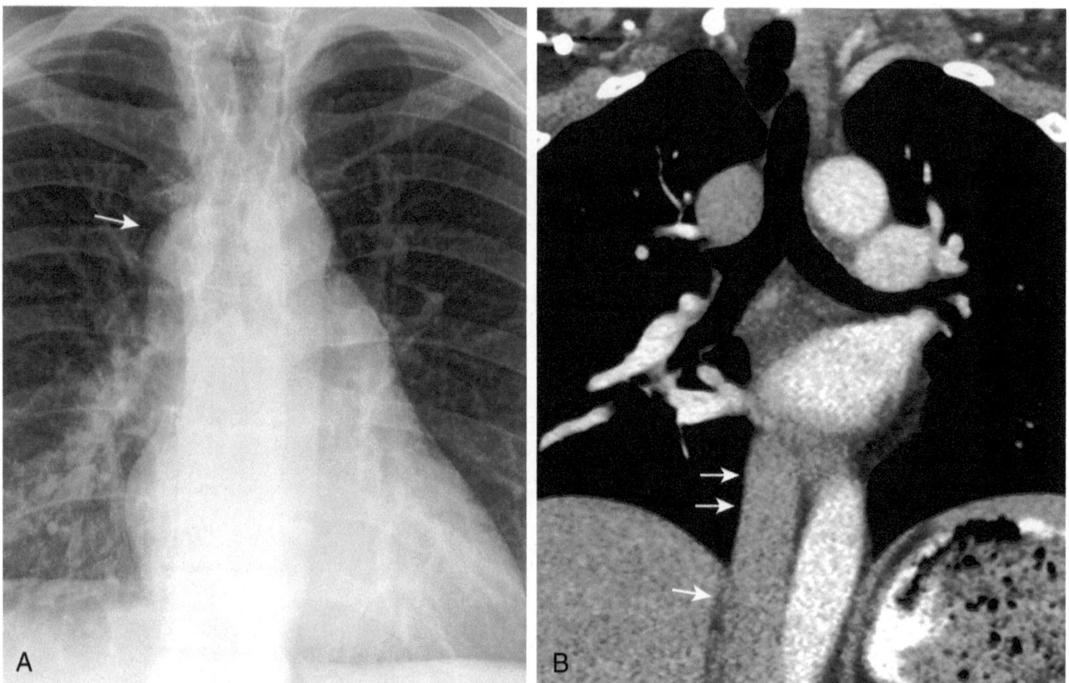

FIGURE 2.20 Dilated azygous arch in the setting of azygous continuation of the inferior vena cava. **A,** Posteroanterior radiograph demonstrates an abnormally dilated azygous arch, measuring greater than 10 mm *(arrow)*. **B,** Coronal computed tomography image reveals that the dilated arch is caused by azygous continuation of the inferior vena cava in this patient *(arrows)*.

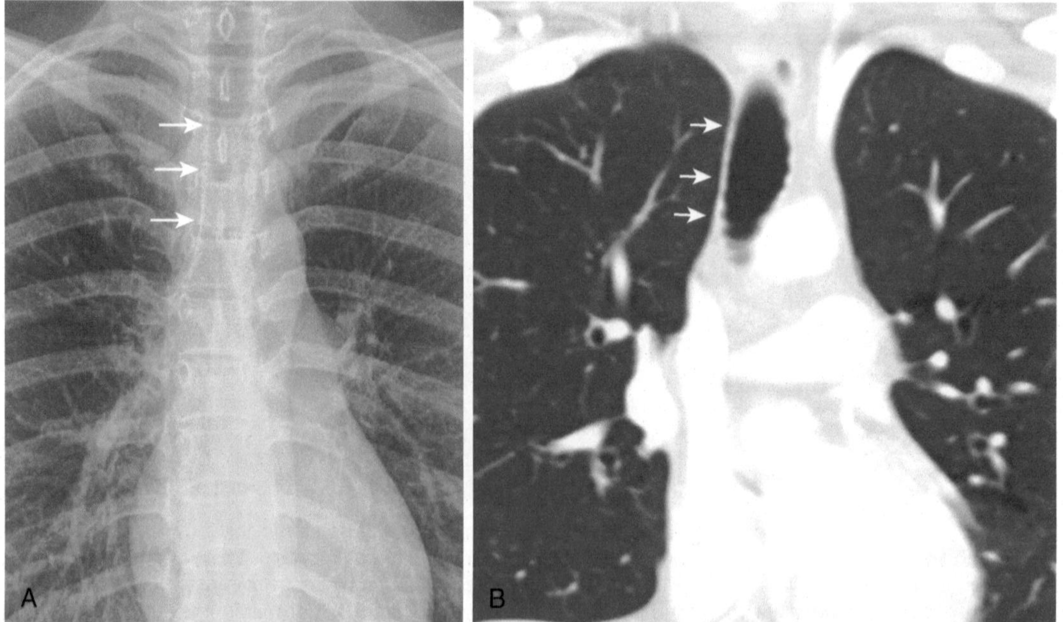

FIGURE 2.21 Right paratracheal stripe. **A,** Posteroanterior radiograph shows the normal thin (<4 mm) right paratracheal stripe extending from the thoracic inlet to the level of the azygous arch *(arrows)*. **B,** Coronal computed tomography image demonstrating the interface between the right upper lobe and right lateral tracheal wall, which forms the stripe *(arrows)*.

interface between the left upper lobe and the left lateral tracheal wall or adjacent mediastinal fat. When visible, the stripe extends from the reflection of the left subclavian artery to the aortic arch in a cranial to caudad direction.

The *anterior junction line* is composed of four pleural layers and represents the approximation of the visceral and parietal pleura of the anterior right and left lung. Often there is a small amount of retrosternal fat or thymus gland interposed between the anterior pleural reflections of the right and left upper lobes. The anterior junction line tends to have an oblique right-to-left course on the PA chest radiograph extending inferiorly from the level of the anterior

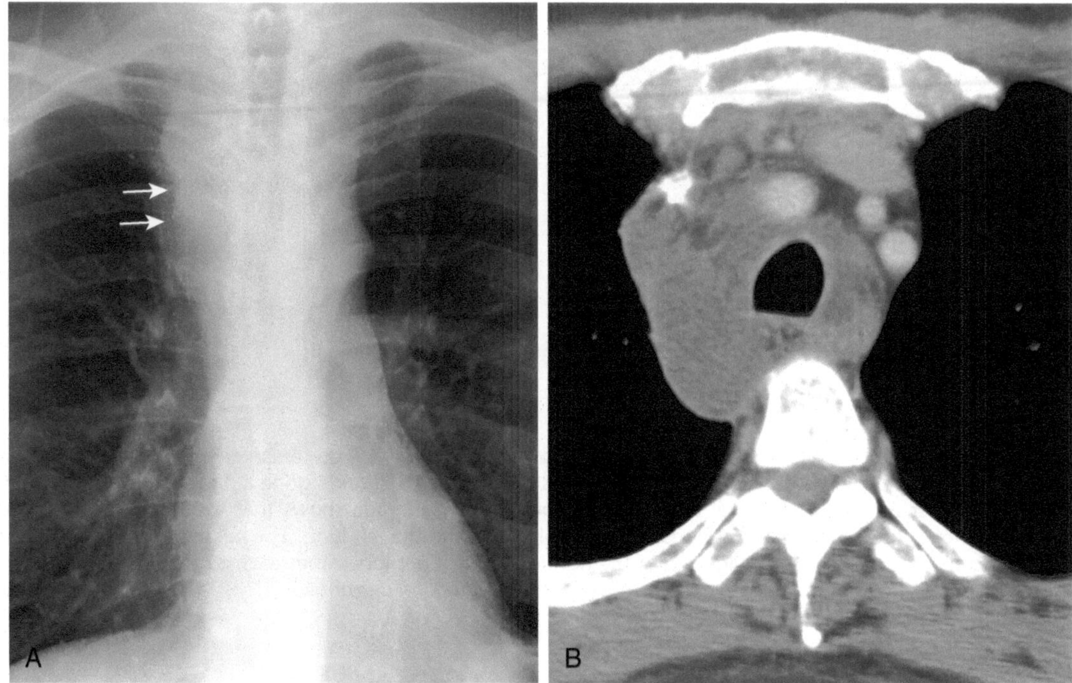

FIGURE 2.22 Thickened right paratracheal stripe caused by mediastinitis. **A,** There is marked thickening of the right paratracheal stripe *(arrows)* on this posteroanterior chest radiograph. **B,** Axial computed tomography image shows abnormal soft tissue in the right paratracheal space, which was caused by mediastinitis.

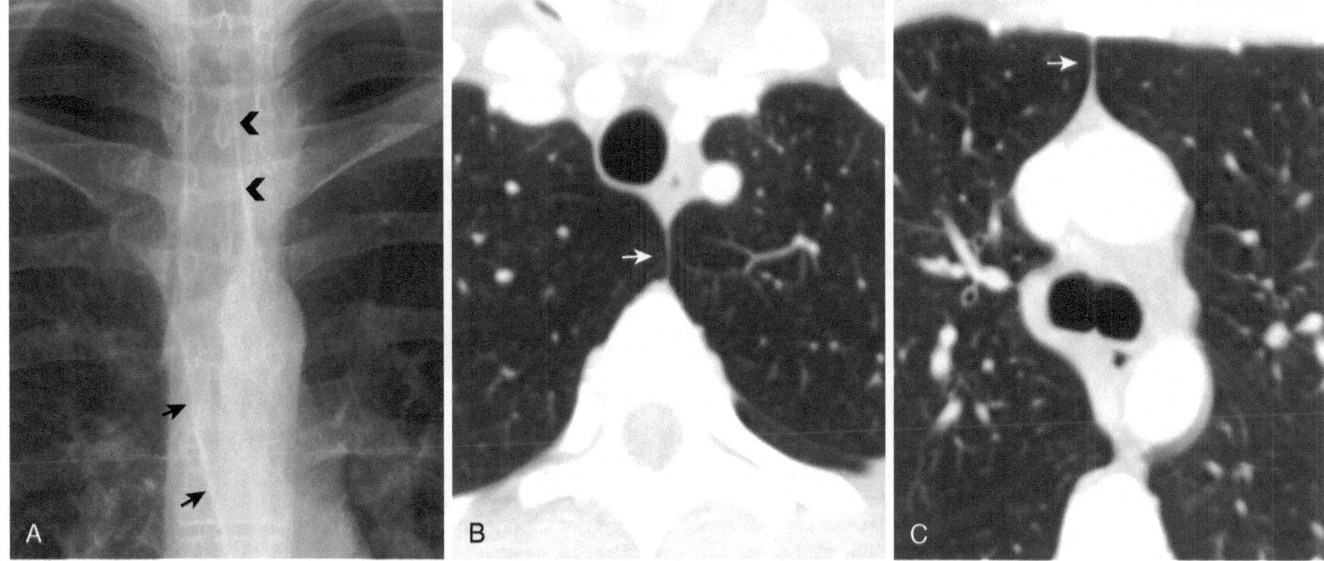

FIGURE 2.23 Anterior and posterior junction lines. **A,** Frontal radiograph demonstrates the posterior and anterior junction lines. The posterior junction line is seen above the aortic arch *(arrowheads)*. The anterior junction line extends from the level of the aortic arch and courses inferiorly and slightly to the left *(arrows)*. **B,** Axial computed tomography (CT) image shows where the right and left upper lobes interface to form the posterior junction line in the retroesophageal prevertebral region, above the level of the aortic arch *(arrow)*. **C,** Axial CT image shows where the right and left upper lobes meet anteriorly to form the anterior junction line *(arrow)*.

mediastinal triangle, which is visible as an inverted triangular opacity. The normal thickness of the anterior junction line is 1 to 3 mm (Fig. 2.23). Volume loss or hyperinflation of the lung can result in displacement of the line (Fig. 2.24).

The *posterior junction line or stripe* refers to the reflection of the right and left lungs posterior to the esophagus and anterior to the thoracic vertebral bodies. Similar to the anterior junction line, it is composed of four pleural layers in addition to mediastinal fat. The posterior junction line extends from the lung apices above the level of the clavicles to the aortic arch on the PA radiograph and is typically visible through the tracheal air column as a vertically oriented line (see Fig. 2.23). The normal thickness of the posterior junction line ranges from several

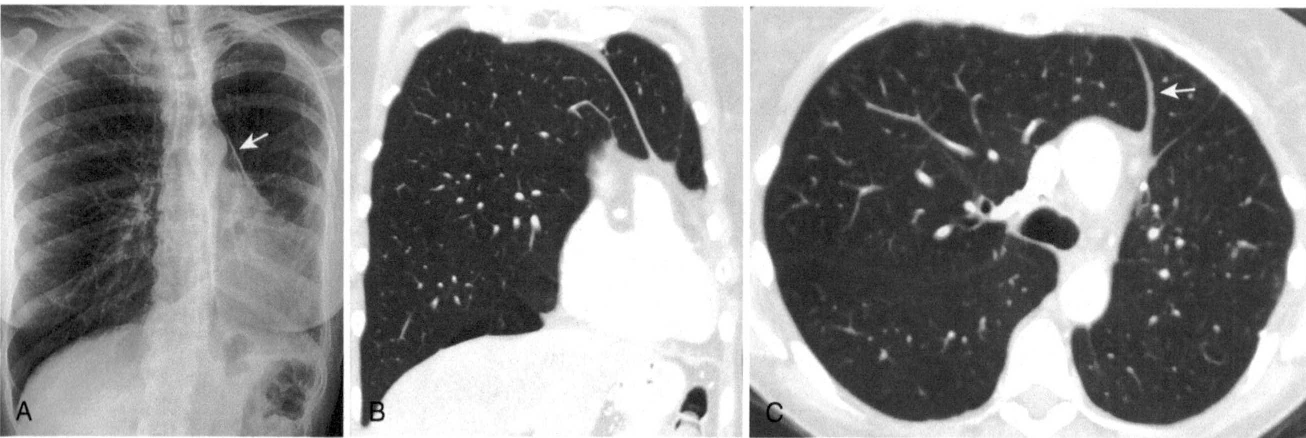

FIGURE 2.24 Displaced anterior junction line after left lower lobectomy. **A,** A posteroanterior radiograph shows that the anterior junction line is displaced to the left in this patient who had undergone a prior left lower lobectomy for lung cancer *(arrow).* **B,** Coronal computed tomography (CT) image shows that the right upper, middle, and lower lobes are hyperinflated as a result of the volume loss in the left lung. The heart and mediastinum are shifted to the left. **C,** Axial CT image shows the right and left upper lobes abut each to the left of the midline where the four layers of opposed pleura form the anterior junction line *(arrow).*

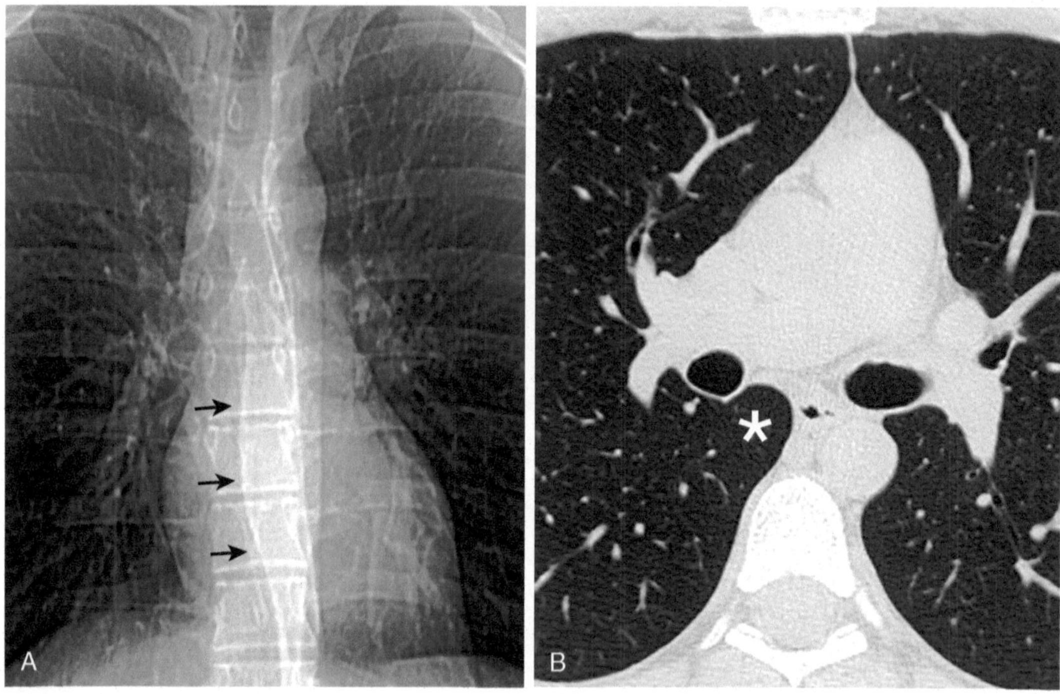

FIGURE 2.25 Azygoesophageal line and recess. **A,** Anteroposterior topogram shows the normal reverse-S–shaped contour of the azygoesophageal line as it descends from the azygous arch to the diaphragmatic hiatus *(arrows).* **B,** Axial computed tomography image demonstrates the azygoesophageal recess where the right lower lobe approximates the lateral wall of azygous vein and esophagus *(asterisk).*

mm to 1 cm owing to the variable amount of intervening mediastinal fat.

In the mid to lower chest, the right lower lobe contacts the right wall of the esophagus and the azygous vein, forming the *azygoesophageal line.* The azygoesophageal line typically has slight reverse-S- or reverse-C-shaped contour. The *azygoesophageal recess* is located posterolateral to the esophagus and anterior to the vertebral bodies, where the right lower lobe interfaces with the retrocardiac mediastinum. The recess extends from the subcarinal space to the aortic hiatus inferiorly (Figs. 2.25 and 2.26).

The supraaortic area is a region of the left mediastinum located posterior to the anterior mediastinum from the aortic arch to the thoracic inlet, superiorly. The left subclavian artery, left lateral tracheal wall, left superior intercostal vein, and mediastinal fat are located within the supraaortic area. A round or triangular opacity less than 4.5 mm in diameter referred to as the *aortic nipple* can occasionally project from the lateral aspect of the aortic arch and is formed by the left superior intercostal vein as it arches from the spine anteriorly along the aortic arch to drain into the left brachiocephalic vein (Figs. 2.27 and 2.28). In the

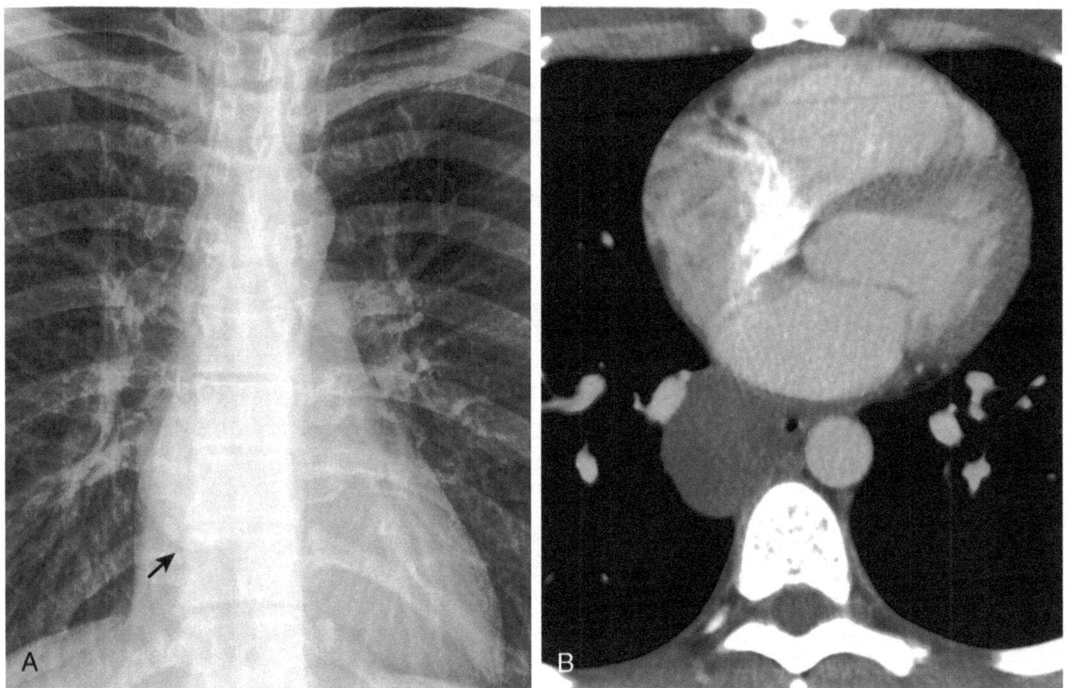

FIGURE 2.26 Abnormal azygoesophageal recess caused by a bronchogenic cyst. **A,** Frontal radiograph shows a rounded opacity in the azygoesophageal recess *(arrow)*. **B,** Axial computed tomography image shows a cystic lesion in the recess, which abuts the azygous vein and esophagus. This lesion was surgically resected and found to represent a bronchogenic cyst.

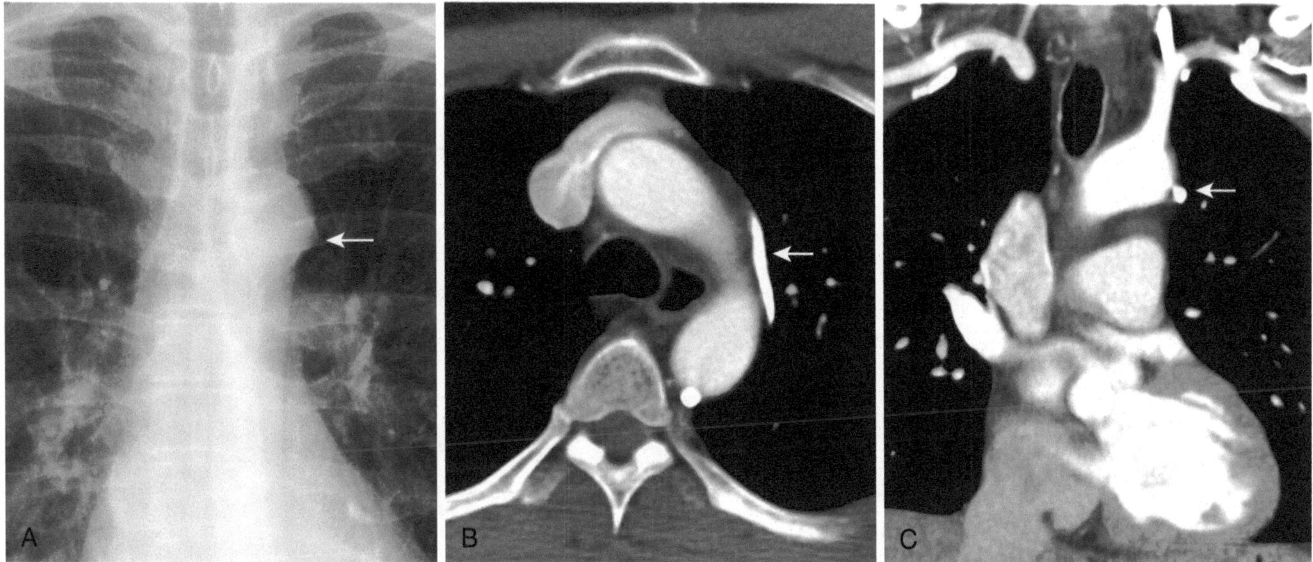

FIGURE 2.27 Left superior intercostal vein: the "aortic nipple." **A,** Frontal radiograph shows a small protuberance along the lateral aspect of the aortic arch, referred to as the "aortic nipple." **B,** Axial computed tomography (CT) image shows the left superior intercostal vein coursing along the lateral aspect of the aortic arch to drain into the brachiocephalic vein *(arrow)*. In most individuals, as in this case, the vein communicates with the superior (accessory) hemiazygous vein. **C,** Coronal CT image demonstrates the left superior intercostal vein imaged end-on *(arrow)*, which creates the appearance of a "nipple" on the posteroanterior radiograph.

setting of SVC or left brachiocephalic vein obstruction, the left superior intercostal vein frequently becomes dilated because it provides collateral flow to hemiazygous and azygous veins in most individuals.

The *aortic-pulmonary reflection* or *aortic-pulmonary stripe* is variably visible on the PA radiograph and represents the interface between the left lung and the adjacent main pulmonary artery and thoracic aorta. The presence of mediastinal fat along the anterolateral margin of the left pulmonary artery and the left anterior border of the aortic arch creates the interface, with the mediastinum appearing relatively more opaque than the more laterally located left lung. The aortic-pulmonary reflection may be straight or minimally convex laterally at the level of the main pulmonary artery, depending on the amount of mediastinal fat, and is most often straight or concave as it projects over the aortic arch (Fig. 2.29).

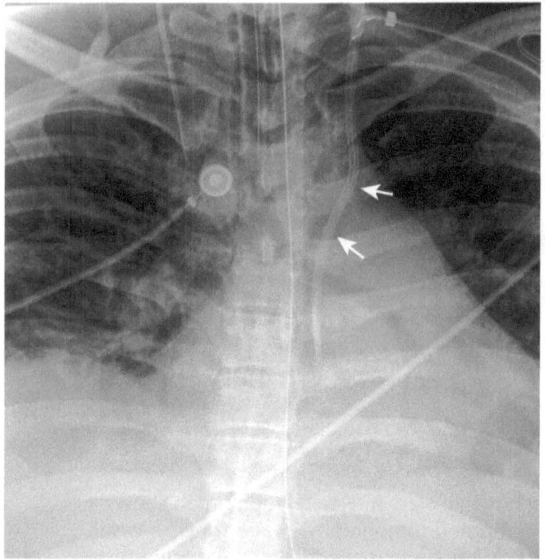

FIGURE 2.28 Malpositioned catheter in the left superior intercostal and superior hemiazygous veins. Portable chest radiograph shows a malpositioned hemodialysis catheter that had traversed the left brachiocephalic vein to enter the left superior intercostal vein and terminate in the left hemiazygous vein *(arrows)*. The catheter course was confirmed with computed tomography.

As the left lung abuts the mediastinum below the aortic arch and superior to the left pulmonary artery, it forms a space known as the *aortopulmonary window (AP window)*. The medial border of the AP window is the ductus ligament, and its lateral boundary is the mediastinal parietal pleura and visceral pleura of the adjacent left upper lobe. The normal contents of the AP window are mediastinal fat, the left recurrent laryngeal nerve, left bronchial arteries, and lymph nodes. A convex aortopulmonary window interface often indicates a mediastinal abnormality in this location, most frequently caused by lymphadenopathy or a saccular thoracic aortic aneurysm. The lateral border is normally concave or sometimes straight (Figs. 2.30 and 2.31).

Inferior to the aortopulmonary stripe, the main pulmonary artery and the heart form the left mediastinal border. The left lower lobe can protrude anterior to the descending aorta and posterior to the heart into the preaortic recess and form an interface known as the *preaortic line*, which is similar to the azygoesophageal recess on the right. The preaortic line is typically thinner and less well seen than the azygoesophageal line.

The left paraaortic interface represents the area of contact between the lateral aspect of the descending thoracic aorta and the adjacent left lung. The contour of the left paraaortic interface can be straight, convex, or concave, depending on the contour of the thoracic aorta (Figs. 2.32 to 2.34).

Normal Mediastinal Contours: The Lateral Projection

On the lateral projection, the length of the trachea descends inferiorly and posteriorly in a vertical orientation. The

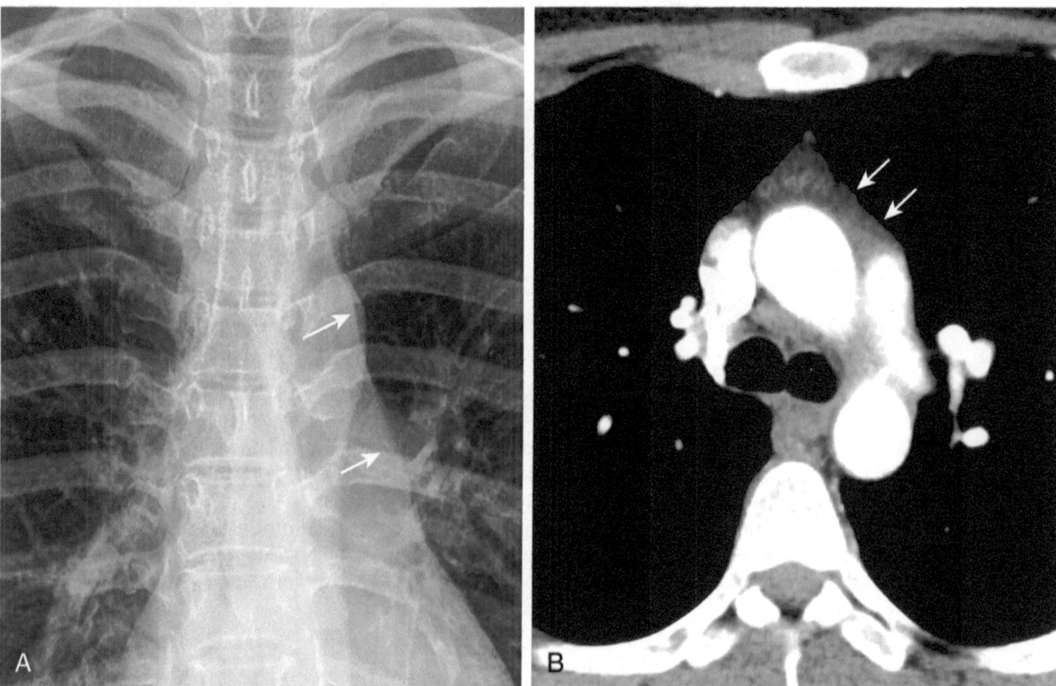

FIGURE 2.29 Aortic-pulmonary reflection or stripe. **A,** Posteroanterior radiograph demonstrates the normal aortic-pulmonary stripe, which in this case has a minimally convex configuration overlying the main pulmonary artery *(lower arrow)* and appears as a straight line at the level of the aortic arch *(upper arrow)*. **B,** Axial computed tomography image shows the presence of mediastinal fat along the anterolateral aspect of the left pulmonary artery and aortic arch, which produces the stripe *(arrows)*.

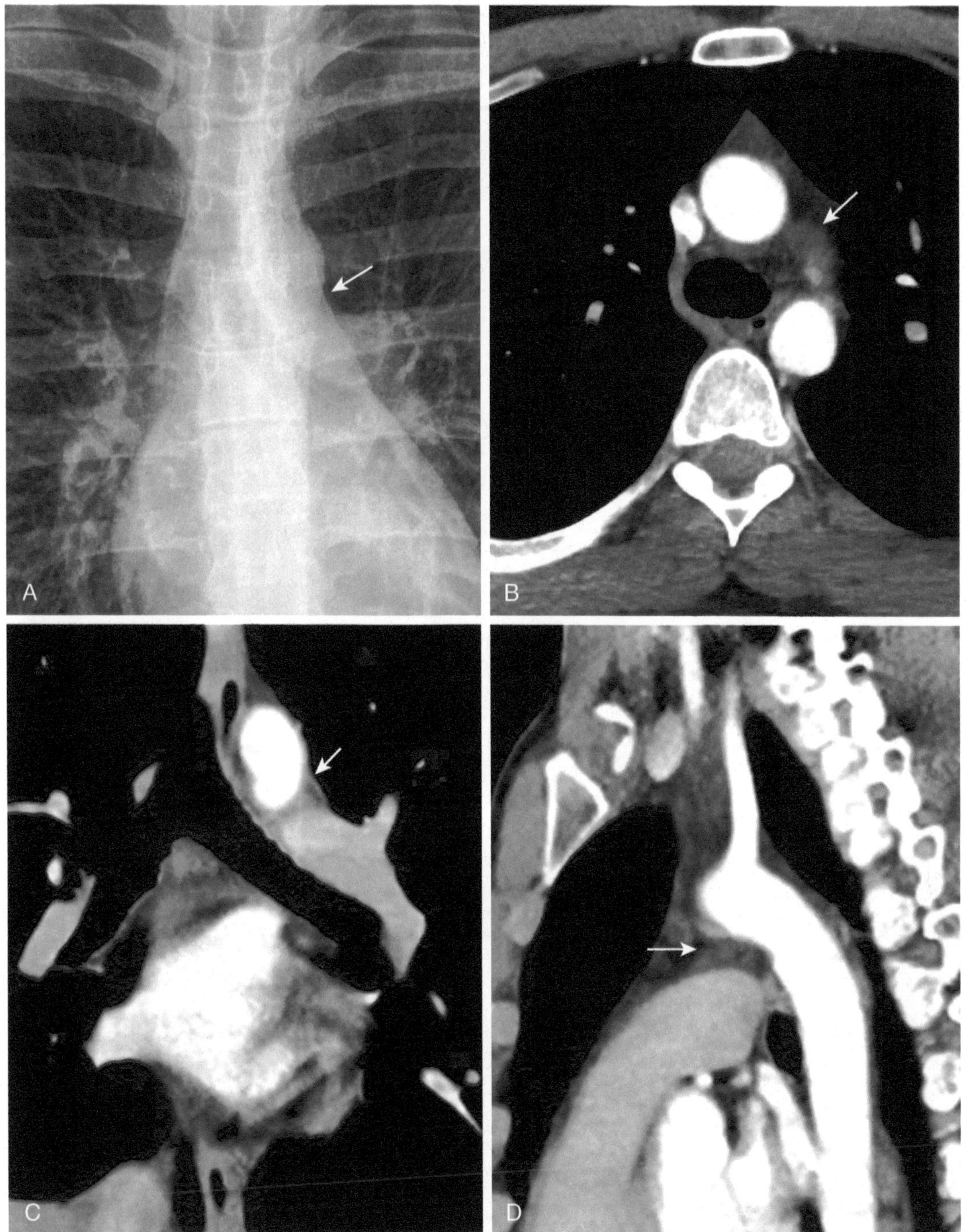

FIGURE 2.30 Aortopulmonary window. **A,** Posteroanterior radiograph demonstrates the normal appearance of the aortopulmonary window, with a concave interface between the aortic arch and left pulmonary artery and the adjacent left lung *(arrow)*. Axial **(B)**, coronal **(C)**, and sagittal **(D)** computed tomography images show the presence of mediastinal fat and occasional lymph nodes that are in the aortopulmonary window *(arrows)*.

anterior wall of the trachea is typically obscured by adjacent mediastinal fat and vessels. The *posterior tracheal band or stripe* is created by the interface of the right upper lobe with the posterior wall of the trachea (Fig. 2.35). In some individuals, the approximation of the anterior esophageal wall with the posterior wall of the trachea and adjacent mediastinal fat creates a thicker interface known as the *tracheoesophageal stripe*. The variability in the relationship of the esophagus with the trachea and the amount of intervening mediastinal fat leads to a range in the normal thickness of the posterior tracheal stripe or tracheoesophageal stripe, which may measure up to 5.5 mm.

The right ventricle and right ventricular outflow tract are the most anteriorly located cardiac structures on the lateral chest radiograph. The interface between the anterior lungs and the retrosternal soft tissues, including fat and internal mammary vessels, represents the *retrosternal stripe*. In most individuals, the stripe measures 7 mm or less in thickness (Fig. 2.36). Inferiorly, the stripe may increase in thickness in normal individuals because of the presence of

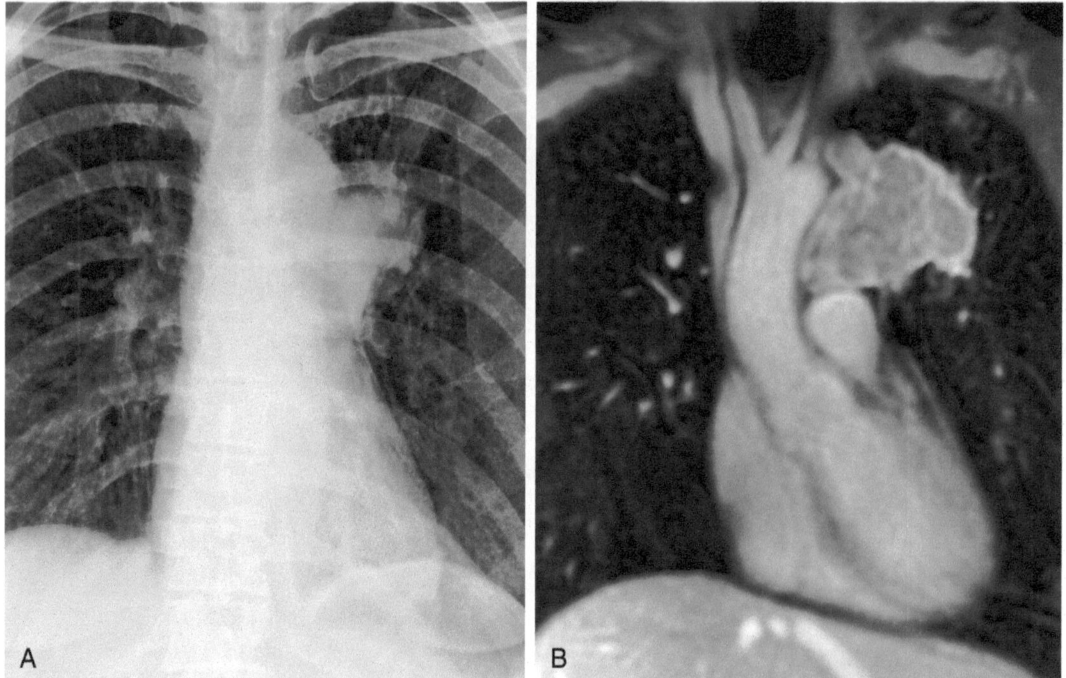

FIGURE 2.31 Aortopulmonary window lymphadenopathy caused by non–small cell lung cancer (NSCLC). **A,** Posteroanterior chest radiograph shows a mass-like opacity obscuring the normal contour of the aortopulmonary window with convex lateral bulging. **B,** Coronal fat-suppressed postcontrast T1-weighted three-dimensional gradient-echo magnetic resonance image shows that the opacity corresponds to extensive aortopulmonary window lymphadenopathy in this patient with NSCLC.

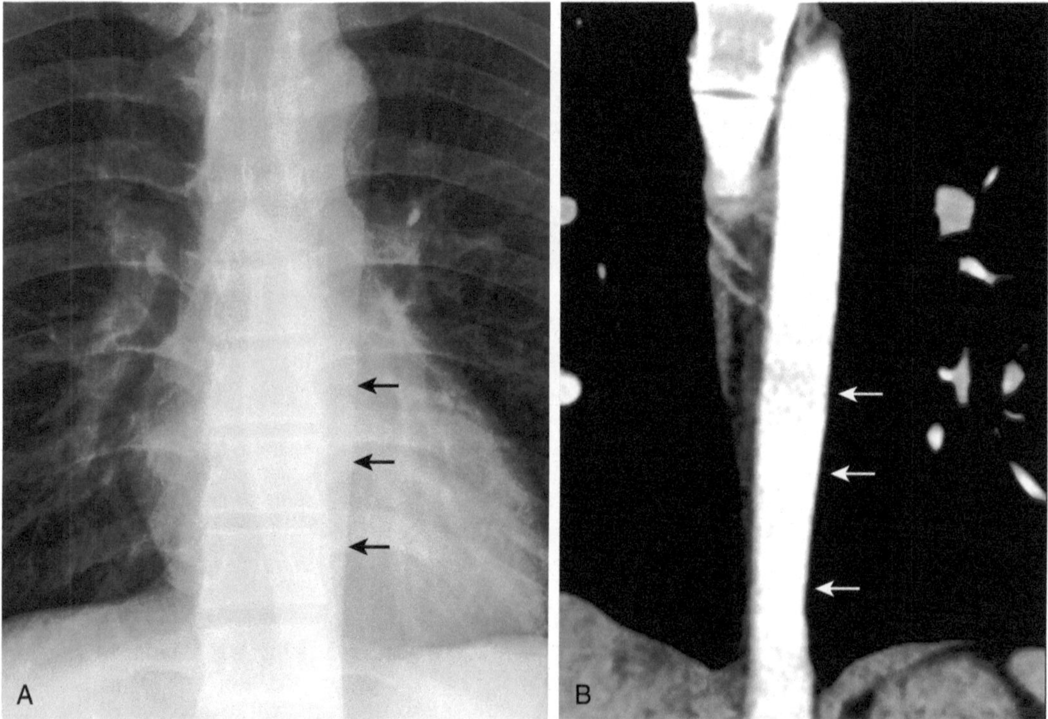

FIGURE 2.32 Left paraaortic interface. **A,** Posteroanterior radiograph shows the left paraaortic interface, where the descending thoracic aorta abuts the lucent left lung *(arrows)*. **B,** Coronal computed tomography image shows the descending thoracic aorta, which in this patient has a relatively straight contour *(arrows)*.

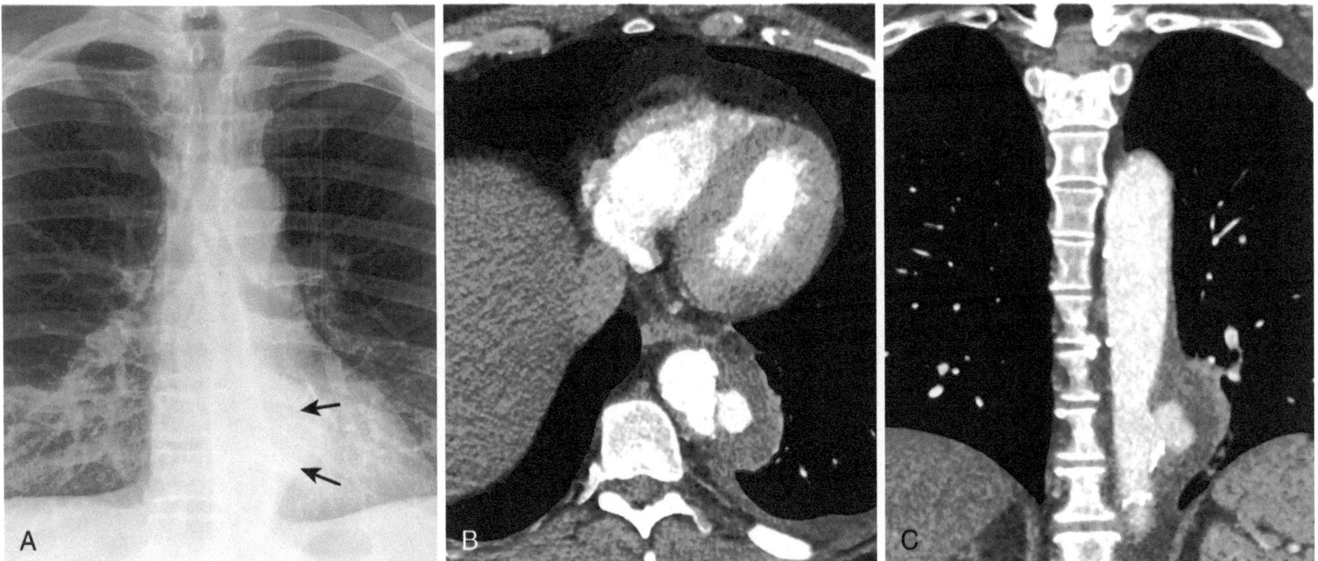

FIGURE 2.33 Abnormal left paraaortic interface from a penetrating aortic ulcer and aortobronchial fistula. **A,** Posteroanterior radiograph demonstrates abnormal convexity of the left paraaortic interface *(arrows)*. Axial **(B)** and coronal **(C)** computed tomography images demonstrate a penetrating ulcer of the descending thoracic aorta that had eroded into adjacent left lower lobe bronchi. The patient presented with hemoptysis.

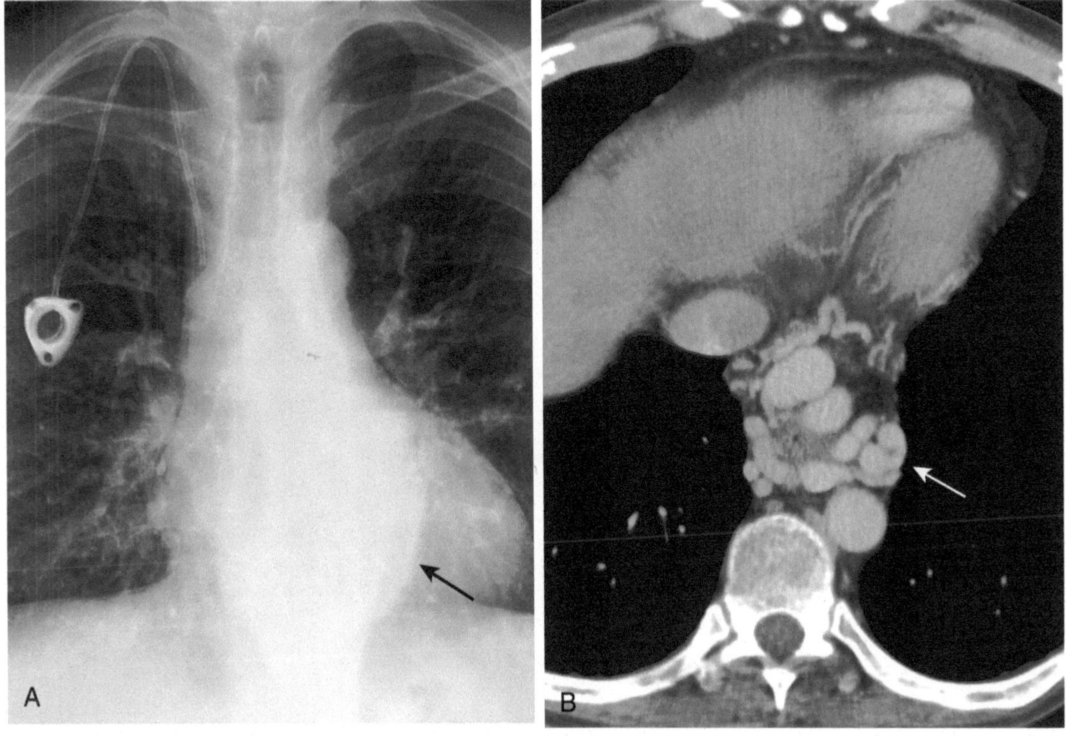

FIGURE 2.34 Abnormal left paraaortic interface caused by paraesophageal varices. **A,** Posteroanterior radiograph shows an abnormal opacity obscuring the left paraaortic interface *(arrow)*. **B,** Axial computed tomography image shows the presence of extensive enhancing paraesophageal varices anterior to the aorta corresponding to the opacity *(arrow)*.

an epicardial fat pad and the adjacent cardiac apex, which prevent the left lung from contacting the sternum and are referred to as the *cardiac incisura*.

The retrosternal clear space, also denoted the anterior clear space, is located anterior to the right ventricle, main pulmonary artery, and ascending aorta and posterior to the sternum. A new opacity in the retrosternal clear space can indicate the presence of a mediastinal mass (Figs. 2.37 and 2.38).

The *retrotracheal triangle,* also known as the Raider triangle, denotes the radiolucent triangle visible on the lateral chest radiograph, which is bounded anteriorly by the posterior wall of the trachea, posteriorly by the thoracic vertebral bodies, and inferiorly by the aortic arch

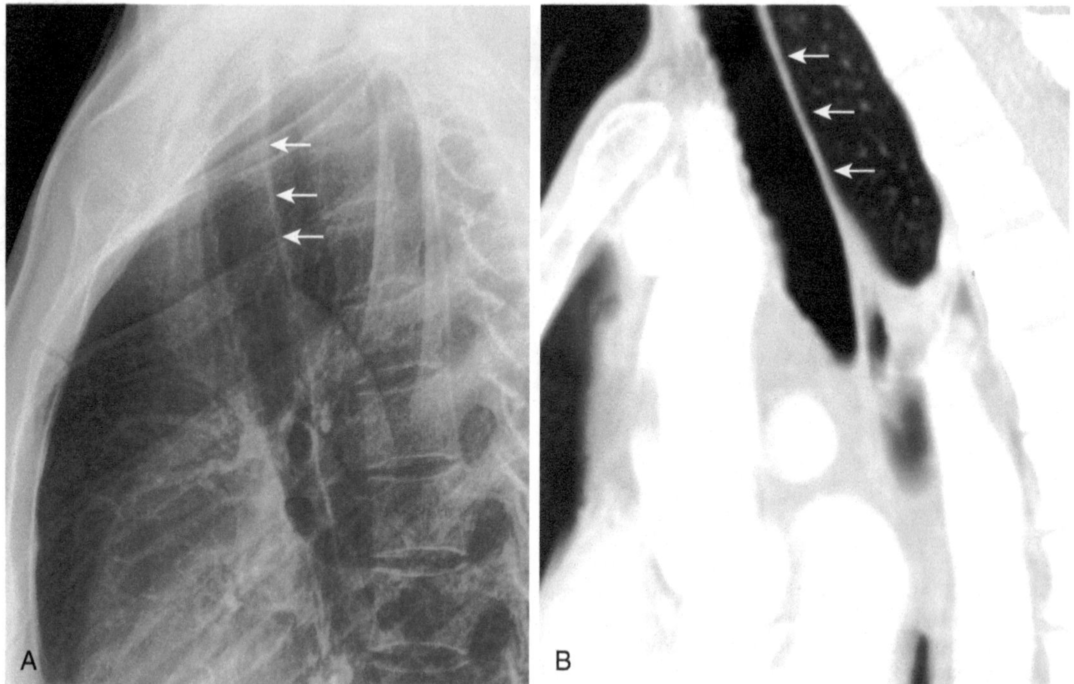

FIGURE 2.35 Posterior tracheal stripe. **A,** Lateral chest radiograph demonstrates the linear opacity of the posterior tracheal stripe *(arrows)* paralleling the tracheal air column. **B,** Sagittal computed tomography image shows the posterior tracheal wall *(arrows)*, which forms the tracheal stripe where it contacts the right upper lobe lung parenchyma *(arrows)*.

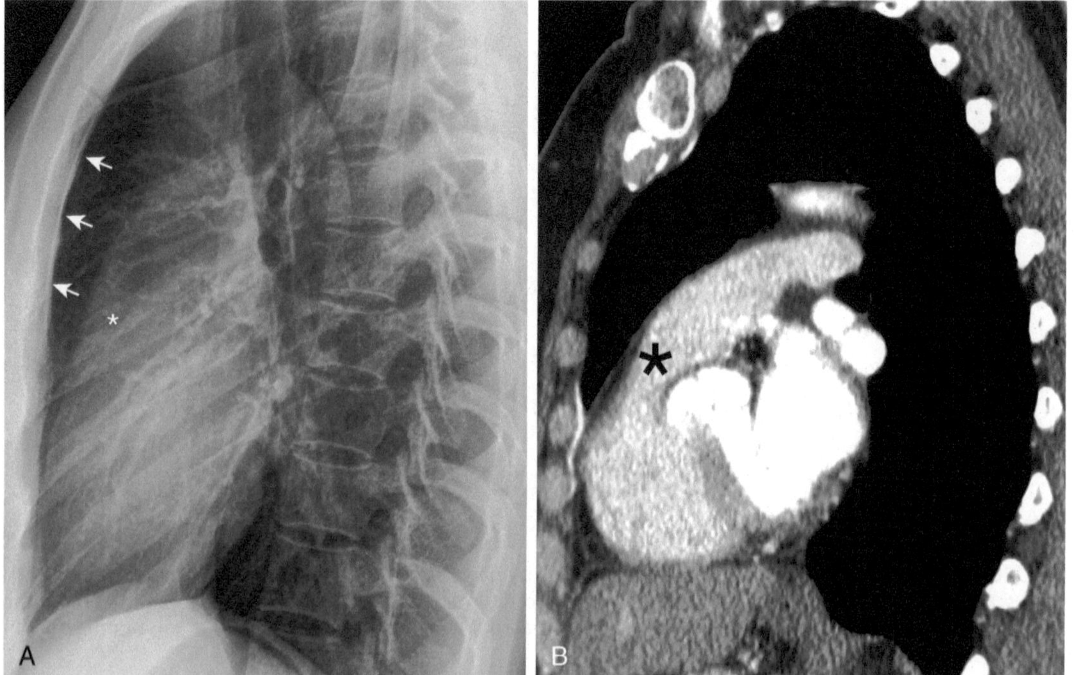

FIGURE 2.36 Retrosternal stripe and right ventricular outflow tract. **A,** Lateral radiograph demonstrates the thin retrosternal stripe where the anterior lungs interface with retrosternal soft tissues *(arrows)*. The right ventricular outflow tract *(asterisk)*, which along with the right ventricle represent the most anteriorly located cardiac structures on the lateral radiograph. **B,** Sagittal computed tomography image shows the anterior location of the right ventricular outflow tract *(asterisk)* and right ventricle.

(Fig. 2.39). The thoracic inlet marks the superior border of the triangle. The contents of the retrotracheal triangle include the thoracic duct, esophagus, left recurrent laryngeal nerve, mediastinal lymph nodes, and lungs. A variety of mediastinal pathologies can result in abnormal opacity or contours within the retrotracheal triangle (Fig. 2.40). The most common pathologic conditions to involve the retrotracheal triangle are vascular in etiology, most frequently an aberrant right subclavian artery.

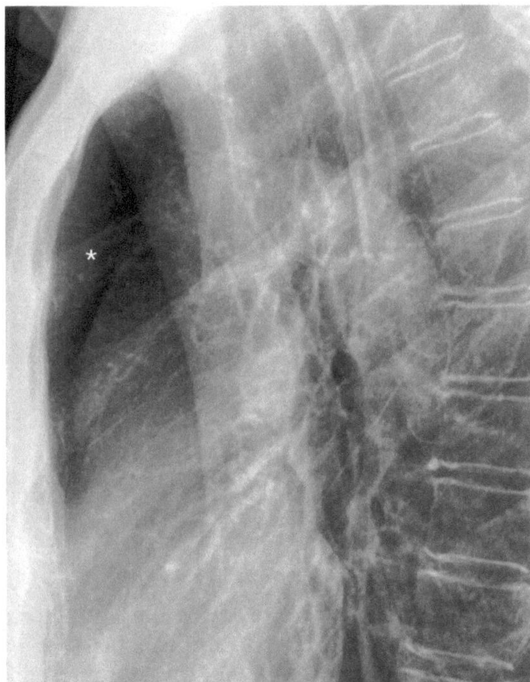

FIGURE 2.37 Retrosternal clear space. Lateral radiograph shows the retrosternal clear space *(asterisk)* located anterior to the right ventricle, right ventricular outflow tract, and ascending aorta and posterior to the sternum.

The Hila: The Frontal Projection

The hila can be divided into upper and lower zones, with specific anatomic structures visible in each zone. On the frontal view, the ***upper portion of the right hilar opacity*** represents the truncus anterior branch of the right pulmonary artery, which is medially located, and the right superior pulmonary vein (Fig. 2.41). The contiguous anterior segmental artery and bronchus are often visible end-on. The ***lower portion of the right hilum*** represents the right interlobar artery, which is vertically oriented, the right superior pulmonary vein along the lateral and superior margin, and their branches. The lucent lumen of the bronchus intermedius is located medial to the interlobar artery. The right inferior pulmonary vein is seen inferior and medial to the hilum. The right inferior venous confluence is a well-recognized pseudotumor (Fig. 2.42).

The main pulmonary artery appears below the aortic arch and superior to the left main bronchus on the frontal radiograph as a radiopaque oval opacity (see Fig. 2.41). The ***upper portion of the left hilar opacity*** is formed by the distal left pulmonary artery, the proximal aspect of the left interlobar artery, the left superior pulmonary vein, and their respective branches. The proximal left pulmonary artery is usually higher than the most superior aspect of the right interlobar artery (see Fig. 2.41). Unlike on the right, the left superior hilum is frequently partially obscured by adjacent mediastinal fat and a portion of the cardiac silhouette. The lower portion of the left hilum is composed of the distal left interlobar artery and lingular artery and vein and the left inferior pulmonary vein inferiorly.

Pulmonary arterial enlargement results in hilar enlargement; however, the hila maintain their vascular configuration. The hilar vessels approximate the lateral aspect of the hila, which is referred to as the hilar convergence sign (see Fig. 2.43). In cases of a hilar mass or lymphadenopathy, the involved hilum may demonstrate increased density or an enlarged, nodular contour (Fig. 2.44).

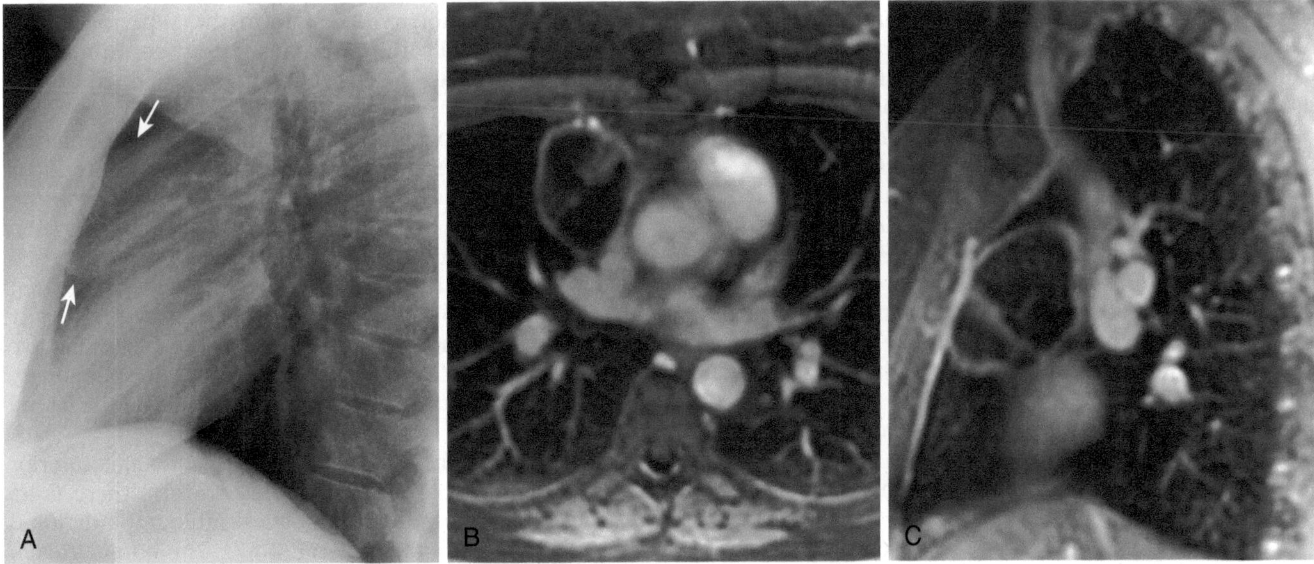

FIGURE 2.38 Abnormal retrosternal clear space in a patient with a mediastinal dermoid. **A,** Lateral radiograph demonstrates a mass-like opacity in the retrosternal anterior mediastinum *(arrows)*. Axial **(B)** and sagittal **(C)** fat-suppressed postcontrast T1-weighted three-dimensional gradient-echo magnetic resonance images show peripheral enhancement of the mass, which was pathologically shown to represent a mediastinal dermoid.

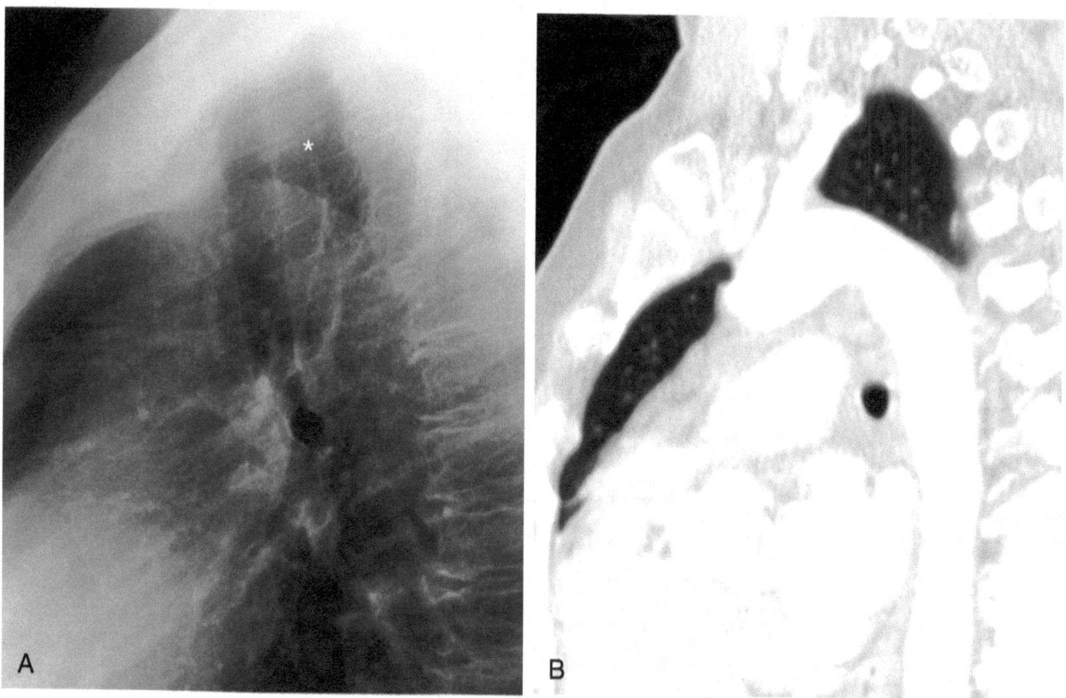

FIGURE 2.39 Retrotracheal space: Raider triangle. **A,** Lateral radiograph shows a lucent triangle posterior to the trachea and anterior to the vertebral bodies, which represents the retrotracheal space *(asterisk)*. The space is bounded inferiorly by transverse portion of the aortic arch and superiorly by the thoracic inlet. **B,** Sagittal chest computed tomography image shows intervening lung, which forms the lucent retrotracheal space on the lateral radiograph.

The Hila: The Lateral Projection

The right and left hilar structures are superimposed on one another on the lateral view. The carina is located at approximately the left of the fourth or fifth thoracic vertebra and can be seen where the tracheal air column tapers. The right upper lobe bronchus is usually less well circumscribed compared with the left upper lobe bronchus because of a lack of adjacent vascular structures. When visible, it is seen as a rounded lucency along the anterior and superior aspect of the intermediate stem line. The tracheal air column ends caudally in a rounded radiolucency, which represents the distal left main bronchus that is continuous with the orifice of the left upper bronchus visible end-on and denoted the ***left main-upper lobe continuum*** (LULC) (see Fig. 2.45).

The posterior wall of the right main and intermediate bronchi forms the ***intermediate stem line,*** seen in 95% of people, which normally measures up to 3 mm in thickness. The intermediate stem line is visible because of the presence of air within the lumen of the bronchus intermedius in addition to the aerated lung in the azygoesophageal recess abutting the posterior wall of the right main and intermediate bronchi. The intermediate stem line projects over the mid or posterior third of the circular LULC, which is seen end-on (Figs. 2.45 and 2.46). The intermediate stem line terminates at the level of the right lower lobe superior segmental bronchus.

The ***left retrobronchial line*** represents the posterior wall of the left main bronchus and proximal left lower lobe bronchus, normally measuring up to 3 mm in thickness and terminating at the left lower lobe superior segmental bronchus. The left retrobronchial line is more posteriorly located than the intermediate stem line and shorter in length. In contrast to the left retrobronchial line in the left hilum, the ***left retrobronchial stripe*** represents the combined thickness of the anterior wall of the esophagus, mediastinal fat, and the left main bronchus posterior wall where it abuts the superior segment of the left lower lobe.

The ***right hilar vascular opacity (RHVO)*** is composed of truncus anterior, the right pulmonary artery, and the interlobar artery. The truncus anterior and transverse portion of the right pulmonary artery form the superior aspect of the RHVO while the interlobar artery contributes to the inferior aspect. The RHVO is often ill defined on the lateral radiograph; however, the right superior pulmonary vein contributes to a more well-delineated anterior margin as it approximates the anterior aspect of the interlobar artery. The left hilar vasculature is visible posterior to the intermediate stem line. The ***left pulmonary artery*** is seen in most individuals as a well-delineated comma-shaped opacity above and posterior to the rounded radiolucent LULC (see Fig. 2.6). The left pulmonary artery is typically marginated by lung superiorly and resembles a miniature aortic arch on the lateral view. The left superior pulmonary vein does not contribute to the hilar contour on the lateral radiograph.

Inferior to the right hilar vascular opacity and anterior to the comma-shaped left pulmonary artery, there is an avascular region on the normal chest radiograph denoted the ***inferior hilar window*** (Fig. 2.47). The boundaries of the inferior hilar window are the right middle lobe bronchus anteriorly and the left lower lobe bronchus posteriorly. This region should not contain nodular opacities greater

Text continued on p. 47

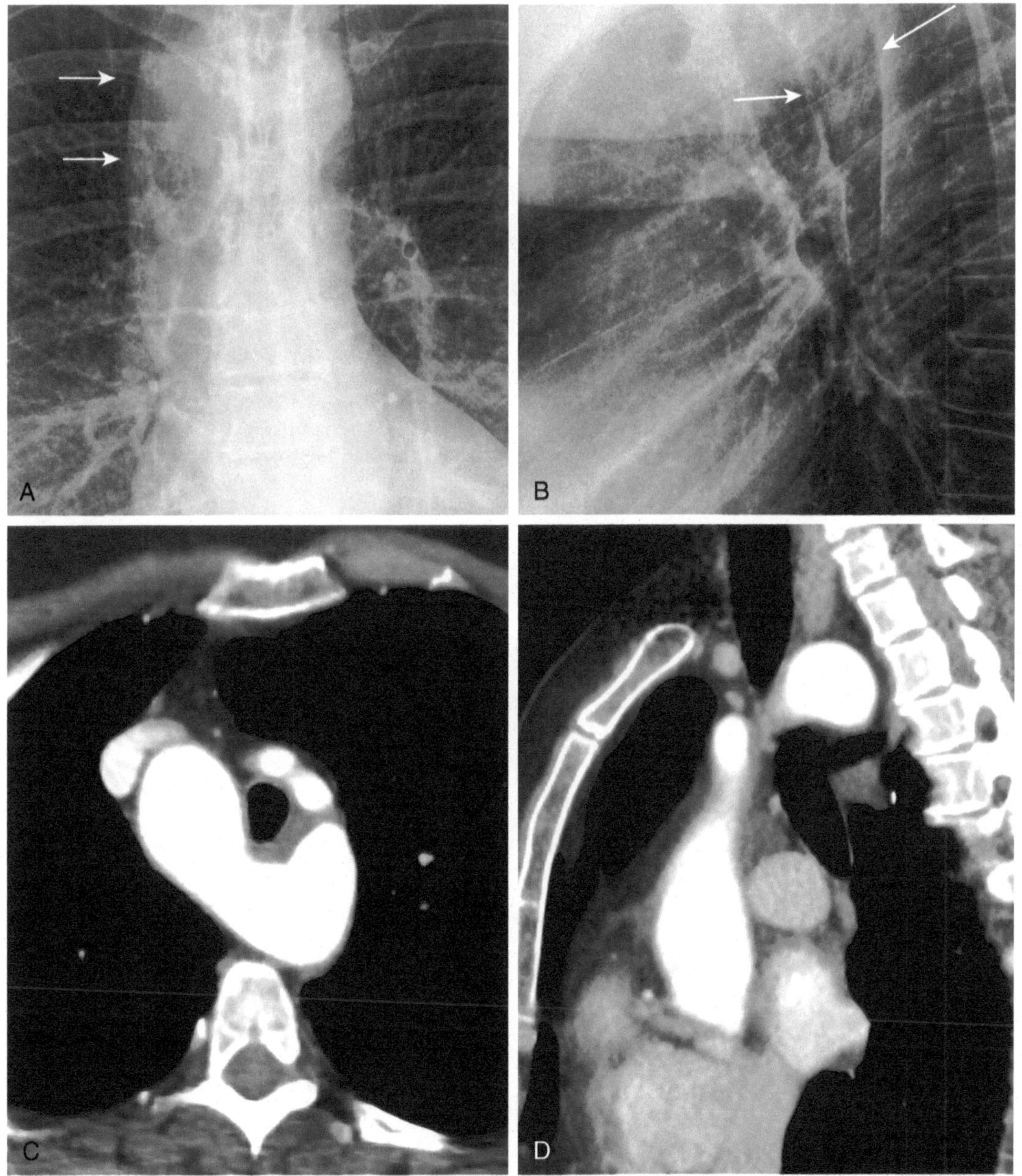

FIGURE 2.40 Abnormal retrotracheal space in patient with an incomplete double aortic arch. **A,** Posteroanterior chest radiograph shows an abnormal widening of the superior mediastinum and an opacity in the right paratracheal space *(arrows)*. **B,** Lateral radiograph reveals that the retrotracheal triangle is partially obscured *(arrows)*. Axial **(C)** and sagittal **(D)** computed tomography images show that the patient has an incomplete double aortic arch with an atretic distal left arch. The right arch has a retrotracheal course as shown, which produces the abnormal opacity in the retrotracheal triangle on the lateral radiograph.

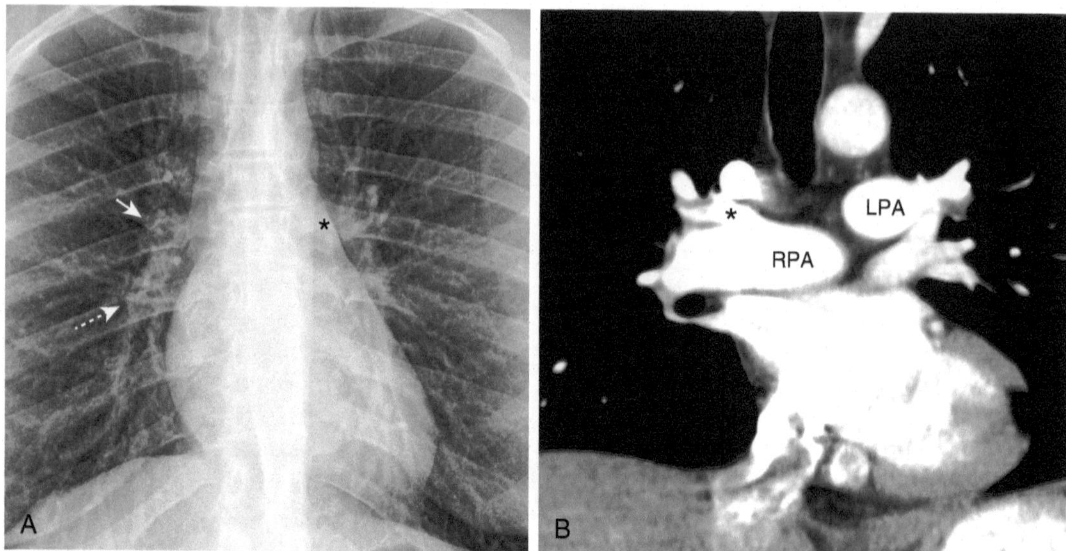

FIGURE 2.41 Hilar vessels. **A,** Posteroanterior radiograph shows the normal appearance of the pulmonary hila. The upper portion of the right hilar vascular opacity is visible *(arrow)* along with the inferior portion (dashed arrow). **B,** Coronal computed tomography image showing the right and left pulmonary arteries. The truncus anterior *(asterisk)* can be seen, which contributes to the superior right hilar vascular opacity and is located anterior to the right upper lobe bronchus. As shown here, the right pulmonary artery (RPA) has a longer and more horizontal course than the left. The left pulmonary artery (LPA) is located slightly more superior than the right.

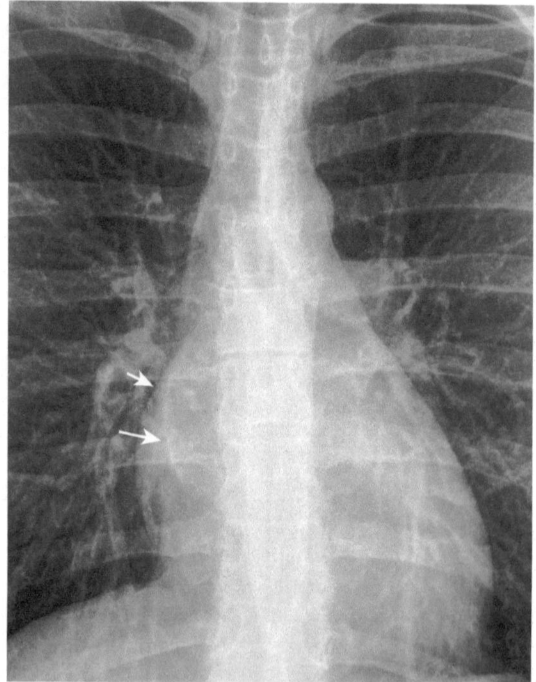

FIGURE 2.42 Right inferior pulmonary venous confluence. Frontal radiograph shows the normal right interior pulmonary venous confluence *(arrows)*, located posterior and medial to the right interlobar pulmonary artery. The linear opacity of the right inferior pulmonary venous confluence may form a mass-like opacity in the retrocardiac right lower lobe that can be mistaken for a lesion.

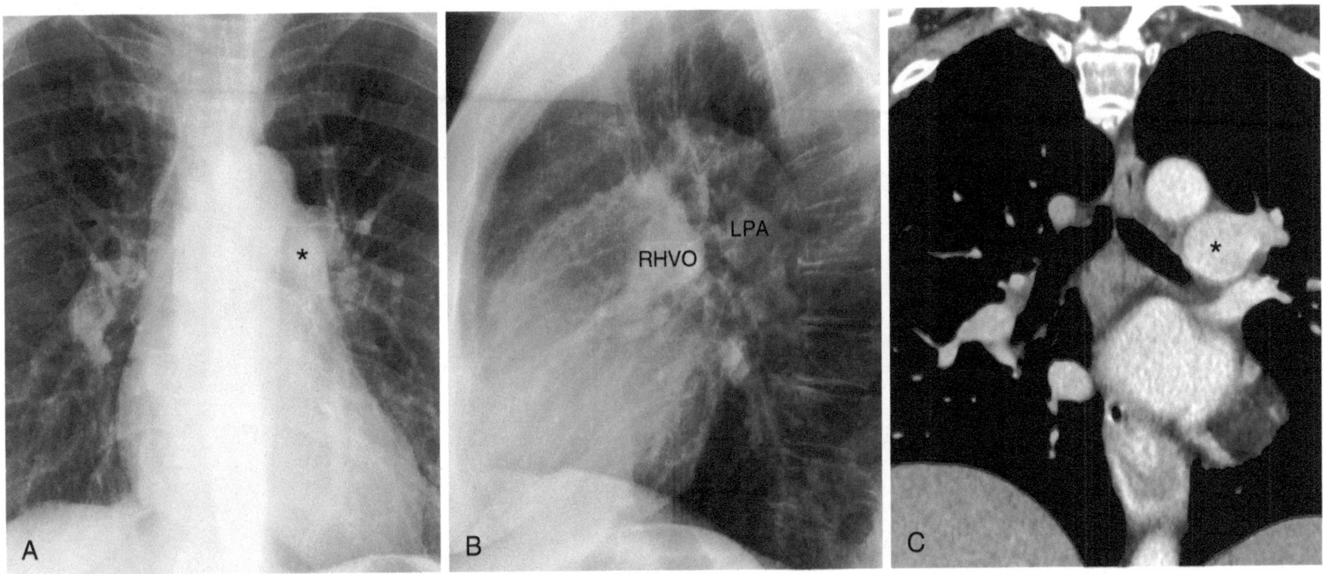

FIGURE 2.43 Hilar convergence sign: pulmonary arterial enlargement in a patient with CREST (calcinosis, Raynaud phenomenon, esophageal dysmotility, sclerodactyly, and telangiectasia) syndrome. **A,** The posteroanterior radiograph shows dilation of the right and left main pulmonary arteries as they converge at the hilum. The main pulmonary artery is also enlarged *(asterisk)*. **B,** Lateral radiograph shows an enlarged right hilar vascular opacity (RHVO) caused by the dilated right pulmonary artery as well as an enlarged "comma-shaped" descending left pulmonary artery (LPA). **C,** Coronal computed tomography image shows the markedly dilated left pulmonary artery *(asterisk)*.

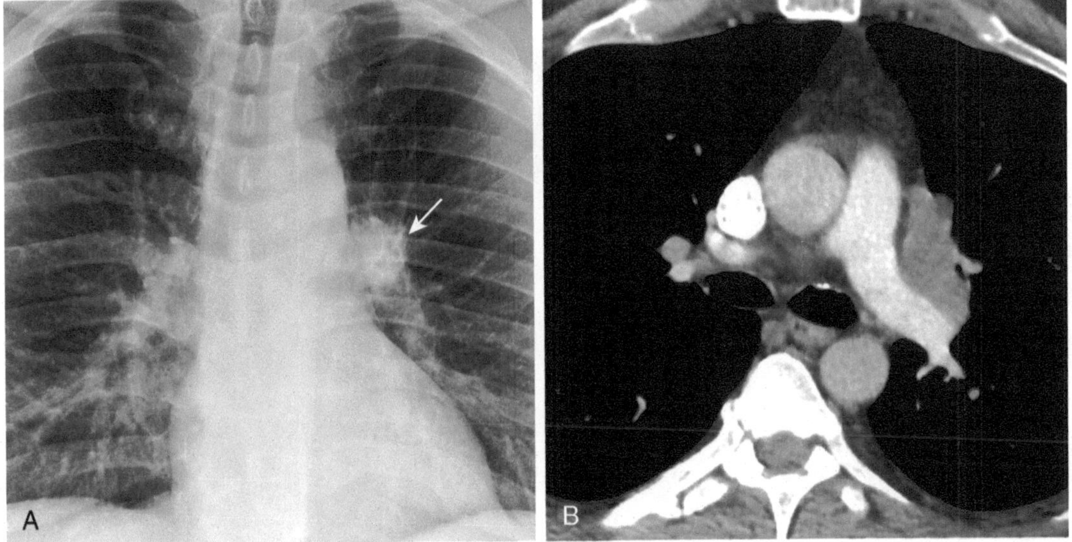

FIGURE 2.44 Abnormal hilar density caused by left hilar lymphadenopathy in the setting of non-Hodgkin lymphoma. **A,** Posteroanterior chest radiograph demonstrates increased density and an abnormal nodular contour of the left hilum *(arrow)*. **B,** Axial computed tomography image from the same patient shows left hilar lymphadenopathy.

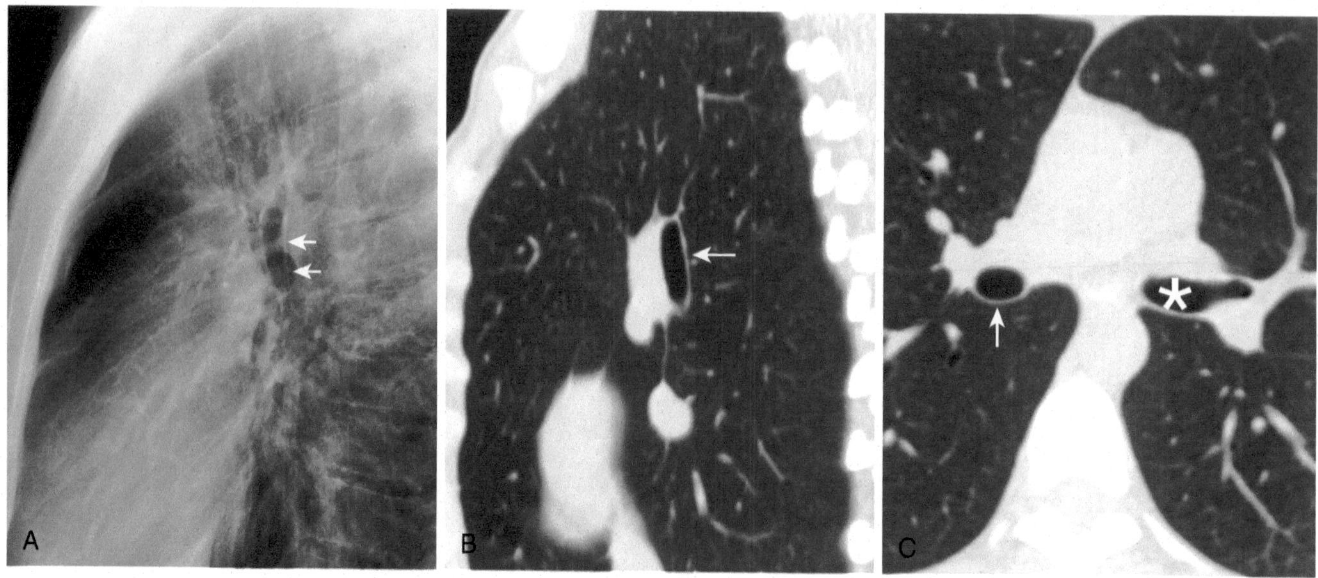

FIGURE 2.45 Intermediate stem line. **A,** Lateral radiograph demonstrates the normal appearance of the intermediate stem line, which appears as a thin line *(arrows)* intersecting the left main–upper lobe continuum (LULC) and terminating at the right lower lobe superior segmental bronchus. **B,** Sagittal computed tomography (CT) image shows the thin posterior wall of the bronchus intermedius *(arrow)*. **C,** Axial CT image shows that the posterior wall of the bronchus intermedius *(arrow)* aligns with the LULC *(asterisk)*, which makes the intermediate stem line visible within the oval of the LULC on the lateral radiograph.

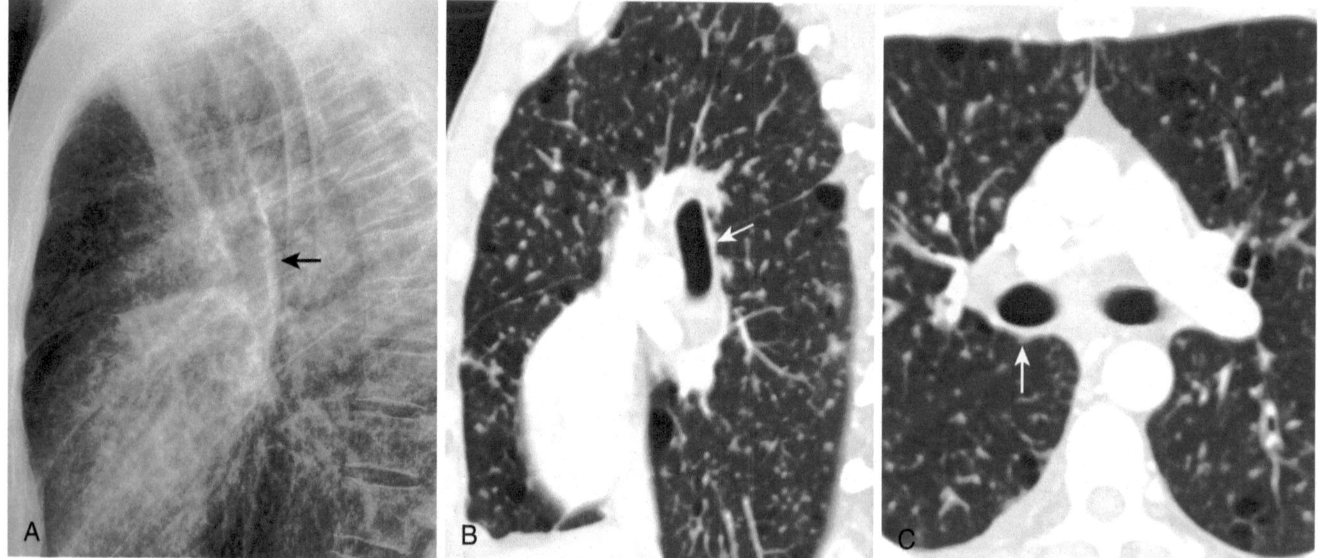

FIGURE 2.46 Thickened intermediate stem in an immunocompromised patient with disseminated coccidioidomycosis. **A,** Lateral radiograph shows a thickened intermediate stem line *(arrow)*. Sagittal **(B)** and axial **(C)** computed tomography images demonstrate diffuse miliary pulmonary nodules and thickening of the posterior wall of the bronchus intermedius *(arrows)*.

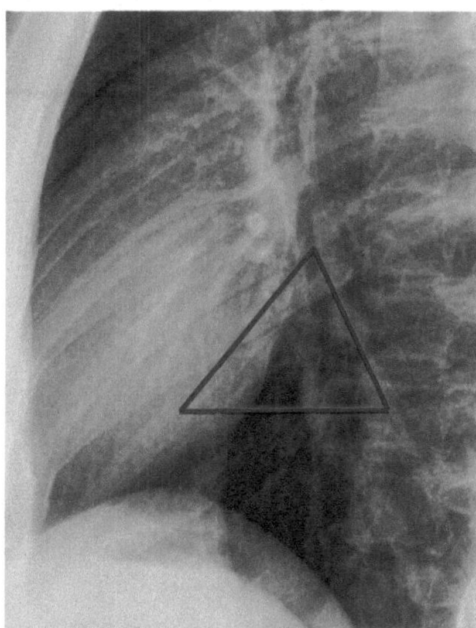

FIGURE 2.47 Inferior hilar window. Lateral radiograph shows the normal appearance of the inferior hilar window *(triangle)*.

than 1 cm. The presence of a nodular opacity of more than 1 cm in the inferior hilar window should raise concern for an infrahilar mass or adenopathy (Fig. 2.48).

ATELECTASIS

Atelectasis derives from the Greek phrase *ateles ektasis,* which means incomplete expansion. The term refers to the process in which diminished aeration of the lung results in decreased volume.

Recognizing atelectasis or a component of atelectasis within consolidated lung is possible by identifying direct and indirect signs of associated volume loss. Direct signs of atelectasis include displacement of interlobar fissures and crowding of the bronchi and/or vessels within atelectatic lung. Indirect signs reflect compensatory mechanisms, including diaphragmatic elevation, mediastinal shift, approximation of the ribs, hilar displacement, and compensatory overinflation.

Mechanisms of Atelectasis

Relaxation (passive) atelectasis occurs when lung volume decreases secondary to the presence of a space-occupying structure such as a pleural effusion, pneumothorax, or pleural mass (Fig. 2.49). In the absence of pleural adhesions or other restrictive pathology, atelectasis of a region of the lung is directly proportional to the amount of air or fluid in the subjacent pleural space. In cases of pneumothorax-induced total lung collapse, the lobar and proximal segmental bronchi typically remain patent and air filled with visible air bronchograms surrounded by airless parenchyma. Failure to identify the presence of air bronchograms within a collapsed lung from presumed relaxation atelectasis should raise suspicion for an endobronchial obstruction. A similar phenomenon is *compressive atelectasis,* which denotes a more confined process where there is focal parenchymal collapse along the margin of a localized space-occupying lesion.

When the communication between the alveoli and airways is obstructed, *resorption atelectasis* results. In the setting of an obstructed airway, the alveolar gas diffuses into the adjacent capillaries and cannot be replenished by inspired air, leading to diminished alveolar volume. The site of airway obstruction may be the trachea, main bronchi, lobar bronchi, or more distal bronchi or bronchioles. In normal lungs, the presence of a central airway obstruction typically leads to a gasless lung within 18 to 24 hours. In resorption atelectasis with obstruction of a main bronchus, the bronchi within the collapsed lung will frequently not remain patent, and air bronchograms will be absent. When the site of airway obstruction is more distal, for example, with bronchiolar obstruction from mucous plugging, air bronchograms are more commonly preserved.

Cicatrization atelectasis denotes the volume loss associated with retraction of fibrotic lung parenchyma. There are typically compensatory signs of chronic volume loss and associated dilation of the involved bronchi and bronchioles as a result of increased elastic recoil leading to traction bronchiectasis and bronchiolectasis (Fig. 2.50). Cicatrization atelectasis can be associated with prior granulomatous infection, particularly tuberculosis.

When surfactant deficiency produces diminished lung volume, *adhesive atelectasis* results. Surfactant limits alveoli collapse by decreasing the surface tension of alveoli as their volume or surface area declines. The most commonly encountered examples of adhesive atelectasis are acute lung injury, respiratory distress syndrome in infants, and acute radiation pneumonitis. Adhesive atelectasis has also been found to occur in some cases of pneumonia, in smoke inhalation, and in the postoperative setting.

Patterns of Atelectasis

Rounded Atelectasis

Rounded atelectasis occurs in association with subjacent pleural thickening or effusion. The atelectatic lung may appear round or elliptical or as an irregular subpleural mass. The atelectatic lung should extensively contact the abnormal pleural surface. There is characteristic curving of the adjacent bronchi and pulmonary vessels as they approach the collapsed portion of lung, which is best identified on CT and resembles that of a comet tail (e.g., the *comet tail sign*) (Figs. 2.51 and 2.52). Enhancement of the collapsed lung parenchyma on CT is typical. As with all forms of atelectasis, there should be evidence of volume loss. The posterior lower lobes are the most frequent site of rounded atelectasis. The mass-like appearance of rounded atelectasis can frequently mimic lung cancer. Asbestos-related pleural disease is a common cause of pleural thickening and fibrosis leading to rounded atelectasis.

Total Collapse of the Lung

With total atelectasis of a lung, the affected hemithorax becomes completely opaque (Fig. 2.53). There is elevation of the ipsilateral hemidiaphragm, which is typically only visible radiographically on the left because of the presence of the stomach bubble. There is compensatory hyperinflation of the contralateral lung, which crosses the midline and creates an enlarged retrosternal air space on the lateral radiograph. The mediastinum and hilum shift to the affected side. In the setting of lung collapse secondary

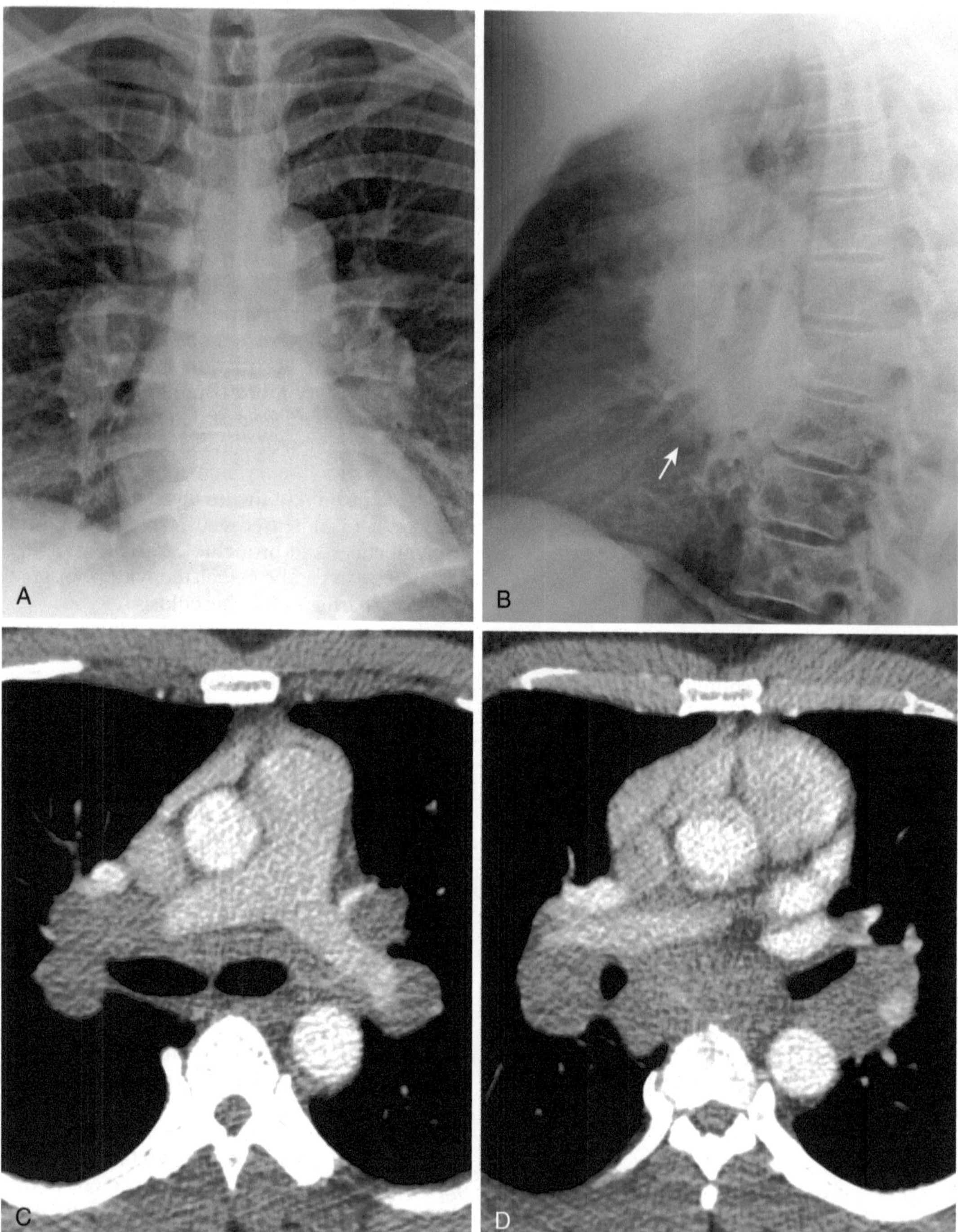

FIGURE 2.48 Abnormal inferior hilar window in a patient with sarcoidosis. **A,** Posteroanterior radiograph shows bilateral hilar enlargement and thickening of the right paratracheal stripe. **B,** Lateral radiograph shows abnormal opacification of the inferior hilar window *(arrow)*. **C** and **D,** Axial computed tomography images show bilateral hilar and subcarinal lymphadenopathy causing opacification of the inferior hilar window.

to a pneumothorax, the lung collapses toward the hilum and mediastinum, which can shift toward the opposite side. The inferior pulmonary ligaments serve as an attachment of the lower lobes to the mediastinum, which cause the lower lobes to collapse medially (Fig. 2.54).

Lobar Collapse

Collapse of a lobe may be complete or partial. The most frequent cause of lobar collapse is central bronchial obstruction. Opacification caused by airlessness and displacement of the interlobar fissures toward the collapsed lobe should be present. If the obstruction of the lobar bronchus is caused by a mass, there may be a bulge in the contour of the collapsed lobe. The atelectatic lobe may have a lobular contour with undulation of the fissure if tumor replaces the lobe. Air bronchograms should be preserved; however, if a central endobronchial tumor is causing the collapse, the bronchi may occlude or become narrowed. After collapse, the affected lobe becomes triangular or pie shaped, with the apex directed centrally toward the hilum.

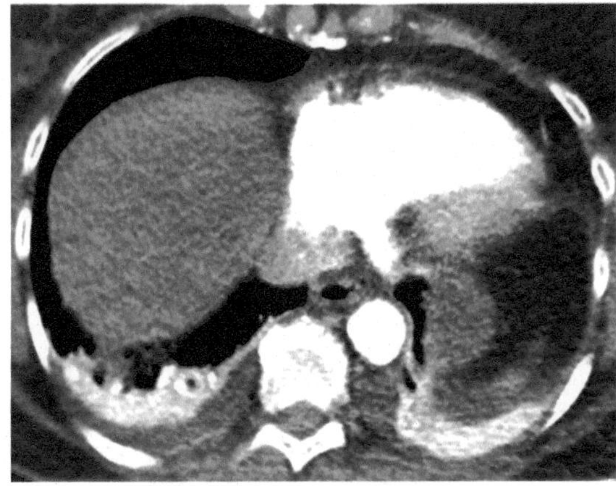

FIGURE 2.49 Relaxation atelectasis. Axial computed tomography image in a patient with small bilateral pleural effusions shows relaxation atelectasis involving the posterior lower lobes. The atelectatic lung demonstrates homogeneous enhancement.

Right Upper Lobe Atelectasis

The right upper lobe collapses superiorly and medially, obscuring the right superior mediastinal contours. The minor fissure is displaced superiorly, and the major fissure is anteriorly displaced. With complete collapse, the lobe is marginated against the mediastinum. If there is a central mass causing the collapse, the lateral aspect of the minor fissure bows upward, and there is a downward convexity of the medial fissure, leading to a reverse S configuration on the PA radiograph, the so-called *reverse S sign of Golden* (Fig. 2.55). An additional sign of upper lobe atelectasis (either right or left) is the *juxtaphrenic peak.* The juxtaphrenic peak is visible on the frontal radiograph as a well-demarcated triangular opacity arising from the medial aspect of the hemidiaphragm with the apex directed superiorly (Fig. 2.56). In most cases, the presence of a juxtaphrenic peak in the setting of an upper lobe collapse represents retraction of an inferior accessory fissure. On the lateral radiograph, the collapsed right upper lobe often appears as an indistinct triangular opacity with the apex abutting the hilum and the base abutting the parietal pleura of the apex of the right hemithorax. On CT, the collapsed right upper lobe appears as a wedge-shaped opacification extending along the mediastinum to the anterior chest wall (see Fig. 2.55). The volume loss leads to superior retraction of the hilum and outward rotation of the bronchus intermedius, which demonstrates a more horizontally oriented course. Hyperinflation of the right middle and right lower lobes occurs, and the right middle lobe occupies the anterior superior hemithorax.

Left Upper Lobe Atelectasis

The absence of a left minor fissure leads to a different appearance of collapse of the left upper lobe compared with the right. With left upper lobe collapse, the major fissure is anteriorly displaced, approximately parallel to the anterior chest wall. On the lateral view, the displaced

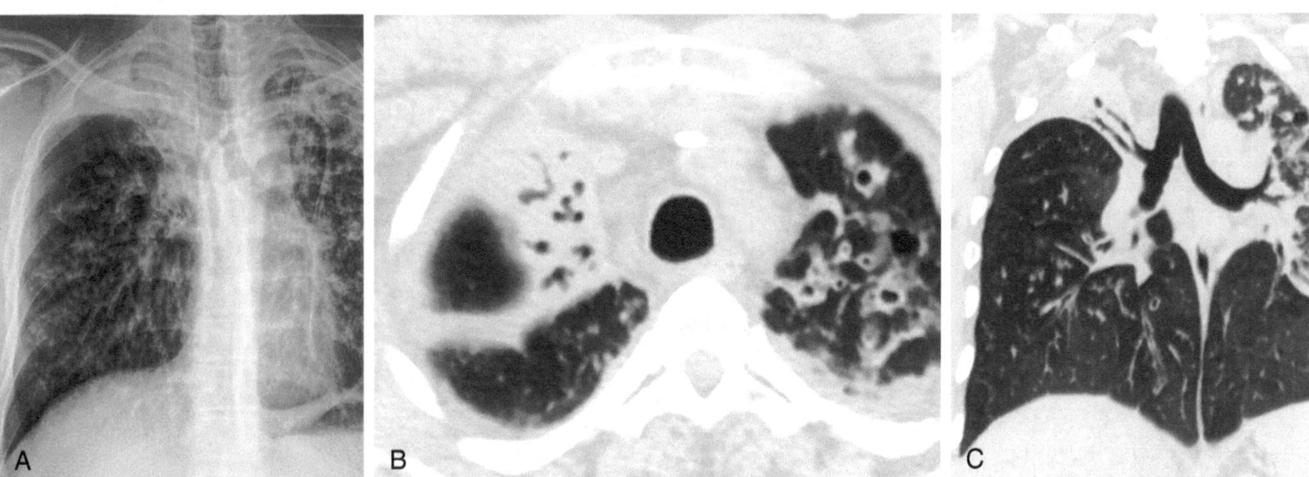

FIGURE 2.50 Cicatrization atelectasis of the right upper lobe in a patient with cystic fibrosis. **A,** Posteroanterior radiograph shows collapse of the right upper lobe with superior retraction of the right hilum. The right hemidiaphragm is elevated. Axial **(B)** and coronal **(C)** computed tomography images show traction bronchiectasis within the collapsed right upper lobe.

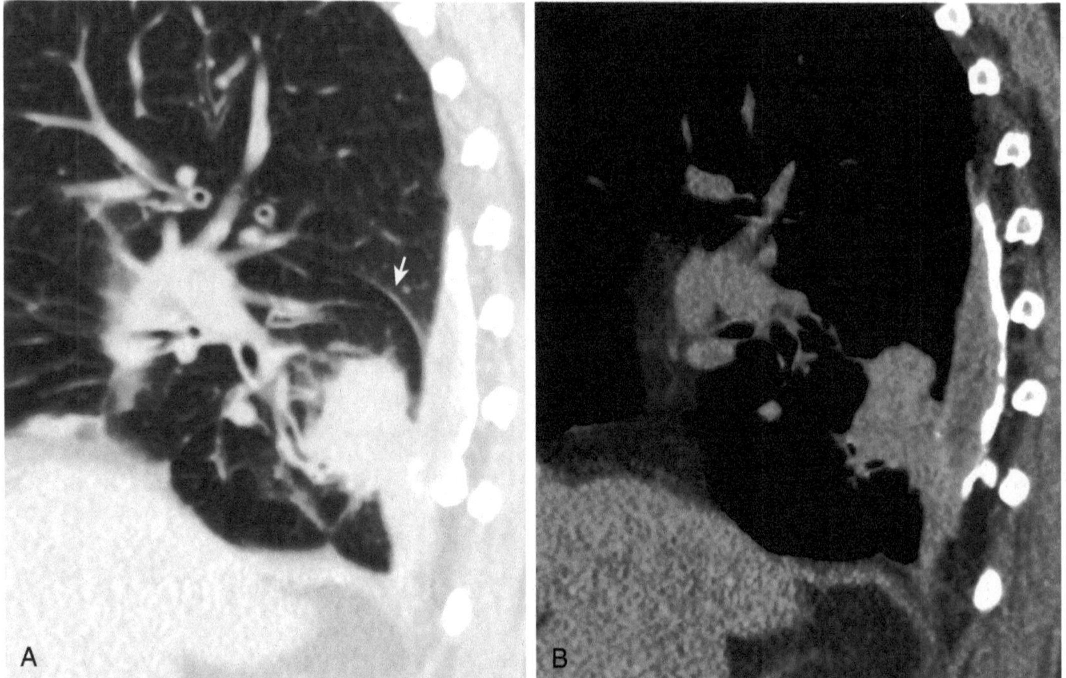

FIGURE 2.51 Rounded atelectasis. **A,** Sagittal computed tomography (CT) image on lung windows shows a subpleural mass-like opacity in the right lower lobe. The curvilinear bronchovascular bundles course toward the opacity (the comet tail sign), and there is evidence of volume loss with inferior displacement of the right major fissure *(arrow)*. **B,** Sagittal CT image on soft tissue windows shows that this area of rounded atelectasis directly contacts the adjacent abnormal pleura, in this patient with chronic pleural thickening from prior asbestos exposure.

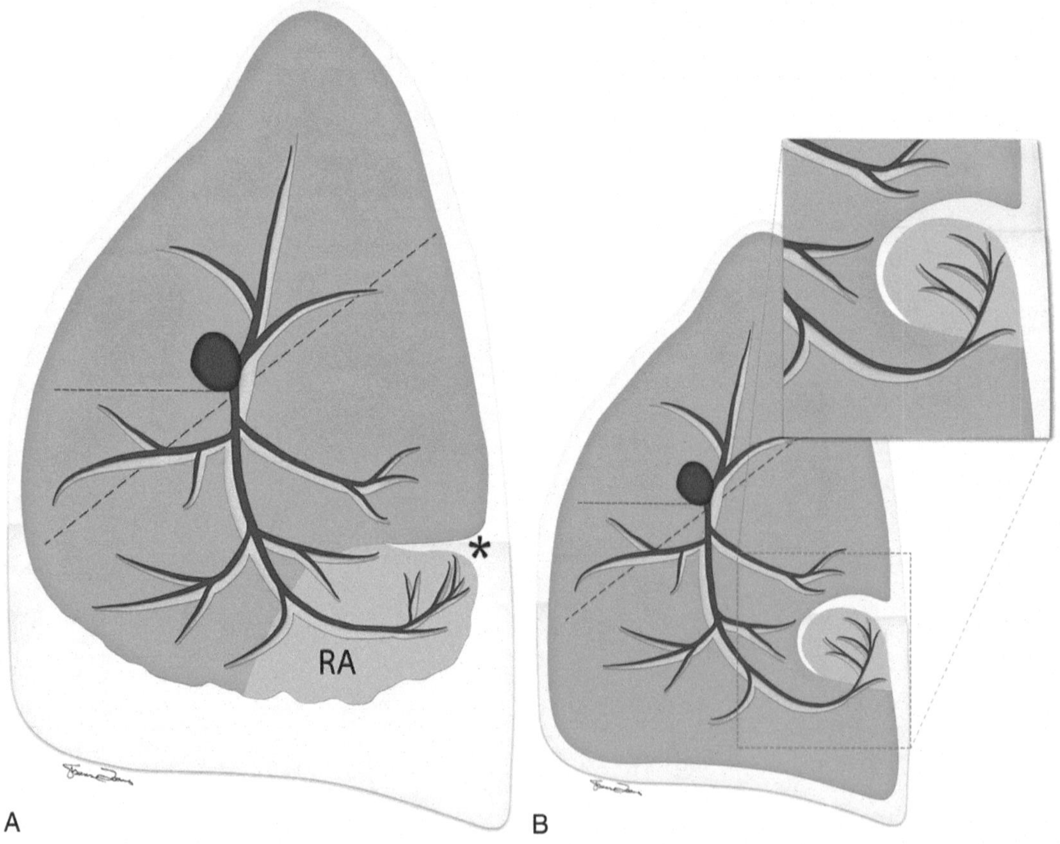

FIGURE 2.52 Mechanism of rounded atelectasis (RA). **A,** An area of pleural thickening or fluid causes tethering of the lung and creates an invagination or pleural groove *(asterisk)* along the margin of RA. **B,** The lung eventually contracts further, and there is an infolding of the lung parenchyma along the adjacent abnormal pleural surface. This creates a rounded opacity along the pleural surface.

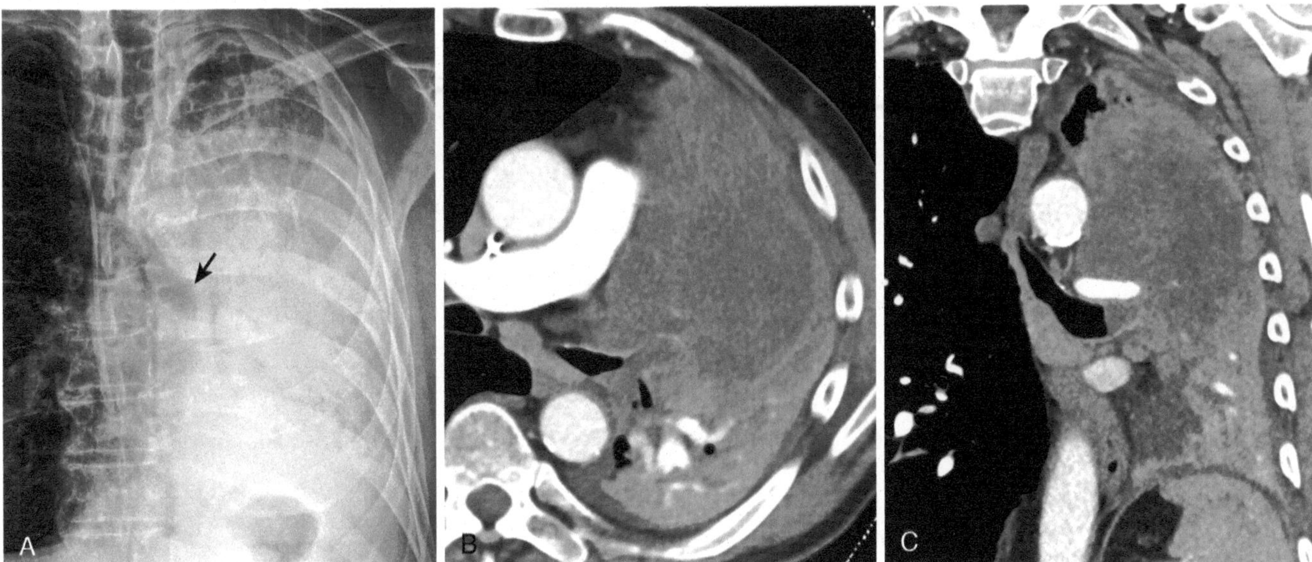

FIGURE 2.53 Left lung collapse secondary to small cell lung cancer. **A,** Posteroanterior radiograph demonstrates near complete collapse of the left lung with an abrupt termination of the distal left main bronchus, the bronchial cut-off sign *(arrow)*. The left hemidiaphragm is completely obscured, and the gastric bubble is elevated. **B,** Axial computed tomography (CT) image shows a necrotic hypoattenuating tumor arising from the left upper lobe and occluding the distal left main bronchus. **C,** Coronal CT image shows tumor extension into the left main bronchus, causing the bronchial cut-off sign.

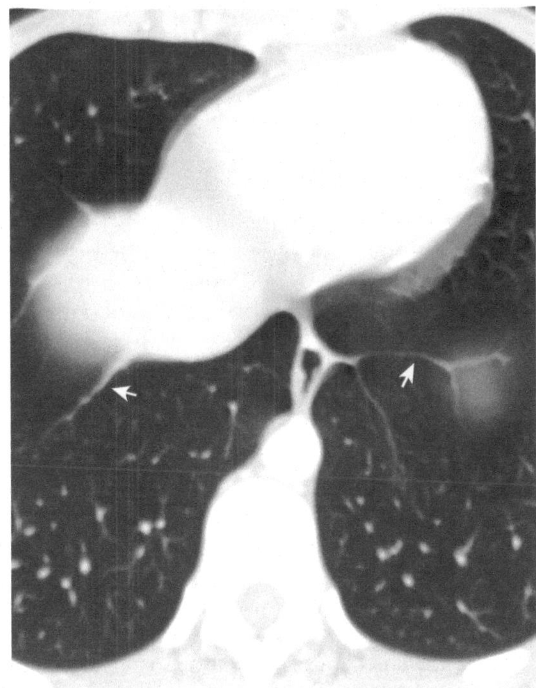

FIGURE 2.54 Inferior pulmonary ligaments. Axial computed tomography image shows the right and left inferior pulmonary ligaments in this patient *(arrows)*. The ligaments are linear structures that extend laterally from the mediastinum in close proximity to the diaphragm.

major fissure can be seen parallel to the sternum (Fig. 2.57). The opacity of the left upper lobe is anterior to the fissure extending from the apex of the lung to the diaphragm. On the frontal chest radiograph, there is hazy opacification of the left hemithorax, which obscures the left heart border and superior mediastinum (i.e., silhouette sign). If aeration of the lingula is maintained, the left heart border will remain distinct. The hyperinflated superior segment of the lower lobe occupies the apex of the lung, which may insinuate between the mediastinum and upper lobe on the frontal radiograph, creating a crescentic lucency along the aortic arch known as the *luftsichel sign* (Fig. 2.58). The lucency of the luftsichel sign can be seen anywhere from the apex of the left hemithorax to the superior pulmonary vein.

Right Middle Lobe Atelectasis

The right middle lobe collapses medially toward the heart with downward displacement of the minor fissure and superior displacement of the major fissure. Associated secondary signs of volume loss such as hilar displacement or compensatory hyperinflation are often less prominent compared with other lobes given the relatively smaller volume of the right middle lobe. The collapsed lobe may appear as an opacity obscuring the right heart border on the PA chest radiograph. On the lateral projection, the collapsed lobe can be seen as a linear band or wedge-shaped triangular opacity with the apex directed toward the hilum and the base approximating the anterior parietal pleura. Right middle lobe atelectasis can be identified on CT as a triangular or trapezoidal opacity with the apex again directed toward the hilum and the hyperinflated right upper lobe displaced anteromedially (Fig. 2.59).

Lower Lobe Atelectasis

The pattern of lower lobe atelectasis is similar on the right and left because of the equivalent anatomy. Both the right and left lower lobes collapse posteromedially and inferiorly. The superior aspect of the major fissure is retracted downward, and the inferior aspect of the fissure moves posteriorly. The inferior pulmonary ligament anchors the medial lower lobe to the adjacent mediastinum (see Fig. 2.54), and as a result, the atelectatic lobe assumes a

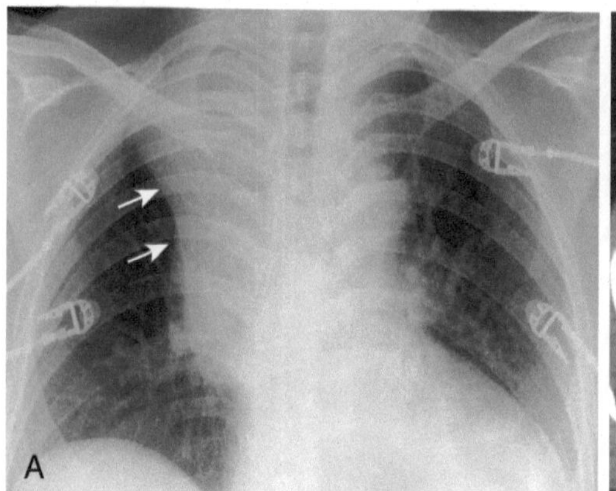

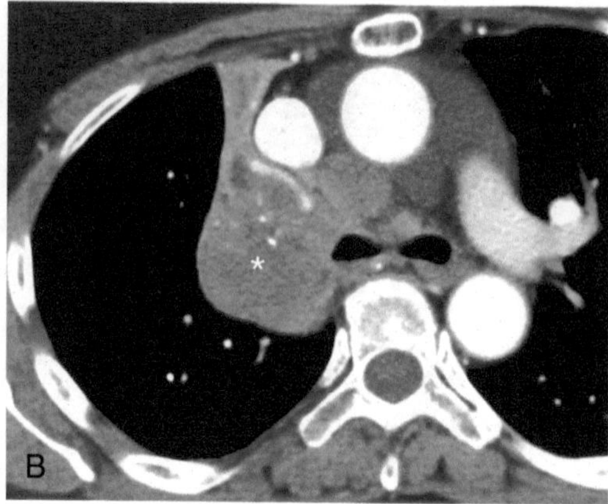

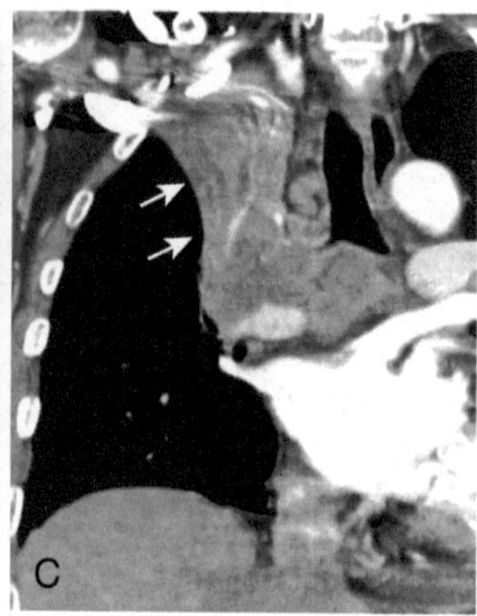

FIGURE 2.55 Right upper lobe collapse caused by lung cancer. **A,** Posteroanterior radiograph shows a right hilar mass with complete opacification of the right upper lobe. The right minor fissure is markedly displaced superiorly *(arrows)*. The minor fissure is concave laterally but the medial portion shows a convex bulge caused by the hilar mass, creating the appearance of a reverse S, which is denoted the S sign of Golden. **B,** Axial computed tomography (CT) image shows the right hilar mass *(asterisk)* occluding the right upper lobe bronchus. **C,** Coronal CT image demonstrates the superior and medial displacement of the right minor fissure.

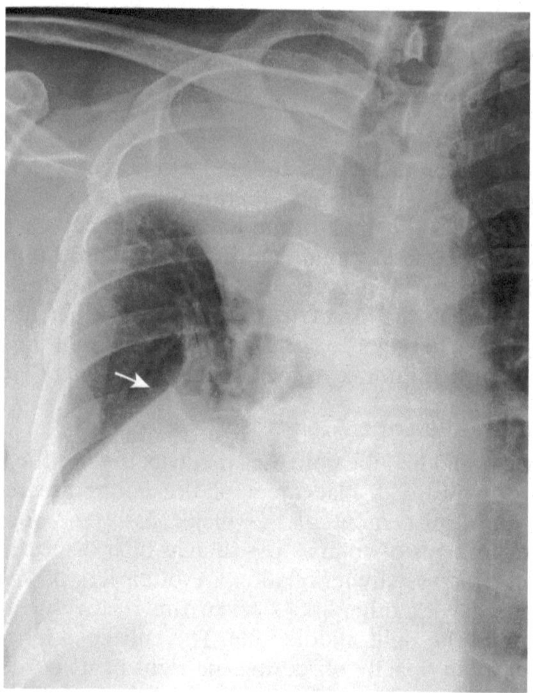

FIGURE 2.56 Juxtaphrenic peak. A portable chest radiograph in a patient with a collapsed right upper lobe shows a prominent juxtaphrenic peak caused by extensive volume loss in the right lung *(arrow)*.

triangular configuration with the apex at the hilum. On a well-penetrated PA radiograph, the atelectatic lower lobe appears as a triangular or rounded opacity in the costovertebral angle. The hilum is displaced inferiorly, and the interlobar artery is typically obscured by adjacent atelectatic lung (Figs. 2.60 and 2.61).

In left lower lobe atelectasis, leftward shift of the heart along with cardiac rotation results in loss of concavity of the left heart border, which appears straight and has been described as the *flat waist sign* (Fig. 2.62). Atelectasis of the right lower lobe causes inferior retraction of the right minor fissure, which can be identified on the PA radiograph. In many instances, a hazy increase in density is seen projecting over the lower thoracic vertebra on the lateral radiograph rather than a discrete opacity. The axial CT appearance of lower lobe atelectasis corresponds to the radiographic findings, with the collapsed lobe contacting the posterior mediastinum and abutting the medial hemidiaphragm.

Combined Right Upper and Right Middle Lobe Atelectasis

The collapse of both the right upper and middle lobes is rare because the bronchi to these lobes are not located in close proximity to one another. However, it can be seen in the setting of a right hilar lesion that obstructs both the right upper and right middle lobe bronchi or in the presence of multiple endobronchial lesions. The PA chest radiograph demonstrates obscuration of both the right superior mediastinum and right heart border because of the collapse of the right upper and middle lobes, respectively (Fig. 2.63). The appearance mimics left upper lobe collapse on the lateral radiograph because both the right upper and right middle lobes are located anterior to the right major fissure.

Combined Right Middle and Right Lower Lobe Atelectasis

An obstructed bronchus intermedius leads to combined right middle and right lower lobe collapse. The major and minor fissures are displaced inferiorly and posteriorly, creating an opacity on the PA view that obscures the dome of the right hemidiaphragm and the right heart border (Fig. 2.64).

Subsegmental Atelectasis

Subsegmental atelectasis appears as linear opacities that are typically 1 to 3 mm thick and approximately 4 to 10 cm in length. They are most frequently found in the lower lung zones and occur in the horizontal plane, parallel to the diaphragm or in an oblique plane. The linear opacities that occur with subsegmental atelectasis are almost invariably associated with conditions that limit diaphragmatic excursion.

Text continued on p. 60

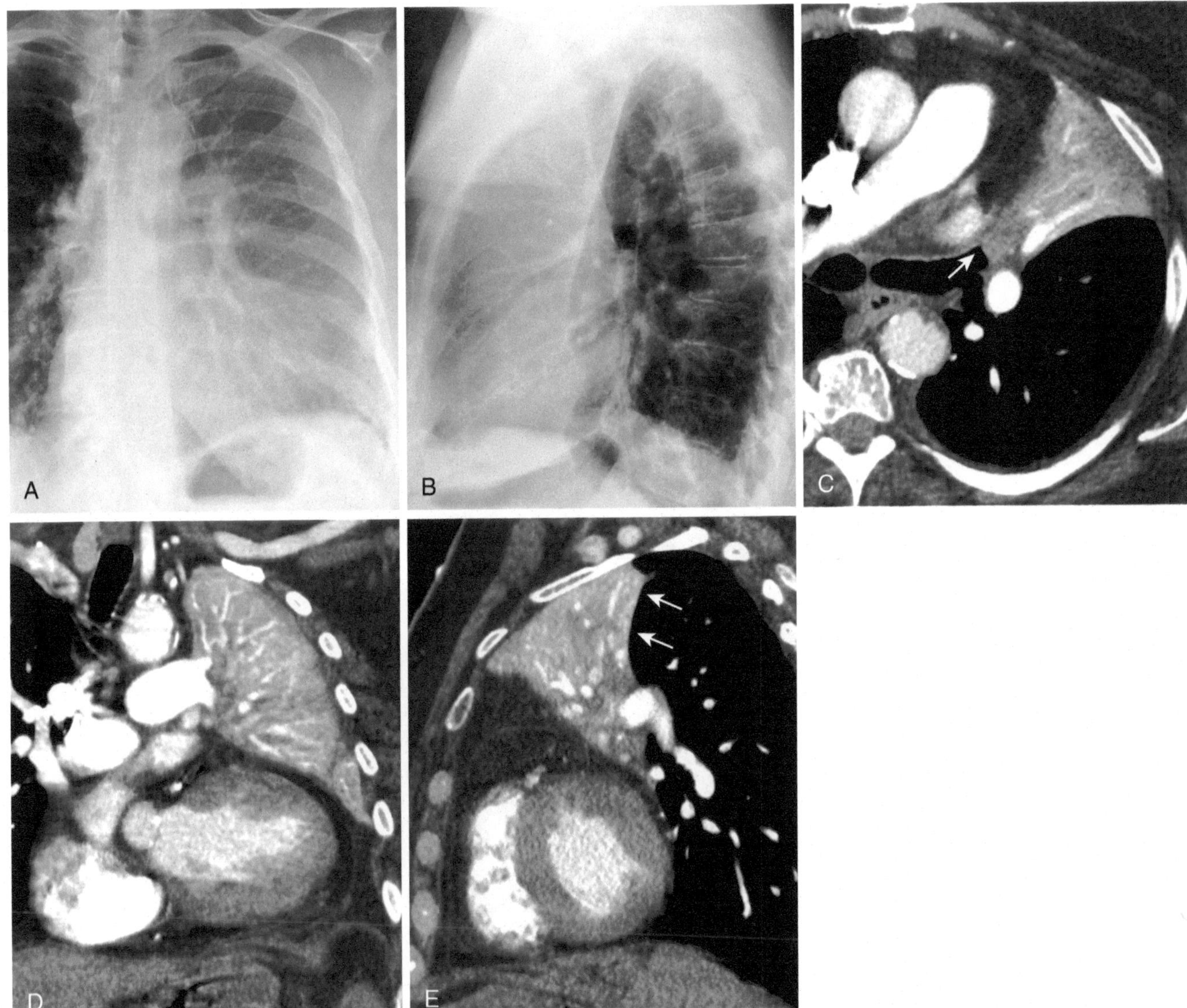

FIGURE 2.57 Left upper lobe collapse caused by an aspirated celery. **A,** The left heart border and left superior mediastinal border are obscured on this posteroanterior radiograph. There is increased opacity in the left hemithorax. **B,** Lateral radiograph shows increased density in the anterior left hemithorax, marginated by the left major fissure posteriorly. **C,** Axial computed tomography (CT) image reveals a low attenuation endobronchial lesion in the left upper lobe bronchus, representing the aspirated celery *(arrow)*. **D,** Coronal CT image shows the collapsed lobe abutting the left heart border and superior mediastinum. **E,** Sagittal CT image shows the anteriorly displaced left major fissure *(arrows)*.

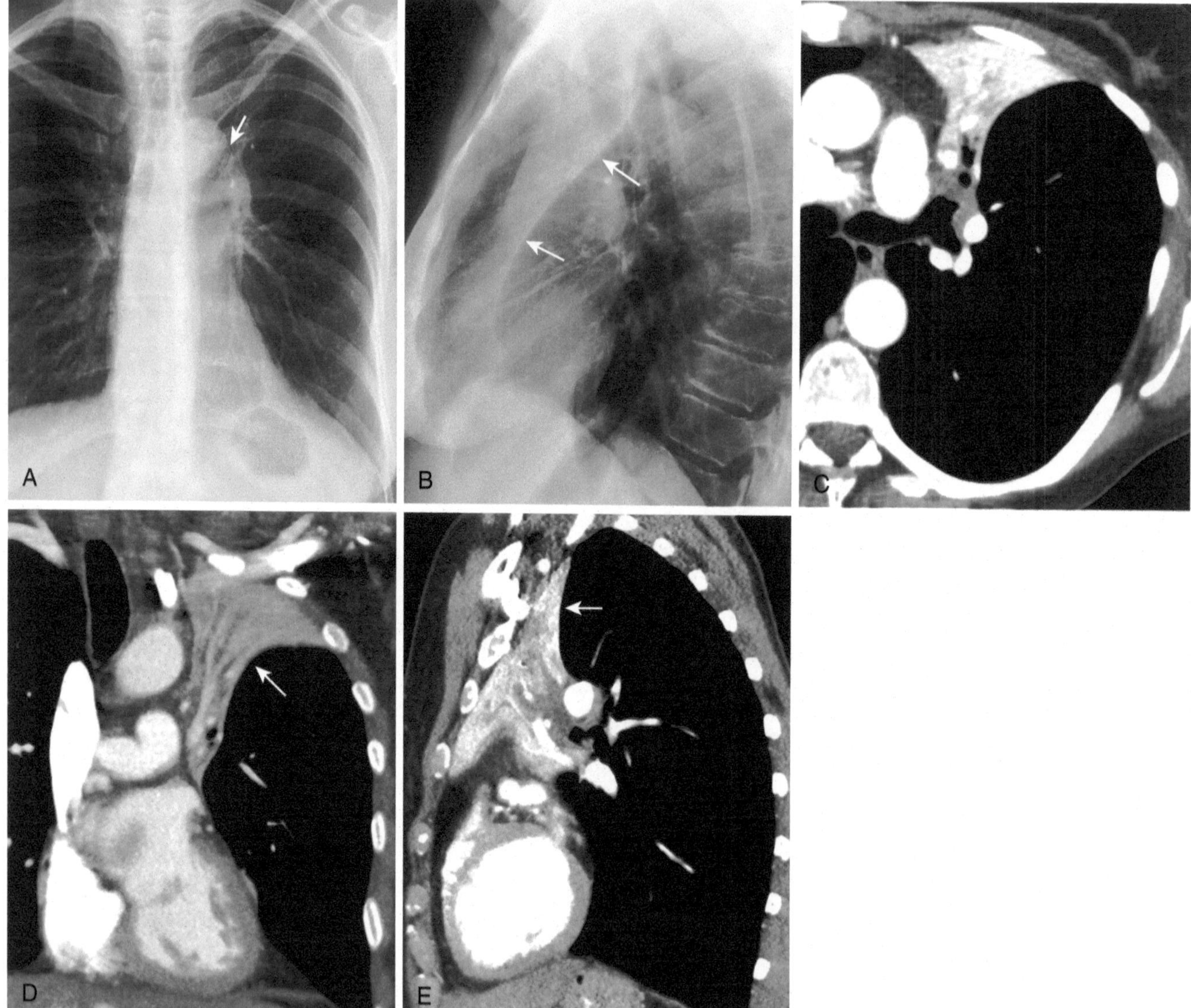

FIGURE 2.58 Left upper lobe collapse associated with an endobronchial hamartoma. **A,** Posteroanterior radiograph shows that the left hilum is elevated. There is a crescentic lucency, the *Luftsichel sign,* adjacent to the aortic arch *(arrow),* representing the hyperinflated left lower lobe superior segment that inserts between the collapsed left upper lobe and the adjacent aortic arch. **B,** Lateral radiograph shows the anterior displacement of the left major fissure *(arrows),* which approximates the plane of the left anterior chest wall. **C,** Axial computed tomography (CT) image at the level of the left upper lobe bronchus shows a low-attenuation lesion occluding the bronchus, which was pathologically shown to represent a hamartoma. Coronal **(D)** and sagittal **(E)** CT images show the anteromedial displacement of the left major fissure marginating the collapsed left upper lobe *(arrows).*

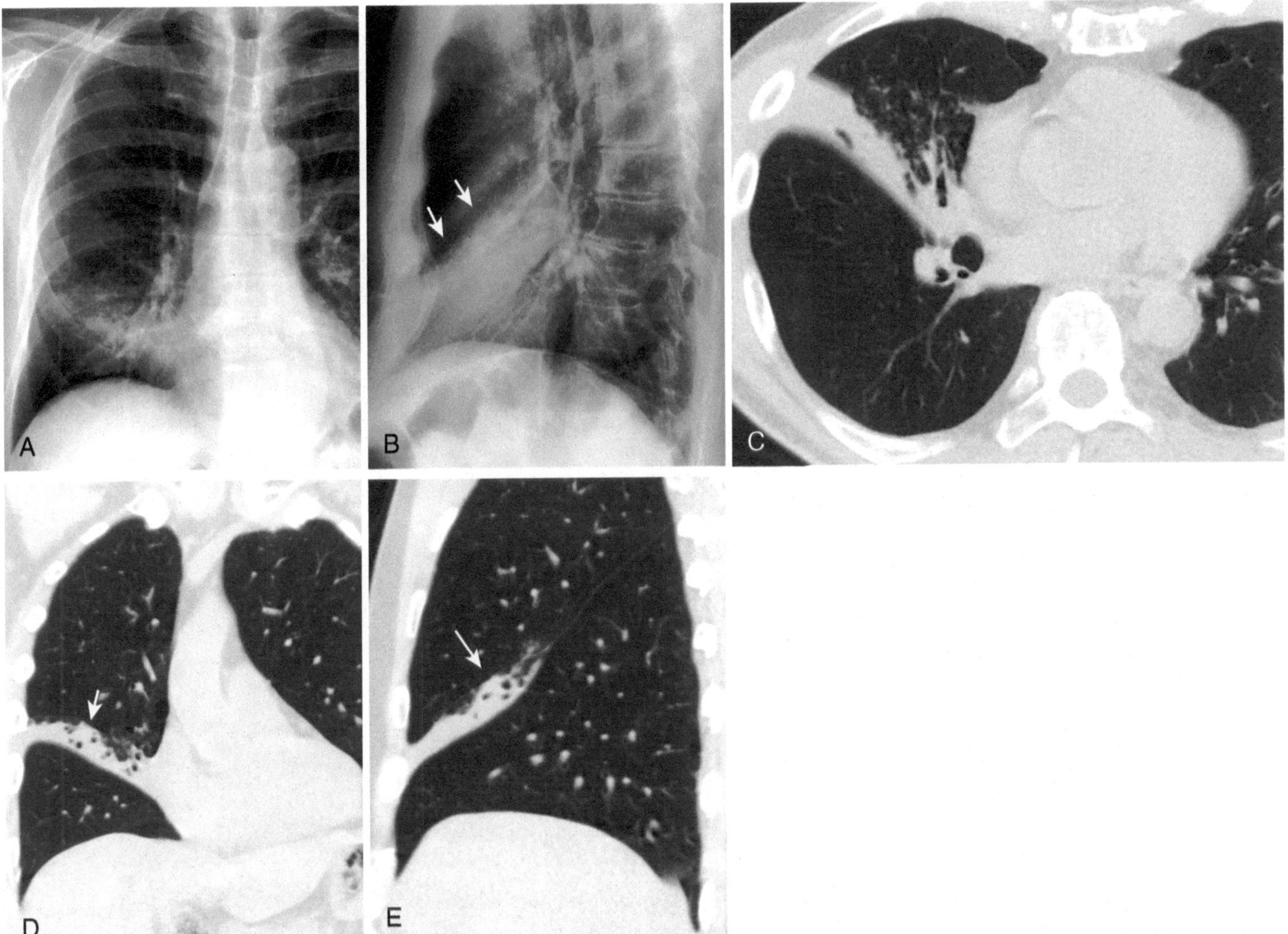

FIGURE 2.59 Right middle lobe atelectasis secondary to an aspirated macadamia nut. **A,** Posteroanterior radiograph shows an ill-defined airspace opacity, which obscures the right heart border. **B,** Lateral radiograph demonstrates inferior displacement of the minor fissure *(arrows)*. The collapsed right middle appears as a thin triangular opacity emanating from the hilum. **C,** Axial computed tomography (CT) image shows tree-in-bud nodules in the aeration portion of the medial segment of the right middle lobe, consistent with postobstructive bronchopneumonia. Coronal **(D)** and sagittal **(E)** CT images show the collapsed middle lobe with inferior displacement of the right minor fissure *(arrows)*.

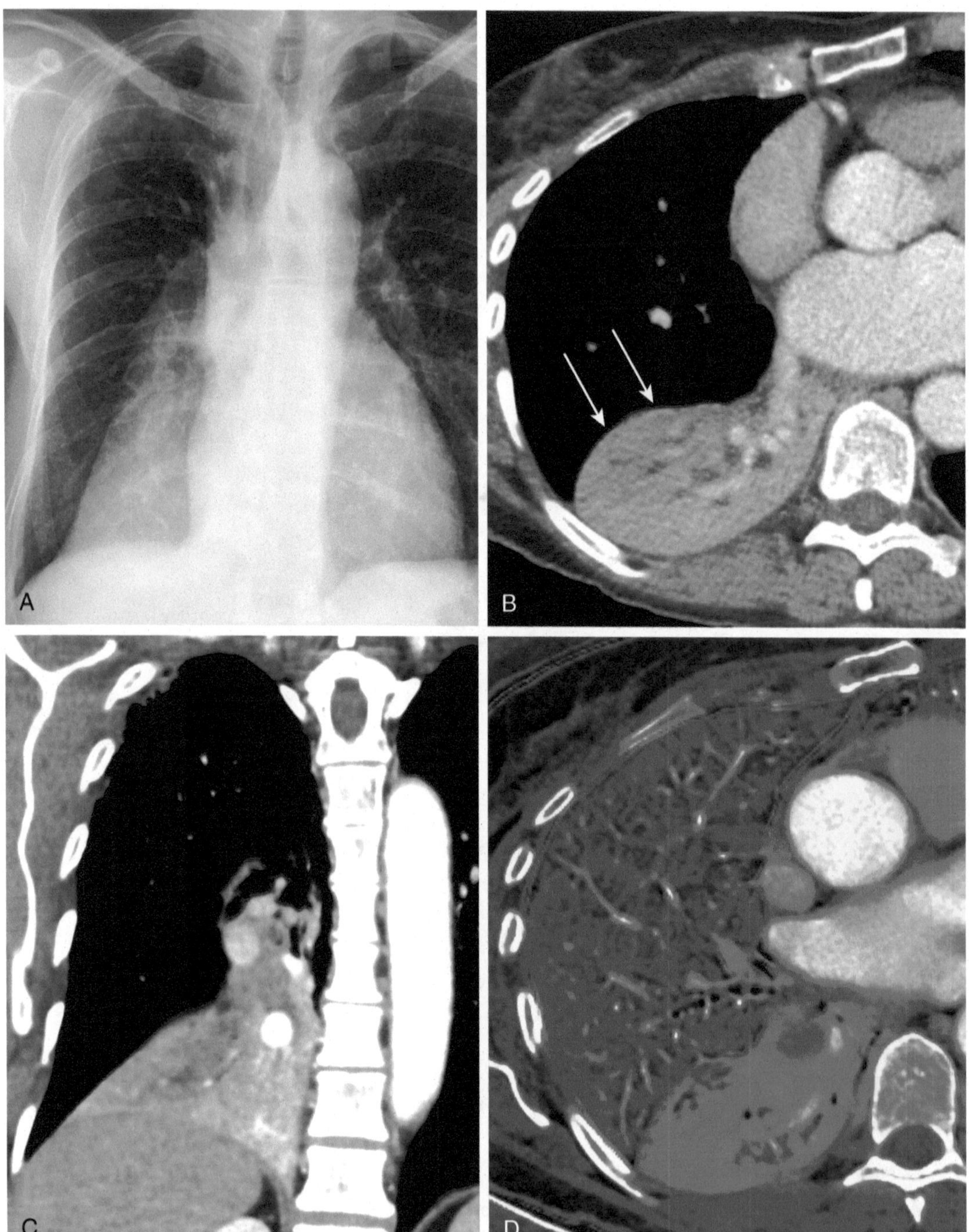

FIGURE 2.60 Right lower lobe collapse caused by mucous secretions in a patient with asthma and *Aspergillus fumigatus* infection. **A,** Posteroanterior radiograph shows a triangular opacity extending inferiorly from the right hilum and partially obscuring the right hemidiaphragm. The right interlobar pulmonary artery is obscured. **B,** Axial computed tomography (CT) image shows the collapsed right lower lobe with posterior displacement of the right major fissure *(arrows)*. **C,** Heterogeneous enhancement of the collapsed right lower lobe is evident on the coronal image, suggestive of postobstructive pneumonia. **D,** Dual-energy iodine density CT image highlights the decreased iodine content within the mucoid impacted bronchi.

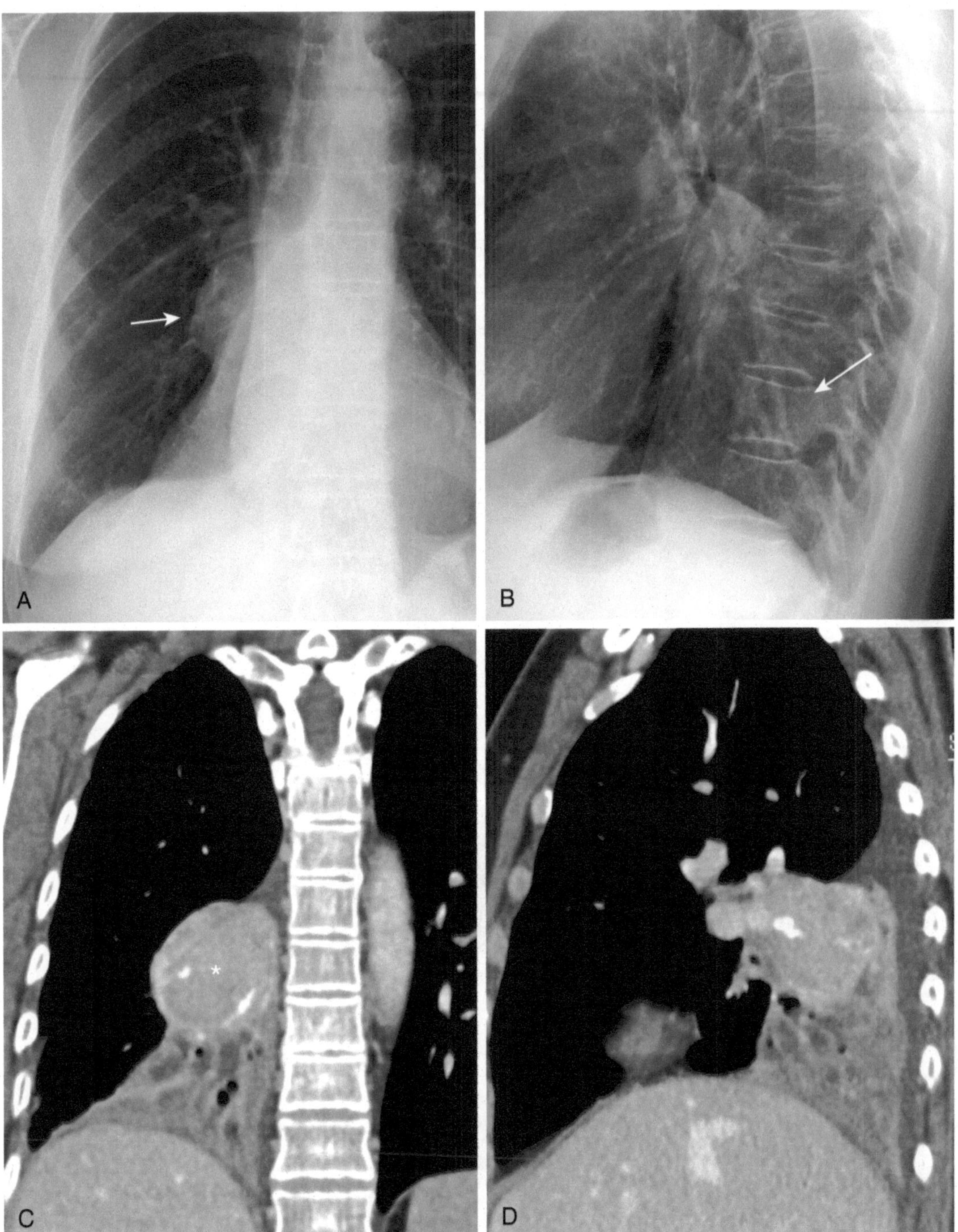

FIGURE 2.61 Right lower lobe collapse caused by a typical carcinoid tumor. **A,** Posteroanterior chest radiograph shows a right perihilar mass *(arrow)* with inferior displacement of the right hilum and obscuration of the right interlobar pulmonary artery. **B,** Lateral radiograph shows an ill-defined opacity overlying the lower thoracic spine *(arrow)* representing the collapsed right lower lobe, an example of the spine sign. Coronal **(C)** and sagittal **(D)** computed tomography images show the partially calcified mass *(asterisk)*, which occludes the right lower lobe bronchus and extends into the bronchus intermedius. There is evidence of postobstructive pneumonia, with low-attenuation fluid within the airways of the collapsed right lower lobe.

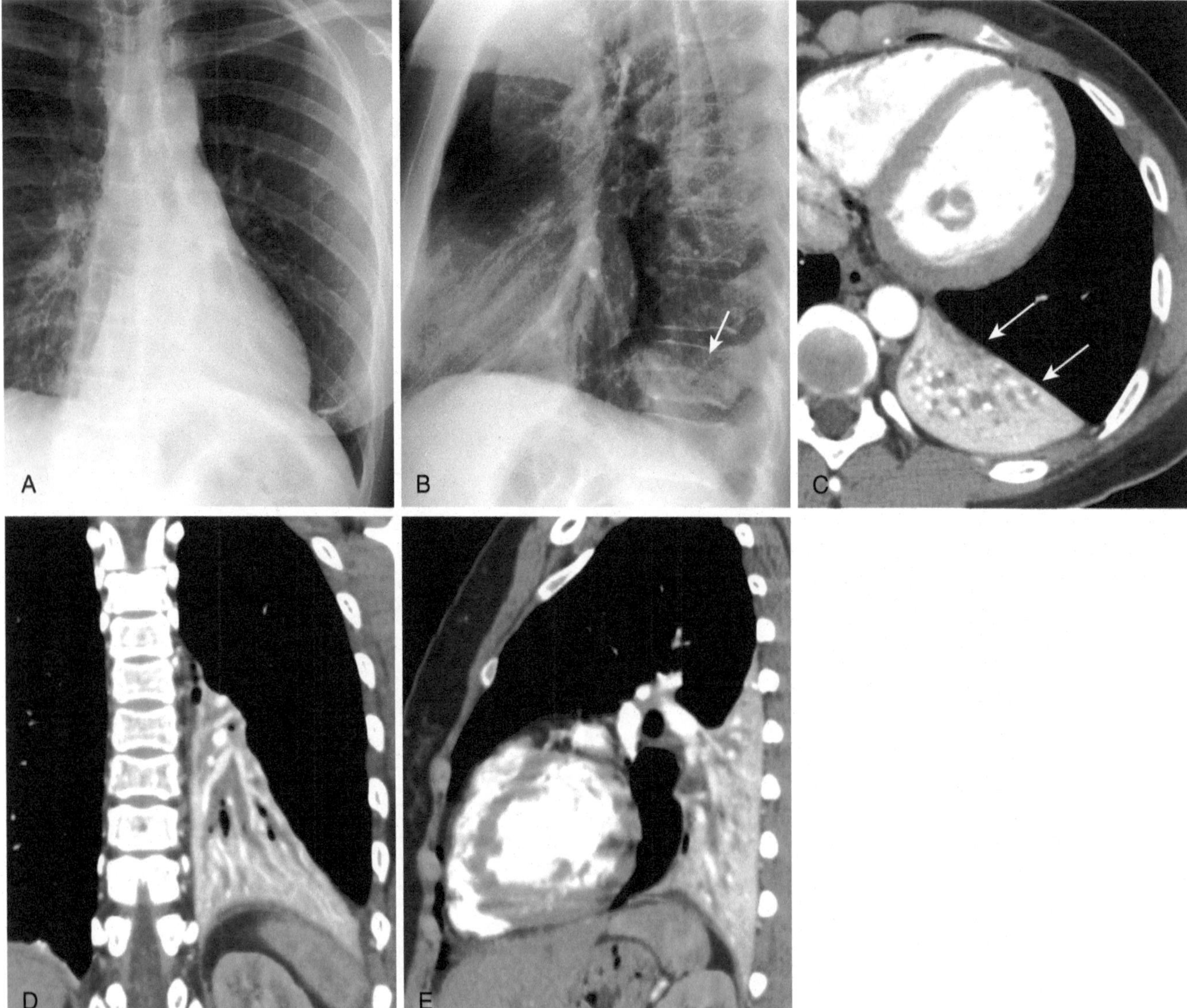

FIGURE 2.62 Left lower lobe collapse caused by mucous secretions. **A,** On the posteroanterior radiograph, there is mild leftward shift of the heart and mediastinum. A triangular opacity representing the collapsed left lower lobe projects adjacent to the descending thoracic aorta and vertebral bodies. The left mediastinal contour caused by leftward rotation of the heart appears flattened, which is denote by the flat waist sign. **B,** Lateral radiograph shows an abnormal opacity projecting over the lower thoracic spine, an example of the spine sign *(arrow)*. **C,** Axial computed tomography (CT) image shows low-attenuation mucus occluding segmental and subsegmental bronchi. The major fissure is displaced posteriorly *(arrows)*. Coronal **(D)** and sagittal **(E)** CT images show homogeneous enhancement of the atelectatic lobe surrounding low-attenuation areas of mucoid impaction.

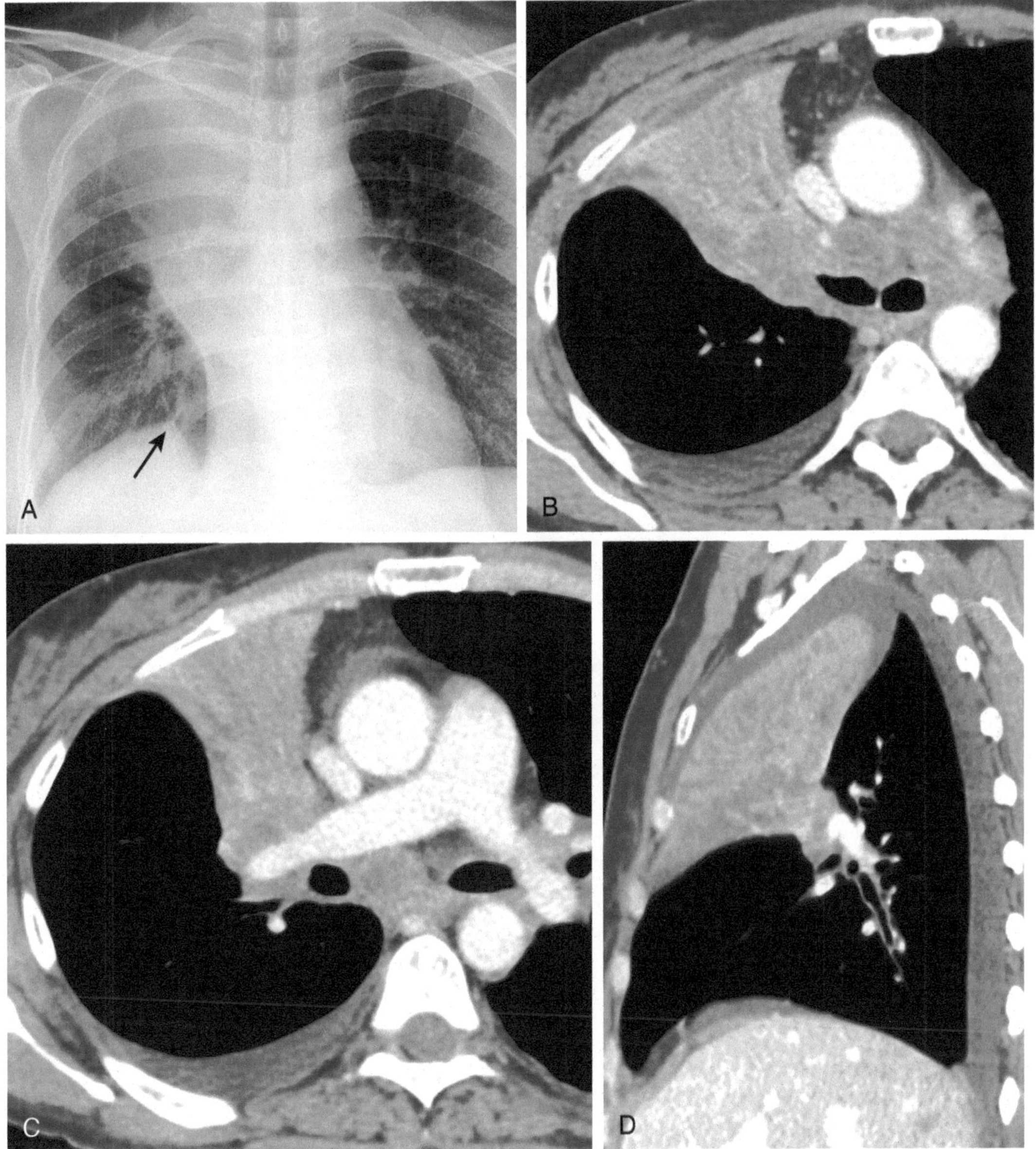

FIGURE 2.63 Right upper and right middle lobe collapse secondary to non–small cell lung cancer. **A,** Frontal radiograph shows a right hilar mass with obscuration of the right heart border and right superior mediastinum. A juxtaphrenic peak is seen on the right caused by the extensive volume loss in the right lung *(arrow)*. **B,** Axial computed tomography (CT) image shows occlusion of the right upper lobe bronchus caused by the right hilar mass. **C,** Axial CT image more inferiorly demonstrates the collapsed right upper lobe at this level. **D,** Sagittal CT image shows the collapsed right upper and middle lobes, which are displaced anteriorly. The right lower lobe is hyperinflated.

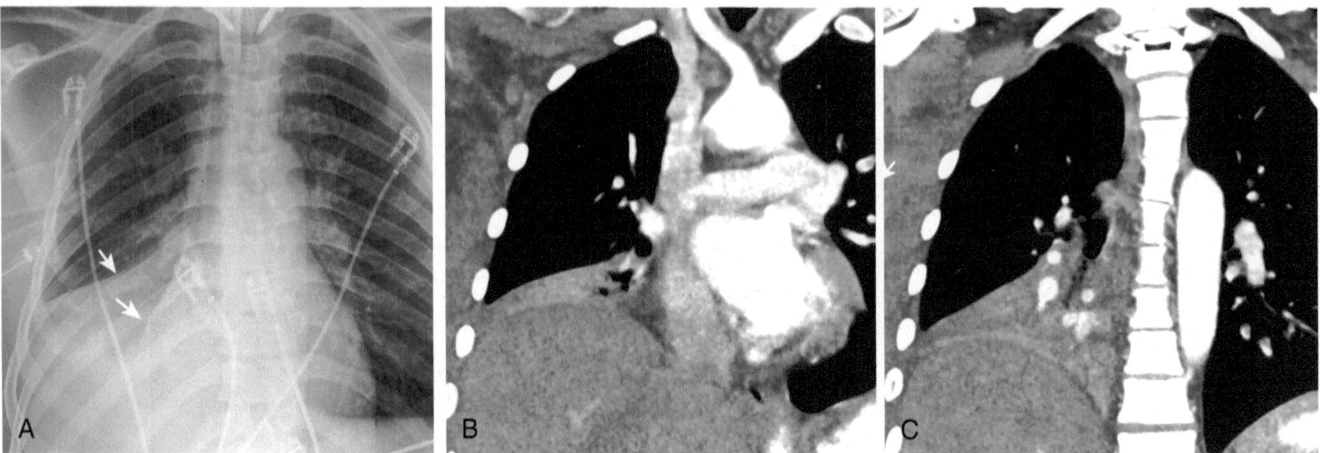

FIGURE 2.64 Right middle and right lower lobe collapse caused by endobronchial secretions, **A,** Portable chest radiograph shows the collapsed right middle and lower lobes obscuring the right heart border and right hemidiaphragm. The right major and minor fissures are inferiorly displaced *(arrows)*. There is rightward shift of the trachea as well as the heart and mediastinum. **B** and **C,** Coronal computed tomography images show the collapsed lobes with secretions in the bronchus intermedius.

SUGGESTED READINGS

Vix VA, Klatte EC. The lateral chest radiograph in the diagnosis of hilar and mediastinal masses. *Radiology*. 1970;96:307-316.

Proto AV, Speckman JM. The lateral chest radiograph of the chest. Part one. *Med Radiogr Photogr*. 1979;55:30-74.

Proto AV, Speckman JM. The lateral chest radiograph of the chest. Part two. *Med Radiogr Photogr*. 1979;56:38-64.

Park CK, Webb WR, Klein JS. Inferior hilar window. *Radiology*. 1991;178:163-168.

Schnur MJ, et al. Thickening of the posterior wall of the bronchus intermedius: a sign on lateral radiographs of congestive heart failure, lymph node enlargement, and neoplastic infiltration. *Radiology*. 1981;139:551-559.

McComb BL. Reflecting upon the left superior mediastinum. *J Thorac Imaging*. 2011;16:56-64.

McComb BL. The chest in profile. *J Thorac Imaging*. 2002;17:58-69.

Landay MJ. Anterior clear space: How clear? How often? How come? *Radiology*. 1994;192:165-169.

Franquet T, et al. The retrotracheal space: normal anatomic and pathologic appearances. *Radiographics*. 2002;22:S231-S246.

Shroff GS, Viswanathan C, Godoy MC, et al. Pitfalls in oncologic imaging: pericardial recesses mimicking adenopathy. *Semin Roentgenol*. 2015;50(3):226-228.

Fraser RG, Muller NL, Fraser RS, et al. *Diagnosis of Diseases of the Chest*. Philadelphia: WB Saunders; 2001.

Batra P, Brown K, Hayashi K, et al. Rounded atelectasis. *J Thorac Imaging*. 1996;11:187-197.

Webb RW, Higgins CB. *Thoracic Imaging*. 2nd ed. Philadelphia: Lippincott, Williams and Wilkins; 2011.

Chapter 3

Thoracic Magnetic Resonance Imaging: Technique and Approach to Diagnosis

Jeanne B. Ackman

INTRODUCTION

Uses of Thoracic Magnetic Resonance Imaging

Chest radiography (CXR) and chest tomography (CT) have been the mainstays of thoracic imaging for decades, and 18-fluorodeoxyglucose positron emission tomography (FDG-PET)–CT has more recently proven its value in staging lung cancer and metastatic disease within the thorax. Upon technical improvements that have addressed challenges related to cardiorespiratory motion, magnetic resonance imaging (MRI) has become appreciated for its capability in tissue diagnosis, without ionizing radiation exposure. The term *thoracic MRI* is defined here to encompass all of thoracic MRI except cardiovascular and breast MRI.

Problem Solving

Magnetic resonance imaging has proven impactful as a problem solver in the thorax when lesions are indeterminate by CT. Although problem solving with MRI has been largely focused on the mediastinum and pleura, its applications in the lung have been increasing, with examples including serial follow-up of patients with cystic fibrosis, tissue characterization of indeterminate but probably benign pulmonary nodules on CT greater than or equal to 1 cm, and discernment of tumor from postobstructive atelectasis.

Full Chest Imaging and Screening

In addition to full chest MRI for mesothelioma, there has been increased use of MR to screen for and follow various disease entities in the thorax without ionizing radiation exposure, such as endometriosis, chronic lymphocytic leukemia and lymphoma in young and pregnant patients (Fig. 3.1), cystic fibrosis, paragangliomas (e.g., SDHD mutation), teratomas (NMDA [*N*-methyl-D-aspartate] receptor antibodies), carcinoid tumors (multiple endocrine neoplasia type 1), and syndromes with high risk for malignancy (e.g., Li-Fraumeni syndrome).

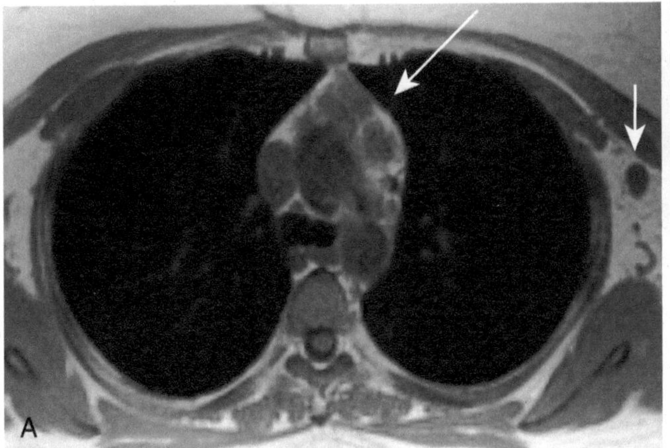

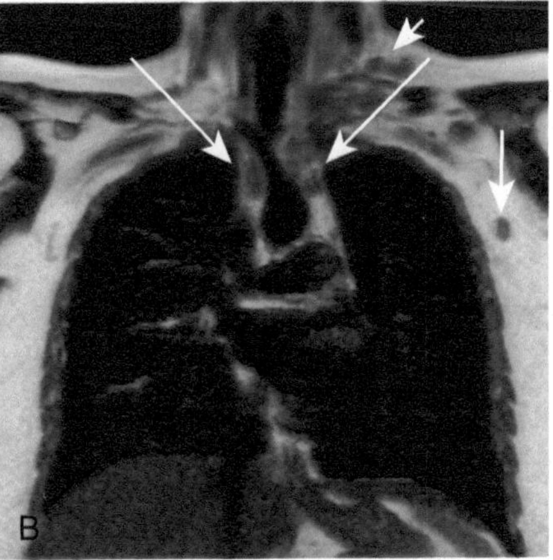

FIGURE 3.1 "No-dose imaging": a 29-year-old woman with Hodgkin disease in need of staging while pregnant. **A** and **B,** Axial in-phase T1-weighted image and coronal single-shot fast spin-echo T2-weighted image show anterior mediastinal *(long arrows)*, left axillary *(medium-sized arrows)*, and left supraclavicular *(short arrow)* lymphadenopathy.

Strengths of Magnetic Resonance Imaging Over Computed Tomography

No Ionizing Radiation

The ability to make a diagnosis and impact clinical management without ionizing radiation exposure is a substantial benefit of MR over CT, provided MR is used for appropriate indications (see Fig. 3.1).

Better Soft Tissue Contrast

The high soft tissue contrast of MRI and chemical composition analysis by this modality offer a multitude of diagnostic benefits, including:

- Better definition of soft tissue planes
  - More accurate determination of the compartment where a lesion resides (Fig. 3.2)

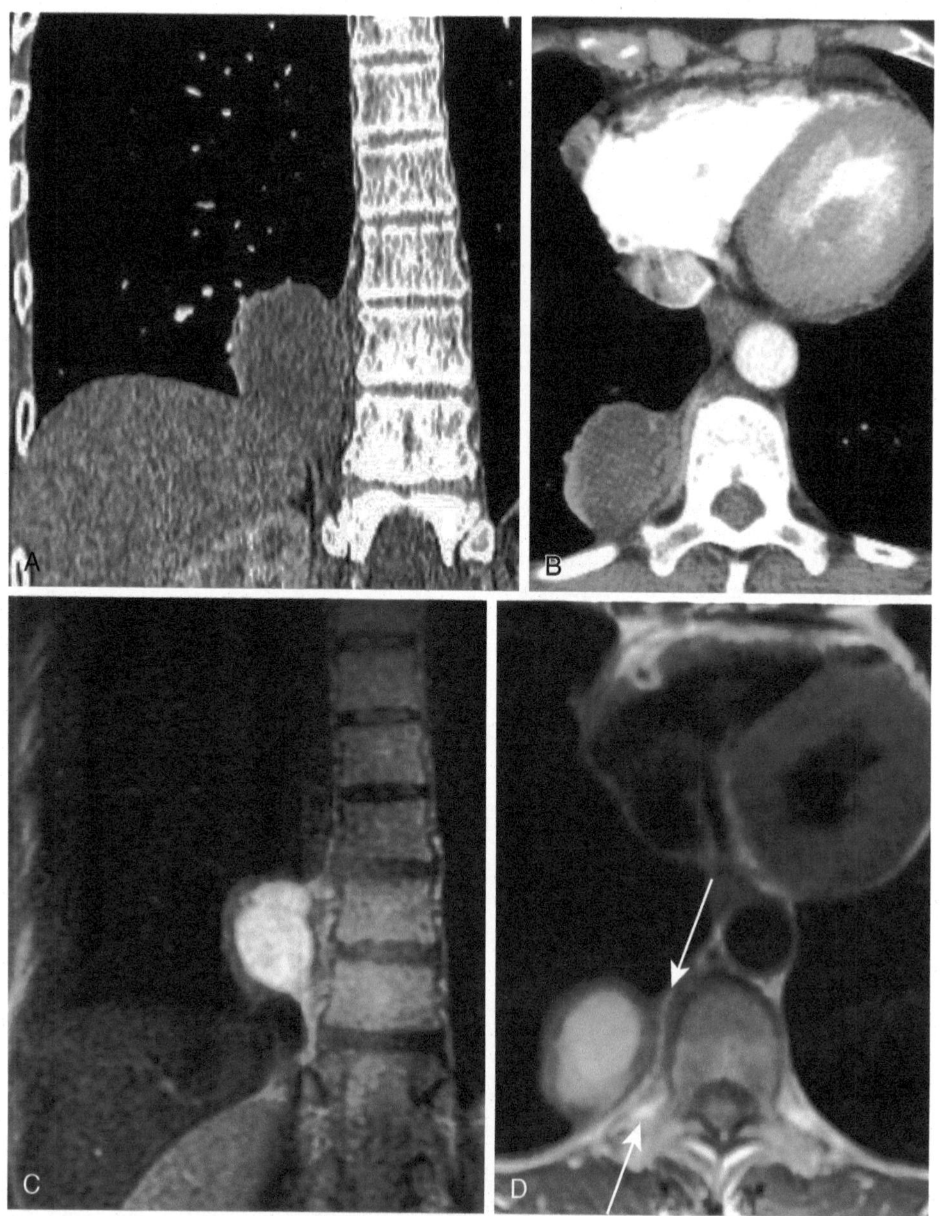

FIGURE 3.2 Accurate compartmental localization aids differential diagnosis. Intrapleural bronchogenic cyst. Coronal **(A)** and axial **(B)** computed tomography (CT) scans demonstrate a complex, cystic hypoattenuating mass in the right posteromedial hemithorax. It is unclear by CT whether this mass resides in the paravertebral mediastinum or the pleural space, with the differential diagnosis including paravertebral masses such as cystic schwannomas and cystic pleural lesions such as extralobar sequestration and intrapleural bronchogenic cyst. Coronal single-shot fast spin-echo T2-weighted **(C)** and axial cardiac-gated double inversion recovery T1-weighted **(D)** magnetic resonance images show this lesion to be T1- and T2-hyperintense (secondary to hemorrhagic or proteinaceous content), thick walled, and septated. The axial T1-weighted MR image **(D)** shows the preserved right paravertebral fat plane *(arrows)* and proves this mass to be outside the paravertebral mediastinum and within the pleural space, excluding neurogenic tumors from the differential diagnosis. The absence of a systemic arterial supply to this lesion favors a rare intrapleural bronchogenic cyst over an extralobar sequestration. Surgical pathology confirmed an intrapleural bronchogenic cyst.

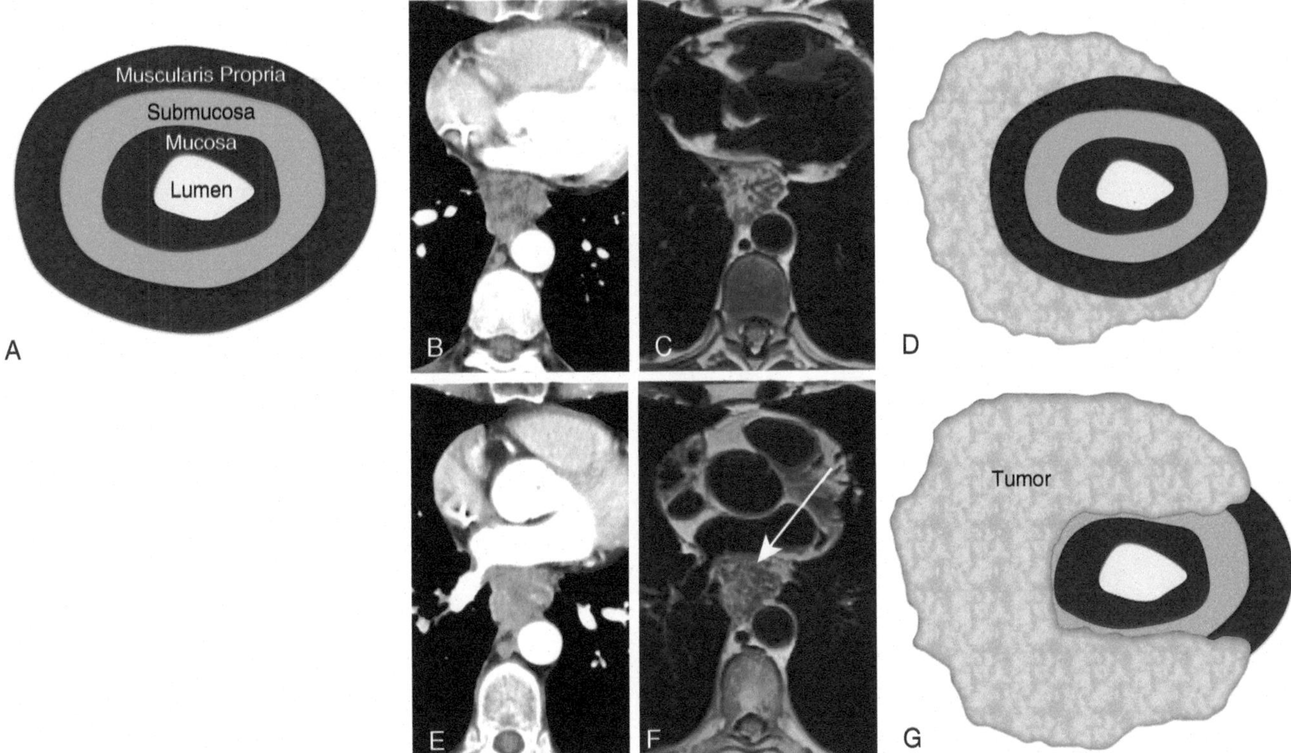

FIGURE 3.3 Detection of invasion: subcarinal metastatic bladder cancer invading the esophagus. **A,** Artistic rendering showing the correlative names for the various high- and low-signal layers of the esophagus. Matched axial computed tomography (CT) **(B)** and axial cardiac-gated (CG) double inversion recovery (IR) T2-weighted **(C)** magnetic resonance images (MRIs) and artistic rendering **(D)** of an amorphous heterogeneous attenuation mass on CT, effacing the fat plane between it and the right half of the esophageal wall. The presence of esophageal wall invasion by the mass is indeterminate by CT. Correlative T2-weighted MRI and artistic rendering reveal partial encasement of the esophagus by tumor without invasion through the laminar wall of the esophagus. Matched axial CT **(E)** and CG double IR T2-weighted **(F)** MR images and artistic rendering **(G)** of the mass at a higher level, again revealing partial encasement of the esophagus and effacement of the fat plane between these two entities on CT. T2-weighted MRI and rendering reveal effacement of a portion of the wall (muscularis propria and submucosa) of the esophagus *(arrow)*, compatible with invasion of these layers of the esophageal wall by tumor.

- Better demonstration of neurovascular, esophageal (Fig. 3.3), and chest wall involvement
- Definitive differentiation of cystic from solid lesions (hyperattenuating hemorrhagic and proteinaceous cystic lesions can be misperceived as solid on CT) (Fig. 3.4)
- More thorough and sensitive depiction of lesion complexity (heterogeneous composition, small nodules, septations, wall asymmetries, and irregularities)
- Detection of microscopic fat (in addition to macroscopic fat), blood products, fibrous tissue, cartilage, and smooth muscle
- Differentiation of muscles from nerves, tendons, and ligaments

Impact on Clinical Decision Making

These strengths of MR regarding tissue characterization and compartmental localization often yield higher diagnostic specificity, more accurate assessment of resectability, guidance to the interventionist regarding optimum (solid, cellular) sites for biopsy for higher diagnostic yield (Fig. 3.5), guidance to the thoracic surgeon regarding the surgical approach, prevention of unnecessary diagnostic intervention, and prevention of unnecessary follow-up imaging and related clinical care.

Value

Used judiciously, MR therefore offers great value, defined by Harvard Business School professor Michael E. Porter as quality divided by cost. Professor Porter puts it simply: "To reduce cost, the best approach is often to spend more on some services to reduce the need for others." He stresses thinking about the *full cost over the care cycle* of the patient, rather than the cost of an individual test. When MRI makes a more precise tissue diagnosis than CT, better defines tissue planes and invasiveness for the surgeon, prevents unnecessary surgery and its associated morbidity and mortality, and prevents unnecessary follow-up imaging, then it has saved a substantial amount *over the care cycle of the patient* and is invaluable.

TISSUE CHARACTERIZATION AND MAGNETIC RESONANCE IMAGING INTERPRETATION

The basic principles of MR tissue characterization in other parts of the body are fully applicable to lesions in the thorax. Generally, the signal intensity of a lesion is described

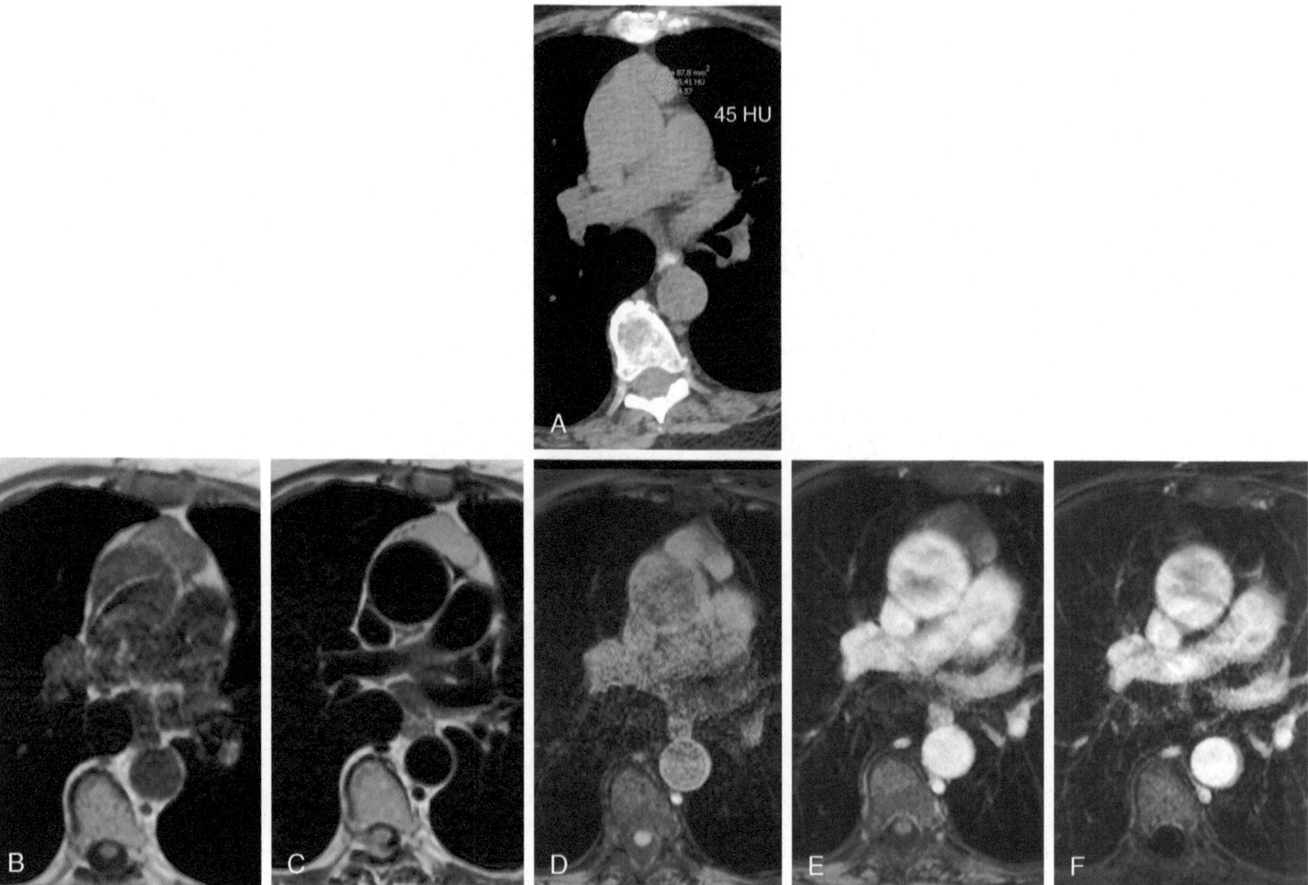

FIGURE 3.4 Distinction of cystic from solid lesions: indeterminate thymic mass on computed tomography (CT) characterized as a unilocular proteinaceous or hemorrhagic cyst by magnetic resonance imaging (MRI). **A,** Axial CT image shows a homogeneous attenuation, 45 HU (Hounsfield units) mass with saccular morphology filling much of the thymic bed. The differential diagnosis includes thymic hyperplasia, thymic cyst, thymic neoplasm, and lymphoma. **B,** Axial in-phase T1-weighted, **C,** Cardiac-gated double-inversion recovery T2-weighted, **D,** Precontrast ultrafast three-dimensional (3D) gradient echo (GRE), fat-saturated T1-weighted, **E,** Postcontrast ultrafast 3D GRE, fat-saturated T1-weighted, and **F** Postcontrast, postprocessed subtracted MR images, respectively, show the mass to be of intermediate T1 signal and homogeneously and markedly T2-hyperintense and to exhibit no internal enhancement, proving the mass to represent a thymic cyst. Thin smooth wall enhancement is present and commonly appreciable in thymic cysts by MRI, albeit seldom by CT.

in reference to skeletal muscle on the same image and referred to as hypointense, isointense, or hyperintense (to muscle). If another reference standard is used besides muscle, it is helpful, when reporting the study, to specify the tissue to which the signal of the lesion is being compared. Table 3.1 lists the typical MR signal characteristics of various lesion tissue types encountered in the thorax (and elsewhere). Knowledge of the classic signal characteristics of these tissue types can markedly narrow the differential diagnosis of a lesion.

Cyst Versus Solid

Cysts and fluid collections are almost always very T2-hyperintense (to muscle) or -isointense to cerebrospinal fluid (CSF) (Fig. 3.6), with the exception of endometriomas and other long-standing hemorrhagic cysts, which may be T2-hypointense, exhibiting "T2-shading" secondary to their highly concentrated iron content (Fig. 3.7). Because cysts contain fluid, they do not internally enhance, with the exception of lymphangiomatous locules into which intravenous (IV) contrast may eventually seep with time. The walls of benign cysts lined by epithelium may exhibit thin, smooth wall enhancement. Unilocular cysts with no wall enhancement or thin smooth wall enhancement are virtually always benign. Inflammatory cyst walls typically enhance. Irregular, nodular, or asymmetric wall enhancement of a cystic lesion or enhancing septations warrant consideration of a more complex benign multilocular lesion (e.g., a multilocular lymphangioma (see Fig. 7.11) or multilocular thymic cyst), an inflammatory lesion, and a cystic neoplasm. The T1 signal of cysts is variable, depending on the nature of the fluid. If the fluid is serous, the T1 signal will be hypointense. Hemorrhagic or proteinaceous fluid and fatty fluid are generally T1-isointense or -hyperintense to muscle. Cysts occasionally exhibit fluid–fluid levels that have been referred to as "hematocrit levels," in the context of hemorrhagic cysts (see Fig. 5.10).

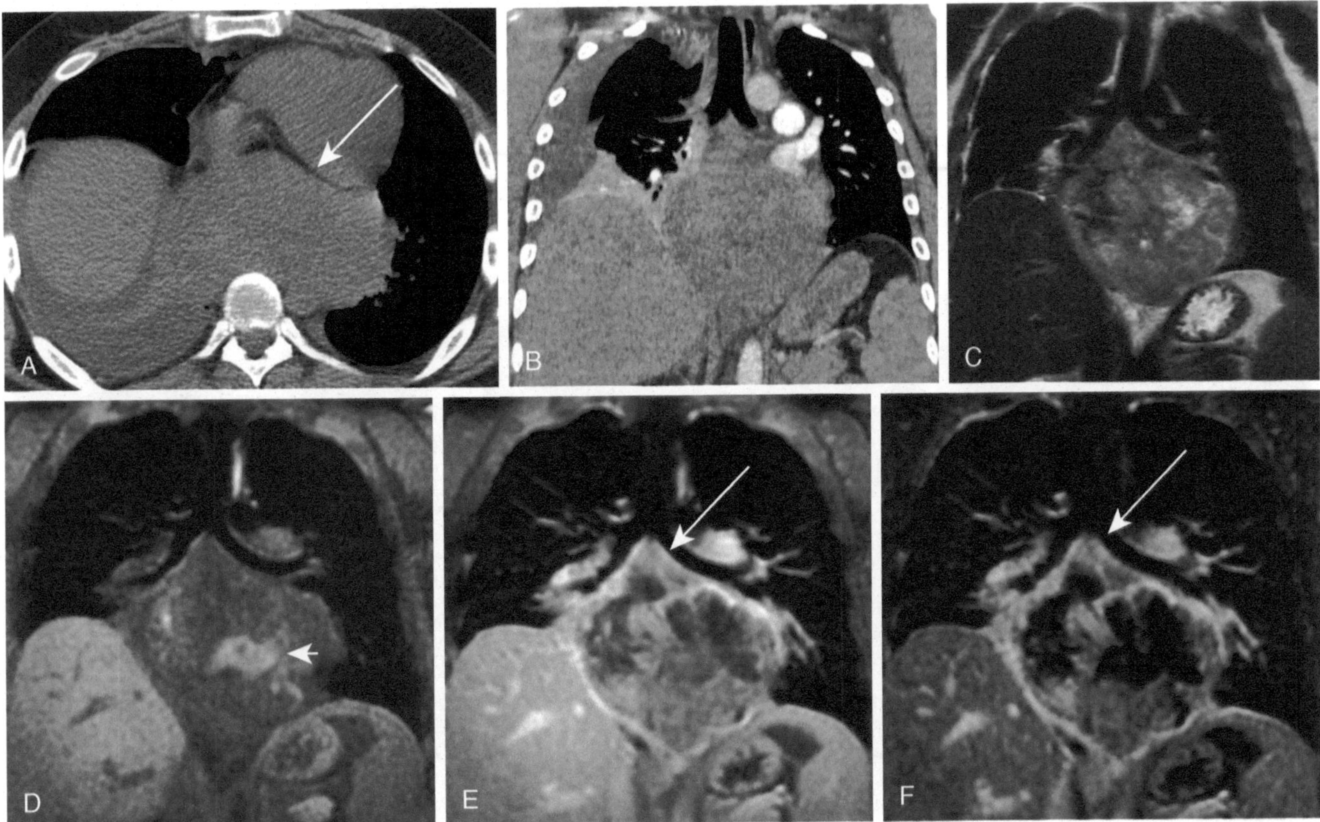

FIGURE 3.5 Magnetic resonance imaging (MRI) differentiates solid tissue from fluid in a mass, guiding biopsy for higher diagnostic yield: indeterminate hemorrhagic mass involving visceral mediastinum on computed tomography (CT), shown to be mixed solid and hemorrhagic–necrotic on MRI. Axial noncontrast **(A)** and coronal contrast-enhanced **(B)** CT images show amorphous, heterogeneous attenuation material in the visceral mediastinum, anteriorly displacing the heart and esophagus *(short arrow)*, with an adjacent or contiguous right pleural effusion and partial right lower lobe relaxation atelectasis. It is unclear by CT whether this finding represents pure hemorrhage or a hemorrhagic mass and, if a hemorrhagic mass, where its solid components are. **C,** Coronal single-shot fast spin-echo T2-weighted, **D,** Precontrast fat-saturated T1-weighted, **E,** Postcontrast ultrafast three-dimensional gradient echo, fat-saturated T1-weighted, **F,** Postcontrast, postprocessed subtraction MR images reveal the indeterminate CT finding to represent a large, well-circumscribed mediastinal mass of heterogeneous T1- and T2-weighted signal, with areas of T1-hyperintensity representing hemorrhage (e.g., *short arrow*). The postcontrast image and, in particular, the subtraction image clearly delineate the solid, cellular, enhancing components of this mass that would be most promising for diagnostic biopsy, including a subcarinal solid component *(long arrow)* accessible to minimally invasive bronchoscopic needle biopsy.

TABLE 3.1 Magnetic Resonance Tissue Characterization Features*

Tissue Type	T1 Signal Intensity	T2 Signal Intensity	Enhancement Pattern	Restricted Diffusion
Serous cyst	Hypointense	Hyperintense	No internal enhancement; may see thin, smooth wall enhancement	No
Proteinaceous or hemorrhagic cyst	Isointense or hyperintense	Hyperintense	No internal enhancement; may see thin, smooth wall enhancement	No, unless old congealed blood or hematoma, which can be restricted
Microscopic fat	Not discernible on in-phase images; hypointense on opposed-phase images	NA	NA	NA
Macroscopic fat	Hyperintense	Hyperintense	No enhancement	No
Cartilage	Hypointense	Hyperintense	Little to no enhancement of cartilage substance; enhancement of scaffolding or rim or septations, however	No
Fibrous tissue	Isointense	Iso- to hypointense (T2-hypointense compared with most lesions)	Gradual, sometimes limited	DWI *hypo*intense (collagen, no water), ADC hypointense
Smooth muscle	Isointense	Isointense (T2-hypointense, compared with most lesions)	Gradual	Variable

*Signal intensity is described *relative to skeletal muscle*. Skeletal muscle is intermediate in signal on T1-weighted images and of low signal on T2-weighted images.
ADC, Apparent diffusion coefficient; *DWI*, diffusion-weighted imaging.

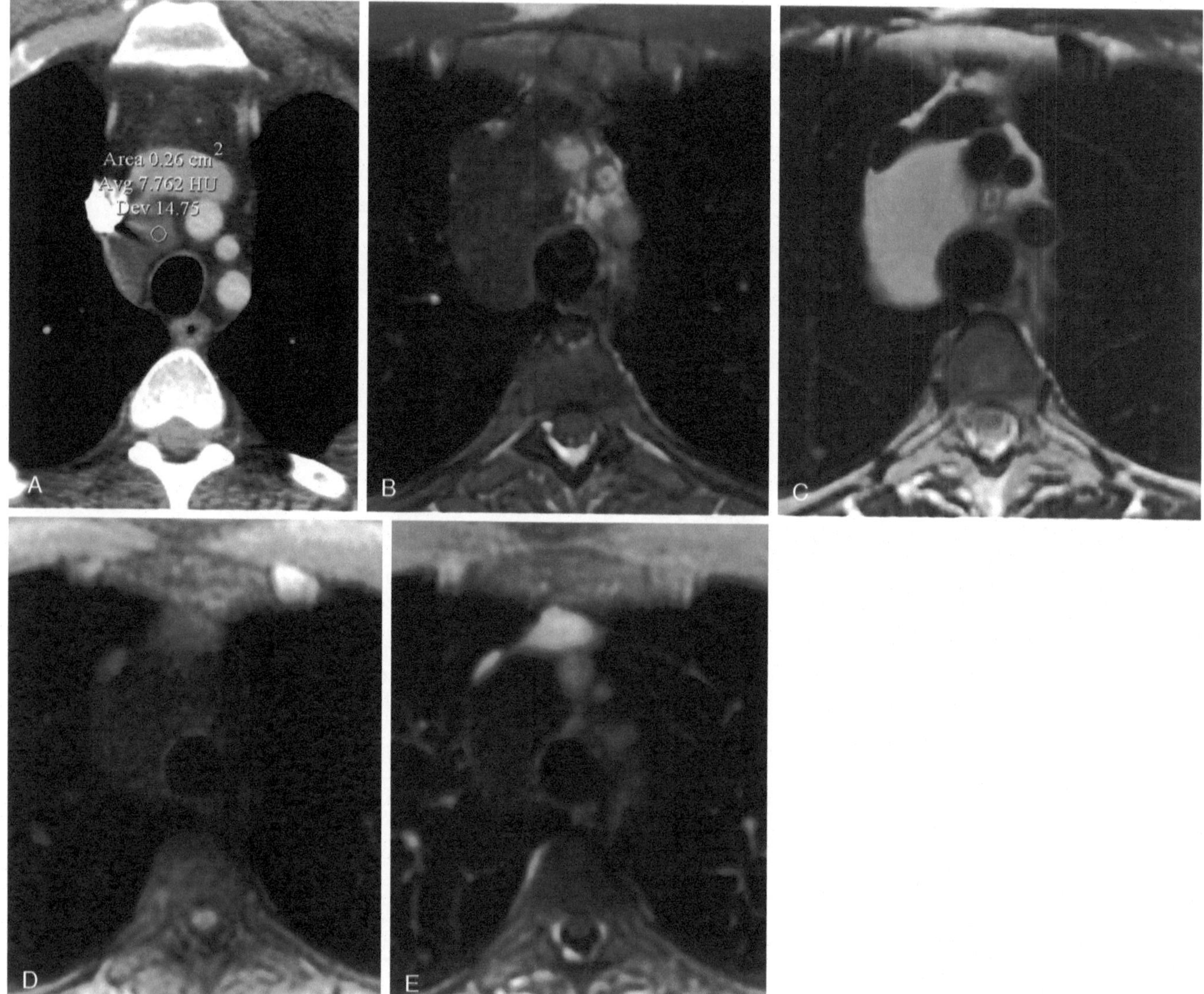

FIGURE 3.6 Classic right paratracheal bronchogenic cyst. **A,** Axial computed tomography (CT) shows a well-circumscribed, homogeneous, water attenuation mass with an imperceptible wall filling the right paratracheal space. These CT features and location are characteristic of a bronchogenic cyst. Although a mesothelial cyst and unilocular lymphangioma could also have this appearance, they are less common in this location. **B,** Axial in-phase T1-weighted, **C,** Cardiac-gated double-inversion recovery T2-weighted, and Pre- **(D)** and postcontrast **(E)** ultrafast three-dimensional gradient echo, fat-saturated T1-weighted images reveal the mass to be homogeneously T1-hypointense (excluding artifacts) and T2-hyperintense (reflecting the serous nature of the fluid), with a thin, smooth wall and no internal enhancement or lesion complexity.

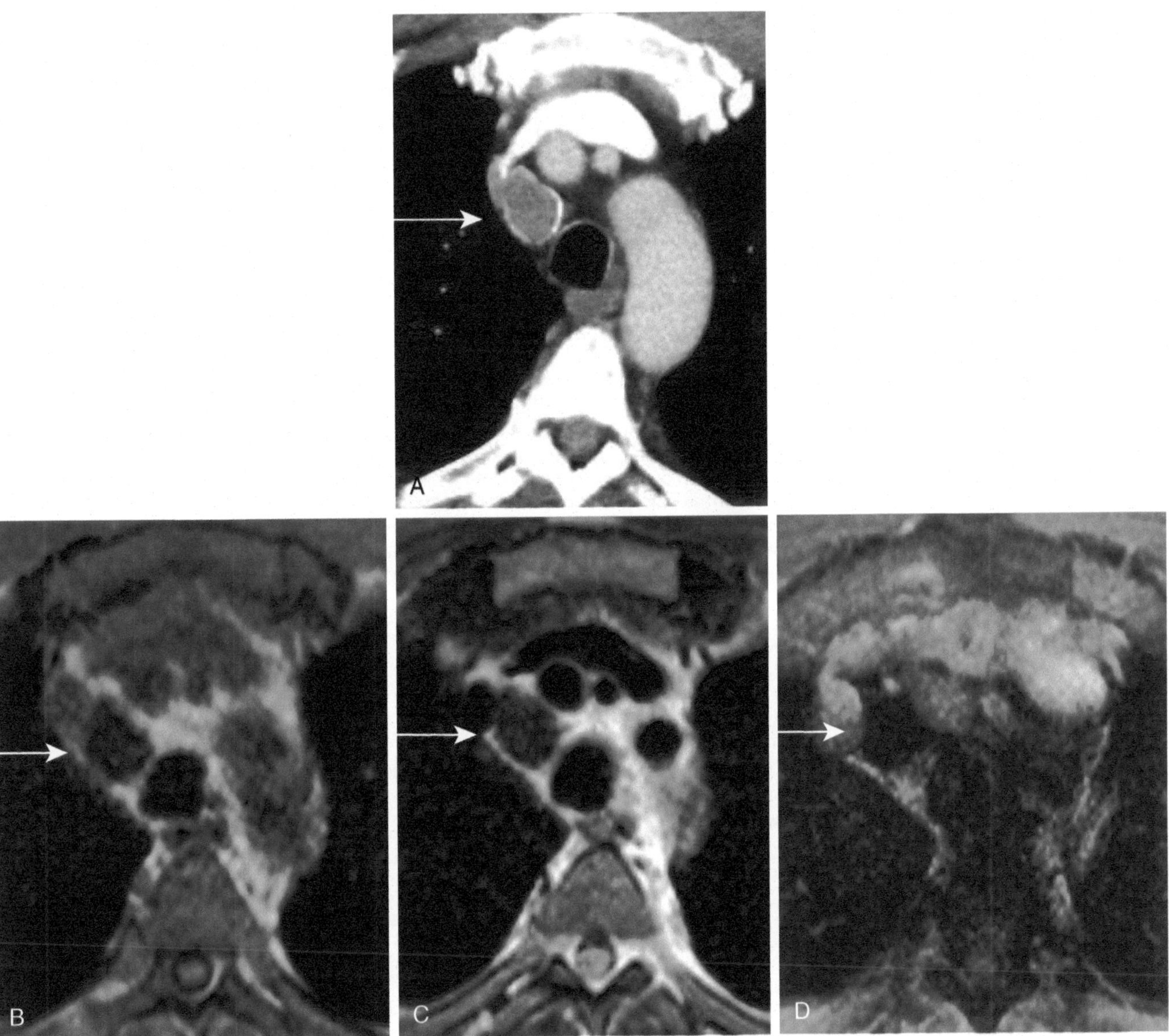

FIGURE 3.7 Low T2 signal secondary to concentrated iron: indeterminate, rim-calcified, soft tissue attenuation right paratracheal mass on computed tomography (CT) shown to be a hemosiderin-laden bronchogenic cyst by magnetic resonance imaging. **A,** Axial CT shows a rim-calcified, ovoid, right paratracheal mass with a slightly irregular contour *(arrow)*. **B,** Axial in-phase T1-weighted image, **C,** Cardiac-gated double-inversion recovery T2-weighted, and **D,** Postcontrast ultrafast three-dimensional gradient echo, fat-saturated T1-weighted images reveal the mass *(arrow)* to be markedly T1- and T2-hypointense and nonenhancing. These features are compatible with an old, contracted, hemorrhagic bronchogenic cyst containing concentrated iron or hemosiderin. Its slightly irregular contour reflects partial contraction over time. A remote neck CT (not shown) of this same patient showed a larger water attenuation, well-circumscribed unilocular cyst in this area at that time.

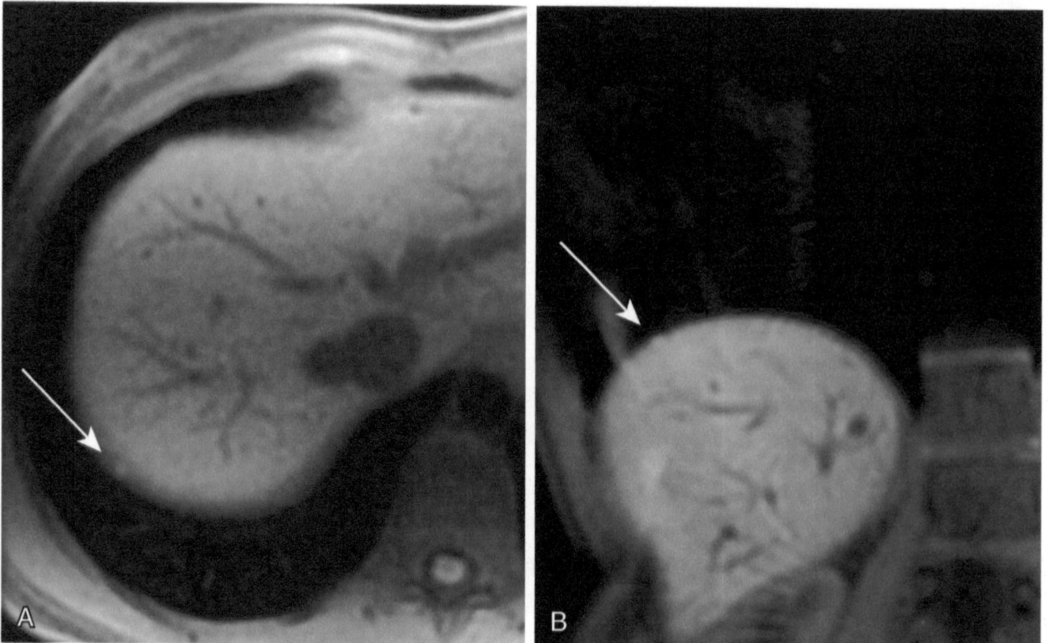

FIGURE 3.8 High sensitivity and specificity of magnetic resonance imaging (MRI) for blood product detection: tiny endometrioma along right hemidiaphragmatic pleura. Axial **(A)** and coronal **(B)** precontrast, ultrafast three-dimensional gradient echo, fat-saturated T1-weighted images reveal a 4-mm, ovoid, well-circumscribed T1-hyperintense nodule *(arrows)* along the diaphragm in this young woman with right upper quadrant and pleuritic chest pain during menses over the past 1 to 2 years. Initially, her full chest screening MRI was negative for endometriomas; however, it was performed when she was not symptomatic. This MR, performed 6 weeks later, during menses, when she was symptomatic, manifested a tiny endometrioma.

Blood Products

Magnetic resonance imaging has higher sensitivity and specificity than CT for the detection of and distinction between blood products. For this reason, it is the test of choice when screening for endometriomas (Fig. 3.8). The signal characteristics of hemorrhage and hematomas vary over time and depend on the age and volume of blood. The most useful signal characteristics of blood products to remember are:

- Methemoglobin is T1-hyperintense, whether intracellular or extracellular, T2-hypointense if intracellular, and T2-hyperintense if extracellular.
- Chronic recurrent hemorrhage within a cyst may yield iron accumulation, with resultant T2-hypointensity or "T2 shading,"
- Hemosiderin is invariably T1- and T2-hypointense.

Calcification

Magnetic resonance imaging cannot readily identify calcification, unlike CT. Nevertheless, when foci or a rim of T2-hypointensity is observed in a lesion in which calcification can occur, the presence of calcification can be suggested.

Macroscopic Fat

Both CT and MRI readily detect macroscopic, or "gross," fat. By MRI, macroscopic fat is T1- and T2-hyperintense unless a saturation pulse is applied to it, in which case its signal "saturates" and becomes hypointense to muscle on both T1- and T2-weighted imaging. This fat saturation technique takes advantage of the difference in precession frequency of protons in fat and water environments. In the absence of a correlative prior CT, fat saturation may be necessary to facilitate the distinction between macroscopic fat and T1-hyperintense blood products within a lesion (Fig. 3.9).

Microscopic Fat

Microscopic fat is not detectable by CT but is detectable by chemical shift MRI or in- and opposed-phase (out-of-phase) gradient echo (GRE) imaging. Microscopic fat suppresses on opposed-phase images. In other words, its signal drops on the opposed-phase image, compared with the in-phase image (Figs. 3.10 and 3.11). Please also see Figs. 5.6, 5.8, and 5.18.

Although it is often possible to qualitatively discern the reduction in signal on chemical shift MRI when microscopic fat is present, it is not possible to discern subtler signal reduction with the naked eye. In such cases, more quantitative techniques can be applied for microscopic fat detection, including simple chemical shift ratio (CSR) and signal intensity index (SII) calculations. To date, the CSR calculation has exclusively been applied in the thorax for detection of microscopic fat within thymic tissue, based on the fact that presence of microscopic fat within thymic tissue proves a histologic diagnosis of normal thymus or thymic hyperplasia, rather than thymic tumors, such as thymoma and lymphoma, which do not contain

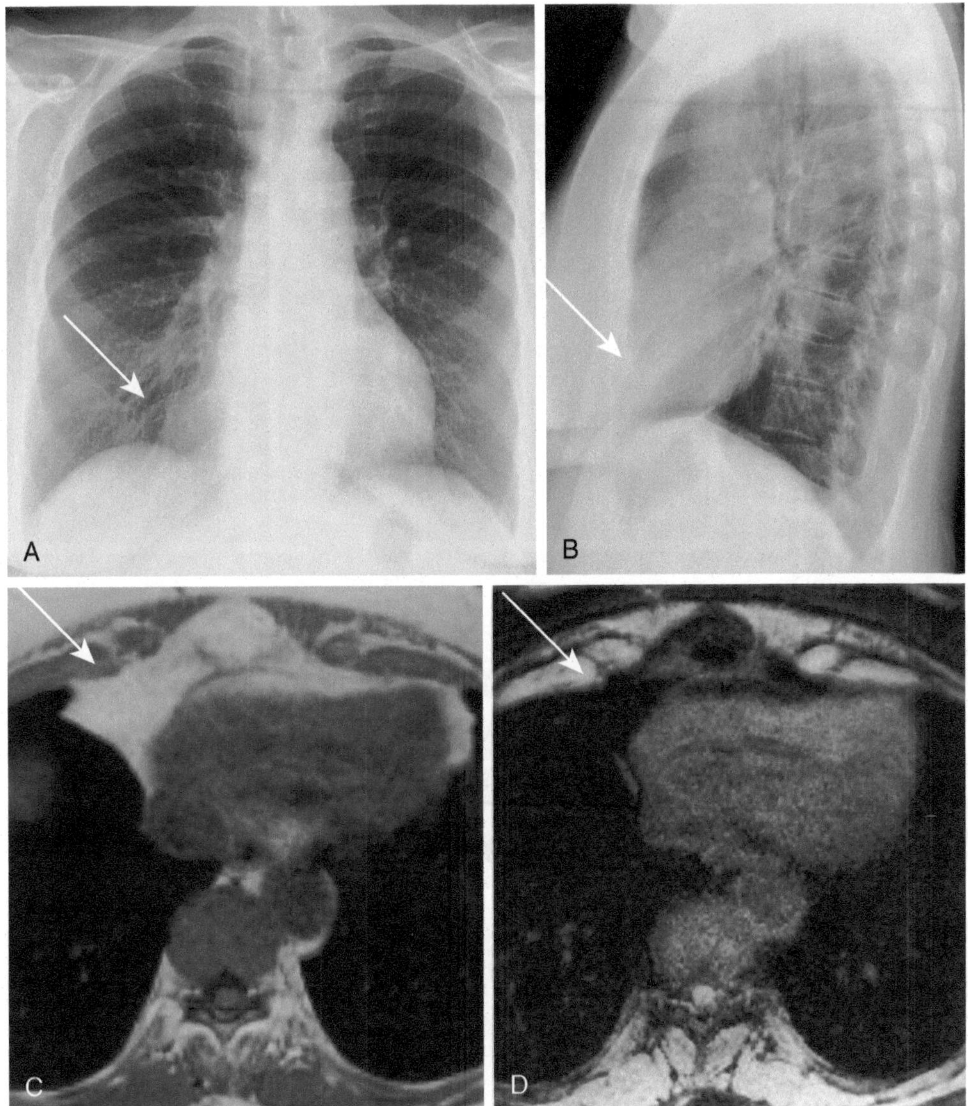

FIGURE 3.9 Detection of macroscopic or gross fat: pericardial fat pad. Indeterminate right cardiophrenic mass on chest radiography in a young woman with concerns about ionizing radiation. Posteroanterior **(A)** and lateral **(B)** chest radiographs show a rounded right cardiophrenic angle mass *(arrows)*, the differential diagnosis of which includes pericardial fat pad, pericardial cyst, lymphoma, and a low-lying thymic neoplasm. **C,** Axial in-phase T1-weighted magnetic resonance image shows this lesion *(arrow)* to be homogeneously isointense to subcutaneous fat. **D,** Axial precontrast three-dimensional ultrafast gradient echo, fat-saturated T1-weighted image shows complete signal dropout or fat saturation of this mass *(arrow)*, proving it to represent a pericardial fat pad, without subjecting the patient to ionizing radiation or unneeded intravenous contrast.

microscopic fat. *Mature* teratomas or dermoid cysts often contain microscopic fat, macroscopic fat, or both; however, their morphology and heterogeneity of signal are quite different from normal thymus and thymic hyperplasia, so these entities are unlikely to be mistaken for one another (see Fig. 5.18).

Chemical Shift Ratio Region-of-Interest Placement and Calculation

To obtain an accurate chemical shift ratio, proper region-of-interest (ROI) placement is critical. ROIs of the same size and shape must be placed over the *same* area of thymic tissue and paraspinal muscle on the same slice (table position) of the in-phase and the out-of-phase chemical shift MR series, avoiding the black lines or chemical shift artifact ("India ink artifact") at the interface between fat and water-containing soft tissue (Fig. 3.12; see also Fig. 5.8). It is best to place ROIs on the thymus and paraspinal muscle on the opposed-phase image first, avoiding the black lines of chemical shift artifact, and then base the in-phase ROI position on the opposed-phase ROI location. If the paraspinal muscle is of heterogeneous signal, usually secondary to partial fatty replacement or atrophy, the ROI should instead be placed on another more homogeneous,

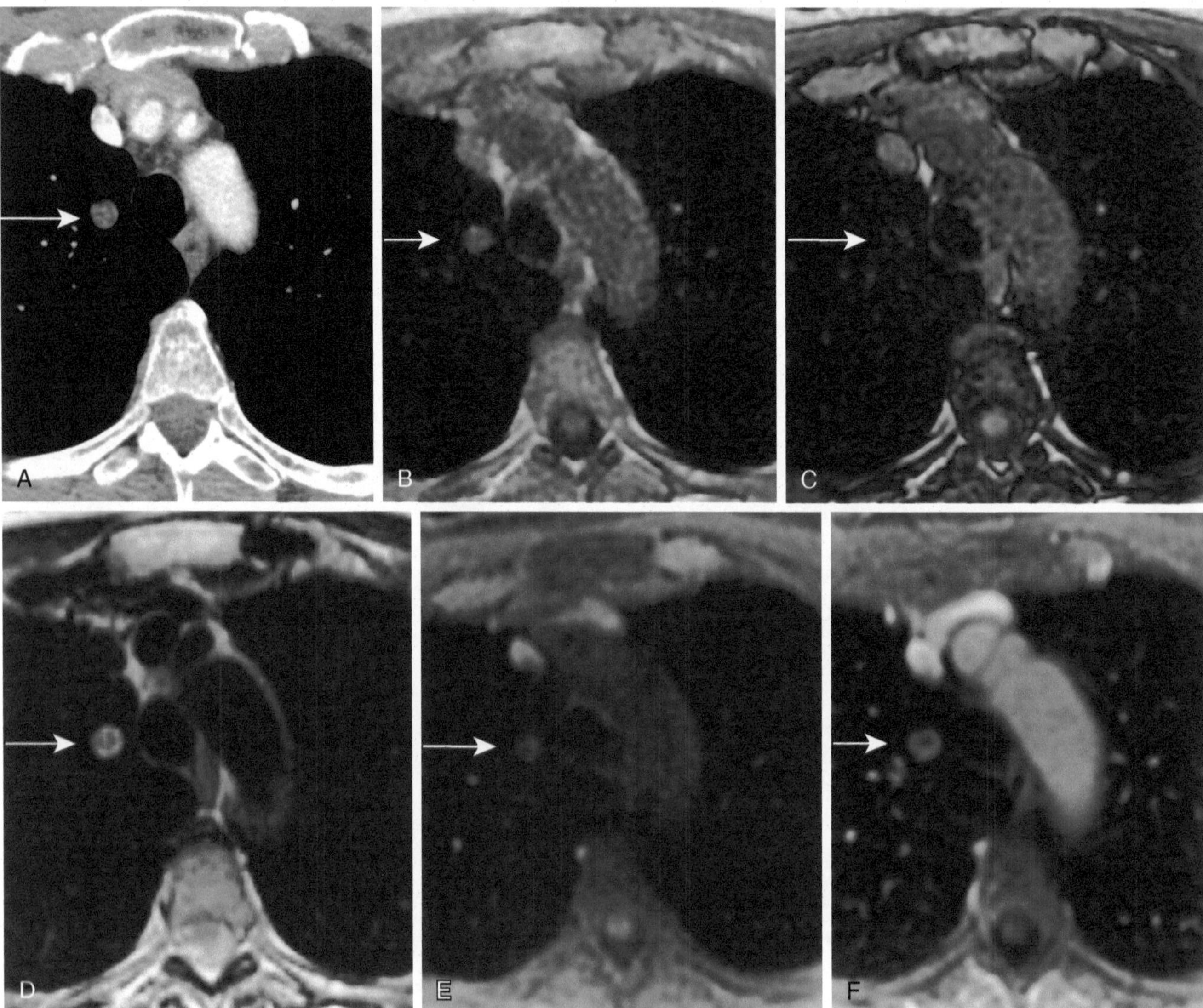

FIGURE 3.10 Detection of microscopic fat: microscopic fat–containing pulmonary hamartoma. **A,** Axial computed tomography scan shows an indeterminate 1-cm right upper lobe pulmonary nodule *(arrow)* with a very broad differential diagnosis. It is unclear whether the punctate low-attenuation foci within this nodule represent image noise or macroscopic fat. **B,** Axial in-phase T1-weighted magnetic resonance image reveals the lesion *(arrow)* to be of intermediate T1 signal and therefore not macroscopically fatty. **C,** Axial opposed-phase T1-weighted image reveals near-complete signal dropout of the nodule *(arrow)*, proving the presence of microscopic fat and that this nodule likely represents a pulmonary hamartoma. It cannot represent a benign inflammatory nodule, a lung cancer, or most metastases because of this microscopic fatty content. Its solitary nature and upper lobe location separately decrease the likelihood of a metastasis. **D,** Axial cardiac-gated double inversion recovery T2-weighted, Pre **(E)** and postcontrast **(F)** ultrafast three-dimensional gradient echo, fat-saturated T1-weighted images show additional characteristics of this hamartoma *(arrows)*, including its T2-hyperintensity, with an even more T2-hyperintense rim, its halo-like enhancement, and relative lack of internal enhancement.

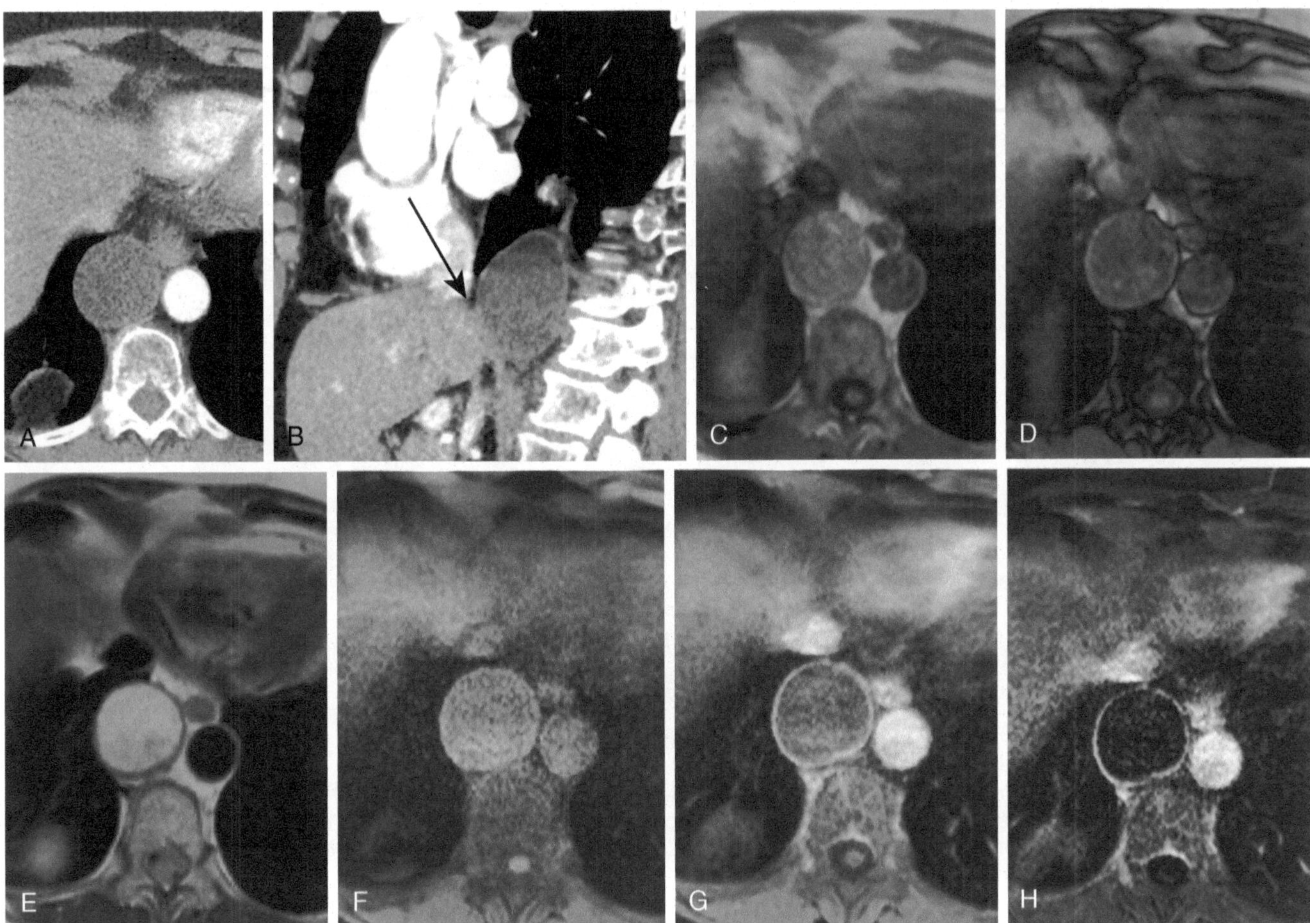

FIGURE 3.11 Detection of microscopic fat and value of subtraction imaging for intrinsically T1-hyperintense lesions: thoracic duct cyst. Axial **(A)** and sagittal **(B)** computed tomography images show a vertically oriented, ovoid, water attenuation visceral mediastinal mass extending inferiorly into the right retrocrural space, with no ancillary findings. The differential diagnosis includes foregut duplication cyst, mesothelial cyst, lymphangioma, thoracic duct cyst, and cystic neoplasm (*black arrow* points to the diaphragm). In- **(C)** and out-of-phase **(D)** T1-weighted magnetic resonance images (MRIs) reveal T1-hyperintensity to muscle and a reduction in signal of the fluid content on the opposed-phase image, particularly within the anterior half of the cystic lesion and to a lesser degree posteriorly, indicating the presence of microscopic fat. **E,** Axial cardiac-gated double-inversion recovery T2-weighted image. Pre- **(F)** and postcontrast **(G)** ultrafast three-dimensional gradient echo, fat-saturated T1-weighted. **H,** Postcontrast, postprocessed subtracted MR images confirm the absence of lesion complexity (no internal septations, wall irregularity, or nodularity). Only the thin, smooth wall of this lesion enhances. The fluid–fluid level in this cyst reflects the differential density of cystic content, most likely secondary to fattier fluid nondependently. The finding of microscopic fat within a unilocular cystic lesion in this location is diagnostic of a thoracic duct cyst.

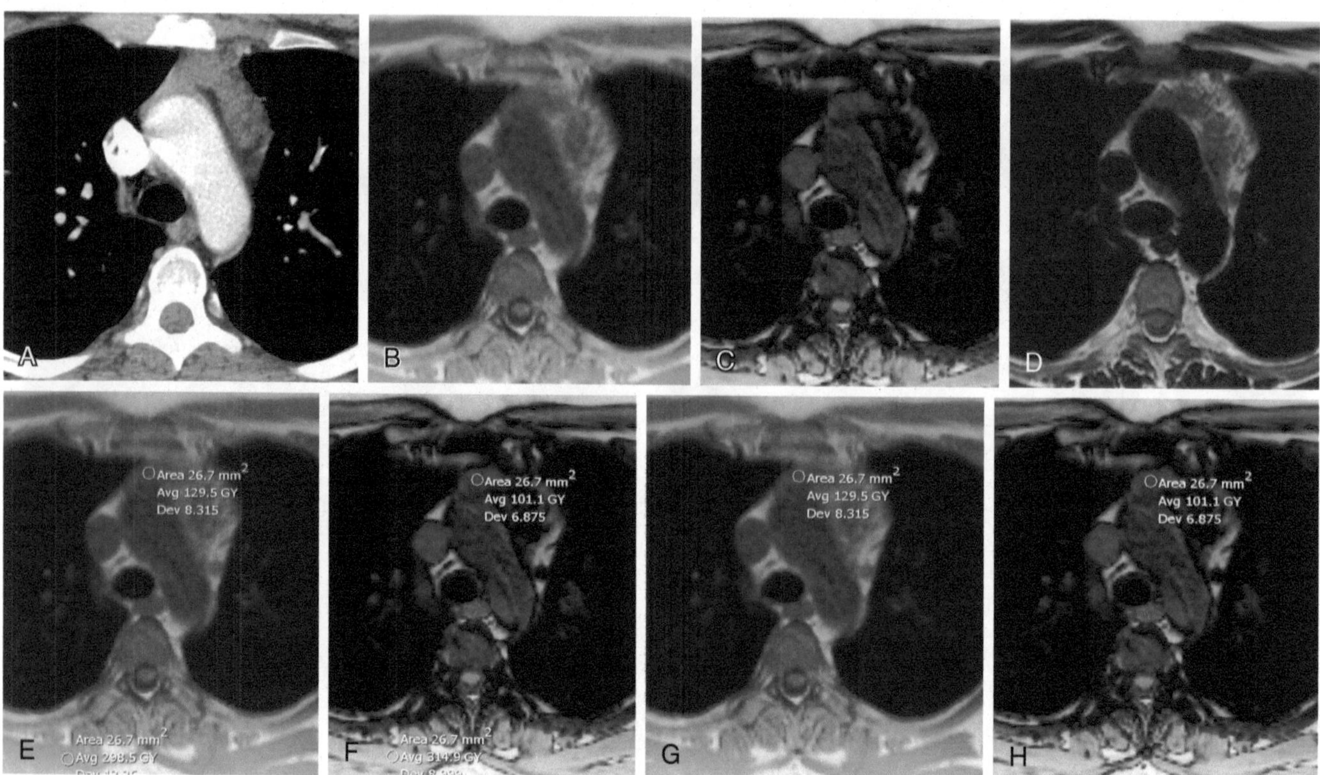

FIGURE 3.12 Region of interest (ROI) placement for chemical shift ratio (CSR) and signal intensity index (SII) calculation and detection of microscopic fat: thymic hyperplasia with nonevenly distributed fatty intercalation. **A,** Axial computed tomography scan reveals borderline excess thymic tissue for age in the thymic bed of this 29-year-old woman (measuring 1.8 cm in maximal thymic lobar thickness), with macroscopic fatty intercalation (or "marbling") of the left thymic bed tissue and with a homogeneous soft tissue attenuation, mass-like appearance in the right thymic bed. In- **(B)** and opposed-phase **(C)** gradient echo T1-weighted magnetic resonance images (MRIs) reveal complete suppression of the nongrossly fatty components of the left thymic bed tissue, indicating the presence of microscopic fat and therefore mildly hyperplastic thymic tissue. The right thymic bed tissue again appears slightly rounded and does not suppress appreciably when viewed with the naked eye. **(D)** Axial cardiac-gated double inversion recovery T2-weighted image shows this tissue to be T2-hyperintense to muscle. **E** and **F,** Proper placement of ROI circles over the least suppressing thymic tissue and paraspinal muscle, avoiding areas of overt chemical shift artifact and macroscopic fat (India ink artifact), yields a CSR of ([101.1/314.9] ÷ [129.5/298.5]) = 0.32/0.43 = 0.7. A CSR of 0.7 or less is compatible with thymic hyperplasia rather than thymic tumor or lymphoma. **G** and **H,** Proper placement of ROIs for calculation of the SII, a quicker, less error-prone method of microscopic fat detection that can be used, provided the in- and opposed-phase MRIs are acquired with dual echo technique. SII = ([129.5 − 101.1]/129.5) × 100 = 22% signal dropout, also compatible with thymic hyperplasia rather than tumor (SII > 9% indicates the presence of microscopic fat).

robust, nonatrophic muscle on the same image. The CSR calculation is as follows.

$$\text{CSR} = \frac{\text{OP SI thymus}/\text{OP SI paraspinal muscle}}{\text{IP SI thymus}/\text{IP SI paraspinal muscle}}$$

IP = in-phase OP = opposed-phase SI = signal intensity as measured by ROI

CSR ≤ 0.7 = normal or hyperplastic thymus

CSR ≥ 1.0 = tumor in *most but not all* cases

CSRs of 0.8 and 0.9 = indeterminate

If results are indeterminate, consider a 3- to 6-month follow-up MRI, depending on the level of suspicion. If the thymic tissue exhibits suspicious morphology, signal, or appearance, then diagnostic intervention should be considered.

Signal Intensity Index Region-of-Interest Placement and Calculation

Use of the SII to detect microscopic fat requires *dual-echo* acquisition of the in- and out-of-phase MR images to ensure that the imaging parameters and table position are identical in all respects except the time to echo (TE). It uses the same method of ROI placement on thymic tissue as the CSR but does not require paraspinal muscle ROI placement. It therefore represents a shorter, simpler, and potentially more accurate method of microscopic fat detection than CSR acquisition.

$$\text{SII} = [(\text{IP SI thymus} - \text{OP SI thymus})/\text{IP SI thymus}] \times 100$$

SII > 9% = normal thymus or thymic hyperplasia rather than tumor

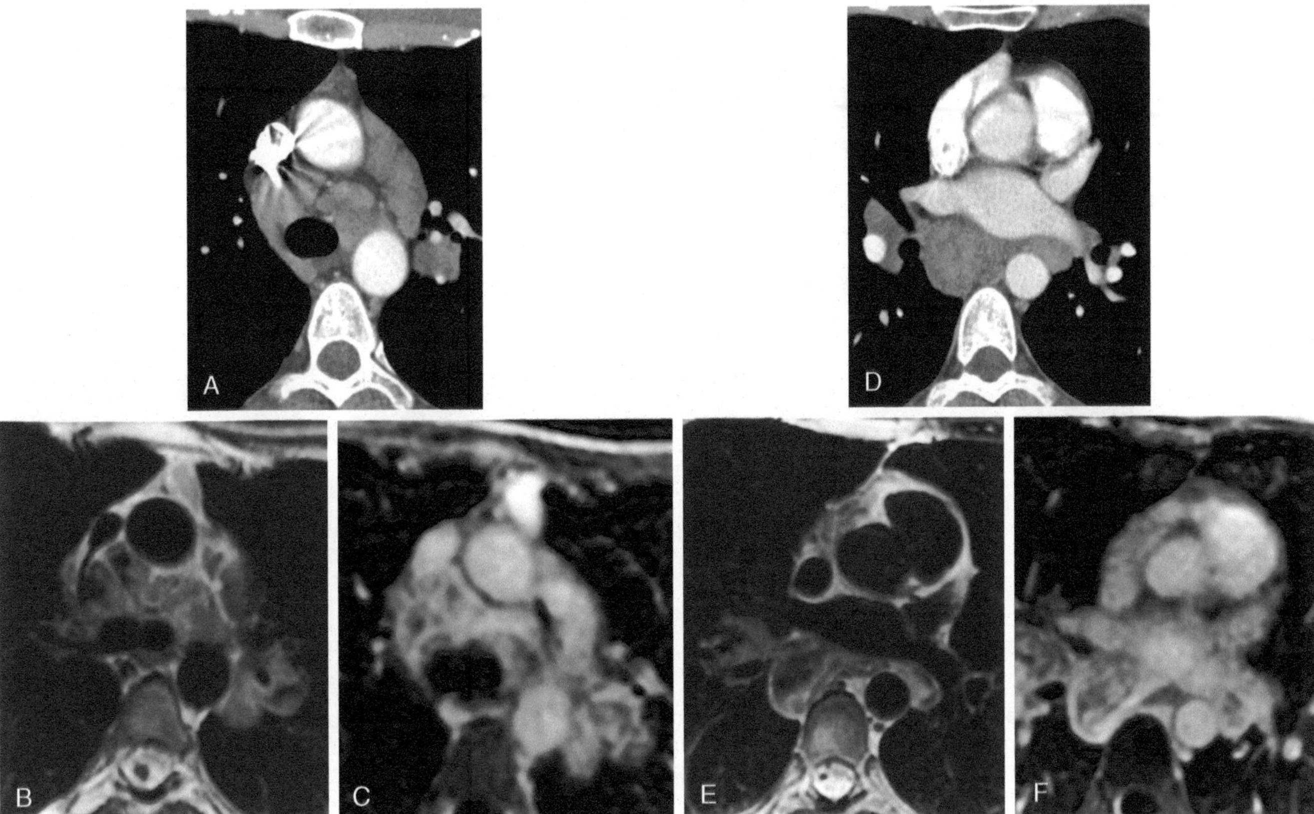

FIGURE 3.13 Dark lymph node sign: sarcoidosis-related lymphadenopathy. Matched axial computed tomography (CT) scan **(A)**, cardiac-gated (CG) double-inversion recovery (IR) T2-weighted magnetic resonance imaging (MRI) **(B)**, and postcontrast ultrafast three-dimensional (3D) gradient echo, fat-saturated T1-weighted **(C)** MR images reveal bilateral hilar and mediastinal lymphadenopathy, without calcification, on the CT. The patchy low T2 signal and relative hypoenhancement or nonenhancement of portions of these lymph nodes on the MRI likely indicate the presence of fibrotic material and strongly favor granulomatous lymph nodes over non-treated lymphoma. After treatment, lymphoma can also exhibit areas of fibrosis, reduced T2 signal, and reduced enhancement. Matched axial CT **(D)**, CG double IR T2-weighted MR **(E)**, and postcontrast ultrafast 3D gradient echo, fat-saturated T1-weighted **(F)** MRI images of the same patient at a lower level, with similar manifestations also compatible with granulomatous lymph nodes and sarcoidosis. It is important to be aware that not all granulomatous or sarcoid-containing lymph nodes will show this sign (they may not yet be hyalinized/fibrosed).

Lymph Nodes, Acute Inflammatory Lesions, and Most Thoracic Neoplasms

Nongranulomatous lymph nodes, acute inflammatory lesions, and most neoplasms in the thorax (including lymphoma) are generally of intermediate T1 signal (unless necrotic, in which case they may contain T1-hypointense signal) and T2-hyperintense to muscle because of their water content. Fibromatosis and fibrosarcomas are also T2-hyperintense to muscle, despite the word root "fibro-" in their name, because of higher water content than purely fibrous tissue. Sarcoid-related lymph nodes and possibly other granulomatous lymph nodes represent an exception in that these lymph nodes, even when noncalcified, *may* demonstrate areas of low T2 signal that are believed to reflect internal fibrous content—the "dark lymph node sign" (Fig. 3.13). Lymph nodes involved by sarcoid may show relative hypoenhancement in the fibrotic areas as well. The "dark lymph node sign" on MRI can be helpful for the diagnostic dilemma that sometimes arises on CT between sarcoidosis and lymphoma and can prevent invasive diagnostic procedures, provided ample clinical correlation and follow-up are performed.

Fibrous Tissue

Because of the densely packed collagen bundles and relative absence of water in fibrous tissue, fibrous tissue is T2-hypointense, unlike most acute inflammatory tissue and virtually all neoplasms except solitary fibrous tumors (see Fig. 7.19), fibromas, and leiomyomas (Fig. 3.14; see also Fig. 5.29). The T2 signal of the tightly packed collagen bundles of fibrous tissue would be expected to be lower than that of the tightly packed smooth muscle cells of leiomyomas because of negligible water content in the former. Chronic fibrosing mediastinitis is therefore T2-hypointense (see Fig. 5.42), unlike acute mediastinitis, an acute inflammatory condition that is T2-hyperintense. Although untreated lymphoma is T2-hyperintense to muscle, successfully treated lymphoma exhibits low T2 signal secondary to fibrosis. Densely fibrotic material restricts diffusion and therefore demonstrates low signal on an

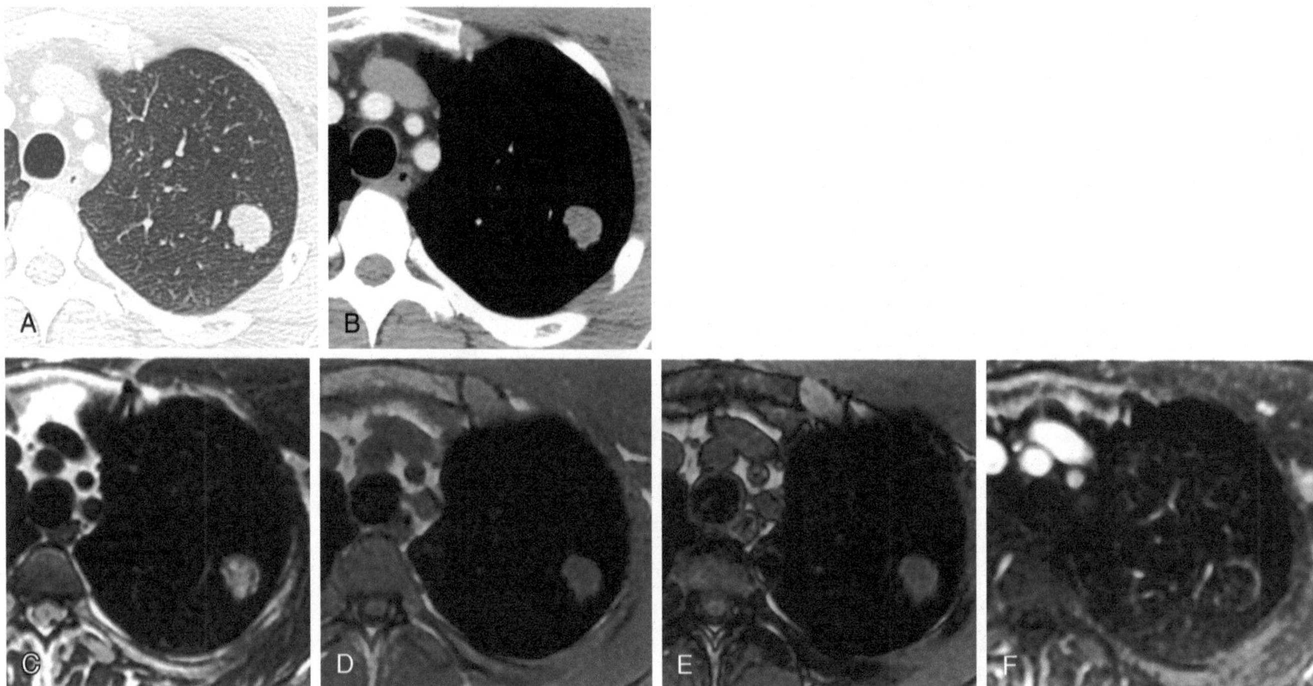

FIGURE 3.14 Cartilage detection by magnetic resonance imaging (MRI). Indeterminate pulmonary nodule on computed tomography (CT) scan; chondroid hamartoma on MRI. Axial **(A)** lung and soft tissue **(B)** windows of CT show a 2-cm, well-circumscribed, lobulated left upper lobe nodule without gross fat or calcification. **C,** Axial cardiac-gated double-inversion recovery T2-weighted MRI reveals heterogeneous, overall T2-hyperintense signal, with foci of particularly T2-hyperintense signal, along with a multicameral appearance of this nodule. Axial in- **(D)** and out-of-phase **(E)** gradient echo T1-weighted images reveal no suppression on the opposed-phase image to indicate the presence of microscopic fat. **F,** Postprocessed, postcontrast ultrafast three-dimensional gradient echo T1-weighted subtraction image again shows the multicameral appearance of this nodule, with rim and internal septal enhancement and little to no enhancement of the interstices of the lesion. This lobulated, well-circumscribed multicameral nodule, with internal T2-hyperintense, nonenhancing interstices, is characteristic of a cartilage-containing or chondroid hamartoma.

apparent diffusion coefficient (ADC) map; however, somewhat atypically, it will also exhibit low signal on diffusion-weighted imaging (DWI) because if its tightly woven collagen bundles, lack of water, and therefore lack of T2 signal. Box 3.1 lists thoracic lesions that are typically T2-hypointense. The finding of T2-hypointensity in a thoracic lesion can substantially narrow the differential diagnosis and often, in conjunction with other findings, yield a specific diagnosis.

BOX 3.1 T2-Hypointense Thoracic Lesions

Chronic fibrosing mediastinitis
Sarcoidosis-related lymphadenopathy (both noncalcified and calcified, but not always)
Hemosiderin or concentrated iron in wall or interior of a hemorrhagic cyst
Treated lymphoma
Solitary fibrous tumor
Mediastinal leiomyoma

Cartilage

Because cartilage has high water content and its main substance is avascular, the MR signal of cartilage within cartilaginous lesions in the thorax, including chondroid hamartomas (see Fig. 3.14) and chondrosarcomas (see Fig. 7.49), resembles that of water—T1-hypointense, T2-hyperintense, and hypoenhancing or nonenhancing. The scaffold or supporting tissues of these lesions do enhance, however.

Smooth Muscle

The well-known T2-hypointensity of classic, nondegenerated uterine leiomyomas is due to their composition primarily of smooth muscle. Leiomyomas, including those in the chest, whether esophageal or rarely arising elsewhere in the mediastinum, are T2-hypointense, relative to most lymph nodes and masses, and T2-isointense or slightly hyperintense to skeletal muscle because of the closely bundled, actin- and myosin-containing smooth muscle cells, which secrete a collagenous extracellular matrix with relatively little extracellular water content compared with that of lymph nodes and most inflammatory and neoplastic lesions (Fig. 3.15; see also Fig. 5.29). It is important to be aware, however, that as leiomyomas grow, they can outstrip their blood supply and degenerate, yielding cystic change and hemorrhage that may increase the T2 (and T1) signal intensity within them.

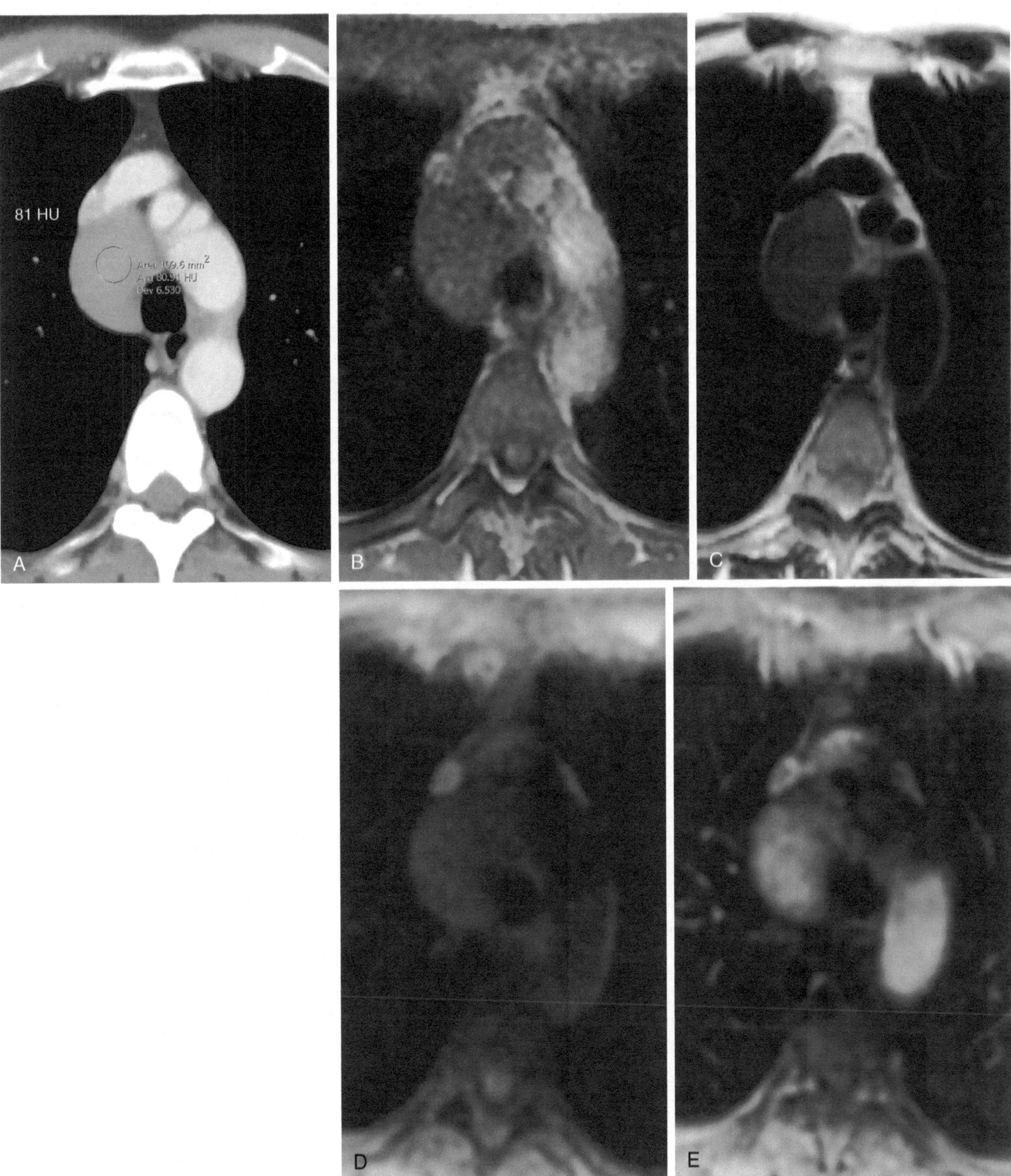

FIGURE 3.15 Diagnostic value of low T2 signal: indeterminate right paratracheal mass on computed tomography (CT) scan, suggested by magnetic resonance imaging (MRI) to represent a leiomyoma or solitary fibrous tumor of the mediastinum. **A,** Axial CT with intravenous contrast shows an 81 HU, well-circumscribed right paratracheal mass of similar morphology to the right paratracheal bronchogenic cyst in Fig. 3.6. Bronchogenic cysts can exhibit attenuation values up to 100 HU because of fluid containing calcium oxalate, hemorrhage, or proteinaceous material. **B,** Axial in-phase T1-weighted image, **C,** Cardiac-gated double-inversion recovery T2-weighted, and **(D)** Pre- and **(E)** Post-contrast ultrafast three-dimensional gradient echo, fat-saturated T1-weighted MR images reveal the mass to be of intermediate T1 signal, homogeneous and relatively low T2 signal (compared with lymph nodes, most tumors, and bronchogenic cysts) and to enhance homogeneously. The solid, low–T2 signal nature of this mass strongly favors a rare mediastinal leiomyoma or mediastinal solitary fibrous tumor as the diagnosis. Surgical pathology confirmed it to represent a leiomyoma. (Copyright permission obtained from Elsevier, License #4035340649175.)

Lesion Vascularity

The nonfibrous components of all solid, cellular lesions enhance on MRI. For example, normal, nonpathologic lymph nodes enhance vividly on MRI. Even muscle mildly enhances on MRI, although this normal muscle enhancement is best appreciated on postcontrast, postprocessed subtraction images. Enhancement of normal lymph nodes is generally not appreciable by CT because of the lower soft tissue contrast of this imaging modality. Hyperenhancing lymph nodes such as those of Castleman disease are recognizable on CT, however (see Fig. 5.22). As on CT, but exaggeratedly so on MRI, carcinoid tumors (Fig. 3.16), whether based in the mediastinum or lung, and paragangliomas hyperenhance. Soft tissue hemangiomas in the thorax exhibit a variable appearance, whether round, lobulated, or "crumbly" in morphology, with variable enhancement. They tend to be of intermediate T1-intensity and T2-hyperintense and may exhibit similar enhancement patterns to their counterparts in the liver, whether uniformly enhancing or exhibiting discontinuous, peripheral nodular enhancement with partial or complete fill-in over time (Fig. 3.17). Dynamic contrast-enhanced (DCE) imaging has been shown to be helpful not only in detection of hemangiomas (see Fig. 3.17) but also in the distinction of low-risk thymomas (Fig. 3.18) from high-risk thymomas, thymic carcinoma (Fig. 3.19), and lymphoma and in the distinction of tumor thrombus from bland thrombus (Fig. 3.20).

Restricted Diffusion

The more restricted the diffusion of water molecules within a lesion, as detected by DWI, the more cellular, fibrous, or viscous the lesion is. The degree of diffusion weighting on MR correlates with the b value at which the images are acquired and increases with increasing b values. A range of 3 or more low to high b values are required to create an adequate ADC map.

Although DWI is T2-weighted, the higher the b value, the more diffusion weighting and the less the risk of misinterpreting a lesion as diffusion-restricted, when it is simply intrinsically T2-hyperintense. It is therefore important to be aware of the b values used to create the DWI undergoing interpretation—that is, the degree of diffusion weighting—so as not to confuse "T2 shine-through" for true restricted diffusion. Low b values in the 0 to 200 range indicate little diffusion weighting and are prone to T2 shine-through. High b values in the 600 to 1000 range are more diffusion-weighted, with decreased T2 shine-through. With the exception of fibrous tissue, whereas lesions with restricted diffusion will remain hyperintense with increasing b values, intrinsically T2-hyperintense lesions without restricted diffusion, but hyperintense at low b values (e.g., 0–200 range), because of T2 shine-through, decrease in signal at higher b values.

Neoplasms, viscous hematomas, and viscous abscesses all restrict the diffusion of water molecules and yield hyperintensity on DWI and hypointensity on the ADC map. Densely fibrous tissue is exceptional—because of its near-complete lack of water content and associated, very low T2 signal, it exhibits low diffusion-weighted signal at any b value (no T2 signal to "shine through") and low ADC values or hypointensity on the ADC map, not because of malignancy but because it essentially contains no water (see Fig. 5.42). In the context of *solid* neoplasms (areas of cystic change and necrosis excepted), the more hypercellular or malignant the lesion, the more restricted its diffusion, with higher diffusion-weighted signal on DWI and lower signal on the ADC map. For example, low-risk thymomas have higher ADC values than high-risk thymomas, thymic carcinoma, and lymphoma, with a proposed cutoff value of 1.25×10^{-3} mm^2/sec for distinguishing low- from high-risk thymic lesions (see Figs. 3.18 and 3.19).

Apparent diffusion coefficient values are obtained by ROI placement over the lesion on the ADC map image, dividing the mean ROI value by 1000, and then adding the following units or "suffix": $\times 10^{-3}$ mm^2/sec.

Concept of Matching Lesions

Because MR uses multiple pulse sequences, including forms of T1-weighted imaging, with or without fat suppression or fat saturation, and T2-weighted imaging, with and without fat saturation, DCE imaging, and DWI, to characterize a lesion, if two lesions in the same patient exhibit the same signal characteristics on multiple distinct pulse sequences, they are likely to be histopathologically identical (Figs. 3.21 and 3.22).

Lesion Measurement

It is best to measure lesions on the highest resolution, highest signal images of a given MR examination. For this reason, some of the best pulse sequences to use for lesion measurement include in-phase T1-weighted, electrocardiography (EKG)-gated double-inversion recovery (IR) T2-weighted or radially acquired, multishot fast spin-echo T2-weighted, and postcontrast three-dimensional (3D) ultrafast GRE fat-saturated T1-weighted sequences, but *only* if these pulse sequences are of high quality and the lesion is clearly depicted on the given image. If lesion margins are blurry for whatever reason, it is best to select a more optimal image of the lesion from another pulse sequence in that particular examination. It is preferable not to measure lesions on pulse sequences containing chemical shift or India ink artifact because the artifact often obscures the actual border of the lesion.

Detection of Pulmonary Nodules

Some pulse sequences are more sensitive than others for pulmonary nodule detection. All nodules greater than or equal to 8 to 10 mm are visible on MR, with optimal pulse sequence selection and performance. The sensitivity of MR for detection of nodules greater than or equal to 4 mm is 80% to 90%, provided the MR examination is optimal. Currently, one of the best pulse sequences for identification and measurement of pulmonary nodules is a postcontrast 3D-ultrafast GRE, fat-saturated T1-weighted sequence. Any other pulse sequence on the given examination that depicts the nodule margins clearly would also be a reasonable choice, including EKG-gated double IR T1-weighted and T2-weighted sequences. In general, in- and opposed-phase images, single-shot fast spin-echo (SSFSE) images, and

Text continued on p. 82

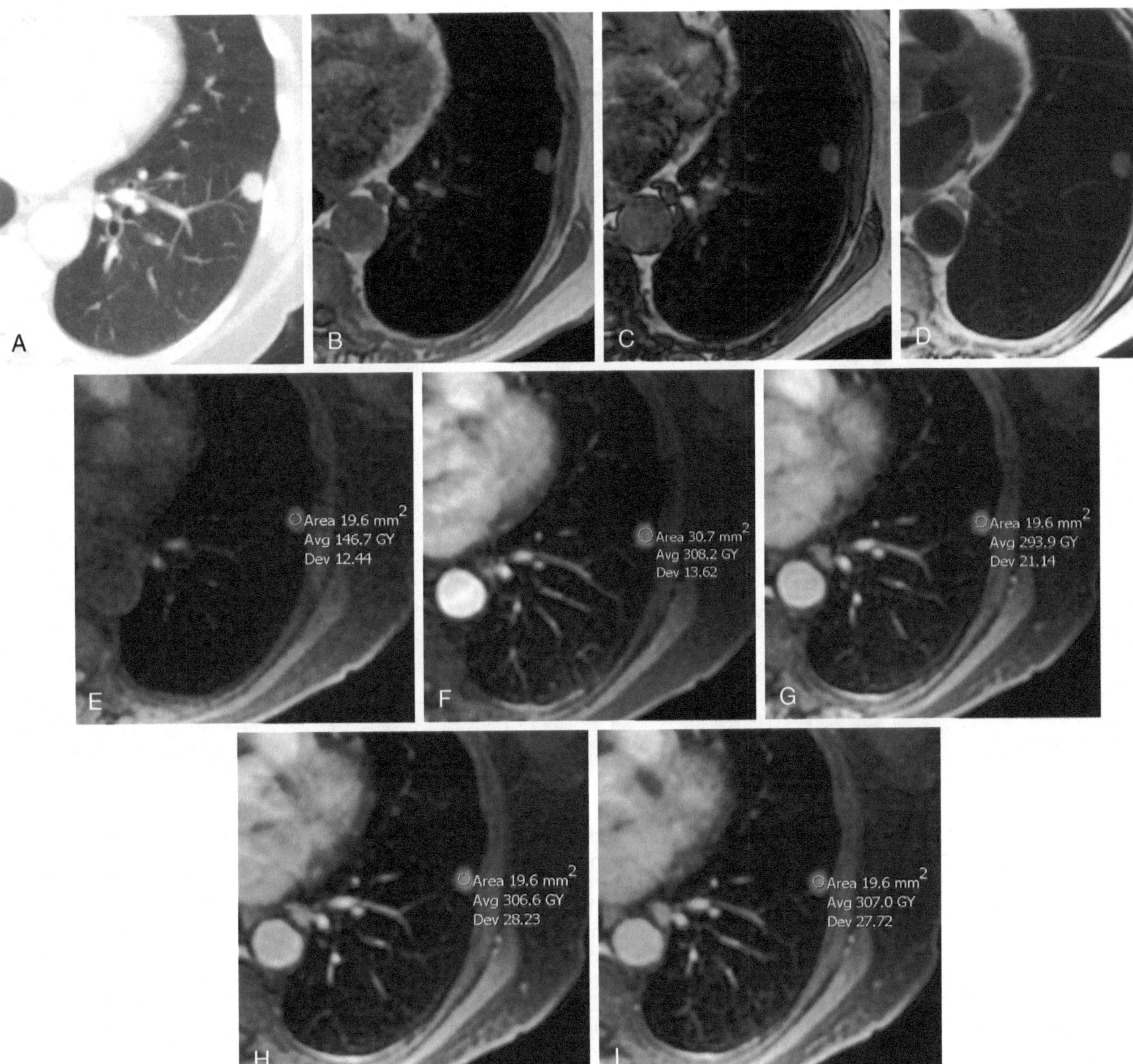

FIGURE 3.16 Diagnostic value of dynamic contrast-enhanced (DCE) magnetic resonance imaging (MRI), narrowing the differential diagnosis of an indeterminate pulmonary nodule on computed tomography (CT) scan: probable carcinoid tumor on MRI. **A,** Axial CT scan demonstrates a round, well-circumscribed, peripheral 1.4-cm pulmonary nodule in the left lower lobe. There was no macroscopic fat or calcification of this mass on the soft tissue windows (not shown). Axial in- **(B)** and opposed-phase **(C)** gradient echo T1-weighted MRIs reveal no isointensity to subcutaneous fat to indicate the presence of a macroscopic fat-containing hamartoma and no suppression of signal on the opposed-phase images, decreasing the likelihood of a microscopic fat-containing hamartoma. **D,** Axial cardiac-gated double inversion recovery T2-weighted image shows no multicameral appearance and no foci of bright T2 signal to raise the possibility of cartilaginous content. Precontrast **(E)** and postcontrast **(F–I)** ultrafast three-dimensional gradient echo, fat-saturated T1-weighted DCE images at 20 seconds **(F)**, 1 minute **(G)**, 3 minutes **(H)**, and 5 minutes **(I)** after intravenous gadolinium administration reveals strong, rapid time-to-peak enhancement at 1 minute and no significant washout over time: precontrast: 147, 20 seconds = 308, 1 minute = 294, 3 minutes = 307, 5 minutes = 307. This vigorous enhancement, without washout, and the well-circumscribed nature of this nodule somewhat favor carcinoid tumor over lung cancer. A non–fat-containing, noncartilaginous hamartoma and nonfibrotic, noncaseating granuloma are also in the differential diagnosis. CT-guided core biopsy and subsequent surgical pathology confirmed this nodule to be a carcinoid tumor.

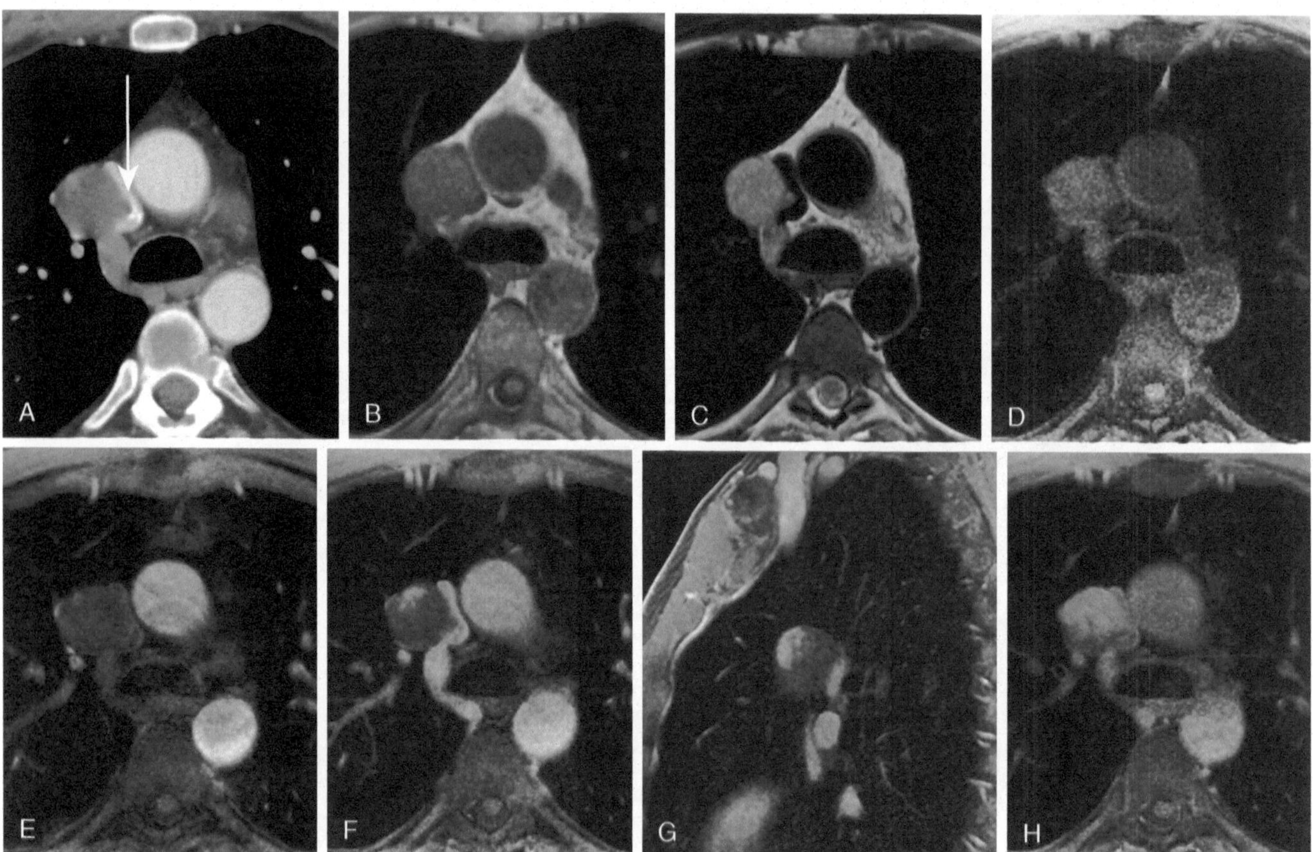

FIGURE 3.17 Diagnostic value of dynamic contrast-enhanced (DCE) magnetic resonance imaging (MRI). Indeterminate right visceral mediastinal mass protruding into the superior vena cava (SVC) on computed tomography (CT); hemangioma on MRI. **A,** Axial CT reveals a round, well-circumscribed mass compressing the SVC, with a focally protruding medial component *(arrow)* indenting or invading the SVC. The mass is of homogeneous attenuation, aside from a focal, hyperattenuating, right anterolateral, peripheral component. The differential diagnosis is broad. **B,** Axial in-phase gradient echo (GRE) T1-weighted image, **C,** Cardiac-gated double-inversion recovery T2-weighted image, and Precontrast **(D)** and postcontrast **(E–H)** ultrafast three-dimensional GRE fat-saturated, T1-weighted DCE MR images reveal this mass to be of intermediate T1 signal and homogeneously and markedly T2-hyperintense (isointense to cerebrospinal fluid) and to exhibit peripheral nodular enhancement with fill-in over time (**E,** 20 sec; **F,** 1 minute axial; **G,** 3 minutes sagittal; and **H,** 5 minutes axial postcontrast MR images). These findings are virtually pathognomonic for a hemangioma. Nevertheless, please note that hemangiomas may have variable appearance within the thorax.

FIGURE 3.18 Diagnostic value of dynamic contrast-enhanced (DCE) magnetic resonance MR imaging (MRI) and apparent diffusion coefficient (ADC) map: low-risk thymoma, temporal enhancement and ADC map characteristics. **A,** Axial computed tomography scan reveals a lobulated, off-midline, solitary soft tissue mass *(arrow)* in the right thymic bed, highly suggestive of a thymic neoplasm in this adult, although the differential diagnosis includes a hyperattenuating multilocular thymic cyst and, less likely, focal thymic hyperplasia. In- and opposed-phase images (not shown) showed no suppression on the opposed-phase images, making thymic hyperplasia even less likely. Precontrast **(B)** and postcontrast **(C–F)** ultrafast three-dimensional gradient echo, fat-saturated T1-weighted DCE MR images reveal rapid time-to-peak enhancement with washout over time with ROIs of (**B,** 92 precontrast; **C,** 181 at 20 seconds; **D,** 174 at 1 minute; **E,** 164 at 3 minutes; **F,** 153 at 5 minutes and **G,** An ADC value of 1.71×10^{-3} mm^2/sec. Given the proposed cutoff between low- and high-risk thymomas and thymic carcinoma of 1.25×10^{-3} mm^2/sec, this tumor's ADC value of 1.7 favors a low-risk thymoma. Its temporal enhancement pattern is also more typical of a low-risk thymoma. High-risk thymoma, thymic carcinoma, and lymphoma are reportedly more apt to gradually enhance over time, rather than enhance rapidly and partially wash out with time.

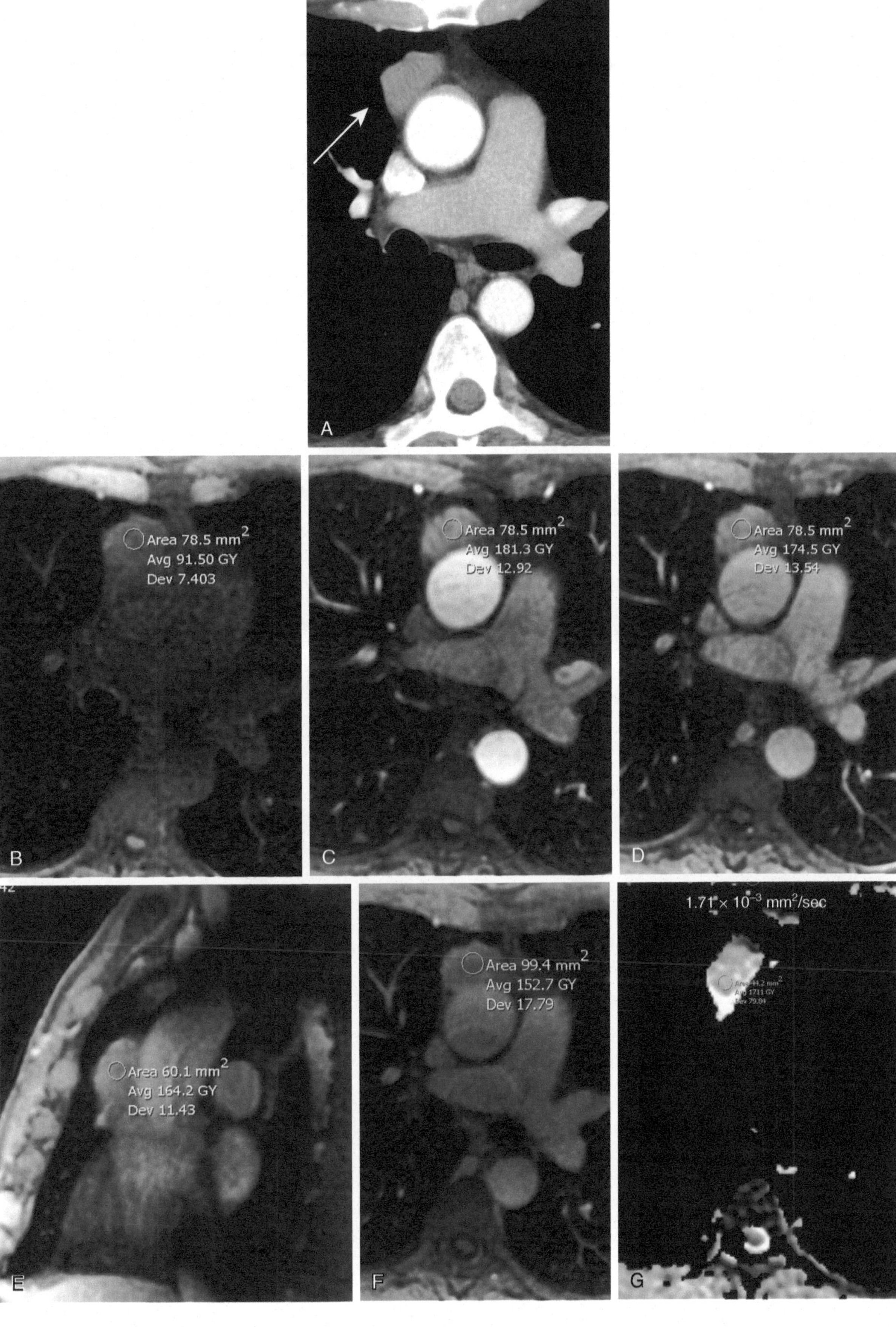
A
Area 78.5 mm2
Avg 91.50 GY
Dev 7.403
B
Area 78.5 mm2
Avg 181.3 GY
Dev 12.92
C
Area 78.5 mm2
Avg 174.5 GY
Dev 13.54
D
Area 60.1 mm2
Avg 164.2 GY
Dev 11.43
E
Area 99.4 mm2
Avg 152.7 GY
Dev 17.79
F
1.71 × 10−3 mm2/sec
G

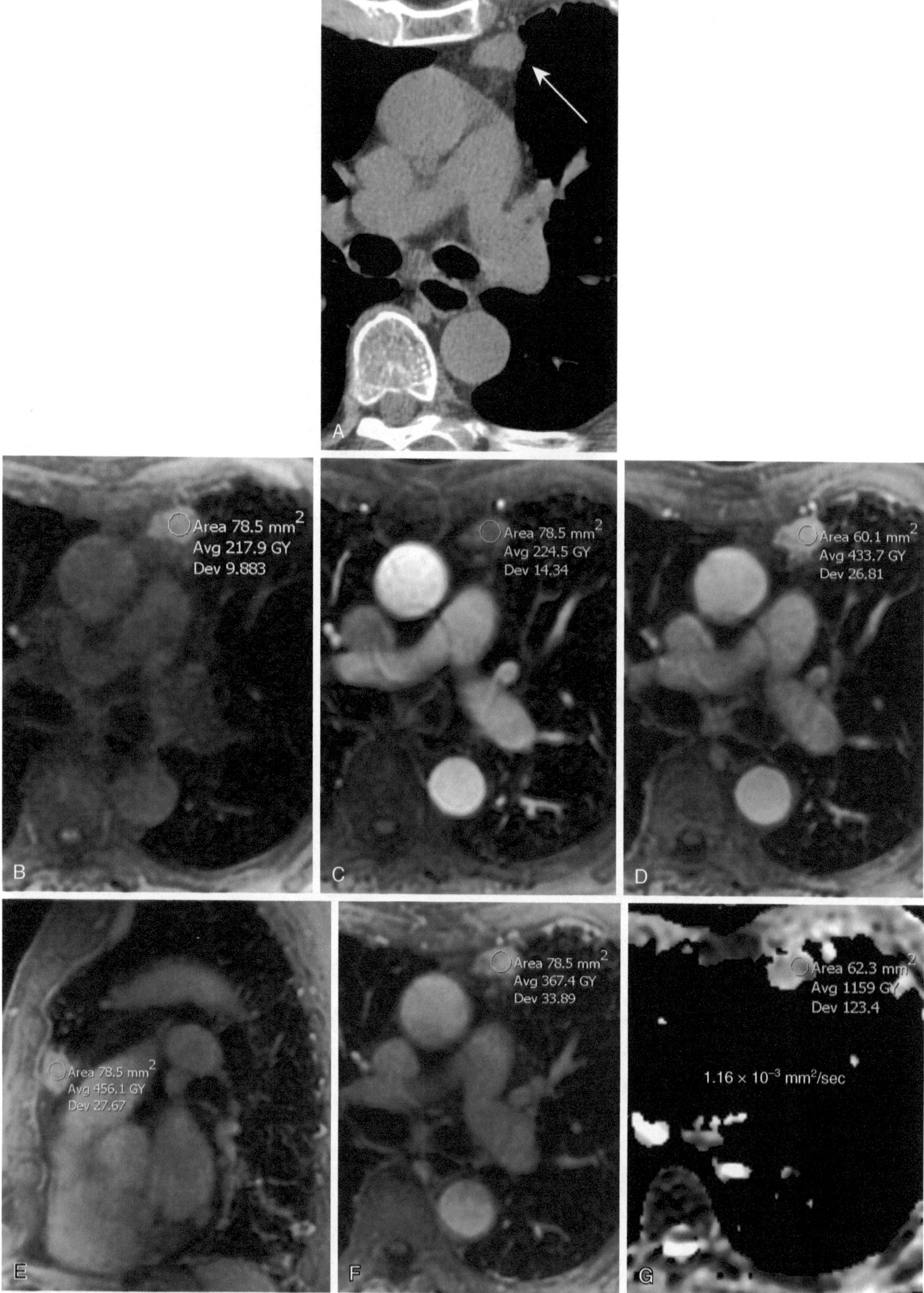

FIGURE 3.19 Diagnostic value of dynamic contrast-enhanced (DCE) magnetic resonance imaging (MRI) and apparent diffusion coefficient (ADC) map: thymic carcinoma—its typical temporal enhancement and ADC map characteristics. **A,** Axial computed tomography scan reveals an irregularly contoured, mildly lobulated, indeterminate mass *(arrow)* centered within the otherwise fatty thymic bed. Precontrast **(B)** and postcontrast **(C–F)** ultrafast three-dimensional gradient echo, fat-saturated T1-weighted DCE MR images reveal increasing enhancement out to 3 minutes in **E**, with some washout at 5 minutes in **F** (20 seconds = 224; 1 minute = 434; 3 minutes sagittal = 456; 5 minutes axial = 367). **G,** ADC map provides an ADC value of 1.16×10^{-3} mm^2/sec. This more sustained temporal enhancement, in combination with the low ADC value of 1.2, favors a high-risk thymoma or thymic carcinoma over low-risk thymoma. Surgical pathology confirmed thymic carcinoma.

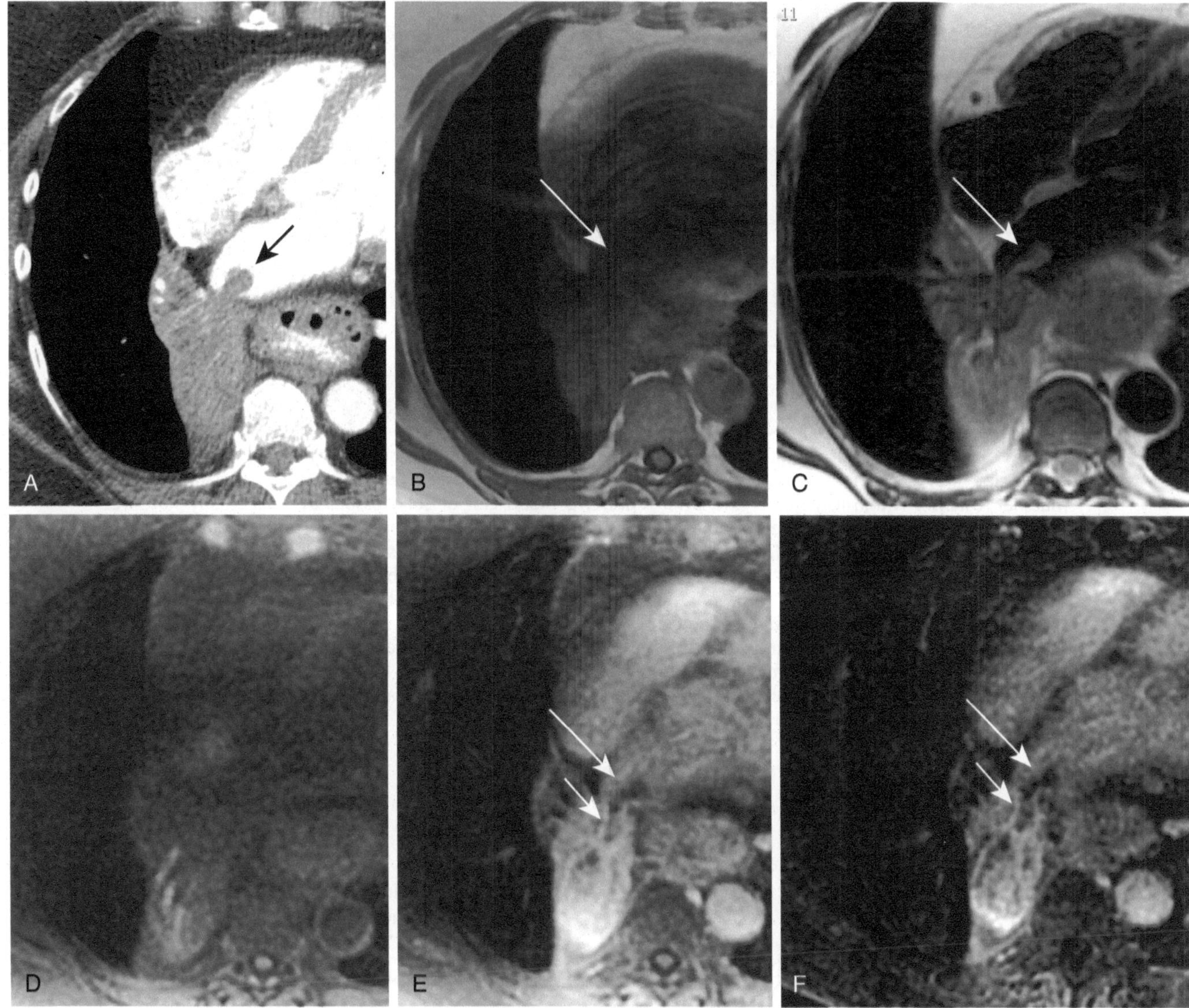

FIGURE 3.20 Bland thrombus versus tumor thrombus in the setting of invasive lung cancer. **A,** Axial computed tomography scan reveals a portion of the known, centrally obstructing right lower lobe mass to demonstrate contiguity with a polypoid mass in the left atrium *(black arrow)*. **B**. In-phase T1-weighted, **C,** Cardiac-gated double-inversion recovery T2-weighted, nongated precontrast **(D)** and postcontrast **(E)** ultrafast three-dimensional gradient echo, fat-saturated T1-weighted, and **F,** Postprocessed subtraction MR images reveal this polypoid lesion *(long arrow)* to be T1-isointense and T2-hyperintense and to exhibit no enhancement. Of note, the vermiform, serpentine structure arising from the tumor and filling the right inferior pulmonary vein does enhance *(short arrow)*, but the enhancement of this tissue ceases at the inferior pulmonary venous ostium or margin with the left atrium. Thus, this MRI shows not only enhancing tumor thrombus filling the right inferior pulmonary vein *(short arrow)*, but also nonenhancing, bland thrombus in the left atrium *(long arrow)*.

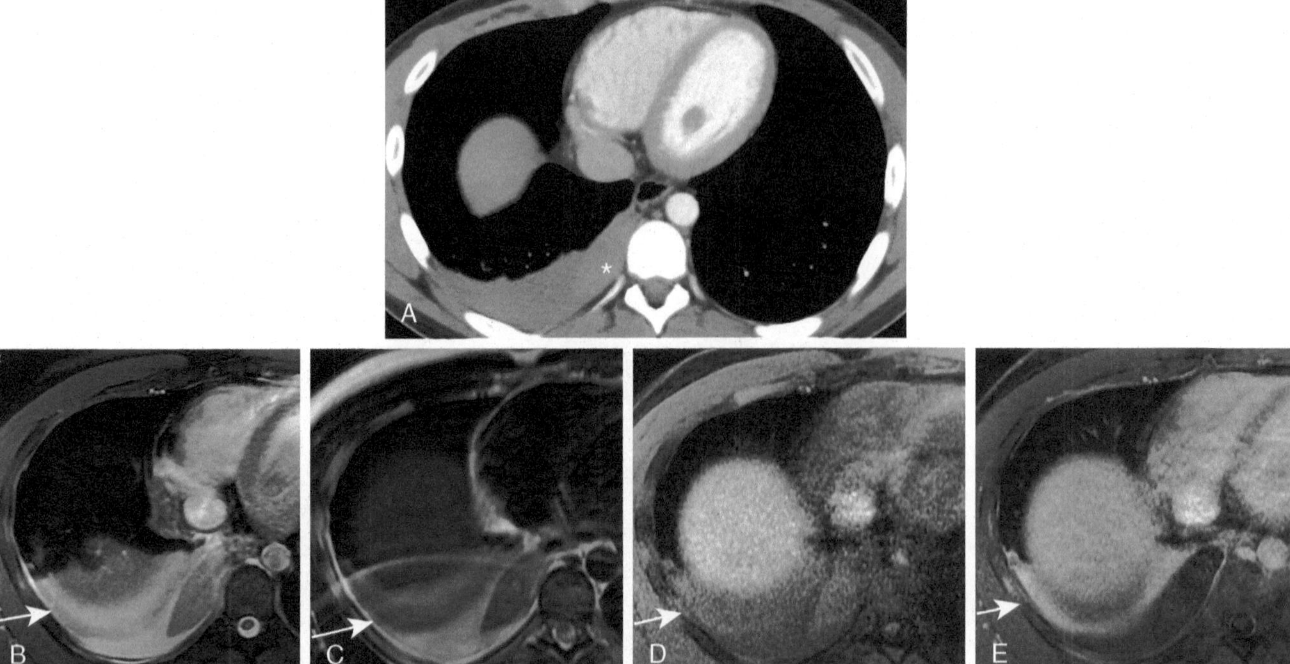

FIGURE 3.21 The concept of matching lesions: torsed, infarcted extralobar sequestration. **A,** Axial computed tomography (CT) scan shows a small, layering right pleural effusion containing medial, relatively hyperattenuating material *(asterisk)* within it, whether the latter represents blood clot or solid tissue. **B.** Axial steady-state free precession (SSFP), **C,** Cardiac-gated double-inversion recovery T2-weighted, and **D,** Precontrast ultrafast three-dimensional (3D) gradient echo (GRE), fat-saturated T1-weighted MR images show the indeterminate, relatively hyperattenuating material within the pleural fluid on CT to be well-circumscribed and lobar in morphology and to match the signal intensity of the adjacent, partially atelectatic right lower lobe *(arrow)* on all pulse sequences, strongly favoring it to be of the same tissue composition—lung. **E,** Postcontrast ultrafast 3D GRE, fat-saturated T1-weighted MRI shows, discordantly, that this mass situated within the pleural space does not enhance, unlike the adjacent atelectasis. No systemic arterial supply was identified at the time of interpretation. It was therefore deduced that this finding represented a torsed, infarcted extralobar sequestration, rather than a blood clot or neoplasm, with this diagnosis proven at surgical pathology.

steady-state free precession (SSFP) images are not as reliable for pulmonary nodule detection and measurement.

THORACIC MAGNETIC RESONANCE PROTOCOLING AND PERFORMANCE

Goals

The goal of thoracic MR protocol design and performance is to answer the clinical question with high-quality imaging in the shortest possible amount of time, using a minimum number of pulse sequences. Because of MR trade-offs between signal and noise, spatial resolution, slice thickness, matrix size, field of view, and acquisition time, it is often desirable to confine imaging exclusively to the area of interest, rather than imaging the entire thorax—in other words, to perform focused imaging exclusively of the lesion.

It is important to remember that the patient experience matters. Best-quality thoracic MRI currently requires breath-hold imaging for nearly all pulse sequences. Multiple serial breath-holds can fatigue both the patient and the technologist who is coaching the patient. Therefore, "positive energy" is required. A comfortable, well-coached, motivated patient who feels supported is more able to cooperate for the duration of the examination, facilitating higher quality motion-free diagnostic images.

Successful Breath-Hold Imaging

Although respiratory gating is a solid backup solution for patients who cannot breath-hold, it is imperfect, and breath-hold imaging remains a superior means of obtaining images free of respiratory motion. With appropriate coaching, virtually all patients sent for a thoracic MR, from preteen up through the mid-90s, are capable of successfully performing serial breath-holds in the 8- to 20-second range.

It is very helpful to inform the patient before he or she lies down on the MR table of the breath-hold instructions and the anticipated range of breath-hold length (8–20 seconds). It is also helpful to practice or do a "breath-hold" rehearsal with the patient. This rehearsal serves two purposes. First, the technologist can ascertain the patient's breath-hold capability and second, the technologist can ask and determine whether "single breathing" or "double breathing" (the latter formerly and inaccurately referred to as "hyperventilation") breath-hold commands will be

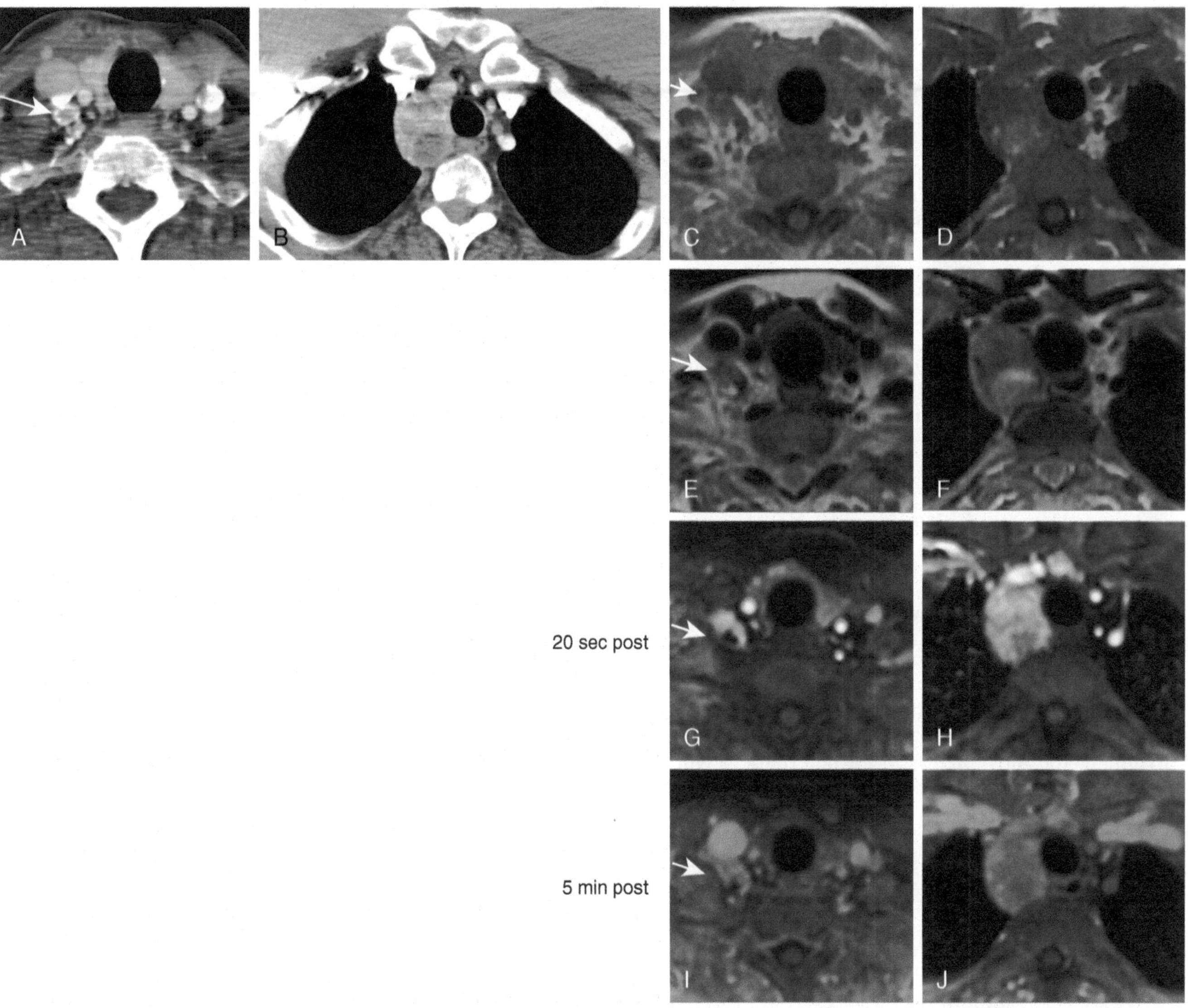

FIGURE 3.22 The concept of matching lesions: metastatic thyroid carcinoma. Axial computed tomography scan at the level of the thyroid gland **(A)** and at the level of the highest right paratracheal space **(B)** show a small subcentimeter heterogeneously enhancing right level IV cervical lymph node *(arrow)* (initially missed) and a heterogeneously enhancing, partially cystic right paratracheal mass. There was no continuity of this mass with the thyroid gland. Paired neck base and upper thoracic In-phase gradient echo (GRE) T1-weighted (**C** and **D**), cardiac-gated double-inversion recovery T2-weighted, (**E** and **F**), 20 seconds postcontrast (**G** and **H**), and 5 minutes postcontrast (**I** and **J**) ultrafast three-dimensional GRE, fat-saturated T1-weighted dynamic contrast-enhanced (DCE) MR images reveal the signal characteristics of the right level IV cervical lymph node *(arrow)*, portions of the thyroid gland, and the solid component of the right paratracheal mass to be identical on all pulse sequences, including the DCE images, virtually proving these three entities to be identical histopathologically. This finding of shared signal characteristics led to a proposed MR diagnosis of metastatic thyroid carcinoma, which was proven upon endobronchial ultrasound-guided fine-needle aspiration of the fluid from the cyst (cyst fluid thyroglobulin = 911) and subsequent surgical resection with lymph node dissection.

more effective. Third, this practice has the effect of preparing and motivating the patient, creating an atmosphere of teamwork between the patient and technologist. The term "single breathing" refers to the breath-hold instruction: "Take a breath in and hold it." The term "double breathing" refers to the breath-hold instruction: "Take a breath in, blow it out, take another breath in, and hold it."

If breath-hold difficulty is anticipated, 2 L of MR-compatible nasal cannula oxygen (NCO_2) can be administered to enhance breath-hold capability. If the patient is on more than 2 L of NCO_2 as an inpatient or outpatient, then at least as much NCO_2, if not more, should be administered during the MRI.

It is critical that the technologist not press the MR image acquisition start button until the patient's chest or abdomen has stopped moving, or even the best of breath-hold efforts will be compromised by respiratory motion at the start of the image acquisition. Breath-hold success is also enhanced by keeping all breath-holds under 20 seconds in length

BOX 3.2 Keys to Successful Breath-Hold Imaging

Coach patient before he or she lies down on table.
Ascertain patient preference regarding double versus single breathing.
Inform of breath-hold length before each pulse sequence.
Keep all breath-holds at 20 seconds or less.
Consider 2 L of NCO_2 (or more if on home O_2 or hospital O_2).
Keep examination as short as possible, avoiding unnecessary pulse sequences.

and adjusting pulse sequence parameters and imaging stack size if needed to keep the image acquisition time short. It is also helpful to inform the patient of the anticipated breath-hold length before each pulse sequence or image acquisition. The basic concept is that a patient who knows what to expect will perform better. Better patient performance means less respiratory motion and higher quality, more diagnostic images for interpretation. Keys to successful breath-hold imaging are summarized in Box 3.2.

Free-Breathing Techniques

With ultrafast imaging techniques such as SSFP, high-quality images of the thorax can be obtained in the coronal and sagittal planes when the patient is breathing quietly and evenly. This technique can be especially useful for observation of diaphragmatic movement and for determining whether mediastinal tumors are, for example, fixed to the chest wall.

The Magnetic Resonance Sniff Test

Although respiratory triggering and breath-hold imaging techniques essentially freeze diaphragmatic motion, free-breathing SSFP MRI exhibits diaphragmatic movement in real-time, much like fluoroscopy. It can therefore be used to assess diaphragmatic movement and rule out diaphragmatic paralysis. In addition to free-breathing instructions, a patient can be coached (outside of the magnet first) and then instructed (while in the magnet) to take several sniffs during a fixed coronal slice SSFP MR acquisition at the level of the diaphragmatic dome. Paradoxical movement of the diaphragm can be easily recognized and recorded for posterity (Fig. 3.23 and Video 3.1).

Cardiac Gating

There are two forms of cardiac gating—EKG gating and peripheral gating. EKG gating requires placement of MR-compatible EKG leads on the patient's chest before scanning, and peripheral gating solely requires photosensor placement on a patient's finger for peripheral pulse detection. EKG gating is superior to peripheral gating because it more precisely times the image acquisition to a specific phase of the cardiac cycle. Although EKG gating creates beautiful high signal-to-noise ratio (SNR), high-resolution images uncompromised by cardiac motion and pulsatility artifact, the trade-off for this substantial benefit is time.

Slice Thickness Selection

With currently available MR hardware and software, slice thicknesses greater than or equal to 4 mm are currently preferable for most pulse sequences in the chest to ensure good signal-to-noise ratio (SNR). An exception is breath-hold 3D ultrafast gradient-echo T1-weighted images, which can be of sufficient image quality in the thorax at 3-mm slice thickness.

BASIC THORACIC MAGNETIC RESONANCE PROTOCOL

Characterizing most lesions by MR generally requires some form of T1-weighted imaging, some form of T2-weighted imaging, and pre- and postcontrast imaging, all of which can be performed with and without fat saturation, depending on the lesion under investigation. DWI and short tau inversion recovery (STIR) imaging may provide additional useful information but are not always required.

To counter the challenges related to cardiorespiratory motion in the thorax, a high-quality thoracic MR protocol consists of a combination of standard breath-hold and respiratory-triggered MRI pulse sequences commonly used for abdominal MRI and one or more breath-hold EKG-gated pulse sequences commonly used for cardiac MRI. These standard pulse sequences are available in all standard MR software packages and have been optimized by vendor for a given MR scanner. Vendor-optimized pulse sequences can be adapted and optimized further by on-site testing on a volunteer.

Commonly used body MRI pulse sequences adopted from abdominal MRI include breath-hold, noncardiac-gated or noncinematic SSFP and SSFSE localizer(s); breath-hold dual-echo in- and out-of-phase GRE T1-weighted sequence; respiratory-triggered, radially acquired, multishot fast spin-echo T2-weighted images without and with fat saturation; breath-hold ultrafast pre- and postcontrast, 3D ultrafast GRE; DCE fat-saturated T1-weighted imaging; and breath-hold or respiratory-triggered DWI with ADC mapping. Commonly used pulse sequences adopted from cardiac MRI include the noncinematic version of SSFP ultrafast bright blood GRE pulse sequence and a breath-hold, EKG-gated IR recovery T2-weighted sequence. The latter is required if elimination of all cardiovascular motion artifact is desired. Table 3.2 illustrates these commonly used thoracic MR pulse sequences, their purposes, and their acquisition times.

When building an MR protocol on a magnet, working with the preoptimized pulse sequences built into the magnet by the given MR vendor is a good starting point. It is nevertheless important to test all pulse sequences, short of IV contrast administration (gadolinium), on a volunteer to optimize them further.

Rationale for Each Pulse Sequence in the Protocol

T1-Weighted Imaging

Breath-hold dual-echo in- and out-of-phase GRE or chemical shift MRI is quite useful as the primary T1-weighted sequence of a thoracic MR protocol because, depending on the scanner, MR software, and size of the patient, this rapid T1-weighted sequence can image half of or even an entire chest in a single 20-second breath-hold and yield sufficient image quality, free of respiratory motion. A breath-hold EKG-gated double IR T1-weighted pulse sequence (which is much slower, acquiring two slices,

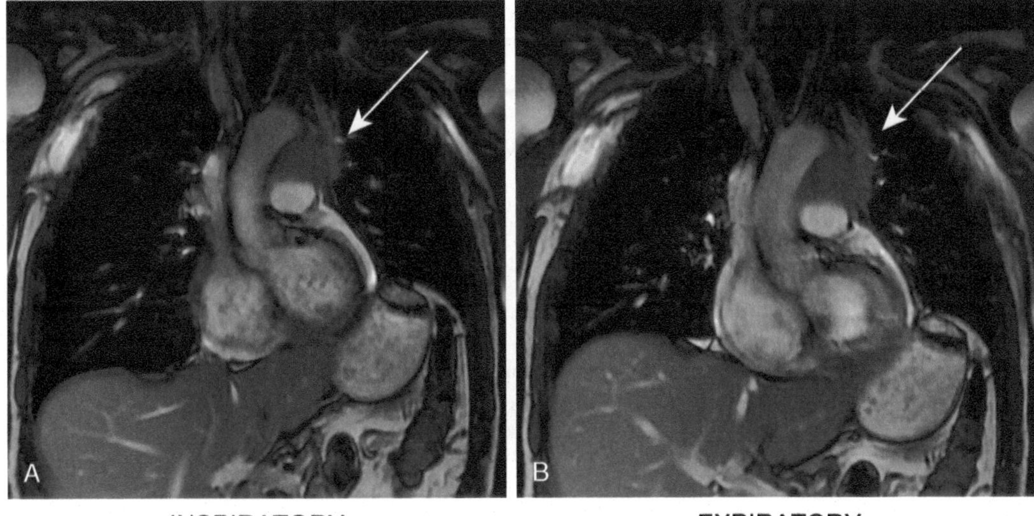

FIGURE 3.23 Free-breathing magnetic resonance imaging (MRI): MR sniff test in setting of a left prevascular mass. Coronal inspiratory **(A)** and expiratory **(B)**, free-breathing steady-state free precession (SSFP) MR images show an intermediate signal left prevascular mass *(arrows)* involving the anteroposterior window, along which the phrenic nerve passes. On inspiration, the right hemidiaphragm moves down appropriately; on expiration, the right hemidiaphragm moves up appropriately, but the left hemidiaphragm moves paradoxically—upward during inspiration and downward during expiration. See the video of cinematic free-breathing SSFP MRIs during sniffing. This constellation of findings is compatible with left hemidiaphragmatic paralysis secondary to involvement of or impingement on the left phrenic nerve by a tumor.

rather than the entire area of interest, in 20 seconds) is almost never needed for clarification, despite the latter's higher signal and lack of both pulsatility artifact and respiratory motion artifact. Chemical shift T1-weighted MRI provides the added bonus of microscopic fat detection, unlike double IR T1-weighted imaging (a spin-echo sequence) and 3D ultrafast GRE T1-weighted imaging, the latter two of which are solely acquired at one TE. On 1.5-Tesla (1.5T) magnets, this chemical shift MR image acquisition can be performed with two-dimensional (2D) technique. On a 3T magnet, chemical shift MRI should only be performed with 3D technique to ensure correct TE selection. This 3D in- and out-of-phase technique provides four types of images in a single 20-second breath-hold: in-phase T1-weighted, opposed-phase T1-weighted, "water only," and "fat only" images. The latter two image types are mathematically calculated and created to yield images with virtually perfect, homogeneous fat saturation (the "water only" images) and water saturation (the "fat only" images).

T2-Weighted Imaging

Best-quality T2-weighted images are best acquired with a breath-hold EKG-gated double IR T2-weighted pulse sequence; however, given that this pulse sequence acquires one slice per 20-second breath-hold instead of many slices, this sequence should be reserved for *no more than 10 to 14 slices of coverage*, whatever the specified slice thickness. More than 10 to 14 serial 20-second breath-holds for one pulse sequence are a "big ask" in terms of patient and technologist effort and image acquisition time. For larger lesions, it is better to perform T2-weighted imaging with respiratory-triggered, radially acquired multishot fast spin-echo T2-weighted images. The radial acquisition and the respiratory triggering of this pulse sequence substantially reduce cardiorespiratory motion artifact, making it "next best" to breath-hold EKG-gated double IR T2-weighted imaging. If there are any focal areas in need of higher signal, higher resolution, motion-free images for diagnostic clarification, breath-hold EKG-gated double IR T2-weighted imaging could be performed over this smaller area. A sample thoracic MR protocol, including optional or supplemental pulse sequences, is provided in Table 3.2.

Dynamic Contrast-Enhanced Imaging

Dynamic contrast-enhanced imaging is helpful to assess the pattern and rate of enhancement and can help differentiate one lesion from another. DCE imaging takes the guesswork out of postcontrast imaging timing, offering multiple snapshots of a lesion as it enhances over time. Whichever imaging planes are desired postcontrast must be performed precontrast to enable visual and occasionally quantitative assessment of change in signal upon contrast administration and to enable postprocessed subtraction. Postprocessed subtraction is critical for ascertaining subtle enhancement, particularly for ascertaining enhancement of intrinsically T1-hyperintense lesions (Figs. 3.4, 3.5, and 3.11). With increased use of DCE imaging in the thorax, other distinguishing features of lesions may be found.

Optional Pulse Sequences

Diffusion-weighted imaging is optional and should be reserved for situations in which further lesion characterization is needed beyond that already achieved with dual-echo T1-weighted, T2-weighted, and fat-saturated DCE MRI—for

TABLE 3.2 Basic Thoracic Magnetic Resonance Imaging Protocol for Focused Imaging*†

Pulse Sequence	Rationale	Acquisition Time‡
BH three-plane localizer	Standard three-plane localizer	15 sec
BH axial SSFP localizers	Rapid white blood GRE technique, water-weighted; good overview	8–10 sec per pulse sequence
BH coronal single-shot fast spin-echo, T2-weighted	Rapid black blood T2-weighted spin-echo technique; good overview; fair signal; somewhat noisy	20 sec per pulse sequence
BH axial dual echo in- and out-of-phase ultrafast GRE T1-weighted	Rapid in- and opposed-phase GRE chemical shift MR technique for rapid, adequate SNR, T1-weighted image acquisition and detection of microscopic fat	20 sec per pulse sequence
BH axial EKG-gated double IR, T2-weighted	Slow, high SNR, black blood T2-weighted technique; freezes cardiac motion; eliminates pulsatility artifact	20 sec per *slice*
BH pre- and postcontrast 3D-ultrafast GRE fat-saturated T1-weighted at 20 sec, 1, 3, and 5 min,§ with automatic postprocessed subtraction (different orthogonal plane at 3 min)	Rapid pre- and post-DCE imaging; postprocessed subtraction helpful for detecting subtle enhancement and particularly helpful when lesions are intrinsically T1-hyperintense	20 sec per pulse sequence
Optional BH or RTr DWI with ADC	Detection of restricted diffusion, which can indicate hypercellularity or viscous fluid	RTr: 3–4 min BH: 20 sec
Optional BH STIR	Most sensitive for detection of marrow edema	20 sec
Optional RTr radially acquired multishot fast spin-echo, T2-weighted	Next best T2-weighted sequence; motion-corrected, high-SNR T2-weighted sequence to EKG-gated double IR T2-weighted imaging	2–5 min, depending on breadth of coverage
Optional 3D ultrafast GRE, T1-weighted (without fat saturation)	Rapid means of acquiring adequate SNR T1-weighted images but does not detect microscopic fat	20 sec
Optional EKG-gated double IR, T1-weighted	Slow, high SNR T1-weighted sequence; use only if in- and out-of-phase T1-weighted images or 3D ultrafast GRE T1-weighted images are inadequate	10 sec per slice or 20 sec per 2 slices

*For full chest imaging, the electrocardiography-gated double-inversion recovery (IR) T2-weighted sequences should be replaced with the respiratory-triggered (RTr) radially acquired multishot fast spin-echo T2-weighted sequence, so as not to subject the patient to 30 to 40 sequential 20-second breath-holds. *Double IR T2-weighted imaging should be reserved for problem solving over a limited area.* A basic rule of thumb is to avoid acquiring more than 10-14 double IR T2-weighted slices.
†Abbreviated thoracic magnetic resonance (MR) protocol for noninvasive lesions.
‡Typical acquisition time; however, this can vary as a function of MR hardware and software, desired imaging coverage, slice thickness, and so on.
§Whichever orthogonal planes are desired postcontrast must be performed precontrast.
ADC, Apparent diffusion coefficient; *BH,* breath-hold; *DCE,* dynamic contrast enhanced; *DWI,* diffusion-weighted imaging; *EKG,* electrocardiography; *GRE,* gradient echo; *SNR,* signal-to-noise ratio; *SSFP,* steady-state free precession; *STIR,* short tau inversion recovery; *3D,* three-dimensional.

example, as an adjunct to weigh a differential diagnosis toward benignity or malignancy and to provide supplemental information if intravenous contrast is contraindicated. Breath-hold or respiratory-triggered STIR imaging can be reserved for situations in which higher sensitivity is needed for bone marrow edema detection. EKG-gated double IR T1-weighted imaging can be reserved for the rare situation in which ultrafast dual-echo GRE T1-weighted imaging is inadequate.

SUGGESTED READINGS

Abdel Razek AA, Khairy M, Nada N. Diffusion-weighted MR imaging in thymic epithelial tumors: correlation with World Health Organization classification and clinical staging. *Radiology*. 2014;268-275.

Ackman JB. A practical guide to nonvascular thoracic magnetic resonance imaging. *J Thorac Imaging*. 2014;29(1):17-29.

Ackman JB. MR imaging of mediastinal masses. *Magn Reson Imaging Clin N Am*. 2015;23(2):141-164.

Ackman JB, Gaissert HA, Lanuti M, et al. Impact of nonvascular thoracic MR imaging on the clinical decision making of thoracic surgeons: a 2-year prospective study. *Radiology*. 2016;280(2):464-474.

Ackman JB, Verzosa S, Kovach AE, et al. High rate of unnecessary thymectomy and its cause. Can computed tomography distinguish thymoma, lymphoma, thymic hyperplasia, and thymic cysts? *Eur J Radiol*. 2015;84(3):524-533.

Biederer J, Mirsadraee S, Beer M, et al. MRI of the lung (3/3)-current applications and future perspectives. *Insights Imaging*. 2012;3(4):373-386.

Biederer J, Schoene A, Freitag S, et al. Simulated pulmonary nodules implanted in a dedicated porcine chest phantom: sensitivity of MR imaging for detection. *Radiology*. 2003;227:475-483.

Chung JH, Cox CW, Forssen AV, et al. The dark lymph node sign on magnetic resonance imaging: a novel finding in patients with sarcoidosis. *J Thorac Imaging*. 29(2):125-129.

Huang SY, Seethamraju RT, Patel P, et al. 2015 Body MR imaging: artifacts, k-space, and solutions. *Radiographics*. 2014;35:1439-1460.

Inaoka T, Takahashi K, Mineta M, et al. Thymic hyperplasia and thymus gland tumors: differentiation with chemical shift MR imaging. *Radiology*. 2007;243(3):869-876.

Khashper A, Addley HC, Abourokbah N, et al. T2-hypointense adnexal lesions: an imaging algorithm. *Radiographics*. 2012;32(4):1047-1064.

Kurihara Y, Matsuoka S, Yamashiro T, et al. MRI of pulmonary nodules. *AJR Am J Roentgenol*. 2014;202(3):W210-W216.

Levesque MH, Aisagbonhi O, Digumarthy S, et al. Primary paratracheal leiomyoma: Increased preoperative diagnostic specificity with magnetic resonance imaging. *Ann Thorac Surg*. 2016;102(2):e151-e154.

McDonald RJ, McDonald JS, Kallmes DF, et al. Intracranial gadolinium deposition after contrast-enhanced MR imaging. *Radiology*. 2015;275(3):772-782.

Ohno Y, Hatabu H, Takenaka D, et al. Solitary pulmonary nodules: potential role of dynamic MR imaging in management initial experience. *Radiology*. 2002;224(2):503-511.

Ohno Y, Koyama H, Yoshikawa T, et al. Pulmonary magnetic resonance imaging for airway diseases. *J Thorac Imaging*. 2011;26(4):301-316.

Porter ME, Teisberg EO. *Redefining Health Care. Creating Value-Based Competition on Results*. Boston: Harvard Business School Press; 2006.

Priola AM, Priola SM, Ciccone G, et al. Differentiation of rebound and lymphoid thymic hyperplasia from anterior mediastinal tumors with dual-echo chemical-shift MR imaging in adulthood: reliability of the chemical-shift ratio and signal intensity index. *Radiology*. 2015;274(1):238-249.

Puderbach M, Eichinger M. The role of advanced imaging techniques in cystic fibrosis follow-up: is there a place for MRI? *Pediatr Radiol*. 2010;40(6):844-849.

Rholl KS, Levitt RG, Glazer HS. Magnetic resonance imaging of fibrosing mediastinitis. *AJR Am J Roentgenol*. 1985;145(2):255–259.

Riddell AM, Hillier J, Brown G, et al. Potential of surface-coil MRI for staging of esophageal cancer. *AJR Am J Roentgenol*. 2006;187(5):1280–1287.

Sakai S, Murayama S, Soeda H, et al. Differential diagnosis between thymoma and non-thymoma by dynamic MR imaging. *Acta Radiol*. 2002;42(3):262–268.

Siegelman ES, Outwater EK. Tissue characterization in the female pelvis by means of MR imaging. *Radiology*. 1999;212(1):5–18.

Westbrook C, Roth CK, Talbot J. *MRI in Practice*. 4th ed. Chichester, West Sussex, UK: Wiley-Blackwell; 2011.

Wu JS, Hochman MG. Soft tissue tumors and tumorlike lesions: A systematic imaging approach. *Radiology*. 2009;253(2):297–316.

Chapter 4

PET-CT and PET-MRI: Technique, Pitfalls, and Findings

Bojan Kovacina and Subba R. Digumarthy

INTRODUCTION

Positron emission tomography (PET) has become an important imaging tool in thoracic oncology over the past 10 to 20 years. It has proven its usefulness in the diagnosis of malignancies, initial staging, assessing response to treatment, and posttreatment monitoring for recurrence. Integration of PET with computed tomography (CT) initially and magnetic resonance (MR) lately has further improved its diagnostic accuracy, which has made it an invaluable factor in clinical decision making at tumor boards and interdisciplinary rounds. Although thoracic PET-CT and PET/MR have mainly been used for staging of non-small cell lung cancer (NSCLC) and lymphoma, their use has increasingly been broadened to many nononcologic conditions in the thorax as well, such as infectious and inflammatory processes.

TECHNIQUE

PET imaging is based on a radionuclide whose decay produces positrons, which themselves emit 511-MeV photons when they encounter electrons. These emitted photons are subsequently captured by detectors in the PET machine. The most commonly used radionuclide in PET imaging is ^{18}F because of its most convenient half-life (110 minutes). Uptake of a radionuclide by the body is usually achieved by coupling of ^{18}F with a biologically active molecule, most commonly glucose. A newly formed 2-deoxy-2-fluoro-D-glucose (^{18}F-FDG) is transported into cells with membrane transporters and becomes intracellularly trapped after it is phosphorylated. Consequential accumulation of ^{18}F-FDG in these cells is detected on PET images. This mechanism of ^{18}F-FDG metabolism is particularly of benefit in oncology because malignant cancer cells have greater energy requirements than adjacent normal tissue and almost uniquely use glucose as their energy source. The degree of ^{18}F-FDG uptake in one specific region may be visually assessed or quantified with the standardized uptake value (SUV). SUV is a ratio between the amount of uptake in a tissue per unit of volume and a normalizing factor. An SUV of 2.5 is usually considered as a differentiating value between a pathologic process and normal uptake, but there can be significant overlap between benign and malignant lesions. It is more practical to subjectively assess the ^{18}F-FDG uptake in thoracic lesions by comparing it with the mediastinal blood pool. The lesion uptake is considered negative if ^{18}F-FDG uptake is less than mediastinal blood and equivocal if equal to the mediastinum. If the ^{18}F-FDG uptake in the lesion is greater than the mediastinum, it is considered positive.

Given the fact that ^{18}F-FDG molecule competes with glucose for transporters across the cell membrane, special preparation is required before PET imaging to decrease the blood glucose levels. Patients are usually instructed to refrain from vigorous physical activity and to follow a low-carbohydrate diet for 24 hours before the test. Furthermore, patients are asked not to eat or drink (except water) for 6 hours before a PET scan. Patients with diabetes are additionally instructed not to take insulin in the morning on the day of the examination; target morning glucose in these patients is between 80 and 180 mg/dL (Fig. 4.1). PET scans performed for assessment of sarcoidosis may require prolonged pretest preparation with a high-fat, low-sugar diet (24–72 hours) and a longer fasting period (12 hours). This prolonged preparation also improves assessment of the myocardium.

PET-CT

The functional and physiologic basis of PET imaging allows greater sensitivity for the detection of pathologic processes in visually normal tissue. However, the intrinsic poor spatial resolution (or ability to precisely localize the pathologic process) of the PET scan has been one of the major problems of this imaging modality, particularly in the past. This problematic issue was in great part corrected with integration of PET with either CT scan or MR. CT and MR components allow anatomic correlation with functional data obtained by PET, thus increasing spatial resolution and accuracy of the imaging modality. PET-CT integration can be achieved by several means, although the most common way these days is a single machine that sequentially obtains both CT and PET images. CT images, usually obtained first, may be of full contrast-enhanced diagnostic quality or of lower quality as part of a low-transmission scan obtained for attenuation correction artifacts. Images from both of these CT types may be fused or superimposed over subsequently obtained PET images, allowing precise anatomic-functional correlation. The ability to obtain CT and PET images almost at the same time has significantly decreased (although not completely eliminated) misregistration artifacts compared with other integration techniques, which required doing PET and CT scans at different dates. Moreover, the integrated machine conveniently obtains CT and PET at the same appointment, eliminating the need for a patient to come back to the radiology department on another day.

PET-MR

Recent technologic advances enabled integration of PET images with MR images in several ways. Similar to PET and CT integration, MR and PET images may be obtained separately (at different times) and then integrated together by fusion software or may be obtained with a combined PET and MR machine. Although preferable, a single integrated PET-MR machine was technically more challenging to create than a PET-CT machine because of potential PET-MR hardware interference. Different manufacturers offer two different types of integrated PET-MR systems: sequential and concurrent. In the former, the MR and PET images are sequentially obtained in individual machines adjacent to each other during the same examination. In the latter, MR and PET images are obtained at the same time by a single combined gantry. The second system, although more expensive and difficult to create, theoretically offers better spatial resolution given even smaller chance of misregistration and motion artifacts. A single, short MR sequence is usually obtained for both anatomic correlation and PET attenuation correction, although additional diagnostic sequences may be performed if time allows (including MR functional imaging, diffusion-weighted imaging, MR spectroscopy, and perfusion-weighted imaging) (Fig. 4.2).

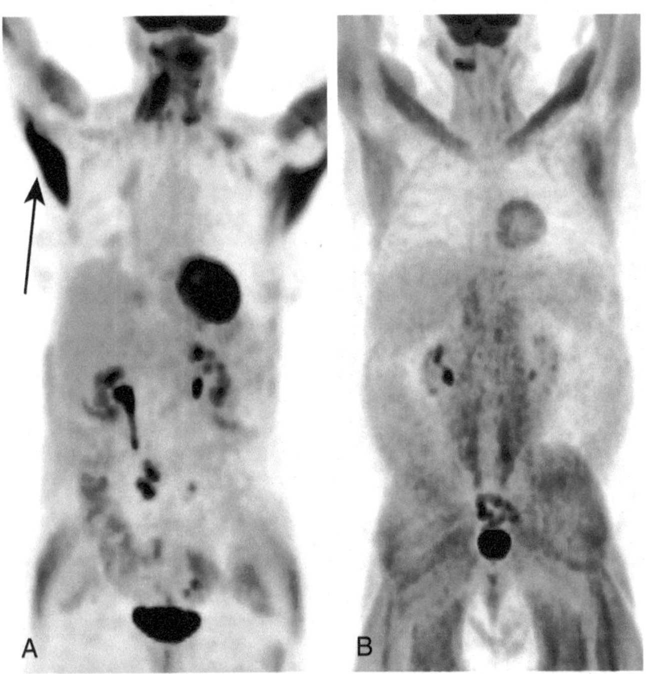

FIGURE 4.1 2-Deoxy-2-fluoro-D-glucose (^{18}F-FDG) uptake in skeletal muscles. **A,** Coronal attenuation–corrected positron emission tomography (PET) image demonstrating increased ^{18}F-FDG uptake in contracting skeletal muscles, best seen in latissimus dorsi muscles *(arrow)*. **B,** Coronal attenuation–corrected PET image demonstrating diffusely ^{18}F-FDG–avid muscles in a diabetic patient treated with insulin.

ADVANTAGES

Although PET-CT scan has also been used for characterization of nononcologic processes, its main indication has been staging of malignancies, particularly lymphoma and NSCLC (Fig. 4.3). It has been demonstrated that PET-CT has a greater value in determining local tumor extent, nodal metastasis, and distal metastasis than PET or CT alone (Fig. 4.4). More precisely, PET-CT may accurately determine the T-stage of NSCLC in 82% of cases; these values are 68% and 55% for CT and PET alone, respectively. Not only can PET-CT scan demonstrate additional areas of tumor invasion compared with CT scan, but it can also precisely determine the size of the tumor if tumor margins are obscured by associated atelectatic lung parenchyma on diagnostic CT images (Fig. 4.5). PET-CT scan is considered the best imaging method to determine nodal staging of a malignancy. Its accuracy is shown to be 78% compared with 56% for PET alone. Whereas PET alone is predominantly limited by poor spatial resolution, CT alone is limited by its use of size criteria

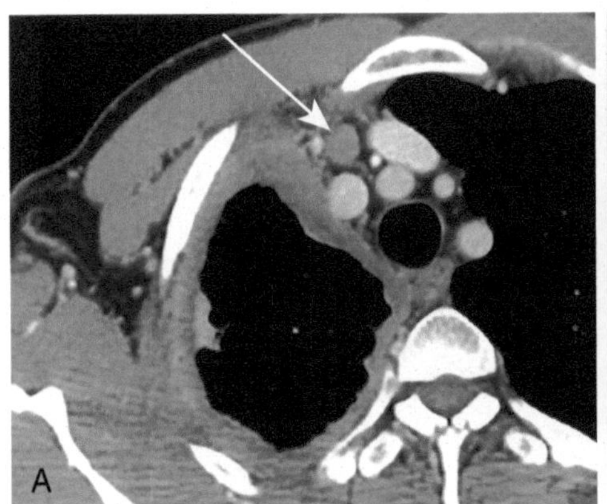

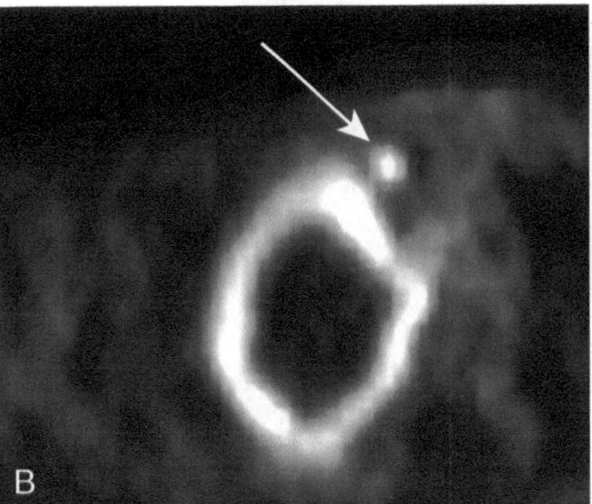

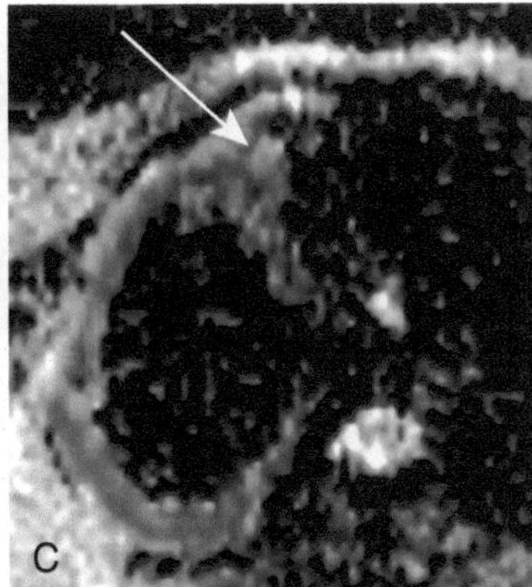

FIGURE 4.2 Diffusion-weighted in positron emission tomography (PET)–magnetic resonance (MR) imaging. Axial image of diagnostic computed tomography (CT) **(A)** and axial image of MR attenuation-corrected PET **(B)** through the upper mediastinum demonstrate a rind of fluorodeoxyglucose-avid soft tissue encasing the right lung and an enlarged right internal mammary lymph node *(arrows)*. **C,** Apparent diffusion coefficient axial MR image demonstrates restricted diffusion within the rind and lymph node.

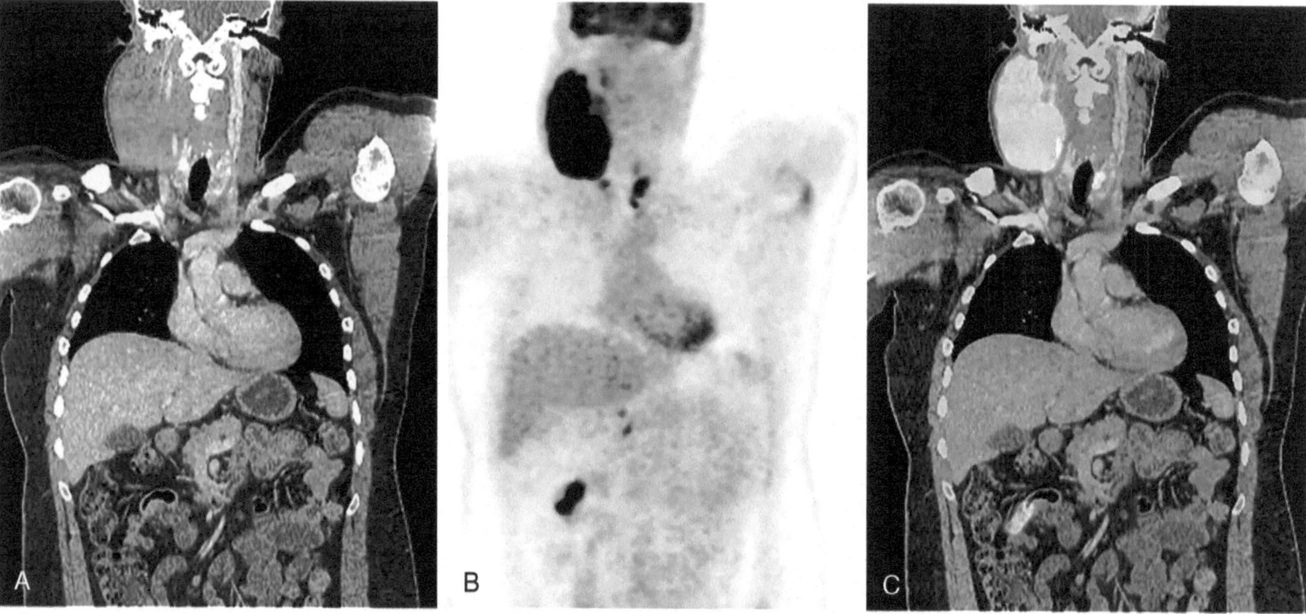

FIGURE 4.3 Upstaging in diffuse large B-cell lymphoma. Diagnostic computed tomography (CT) **(A)**, attenuation-corrected positron emission tomography (PET) **(B)**, and fused PET-CT coronal images **(C)**. There is increased fluorodeoxyglucose uptake in the clinically noted large right neck mass and unsuspected bowel lymphoma in the right mid abdomen.

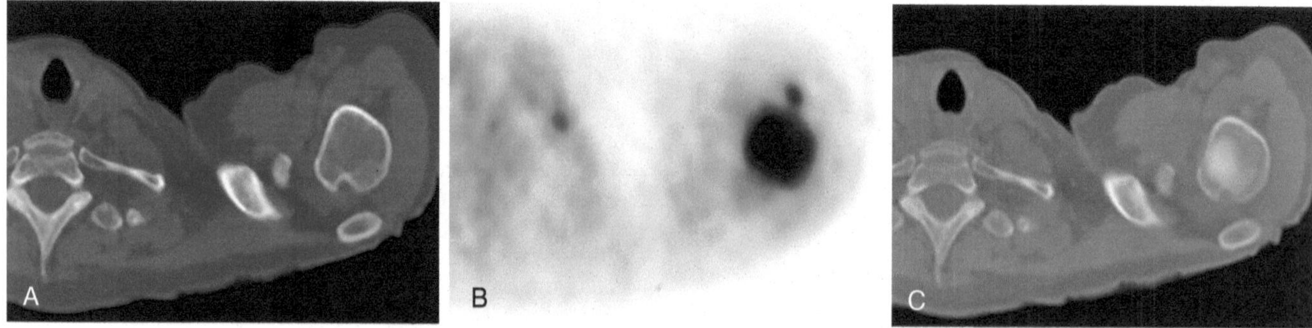

FIGURE 4.4 Occult bone disease in lymphoma. Diagnostic computed tomography (CT) **(A)**, attenuation-corrected positron emission tomography (PET) **(B)**, and fused PET-CT axial images **(C)**. There is increased fluorodeoxyglucose uptake in left humeral head without CT abnormality. This was confirmed to be non-Hodgkin lymphoma.

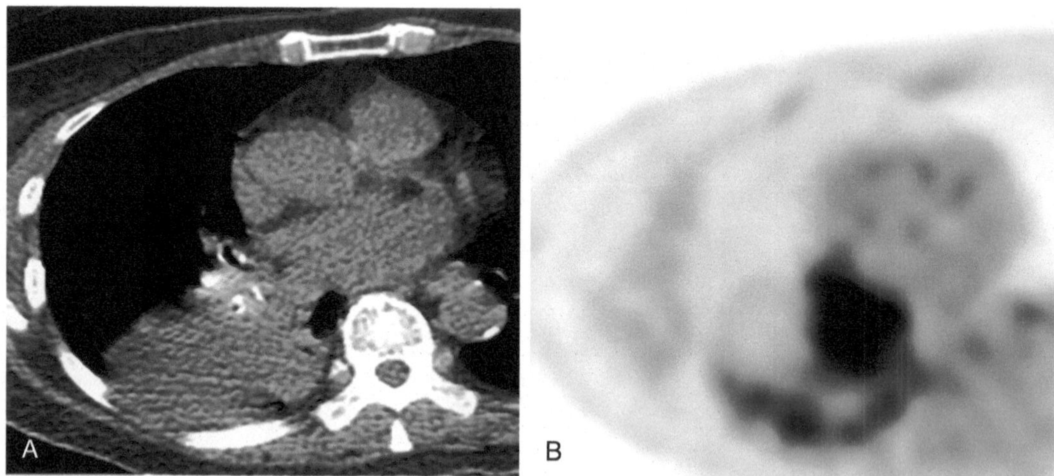

FIGURE 4.5 Non–small cell lung cancer. **A,** Axial image of low-transmission computed tomography scan demonstrates large right hilar mass with collapse of right lower lobe. Mass is indistinguishable from collapsed lung parenchyma. **B,** Attenuation-corrected axial positron emission tomography image delineates the hilar mass with increased fluorodeoxyglucose uptake.

for detection of nodal metastasis. In fact, nodal metastasis may be detected in intrathoracic lymph nodes measuring less than 1 cm in size in short axis by PET scan; those same lymph nodes would not be considered significant as per CT size criteria (Fig. 4.6). Conversely, lymph nodes greater than 1 cm in size may be metastasis-free on pathology but considered metastatic on CT scan according to their size, therefore falsely increasing N stage. Compared with CT alone, PET-CT also has a higher rate of detecting distant metastases, most commonly affecting the brain, adrenal glands, bone, liver, and lungs in the context of lung cancer (Fig. 4.7). Some bone metastases may not be seen on CT images alone, particularly if they do not involve or destroy the cortex, but they can be detected on PET-CT because of their internal increased FDG uptake (see Fig. 4.4). Furthermore, recurrent lung cancer at surgical resection sites (bronchial stumps or parenchymal staple lines) may be detected on PET-CT before there is any measurable morphologic anomaly on anatomic images. Finally, PET-CT may characterize a pleural effusion as malignant if diffuse increased FDG uptake is demonstrated, even if definite pleural deposits are not morphologically seen on CT (Fig. 4.8).

Given its superior soft tissue contrast, MR has been shown to be of particular benefit in assessment of tumors in brain, liver, breasts, spinal cord, and neck. Several studies also demonstrated that PET-CT and PET-MR revealed comparable lesion characterization and nodal staging for the evaluation of NSCLC. PET-MR may have slight advantage over PET-CT in detecting distant metastasis, mainly because of its higher accuracy in identifying and characterizing lesions in the liver and brain, both common places for

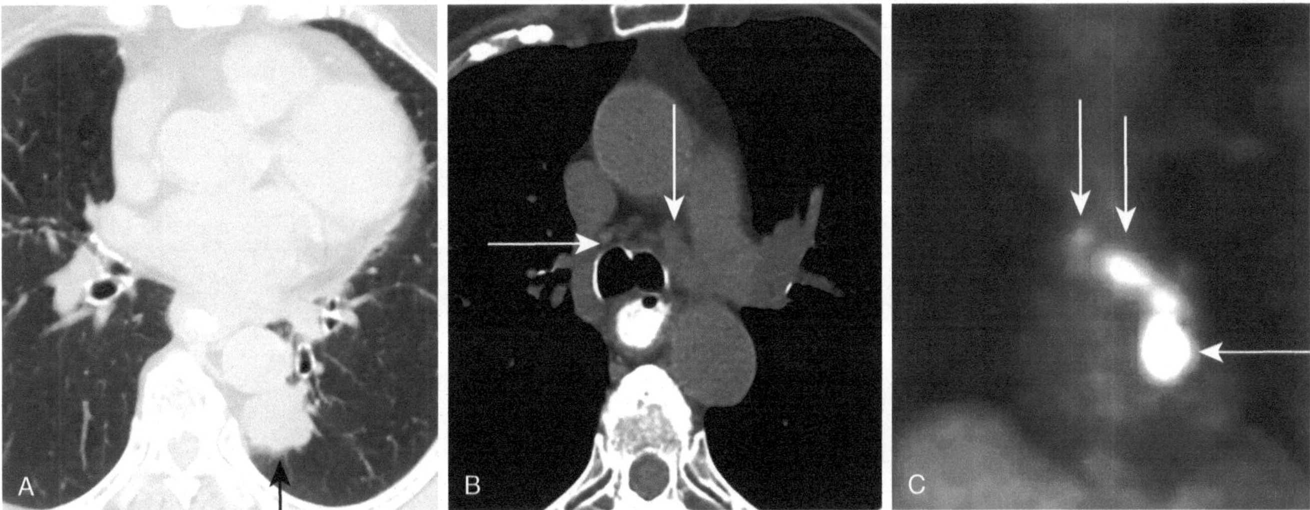

FIGURE 4.6 Non–small cell lung cancer. Lung window **(A)** and soft tissue window **(B)** axial images of chest computed tomography (CT) scan demonstrate a left lower lobe paravertebral mass (*arrow* in **A**) with enlarged left lower paratracheal nodes and small right lower paratracheal nodes, presumed N2 disease on CT (*arrows* in **B**). **C,** Coronal image of attenuation-corrected positron emission tomography (PET) shows corresponding increased fluorodeoxyglucose (FDG) uptake in the left lower lobe mass and enlarged left lower paratracheal nodes *(arrows)*. PET also demonstrated FDG avidity in small contralateral right lower paratracheal nodes, concerning for N3 disease, later confirmed by biopsy.

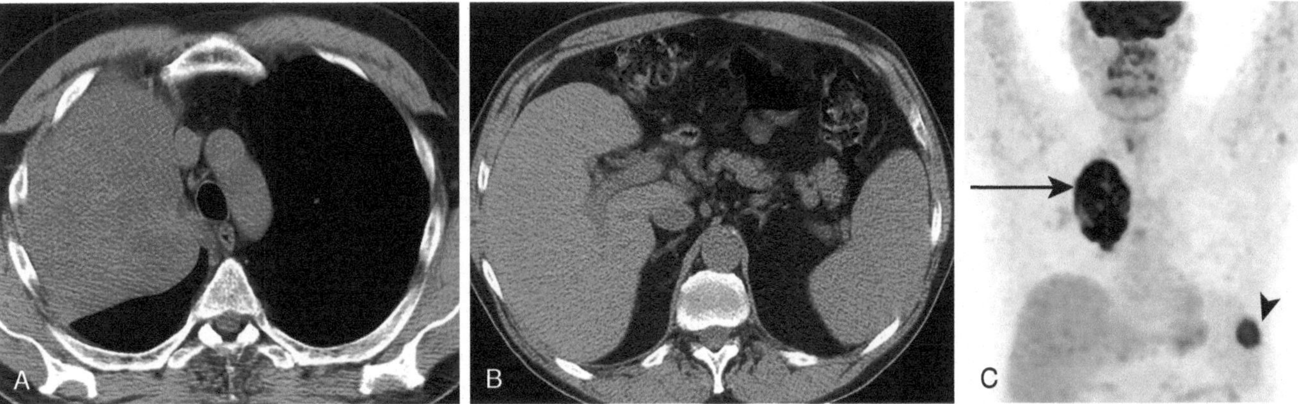

FIGURE 4.7 Small cell lung cancer. **A,** Axial image of chest computed tomography (CT) scan demonstrates a large central mass in the right upper lobe with occlusion of right upper lobe bronchus. **B,** Axial image of chest CT scan through the upper abdomen does not show metastasis in the upper abdomen. **C,** Coronal image of attenuation-corrected positron emission tomography demonstrates increased focal fluorodeoxyglucose uptake in the right upper lobe mass *(arrow)* and unsuspected solitary splenic metastasis *(arrowhead)*.

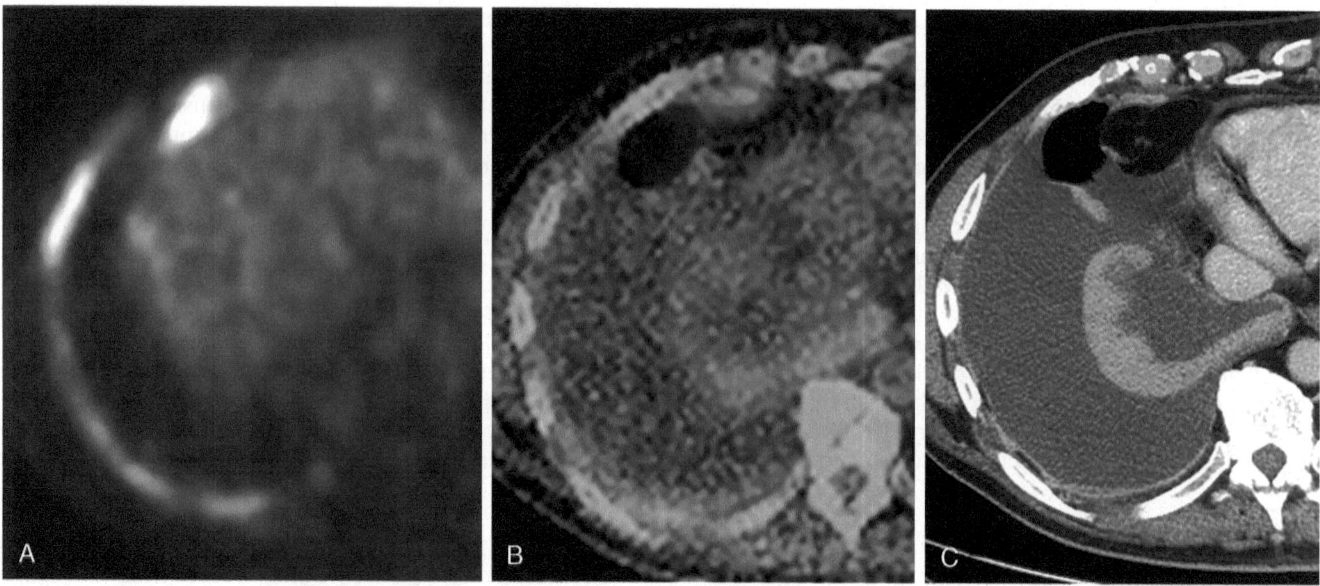

FIGURE 4.8 Malignant right pleural effusion. Attenuation-corrected positron emission tomography (PET) **(A)**, fused computed tomography (CT)–positron emission tomography **(B)**, and diagnostic CT axial **(C)** images demonstrate diffuse increased fluorodeoxyglucose uptake in right pleural thickening.

NSCLC metastasis. Functional MR imaging, obtainable with hybrid PET-MR machines, includes but is not limited to MR spectroscopy and MR perfusion sequences. This type of imaging adds supplemental information about a malignant lesion that can be beneficial in determining prognosis, treatment planning, selecting appropriate medication, and predicting tumor response to treatment. Finally, compared with PET-CT scan, radiation dose to a patient is smaller with PET-MR, which makes it a preferable imaging tool in the pediatric population and in patients requiring multiple follow-up studies (Table 4.1).

PITFALLS

PET imaging is associated with several pitfalls that need to be recognized to avoid misinterpretation of findings and selection of the wrong management (Table 4.2). Despite markedly improved PET-CT and PET-MR combination techniques over recent years, misregistration artifacts are still encountered (Fig. 4.9). These artifacts represent improper superposition of functional and anatomic images caused by sequential (nonsimultaneous) acquisition of data. Misregistration artifacts may occur anywhere in the body but are most common in the thorax and upper abdomen because of continual cardiac and diaphragmatic motion.

False-negative findings are rare and usually are related to the size or the degree of physiologic activity of target lesions. For example, neoplastic pulmonary nodules and lymph nodes smaller than 1 cm in size may falsely demonstrate lack of increased ^{18}F-FDG uptake on PET. As well, some neoplasms are characterized by low metabolic activity and typically do not demonstrate abnormal ^{18}F-FDG uptake even if they are larger than 1 cm in size. Such tumors include carcinoid tumor, adenocarcinoma in situ and minimally invasive adenocarcinoma of the lung (formerly known as bronchoalveolar carcinoma), and metastasis from mucin-producing primary tumors of breast and gastrointestinal origin (Fig. 4.10). The metastases from renal cell carcinoma are usually negative on PET. Finally, serum hyperglycemia is a known condition that may cause false-negative results on PET. In the context of high blood glucose, tumor cell membrane transporters may get saturated by glucose. Consequently, the transporters will be unable to uptake ^{18}F-FDG into tumor cells, resulting in negative PET findings.

TABLE 4.1 Comparison of PET-CT and PET-MR

	PET-CT	PET-MR
Advantages	Faster imaging	Lower radiation
	Easier accessibility	Superior soft tissue contrast resolution
	Better spatial resolution for lungs	Availability of multiplanar image acquisition
	No definite contraindications	Capability for additional functional imaging (DWI, MR spectroscopy, perfusion imaging)
Disadvantages	Radiation	Expensive and challenging to build
	Lower contrast resolution for certain areas (pleura, heart, liver, brain, bone marrow)	Cannot be performed in patients with definite MR contraindications
	Higher chance of misregistration artifacts	

DWI, Diffusion-weighted imaging; *MR*, magnetic resonance; *PET*, positron emission tomography.

TABLE 4.2 Common Pitfalls of Thoracic Oncology Positron Emission Tomography Imaging

	Pitfalls	
	Pulmonary	**Extrapulmonary**
False positive	Infection	Infection
	Tuberculosis and non-TB mycobacteria	Tuberculosis and non-TB mycobacteria
	Histoplasmosis and other endemic fungi	Histoplasmosis and other endemic fungi
	Bacterial pneumonia	Sarcoidosis
	Abscess	Reactive intrathoracic lymph nodes
	Pneumocystis jiroveci	Normal uptake in myocardium, brown fat, and bowel
	Sarcoidosis	Iatrogenic metal objects (e.g., stents) Talc pleurodesis
	Active pulmonary fibrosis	Silicone granulomas
	Progressive massive fibrosis	Thymic hyperplasia Vocal cord motion or prosthesis Vasculitis
	Radiation pneumonitis Aspiration pneumonitis	Misregistration artifacts
	Drug-induced pneumonitis	
	Postsurgical changes	
	Connective tissue diseases (RA, vasculitis)	
	Round atelectasis	
	Misregistration artifacts	
False negative	Pulmonary nodules <1 cm in size	High normal physiologic uptake in mediastinum
	Carcinoid	Preventing detection of pathology
	Adenocarcinoma in situ	Misregistration artifacts
	Misregistration artifacts	Hyperglycemia
	Hyperglycemia	

RA, Rheumatoid arthritis; *TB*, tuberculosis.

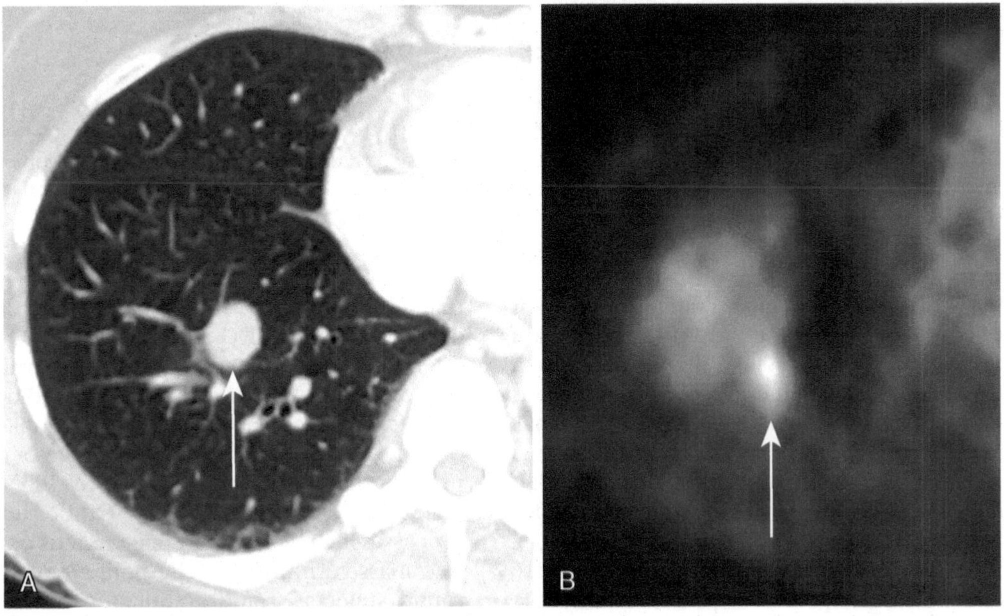

FIGURE 4.9 Misregistration artifact. **A,** Axial image of diagnostic computed tomography scan shows metastatic nodule in the right lower lobe from melanoma. **B,** Axial image of attenuation-corrected positron emission tomography. The fluorodeoxyglucose-avid lung metastasis is seen projecting on the liver because of misregistration caused by respiratory motion.

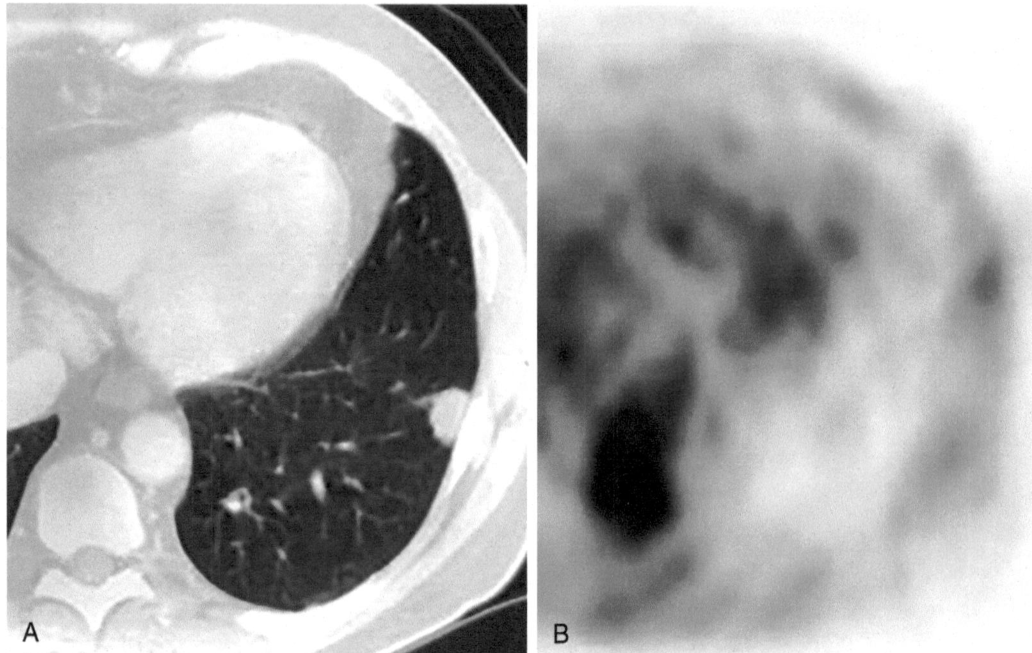

FIGURE 4.10 Carcinoid tumor. **A,** Fused positron emission tomography (PET)–computed tomography axial image shows a 1.5-cm nodule in the left lower lobe without increased fluorodeoxyglucose (FDG) uptake. **B,** Attenuation-corrected PET axial image also demonstrates absence of increased FDG uptake in the nodule.

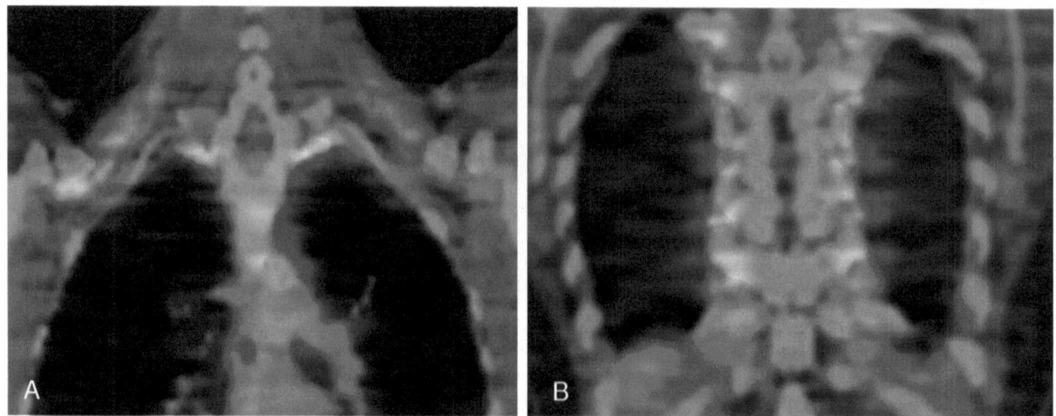

FIGURE 4.11 Brown fat. Coronal images of fused positron emission tomography–computed tomography image demonstrate symmetric increased fluorodeoxyglucose uptake in neck and axillae **(A)** and paravertebral regions **(B)** corresponding to distribution of brown fat.

False-positive PET findings are more common than their false-negative counterparts. Several normal tissues are known to demonstrate ^{18}F-FDG uptake that is higher than background; in addition, several nonneoplastic conditions characteristically demonstrate high ^{18}F-FDG uptake and may be confused with a neoplasm. For example, hamartoma may demonstrate moderate uptake. Normal tissue that generally demonstrates increased ^{18}F-FDG uptake includes myocardium, brown fat, liver, bowel, and brain (Fig. 4.11). Iatrogenic metallic objects in the thorax may also create apparent increased ^{18}F-FDG uptake in adjacent normal tissue because of attenuation-related artifacts. Nonneoplastic conditions that can give false-positive PET findings are characterized by activation of inflammatory cells, such as neutrophils and microphages, and are broadly separated into infectious and inflammatory processes. Infections that are commonly associated with increased pulmonary or mediastinal ^{18}F-FDG uptake include tuberculosis; fungal infections such as histoplasmosis, aspergillosis, and cryptococcosis; and other infections, including *Pneumocystis jiroveci* pneumonia, bacterial pneumonia, and abscesses (Fig. 4.12). Sarcoidosis is one example of an inflammatory process that is typically positive on PET and may mimic metastatic disease (Fig. 4.13). Other such inflammatory processes include radiation pneumonitis or fibrosis, progressive massive fibrosis in the context of pneumoconiosis, round atelectasis, and granulation tissue in or around a tumor. Thymic hyperplasia, silicone granulomas from extravasated silicone in the context of ruptured breast implants, and talc granulomas after talc pleurodesis are other circumstances that may cause increased ^{18}F-FDG uptake and be falsely presumed to represent a neoplasm (Fig. 4.14).

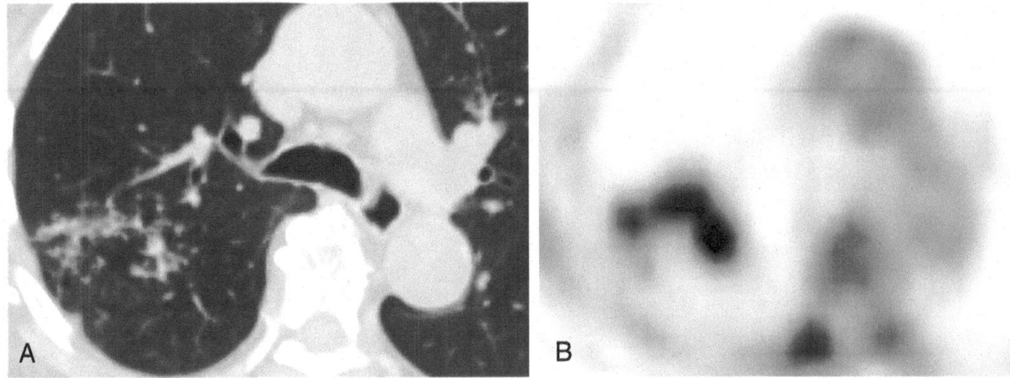

FIGURE 4.12 Tuberculosis. Diagnostic computed tomography **(A)** and attenuation-corrected positron emission tomography axial **(B)** images demonstrate tree-in-bud nodules in the posterior right upper lobe with corresponding increased fluorodeoxyglucose uptake.

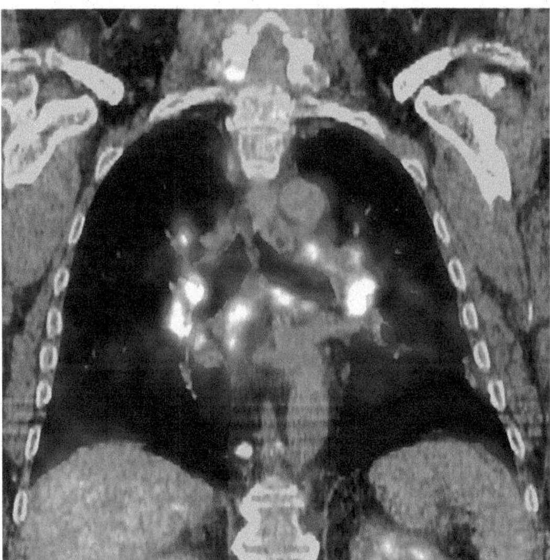

FIGURE 4.13 Sarcoidosis. Increased fluorodeoxyglucose uptake in symmetric mediastinal and hilar lymph nodes on a coronal fused positron emission tomography–computed tomography image. This can mimic malignancy.

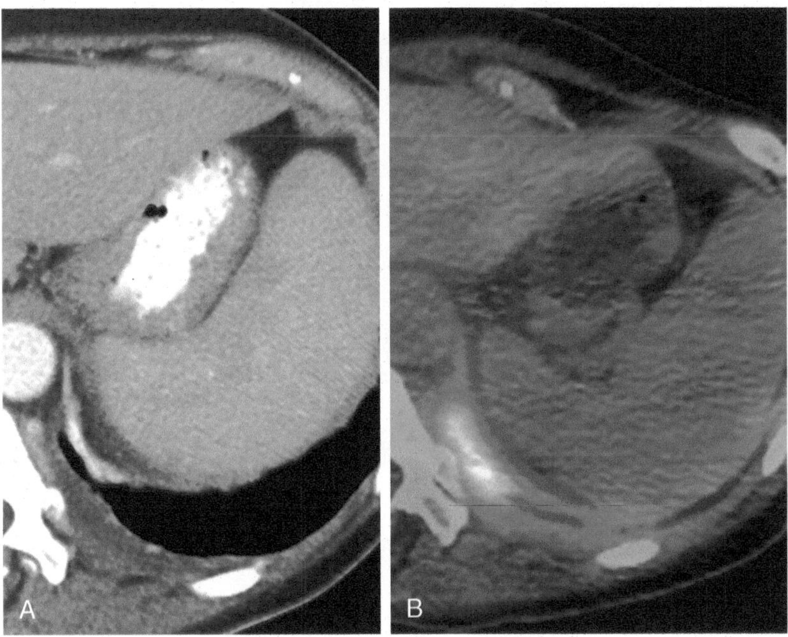

FIGURE 4.14 Talc pleurodesis. **A,** Axial image of diagnostic computed tomography (CT) demonstrates high-attenuation nodularity and thickening in the left basilar pleura after talc pleurodesis. **B,** Axial image of fused positron emission tomography–CT shows corresponding increased pleural fluorodeoxyglucose uptake corresponding to talc deposition.

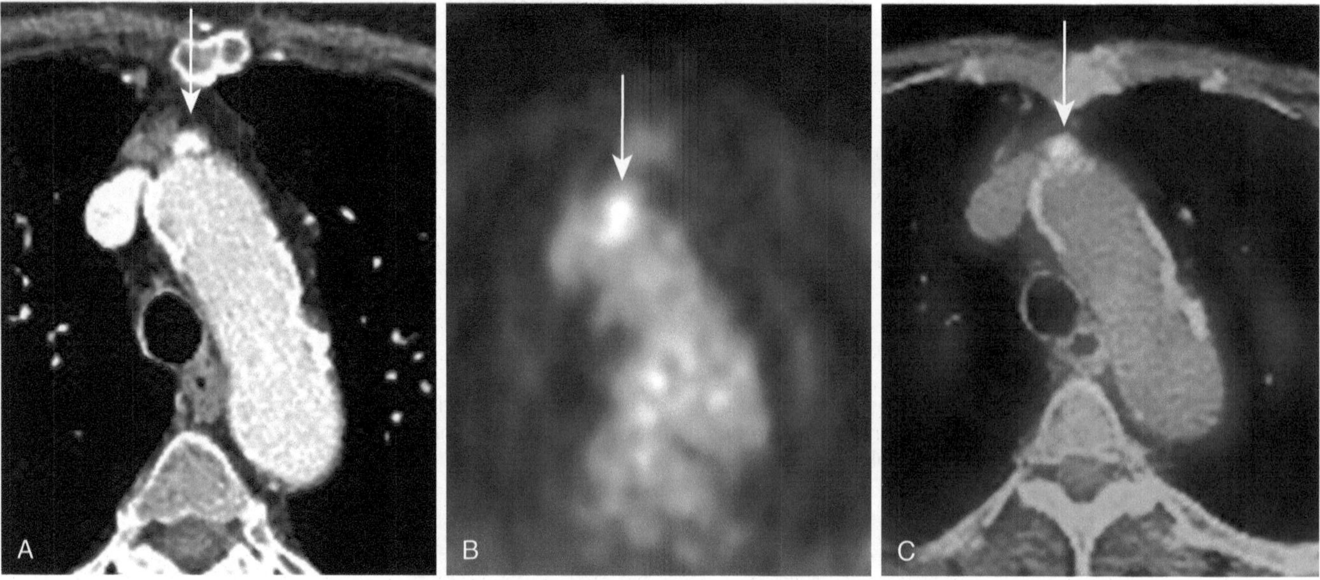

FIGURE 4.15 Inflammatory atherosclerotic plaque. Diagnostic computed tomography (CT) **(A)**, attenuation-corrected positron emission tomography (PET) **(B)**, and fused PET-CT axial **(C)** images demonstrate calcific and noncalcific atherosclerotic plaques in the aortic arch with focal increased fluorodeoxyglucose uptake in one of the plaques in the anterior wall *(arrows)* of the aorta.

Inflammatory processes in the vessel walls related to vasculitis and atherosclerosis can have increased FDG uptake and can be mistaken for uptake in mediastinal nodes (Fig. 4.15). The accurate diagnosis requires correlation with anatomic imaging on CT or MRI and comparison with older studies in conjunction with clinical history.

SUGGESTED READINGS

Antoch G, Vogt FM, Freudenberg LS, et al. Whole-body dual-modality PET-CT and whole-body MRI for tumor staging in oncology. *JAMA*. 2003;290:3199-3206.

Cerfolio RJ, Ojha B, Bryant AS, et al. The accuracy of integrated PET-CT compared with dedicated PET alone for the staging of patients with nonsmall cell lung cancer. *Ann Thorac Surg*. 2004;78:1017-1023.

Chang JM, Lee HJ, Goo JM, et al. False positive and false negative FDG-PET scans in various thoracic diseases. *Korean J Radiol*. 2006;7:57-69.

De Wever W, Ceyssens S, Mortelmans L, et al. Additional value of PET-CT in the staging of lung cancer: comparison with CT alone, PET alone and visual correlation of PET and CT. *Eur Radiol*. 2007;17:23-32.

Heusch P, Buchbender C, Kohler J, et al. Thoracic staging in lung cancer: prospective comparison of ^{18}F-FDG PET/MRI and ^{18}F-FDG PET/CT. *J Nucl Med*. 2014;55:1-6.

Lardinois D, Weder W, Hany TF, et al. Staging of non-small-cell lung cancer with integrated positron-emission tomography and computed tomography. *N Engl J Med*. 2003;348:2500-2507.

Kligerman S, Digumarthy S. Staging of non-small cell lung cancer using integrated PET/CT. *AJR Am J Roentgenol*. 2009;193:1203-1211.

Roberts PF, Follette DM, von Haag D, et al. Factors associated with false-positive staging of lung cancer by positron emission tomography. *Ann Thorac Surg*. 2000;70:1154-1160.

Schwenzer NF, Schraml C, Muller M, et al. Pulmonary lesion assessment: comparison of whole-body hybrid MR/PET and PET/CT imaging-pilot study. *Radiology*. 2012;264:551-558.

Taira AV, Herfkens RJ, Gambhir SS, et al. Detection of bone metastases: assessment of integrated FDG PET/CT imaging. *Radiology*. 2007;243:204-211.

Torigian DA, Zaidi H, Kwee TC, et al. PET/MR imaging: technical aspects and potential clinical applications. *Radiology*. 2013;267:26-42.

Truong MT, Pan T, Erasmus JJ. Pitfalls in integrated CT-PET of the thorax: implications in oncologic imaging. *J Thorac Imaging*. 2006;21:111-122.

Zaidi H, Del Guerra A. An outlook on future design of hybrid PET/MRI systems. *Med Phys*. 2011;38:5667-5689.

Chapter 5

The Mediastinum

Lan Qian (Lancia) Guo and Jeanne B. Ackman

INTRODUCTION

The mediastinum is bounded anteriorly by the sternum, posteriorly by the thoracic spine, laterally by the mediastinal pleura, superiorly by the thoracic inlet, and inferiorly by the diaphragm. It contains vital intrathoracic structures and organs, including the heart, aorta, great vessels, major lymphatic structures, trachea and mainstem bronchi, esophagus, thymus, and major nerves. The mediastinum can be affected by a wide variety of both focal and diffuse disease processes. Frequently used imaging modalities for mediastinal imaging include chest radiography (CXR) and chest computed tomography (CT). Advances in positron emission tomography-computed tomography (PET-CT) and magnetic resonance imaging (MRI) have further improved our ability to detect, define, and characterize mediastinal abnormalities.

MEDIASTINAL LANDMARKS

Radiographic landmarks, including lines, stripes, and interfaces, play an important role in the detection of mediastinal abnormalities. Recognition that a chest radiograph is abnormal because of displacement or deformation of one of these lines or stripes often prompts the recommendation for a chest CT for further evaluation. Therefore, radiologists must have a command of these normal mediastinal landmarks. Please refer to Chapter 2 for a detailed description of these radiographic anatomic findings.

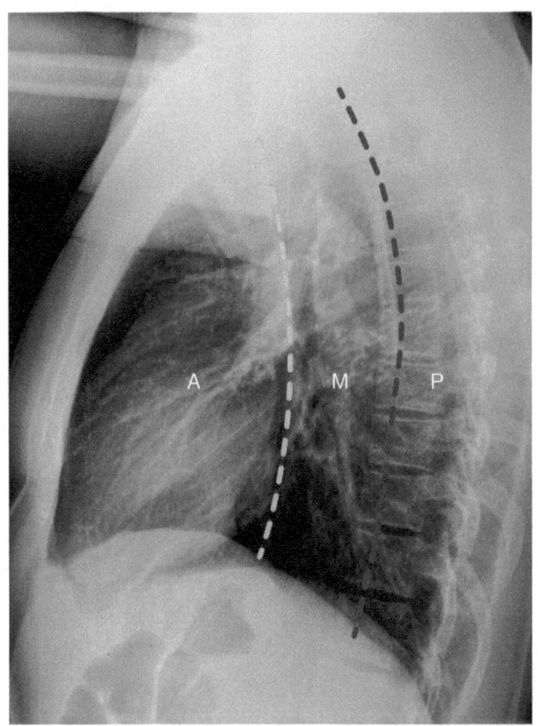

FIGURE 5.1 Felson diagram of the three mediastinal compartments. Lateral chest radiograph shows the anterior (A), middle (M), and posterior (P) mediastinal compartments. The yellow dashed line divides the anterior mediastinum from the middle mediastinum. The magenta dashed line divides the middle mediastinum from the posterior mediastinum.

MEDIASTINAL COMPARTMENTS AND THEIR ASSOCIATED LESIONS

The division of the mediastinum into specific compartments allows generation of a more specific differential diagnosis; aids in biopsy and surgical planning; and facilitates communication among radiologists, clinicians, and pathologists. There are several traditional mediastinal division schemes that are based on arbitrary landmarks on lateral chest radiographs, for example, the scheme proposed by Felson (Fig. 5.1).

Recently, the International Thymic Malignancy Interest Group (ITMIG) developed a more anatomically and CT-based scheme of mediastinal division. The ITMIG model divides the mediastinum into the prevascular (anterior), visceral (middle), and paravertebral (posterior) compartments (Fig. 5.2 and Table 5.1).

The Prevascular Compartment or Anterior Mediastinum

The prevascular compartment contains the thymus, fat, lymph nodes, and the left innominate vein. Therefore, the most common masses encountered in the prevascular compartment include thymic lesions, lymphoma and metastatic lymphadenopathy, intrathoracic thyroid masses, and germ cell neoplasms.

The Visceral Compartment or Middle Mediastinum

The contents of the visceral compartment fall into two major categories: (1) vascular structures, including the heart, superior and inferior venae cavae, entire thoracic aorta, intrapericardial pulmonary arteries and veins, and thoracic duct, and (2) nonvascular structures, including the trachea and mainstem bronchi, esophagus, and lymph nodes. Lesions in the visceral compartment include lymphoma and metastatic lymphadenopathy, foregut duplication cysts, tracheal lesions, esophageal lesions, and lesions of the heart and great vessels (including aortic aneurysms and vascular tumors).

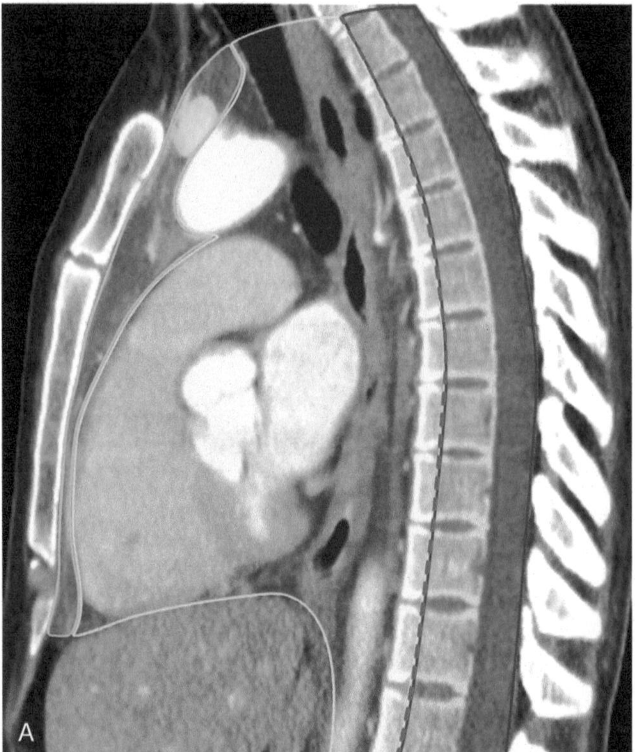

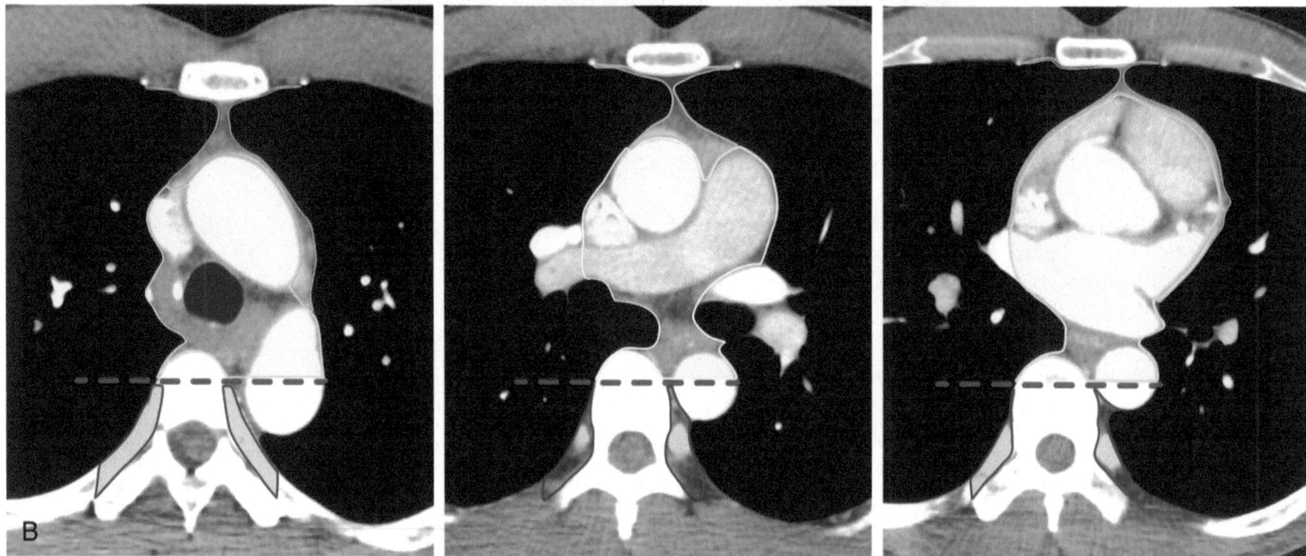

FIGURE 5.2 International Thymic Malignancy Interest Group diagram of the three mediastinal compartments. **A** and **B,** Sagittal and serial, cranial-to-caudal, axial computed tomography images, respectively, highlighting the prevascular *(green)*, visceral *(yellow)*, and paravertebral *(indigo)* compartments. The *magenta solid* and *dashed lines* divide the visceral compartment from the paravertebral compartment at the junction of the anterior and middle thirds of the thoracic vertebral body.

The Paravertebral Compartment or Posterior Mediastinum

The paravertebral compartment contains the thoracic spine and paravertebral soft tissues, including fat, lymphatics, and nerves. Therefore, neurogenic tumors feature prominently in this area, in addition to soft tissue masses arising from spinal infection (discitis, osteomyelitis), extramedullary hematopoiesis, and trauma (e.g., hematoma).

Multicompartment Lesions

In addition to lymphadenopathy, lymphangiomas and hemangiomas can occur anywhere in the mediastinum, although the latter are rare. Lymphangiomas, when large, classically present in the pediatric population, more often in the neck than in the thorax. Mesothelial cysts (i.e., pleuropericardial or pericardial cysts) can occur anywhere that mesothelium exists and therefore can present in any

TABLE 5.1 The Three Mediastinal Compartments Reclassified by the International Thymic Malignancy Interest Group Using Computed Tomography Landmarks

Compartment	Anatomic Boundaries	Major Contents	Common Lesions
Prevascular (anterior)	*Superior:* thoracic inlet *Inferior:* diaphragm *Anterior:* sternum *Posterior:* anterior aspect of the pericardium, back to the anterior margins of the superior and inferior pulmonary veins *Lateral:* mediastinal pleura and lateral margins of the internal mammary vessels	Thymus Fat Lymph nodes Left innominate vein	Lymphadenopathy Pericardial cyst Morgagni hernia Intrathoracic multinodular thyroid gland Thymic lesions Germ cell tumors
Visceral (middle)	*Superior:* thoracic inlet *Inferior:* diaphragm *Anterior:* posterior boundary of the prevascular compartment *Posterior:* vertical line drawn 1 cm posterior to the anterior margin of the thoracic spine	Vascular structures: heart, aorta, intrapericardial pulmonary arteries and veins, SVC, azygous vein, thoracic duct Nonvascular structures: trachea, carina, esophagus, lymph nodes	Hiatal hernia Lymphadenopathy Esophageal tumors Tracheal lesions Cardiac lesions Thoracic aortic aneurysm
Paravertebral (posterior)	*Superior:* thoracic inlet *Inferior:* diaphragm *Anterior:* posterior boundary of the visceral compartment *Posterior:* vertical line drawn along the posterior margin of the chest wall at the lateral margin of the thoracic spinal transverse process	Thoracic spine Paravertebral soft tissues	Bochdalek hernia Lymphadenopathy Trauma Infection Neurogenic tumors

SVC, Superior vena cava.
Modified from Carter BW, Tomiyama N, Bhora FY, et al. 2014 A modern definition of mediastinal compartments. J Thorac Oncol. 2014 9(9 Suppl 2):S97-101.

compartment of the mediastinum but most typically in the right cardiophrenic angle, where they are most commonly referred to as pericardial cysts. Mediastinitis can also affect any or all compartments of the mediastinum.

IMAGING WORKUP

Chest Radiography

Plain chest radiography is typically the first imaging examination requested for suspected mediastinal pathology and is often the source of incidentally discovered mediastinal masses. Radiographic detection of mediastinal pathology relies on either opacification of a relatively lucent anatomic region or abnormal widening, displacement, or obliteration of previously described mediastinal lines, stripes, and interfaces. Recognition of these mediastinal landmarks on CXR facilitates localization of the mediastinal mass to a specific compartment and narrows the differential diagnosis. For example, obliteration of the retrosternal clear space, deformation or widening of the anterior junction line, and silhouetting of cardiac borders are indicative of a prevascular or anterior mediastinal process (Fig. 5.3). A mass in the visceral (middle) mediastinum may present as a thickened paratracheal stripe (Fig. 5.4), convexity of the aortopulmonary stripe or anteroposterior (AP) window, silhouetting of cardiac borders or abnormal rightward convexity of the azygoesophageal interface. Deformation or widening of the posterior junction line and displacement of the paraspinal lines are often caused by the presence of a paravertebral (posterior) mediastinal mass, such as a neurogenic tumor or paraspinal hematoma (Fig. 5.5).

Fluoroscopy

In today's radiology practice, fluoroscopy has a limited role in the assessment of mediastinal pathology, owing to widespread use of CT. The esophagram remains the initial imaging modality of choice for suspected esophageal perforation. When esophageal perforation is of concern, initially a water-soluble isoosmolar or low-osmolar oral contrast is administered to exclude a leak because it is disposed of fairly readily by the body. Barium can harden and remain indefinitely in the lungs or pleural space if aspirated or leaked. If no leak is demonstrated with a water-soluble agent and concern remains, then barium can be administered for more definitive confirmation and increased sensitivity for detection of mucosal pathology because it is thicker, more adherent to pathology, more opaque than water-soluble contrast agents, and does not wash away as quickly. Alternatively, the patient can be sent for CT immediately after an esophagram to probe further and obtain additional information. Fluoroscopy is also frequently used during a "sniff test" to evaluate diaphragmatic motion and exclude diaphragmatic paralysis (see Chapter 7; see also Fig. 3.23).

Computed Tomography

Computed tomography is the workhorse for image-based diagnosis of mediastinal pathology because of its ability to detect, delineate, and characterize mediastinal pathology better than radiography alone. CT usually allows accurate anatomic localization of the mediastinal lesion suspected on chest radiographs and offers superior soft tissue contrast to radiography, differentiating tissue such as air, fat, serous fluid, soft tissue, and calcification based on differences in CT attenuation, the latter measured in Hounsfield units (HU). CT has difficulty, however, differentiating soft tissue attenuation caused by bona fide solid soft tissue from soft tissue attenuation caused by hyperattenuating fluid. Indications for CT include, but are not limited to, radiographic abnormalities such as widened mediastinum, pneumomediastinum, pneumopericardium, an apparent

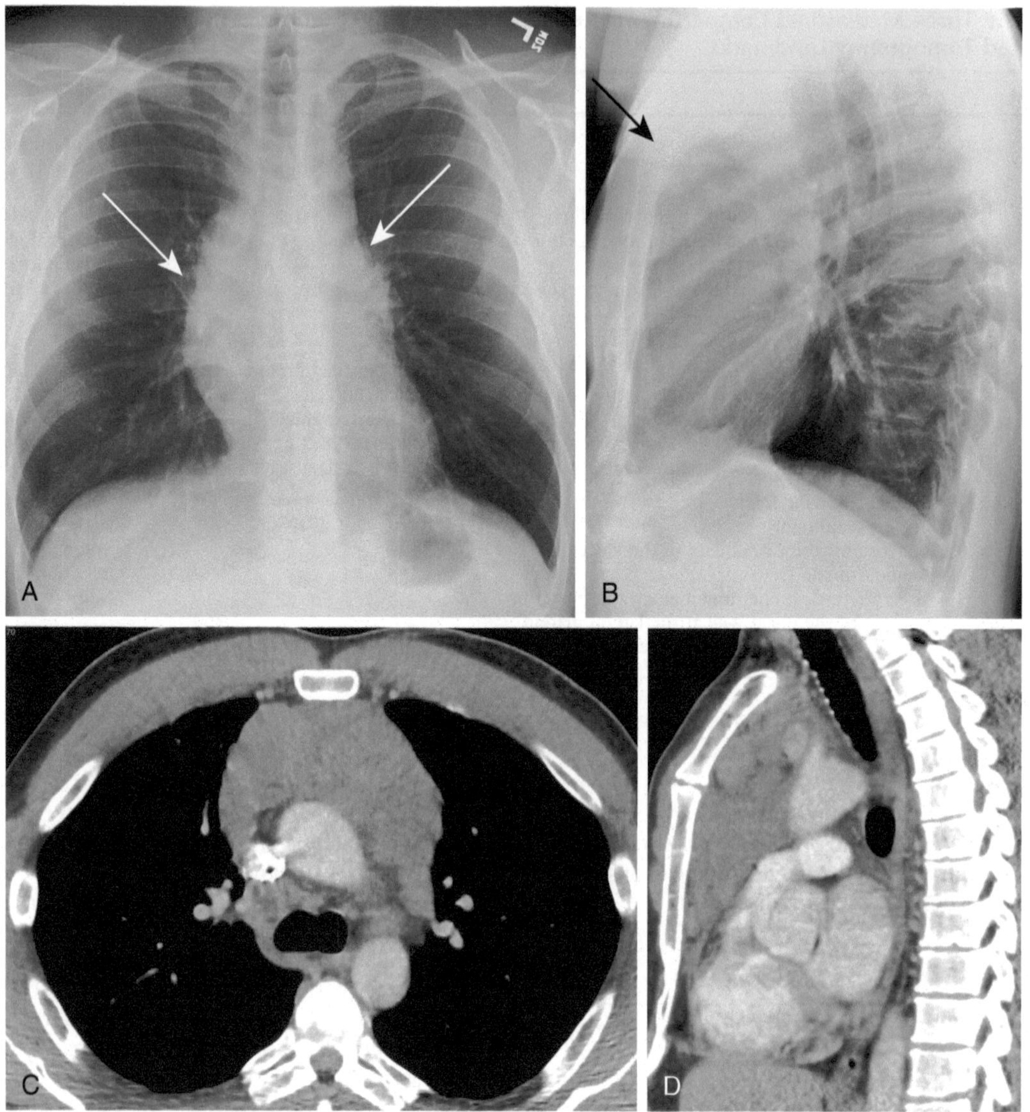

FIGURE 5.3 Prevascular mediastinal mass: Hodgkin lymphoma, nodular sclerosis type. **A,** Posteroanterior radiograph shows a widened mediastinum *(white arrows)*, with partial fill-in of the anteroposterior window and no silhouetting of the paraspinal line or descending thoracic aorta. **B,** Lateral radiograph shows complete opacification of the retrosternal clear space *(black arrow)*. These chest radiographic findings indicate the presence of a large prevascular mass. **C** and **D,** Correlative axial and sagittal intravenous contrast-enhanced computed tomography images showing a large, biconvex, lobulated, multinodular, soft tissue attenuation mass distributed fairly evenly throughout the prevascular mediastinum. These combined features strongly favor lymphoma over thymoma and other mediastinal masses.

mediastinal mass on CXR, and staging and restaging of malignancy. Please see Chapter 1 regarding CT techniques.

Magnetic Resonance Imaging

Recognition of the value of MRI for mediastinal lesion evaluation has increased upon mastery of earlier technical challenges related to cardiorespiratory motion. MRI offers superior soft tissue contrast to CT, allowing for both superior tissue characterization and more precise mediastinal compartmental localization, yielding higher diagnostic specificity. Exploiting the differences in T1- and T2-weighted signal characteristics and enhancement patterns enables detection of and distinction between serous and hemorrhagic or proteinaceous fluid content, macroscopic and microscopic fat, fibrous tissue, smooth muscle, and cartilage. By CT, it can often be quite difficult to distinguish a hyperattenuating cystic lesion from a solid lesion because hyperattenuating mediastinal cysts can reach attenuation values as high as 100 HU. The sole tissue characterization deficit of MR, relative to CT, is its inability to definitively demonstrate calcification. Because of its higher soft tissue contrast, MR can provide superior anatomic delineation of the relationship between a mediastinal lesion and adjacent structures, whether muscle, pericardium, neurovascular structures, or bone, and is more sensitive for the detection of bone marrow involvement by edema, infection, and malignancy. MR can therefore more precisely assist in the staging of mediastinal tumors.

Dynamic contrast-enhanced (DCE) MRI offers further benefit with regard to tissue distinction, not only distinguishing cystic from solid lesions and gauging lesion complexity,

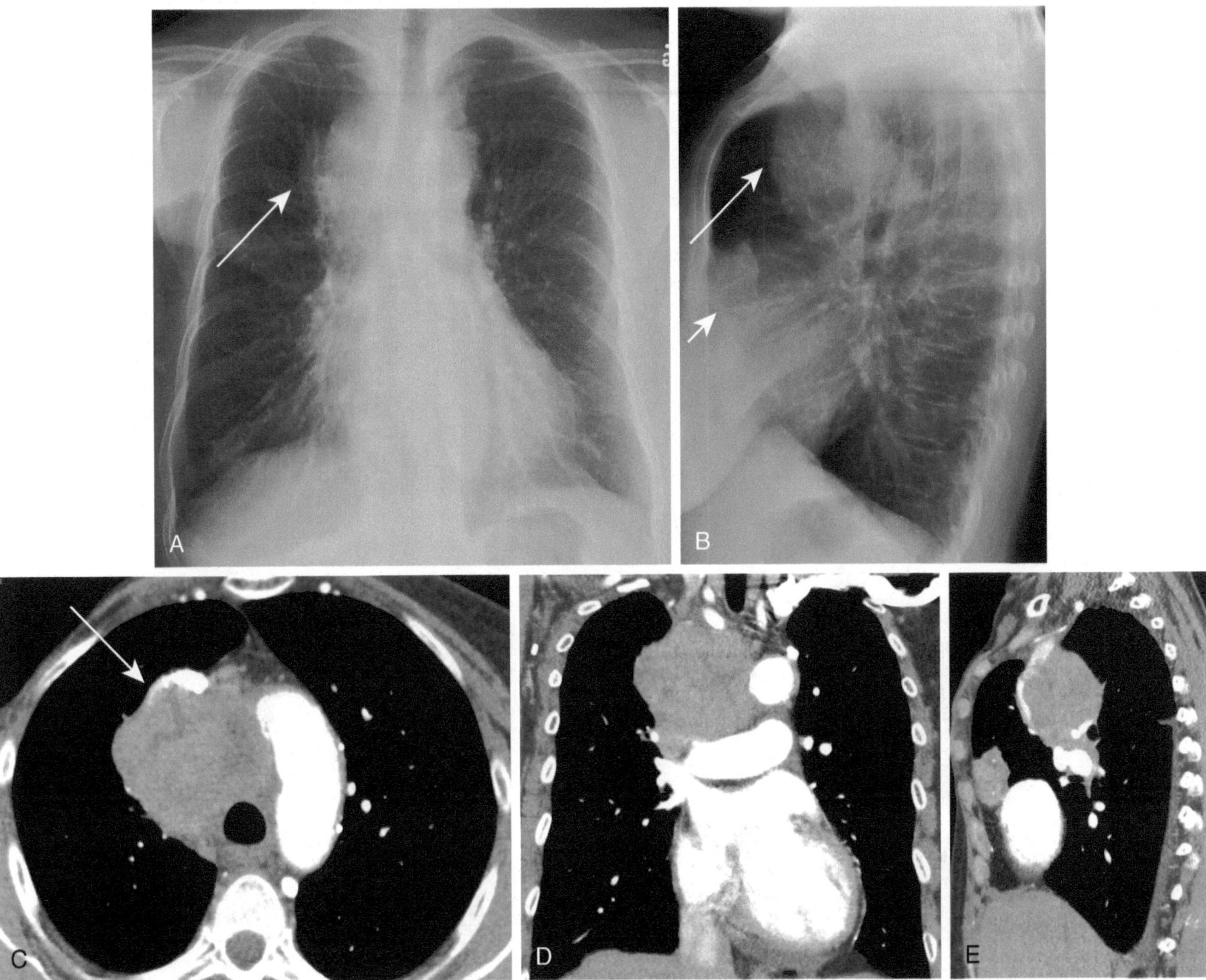

FIGURE 5.4 Visceral mediastinal mass: small cell carcinoma. **A,** Posteroanterior radiograph shows a rounded right paratracheal soft tissue mass silhouetting the right paratracheal stripe and widening the right side of the mediastinum *(arrow)*. **B,** Lateral radiograph confirms the visceral mediastinal location of this mass *(arrow)*, which partially overlies the trachea and silhouettes the aortic arch and more anterior great vessels. This lateral radiograph better demonstrates a concurrent anterior right middle lobe mass *(short arrow)* representing the primary tumor. **C** to **E,** Axial, coronal, and sagittal computed tomography images through this large right paratracheal mass show anterior displacement, compression, and invasion of the superior vena cava (SVC) *(arrow)* by this heterogeneously enhancing mass of confluent lymphadenopathy, predisposing toward SVC syndrome. The areas of low attenuation within this mass represent necrosis. The concurrent right middle lobe primary mass is again demonstrated (**E**).

but also assisting in the distinction of low risk thymomas from high risk thymoma, thymic carcinoma, and lymphoma and in differentiating mediastinal hemangiomas from lymph nodes. Diffusion-weighted MRI with apparent diffusion coefficient (ADC) mapping may also contribute to diagnostic specificity, with examples including the higher restricted diffusion of high-risk thymic tumors, thymic carcinoma, and lymphoma when compared with low-risk thymomas and the absence of restricted diffusion in most benign lesions. Abscesses and hematomas may restrict the diffusion of water, however, because of the thick, tenacious, congealed nature of their content. In such cases, the T1 and T2 signal and lack of enhancement of these benign lesions on MRI facilitates the correct diagnosis.

When CT localization of a mass is indeterminate, MRI can more precisely localize the lesion within an intrathoracic compartment. For example, MRI can often better show whether a mass resides in the paravertebral mediastinum or pleural space (see Fig. 3.2)—an important distinction because the differential diagnosis of the former includes neurogenic tumors and the differential diagnosis of the latter does not. See Chapter 3 for more information about thoracic MRI.

Positron Emission Tomography

In the mediastinum, PET, using the isotope 18-fluorodeoxyglucose (^{18}FDG) is primarily of value for detection and staging of mediastinal involvement by malignancies such as lung cancer, breast cancer, lymphoma, and melanoma. PET detects metastatic lymph nodal involvement with higher sensitivity than CT and is of particular value in

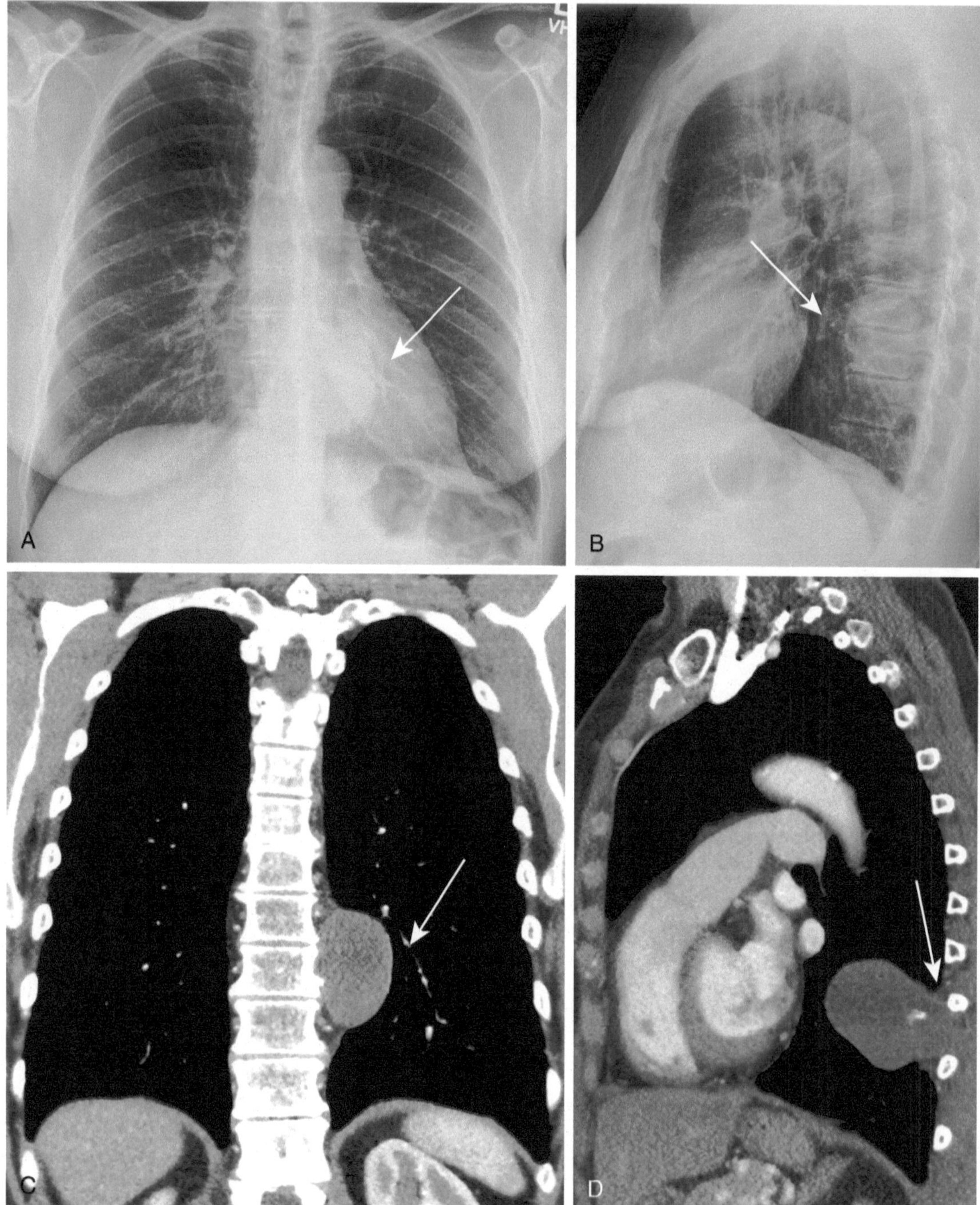

FIGURE 5.5 Paravertebral mediastinal mass—chondrosarcoma. **A,** Posteroanterior radiograph reveals a rounded, inferior left paravertebral mass *(arrow)* silhouetting the left paraspinal line and lateral margin of the descending thoracic aorta. **B,** Lateral radiograph shows the mass *(arrow)* to overlie the lower thoracic spine. **C** and **D,** Coronal and sagittal contrast-enhanced computed tomography images show this mass to be mildly and homogeneously hypoattenuating to muscle, to partially erode the left lateral margin of T10 *(arrow)*, and to contain calcification *(arrow)*. The presence of calcification decreases the likelihood of most neurogenic tumors (which are more common in this compartment) and, in conjunction with the lack of hypervascularity, favors chondrosarcoma over paraganglioma and hemangioma.

detection of malignancy within lymph nodes that are not enlarged based on standard CT size criteria. Nevertheless, detection of metastatic involvement within lymph nodes less than 5 mm in short axis is limited. False positives can occur when lymph nodes are involved by an active inflammatory process such as granulomatous disease, including sarcoidosis, histoplasmosis, tuberculosis, and other infection. Definitive diagnosis of lymph nodal metastases often requires biopsy via mediastinoscopy or endobronchial ultrasonography (EBUS). ^{18}FDG-PET imaging is of limited value for thymic evaluation because normal thymus, thymic hyperplasia, and thymic neoplasms can be FDG-PET avid and have demonstrated overlapping standardized uptake values (SUVs). See Chapter 4 for more information about PET imaging.

MEDIASTINAL MASSES

Prevascular and Anterior Mediastinal Masses

Thymic Lesions

Normal Thymus. The thymus is composed of lymphoepithelial tissue and plays an important role in the maturation of T cells and recognition of self. It is disproportionately larger in infants, reaches maximal weight at puberty, and gradually involutes with age, becoming increasingly intercalated with fat. The rate of fatty atrophy of the thymus varies among individuals and has been shown to vary between the sexes as well (Fig. 5.6). The thymus is largely fatty by the fifth decade of life and almost completely fatty by the seventh decade. Reticulonodular strands of thymic soft tissue and residual islands of thymic tissue measuring up to 7 mm may remain in older individuals, however.

Because of the embryologic descent of the thymus from the third pharyngeal pouch of the neck, normal thymic tissue and thymic pathology, although most commonly found in the middle to upper prevascular mediastinum, may also be found anterosuperior to the left innominate vein and in the base of the neck. Thymic tissue, and therefore thymic pathology, may also rarely be found as low as the cardiophrenic angle. In adults, the thymus is classically bilobed, bipyramidal, or arrowhead-shaped, but it can be unilobar and quadrilateral as well. To avoid misinterpretation of normal thymus as a thymic mass in young men and women, it is important to be aware of a sex difference in normal thymic appearance. The thymuses of young women tend to be fuller and more quadrilateral in shape and more attenuating than those of men and therefore risk misinterpretation as thymic hyperplasia, thymic neoplasm, and lymphoma. In the 20- to 30-year age

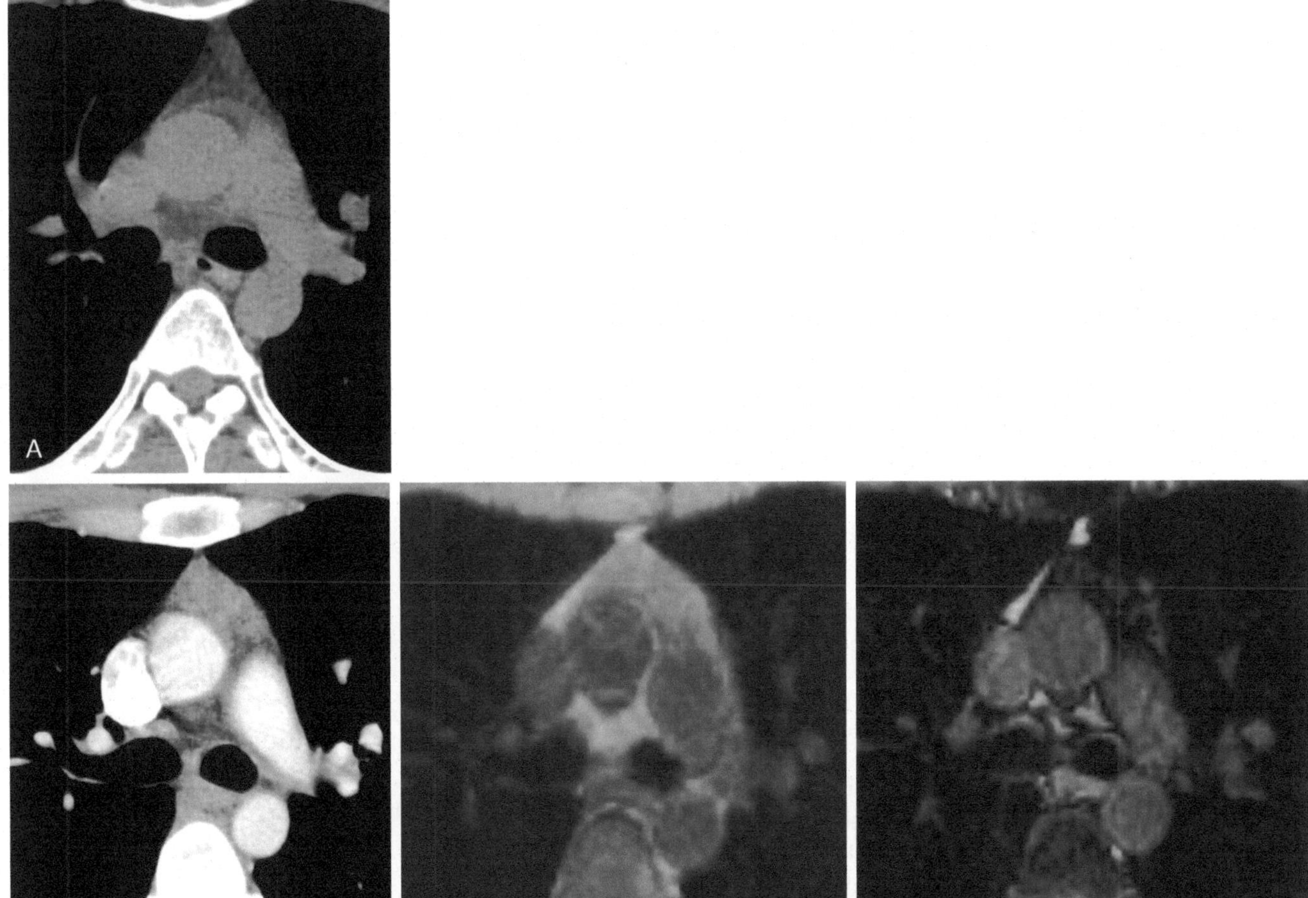

FIGURE 5.6 **A,** Normal thymus in a 28-year-old man. Axial computed tomography (CT) scan shows diffuse fatty intercalation throughout atrophic thymic tissue in the thymic bed. **B** to **D,** Normal thymus in a 30-year-old woman. **B,** Axial CT shows levoconvex, grossly fatty intercalated soft tissue filling the thymic bed. **C** and **D,** In- and opposed-phase chemical shift magnetic resonance images, respectively, show loss or suppression of signal of this tissue on the opposed-phase image, indicative of the presence of microscopic fat. Given the normal thymic thickness and morphology for age, this finding represents normal, rather than hyperplastic, thymus.

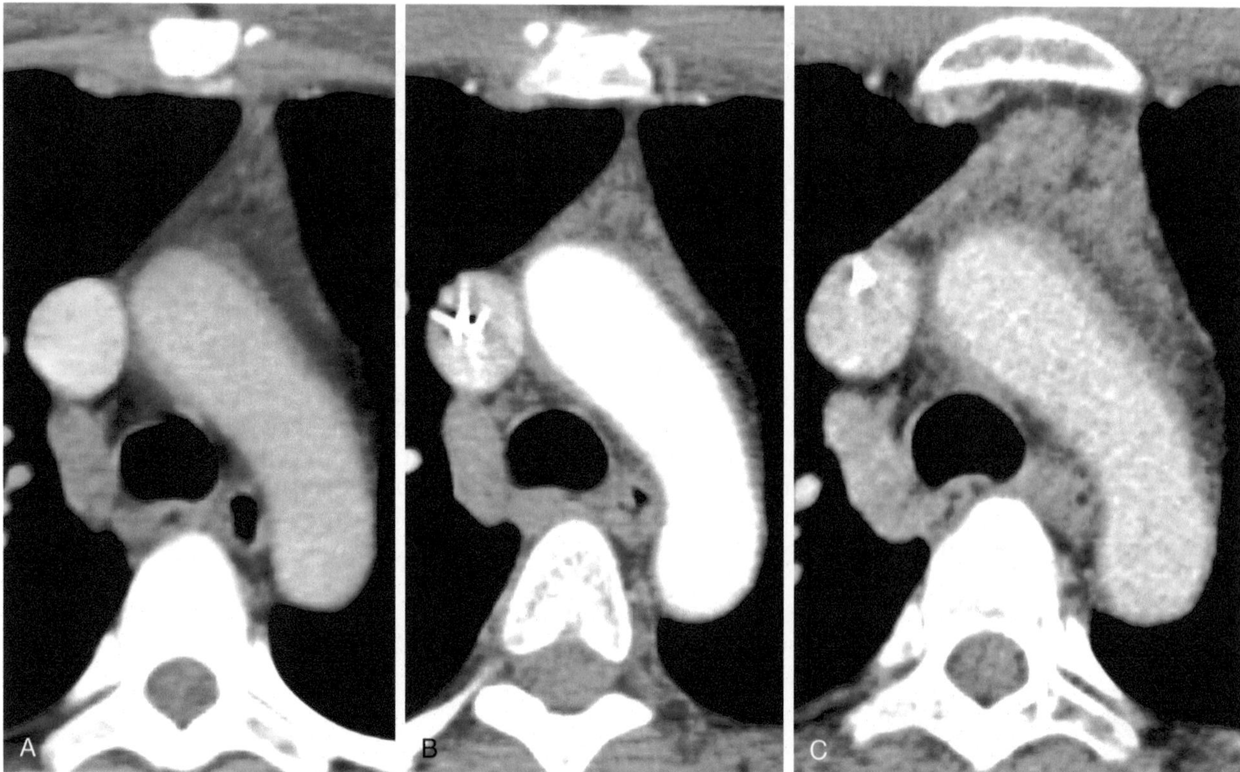

FIGURE 5.7 Rebound thymic hyperplasia in a 49-year-old woman 3 months after completion of 6 cycles of chemotherapy for peritoneal carcinoma. **A,** Baseline computed tomography (CT) scan 3 years before chemotherapy at age 46 years, revealing normal, primarily fatty thymic tissue for age. **B,** CT acquired a few weeks after completion of 6 cycles of chemotherapy, showing slightly increased attenuation of thymic tissue when compared with baseline. **C,** Axial CT scan performed 4 months after chemotherapy cessation reveals interval development of abundant, bipyramidal thymic soft tissue, representing thymic rebound.

group, a triangular or arrowhead thymus may measure up to 1.6 cm in maximal thymic lobe thickness and a quadrilateral thymus may measure up to 2.2 cm in maximal thymic lobe thickness. These figures are higher than the figure of 1.3 cm reported in the mid-1980s for maximal thymic lobe thickness in adults older than 20 years of age in the era of nonhelical CT and 10-mm slice acquisition.

The thymus is sensitive to a variety of stressors, including systemic infection, corticosteroid therapy, burns, surgery, radiation, and chemotherapy. In response to stress, it can atrophy at unknown rates in humans, only to regrow to its original size or even larger when the inciting physiologic stressor resolves, with the latter referred to as thymic rebound or rebound thymic hyperplasia (Fig. 5.7).

Thymic Hyperplasia. There are two main types of thymic hyperplasias: true thymic hyperplasia, in which there is increased size and weight of the thymus for age, with preservation of normal histology, and lymphoid follicular thymic hyperplasia (LFH), in which the number of lymphoid germinal centers are increased. In LFH, the thymus may or may not be enlarged. Clinically, a wide variety of conditions may lead to thymic hyperplasia (Table 5.2). On CT, a hyperplastic thymus may manifest as a diffusely enlarged gland with increased maximal thymic lobe thickness, unilateral or bilateral convexity, more nonfatty soft tissue in the thymic bed than expected for age or sex, or as a focal mass; it is not infrequently confused for neoplasm. In a fairly recent study, LFH was found to be more attenuating than true thymic hyperplasia on CT, with a cut-off value of 41 HU proposed as a means of differentiating these entities; however, this cutoff could theoretically vary with age and sex as well and therefore can only be used as a rough guide. LFH can occasionally be found amidst predominantly fatty thymic tissue.

TABLE 5.2 Conditions Associated With the Two Main Types of Thymic Hyperplasias

	True Thymic Hyperplasia	Lymphoid Follicular Hyperplasia
Etiology	Idiopathic Hyperthyroidism or Graves disease Sarcoidosis Red blood cell aplasia Rebound or recovery from recent physiologic stress, such as*: • Systemic infection • Corticosteroid therapy • Surgery • Burns • Chemotherapy • Radiation	Autoimmune diseases including: • Myasthenia gravis • Hyperthyroidism or Graves disease • Systemic lupus erythematosus • Scleroderma • Rheumatoid arthritis • Polyarteritis nodosa • Hashimoto thyroiditis • Addison disease • Autoimmune hemolytic anemia • Behçet disease HIV infection

*The thymus may also be of normal weight or nonhyperplastic in thymic rebound.

Chemical shift MRI can be used to differentiate normal and hyperplastic thymus from thymic neoplasm in adults

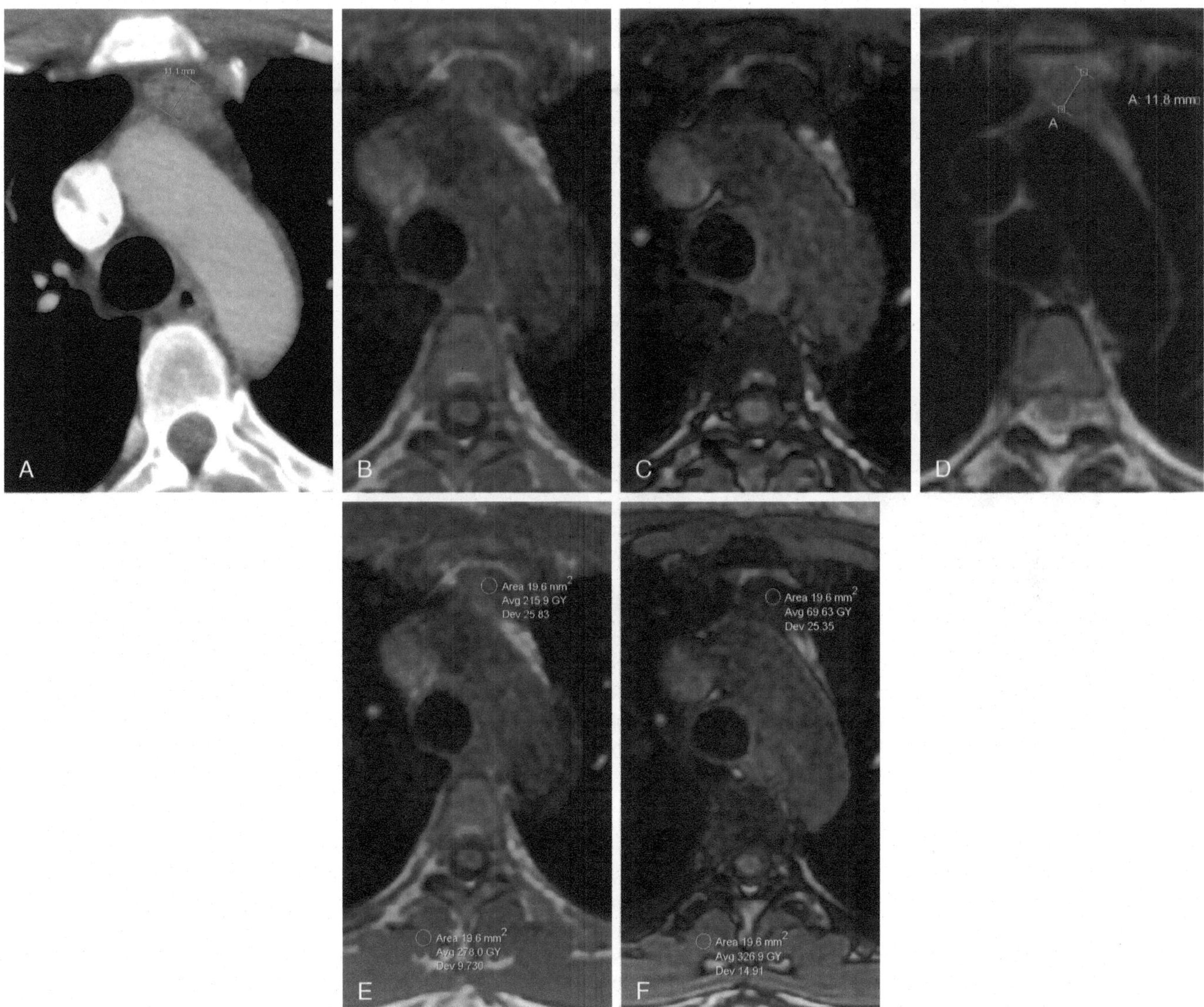

FIGURE 5.8 Thymic hyperplasia in a 45-year-old woman. **A,** Axial computed tomography scan shows abnormal, excess, lobulated soft tissue for age within the thymic bed. **B** and **C,** In- and out-of-phase chemical shift magnetic resonance images (MR images) reveal marked signal suppression throughout this tissue on the opposed-phase image, proving the presence of microscopic fat and that this finding represents thymic hyperplasia. **D,** Electrocardiography (ECG)-gated double-inversion recovery (black blood) T2-weighted MRI reveals expected T2 hyperintensity of this hyperplastic thymic tissue relative to muscle (not relative to gross or macroscopic fat). **E** and **F,** In- and opposed-phase MR images showing proper region-of-interest (ROI) placement on the thymic tissue and paraspinal musculature, yielding a chemical shift ratio (CSR) of 0.3 and a signal intensity index (SII) of 68%. A CSR of 0.7 or less or an SII of 9% or greater indicates the presence of microscopic fat, proving either normal thymus or thymic hyperplasia, depending on patient age, rather than thymic tumor.

because it capitalizes on the fact that microscopic fat is usually present in normal and hyperplastic thymuses and not present in thymic tumors. Suppression of thymic soft tissue signal on the opposed-phase images indicates the presence of microscopic fat and excludes tumor, unless the suppression of signal is observed within a cystic thymic lesion, in which case a cystic teratoma or dermoid tumor should be considered. The chemical shift ratio (CSR) is calculated by placing a region of interest (ROI) over the least suppressing thymic tissue and the paraspinal muscle or, if partially fatty replaced, the least atrophic muscle on the same opposed-phase image and then placing comparable ROIs in size, shape, and location over the thymus and paraspinal muscle on the in-phase image at the same level. A CSR of 0.7 or less is consistent with normal or hyperplastic thymus (Fig. 5.8). A CSR of 1.0 or greater is indicative of thymic neoplasm in most cases, with 0.8 and 0.9 representing indeterminate values.

Chemical shift ratio calculation:

$$\frac{\text{OP SI thymus/OP SI paraspinal muscle}}{\text{IP SI thymus/IP SI paraspinal muscle}}$$

Alternatively, provided the in- and opposed-phase images are obtained by a *dual-echo* chemical shift MR acquisition,

IP = in-phase; OP = opposed-phase; SI = signal intensity as measured by ROI.

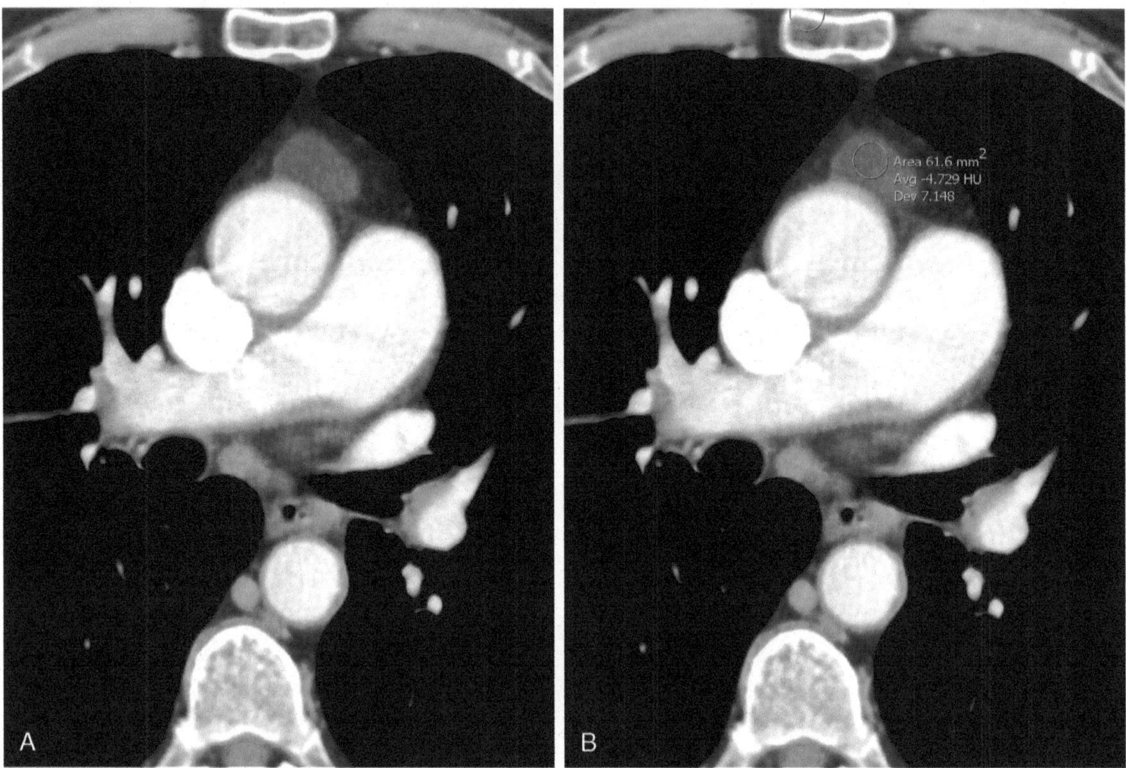

FIGURE 5.9 Thymic cyst, water attenuation. **A,** Axial computed tomography scan reveals a well-circumscribed saccular water attenuation (–5 HU) mass with a barely perceptible wall in the thymic bed, representing a thymic cyst. **B,** Region of interest over lesion.

a signal intensity index (SII) can be calculated to assess the degree of fat suppression (see below) and solely requires ROI placement over the thymus, not the paraspinal musculature. An SII (or signal dropout) greater than 9% has been proposed as indicative of normal thymus or thymic hyperplasia, rather than tumor.

$$\text{SII} = \left(\frac{[\text{IP SI thymus} - \text{OP SI thymus}]}{[\text{IP SI thymus}]} \right) \times 100$$

There are several important caveats with regard to chemical shift MR evaluation of the thymus. There have been cases of nonsuppressing normal and hyperplastic thymic tissue in adults. Therefore, if suppression of thymic tissue is observed on the opposed-phase images, one can be confident that the thymus is normal or hyperplastic. If there is no suppression on opposed-phase imaging, one must be circumspect and determine whether the thymic morphology and MR signal are otherwise normal; if so, confirmation of stability or regression or suppression of the thymic tissue can be made over time by follow-up MRI. In addition, normal, macroscopically fatty thymus and thymic cysts do not suppress on opposed-phase images because they do not contain microscopic fat. *Macroscopic or gross fat saturates on fat-saturated MRI but does not suppress on chemical shift MRI.*

Thymic Cysts. Thymic cysts may be congenital or acquired. Acquired thymic cysts have been associated with prior chemotherapy, radiation, thoracotomy, and infection (including HIV infection). Thymic cysts can also accompany thymic hyperplasia and thymic neoplasms.

On CT and MRI, thymic cysts typically demonstrate homogeneous attenuation and signal, respectively, along with a well-circumscribed saccular, round, or oval shape, infrequently with rim calcification (calcification is definitively recognizable by CT, not MRI). Thymic cysts do not enhance internally, but they may demonstrate thin, smooth wall enhancement on MRI. Although they may be of water attenuation (Fig. 5.9), they may also be hyperattenuating (Fig. 5.10). A mean attenuation of 23 HU, with attenuation values reaching as high as 61 HU, on CT was reported for a series of thymic cysts that underwent thymectomy, reflecting the frequent presence of proteinaceous or hemorrhagic material in these cysts. Thymic cysts with attenuation values of up to 97 HU have been found. The hyperattenuation of thymic cysts on CT has led to frequent misinterpretation of these lesions on CT as solid and therefore as thymic neoplasms or lymph nodes. On MRI, these lesions may be of low, intermediate, or high T1signal (because of variable serous, proteinaceous, and hemorrhagic content) and are usually markedly T2-hyperintense (isointense to cerebrospinal fluid [CSF]). Postprocessed subtraction after DCE MRI can be quite helpful to discern any enhancing tissue within these thymic lesions from intrinsically T1-hyperintense fluid (see Fig. 5.10). Because thymic cysts can fluctuate in size and attenuation over time, a finding of interval enlargement or increased attenuation of a cyst upon follow-up should not elicit concern that it represents a neoplasm. Provided the lesion exhibits no abnormal enhancing wall thickening, nodularity, or septations on MRI without and with dynamic intravenous (IV) contrast administration and with postprocessed subtraction, it should be considered

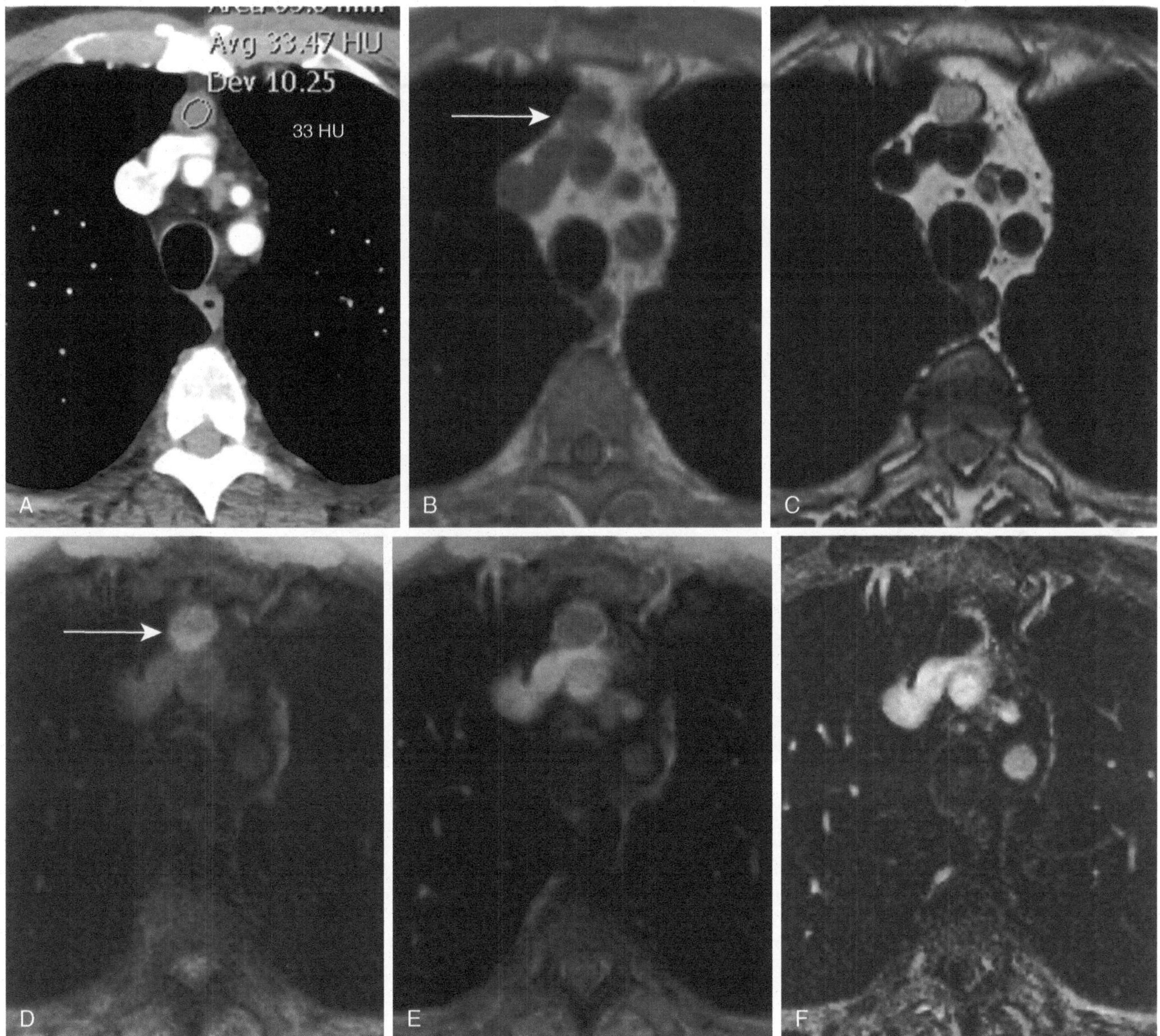

FIGURE 5.10 Thymic cyst, hemorrhagic. **A,** Axial computed tomography scan shows a 33 HU (Hounsfield units), well-circumscribed, ovoid nodule in the thymic bed at risk for being mistaken for a solid thymic neoplasm such as a thymoma. **B** to **F,** Axial T1-weighted, T2-weighted, pre- and postcontrast fat-saturated T1-weighted, and postprocessed subtraction magnetic resonance images, respectively, reveal this lesion to exhibit a fluid–fluid level or hematocrit level on the T1-weighted image *(arrows)*, with T1-hyperintensity dependently and T1-hypointensity anteriorly, suggesting recent spontaneous hemorrhage. This finding, in conjunction with T2-hyperintensity, absence of internal enhancement, and thin, smooth wall enhancement, is consistent with a hemorrhagic thymic cyst. Note that although thymic cysts commonly hemorrhage spontaneously and asymptomatically, fluid–fluid levels are an infrequent finding. The T1-hyperintensity of the cyst fluid, by itself, indicates either proteinaceous or hemorrhagic content.

benign and, if deemed necessary, followed by MRI in 6 to 12 months to confirm continued benign features. If these more complex features are present, then *both* inflammatory and neoplastic cystic thymic lesions, including granulomatous processes, cystic thymoma, and other cystic neoplasms, should be considered.

Thymolipoma. A thymolipoma is a rare, benign, encapsulated, grossly fatty, noninvasive thymic neoplasm containing strands of normal thymic tissue and fibrous septa. Because of their soft, pliable texture, thymolipomas are usually asymptomatic, although patients may present with symptoms related to tumor mass effect. Thymolipomas are often large, conforming to adjacent structures, extending to the cardiophrenic angles, and occupying much of the hemithorax. On CXR, thymolipomas may mimic an enlarged cardiac silhouette, a large pericardial fat pad, lobar collapse, and diaphragmatic elevation. Identification of a macroscopically fatty mass, contiguous with the thymic bed, containing strands of soft tissue attenuation or signal within the mass on CT or MRI is often diagnostic (Fig. 5.11).

Thymic Epithelial Tumors. Thymic epithelial tumors, including both thymoma and thymic carcinoma, demonstrate

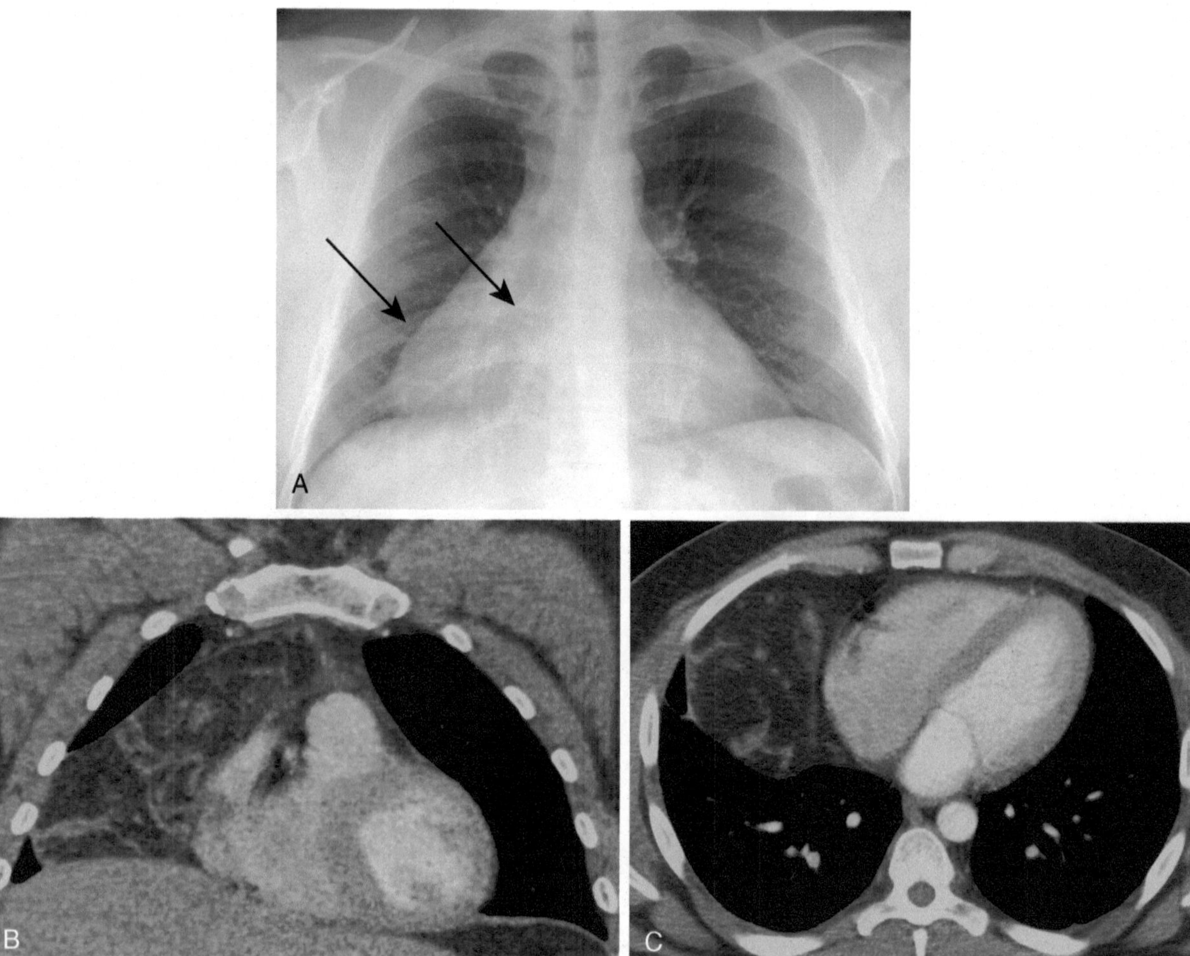

FIGURE 5.11 Thymolipoma. **A,** Posteroanterior radiograph reveals a large, well-circumscribed, fairly lucent, teardrop-shaped (rather than round) mass along the right cardiomediastinal border. **B** and **C,** Coronal and axial computed tomography images show this mass to extend from the thymic bed to the diaphragm, draping around the right cardiomediastinal border, and to be largely comprised of fat, interspersed with strands of soft tissue attenuation. These findings are characteristic of a thymolipoma.

a wide range of histologic features and biological behavior. The 2004 World Health Organization (WHO) classification scheme classifies thymic epithelial tumors based on their cellular morphology and the ratio of lymphocytes to epithelial cells: types A, AB, and B1 are considered low-risk thymomas and types B2 and B3 are considered high-risk thymomas in terms of their prognosis. The 2004 WHO classification discarded the term *type C thymoma* (referred to as thymic carcinoma), which had been in its 1999 classification because the WHO had come to recognize thymic carcinoma as a different entity from thymoma. It is important to be aware that thymomas are often histologically heterogeneous and often contain more than one WHO histologic subtype. Therefore, needle biopsy specimens may not be representative of the most aggressive subtype of the tumor. The Masaoka-Koga clinical staging system, based on surgical findings, is also widely used and better correlates with prognosis or 5-year survival rates after surgical resection than the 2004 WHO classification (Table 5.3).

A classification scheme still used by radiologists divides thymic epithelial tumors into noninvasive thymoma, invasive thymoma, and thymic carcinoma. Noninvasive thymoma is encapsulated and nonaggressive-appearing, but invasive thymoma invades adjacent structures, such as the pericardium, heart and great vessels, pleura, and lung, and may metastasize to the pleura.

TABLE 5.3 **Simplified Version of Masaoka-Koga Staging System for Thymoma**

Stage	Description
I	Encapsulated, noninvasive
II	Capsular invasion
III	Invasion of adjacent organs, including the pericardium, heart and great vessels, and lung
IVA	Pleural or pericardial metastases ("drop metastases")
IVB	Distant metastases

Thymoma is the most common thymic epithelial neoplasm and the most common primary anterior mediastinal neoplasm in adults. Thymoma rarely presents in childhood. A variety of diseases can be seen in association with thymoma, with myasthenia gravis most frequent. Myasthenia gravis affects one third to half of patients with thymoma and 10%

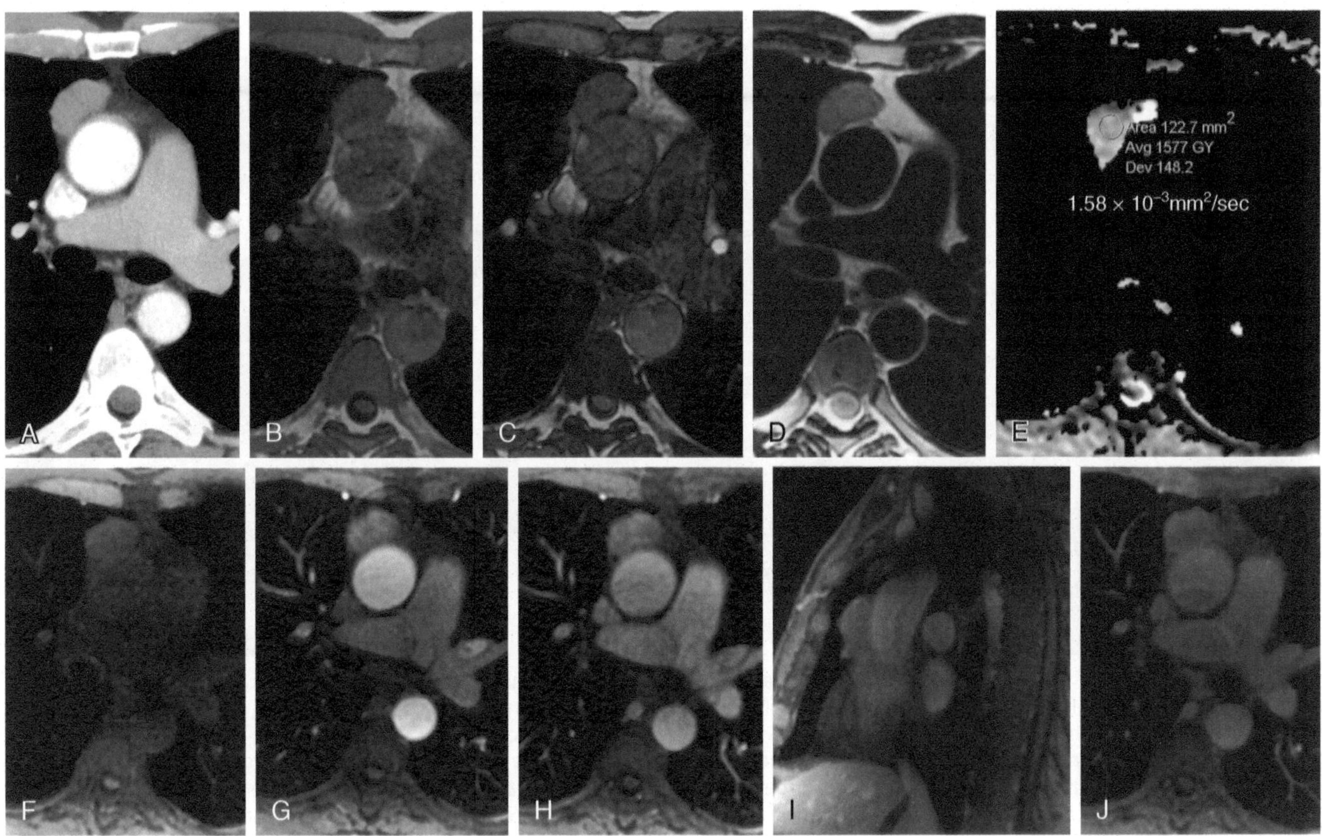

FIGURE 5.12 Thymoma, type AB. **A,** Axial computed tomography scan shows an ovoid, well-circumscribed, off-midline, homogeneous soft tissue attenuation mass in the right thymic bed. **B** and **C,** In- and opposed-phase T1-weighted magnetic resonance images show the lesion to be T1-isointense to muscle and to not suppress, indicating the absence of microscopic fat. **E,** Apparent diffusion coefficient (ADC) map provides an ADC value of 1.6×10^{-3} mm^2/sec, which is fairly typical of low-risk thymomas. Precontrast **(F)** and postcontrast fat-saturated T1-weighted images at 20 seconds **(G)**, 1 minute **(H)**, 3 minutes **(I)**, and 5 minutes **(J)** show qualitative rapid time-to-peak enhancement at 1 minute with partial washout over time, also typical of low-risk thymoma.

to 20% of patients with myasthenia gravis have thymoma. Additional disease entities, such as red blood cell aplasia, hypogammaglobulinemia, rheumatoid arthritis, systemic lupus erythematosus, inflammatory bowel disease, and nonthymic malignancies, can be associated with thymoma.

On CXR, thymoma may present as a prevascular (anterior) mediastinal mass silhouetting anterior mediastinal structures on frontal and lateral projections and as a soft tissue attenuation structure in the retrosternal clear space on the lateral projection. It may occasionally be recognized because of a thickened anterior junction line on frontal CXR as well. Nevertheless, small masses may go undetected on plain radiographs and are better demonstrated on cross-sectional imaging.

On cross-sectional imaging, thymomas typically present as off-midline, round or oval, prevascular masses in the thymic bed, usually without lymphadenopathy or pleural effusion (Fig. 5.12). Calcifications may be present in both early- and advanced-stage thymomas and are not predictive of outcome. More advanced thymomas tend to be more lobulated and heterogeneous in CT attenuation and MR signal; cross midline; exhibit cystic change and necrosis; and invade through the capsule into the adjacent mediastinal fat, pericardium, pleura, lung, and great vessels. Pleural seeding may be detected in the form of nodules and thickening (Fig. 5.13). A pleural effusion is infrequent in invasive and metastatic thymoma and more typical of metastatic adenocarcinoma to the pleura, pleural lymphoma, and mesothelioma.

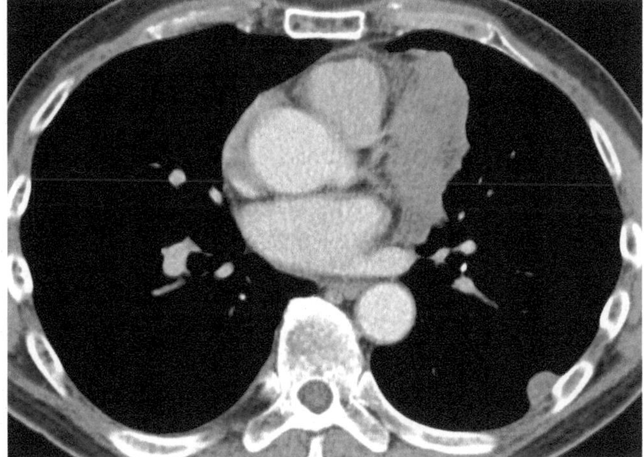

FIGURE 5.13 Thymoma with drop metastasis. Axial chest computed tomography scan with intravenous contrast shows a large, heterogeneous attenuation left prevascular mass and a small left posterolateral pleural nodule *(arrow)*.

On MRI, thymoma is typically intermediate in T1 signal and T2-hyperintense (5-12). In contrast to thymic hyperplasia in adults, which usually exhibits a CSR of 0.7 or less,

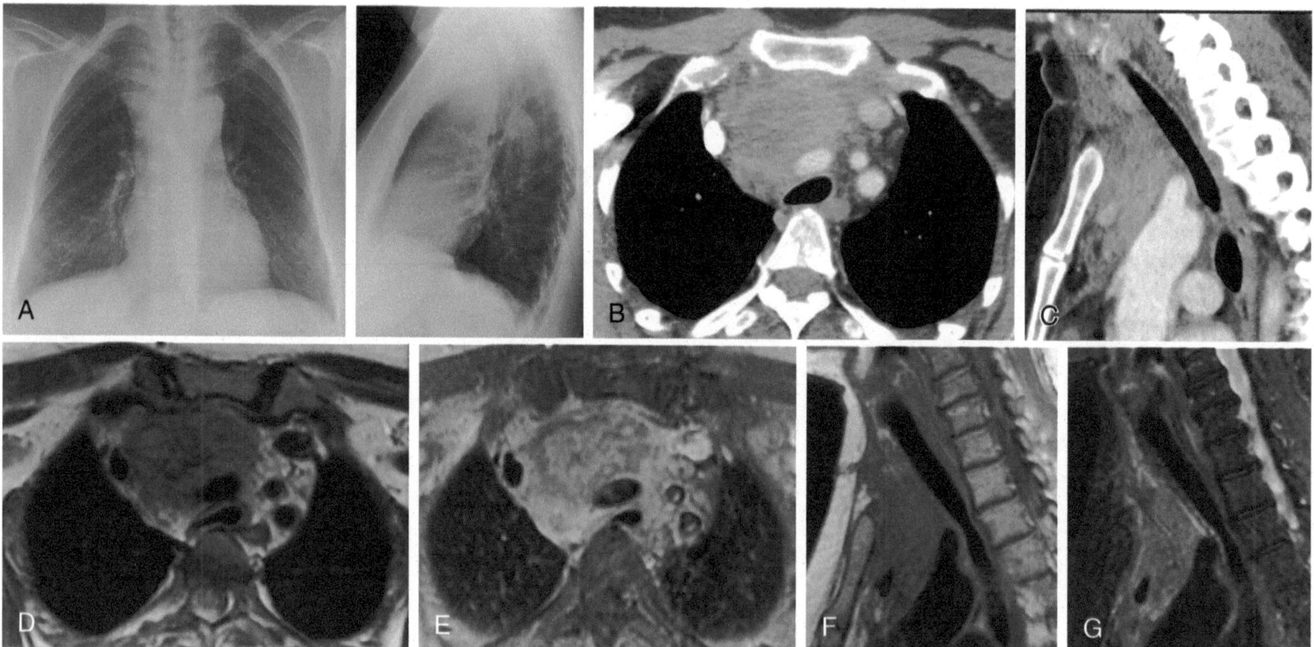

FIGURE 5.14 Thymic carcinoma. **A,** Posteroanterior and lateral radiographs reveal a right paratracheal mass extending anteriorly into and thereby opacifying the upper retrosternal space. **B** and **C,** Axial and sagittal computed tomography image. **D** to **G,** Axial T2-weighted, axial postcontrast, axial T1-weighted, and sagittal precontrast and postcontrast T1-weighted magnetic resonance images show this mass to be centered in the upper right thymic bed and to exhibit ill-defined, irregular contour, amorphous shape, and heterogeneous enhancement. The lesion insinuates between and splays great vessels, retrodisplaces and exerts mass effect on the trachea and esophagus, and tracks upward toward the neck. Its irregular, infiltrative, aggressive appearance somewhat favors thymic carcinoma over high-risk thymoma and makes a low-risk thymoma highly unlikely. The lack of distinct lymphadenopathy elsewhere decreases the likelihood of lymphoma.

the CSR of thymoma is greater than 0.9 because of the absence of microscopic fat in this tumor. MRI offers great advantage in differentiating thymomas from hyperattenuating thymic cysts that mimic solid lesions on CT. Low-risk thymomas tend to exhibit more rapid time to peak enhancement on DCE MRI and less restricted diffusion than high-risk thymomas, thymic carcinoma, and lymphoma.

Thymic carcinoma typically exhibits more irregular, ill-defined margins (Fig. 5.14) and more infiltrative, invasive, and aggressive behavior than thymoma. It often metastasizes to lymph nodes and may metastasize to other sites in the body, including the lung, liver, brain, and bone. Although PET-CT has a limited role in the evaluation of thymic lesions because of overlapping SUVs between normal thymus, thymic hyperplasia, and thymic tumors, SUVs for thymic carcinoma tend to be significantly greater than those of low-risk thymomas.

Thymic Neuroendocrine Tumors. Thymic neuroendocrine tumors, formerly referred to as thymic carcinoid tumors, are rare and are thought to arise from cells of neural crest origin within the thymus. These tumors exhibit more atypia at histology and behave more aggressively than carcinoid tumors within the lung and tracheobronchial tree. Patients may present with endocrine derangements, including Cushing syndrome, syndrome of inappropriate antidiuretic hormone secretion (SIADH), hyperparathyroidism, and multiple endocrine neoplasia types 1 and 2 (MEN1 and MEN2). Approximately 50% of thymic neuroendocrine tumors are invasive at the time of diagnosis and local recurrence is common after resection.

Thymic neuroendocrine tumors tend to demonstrate more irregular margins and more heterogeneous attenuation or signal intensity than low-risk thymomas, manifesting similarly to thymic carcinoma, but can alternatively be round and well circumscribed. Similar to thymic carcinoma, they are more commonly associated with lymphadenopathy and distant metastatic disease than thymomas (Fig. 5.15). Nuclear medicine studies with radiolabeled somatostatin or MIBG (metaiodobenzylguanidine) may show abnormal uptake in these lesions. Although there are no definitive CT or MR imaging features to differentiate thymic neuroendocrine tumors from thymic carcinomas, a coexistent endocrine abnormality may help clinch the diagnosis.

Thyroid Lesions

Thyroid abnormalities account for the majority of thoracic inlet masses in adults and can be both benign and malignant. Most mediastinal masses of thyroid origin represent multinodular thyroid glands or thyroid goiters, which occur primarily in middle-aged and older women. Most are asymptomatic, but some may present with symptoms related to compression of the trachea or esophagus. An enlarged multinodular thyroid gland may extend into the visceral mediastinum, in addition to the prevascular mediastinum, in the right or left paratracheal space, and retrotracheal space.

On CXR, a large thyroid goiter often presents as a substernal or anterior mediastinal mass. Extension posterior to the trachea can occur in up to 25% of cases, resulting in obliteration of the retrotracheal clear space or Raider triangle (Fig. 5.16). If an anterior mediastinal mass demonstrates

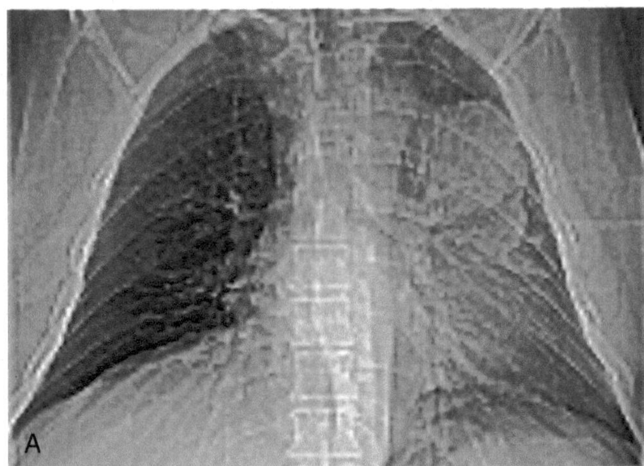

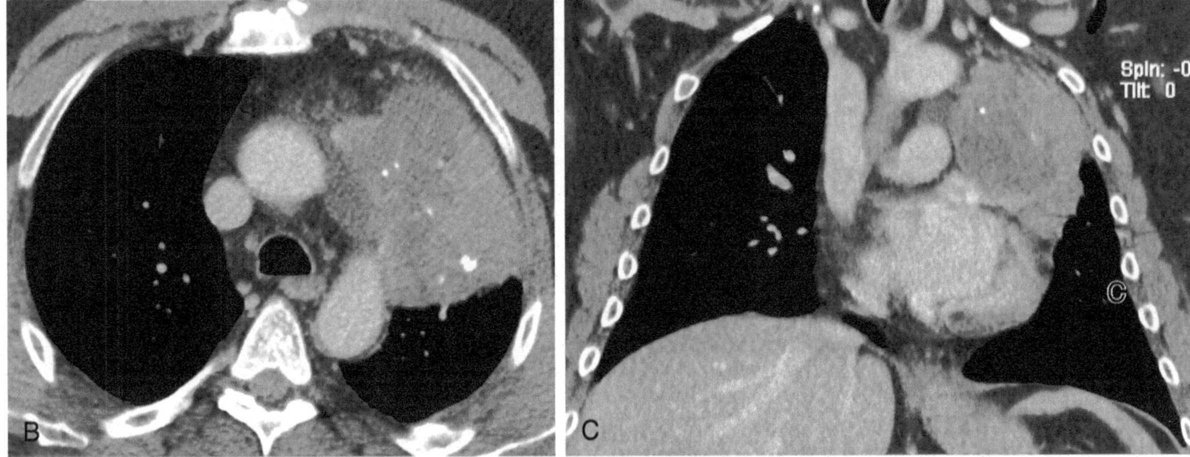

FIGURE 5.15 Thymic neuroendocrine tumor. **A,** Anteroposterior scout view from computed tomography (CT) demonstrates a large, lobulated left prevascular mass silhouetting the left cardiomediastinal border and overlying the left mid-to-upper lung. **B** and **C,** Axial and coronal CT scans show this mass to enhance heterogeneously, with areas of low attenuation that represent necrosis and with scattered coarse calcifications. The mass exhibits a broad base on the pericardium and costal pleura, which neither proves nor excludes the presence of pleuro-pericardial invasion.

continuity with the thyroid gland on cross-sectional imaging, it has likely arisen from the thyroid gland, whether it represents a thyroid goiter or neoplasm. Occasionally, normal and multinodular thyroid tissue is discontinuous with the tissue in the thyroid bed. Unconnected multinodular thyroid tissue is usually isoattenuating to thyroid tissue on CT without and with IV contrast and isointense to thyroid tissue on MRI on all MR pulse sequences, including DCE imaging (see Figure 3.22). In ambiguous cases, a thyroid scan with radioiodine can help confirm the thyroid origin of the unconnected mediastinal component, demonstrating radioiodine uptake in both components.

Mediastinal Lymphoma

Primary mediastinal lymphoma arises from the thymus or from lymph nodes and therefore most typically presents in the prevascular or visceral mediastinum (or both). Lymphoma is generally classified as Hodgkin or non-Hodgkin (Table 5.4), with non-Hodgkin lymphoma the more common of the two. Hodgkin lymphoma most commonly arises in the prevascular mediastinum. An updated staging system for lymphoma is provided in Table 5.5.

On chest radiographs, lymphoma often presents as an anterior mediastinal mass, with widening of the mediastinum on the frontal projection and obliteration of the retrosternal clear space on the lateral projection.

On CT, lymphoma often demonstrates homogeneous soft tissue attenuation; however, it can be of heterogeneous attenuation in the presence of cystic change and necrosis. Calcifications are rare in untreated lymphoma. Extrathoracic lymphadenopathy may be present. Lymphoma can invade the adjacent lung parenchyma and the chest wall (Fig. 5.17). With successful treatment, lymphoma not only decreases in size but also in attenuation on CT, with eventual calcification in some, but not all, cases. On MRI, response to therapy may initially yield increased T2 signal from tumor necrosis and eventually, substantially decreased T2 signal secondary to fibrosis, whether or not calcification develops.

^{18}FDG-PET-CT plays an important role in staging and restaging of lymphoma. Use of whole-body MRI with diffusion-weighted imaging and PET-MRI as an alternative means of serial imaging follow-up for lymphoma will likely increase with time and will reduce ionizing radiation exposure to these patients.

Certain imaging features can help differentiate between mediastinal lymphoma and other anterior mediastinal masses such as thymic epithelial lesions. The finding of a round or oval, well-circumscribed, off-midline mass on CT or MR

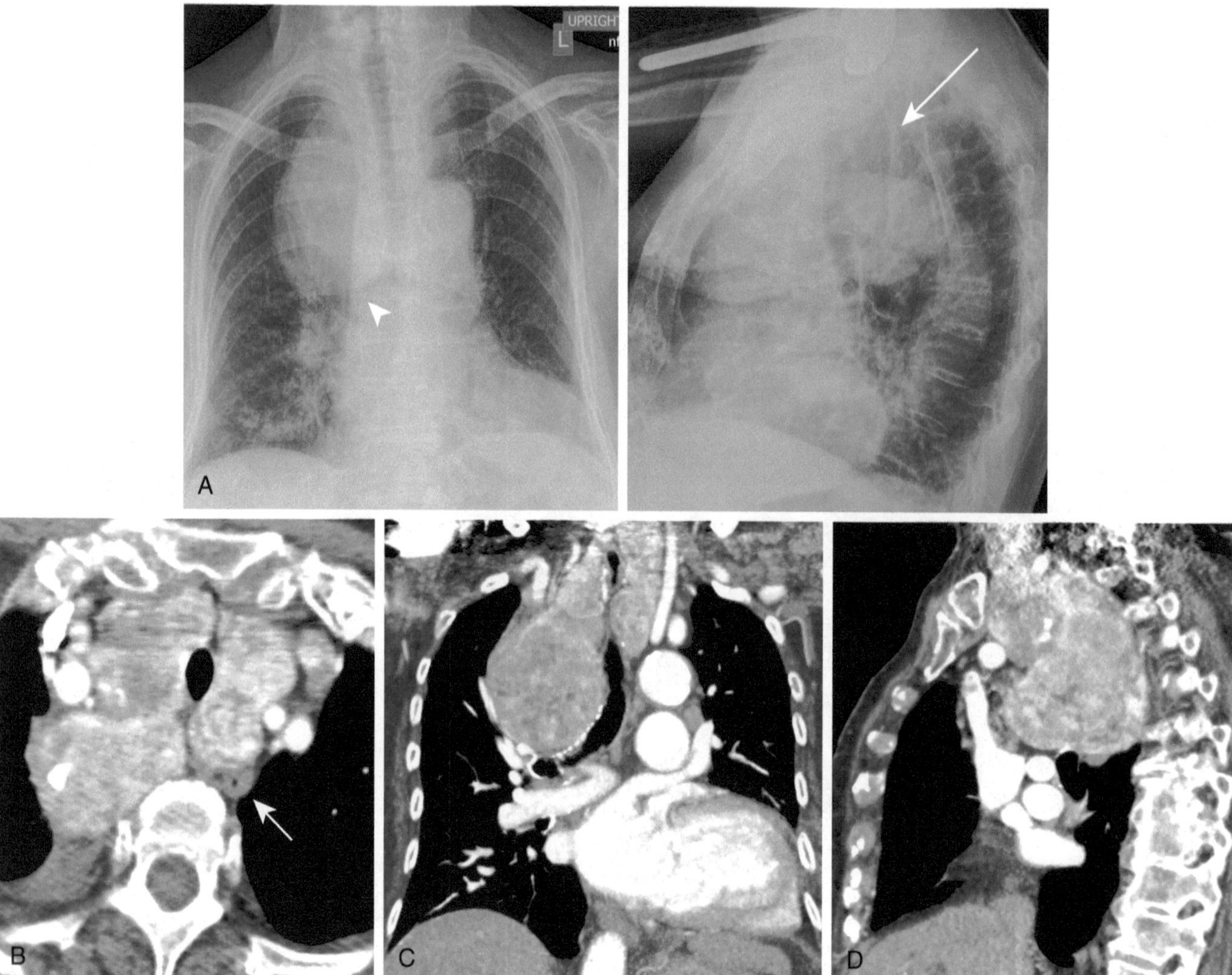

FIGURE 5.16 Substernal thyroid goiter. **A,** Posteroanterior (PA) and lateral radiographs show a large, lobulated prevascular and visceral mediastinal mass widening the right paratracheal stripe on the PA radiograph and overlying the aortic arch on the lateral radiograph. The mass depresses and distorts the right mainstem bronchus *(arrowhead)* and opacifies the retrotracheal space or Raider triangle *(long arrow)*. Axial **(B)**, coronal **(C)**, and sagittal **(D)** computed tomography images reveal this mass to represent a massively enlarged, heterogeneously enhancing, multinodular thyroid gland or goiter, narrowing the trachea and slightly displacing it to the left, laterally displacing great vessels, and displacing the esophagus posteriorly and to the left *(short arrow)*.

TABLE 5.4 Hodgkin Lymphoma Versus Non-Hodgkin Lymphoma

	Hodgkin Lymphoma	Non-Hodgkin Lymphoma
Clinical features	Bimodal age distribution • Young adults • Elderly men	Occurs across all age groups Immunocompromised hosts • Patients with AIDS • Transplant recipients
	Systemic symptoms (B symptoms) common	Older patients may be asymptomatic and require no treatment
	Thoracic involvement in 85% of cases	Thoracic involvement in fewer than 50% of cases at presentation
Radiographic features	Most common location: anterior mediastinum Contiguous involvement of multiple nodal stations	Posterior mediastinal, chest wall, pleural, and lung parenchymal involvement more common than in Hodgkin lymphoma

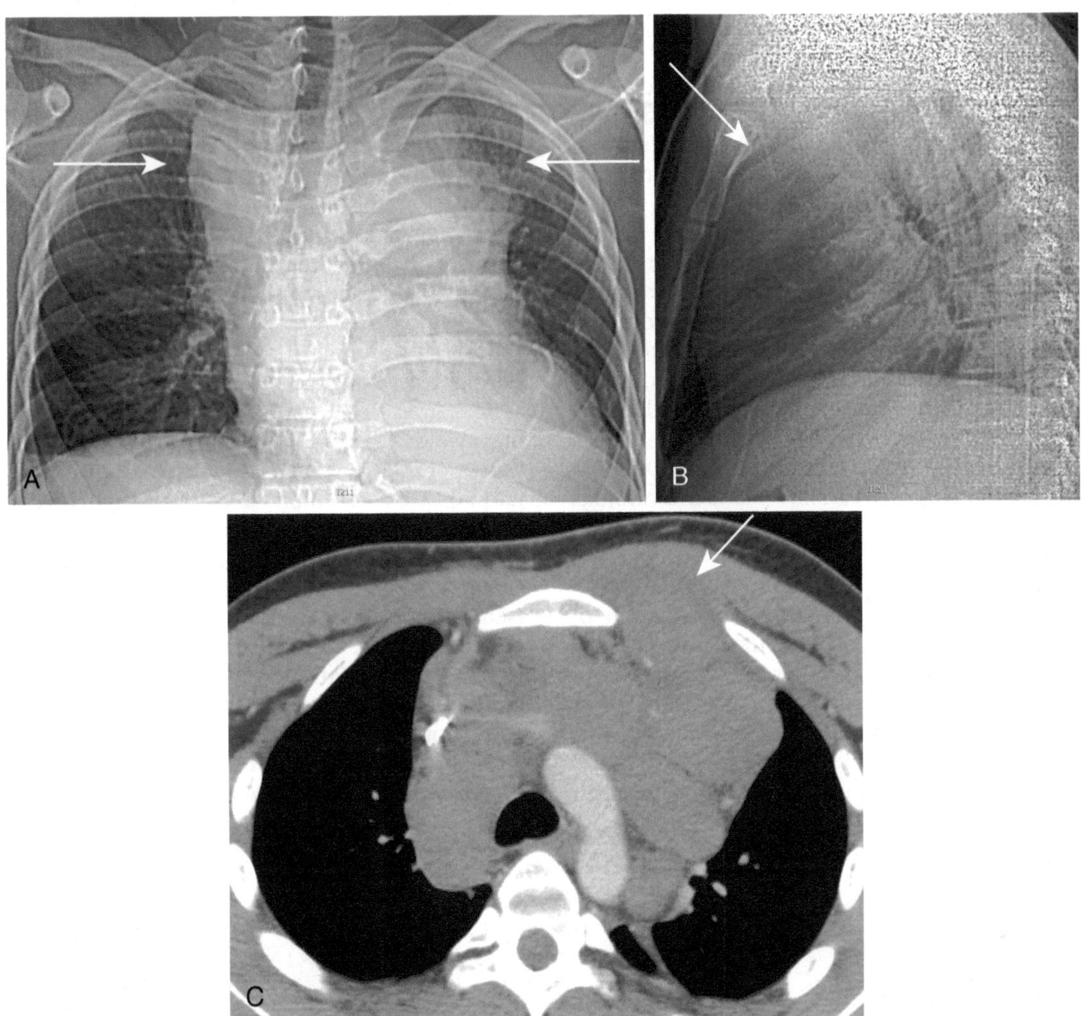

FIGURE 5.17 Lymphoma invading the chest wall (Hodgkin lymphoma). **A** and **B,** Anteroposterior and lateral scout views show a large prevascular mediastinal mass, bilaterally widening the mediastinum *(transverse arrows)*, opacifying the retrosternal clear space *(oblique arrow)*, and retrodisplacing the trachea. **C,** Axial computed tomography image shows a corresponding large, lobulated, multinodular prevascular and visceral mediastinal mass of homogeneous attenuation and near isoattenuation to muscle. There is focal invasion of the chest wall via a left parasternal intercostal space *(arrow)*.

TABLE 5.5 **Revised Staging System for Primary Nodal Lymphomas (Hodgkin and Non-Hodgkin) Based on the 2014 Lugano Classification**

Stage*	Involvement	Extranodal (E) Status
Limited		
Stage I	One node or a group of adjacent nodes	Single extranodal lesion without nodal involvement
Stage II	Two or more nodal groups on the same side of the diaphragm	Stage I or II by nodal extent with limited contiguous extranodal involvement
Stage II bulky†	Stage II, as above, with "bulky" disease	Not applicable
Advanced		
Stage III	Nodes on both sides of the diaphragm or Nodes above the diaphragm with spleen involvement	Not applicable
Stage IV	Additional noncontiguous extralymphatic involvement	Not applicable

*Positron emission tomography computed tomography (CT) is used to determine extent of disease for fluorodeoxyglucose (FDG)-avid lymphomas and CT is used to determine extent of disease for non-FDG-avid lymphomas.

†Definition of "bulky" disease for Hodgkin lymphoma is the largest mass is ≥10 cm in diameter or greater than one third of the transverse thoracic diameter. For non-Hodgkin lymphoma, no consistent definition for bulky disease has been determined. Stage II bulky disease may be treated as limited or advanced, depending on histology and various prognostic factors.

favors thymoma over lymphoma. In contrast, if the mass is lobulated, multinodular, and/or amorphous, and is midline or crosses midline, lymphoma is favored, especially if concurrent lymphadenopathy is present. Additionally, lymphoma is more apt to exert significant mass effect and may involve the pericardium more often than thymoma.

Mediastinal Germ Cell Tumors

Primary germ cell neoplasms arise from rests of primitive germ cells deposited in the mediastinum during their embryonic migration to the urogenital ridge and are less common than thymomas in the anterior mediastinum in adults. The prevascular (anterior) mediastinum is the most common extragonadal site of primary germ cell tumors. Mediastinal germ cell neoplasms may be benign or malignant, with mature teratoma the most common histologic type. Dermoid cysts are a form of mature teratoma. Mature teratomas are often asymptomatic and incidentally discovered as an anterior mediastinal mass on CXR and CT. CT and MR demonstrate a well-circumscribed, heterogeneous attenuation or signal mass that may contain a combination of cystic, soft tissue, fatty, and calcified elements (Fig. 5.18). A fat-fluid level occurs in 10% of cases. Rarely, a tooth is seen. Unlike CT, MR cannot precisely identify calcifications but often shows very low T2 signal at sites of calcification. MR demonstrates not only macroscopic fat with standard T1- and T2-weighted images and fat saturation techniques but can also demonstrate microscopic fat, unlike CT. Microscopic fat within dermoid cysts suppresses on opposed-phase chemical shift gradient-echo images (see Fig. 5.18).

Malignant germ cell tumors are more common in young men. Seminoma is the most common pure histopathologic cell type. Seminomas tend to be more homogeneous in attenuation and signal than nonseminomatous malignant germ cell tumors, and both types may enhance heterogeneously. Malignant germ cell tumors tend to grow rapidly and invade adjacent mediastinal structures.

Pericardiophrenic Masses

Cardiophrenic angle masses present as well-defined opacities silhouetting the heart border on a frontal radiograph and may yield a double density overlying the anteroinferior aspect of the heart on a lateral radiograph. Large pericardial fat pads are a common cause of this radiographic pattern. The differential diagnosis for this finding includes loculated pleural fluid, a pericardial cyst, a Morgagni hernia (see Chapter 7), lymphadenopathy, and a solitary fibrous tumor (whether of pleural or rare mediastinal origin). Thymomas may rarely arise in this location as well (Box 5.1).

Pericardial Fat Pads. Enlarged pericardial fat pads are more common in the setting of obesity, Cushing syndrome, and chronic steroid therapy. Pericardial fat pads are typically more lucent than other cardiophrenic angle masses. *The upper margin of a pericardial fat pad can mimic the*

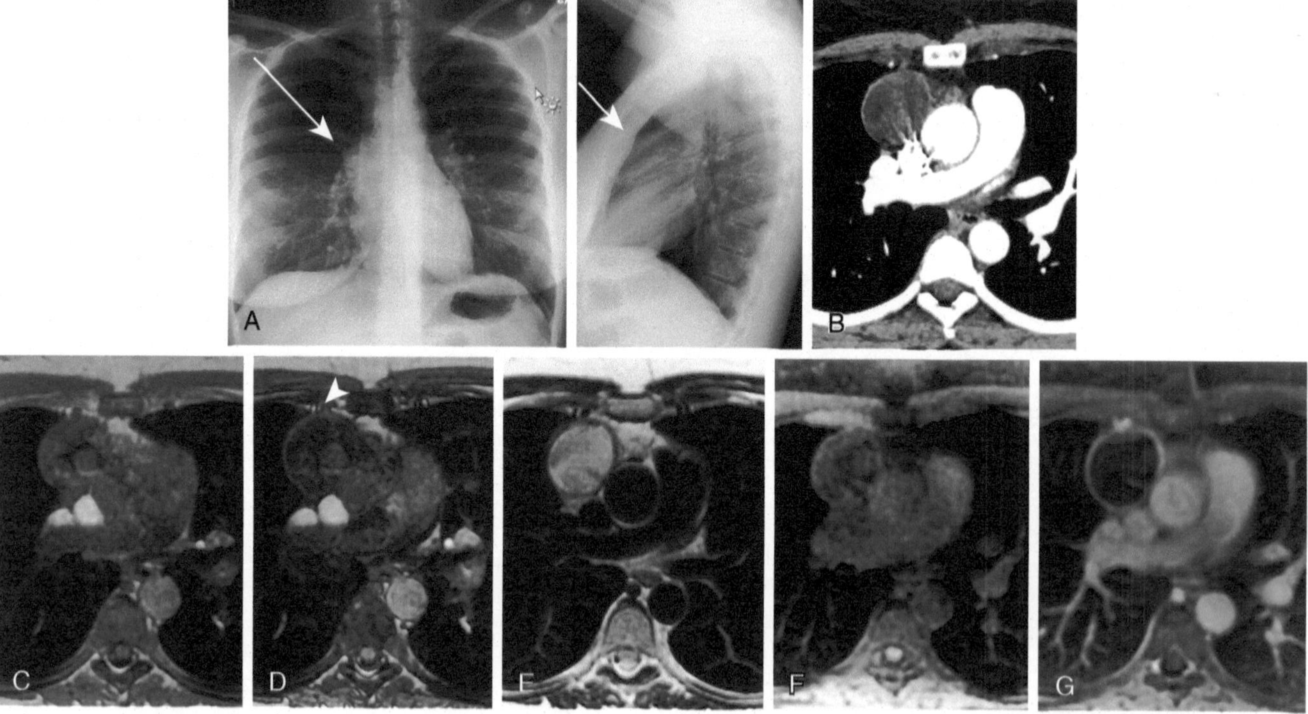

FIGURE 5.18 Mature cystic teratoma. **A,** Posteroanterior and lateral radiographs show a round right prevascular mass *(arrows)* at the level of the mid-hila. **B,** Computed tomography scan shows this mass to be round and well circumscribed, with heterogeneous, isoattenuating, and hypoattenuating content and no gross fat. **C** and **D,** In- and opposed-phase magnetic resonance images show suppression of some internal content on the opposed-phase image, indicating the presence of microscopic fat *(arrowhead)*. **E,** Electrocardiography (ECG)-gated double inversion recovery T2-weighted image shows markedly T2-hyperintense internal content and a smooth, mildly thickened wall. **F** and **G,** Pre- and postcontrast fat-saturated T1-weighted images show smooth wall enhancement and no internal enhancement, aside from that of a septum. The cystic nature of this prevascular mass and its microscopically fatty internal content prove it to be a dermoid cyst or cystic teratoma. Its round, well-circumscribed, largely cystic nature favors a mature, over an immature, teratoma.

meniscus of a pleural effusion on a low-volume, AP portable CXR, particularly on the left. Although CT is diagnostic (Fig. 5.19), a noncontrast MRI with rapid breath-hold sequences such as single-shot fast spin-echo (SSFSE) imaging without and with fat saturation can also diagnose gross fat upon an indeterminate CXR if avoidance of ionizing radiation is sought and there are no old radiographic or CT studies of this area to confirm stability or the presence of fat in this location (see Fig. 3.9).

BOX 5.1 Costophrenic Angle Mass

DIFFERENTIAL DIAGNOSIS

- Prevascular mediastinal mass
  - Pericardial fat pad
  - Pericardial cyst
  - Pericardiophrenic lymphadenopathy
  - Thymic mass
  - Morgagni hernia
- Nonmediastinal mass
  - Pleural mass
    - Loculated pleural fluid
    - Large pleural mass (e.g., solitary fibrous tumor of pleura)
  - Pulmonary mass (e.g., lung cancer)

Pericardial Cysts. Pericardial cysts are congenital, mesothelial-lined cysts or mesothelial cysts that occur in the right cardiophrenic angle. Most are asymptomatic and discovered incidentally on chest radiographs. On CT, pericardial cysts typically demonstrate homogeneous water attenuation, with a thin or imperceptible wall. On MRI, their signal characteristics are therefore those of serous fluid, with homogeneous T1 hypointensity and marked T2 hyperintensity (isointense to CSF) (Fig. 5.20). There is no internal enhancement and occasionally thin smooth wall enhancement of these lesions on MRI.

Pericardiophrenic Lymphadenopathy. Bulky pericardiophrenic lymphadenopathy, generally from lymphoma and metastatic cancer, may also present as a cardiophrenic angle mass on imaging.

Visceral and Middle Mediastinal Masses and Common Vascular Lesions

Lymphadenopathy

Lymphadenopathy is the most common cause of a visceral (middle) mediastinal mass. Common causes include

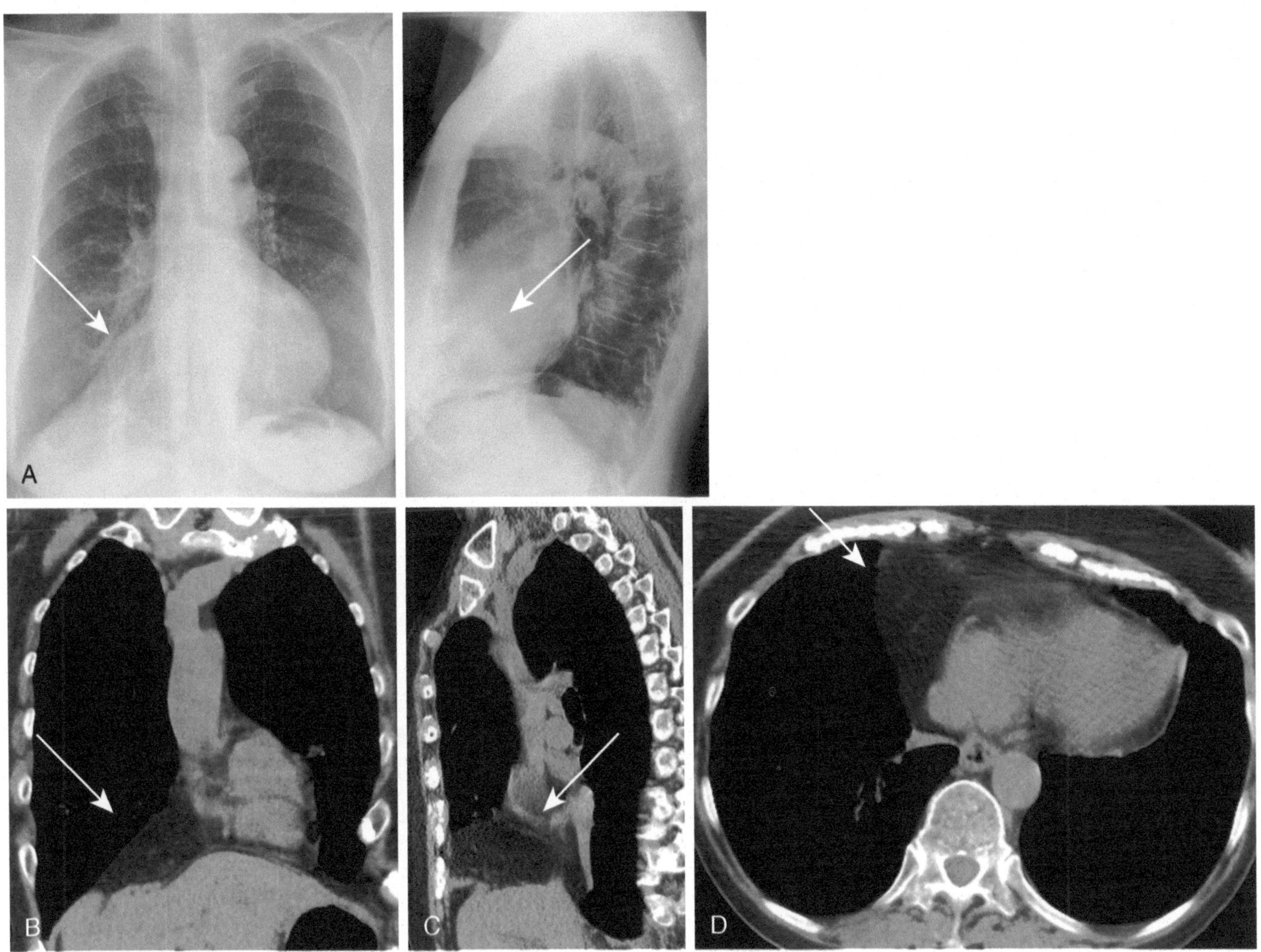

FIGURE 5.19 Pericardial fat pad. **A,** Posteroanterior and lateral radiographs demonstrate a fairly lucent right anterior cardiophrenic angle mass *(arrows)*. Coronal **(B)**, sagittal **(C)**, and axial **(D)** computed tomography images reveal an exclusively fatty attenuation right cardiophrenic angle mass *(arrows)*.

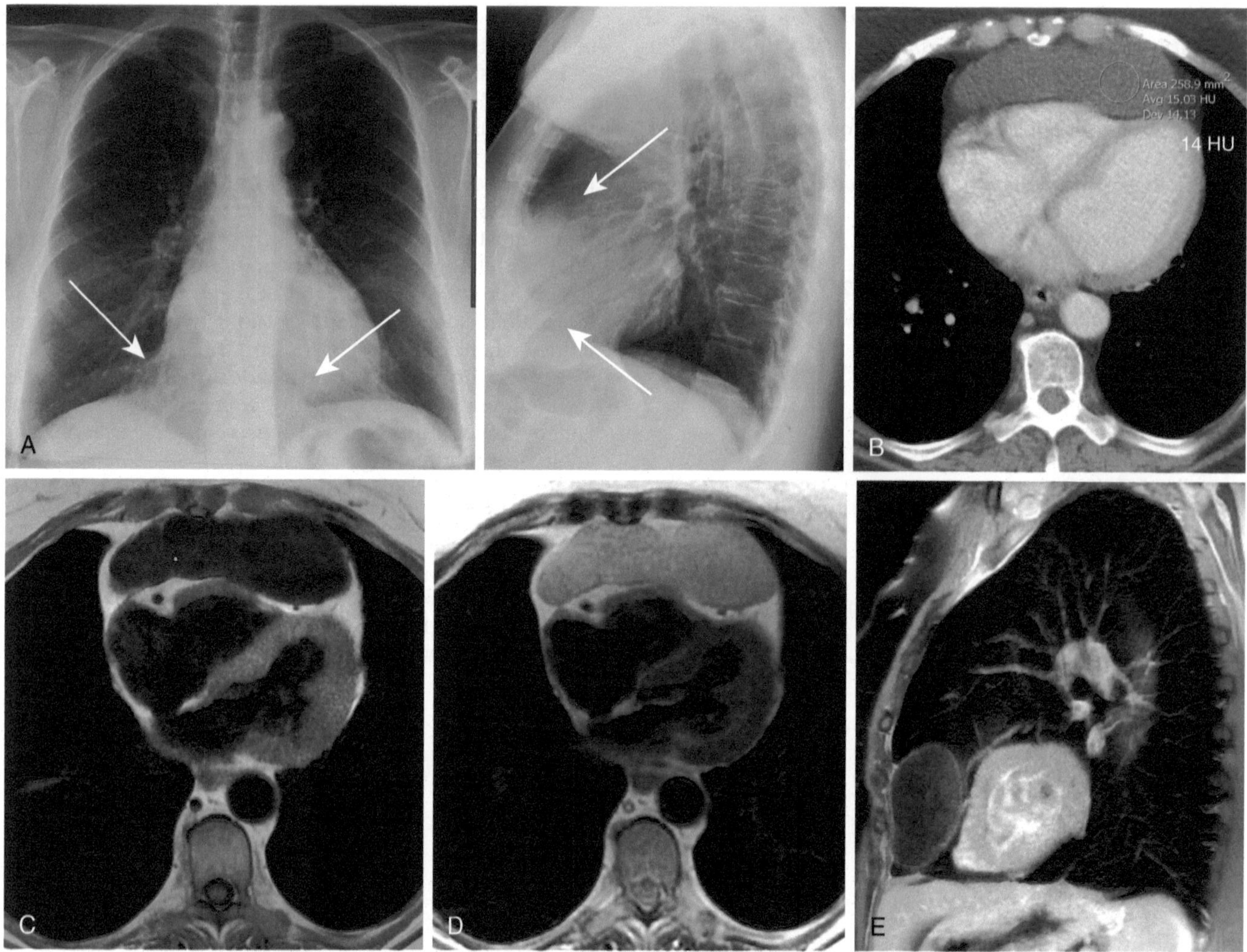

FIGURE 5.20 Pericardial cyst. **A,** Posteroanterior and lateral radiographs show an inferiorly located prevascular mass *(arrows)*. **B,** Axial computed tomography (CT) scan shows this mass to be well circumscribed and of water attenuation (14 Hounsfield units), with a barely perceptible wall. **C** to **E,** Electrocardiography (ECG)-gated axial double inversion recovery T1-weighted and T2-weighted and sagittal postcontrast T1-weighted MR images show this lesion to be uniformly T1-hypointense and T2-hyperintense, with no internal enhancement. There is thin, smooth wall enhancement and no internal lesion complexity (no wall irregularity, wall thickening, nodules, or septations). The CT and MRI findings prove this lesion to represent a simple cyst, whether a pericardial cyst or unilocular lymphangioma, with the former more common in adults, particularly in this location. This lesion was excised and pathologically proven to be a pericardial cyst.

neoplastic (lymphoproliferative and metastatic), infectious, and inflammatory entities. Chronic heart failure is also a common, underrecognized cause of mediastinal lymphadenopathy (Box 5.2). Typically, lymphadenopathy manifests as multiple well-circumscribed nodules or masses at several lymph nodal stations (e.g., AP window, paratracheal, and subcarinal). See Chapter 24 for more details regarding lymph node station nomenclature.

On CXR, common presentations of mediastinal lymphadenopathy include a thickened right paratracheal stripe (Fig. 5.21), an abnormal bulging contour to the AP window, abnormal rightward convexity of the azygoesophageal recess, and soft tissue fullness in the infrahilar window or subcarinal space on the lateral radiograph.

Computed tomography and MRI offer improved detection and characterization of mediastinal lymph nodes, which often demonstrate homogeneous soft tissue attenuation or signal, excluding their fatty hila. Nevertheless, the attenuation and signal of lymph nodes may be heterogeneous because of pathology, and some of their features may help narrow the differential diagnosis. For example, densely calcified lymph nodes may reflect prior granulomatous disease, such as tuberculosis or endemic fungal infections (notably histoplasmosis). Peripheral calcification, often referred to as eggshell calcification, may be seen in pneumoconioses such as silicosis and coal workers pneumoconiosis, sarcoidosis, histoplasmosis, blastomycosis, amyloidosis, and treated Hodgkin disease. Lymph nodal calcifications in sarcoidosis and these other entities may alternatively be more central. Lymphadenopathy in patients with anthrax may demonstrate characteristic high attenuation on CT because of hemorrhage. Lymph nodes with central low attenuation may reflect necrosis, which can be seen in tuberculosis and nontuberculous mycobacterial infections and in necrotic metastatic disease. Low attenuation and fatty lymph nodes have been described in patients with

BOX 5.2 Mediastinal Lymphadenopathy

DIFFERENTIAL DIAGNOSIS

- Reactive
  - Infection
  - Inflammation (e.g., interstitial lung disease)
- Edematous lymph nodes (e.g., congestive heart failure)
- Granulomatous disease
  - Sarcoidosis
  - BeryIliosis
  - Silicosis and other pneumoconioses
  - Histoplasmosis
  - Tuberculosis
- Lymphoproliferative disease
  - Lymphoma
  - Chronic lymphocytic leukemia
  - Castleman disease
  - Kaposi sarcoma
- Primary lung cancer
- Metastatic disease
  - Lung cancer
  - Breast cancer
  - Renal cancer
  - Thyroid cancer
  - Esophageal cancer
  - Colon cancer
  - Melanoma
- Drug therapy (e.g., phenytoin)

Whipple disease. Hypervascular lymph nodal metastases, such as those from melanoma, renal cell carcinoma, thyroid carcinoma, and Kaposi sarcoma, often demonstrate avid enhancement on postcontrast CT and MR. The differential diagnosis for hyperenhancing lymph nodes also includes Castleman disease (Fig. 5.22). Unlike CT, all lymph nodes, including benign and reactive lymph nodes, appreciably enhance to some degree on MRI. This trait of normal lymph nodes is perceptible on MRI because of its higher soft tissue contrast than CT.

Magnetic resonance imaging can also demonstrate lymph nodal size, morphology, distribution, and necrosis. T2-weighted MRI may also be used to help differentiate sarcoidosis-related lymphadenopathy from lymphoma. If patchy low T2 signal is demonstrated within the lymphadenopathy, the so-called dark lymph node sign, it infers the presence of fibrosis or calcification within these lymph nodes and strongly favors sarcoidosis, or at least a fibrotic or granulomatous process, over untreated lymphoma (see Chapter 3 and Fig. 3.13). In response to treatment, lymphomatous lymphadenopathy will drop in T2 signal as it fibroses or becomes calcified. Normal lymph nodes are at least mildly T2-hyperintense. Cystic or necrotic components of lymph nodes demonstrate even higher T2 signal, as do malignant lymph nodes. Both benign and malignant lymph nodes may restrict diffusion on diffusion-weighted MRI.

Congenital-Developmental Cysts

Congenital middle mediastinal cysts include foregut duplication cysts (e.g., bronchogenic cysts and esophageal duplication cysts) and pleuropericardial or mesothelial cysts.

Bronchogenic cysts result from abnormal budding or branching of the tracheobronchial tree during embryogenesis and are therefore lined with pseudostriated columnar respiratory epithelium. They most commonly occur in the visceral mediastinum, near the carina, classically in the subcarinal and right paratracheal spaces, although they may very rarely occur within the lung parenchyma and pleura. Clinical manifestations of bronchogenic cysts are variable, from asymptomatic to chest pain, cough, dyspnea, fever, and sputum production. When complicated by infection or hemorrhage, they may rapidly enlarge and become symptomatic. They may alternatively slowly enlarge over time and eventually exert mass effect on adjacent mediastinal structures. Esophageal duplication cysts occur along the esophagus and may be more oblong and vertically-oriented than bronchogenic cysts. The smooth wall of esophageal duplication cysts may also be slightly thicker on account of greater smooth muscle content. Histopathology is needed for definitive distinction.

On chest radiographs, mediastinal cysts typically manifest as sharply marginated round masses. On CT, these appear as well-demarcated round or oval cystic lesions of variable but typically homogeneous attenuation (0–100 HU), with smooth, thin, or imperceptible walls. Their attenuation varies with fluid composition, increasing in the presence of proteinaceous and hemorrhagic content and in the presence of calcium oxalate. When infected, the cyst may become air-filled or demonstrate an air–fluid level. MRI is superior to CT for differentiating cystic from solid mediastinal lesions. Benign mediastinal cysts are of variable T1-intensity, depending on fluid composition, and are homogeneously and markedly T2-hyperintense. The presence of serous content yields T1-hypointensity, and the presence of proteinaceous or hemorrhagic content yields intermediate to high T1 signal (Fig. 5.23). Benign mediastinal cysts may exhibit smooth thin wall enhancement on MRI; however, they should not manifest enhancing, irregular mural thickening, nodularity, or septations unless they are or have been inflamed or infected.

Tracheal Lesions

See Chapter 6.

Esophageal Lesions

Esophageal lesions, when sufficiently large, present as visceral mediastinal masses.

Achalasia. Achalasia is a primary dysmotility disorder of the esophagus, resulting in a diffusely aperistaltic esophagus distended with retained food contents, secretions, and air. On CXR, achalasia may manifest as a wide, cylindrical middle mediastinal mass traversing the thorax craniocaudally, an abnormal rightward convexity of the azygoesophageal recess, and a thickened tracheoesophageal stripe on the lateral projection. An air–fluid level within the mass and the absence of air in the expected location of the stomach bubble strongly suggest achalasia (Fig. 5.24). A barium swallow typically demonstrates an aperistaltic, markedly dilated esophagus with a characteristic "bird beak" appearance to the distal esophagus. It is always important to consider the possibility of *secondary* achalasia, which can result from distal esophageal obstruction by tumor.

Esophagitis. Esophagitis is a common cause of noncardiac chest pain. Its causes include gastroesophageal reflux disease, caustic ingestion, infection, radiation, and certain medications and foods. Barium esophagography and upper endoscopy are the preferred diagnostic modalities, although CT may be performed in the workup of

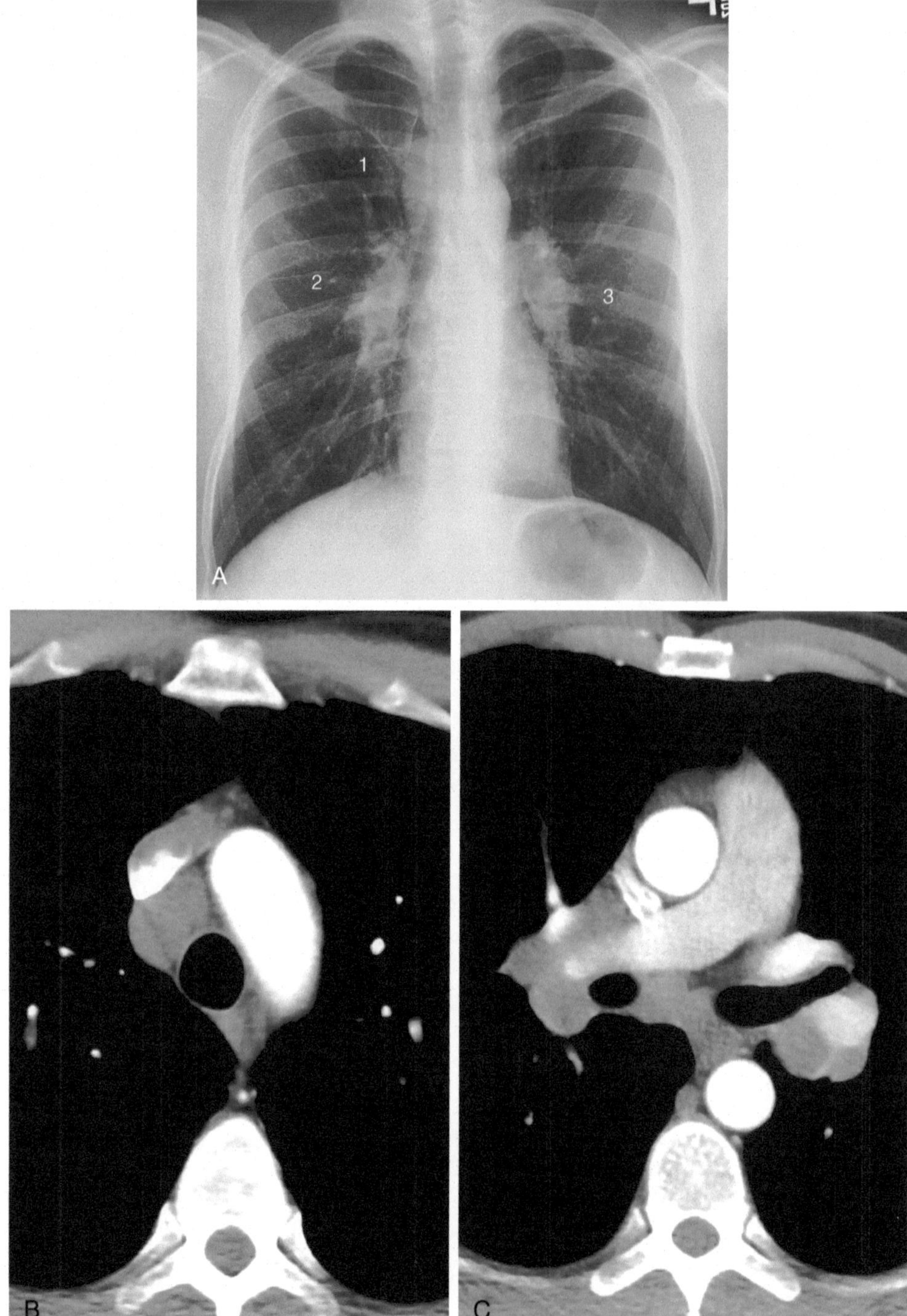

FIGURE 5.21 Lymphadenopathy, sarcoidosis. **A,** Posteroanterior radiograph reveals enlarged, lobulated hila and low right paratracheal soft tissue fullness, compatible with lymphadenopathy and representing the "1-2-3 sign" of sarcoidosis. **B** and **C,** Two axial computed tomography levels show low right paratracheal and bilateral hilar lymphadenopathy.

atypical chest pain or when a complication is suspected. Diffuse esophageal wall thickening, mural edema, and mucosal hyperenhancement may be seen on CT and MRI in cases of severe esophagitis.

Esophageal Injury. Esophageal injury ranges from non-transmural mucosal laceration (Mallory-Weiss tear), intramural dissection, and intramural hematoma to transmural perforation. The latter has a high mortality rate. Causes of esophageal perforation include surgery or instrumentation (e.g., endoscopy) (Fig. 5.25), foreign body impaction, violent and forceful vomiting and retching (Boerhaave syndrome), caustic ingestion, barotrauma, thermal injury related to pulmonary venous ablation for atrial fibrillation, and esophageal malignancy. The left posterolateral wall of the distal third of the esophagus is the most common site of spontaneous esophageal rupture. Esophageal rupture classically results in pneumomediastinum (Fig. 5.26), a left pleural effusion, and cervical and chest wall subcutaneous

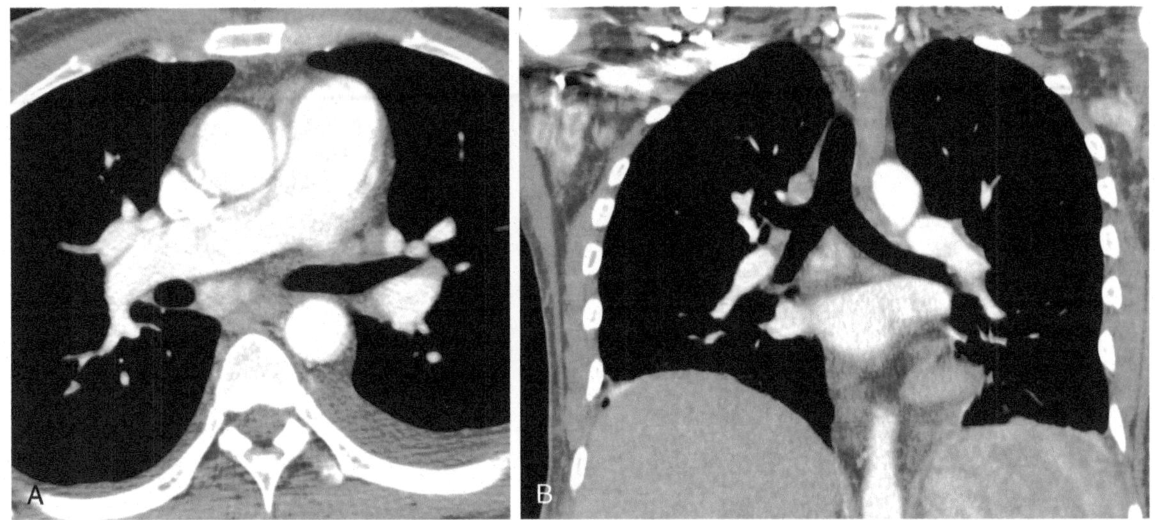

FIGURE 5.22 Lymphadenopathy, Castleman disease. Axial **(A)** and coronal **(B)** computed tomography images show hyperenhancing subcarinal and bilateral axillary lymphadenopathy. Small bilateral layering pleural effusions are also visible on the axial image.

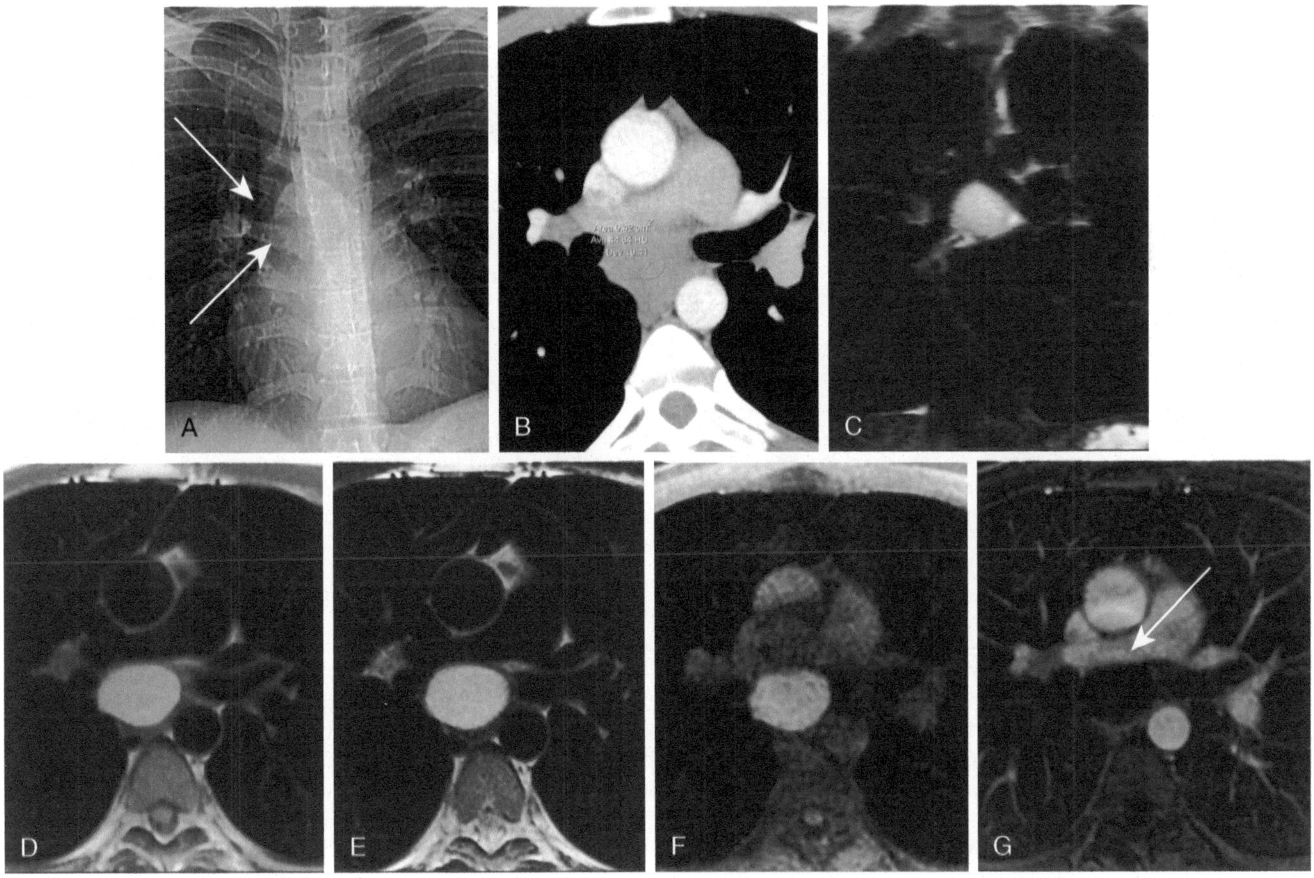

FIGURE 5.23 Bronchogenic cyst. **A,** Anteroposterior computed tomography (CT) scan shows splaying of the mainstem bronchi by a round visceral mediastinal mass *(arrow)*. **B,** Axial CT scan shows a 45 HU mass, which may be cystic or solid, in the subcarinal space. Coronal T2-weighted **(C)**, axial T1-weighted **(D)**, axial T2-weighted **(E)**, and precontrast **(F)** fat-saturated T1-weighted magnetic resonance images reveal this mass to be ovoid, well-circumscribed, and markedly and homogeneously T1- and T2-hyperintense. **G,** Postcontrast, fat-saturated, subtracted MRI reveals no internal enhancement of this lesion *(arrow)*, which therefore likely represents a foregut duplication cyst. The apparent asymmetric wall enhancement of this lesion is due to slight shift in location of structures between the pre- and postcontrast images or "misregistration" upon subtraction. A bronchogenic cyst was confirmed at surgical resection.

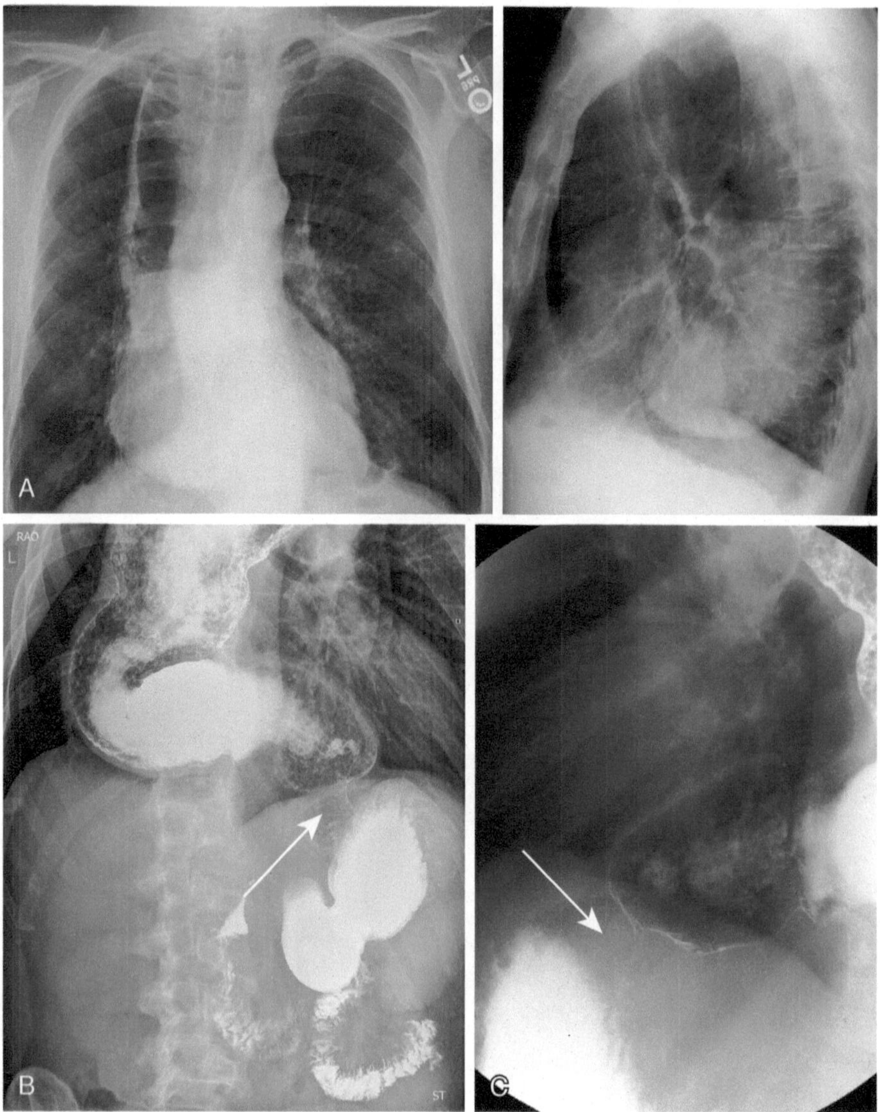

FIGURE 5.24 Achalasia. **A,** Posteroanterior and lateral radiographs show massive, diffuse dilation of the air–fluid-level–containing esophagus throughout its course in the visceral mediastinum. **B** and **C,** Fluorographic image centered at the gastroesophageal junction and subsequent coned-down and magnified image acquired during esophagography reveal oral contrast outlining this diffuse esophageal dilation the latter terminating immediately above a focal beak-like narrowing *(arrow)* of the distal esophagus. Although these findings strongly support the diagnosis of achalasia, the possibility of obstruction secondary to tumor or secondary achalasia must be excluded.

emphysema. When esophageal perforation is suspected, an esophagram is often the study of choice. It is generally performed with isoosmolar or low-osmolar water-soluble oral contrast because of its rapid clearance. Extraluminal contrast leakage is diagnostic. On CT, esophageal wall thickening with extraluminal foci of air and oral contrast material may be seen (see Figs. 5.25 and 5.26). If no extraluminal contrast leak is demonstrated with these isoosmolar or low-osmolar contrast agents, then barium can be administered to increase sensitivity for detection of a small tear.

Esophageal Diverticula. An esophageal diverticulum is a focal outpouching arising from the esophagus. There are three main types, classified based on the location.

Upper esophageal diverticula include the Zenker diverticulum and the Killian-Jamieson diverticulum. A Zenker diverticulum is technically a pulsion pseudodiverticulum and arises posteriorly from the hypopharyngeal midline just above the cricopharyngeus muscle and uppermost esophagus, at the C4–5 or C5–6 level. This is to be distinguished from a Killian-Jamieson diverticulum, which arises below the cricopharyngeal muscle and is often anterolateral in location. Although patients with a Zenker diverticulum may present with dysphagia, halitosis, and regurgitation of food particles, the Killian-Jamieson diverticulum is usually smaller and asymptomatic. Barium esophagography is the diagnostic modality of choice for diagnosing a Zenker diverticulum; this focal outpouching is best demonstrated during swallowing on the lateral projection (Fig. 5.27). Chest CT may demonstrate a focal outpouching with an air-fluid level posterior to the uppermost esophagus.

Middle esophageal diverticula can be divided in to traction diverticula and pulsion diverticula. A traction diverticulum is a true diverticulum, which often occurs because

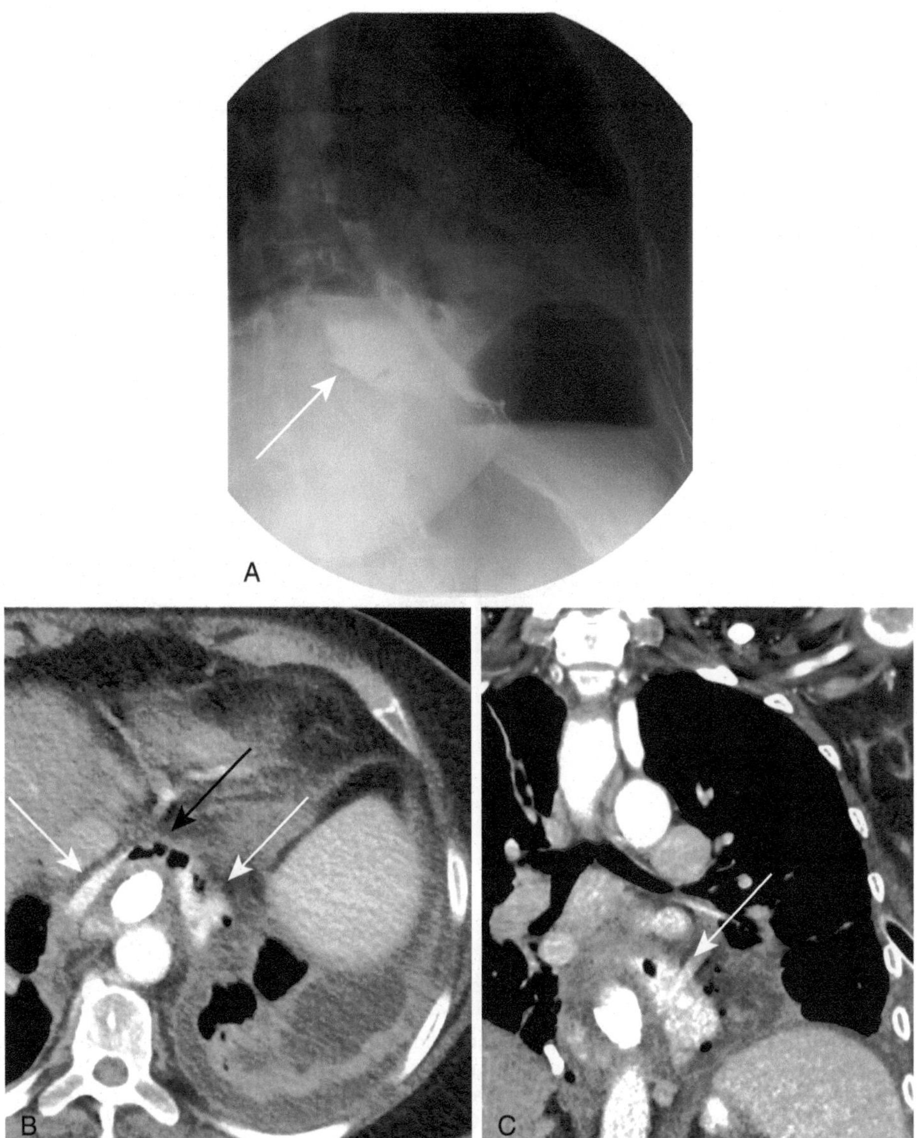

FIGURE 5.25 Iatrogenic esophageal perforation by upper endoscopy. **A,** Fluoroscopic spot image of leaked contrast *(arrow)* along the posterior aspect of the oral contrast-opacified esophagus. **B** and **C,** Axial and coronal computed tomography images show extraluminal contrast leakage *(white arrows)* adjacent to the distal esophagus *(black arrow)*. A left pleural effusion and partial left lower lobe atelectasis are also present. The fat planes are obliterated by fluid and inflammation.

of postinflammatory scarring and fibrosis retracting the esophageal wall, for example, in the setting of tuberculous adenitis and histoplasmosis. A pulsion diverticulum is a false diverticulum and occurs secondary to abnormally increased intraluminal pressure in the esophagus, resulting in herniation of the mucosal and submucosal layers through the muscularis.

Lower esophageal or epiphrenic diverticula are typically pulsion diverticula, often related to esophageal dysmotility. They are located just proximal to the lower esophageal sphincter and most often arise from the right posterolateral wall of the esophagus. Barium esophagography with single-contrast technique is the modality of choice in demonstrating the abnormal focal outpouching and in assessing for any associated esophageal motility disorders and hiatal hernia.

Esophageal Varices. Esophageal and paraesophageal varices most often develop in the setting of portal hypertension and typically occur in or along the lower third of the esophagus because veins in this esophageal segment drain via the left gastric vein into the portal vein, unlike the veins in the upper two-thirds of the esophagus, which drain via the azygous vein into the superior vena cava (SVC). On contrast-enhanced CT and MRI, these dilated vessels may be visible within the wall of the esophagus or along the esophagus, respectively.

Hiatal Hernia. A hiatal hernia results from passage of the stomach into the thorax through the esophageal hiatus. It is divided into sliding and paraesophageal subtypes, with the latter carrying a higher risk of potential complication. A paraesophageal hernia is defined as one in which at least some of the stomach and occasionally

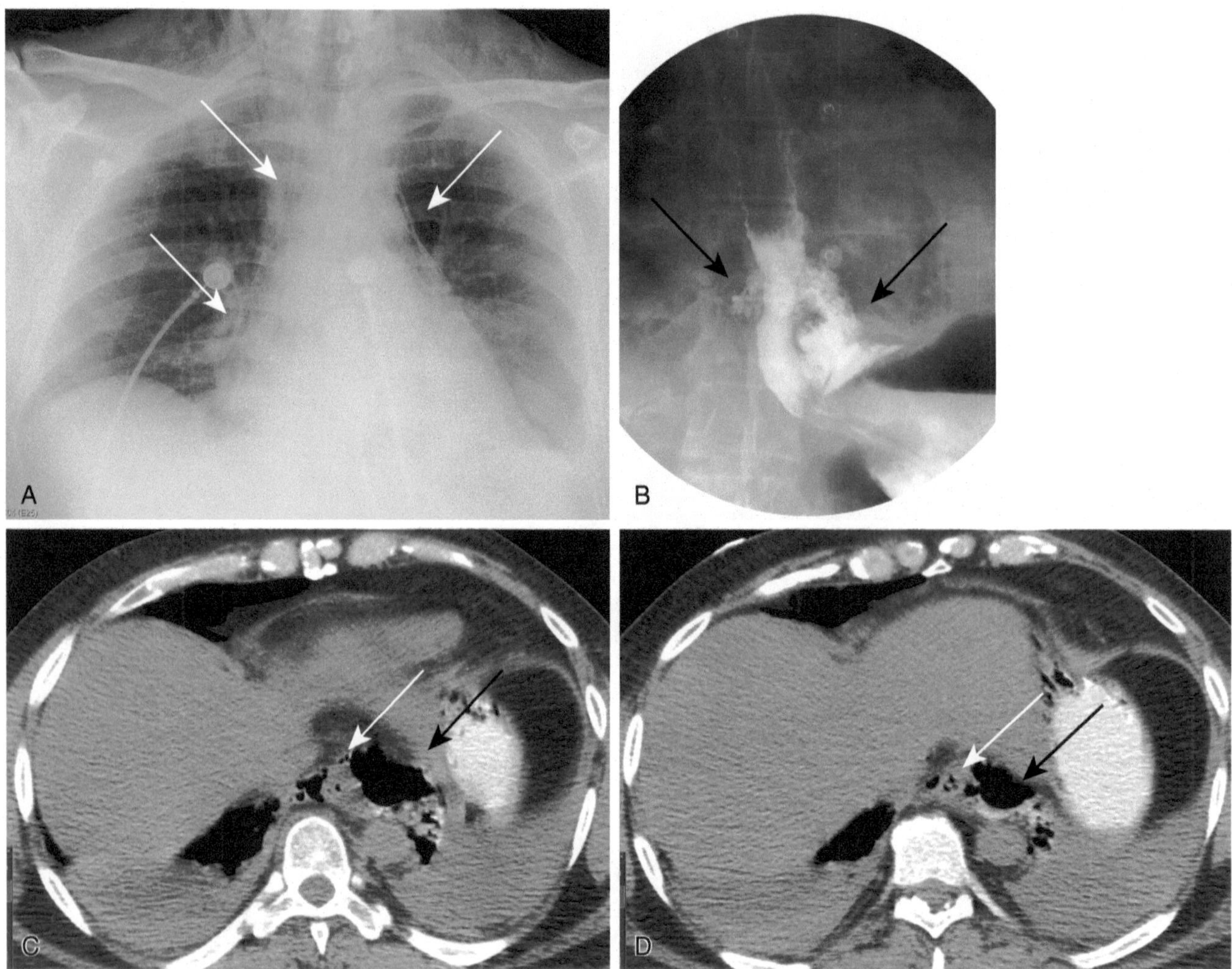

FIGURE 5.26 Boerhaave syndrome. **A,** Anteroposterior radiograph shows bilateral streaky lucencies along the heart and mediastinum representing pneumomediastinum *(white arrows).* There is bilateral subcutaneous emphysema in the neck. **B,** Fluoroscopic spot image from an esophagram shows leakage of oral contrast *(black arrows)* along both sides of the air- and contrast-filled distal esophagus. **C** and **D,** Axial computed tomography images demonstrate bilateral leakage of contrast and air *(black arrows)* along the esophagus *(white arrows).* Pneumomediastinum almost completely outlines the slightly thickened esophageal wall in *C* and partially outlines the esophageal wall in *D,* with the latter representing the suspected level of perforation. There are bilateral mixed attenuation pleural effusions, with the mixed attenuation either due to hemorrhage or spilled ingested material.

additional abdominal contents herniate upward into the chest next to the esophagus rather than simply below it. A true paraesophageal hernia is rare and requires that the gastroesophageal junction (GEJ) remains in its usual place. Usually paraesophageal hernias are a mixture of sliding hiatal and paraesophageal hernias, with the GEJ elevated. When moderate in size, a hiatal hernia typically presents as a retrocardiac opacity, often causing a focal dextroconvex bulge of the inferior aspect of the azygoesophageal line. An air-fluid level within this bulging tissue is virtually diagnostic (Fig. 5.28). A single-contrast barium esophagram or an air-contrast upper GI series can be performed for confirmation. This finding is readily visible by CT and MRI.

Esophageal Neoplasms. Leiomyomas are the most common benign tumors of the esophagus and are intramural rather than mucosal in origin. These lesions may therefore be difficult to detect by upper endoscopy and by esophagography, although an intramural and rarely an exophytic lesion may be inferred by its mass effect, with resultant distortion of the oral contrast column on esophagography. On CT, these tumors usually manifest as homogeneous soft tissue attenuation, round, well-circumscribed exophytic lesions and may mimic adjacent lymphadenopathy and hyperattenuating foregut duplication cysts. Leiomyomas are occasionally cystic. MRI can differentiate between these lesions because leiomyomas tend to be of intermediate to low T2 signal secondary to their tightly bundled smooth muscle fascicles (Fig. 5.29). Lymph nodes tend to be at least mildly T2-hyperintense, and foregut duplication cysts are usually markedly T2-hyperintense. The higher soft tissue contrast of MR may also better demonstrate whether a lesion is truly arising from the esophageal wall or simply next to it.

Malignant esophageal neoplasms are more common in older men and are associated with alcohol use disorder and smoking. Patients may present with dysphagia. CXR may show an air-fluid level in the esophagus caused by distal

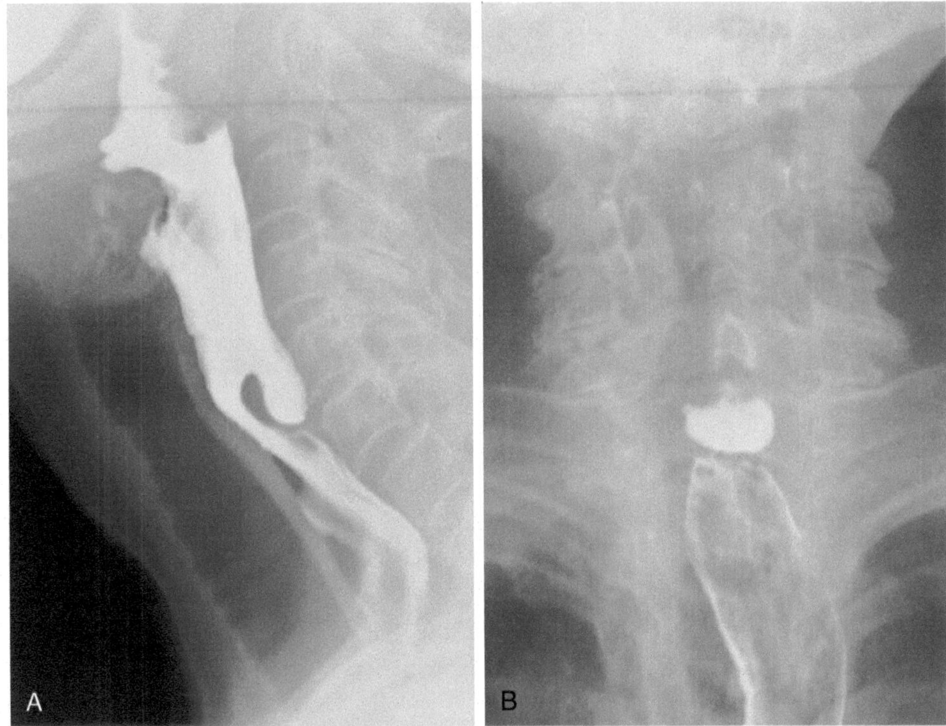

FIGURE 5.27 Zenker diverticulum. Lateral **(A)** and anteroposterior (AP) **(B)** fluoroscopic images during esophagography reveal oral contrast passing into a posterior outpouching at the C5 level, which represents a Zenker diverticulum. Oral contrast is shown to linger in this diverticulum on the AP spot view.

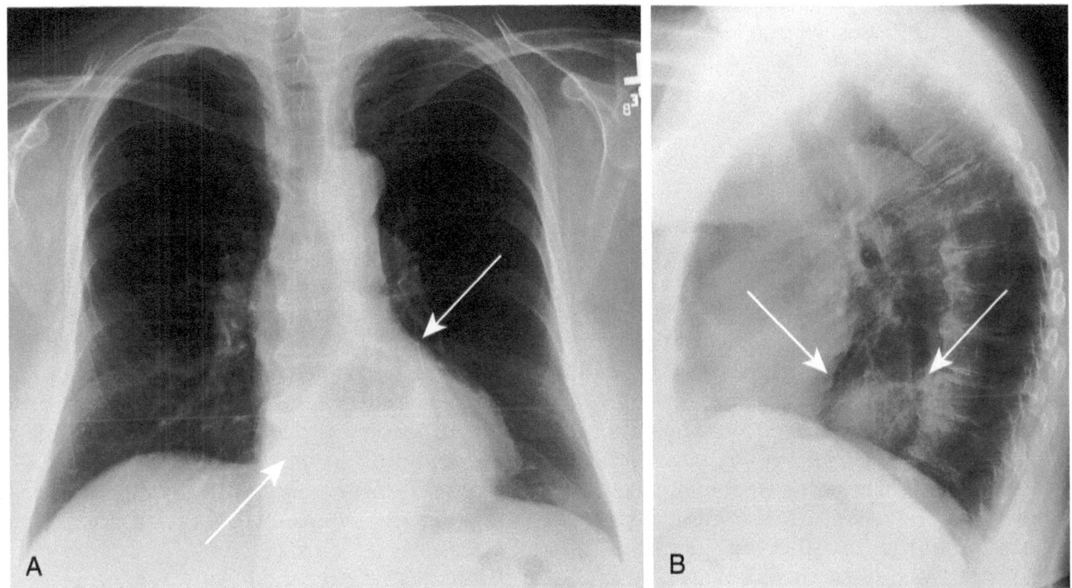

FIGURE 5.28 Hiatal hernia. Posteroanterior **(A)** and lateral **(B)** radiographs show a round mass with an air–fluid level in the lower, visceral mediastinum, yielding a double density over the heart on the frontal radiograph *(arrows)* and a retrocardiac air–fluid level on the lateral radiograph *(arrows)* and representing a moderate-sized hiatal hernia.

obstruction and an abnormally thickened tracheoesophageal stripe. CT may demonstrate abnormal wall thickening or a soft tissue mass involving the esophagus (Fig. 5.30). The appearance of the esophagus on CT may alternatively be normal, however, if the lesion does not appreciably thicken the wall or exclusively involves the mucosa. Unfortunately, underdistention and collapsed folds may mimic true wall thickening on CT, confounding interpretation and further compromising the sensitivity and specificity of CT for detection of esophageal lesions. High-resolution T2-weighted MRI, with techniques that freeze or diminish cardiorespiratory motion, offers better soft tissue contrast and can demonstrate the loss of the normal mural stratification of the esophagus when primary or metastatic tumors involve its different layers (see Fig. 3.3). Both CT and MR may demonstrate associated lymphadenopathy.

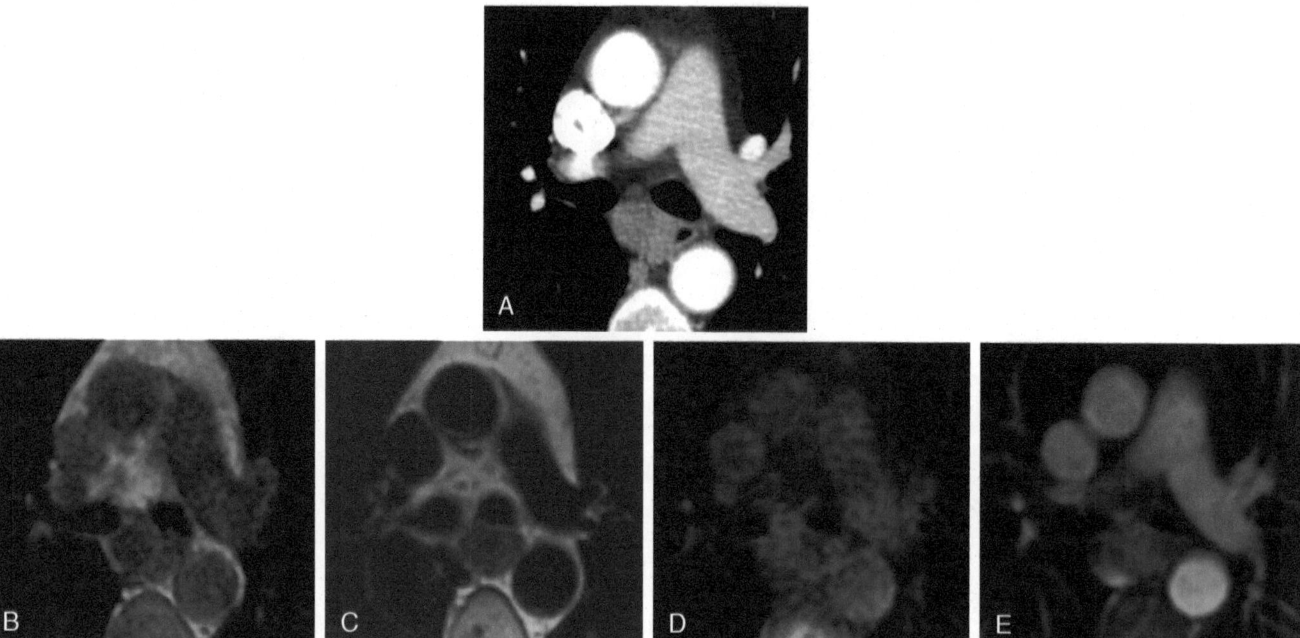

FIGURE 5.29 Esophageal leiomyoma. **A,** Axial computed tomography scan in a woman with breast cancer, believed to be in remission, reveals a soft tissue attenuation, rounded lesion in the posterior subcarinal or mid-paraesophageal space. It is unclear whether it represents lymphadenopathy, a hyperattenuating foregut duplication cyst, or an exophytic esophageal lesion. Axial T1-weighted **(B)**, T2-weighted **(C)**, precontrast fat-saturated T1-weighted **(D)**, and postcontrast T1-weighted **(E)** MR images reveal this lesion to be T1- and T2-hypointense relative to the small nonspecific mediastinal lymph nodes elsewhere and to mildly enhance. The lesion exhibits an intimate relationship with the right lateral wall of the esophagus and likely arises therefrom. Its T2-hypointensity and mild enhancement reflect the presence of smooth muscle or fibrous tissue and exclude a foregut duplication cyst and nongranulomatous lymphadenopathy. These tissue characteristics, in conjunction with the exophytic esophageal origin of this lesion, strongly favor an esophageal leiomyoma (composed of smooth muscle) as the diagnosis, as proven upon endoscopic fine-needle biopsy.

Selected Vascular Lesions

See Chapter 13 and the separate *Requisites: Cardiac Imaging* textbook for a more comprehensive review.

Aortic Aneurysm. A thoracic aortic aneurysm is an abnormal dilation of the aorta. Aneurysms may be classified based on several features, including integrity of the layers of the aortic wall, aneurysm shape, and aneurysm location. Based on the integrity of the aortic wall, aneurysms may be classified as true aneurysms, characterized by an intact aortic wall, or false aneurysms or pseudoaneurysms, characterized by a disrupted aortic wall, in which case the aneurysm is contained exclusively by adventitia or surrounding tissues.

Aneurysms may be further classified by their shape as fusiform or saccular. Whereas a fusiform aneurysm is characterized by cylindrical dilation of the entire aortic circumference, a saccular aneurysm is characterized by a focal outpouching of the aorta.

Most thoracic aortic aneurysms are atherosclerotic and are true aneurysms. Because atherosclerosis usually affects long segments of the aorta, atherosclerotic aneurysms are usually fusiform and may demonstrate both calcified and noncalcified plaques, with occasional mural thrombus.

There is inconsistency across institutions and clinical services regarding the definitions of fusiform aortic ectasia and aortic aneurysm. The thoracic aorta is typically considered ectatic when its diameter is greater than or equal to 4 cm and less than 5 cm; however, some institutions deem a 4.5-cm ascending aorta aneurysmal. Fusiform aortic dilation greater than 5 cm is universally considered a thoracic aortic aneurysm.

By location, aneurysms may be classified as ascending, transverse, or descending. Aneurysms that classically involve the ascending aorta include those caused by cystic medial necrosis from connective tissue diseases such as Marfan syndrome and Ehlers-Danlos syndrome and those caused by syphilis and associated with Turner syndrome. Complications of ascending aortic aneurysms include rupture, dissection, aortic insufficiency, and pericardial tamponade. Aneurysms that commonly involve the descending thoracic aorta include atherosclerotic, posttraumatic, and mycotic aneurysms.

Infected aortic aneurysms are often referred to as "mycotic." Mycotic aneurysms are technically pseudoaneurysms, lacking a true aortic wall. They typically exhibit a saccular configuration (Fig. 5.31) and may be accompanied by periaortic inflammation and abscess.

Aortic aneurysms may also arise from other inflammatory conditions, including the large vessel vasculitides Takayasu arteritis and giant cell or temporal arteritis.

On CXR, an aortic aneurysm should be suspected whenever a mediastinal mass is in the vicinity of the aorta and particularly when the border of the mass is indistinguishable from (or silhouettes) the aortic contour. Peripheral calcification within such a mass is supportive evidence, particularly in atherosclerotic aneurysms. CT, MRI, or angiography can

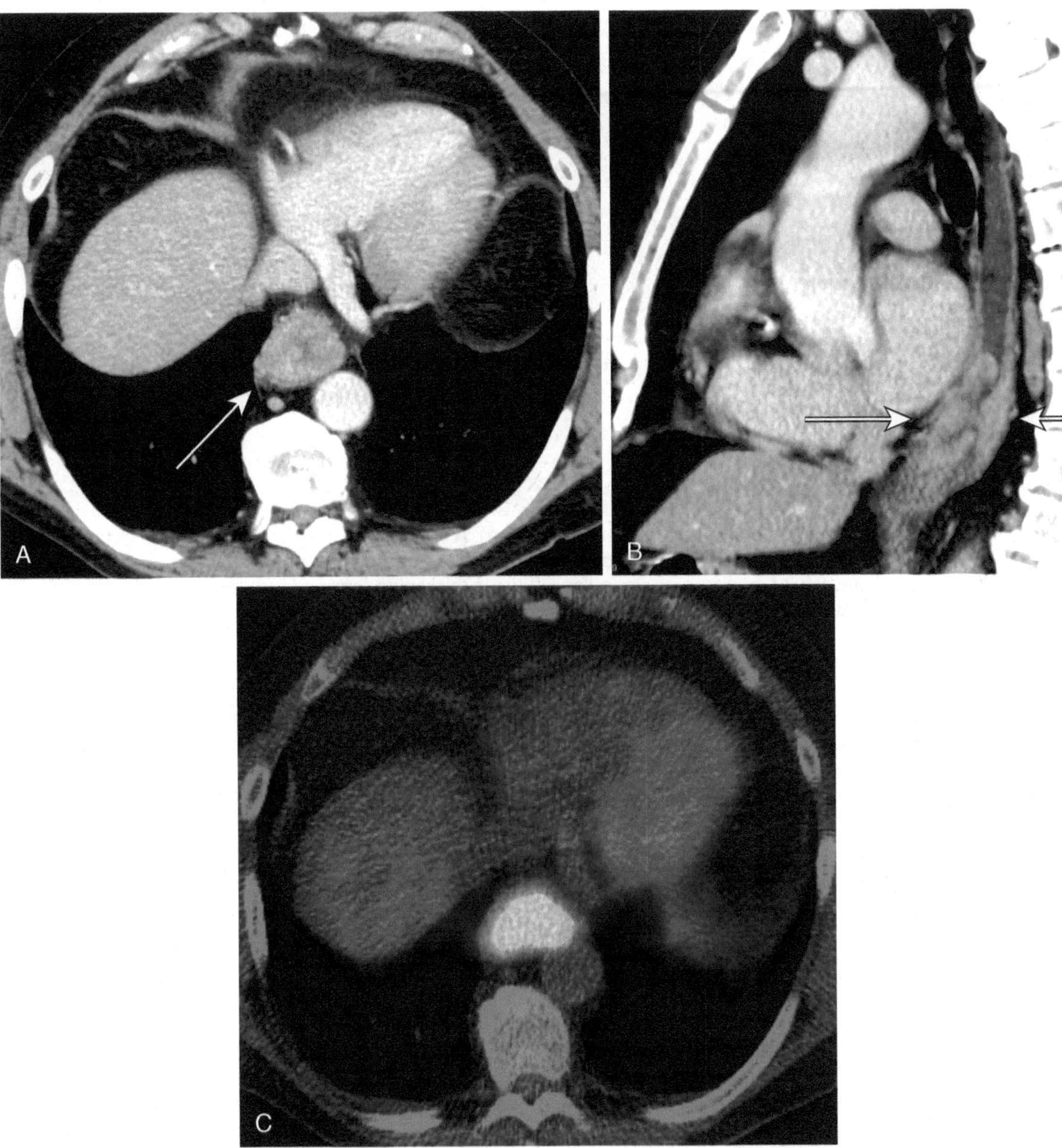

FIGURE 5.30 Esophageal cancer. **A** and **B**, Axial and sagittal computed tomography images show abnormal, heterogeneously enhancing, irregular, segmental distal esophageal wall thickening *(arrows)*. **C**, Fused axial 18-fluorodeoxyglucose (^{18}FDG) positron emission tomography (PET) image shows the intense FDG-PET avidity of this lesion.

confirm the diagnosis. Contrast-enhanced CT and MRI play an important role in imaging aortic aneurysms. Although catheter angiography was historically the method of choice for the evaluation of acute posttraumatic aortic transection, CT angiography has largely replaced catheter angiography for this indication. See Chapter 13 for additional information regarding traumatic aortic injury.

It is important to accurately measure the maximal diameter of an aortic aneurysm and document the rate of dilation because the incidence of rupture correlates with the size of the aneurysm and increases significantly for aneurysms greater than 5 cm in diameter. For these reasons, elective surgical repair has been recommended for ascending aortic aneurysms of 5 to 5.5 cm and for descending thoracic aortic aneurysms 5.5 to 6.5 cm in diameter.

Traumatic Aortic Pseudoaneurysm. See Chapter 13.

Aortic Dissection. Aortic dissection is a life-threatening condition characterized by a tear in the intima of the aortic wall followed by separation of the tunica media that creates two channels for the passage of blood: a true lumen and a false lumen. Aortic dissection is most commonly associated with systemic hypertension, with other risk factors including bicuspid aortic valve, cystic medial necrosis (e.g., Marfan syndrome), syphilitic aortitis, aortic coarctation, Turner syndrome (associated with bicuspid valve and aortic coarctation), and rarely, pregnancy. Affected patients most often present with acute onset of chest and back pain, and they are usually hypertensive.

Chest radiograph findings suggesting aortic dissection include widening of the mediastinum, inward displacement

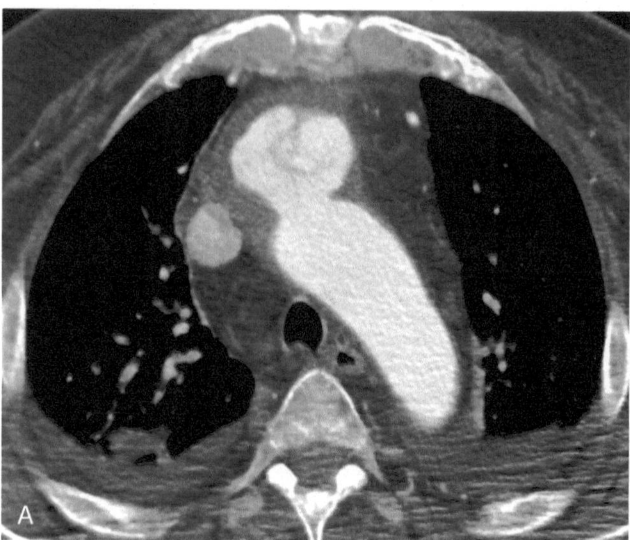

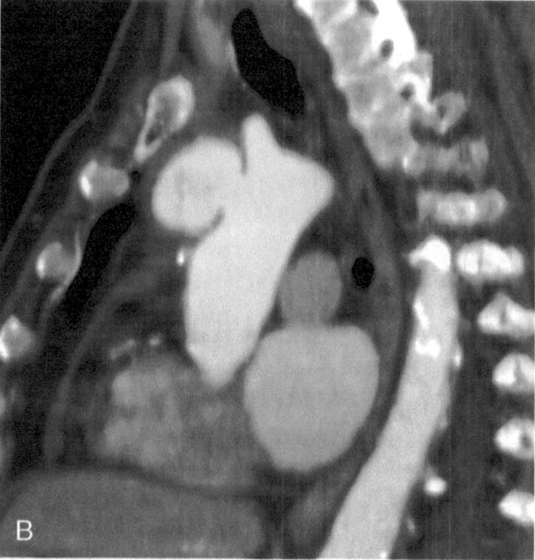

FIGURE 5.31 Mycotic aneurysm (technically, a pseudoaneurysm). **A** and **B,** Axial and sagittal computed tomography images show an irregular, intravenous contrast–containing saccular outpouching from the anterior aspect of the aortic arch into the prevascular mediastinum. Irregular soft tissue thickening forms a false wall around this contrast-containing pseudoaneurysm.

of intimal calcifications, and diffuse aortic enlargement. The best way to appreciate these findings is by an interval change in appearance compared with previous chest radiographs. The definitive diagnosis of dissection depends on identification of an intimal flap, for which contrast-enhanced CT (Fig. 5.32), MRI, transesophageal echocardiography, and conventional angiography are useful.

It is important to accurately localize the site of dissection because management depends on the site of involvement. Because of the propensity of dissections involving the ascending aorta (Stanford type A dissections) to rupture across the coronary ostia and into the aortic valve and pericardium, ascending aortic dissections are treated surgically. Dissections that begin distal to the origin of the left subclavian artery (Stanford type B dissections) are usually treated medically by controlling the patient's hypertension.

Aberrant Subclavian Artery. An aberrant right subclavian artery is a relatively common normal variant, occurring in approximately 1% of the population. The anomalous artery arises as the last branch of a left aortic arch and courses obliquely from left to right, posterior to the esophagus, as it ascends superiorly. This entity is difficult to appreciate by CXR. A barium esophagram may nicely demonstrate the oblique indentation on the posterior wall of the esophagus by the aberrant artery. This finding is readily identified on CT (Fig. 5.33) and MRI. A diverticulum of Kommerell refers to bulbous dilation of the origin of the aberrant vessel as it arises from the aortic arch. Most patients with an aberrant right subclavian artery are asymptomatic, although some may experience symptoms related to mass effect on the esophagus (dysphagia lusoria) or trachea, which can worsen with atherosclerotic change and aneurysm formation. An aberrant left subclavian artery may arise from a right aortic arch (Fig. 5.34), also passing posterior to the esophagus.

Azygous Continuation of the Inferior Vena Cava. Azygous continuation of the inferior vena cava (IVC) represents a rare and usually asymptomatic vascular anomaly in which the hepatic segment of the IVC is absent, the renal segment of the IVC continues retrocrurally as a dilated azygous vein, and the hepatic veins drain directly into the right atrium (Fig. 5.35). It represents one of the many causes of a widened mediastinum, particularly in the right paratracheal space, and should not be mistaken for a mass in this space or in the right retrocrural space. Although it has been associated with congenital heart disease and asplenia and polysplenia syndromes, this finding is more often found incidentally, in the absence of these congenital anomalies.

Paravertebral and Posterior Mediastinal Masses

Neurogenic Tumors

Neurogenic tumors are the most common cause of paravertebral (posterior) mediastinal masses. These are grouped into three major categories based on their site of origin—peripheral nerve, sympathetic ganglion, or paraganglion. Although these tumors are often asymptomatic, patients may experience neurologic symptoms, including radiculopathy and paresthesias.

Peripheral Nerve Sheath Tumors. Peripheral nerve sheath tumors are the most common paravertebral mass, accounting for the majority of mediastinal neurogenic tumors. These include schwannoma (most common), neurofibroma, and malignant peripheral nerve sheath tumor (MPNST). On CXR, CT, and MRI, these tumors may present as well-circumscribed paravertebral masses; however, they can occur at sites of other peripheral nerves in the mediastinum, including the phrenic, vagus, and recurrent laryngeal nerves, which reside in the visceral mediastinum. Peripheral nerve sheath tumors tend to be more rounded in configuration than neurogenic tumors arising from the sympathetic chain, which tend to be more fusiform in shape and vertically-oriented. On CT, neurofibromas and schwannomas are often hypoattenuating, relative to muscle. MRI is the preferred imaging modality for evaluation and diagnosis of these lesions because its superior soft tissue contrast aids in differentiating these

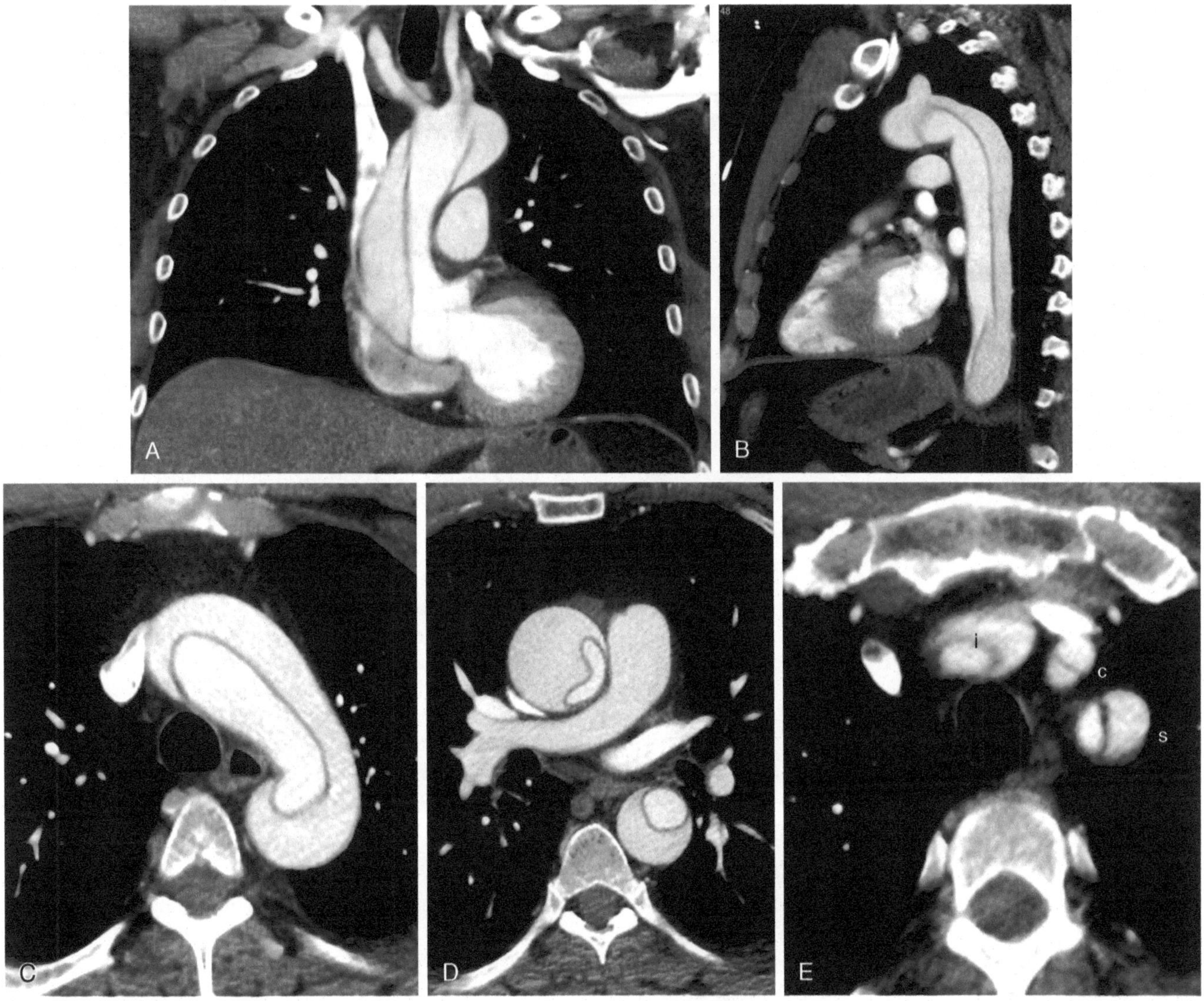

FIGURE 5.32 Aortic dissection, Stanford type A. Coronal **(A)** and sagittal **(B)** computed tomography (CT) images show an extensive intimal flap involving all of the ascending aorta, aortic arch, and descending thoracic aorta and extending into the great vessels. Correlative axial CT images at the level of the aortic arch **(C)**, ascending and descending thoracic aorta **(D)**, and great vessels **(E)**. In this patient, there was extension of the intimal flap into the left subclavian (s), left common carotid (c), and innominate (i) arteries.

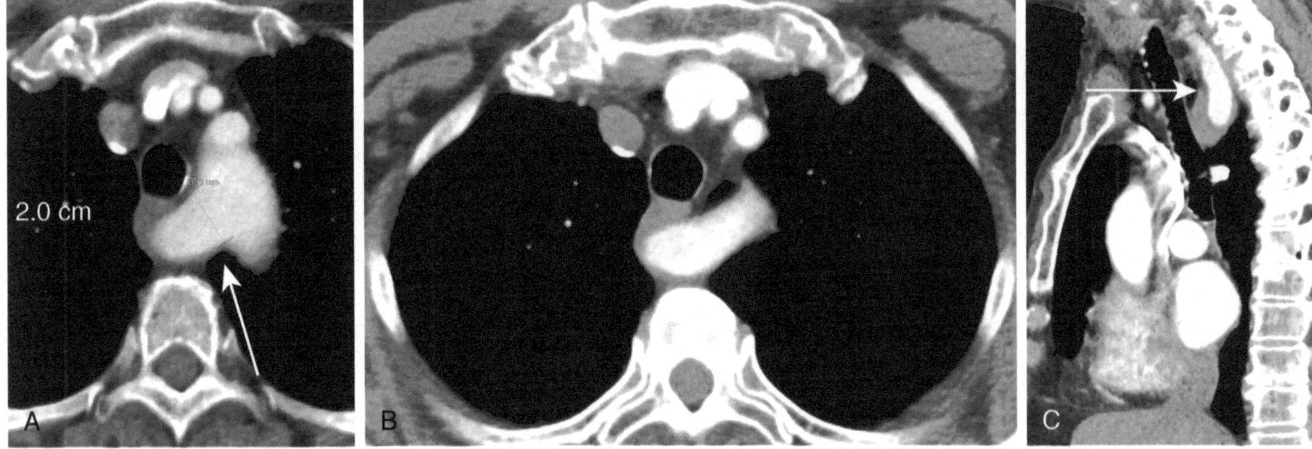

FIGURE 5.33 Left aortic arch with aberrant right subclavian artery. **A** and **B,** Axial computed tomography (CT) images demonstrate a dilated 2-cm aberrant right subclavian artery origin (*arrow,* diverticulum of Kommerell) from the medial margin of the aortic arch posterior to the left subclavian artery origin. From here, it passes between the esophagus and the spine to ascend superolaterally toward the right upper extremity. **C,** Sagittal CT image show this vessel's ascent toward the right upper extremity *(arrow).*

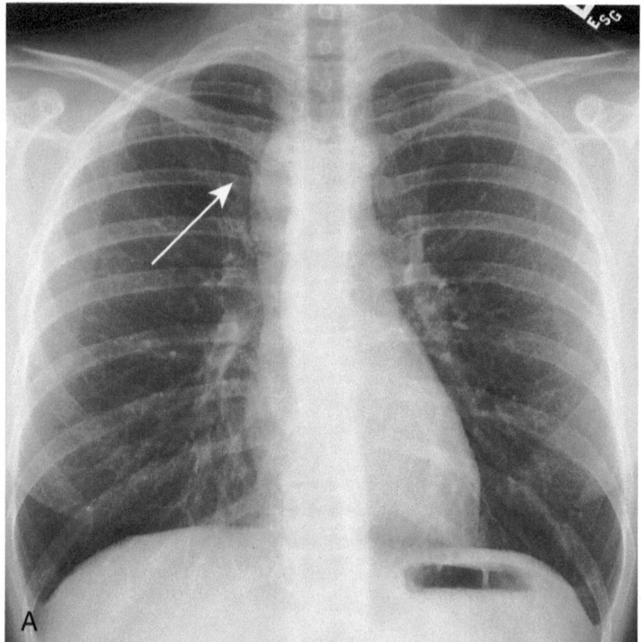

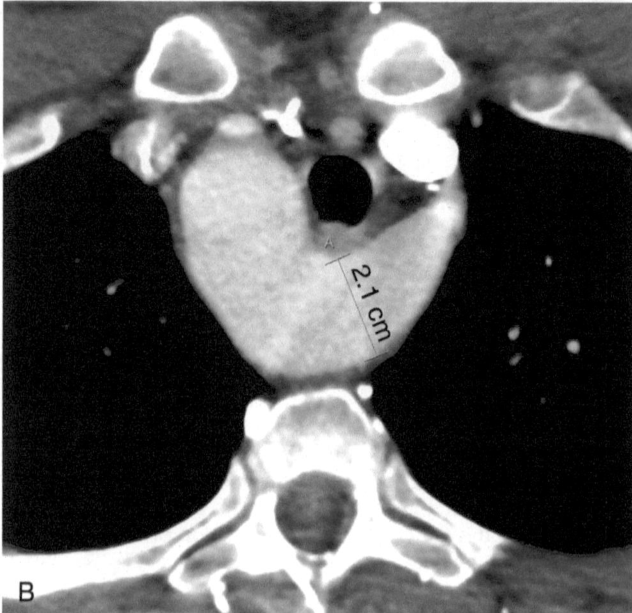

FIGURE 5.34 Right aortic arch with aberrant left subclavian artery. **A,** Posteroanterior radiograph shows a right aortic arch *(arrow)* and no left aortic arch. **B,** Axial computed tomography image revealing aberrant origin of a dilated, 2.1-cm aberrant right subclavian artery (diverticulum of Kommerell) from the right aortic arch.

lesions and better assesses their relationship with the spine and chest wall. These tumors can assume a "dumbbell" or "hourglass" configuration when involving an intervertebral neural foramen. Smooth pressure erosion and scalloping of the adjacent ribs and vertebrae may develop because of their slow growth. Neurofibromas and schwannomas can often be differentiated on MR by their signal characteristics. Compared with schwannomas, neurofibromas typically have lower T2 signal centrally and high T2 signal peripherally, giving rise to the "target sign" (Fig. 5.36). Schwannomas are more often centrally T2-hyperintense, whether or not they are cystic (Fig. 5.37). Findings concerning for malignant transformation of a peripheral nerve sheath tumor or an MPNST include increased heterogeneity of attenuation or signal secondary to tumor degeneration, irregular cystic change and necrosis, irregular peripheral enhancement, and adjacent tissue invasion and bone destruction.

Sympathetic Ganglion Tumors. Sympathetic ganglion tumors are less common neurogenic tumors and include ganglioneuroma, ganglioneuroblastoma, and neuroblastoma. Whereas ganglioneuroma is a rare, benign tumor that occurs in children and young adults, ganglioneuroblastoma and neuroblastoma are malignant tumors that present almost exclusively in children. These tumors are classically more fusiform than round and more vertical in orientation than peripheral nerve sheath tumors. On CT, ganglioneuromas are well-circumscribed masses that are typically hypoattenuating to muscle. On T1- and T2-weighted MRI, ganglioneuromas may exhibit low signal curvilinear bands or nodules amid a homogeneous intermediate signal referred to as a "whorled appearance" (Fig. 5.38). Ganglioneuroblastomas and neuroblastomas tend to exhibit more heterogeneous T2 signal and a more heterogeneous enhancement pattern than ganglioneuromas because of tumor necrosis.

Paragangliomas. Paragangliomas are rare neurogenic tumors of chromaffin cell origin. A total of 1% to 2% of all extraadrenal paragangliomas occur in the thorax. Their most common locations in the mediastinum are along the great vessels and base of the heart (aortopulmonary paraganglia) and along the sympathetic chain in the paravertebral mediastinum, which tracks vertically along the neck of the ribs (aortosympathetic paraganglia). On CT and MRI, these soft tissue masses typically exhibit intense contrast enhancement. On MRI, paragangliomas often exhibit very high T2 signal intensity, although heterogeneous T2 signal intensity may be present if they contain internal hemorrhage or necrosis. When large, these hypervascular tumors may demonstrate a "salt and pepper" appearance on T1-weighted images because of internal curvilinear or punctate flow voids ("pepper"), in conjunction with high signal intensity ("salt") caused by hemorrhagic products.

Other Paravertebral and Vertebral Lesions

Occasionally, a posterior mediastinal mass may be congenital or caused by an infectious, inflammatory (e.g., pancreatic pseudocyst), traumatic, or neoplastic process involving the thoracic spine and paraspinal soft tissues.

Neuroenteric Cysts. Neuroenteric cysts are a rare subtype of foregut duplication cyst and can be pathologically identical to esophageal duplication cysts. They may be symptomatic, eliciting local pain, radiculopathy, or myelopathy, and typically present in childhood. Neuroenteric cysts often have a fibrous or CSF-containing connection to the intradural extramedullary space of the thoracic spine and are typically ventral in location. These cysts can be associated with congenital vertebral body anomalies such as butterfly vertebra and hemivertebra. On CXR, neuroenteric cysts manifest as well-circumscribed posterior mediastinal masses, with a CT and MR appearance similar to that of other foregut duplication cysts, although connection with the spinal canal may be demonstrated. When these cysts communicate with the subarachnoid space, they demonstrate contrast opacification on CT myelography.

Meningoceles. Thoracic meningoceles are protrusions of meninges through the spinal neural foramina and are

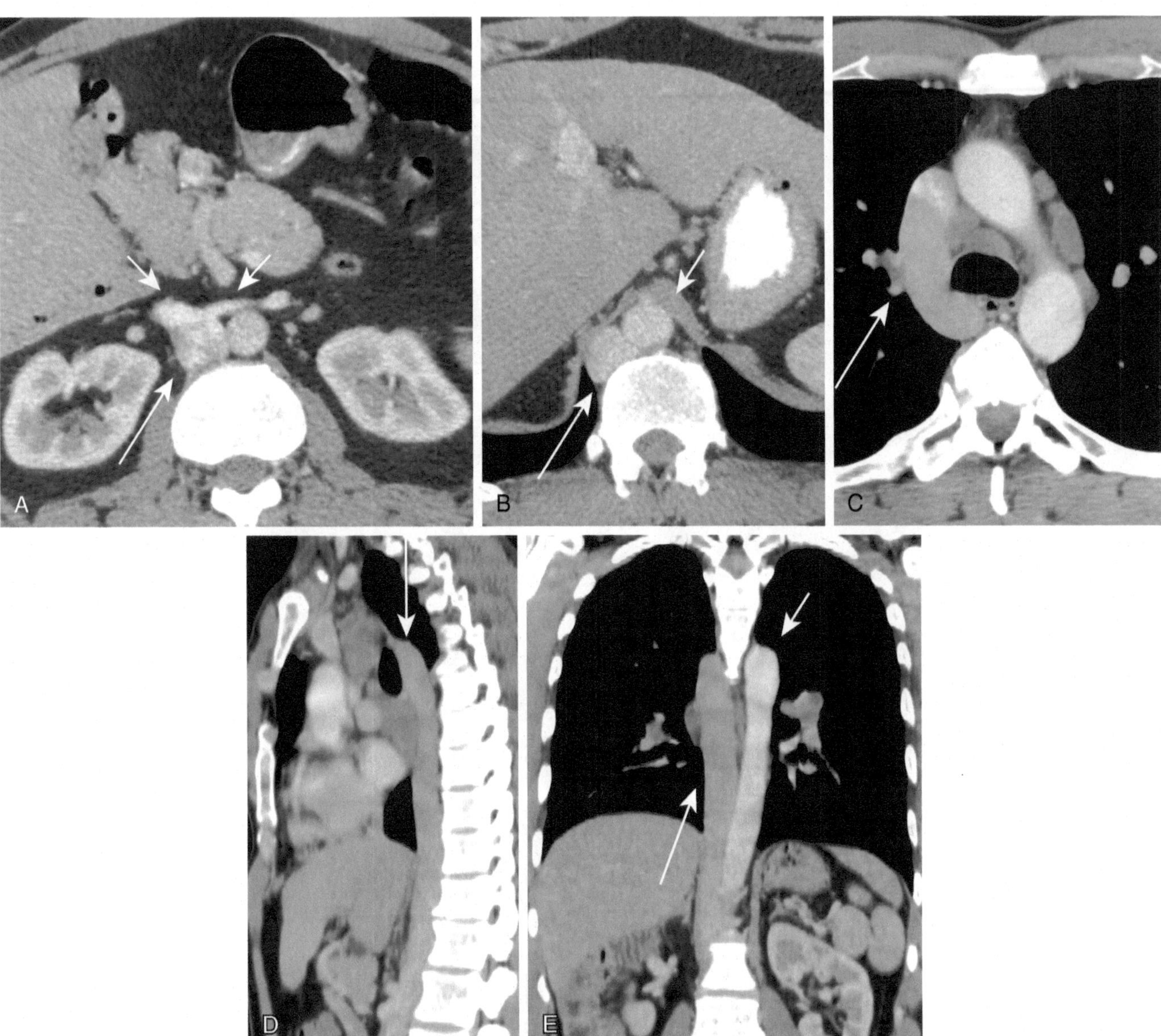

FIGURE 5.35 Azygous continuation of the inferior vena cava (IVC). **A,** Axial computed tomography (CT) image at the level of the bilateral renal upper poles shows confluence of the bilateral renal veins *(short arrows)* as they merge into the IVC *(long arrow)*. **B,** Axial CT image at the retrocrural level reveals azygous continuation of the IVC *(long arrow)*, not to be mistaken for retrocrural lymphadenopathy. The *short arrow* demarcates the aorta. In the absence of this congenital anomaly (or central venous obstruction), the azygous vein would not be so dilated. **C,** Axial CT image at the level of the bridging azygous vein *(arrow)* highlights its dilation and course and is not to be mistaken for a paratracheal mass. **D** and **E,** Sagittal and coronal CT images display the craniocaudal extent and dilation of the azygous vein *(long arrows)*, with the *short arrow* highlighting the location of the descending thoracic aorta, which the azygous vein parallels.

most commonly associated with neurofibromatosis type 1. On CXR, meningoceles manifest as well-marginated posterior mediastinal masses. Smooth, well-corticated pressure erosion and scalloping of the adjacent vertebrae and ribs, widening of the neural foramen, and kyphoscoliosis of the thoracic spine can occur. CT and MRI are virtually diagnostic when they demonstrate a direct relationship to the CSF space, internal CSF attenuation and signal intensity, and a barely perceptible wall. Meningoceles opacify readily at CT myelography.

Extramedullary Hematopoiesis. Extramedullary hematopoiesis is rare and represents paravertebral bone marrow expansion in the setting of severe anemia—notably, thalassemia, hereditary spherocytosis, and sickle cell disease. Chronic myelofibrosis may also yield this entity. It can manifest as multiple, bilateral, lobulated paravertebral masses (Fig. 5.39). Hematopoietic marrow replacement may accompany these findings on MRI. Clinical history helps establish the diagnosis.

Traumatic Lesions. See Chapter 13.

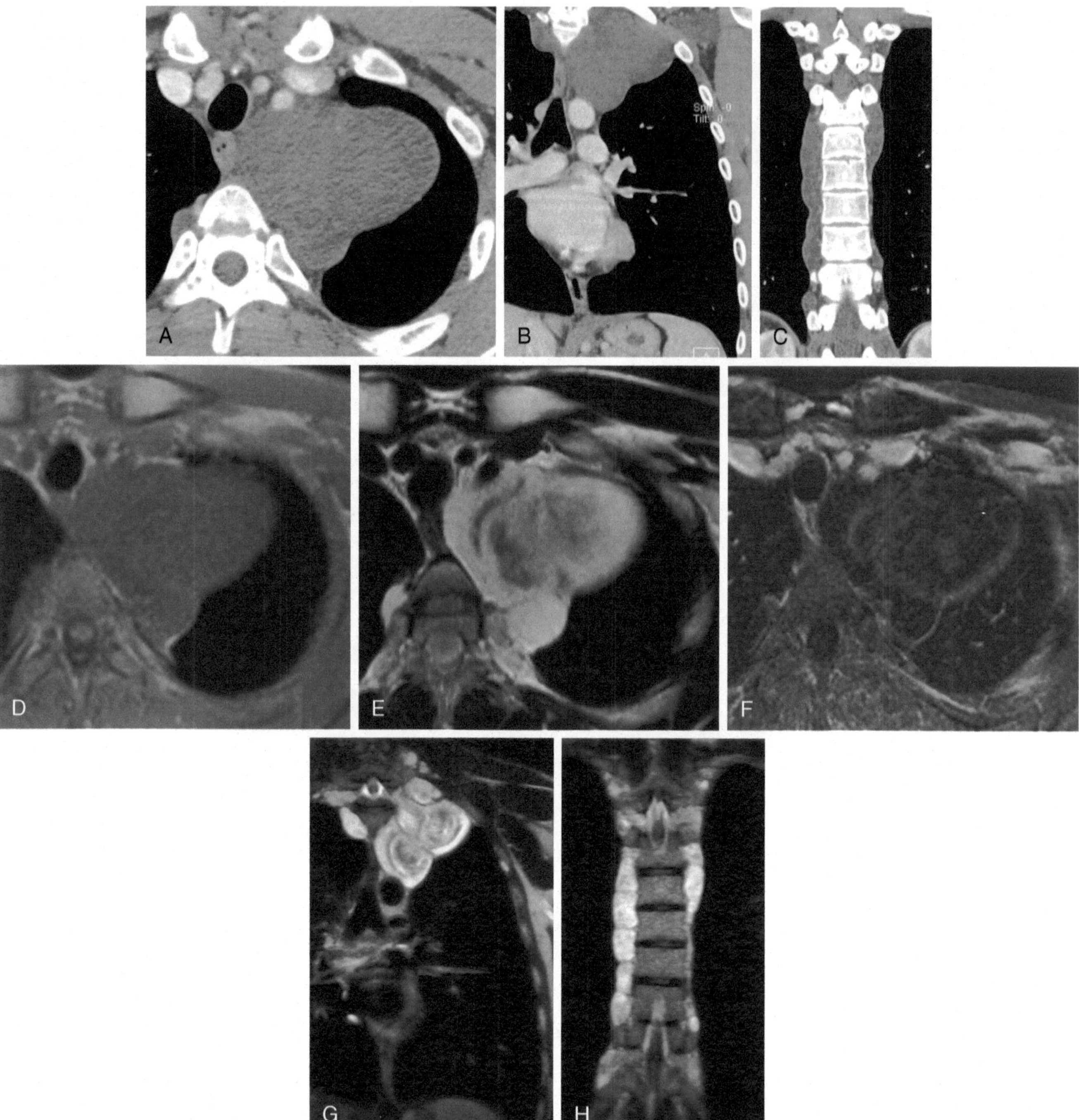

FIGURE 5.36 Neurofibromatosis. Axial **(A)**, anterior coronal **(B)**, and posterior **(C)** coronal computed tomography images show a large, well-circumscribed, lobulated, slightly hypoattenuating mass in the left upper hemithorax, spanning the paravertebral and visceral compartments, in addition to multiple smaller bilateral paravertebral masses arising at multiple thoracic spinal levels. Axial T1-weighted **(D)**, axial T2-weighted **(E)**, and axial postcontrast **(F)** subtracted MR images reveal a large, well-circumscribed, lobulated left paravertebral mass of intermediate to low T1 signal, heterogeneous T2 signal, and little enhancement. The patchy central T2-hypointensity and marked peripheral T2-hyperintensity, the so-called target sign on MRI, are characteristic of neurofibromas and virtually exclude schwannomas. The minimal enhancement, with little heterogeneity and no cystic change, favors a benign neurofibroma that has not malignantly transformed. A similar, albeit much smaller, right paravertebral lesion is present. More anterior **(G)** and more posterior **(H)** coronal T2-weighted MRIs show multiple bilateral paravertebral lesions bearing the "target sign" and representing neurofibromas.

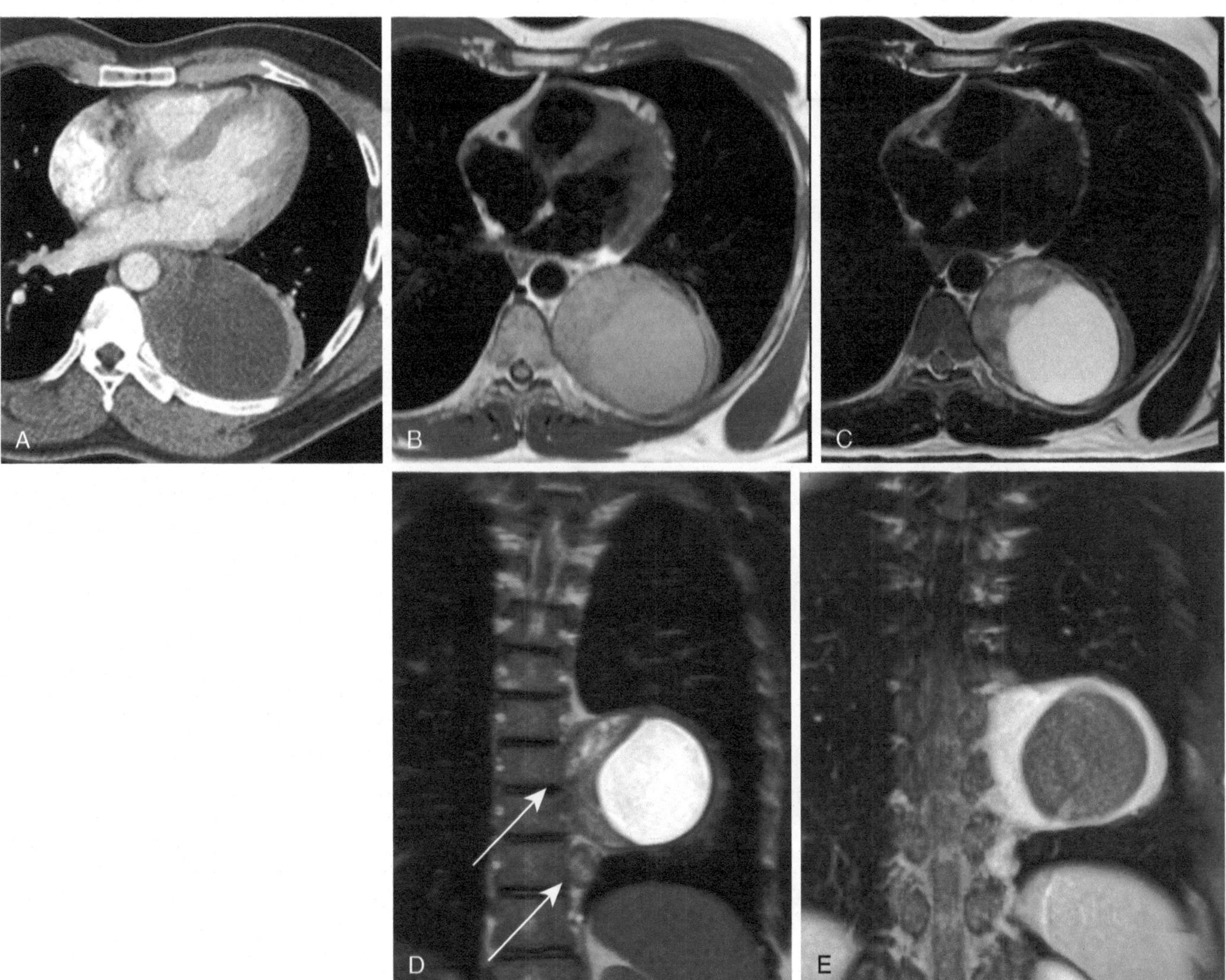

FIGURE 5.37 Tandem schwannomas. **A,** Axial computed tomography scan shows a complex, loculated collection of fluid, whether in the pleural or paravertebral mediastinal space. Mild crescentic, homogeneously enhancing compressive atelectasis drapes over this mass. Axial electrocardiography-gated T1- **(B)** and T2- **(C)** weighted MR images show this lesion to represent an asymmetrically thick-walled cyst. **D,** Coronal T2-weighted MRI reveals the presence of two lesions *(arrows)*, with their solid portions demonstrating identical T2 signal with paravertebral fat wrapping entirely around the smaller more inferiorly located lesion and partially around the upper lesion. These lesions have therefore arisen from the paravertebral space, not the pleural space. **E,** Coronal postcontrast fat-saturated T1-weighted MRI shows marked, homogeneous enhancement of the solid portion of the cystic lesion and diffuse enhancement of the smaller solid lesion. The intimate relationship of both lesions to exiting spinal nerve roots is also demonstrated. The combination of their posterior mediastinal location and signal characteristics on MRI (central T2-hyperintensity and relative peripheral T2-hypointensity, whether cystic or solid) confirm the diagnosis of tandem schwannomas (over neurofibromas), with the upper one cystic and the lower one solid.

DIFFUSE MEDIASTINAL PROCESSES

Diffuse mediastinal processes involve more than one mediastinal compartment, with examples including mediastinal lipomatosis, acute mediastinitis, chronic mediastinitis, and pneumomediastinum.

Mediastinal Lipomatosis

Mediastinal lipomatosis or excess, nonencapsulated fat throughout the mediastinum, is a very common cause of mediastinal widening on imaging (Fig. 5.40). It is precipitated by exogenous and endogenous steroids and obesity.

Acute Mediastinitis

Acute mediastinitis is a life-threatening condition with high morbidity and mortality. It results from acute infection or inflammation of mediastinal structures and the surrounding fat and connective tissue. Acute mediastinitis may be postoperative, posttraumatic, secondary to esophageal perforation, or infectious, whether primary mediastinal,

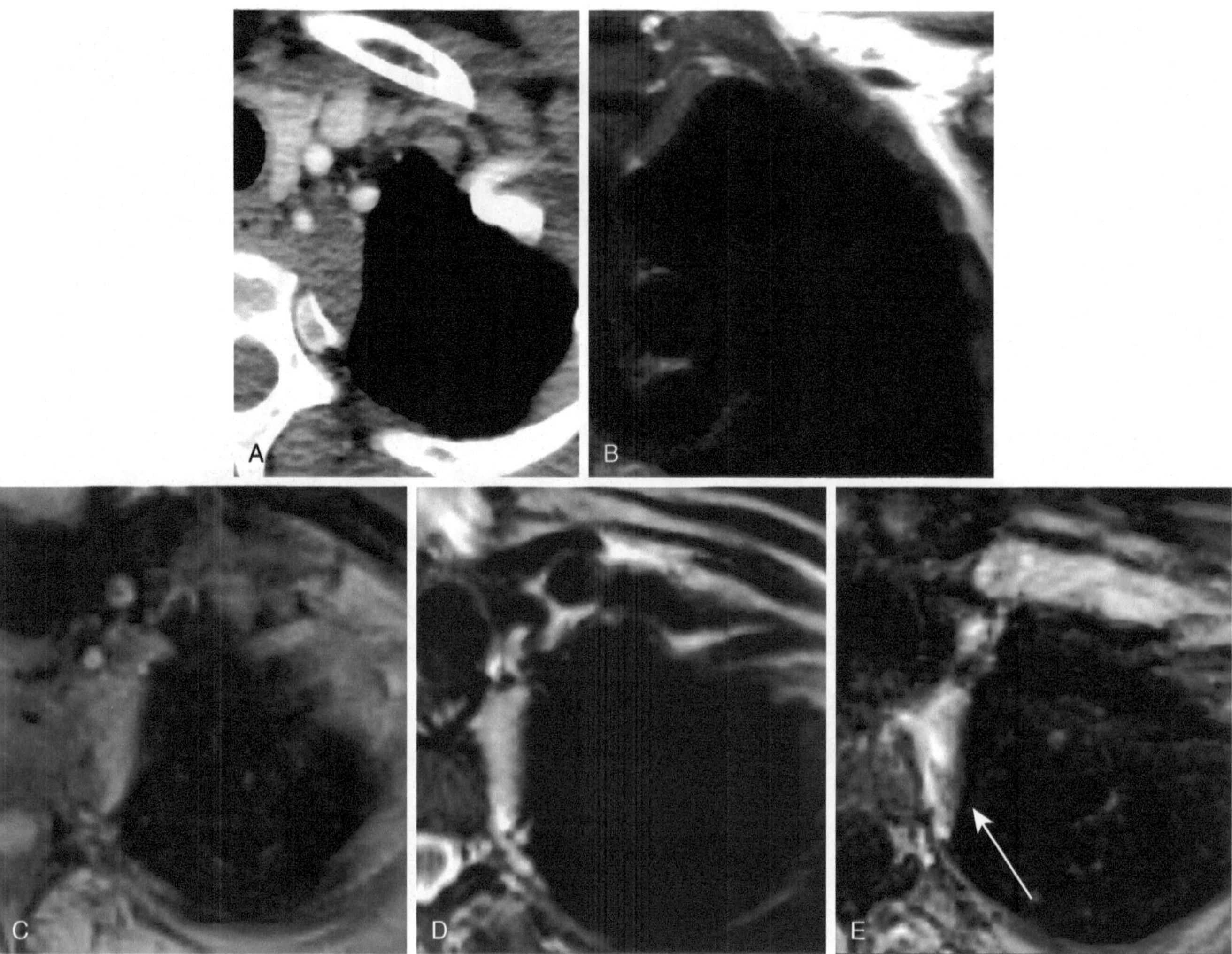

FIGURE 5.38 Ganglioneuroma. **A,** Axial computed tomography scan shows an indeterminate, plaque-like, soft tissue attenuation lesion in the medial left hemithoracic apex, with possible mediastinal fat invasion. It is not clear whether this lesion is arising from the paravertebral mediastinum, pleura, or lung. **B,** Coronal T2-weighted magnetic resonance image reveals this lesion to be oblong and well circumscribed and to be largely enveloped by mediastinal fat, placing it in the paravertebral mediastinum and excluding pleural and pulmonary parenchymal lesions from the differential diagnosis. Its orientation is more vertical than horizontal. Axial fat-saturated T1-weighted **(C)**, T2-weighted **(D)**, and postcontrast fat-saturated T1-weighted **(E)** MR images show this lesion to exhibit intermediate T1 signal, slightly heterogeneous T2-weighted signal, and heterogeneous enhancement with a "whorled appearance, *(arrow)*" which in conjunction with its more vertical orientation, favor ganglioneuroma over other neurogenic tumors.

extending inferiorly from the head and neck, extending superiorly from complications of pancreatitis, caused by contiguous involvement from adjacent osteomyelitis, or caused by hematogenous spread of infection. See Box 5.3. Clinically, patients with acute mediastinitis are very ill, with high fevers, chest pain, dyspnea, and leukocytosis.

On CXR, there may be widening of the mediastinum with distortion of normal mediastinal lines, stripes, and interfaces. CT is the imaging modality of choice because it is widely available and can be done in a timely fashion. CT also helps confirm the diagnosis and delineate the extent of involvement. Common CT findings of acute mediastinitis include increased attenuation or soft tissue stranding of mediastinal fat, loculated fluid collections or abscesses, locules of mediastinal gas, and associated pleural effusion or empyema (Fig. 5.41). Similar findings may be found on MRI. Acute mediastinitis is typically T2-hyperintense, unlike chronic or fibrosing mediastinitis.

Fibrosing Mediastinitis

Chronic mediastinitis, also known as fibrosing mediastinitis, is a rare condition with sometimes extensive fibrotic reaction within the mediastinum. Patients may be asymptomatic or present with symptoms related to obstruction or compression of vital mediastinal structures by the fibrotic tissue, including central systemic veins such as the SVC, the pulmonary veins and arteries, esophagus, and central airways. The most common cause of fibrosing mediastinitis is infection—in particular, granulomatous infections such as histoplasmosis and tuberculosis. Noninfectious causes include autoimmune diseases such as IgG4-related disease,

Behçet disease, and sarcoidosis and neoplasms such as Hodgkin disease. Iatrogenic causes have also been recognized, including radiation and methysergide therapy.

On CXR, fibrosing mediastinitis may manifest as abnormal widening of the mediastinum, with distortion or obliteration of recognizable mediastinal lines, stripes, and interfaces. Calcified and noncalcified, focal and multifocal masses or lymph nodes may be observed. On CT, fibrosing mediastinitis often manifests as an infiltrative soft tissue attenuation mass with associated distortion or obliteration of normal anatomic fat planes. There may be encasement, narrowing, and even occlusion of bronchovascular structures. It most commonly affects the visceral (middle) mediastinum. Two patterns of involvement can be seen on CT: (1) focal or multifocal and (2) diffuse, infiltrative. The focal or multifocal form is much more common and manifests as a soft tissue attenuation mass (or masses), with frequent calcification. In the United States, chronic fibrosing mediastinitis is most frequently caused by histoplasmosis. The diffuse infiltrative pattern, seen in the remaining cases, is likely due to other causes, such as IgG4-related disease, in association with retroperitoneal fibrosis. Chronic fibrosing mediastinitis is more typically T2-hypointense, unlike acute mediastinitis, even when no lymph nodal calcification is present (Fig. 5.42).

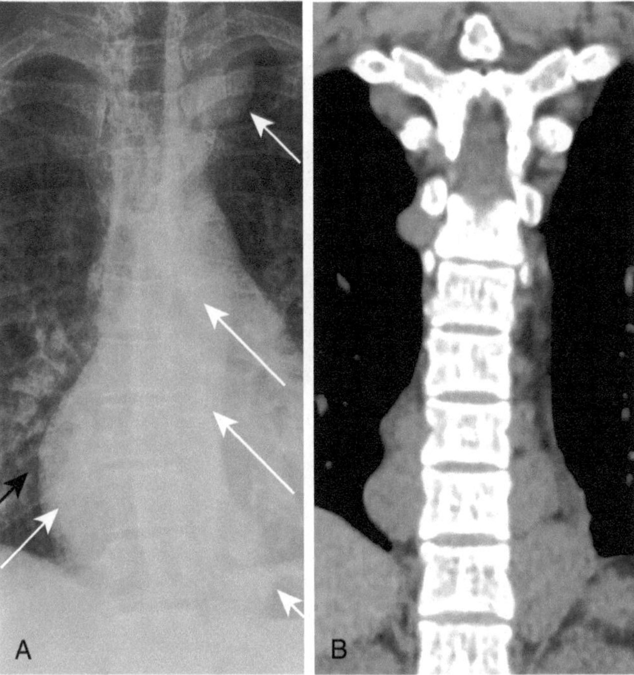

FIGURE 5.39 Extramedullary hematopoiesis in a 26-year-old man with thalassemia major. **A,** Anteroposterior radiograph reveals multiple, bilateral, lobulated paravertebral masses, bulging the paraspinal lines bilaterally *(white arrows).* Note the distinct right heart border *(black arrow).* **B,** Coronal computed tomography scan confirms the presence of multiple, bilateral, lobulated soft tissue masses of varying size that do not demonstrate origination from the neural foramina (latter not shown). In the setting of thalassemia major, this finding is highly likely to represent extramedullary hematopoiesis.

BOX 5.3 Acute Mediastinitis

CAUSES

- Head and neck
  - Oropharyngeal infection
    - Pharyngitis
    - Dental abscess
  - Retropharyngeal infection
  - Epiglottitis
- Esophageal perforation
  - Traumatic
  - Iatrogenic
  - Ulceration from infection, severe reflux esophagitis, or caustic ingestion
  - Boerhaave syndrome
- Postsurgical infection (e.g., sternotomy wound)
- Chest wall septic arthritis (e.g., sternoclavicular joint)
- Pancreatitis with ascending pseudocyst, phlegmon

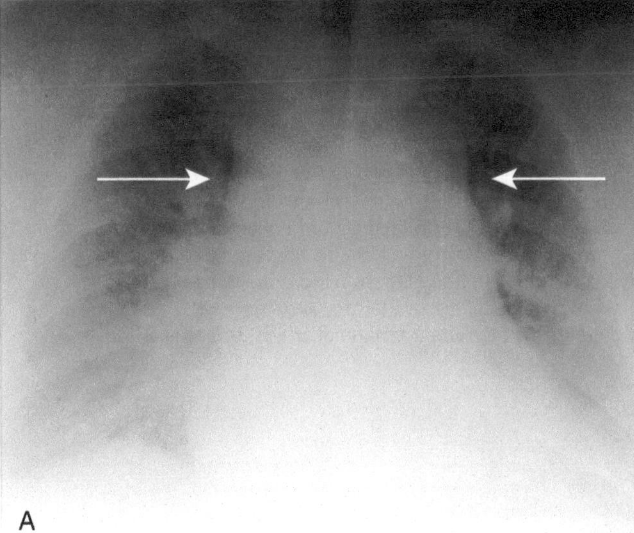

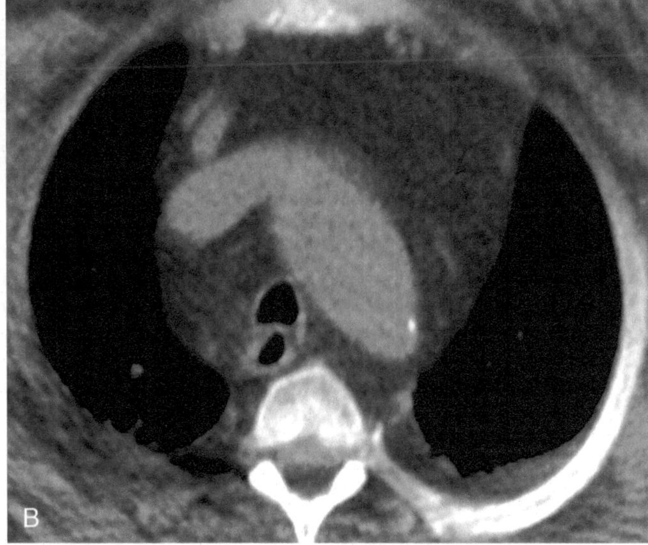

FIGURE 5.40 Mediastinal lipomatosis. **A,** Anteroposterior radiograph reveals moderate mediastinal widening *(arrows)* in the setting of large body habitus (latter compromises x-ray penetration). **B,** Axial computed tomography scan shows this mediastinal widening to be due to excessive mediastinal fat, rather than a mediastinal mass.

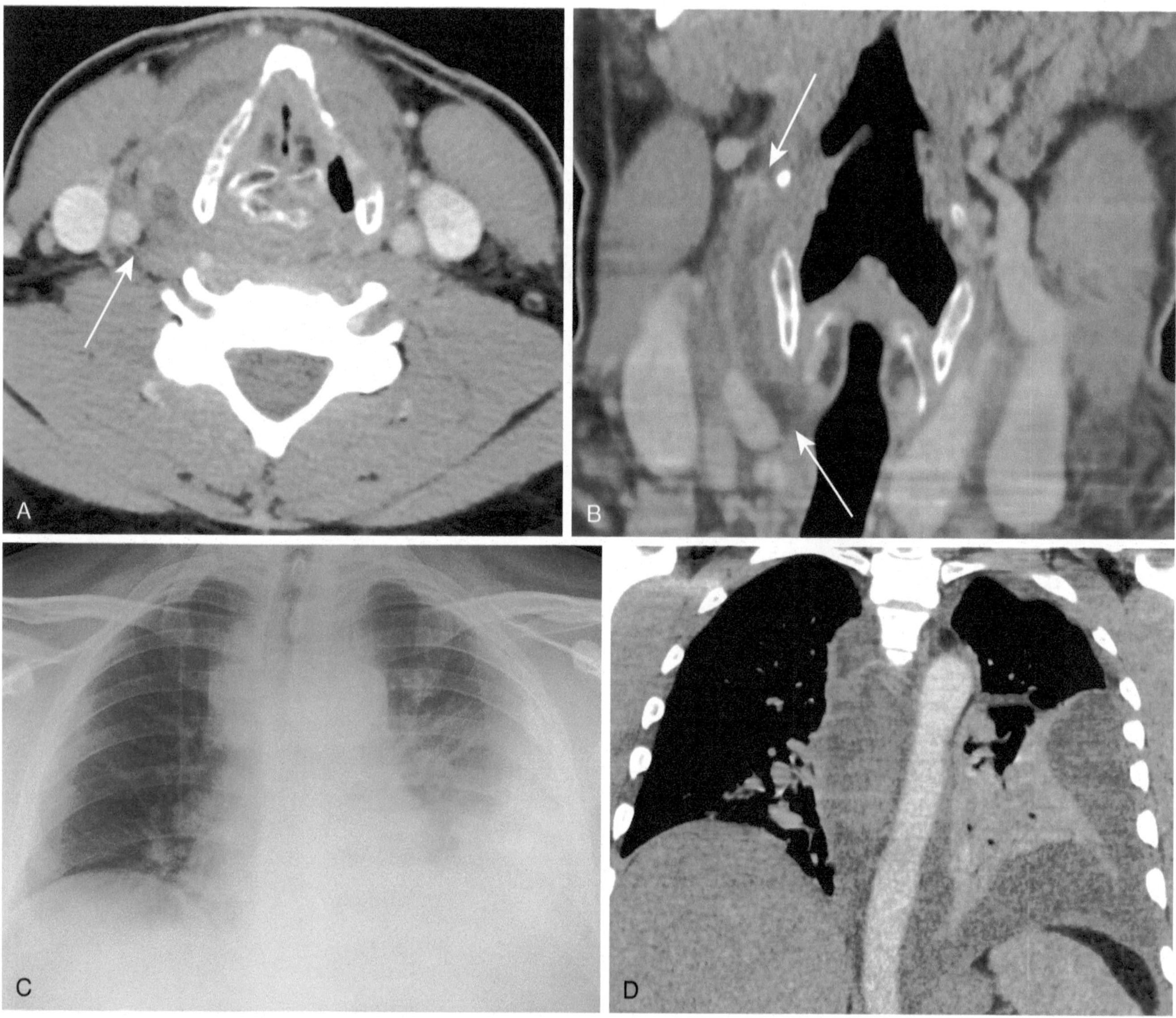

FIGURE 5.41 Acute mediastinitis in a 39-year-old man presenting with neck pain and shortness of breath. **A** and **B,** Axial and coronal computed tomography (CT) images show a rim-enhancing fluid collection *(arrows)* extending from the right parapharyngeal space inferiorly between the thyroid cartilage and right common carotid artery. Anteroposterior **(C)** radiograph and correlative coronal CT image **(D)** showing diffuse mediastinal widening caused by a diffuse mediastinal fluid collection, with an associated moderate, loculated left pleural effusion and partial left lung relaxation atelectasis and consolidation (low attenuation material amidst the otherwise homogeneously enhancing atelectasis).

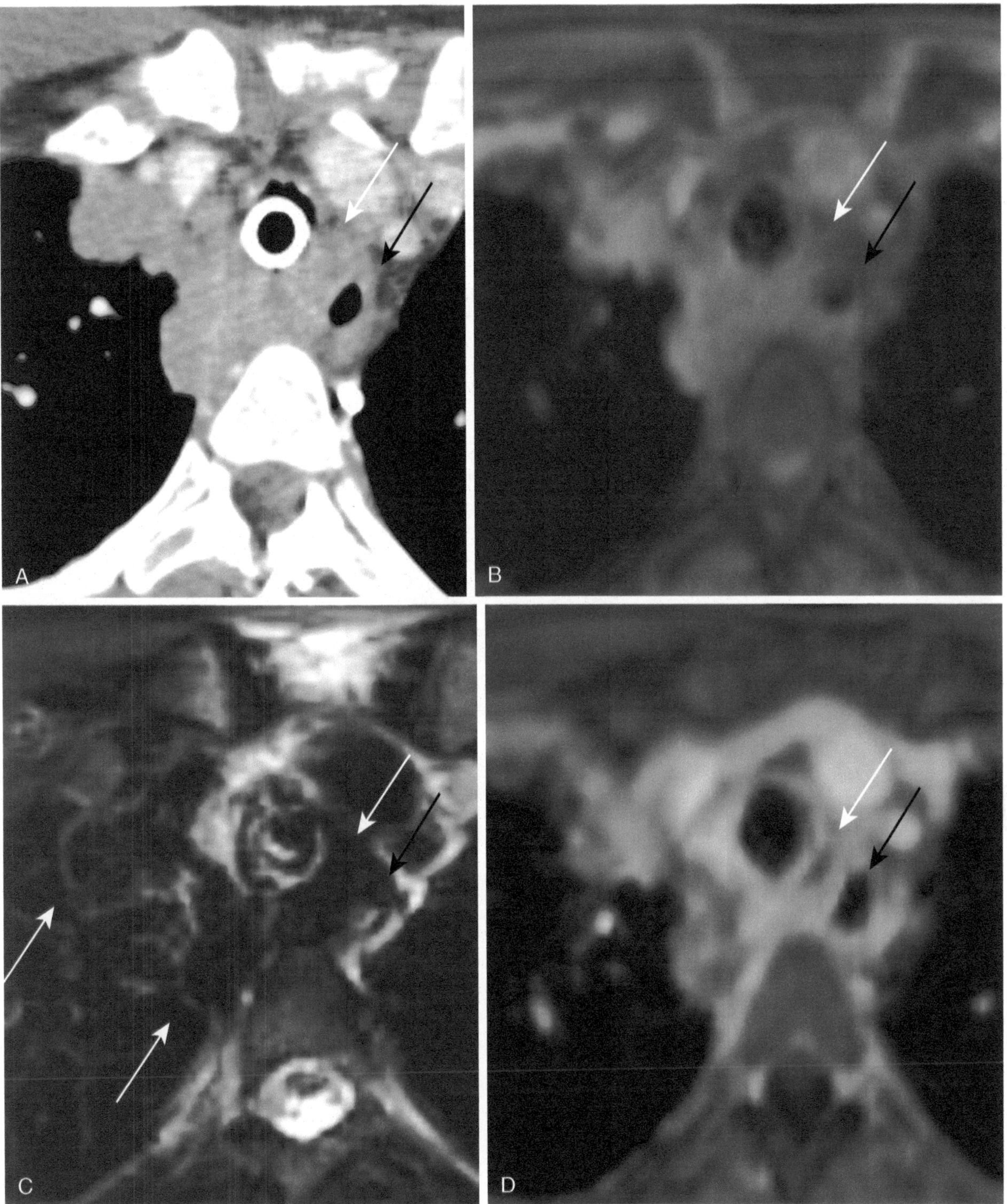

FIGURE 5.42 Chronic fibrosing mediastinitis in a young Haitian woman who presented with severe tracheal stenosis and dysphagia secondary to a contiguous neck and mediastinal mass. **A,** Axial computed tomography (CT) scan with intravenous contrast reveals a tracheostomy tube within the trachea (severe stenosis above level imaged). Isoattenuating soft tissue tracks partially around and between *(white arrow)* the trachea and esophagus *(black arrow)* and protrudes into the medial right lung apex; the composition of this tissue is indeterminate by CT. Axial fat-saturated T1-weighted **(B)**, T2-weighted **(C)**, and fat-saturated postcontrast T1-weighted **(D)** MR images show this tissue to be slightly T1-hyperintense and markedly T2-hypointense and to enhance mildly and heterogeneously. The marked T2-hypointensity and solidity of this mass elucidate its fibrous composition, strongly favoring chronic fibrous mediastinitis over infiltrative tumors such as untreated lymphoma, which would be T2-hyperintense, and alerting interventionalists as to the potentially hard, resistant texture of this mass. Unfortunately, this MRI was requested after nondiagnostic endoscopic and needle biopsies, the former of which yielded an iatrogenic tracheoesophageal fistula (above the level shown). The cause of this fibrosing mediastinitis was not found.

Pneumomediastinum

See Fig. 5.26 and Chapter 10.

SUGGESTED READINGS

Abdel Razek AA, Khairy M, Nada N. Diffusion-weighted MR imaging in thymic epithelial tumors: correlation with World Health Organization classification and clinical staging. *Radiology*. 2014;273(1):268-275.

Ackman JB. A practical guide to nonvascular thoracic magnetic resonance imaging. *J Thorac Imaging*. 2014;29(1):17-29.

Ackman JB. MR imaging of mediastinal masses. *Magn Reson Imaging Clin N Am*. 2015;23(2):141-164.

Ackman JB, Gaissert HA, Lanuti M, et al. Impact of nonvascular thoracic MRI on the clinical decision-making of thoracic surgeons and impact on their patients: a two-year prospective study. *Radiology*. 2016;280(2):464-474.

Ackman JB, Kovacina B, Carter BW, et al. Sex difference in normal thymic appearance in adults 20-30 years of age. *Radiology*. 2013;268(1):245-253.

Ackman JB, Verzosa S, Kovach AE, et al. High rate of unnecessary thymectomy and its cause. Can computed tomography distinguish thymoma, lymphoma, thymic hyperplasia, and thymic cysts? *Eur J Radiol*. 2015;84(3):524-533.

Akman C, Kantarci F, Cetinkaya S. Imaging in mediastinitis: a systematic review based on aetiology. *Clin Radiol*. 2004;59(7):573-585.

Araki T, Sholl LM, Gerbaudo VH, et al. Imaging characteristics of pathologically proven thymic hyperplasia: identifying features that can differentiate true from lymphoid hyperplasia. *AJR Am J Roentgenol*. 2014;202(3):471-478.

Carter BW, Tomiyama N, Bhora FY, et al. A modern definition of mediastinal compartments. *J Thorac Oncol*. 2014;9(9 suppl 2):S97-S101.

Cheson BD, Fisher RI, Barrington SF, et al. Recommendations for initial evaluation, staging, and response assessment of Hodgkin and non-Hodgkin lymphoma: the Lugano classification. *J Clin Oncol*. 2014;32(27):3059-3068.

Gibbs JM, Chandrasekhar CA, Ferguson EC, et al. Lines and stripes: where did they go?-From conventional radiography to CT. *Radiographics*. 2007;27(1):33-48.

Guan YB, Zhang WD, Zeng QS, et al. 2012 CT and MRI findings of thoracic ganglioneuroma. *Br J Radiol*. 2012;85(1016):e365-e372.

Hansell DM, Lynch DA, McAdams HP, et al. *Imaging of Diseases of the Chest*. St. Louis: Mosby-Elsevier; 2010.

Inaoka T, Takahashi K, Mineta M, et al. Thymic hyperplasia and thymus gland tumors: differentiation with chemical shift MR imaging. *Radiology*. 2007;243(3):869-876.

Jeung MY, Gasser B, Gangi A, et al. Imaging of cystic masses of the mediastinum. *Radiographics*. 22 Spec No:S79-93.Marom EM. 2013 Advances in thymoma imaging. *J Thorac Imaging*. 2002;28(2):69-80.

Nakazono T, White CS, Yamasaki F, et al. MRI findings of mediastinal neurogenic tumors. *AJR Am J Roentgenol*. 2011;197(4):W643-W652.

Nasseri F, Eftekhari F. Clinical and radiologic review of the normal and abnormal thymus: pearls and pitfalls. *Radiographics*. 2010;30(2):413-428.

Nishino M, Ashiku SK, Kocher ON, et al. The thymus: a comprehensive review. *Radiographics*. 2006;26(2):335-348.

Priola AM, Priola SM, Ciccone G, et al. Differentiation of rebound and lymphoid thymic hyperplasia from anterior mediastinal tumors with dual-echo chemical-shift MR imaging in adulthood: reliability of the chemical-shift ratio and signal intensity index. *Radiology*. 2015;274(1):238-249.

Rossi SE, McAdams HP, Rosado-de-Christenson ML, et al. Fibrosing mediastinitis. *Radiographics*. 2001;21(3):737-757.

Sakai S, Murayama S, Soeda H, et al. Differential diagnosis between thymoma and non-thymoma by dynamic MR imaging. *Acta Radiol*. 2002;43(3):262-268.

Sung YM, Lee KS, Kim BT, et al. 18F-FDG PET/CT of thymic epithelial tumors: usefulness for distinguishing and staging tumor subgroups. *J Nucl Med*. 2006;47:1628-1634.

Young CA, Menias CO, Bhalla S, et al. CT features of esophageal emergencies. *Radiographics*. 2008;28(6):1541-1553.

Chapter 6
The Airways

Brett W. Carter, Jo-Anne O. Shepard, Mylene T. Truong, and Carol C. Wu

NORMAL ANATOMY

Trachea

The trachea is a tubular structure that extends from the cricoid cartilage superiorly to the carina inferiorly and is purely gas conducting. It is typically cylindrical in shape with slight flattening along its posterior aspect. The trachea measures approximately 11 cm in length and 2 to 2.5 cm in side-to-side diameter. Two specific segments can be identified, a shorter extrathoracic segment and a longer intrathoracic segment, based on the location of the trachea relative to the upper border of the manubrium. The trachea is composed of hyaline cartilage, fibrous tissue, muscular fibers, mucous membranes, and glands. The cartilages form incomplete C-shaped rings that occupy the anterior two thirds of the trachea. The posterior wall of the trachea is membranous and composed of fibrous tissue and nonstriated muscle fibers.

Bronchi

The trachea divides into two (left and right) primary or main bronchi, which branch into the lobar bronchi, which in turn divide into the segmental and intrapulmonary bronchi and bronchioles. Approximately 23 divisions exist from the trachea to the alveoli, and bronchioles are typically encountered after 6 to 20 divisions from the segmental bronchi. These airways are classified as either purely conducting or gas-exchanging regions separated by a transitional zone. The extrapulmonary bronchi are composed of hyaline cartilage, fibrous tissue, muscular fibers, mucous membranes, and glands. Compared with the cartilage of the trachea, the bronchial cartilages are shorter and narrower but maintain the same shape and arrangement. The bronchioles lack cartilage. The last generation of purely conducting airways is the terminal bronchiole. The respiratory bronchioles are the transitional branches that lead to gas-exchanging alveolar ducts, alveolar sacs, and alveoli. An acinus is lung parenchyma distal to a terminal bronchiole, and it is composed of two to five generations of respiratory bronchioles, alveolar ducts, alveolar sacs, and alveoli. Airways that are less than 2 mm in diameter are called small airways.

The secondary pulmonary lobule is the smallest portion of the lung that is surrounded by connective tissue septa, and it is described in detail in Chapter 17.

IMAGING OF THE AIRWAYS

General

A wide variety of imaging modalities are available to evaluate the airways in the clinical setting, including radiography, fluoroscopy, computed tomography (CT), magnetic resonance imaging (MRI), and 18-fluorodeoxyglucose (^{18}FDG) positron emission tomography (PET)/CT. The commonly accepted indications for each of these modalities are listed in Table 6.1.

Radiography

Posteroanterior and lateral chest radiography (CXR) is the most commonly performed radiologic procedure and may be the first imaging modality to evaluate patients presenting with respiratory symptoms. To reduce the visibility of the bony thorax and improve visualization of the various mediastinal interfaces, a high-kilovoltage (140 kVp) technique should be used. Bilateral, oblique radiographs improve visibility of the central airways by rotating the thoracic spine so that it is not superimposed on the trachea and

TABLE 6.1 Imaging Approach to the Airways

Imaging Modality	Clinical Indication
Chest radiography (posteroanterior, lateral, oblique)	Screening examination
Fluoroscopy	Tracheomalacia Air trapping caused by airway obstruction
Multidetector computed tomography	Identification and characterization of airway neoplasms Airway diameter, wall thickness Tracheomalacia Airway compression Tracheobronchial injury
Magnetic resonance imaging	Airway obstruction caused by vascular rings
18-Fluorodeoxyglucose (^{18}FDG) positron emission tomography/computed tomography image	Staging and restaging of airway neoplasms

main bronchi. The tracheal and proximal bronchial air columns should be identified and closely evaluated on all chest radiographs, especially when adult patients present with clinical symptoms such as stridor, wheezing, adult-onset "asthma," recurrent pneumonia, or hemoptysis. However, abnormalities involving the airways may not be readily apparent on CXR, and further evaluation with cross-sectional imaging is typically necessary.

Multidetector Computed Tomography

Computed tomography is the imaging modality of choice for evaluating the trachea and bronchi because it directly demonstrates the normal anatomy of the airways; adjacent structures such as the mediastinum, hila, and lungs; and a wide variety of abnormalities involving the tracheobronchial tree. CT is superior to CXR in demonstrating the relationship between the airways and mediastinal soft tissues, which becomes important in the setting of mediastinal masses abutting or invading the airways and primary airway neoplasms extending into the adjacent mediastinum. Additionally, CT effectively reveals the morphology of airway lesions, particularly neoplasms with fatty components, calcification, or vascular enhancement.

Modern CT scanners enable visualization and characterization of the trachea and main bronchi in a few seconds over the course of a single breath-hold. Thin section images (1-2.5 mm) can be used to generate high-resolution multiplanar reconstructions, which better delineate the craniocaudally oriented trachea and bronchi and many airway abnormalities such as neoplasms. Recent advances such as volumetric imaging, dynamic airway imaging, and other techniques such as two-dimensional (2D) minimum intensity projection (MIP) and three-dimensional (3D) volume imaging have enhanced the ability of radiologists to evaluate the airways. For instance, dynamic imaging performed during expiration and coughing is more sensitive in demonstrating specific abnormalities such as tracheomalacia than paired inspiratory and expiratory CT imaging. The two most commonly used 3D techniques include external volume rendering of the airways and internal rendering or virtual bronchoscopic images, which supplement but do not replace routine axial CT imaging and enable identification of subtle abnormalities, better demonstrate the craniocaudal extent and shape of lesions, and assist in the planning of interventions (see Chapter 1).

Patients may undergo CT scanning to evaluate the airways for a number of reasons, particularly individuals in whom occult airway disease is suspected based on the presence of clinical symptoms such as chronic cough, wheezing, dyspnea, or hemoptysis and patients with abnormalities on CXR that necessitate further delineation with cross-sectional imaging, such as chronic airspace opacities or consolidations or atelectasis. Other indications include discrepancy between clinical presentation and pulmonary function test (PFT) results and to evaluate potential candidates for interventional bronchoscopic procedures.

Magnetic Resonance Imaging

The role of MRI in the evaluation of the airways is limited. Although the large airways (trachea and main bronchi) are easily identified on standard spin-echo sequences, the segmental bronchi are difficult to visualize because of the relatively low spatial resolution of MRI compared with CT. One of the key advantages of MRI is the lack of ionizing radiation, which can be significant in children and young adults who require repeated imaging to decrease the risks associated with radiation exposure. MRI is beneficial in evaluating patients with vascular rings or tracheal compression by vascular anomalies and other mediastinal abnormalities (see Chapter 3).

FDG PET/CT

The role of FDG PET/CT in the evaluation of the airways is primarily limited to the staging of patients with tracheobronchial malignancies (see Chapter 4).

ABNORMALITIES OF THE TRACHEA

Tracheal Diverticula

Focal outpouchings from the tracheal wall are known as tracheal diverticula, which may be congenital or acquired, and are present in approximately 1% of individuals. Acquired diverticula may be single or multiple, usually in the upper right paratracheal region, and are associated with increased intraluminal pressure and chronic cough. Most patients are asymptomatic, and these abnormalities are usually detected incidentally. However, some individuals may report signs and symptoms related to recurrent airway infections and chronic cough.

Small tracheal diverticula are often not visible on CXR but are readily identified on CT, with thin-section, multiplanar, and 3D reconstructions establishing the connection between the diverticula and the trachea (Fig. 6.1). CT effectively distinguishes diverticula from other paratracheal air collections, including laryngocele, pharyngocele, Zenker diverticulum, and apical bullae or blebs.

Tracheal Stenosis

Tracheal narrowing may be idiopathic, iatrogenic, or posttraumatic in etiology or caused by a wide variety of disease

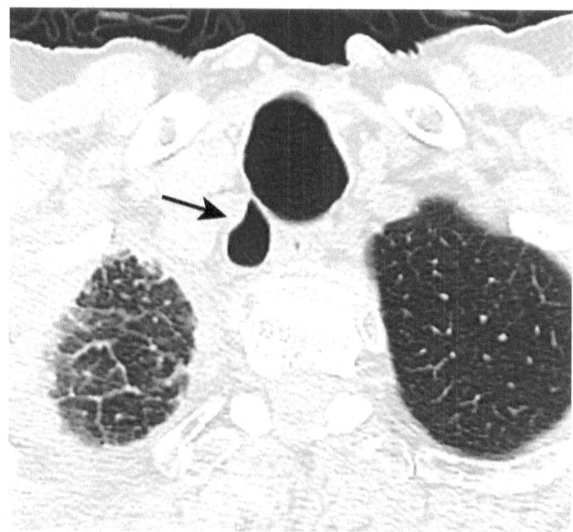

FIGURE 6.1 Tracheal diverticulum. Axial unenhanced computed tomography image demonstrates a large diverticulum connected to the trachea by a narrow neck *(arrow)*.

TABLE 6.2 **Diffuse Tracheal Stenosis**

Etiology	Airway Findings	Associated Abnormalities
Idiopathic	Smooth, tapered, irregular, lobulated, or eccentric narrowing 2–4 cm in length Subglottic airway typical	± Involvement of larynx
Postintubation injury	Smooth narrowing (hourglass configuration)	
Posttraumatic	Smooth narrowing (hourglass configuration)	± Osseous fractures (sternum, upper ribs)
Saber sheath	Smooth narrowing of intrathoracic trachea Coronal diameter half of sagittal diameter	Emphysema Hyperinflated lungs Diffuse bronchial wall thickening
Tracheopathia osteochondroplastica	Submucosal nodularity and ossification Anterolateral walls of trachea and main bronchi affected	
Relapsing polychondritis	Airway wall thickening sparing the posterior wall Diffuse narrowing of trachea and main bronchi ± Airway wall calcification ± Tracheobronchomalacia	Nasal and auricular chondritis Arthritis
Granulomatosis with polyangiitis	Focal or diffuse wall thickening and narrowing ± Enlarged calcified cartilages	Renal and pulmonary involvement
Amyloidosis	Diffuse wall thickening and narrowing Focal nodular masses that enhance and slowly progress ± Nodule calcification	± Lymphadenopathy ± calcification
Sarcoidosis	Airway wall thickening Smooth, irregular, or nodular stenosis Lymph nodes may compress airways	± Lymphadenopathy ± calcification Pulmonary involvement
Rhinosclerosis	Nodular masses or diffuse, symmetric narrowing of trachea and main bronchi Slowly progressive	
Tuberculosis	Hyperplastic stage: irregular wall thickening and narrowing Fibrostenotic stage: smooth narrowing	Mediastinal or hilar lymphadenopathy ± calcification Pulmonary involvement

processes, including chronic obstructive pulmonary disease (COPD), tracheopathia osteochondroplastica, relapsing polychondritis, granulomatosis with polyangiitis, amyloidosis, sarcoidosis, or infection (Table 6.2).

Idiopathic Laryngotracheal Stenosis

Idiopathic narrowing of the laryngeal and subglottic trachea is typically encountered in middle-aged women without a history of endotracheal intubation, traumatic injury, infection, or systemic disorder. The most common clinical symptoms include progressive shortness of breath and associated wheezing, stridor, or hoarseness.

Regions of stenosis measure 2 to 4 cm in length and result in severe compromise of the airway lumen, with affected sites measuring 5 mm or less at the point of greatest narrowing. On CT, the appearance of idiopathic laryngotracheal stenosis is highly variable and ranges from smooth and tapered regions of narrowing to irregular, lobular, and eccentric forms (Fig. 6.2).

Stenoses may be treated conservatively with a wide variety of techniques such as dilation, endotracheal intubation, airway stenting, steroid injection, cryotherapy, or electrocoagulation, or they may be treated surgically.

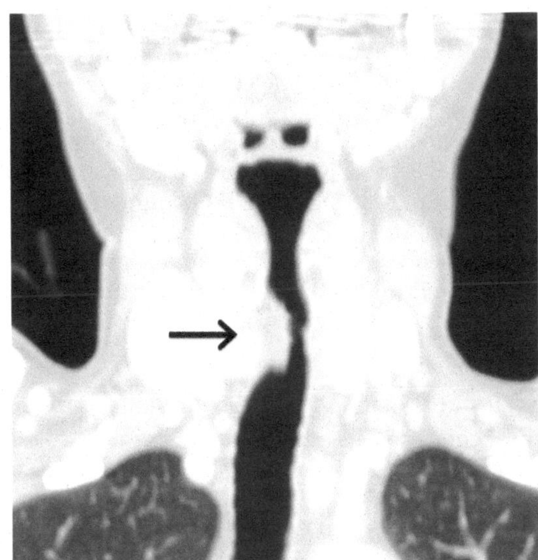

FIGURE 6.2 Idiopathic laryngotracheal stenosis. Coronal contrast-enhanced computed tomography image of the neck shows focal, eccentric, and lobulated soft tissue mass causing stenosis *(arrow)* of the proximal trachea.

Postintubation Injury

Endotracheal intubation and tracheostomy placement are the most common causes of acquired focal tracheal stenosis. Tracheal stenosis and other complications of endotracheal intubation, such as tracheoesophageal fistula and tracheoarterial fistula, are typically caused by cuff injury, specifically pressure necrosis. When the cuff pressure exceeds that of the capillaries, blood supply to the tracheal mucosa becomes compromised, and ischemic necrosis can occur, leading to softening and dissolution of the cartilage and, ultimately, tracheomalacia or scarring and stenosis. The trachea 3

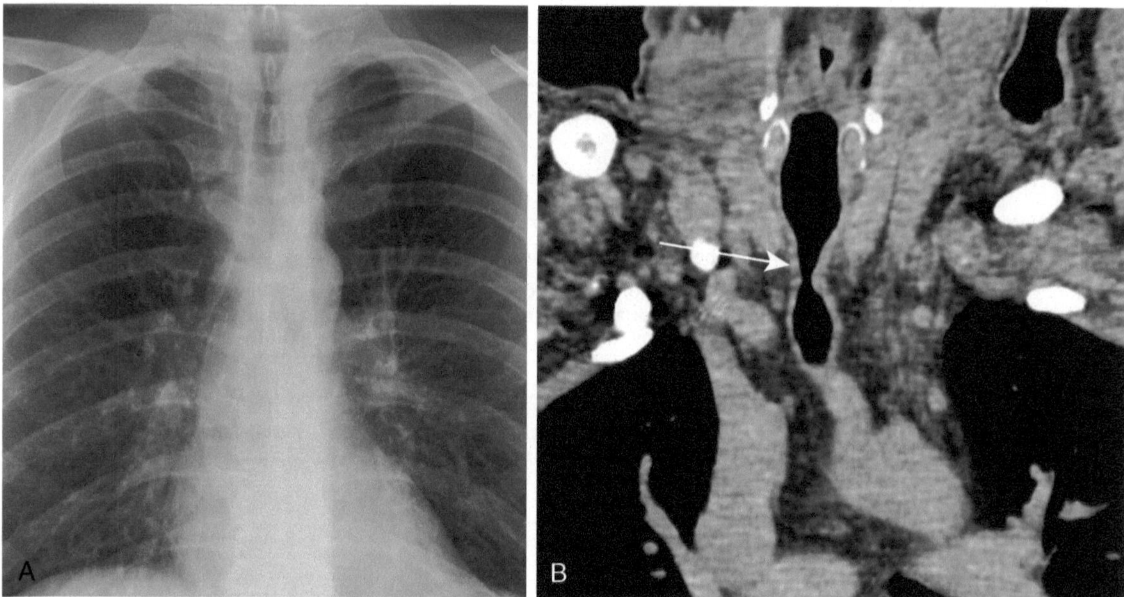

FIGURE 6.3 Postintubation tracheal stenosis. Posteroanterior chest radiograph **(A)** demonstrates marked narrowing of the trachea at the thoracic inlet. Coronal contrast-enhanced computed tomography image **(B)** of the same patient shows tracheal stenosis *(arrow)* in the classic hourglass configuration.

to 4 cm below the cricoid cartilage is typically affected, corresponding to the level of the cuff of the endotracheal or tracheotomy tube. Less commonly, regions of tracheal stenosis may arise at the level of the tracheostomy stoma or at the site of tube tip impingement on the tracheal mucosa. Clinical symptoms of tracheal stenosis typically develop 2 to 6 weeks after extubation, although patients may present months later.

Tracheal stenosis may manifest as focal luminal narrowing on CXR. On multidetector computed tomography (MDCT), postintubation stenosis results in smooth, gradual narrowing with an hourglass configuration that is better demonstrated on coronal and sagittal reformations than axial images (Fig. 6.3). Concentric or eccentric soft tissue thickening, representing edema and granulation tissue, may be present in acute stenosis. Focal expiratory airway collapse caused by destruction of airway cartilage may be identified in chronic stenosis. Stenoses are treated with surgical resection of the damaged region and end-to-end anastomosis.

Posttraumatic Tracheal and Bronchial Stenosis

The most common causes of posttraumatic tracheal stenosis include penetrating injuries, strangulation, and motor vehicle collisions. Iatrogenic airway stenosis may occur following airway anastomoses (see Chapter 12). Posttraumatic tracheal or bronchial stenosis results from healing of an untreated partial laceration or tear, which may be missed initially on imaging because of the lack of associated findings such as pneumomediastinum or pneumothorax in the setting of preservation of the peritracheal or peribronchial connective tissue or occlusion of the tear by a cuff or fibrin deposition. The typical hourglass configuration is usually visible on CT. In contrast, acute laceration of the trachea can occur after traumatic intubation or penetrating or decelerating injuries, discussed in more detail in Chapter 13.

Saber-Sheath Trachea

Saber-sheath trachea is an abnormal configuration of the intrathoracic trachea characterized by narrowing of the transverse diameter that typically begins at the level of the thoracic inlet. Male smokers with COPD are typically affected. In late-stage disease, the entire length of the intrathoracic trachea may be affected. The trachea is characteristically narrowed in the coronal dimension such that it is two thirds or less of the sagittal dimension (Fig. 6.4). It is important to note that the main bronchi are not affected, and tracheal wall thickness is normal.

Tracheopathia Osteochondroplastica

Tracheopathia osteochondroplastica is a rare, idiopathic benign disorder characterized by the presence of osteocartilaginous nodules in the submucosa of the large airways and thickening of tracheal rings. These nodules are connected to the perichondrium of the tracheal rings and protrude into the airway lumen. It is most common in men older than 50 years of age. The anterolateral tracheal walls are affected with a predilection for the upper two thirds of the trachea. Because the posterior wall of the trachea is membranous and lacks cartilage, it is characteristically spared. Most patients with tracheopathia osteochondroplastica are asymptomatic; however, clinical symptoms such as wheezing, cough, and hemoptysis have been reported at clinical presentation.

The most common abnormalities on CXR include nodular thickening and irregularity of the tracheal wall and luminal narrowing. CT effectively demonstrates these mural nodules, which can be seen to protrude into the airway lumen, frequently demonstrate calcification, and spare the membranous wall (Fig. 6.5).

Relapsing Polychondritis

Relapsing polychondritis is a rare autoimmune disorder involving the cartilage of the ears, nose, upper respiratory

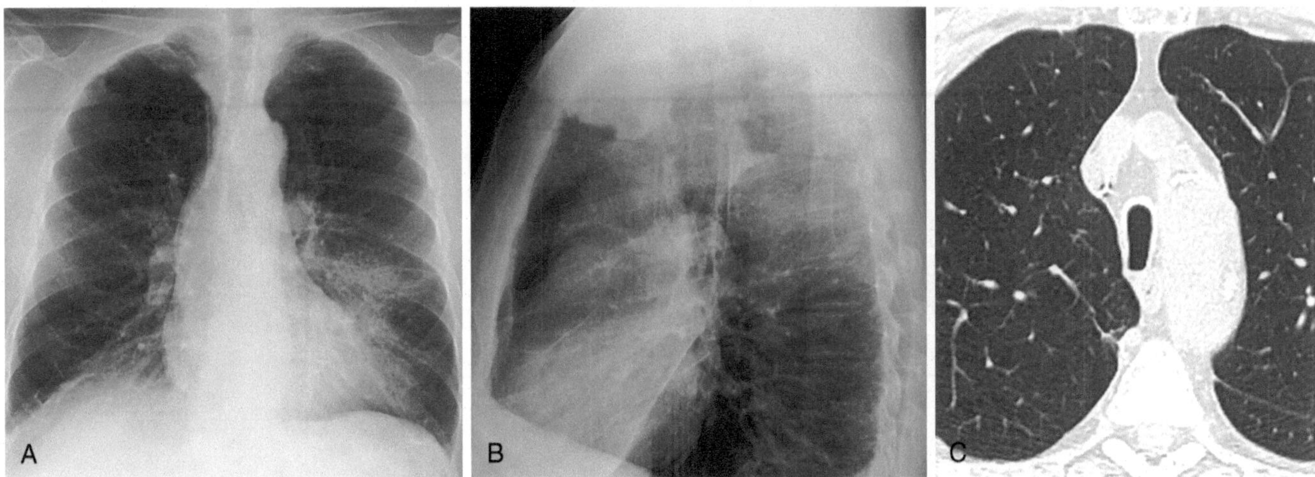

FIGURE 6.4 Saber-sheath trachea. Posteroanterior **(A)** and lateral **(B)** chest radiographs demonstrate narrowing of the trachea in the coronal plane but increased diameter in the sagittal plane and hyperinflated lungs. Axial unenhanced computed tomography image **(C)** of the same patient shows an increased anteroposterior diameter and decreased transverse diameter of the trachea.

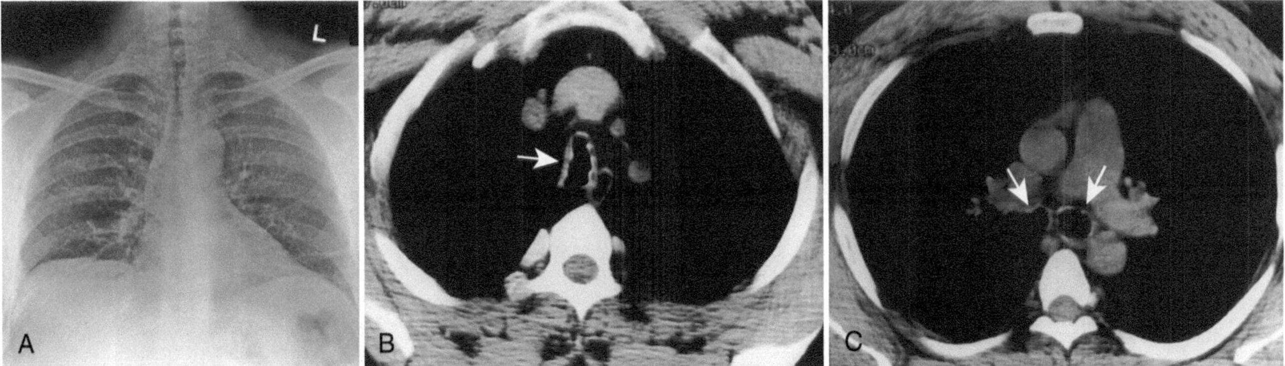

FIGURE 6.5 Posteroanterior chest radiograph **(A)** shows diffuse narrowing of the cervical and thoracic trachea. Axial computed tomography images **(B, C)** show nodularity *(arrows)* of the anterolateral cartilaginous wall of the trachea and main bronchi. Note the associated ossification and sparing of the posterior membranous tracheal wall.

tract, and joints that results in inflammation and destruction. Granulomatous tissue or fibrosis replaces the destroyed cartilage. Up to 50% of patients with the disease experience airway involvement. Associations with other autoimmune disorders such as autoimmune thyroiditis, rheumatoid arthritis, systemic lupus erythematosus, systemic vasculitis, Sjögren syndrome, and inflammatory bowel disease have been described. Airway involvement is more common in women than men, and the average age of presentation is 50 years.

On CXR, the tracheobronchial walls are diffusely thickened, and the trachea and main bronchi show diffuse, smooth narrowing. CT demonstrates diffuse, smooth thickening of the tracheobronchial tree with characteristic sparing of the posterior or membranous segment (Fig. 6.6). Stenosis of the trachea and main bronchi are usually present, and involvement of the smaller airways, including the segmental and subsegmental bronchi, can be seen. Associated findings include calcifications and distal postobstructive bronchiectasis. Dynamic imaging with CT may demonstrate excessive expiratory airway collapse caused by inflammation and destruction of cartilage, often in association with air trapping.

Early detection and treatment of the disease are necessary to delay cartilage destruction. Severe airway involvement is associated with a poor prognosis. Corticosteroids and immunosuppressive medications are the mainstay of medical therapy. Continued positive airway pressure, bronchoscopic interventions such as laser therapy, balloon dilation, and stenting, and tracheostomy in cases of severe stenosis involving the upper trachea can improve clinical symptoms.

Granulomatosis With Polyangiitis

Granulomatosis with polyangiitis (GPA), formerly known as Wegener granulomatosis, is an autoimmune, systemic vasculitis characterized by the presence of cytoplasmic antineutrophil cytoplasmic antibodies (cANCAs) in serum and granuloma formation. Small and medium-sized vessels are typically affected, and up to 50% of patients have involvement of the tracheobronchial tree. The upper and lower portions of the respiratory tract are affected in combination with the kidneys and other visceral organs. When airway involvement is present, the laryngeal and subglottic trachea is typically affected. Diffuse involvement of the tracheobronchial tree is less common and usually encountered in late-stage disease.

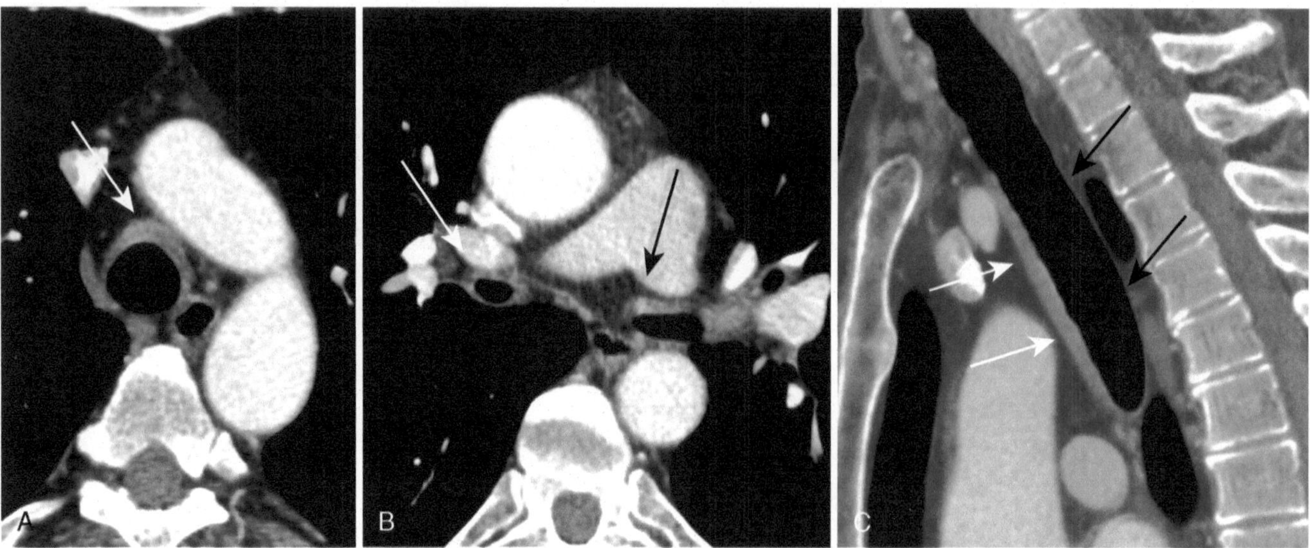

FIGURE 6.6 Relapsing polychondritis. Axial contrast-enhanced computed tomography (CT) images (**A** and **B**) show smooth wall thickening *(arrows)* involving the anterior and lateral walls of the trachea and bronchi. Sagittal contrast-enhanced CT image **(C)** of the same patient demonstrates smooth, long segment thickening involving the anterior tracheal wall *(white arrows)* and sparing of the posterior wall *(black arrows).*

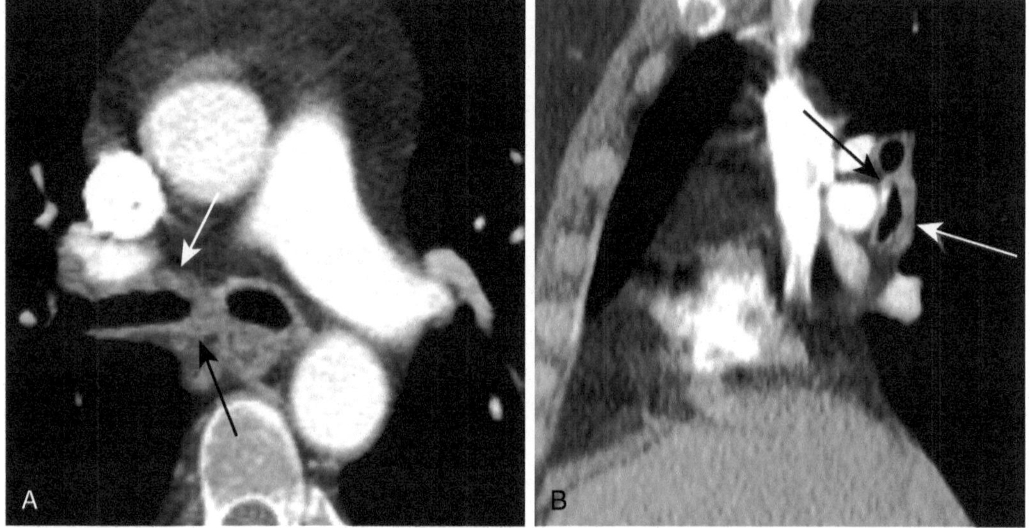

FIGURE 6.7 Granulomatosis with polyangiitis. Axial contrast-enhanced computed tomography (CT) image **(A)** shows smooth wall thickening *(arrows)* involving the anterior *(white arrow)* and posterior walls of the right mainstem bronchus. Sagittal formatted contrast-enhanced CT **(B)** of the same patient demonstrates thickening and calcification of the anterior wall *(black arrow)* and thickening of the posterior wall *(white arrow)* of the bronchus intermedius.

Chest radiography may demonstrate airway wall thickening, focal or diffuse wall irregularity, and luminal narrowing. On CT, involvement of the large airways results in smooth or nodular tracheobronchial wall thickening, which may progress to single or multiple regions of stenosis. Unlike in relapsing polychondritis, airway wall thickening of GPA can be circumferential, without sparing of the posterior wall (Fig. 6.7). Irregular calcification of the cartilage rings, postobstructive atelectasis in the setting of airway obstruction caused by granulation tissue, and bronchiectasis may be present.

Corticosteroids and immunosuppressive medications are used for the medical treatment of GPA. In the setting of persistent airway obstruction, dilation, stent placement, laser ablation, tracheostomy, or surgical resection can improve clinical symptoms.

Amyloidosis

Amyloidosis is a disease characterized by the extracellular accumulation of abnormal proteinaceous, insoluble fibrils that stain with Congo red. These fibrils disrupt the normal airway architecture, act as space-occupying masses, and may have cytotoxic effects. Several types of amyloidosis have been described. In systemic amyloidosis, involvement of the respiratory tract is frequent, but patients are usually asymptomatic, and the manifestations of the disease are

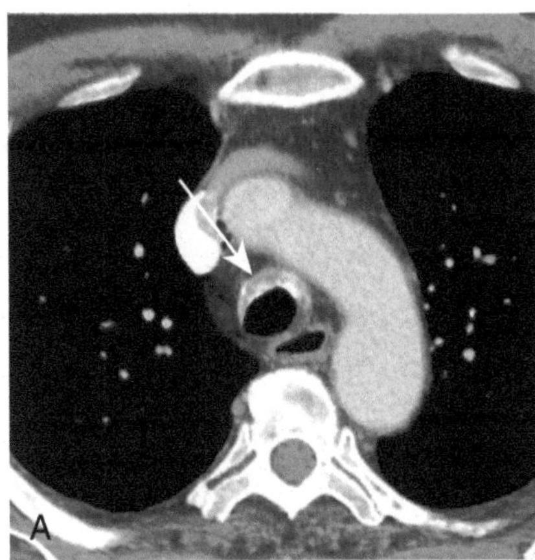

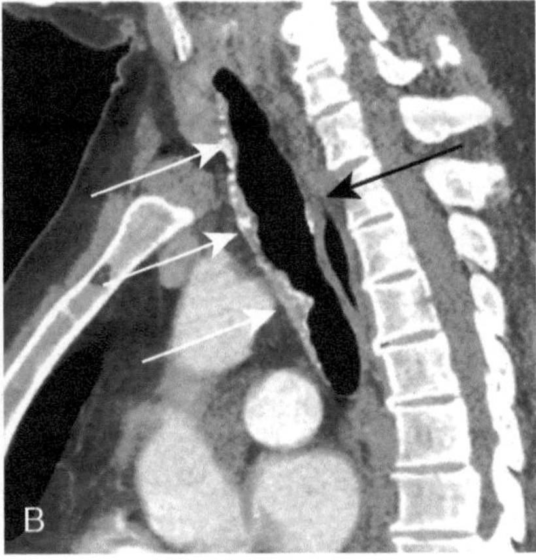

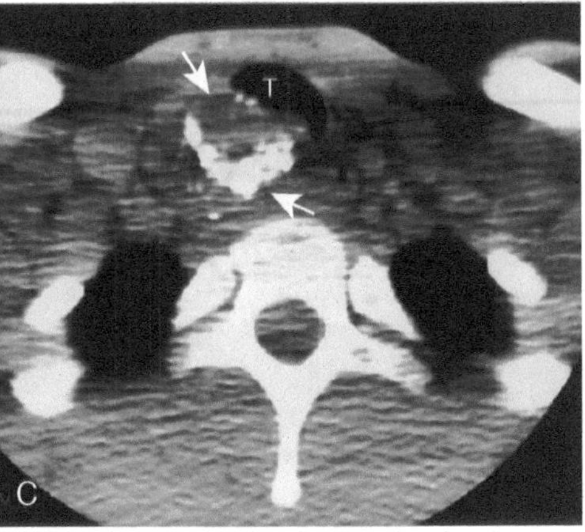

FIGURE 6.8 Amyloidosis. Axial contrast-enhanced computed tomography (CT) image **(A)** shows wall thickening with calcification *(arrow)* involving the anterior and lateral walls of the trachea. Sagittal contrast-enhanced CT **(B)** of the same patient demonstrates thickening and nodularity with calcification involving the anterior *(white arrows)* and posterior *(black arrow)* walls of the trachea. Involvement of the posterior wall distinguishes entities such as amyloidosis from entities such as tracheopathia osteochondroplastica and relapsing polychondritis. Axial noncontrast CT of a different patient **(C)** demonstrates a large, calcified soft tissue mass arising from the posterolateral wall of the trachea **(T)**.

incidentally detected. Localized amyloidosis of the tracheobronchial tree is rare. The trachea and central bronchi are the most common sites of disease, although any portion of the tracheobronchial tract may be affected. Airway involvement may be diffuse or focal, and the lesions tend to grow slowly over time. Tracheobronchial amyloidosis often progresses to respiratory distress, with one third of patients dying of pneumonia or respiratory insufficiency.

On CT, the affected airways demonstrate focal and nodular or diffuse narrowing of the trachea and bronchi caused by submucosal deposits of amyloid, which may project into the airway lumen. Wall thickening is usually present, and internal regions of calcification or ossification may be associated with some foci (Fig. 6.8). Focal deposits of amyloid demonstrate enhancement after the administration of intravenous (IV) contrast. Associated findings such as intrathoracic lymphadenopathy may be present.

Treatment options include debridement, laser ablation, balloon dilation, and stent placement. In the case of localized disease, surgical resection can be performed.

Sarcoidosis

Sarcoidosis is an idiopathic systemic granulomatous disease characterized by the presence of noncaseating epithelioid granulomas. Whereas involvement of the trachea and main bronchi is rare, involvement of the lobar and segmental bronchi is more common. Mucosal and submucosal inflammation and noncaseating granulomas are present in the early stages of the disease and may result in airway narrowing that is smooth, irregular, or nodular in configuration. The late stages are characterized by fibrotic parenchymal abnormalities that result in distortion of the airways and traction bronchiectasis.

Narrowing of the trachea or main bronchi may be visible on CXR. On CT, the most common findings include smooth, irregular, or nodular wall thickening, representing granulomas in the bronchial mucosa and along the peribronchovascular interstitium, and luminal narrowing. Mediastinal lymphadenopathy resulting in airway compression may also be seen. In some cases, air trapping can be seen on expiratory images caused by compression of small airways by peribronchiolar granuloma.

Infection

Rhinosclerosis. Rhinosclerosis is a chronic granulomatous disease associated with *Klebsiella rhinoscleromatis*, a gram-negative bacterium that affects the upper respiratory tract. Although the nose, paranasal sinuses, and pharynx are the most commonly affected anatomic sites, the airways may also be involved. The proximal trachea is involved in fewer than 10% of cases, and the entire tracheobronchial tree may be affected in some patients. Common clinical symptoms of rhinoscleroma include chronic nasal obstruction, rhinorrhea, and epistaxis, which may be encountered in association with absence of the uvula and nasal deformities. Other symptoms such as dyspnea and stridor may be encountered in the presence of airway lesions such as granulomatous nodules and dense fibrotic stenosis.

On CT, rhinosclerosis manifests as nodular masses in the airways or diffuse, symmetric luminal narrowing. Because slow progression over a period of 20 years is typical, most patients are treated with a prolonged course of antibiotics; however, recurrence is common. Associated airway abnormalities are typically treated with bronchoscopic dilation and laser ablation.

Tuberculosis. Tracheobronchial stenosis related to tuberculous infection may be caused by granulomatous changes within the airway wall or extrinsic compression by peribronchial or paratracheal lymphadenopathy. *Mycobacterium tuberculosis* results in wall thickening and luminal narrowing. Multifocal involvement of the large airways is typical, especially the distal trachea and proximal main bronchi.

Several stages of disease have been described based on histopathologic and imaging findings. The hyperplastic stage is reversible and characterized by tubercle formation within the submucosal layer and ulceration and necrosis of the airway wall. On CT, the hyperplastic stage manifests

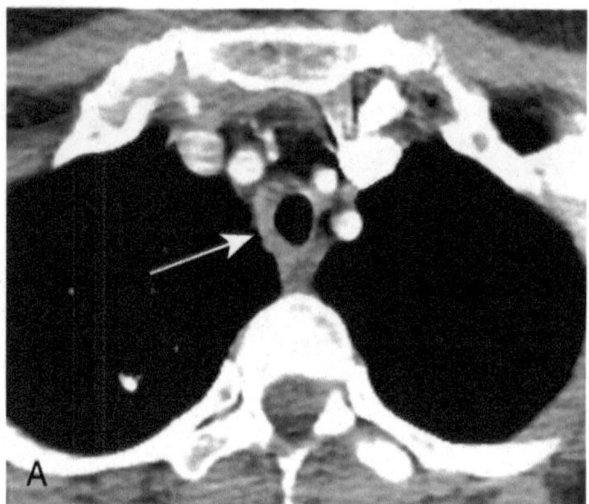

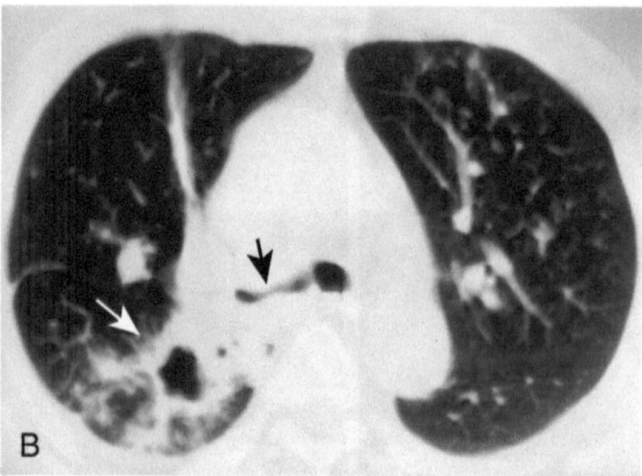

FIGURE 6.9 Tracheobronchial stenosis related to tuberculosis infection. Axial contrast-enhanced computed tomography (CT) image **(A)** shows circumferential tracheal wall thickening with associated luminal narrowing *(arrow)* caused by chronic stenosis. A right upper lobe calcified granuloma is present. Axial CT image of a different patient **(B)** shows irregular thickening and narrowing of the right upper lobe bronchus in the hyperplastic stage of stenosis *(black arrow)* with coexisting right lower lobe cavitation *(white arrow)*.

as irregular thickening with varying degrees of luminal narrowing. Associated abnormalities such as mediastinal or hilar lymphadenopathy and cavitary lesions in the lung parenchyma may be present. The fibrostenotic stage is irreversible and characterized by regions of airway stenosis. On CT, stenoses involving the trachea and bronchi are present, with smooth wall thickening (Fig. 6.9). Associated pulmonary parenchymal findings such as scarring, calcification, bronchiectasis, and atelectasis may be identified. Cases of severe stenosis may be treated with bronchoscopic dilation and stenting (see Chapter 16).

Tracheobronchomegaly (Mounier-Kuhn Syndrome)

Mounier-Kuhn syndrome, also known as congenital tracheobronchomegaly, is a rare disorder characterized by diffuse dilation of the trachea and main bronchi. A characteristic feature of the disease is abrupt transition to normal-sized peripheral airways at the segmental level. Men are primarily affected in the third or fourth decade of life. Most patients with tracheobronchomegaly present clinically with recurrent respiratory infections.

Diffuse dilation of the trachea and main bronchi is usually readily apparent on CXR. CT and MRI imaging demonstrate protrusion of the trachealis muscle between the cartilaginous rings, resulting in a scalloped or corrugated appearance of the airways (Fig. 6.10). Bronchiectasis may be present in patients with repeated respiratory infections.

Tracheal Neoplasms

Malignant Neoplasms

The majority of neoplasms involving the trachea are malignant, typically the result of direct invasion by primary malignancies arising from the thyroid gland, larynx, esophagus, and lung. Primary airway malignancies and metastases from breast, colorectal, and renal cancers or melanoma are less common. The most frequent primary malignant neoplasms arising from the trachea include squamous cell carcinoma (SCC) and adenoid cystic carcinoma. In general, malignant lesions tend to be flat or polypoid in morphology, measure more than 2 cm, and have lobulated or irregular margins. Extension outside of the large airways into the adjacent mediastinal structures or lung indicates advanced disease.

Squamous Cell Carcinoma. Squamous cell carcinoma is the most common primary malignant neoplasm of the trachea, is strongly associated with smoking, and typically affects men 50 to 60 years of age. Almost 40% of patients develop synchronous or metachronous malignancies of the head or neck or lung. One third of patients with SCC present with mediastinal lymphadenopathy or pulmonary metastases (or both) at diagnosis.

On CT, SCC typically appears as a polypoid intraluminal mass, the margins of which may be variable and appear smooth, lobular, or irregular. Any portion of the tracheobronchial tree may be affected, although there is preference for the posterior wall of the lower two thirds of the trachea. When involving the bronchi, the tumor is usual central in location. Tumors may be confined to the affected portion of the airway or result in extraluminal extension into the adjacent mediastinum or lung (Fig. 6.11). Mediastinal structures such as the esophagus may become involved, leading to complications such as tracheoesophageal or bronchoesophageal fistula. Alternatively, SCC may primarily result in focal or circumferential airway wall thickening. On FDG PET/CT, SCC typically demonstrates increased FDG uptake because of the high metabolic activity of the tumor.

Adenoid Cystic Carcinoma. Adenoid cystic carcinoma is the second most common primary malignant neoplasm of the trachea and arises from submucosal minor salivary glands. In contrast to SCC, there is no known association with smoking. Men and women are affected equally, and patients are typically in the fourth decade of life at the time of diagnosis. Approximately 10% of patients present with regional lymph node involvement.

On CT, adenoid cystic carcinoma appears as a focal intraluminal soft tissue mass or diffuse or circumferential thickening of airway walls, which may or may not result in luminal stenosis. The lower trachea and main bronchi are the most commonly affected regions of the tracheobronchial tree. Because of the tendency for adenoid cystic carcinoma to result in submucosal and perineural spread, the full extent of disease can be underestimated on axial imaging;

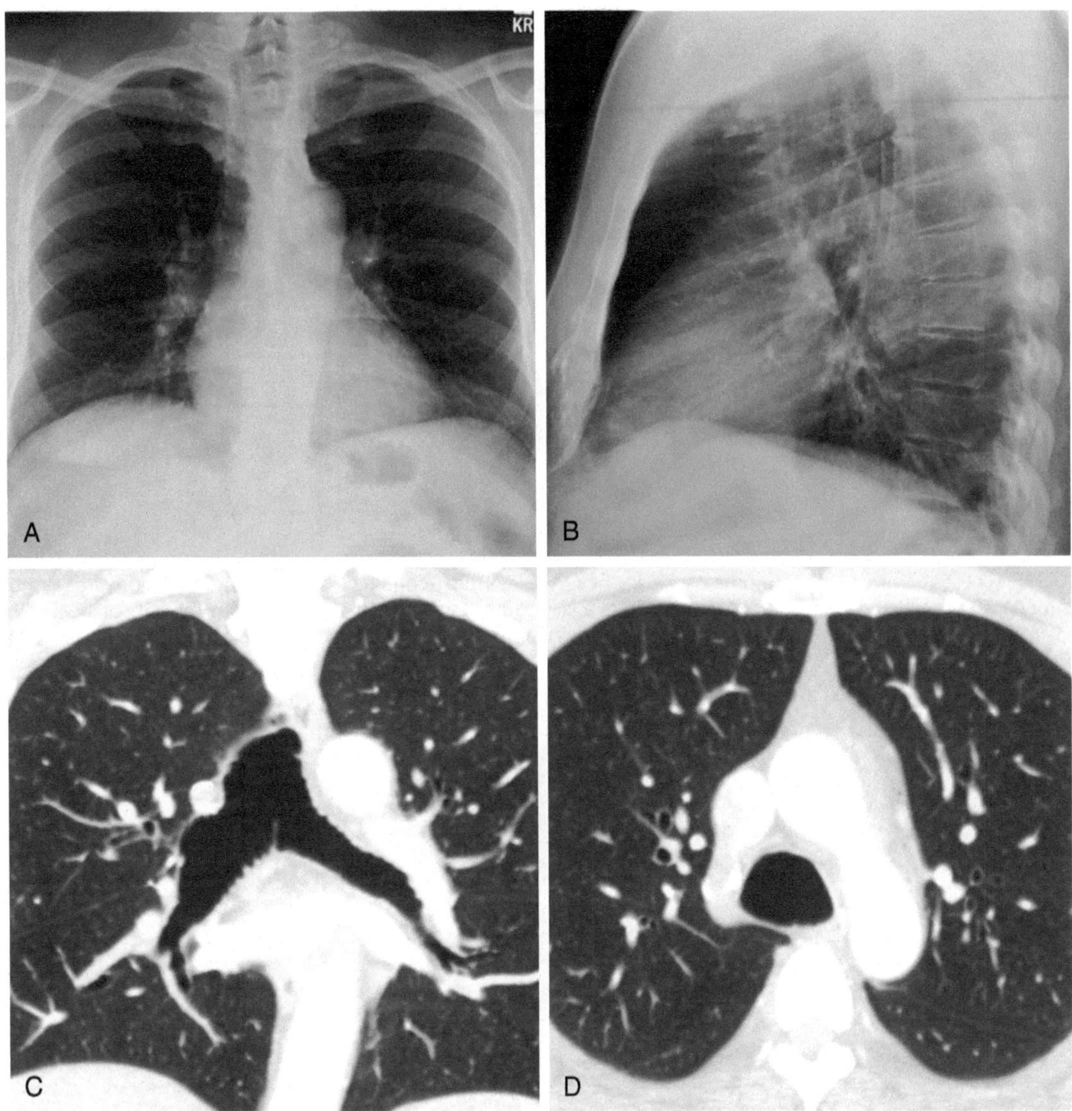

FIGURE 6.10 Mounier-Kuhn syndrome. Posteroanterior **(A)** and lateral **(B)** chest radiographs demonstrate increased transverse and anteroposterior diameters of the trachea. Coronal contrast-enhanced computed tomography (CT) **(C)** demonstrates pronounced dilation of the trachea and main bronchi and a scalloped or corrugated appearance of the airways caused by protrusion of the mucosa between cartilaginous rings. Axial contrast-enhanced CT image **(D)** shows marked dilation of the trachea proximal to the carina.

thus, sagittal and coronal reformations are more effective in demonstrating longitudinal spread of tumor (Fig. 6.12). Because most tumors demonstrate slow growth, FDG uptake on PET/CT can be highly variable, with high-grade tumors tending to demonstrate greater FDG uptake.

Benign Neoplasms

Primary benign neoplasms of the trachea are much less common than malignant tumors. In contrast to malignant neoplasms, benign tumors are typically well defined, round and smooth in configuration, measure less than 2 cm, and do not invade the airway wall. The most common benign lesions include papilloma and hamartoma (Table 6.3). Other neoplasms such as leiomyoma, lipoma, chondroma, and neurogenic neoplasms are less common.

Squamous Cell Papilloma and Tracheobronchial Papillomatosis. Squamous cell papilloma is the most common benign neoplasm of the airways and is composed of a core of fibrovascular tissue surrounded by stratified squamous epithelium. These lesions are associated with smoking, and men are affected more frequently than women. Papillomas may be found in solitary form or as tracheobronchial papillomatosis when multiple lesions exist. Tracheobronchial papillomatosis results from infection with human papillomavirus types 6 and 11, usually acquired from an affected mother during vaginal delivery. Although the majority of these lesions are benign, malignant transformation to SCC can occur.

On CT, squamous cell papilloma manifests as a solitary small nodule projecting into the airway lumen without extraluminal extension. Most lesions originate from a lobar bronchus; involvement of a main bronchus or the trachea is less common. Tracheobronchial papillomatosis appears as multiple intraluminal polypoid nodules in the trachea (Fig. 6.13). The central airways are affected in 5% of cases, and the small airways and lungs are involved in fewer than

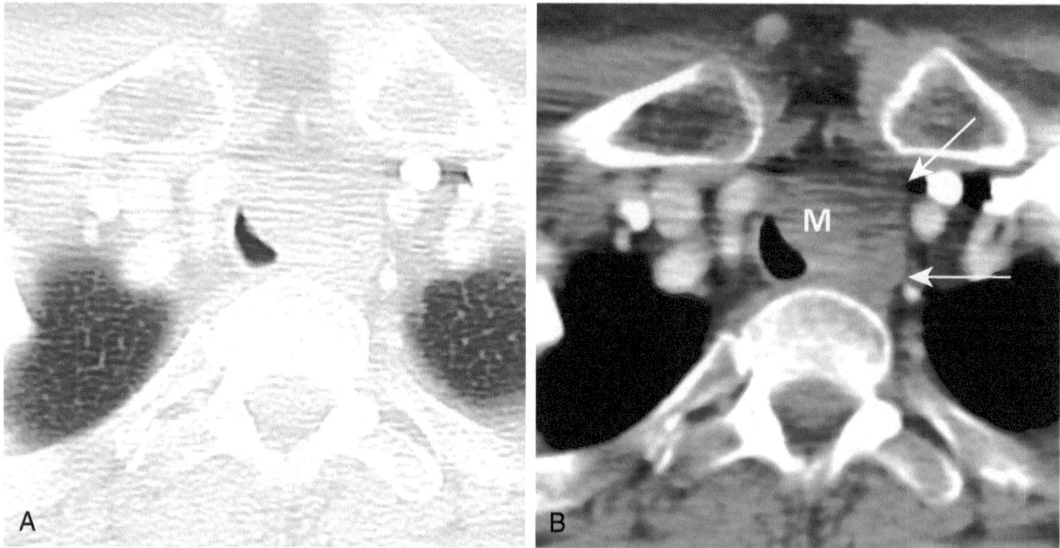

FIGURE 6.11 Squamous cell carcinoma of the trachea. Axial contrast-enhanced computed tomography images in lung **(A)** and soft tissue **(B)** windows demonstrate a large soft tissue mass (M) arising from the left tracheal wall that results in leftward shift and narrowing of the trachea. Note the invasion of the adjacent left mediastinum *(arrows)*.

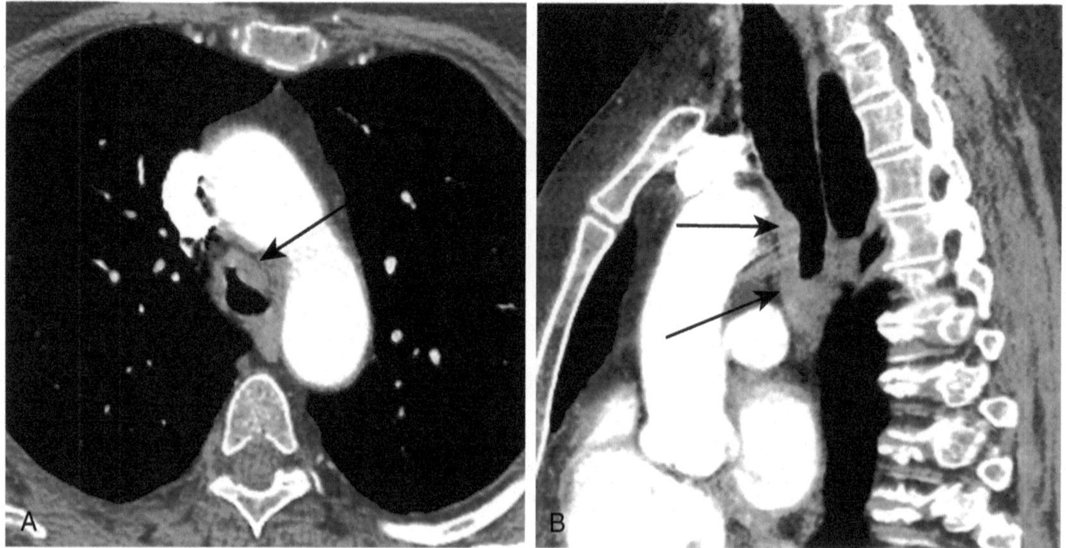

FIGURE 6.12 Adenoid cystic carcinoma of the trachea. Axial contrast-enhanced computed tomography (CT) image **(A)** shows thickening and nodularity of the anterolateral tracheal walls *(arrow)*. Sagittal contrast-enhanced CT **(B)** of the same patient demonstrates the craniocaudal extent of disease *(arrows)*.

1%. When it spreads to the lungs, nodules may cavitate and demonstrate air-fluid levels. These nodules typically present in the posterior half of the chest in the dependent portion of the lung; 2% of patients with pulmonary involvement have been reported to develop SCC.

Tracheobronchomalacia

Tracheobronchomalacia is characterized by weakness of the airway walls and supporting cartilages with subsequent collapsibility that becomes most apparent during coughing or forced expiration. Primary tracheobronchomalacia is caused by a deficiency of airway cartilage. Secondary or acquired tracheobronchomalacia may be idiopathic or caused by a wide variety of disease processes, including endotracheal intubation, trauma, COPD, relapsing polychondritis, or infection. Compression of the airways from mediastinal masses, thyroid goiters, and vascular abnormalities such as aneurysms or aberrant pulmonary vessels may result in focal tracheobronchomalacia. Patients may be symptomatic with retained mucus, respiratory infections, and bronchiectasis caused by an inefficient cough mechanism.

Tracheobronchomalacia is best evaluated with dynamic CT or inspiratory and expiratory CT imaging. In normal patients, expiration or coughing results in narrowing of the tracheobronchial lumen by 10% to 30%; however, in patients with tracheobronchomalacia, the airway lumen decreases by more than 70% (Fig. 6.14). For patients with severe disease, treatment options include stent placement, tracheostomy, and tracheoplasty.

ABNORMALITIES OF THE BRONCHI

Bronchial Neoplasms

Carcinoid Tumors

Carcinoid tumors are classified as neuroendocrine neoplasms and originate from bronchial Kulchitsky cells. Carcinoid tumors are the most common endobronchial neoplasm in children and adolescents. Typical carcinoids tend to affect patients 40 to 50 years of age and manifest as smooth, round, well-defined masses arising from the central bronchi (Fig. 6.15). Atypical carcinoids affect patients 50 to 60 years of age and are more common in men and smokers. These tumors tend to be larger at diagnosis (Fig. 6.16), may be centrally or peripherally located, and have a tendency to metastasize to hilar or mediastinal lymph nodes (see Chapter 21).

TABLE 6.3 Etiologies of Bronchiectasis

Category	Entities
Infection	Viruses (respiratory syncytial virus, adenovirus) Acute bacterial infection (*Bordetella pertussis, Mycoplasma* spp.) Tuberculosis and atypical mycobacteria Chronic or recurrent bacterial infections Recurrent aspiration pneumonia
Impaired host defense	Agammaglobulinemia Granulomatous disease of childhood Acquired immunodeficiency syndrome
Cartilage abnormalities	Williams-Campbell syndrome
Abnormal mucus production	Cystic fibrosis
Abnormal ciliary clearance	Primary ciliary dyskinesia Kartagener syndrome
Traction	Radiation fibrosis Sarcoidosis Idiopathic interstitial pneumonias
Other	Bronchial obstruction Allergic bronchopulmonary aspergillosis Noxious fume inhalation

Mucoepidermoid Carcinoma

Mucoepidermoid carcinoma is a rare primary malignancy of salivary gland origin that represents 0.1% to 0.2% of all pulmonary neoplasms. Metastatic disease is present in 10% of patients at diagnosis. Patients younger than 40 years of age are most frequently affected.

The most common CT appearance of mucoepidermoid carcinoma is an intraluminal soft tissue nodule with mild to marked heterogeneous enhancement after the administration of IV contrast (Fig. 6.17). Thus, these lesions may be indistinguishable from carcinoid tumors on CT. Small internal foci of calcification have been reported in up to 50% of cases. Although any portion of the tracheobronchial tree can be affected, 45% arise from the central airways (the main bronchi more commonly than the trachea), and 55% arise from the distal airways (usually a segmental bronchus). Variable FDG uptake on PET/CT has been reported; whereas low-grade tumors tend to result in low FDG uptake, high-grade tumors show increased FDG uptake.

Hamartoma

Hamartomas are slow-growing benign neoplasms that contain normal airway components such as cartilage, fat, fibrous tissue, and epithelium but arranged in a disorganized fashion. The presence of fat or popcorn calcification in an endobronchial lesion on CT is suggestive of the diagnosis (Fig. 6.18). Calcification is present in approximately 25% of hamartomas and is more common in larger lesions. Distal atelectasis or pneumonia may be identified when endobronchial lesions result in airway obstruction.

Lipoma

Airway lipoma is very rare benign tumor arising from the submucosal adipose tissue. These tumors are usually located

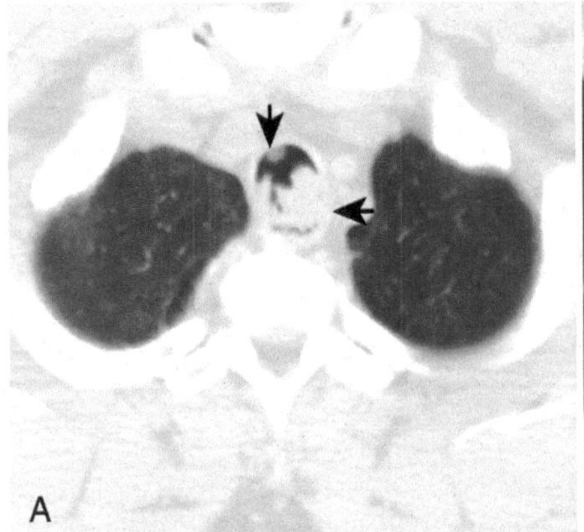

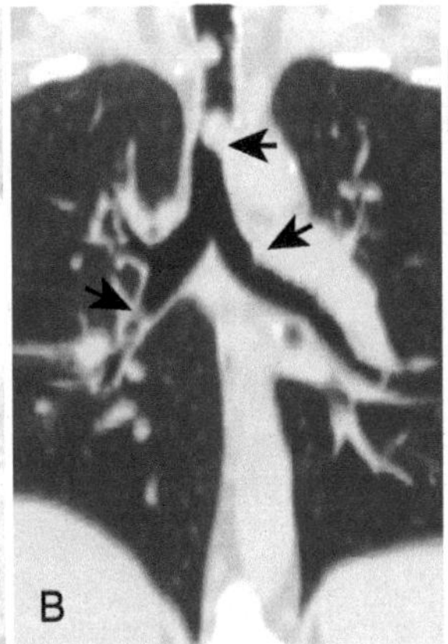

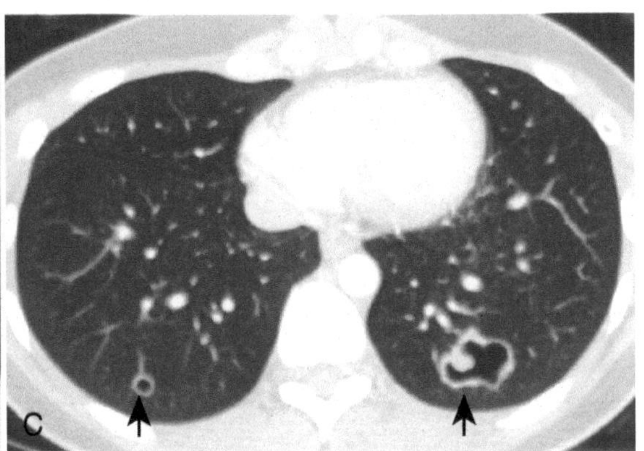

FIGURE 6.13 Tracheobronchial papillomatosis. Axial **(A)** and coronal **(B)** computed tomography (CT) images demonstrate polypoid and sessile nodules within the trachea and left main bronchus *(arrows)*. Axial CT image **(C)** reveals cavitary nodules in the lower lobes that represent lung involvement *(arrows)*.

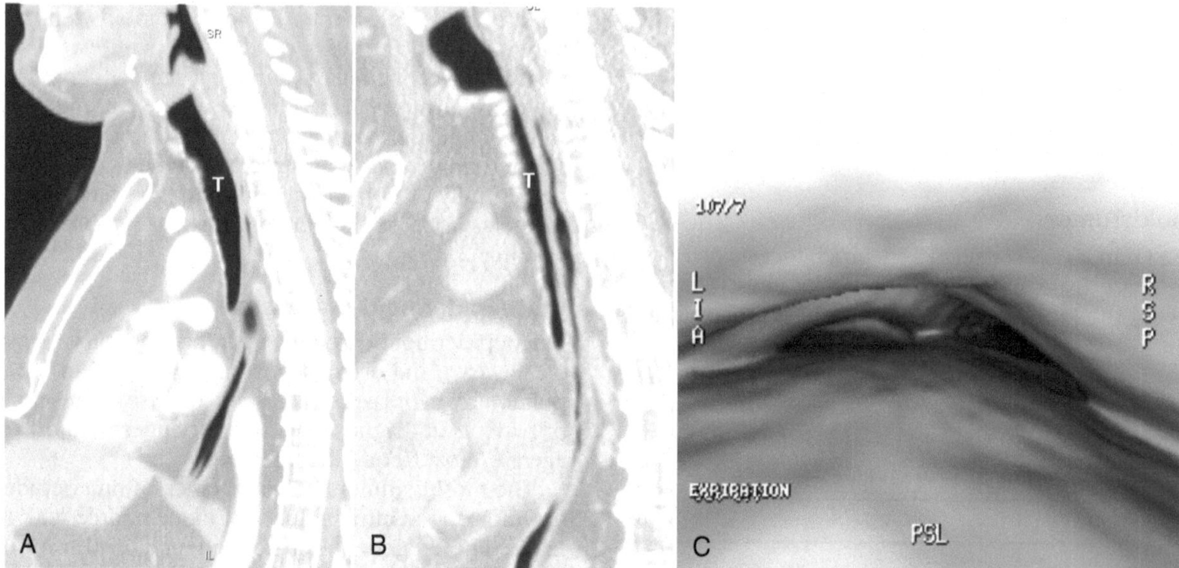

FIGURE 6.14 Tracheobronchomalacia. Sagittal contrast-enhanced computed tomography images through the trachea on inspiration **(A)** and expiration **(B)** demonstrate abnormal collapse of the tracheal wall and a pronounced decrease in the tracheal lumen *(T)* on expiration. The three-dimensional bronchoscopic view **(C)** reveals increased collapsibility of the trachea and main bronchi and a narrowed anteroposterior diameter.

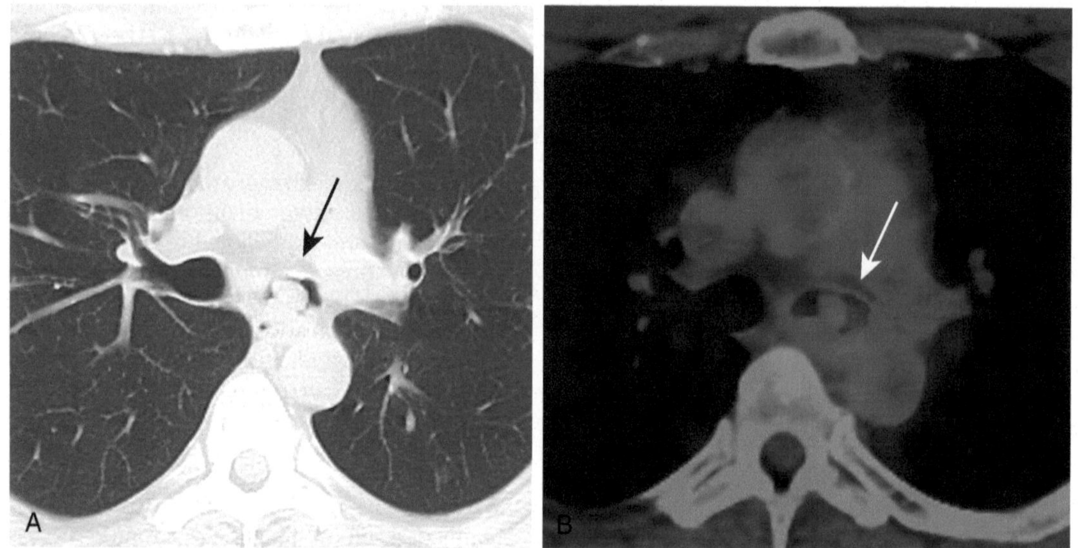

FIGURE 6.15 Typical carcinoid tumor. Axial unenhanced computed tomography image **(A)** demonstrates a lobulated soft tissue nodule in the left main bronchus *(arrow)*. Bronchoscopic biopsy revealed a typical carcinoid tumor. 18-Fluorodeoxyglucose (^{18}FDG) positron emission tomography/computed tomography image **(B)** of the same patient shows low-grade FDG uptake in the tumor *(arrow)*.

in the first three subdivisions of the tracheobronchial tree and consist entirely of fat density or intensity on CT (Fig. 6.19) and MRI. Surgical resection and laser therapy have been successfully used to treat these lesions.

Other Endobronchial Lesions

Broncholithiasis

Broncholithiasis is characterized by calcified material within or adjacent to a bronchus with associated distortion of the airway lumen. Broncholiths arise from calcified peribronchial lymph nodes that erode into the adjacent bronchi, many of which are caused by *Histoplasma capsulatum* infection. Other disease processes that may predispose to the development of broncholiths include fungal infections, tuberculosis (TB), sarcoidosis, and silicosis. Common clinical symptoms at presentation include hemoptysis, wheezing, and coughing. Lithoptysis, or the expectoration of stones, is diagnostic but very rare.

On CXR, a calcified endobronchial lesion or peribronchial lymph node without associated soft tissue is present and may be associated with findings of bronchial obstruction such as atelectasis, postobstructive pneumonia, bronchiectasis, and air trapping. CT readily demonstrates the presence of a broncholith, the segment of airway affected, and any associated abnormalities (Fig. 6.20).

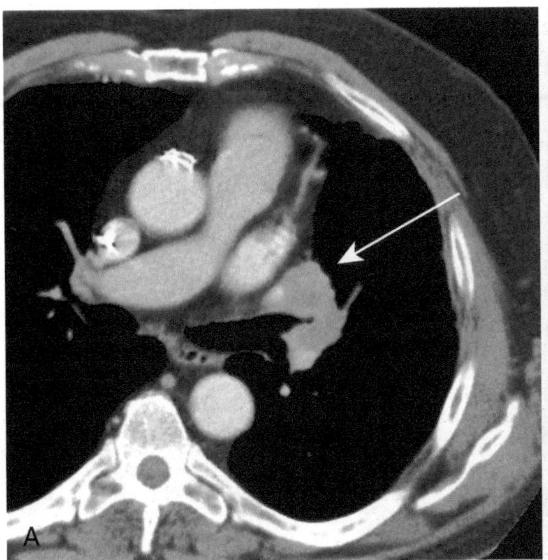

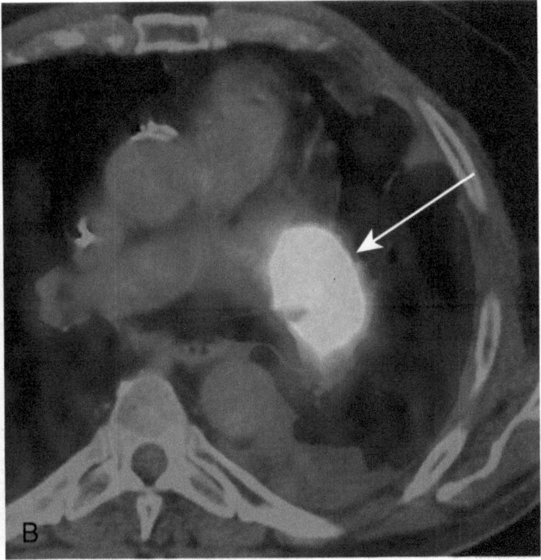

FIGURE 6.16 Atypical carcinoid tumor. Axial contrast-enhanced computed tomography (CT) image **(A)** shows a large soft tissue mass arising from the distal left main bronchus and extending into the left hilar region *(arrow)*. Bronchoscopic biopsy demonstrated atypical carcinoid tumor. 18-Fluorodeoxyglucose (^{18}FDG) positron emission tomography/computed tomography image **(B)** of the same patient demonstrates increased FDG uptake within the lesion due to high metabolic activity *(arrow)*.

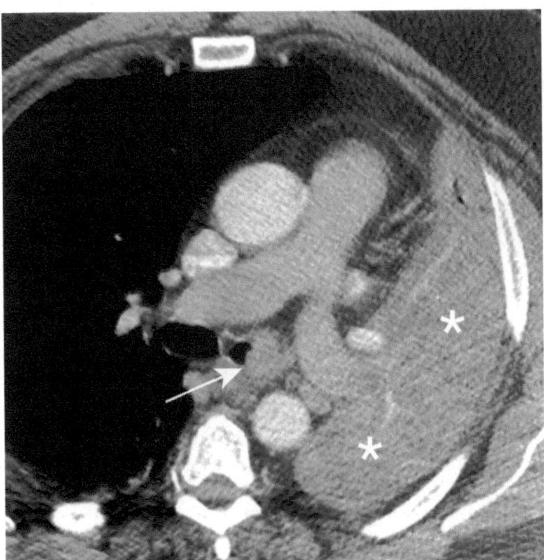

FIGURE 6.17 Mucoepidermoid carcinoma. Axial contrast-enhanced computed tomography image demonstrates a slightly enhancing soft tissue nodule *(arrow)* in the left main bronchus that results in complete atelectasis of the left lung *(asterisks)*.

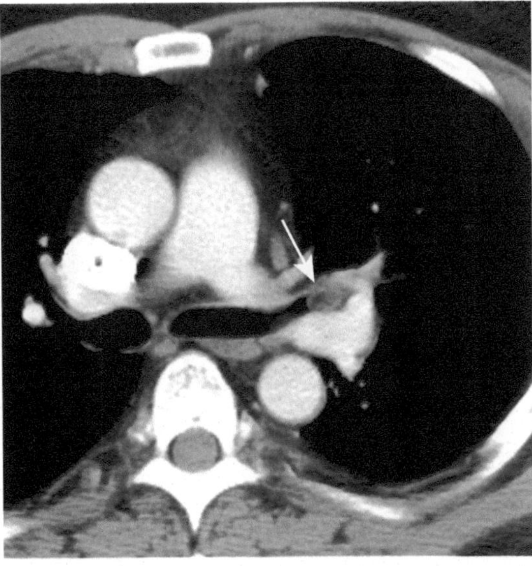

FIGURE 6.18 Bronchial hamartoma. Axial contrast-enhanced computed tomography image shows a well-defined nodule *(arrow)* in the left main bronchus composed of fat and soft tissue diagnostic of a hamartoma.

Foreign Bodies

The majority of aspirated foreign bodies occur in young children, with 50% affecting children younger than 3 years of age. When encountered in adults, altered mental status or poor dentition is frequently coexistent. Most foreign bodies are of vegetable origin, including items such as peanuts, or result from broken teeth or dental fixtures, and tend to become aspirated into the lower lobe bronchi. The right-sided airways are more frequently affected than the left-sided airways because of the more direct angle of the right main bronchus with the trachea (see Chapter 2).

After acute foreign body aspiration, the most common abnormality on imaging studies is air trapping caused by bronchial obstruction and a resultant check-valve mechanism. Expiratory CXR, decubitus CXR, and expiratory CT imaging are the most effective methods of detecting air trapping. In normal patients, the lungs become more opaque after expiration; however, in the setting of air trapping, the obstructed lobe or lung remains lucent and does not decrease in volume upon expiration. On decubitus radiography, the normal, dependent lung is hypoinflated and more opaque; in the setting of air trapping, if the affected lung is in a more dependent position, the mediastinum will shift away from

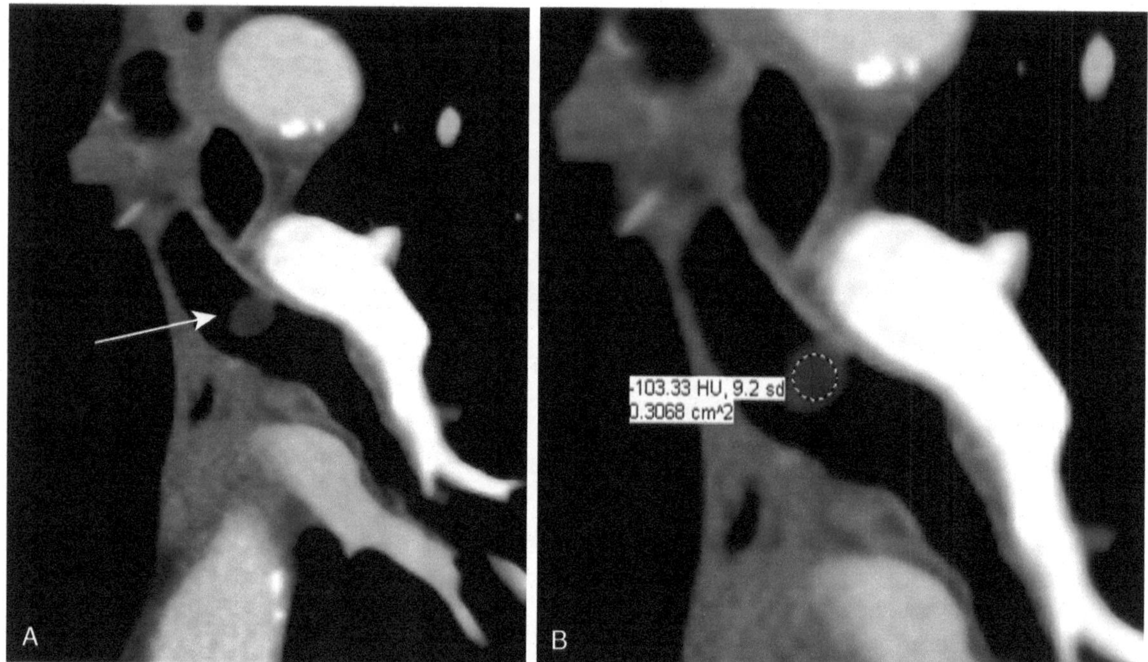

FIGURE 6.19 Bronchial lipoma. Coronal reformation computed tomography image shows a circumscribed nodule (*arrow* in **A**) in the left main bronchus, entirely of fat attenuation (–103 HU in **B**), consistent with a lipoma.

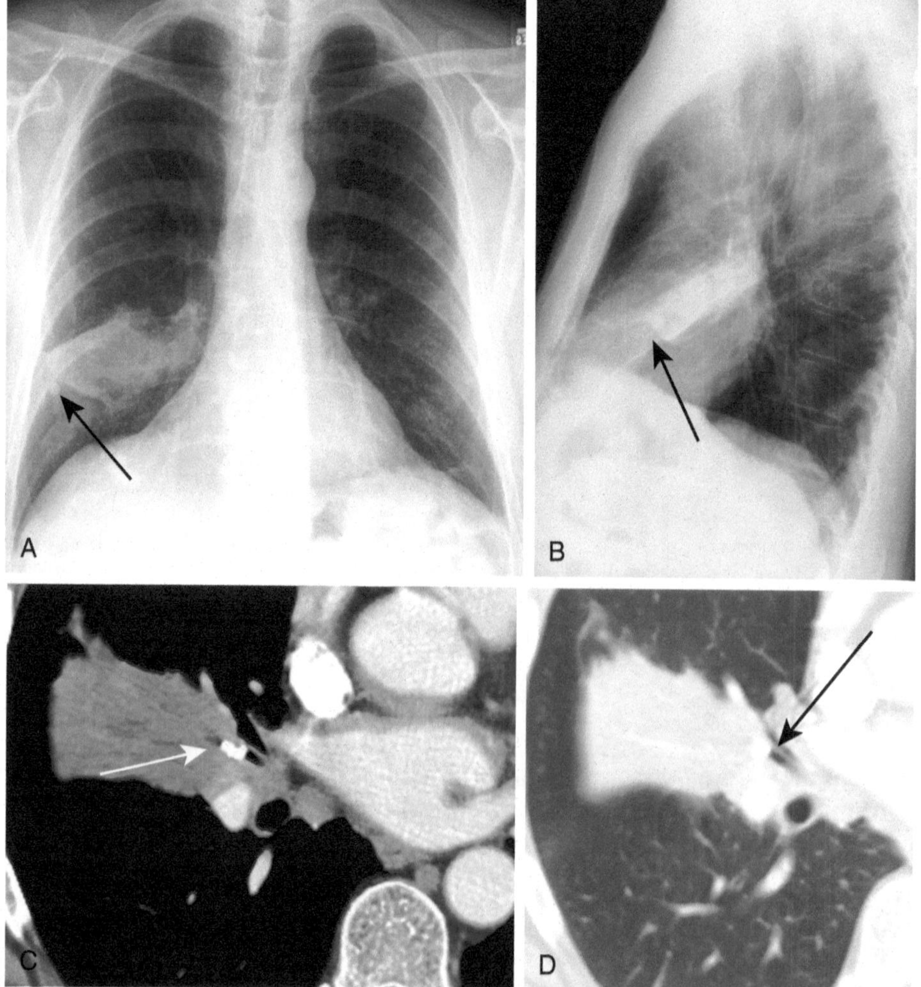

FIGURE 6.20 Broncholithiasis. Posteroanterior **(A)** and lateral **(B)** chest radiographs show right middle lobe collapse and a right middle lobe calcified granuloma *(arrows)*. Axial contrast-enhanced computed tomography images in soft tissue **(C)** and lung windows **(D)** show broncholithiasis *(arrows)* in the right middle lobe bronchus resulting in postobstructive atelectasis.

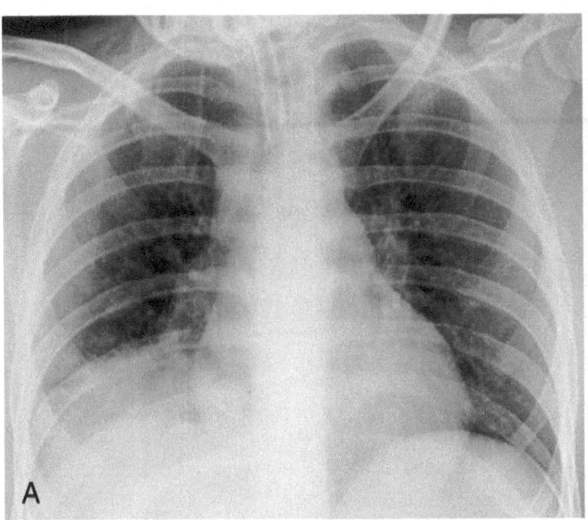

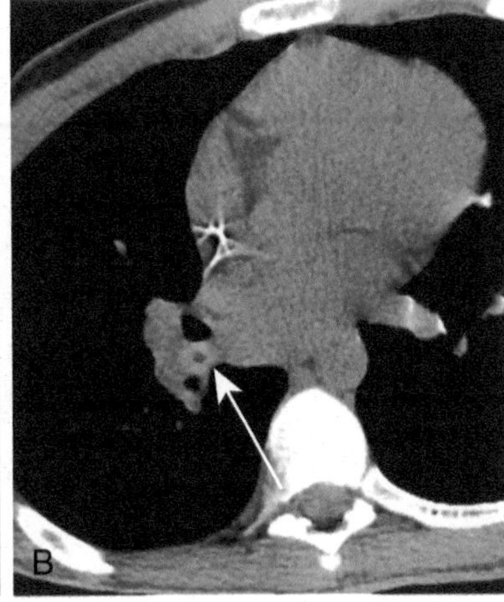

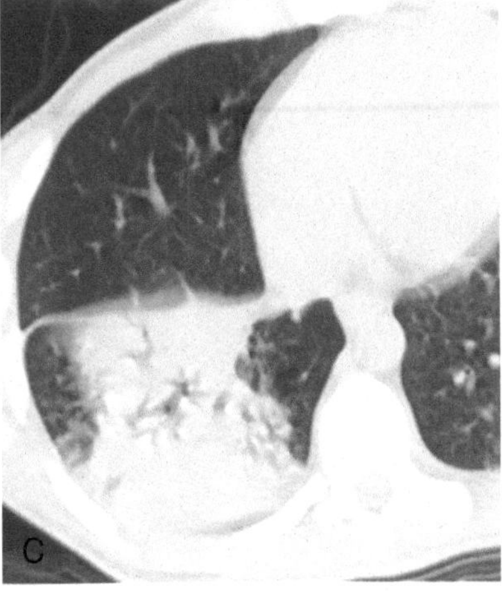

FIGURE 6.21 Foreign body aspiration. Posteroanterior **(A)** chest radiograph demonstrates right lower lobe consolidation and volume loss. Non–contrast-enhanced axial computed tomography images in soft tissue **(B)** and lung **(C)** windows show a hyperattenuating focus with central lucency in the right lower lobe bronchus *(arrow)* and associated right lower lobe postobstructive pneumonia. Bronchoscopy revealed a cotton tip swab lodged in the right lower lobe bronchus.

the side of air trapping. Obstruction may produce hypoxic vasoconstriction, appearing as hyperlucency of the lung and attenuation of the pulmonary vessels. Chronic obstruction may result in atelectasis, recurrent pneumonia (Fig. 6.21), hemoptysis, or bronchiectasis. CT readily demonstrates the presence and etiology of an aspirated foreign body and can be used to localize the abnormality to a specific region of the airway. Foreign bodies that demonstrate high attenuation suggest bone, metallic foreign body, or teeth. Vegetable material has soft tissue density and occasionally has fat density. MRI may be beneficial in identifying peanuts, which typically demonstrate high signal intensity on T1-weighted images.

Airway Fistulas

Esophagorespiratory Fistulas

Esophagorespiratory fistulas may be congenital or acquired. Congenital fistulas are discussed in Chapter 8. Acquired fistulas are typically secondary to neoplasms of mediastinal structures such as the esophagus, tracheobronchial tree, lymph nodes, or the thyroid gland. Nonneoplastic causes include infection, such as histoplasmosis, TB, actinomycosis, and syphilis; trauma; and radiation therapy. The most common clinical symptom reported by patients at presentation is a sense of strangulation after the ingestion of solids or liquids.

Esophagorespiratory fistulas are difficult to visualize on CXR; however, secondary findings related to pneumonia or aspiration may be present, particularly in the lower lobes. Contrast esophagography can be used to establish the diagnosis; high-osmolar contrast should be avoided because of the risk of pulmonary edema if contrast reaches the lungs. CT can demonstrate the presence, cause, and site of esophagorespiratory fistula. Sometimes the fistulous connection is not readily apparent on CT, but focal distention of the esophagus with air near the level of the fistula and signs of aspiration such as mucous plugging of distal airways, atelectasis, or tree-in-bud opacities are often present. Further evaluation with bronchoscopy and esophagoscopy can often enable histologic, cytologic, and bacteriologic examination of fistulas (Figs. 6.22 and 6.23). In challenging cases, methylene blue installation in the esophagus can be used to identify small esophago-airway fistulas during bronchoscopy.

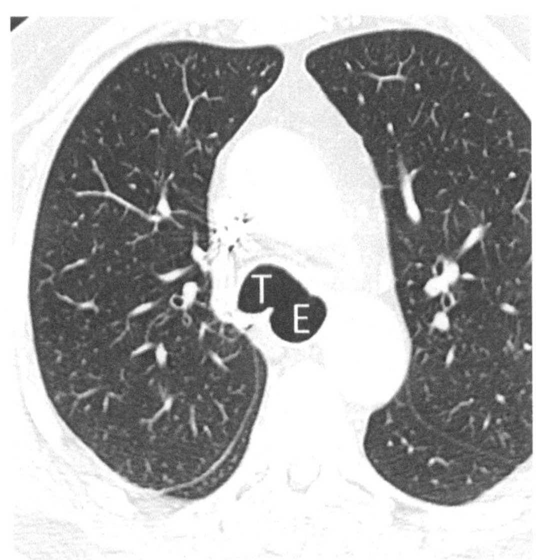

FIGURE 6.22 Tracheoesophageal fistulas. Axial contrast-enhanced computed tomography image of a patient previously treated with radiation therapy for esophageal carcinoma demonstrates complete communication between the trachea *(T)* and the esophagus *(E)* below the aortic arch. Note that the esophageal lumen is distended with air.

Esophagorespiratory fistulas may be treated with surgical isolation of the fistula and closure. Esophageal stents are typically placed in the setting of fistula caused by malignancy.

Other Fistulas

Aortobronchial fistulas typically result from previous surgical graft treatment for aortic coarctation or a chronic aneurysm of the aorta. Most patients present with hemoptysis; other

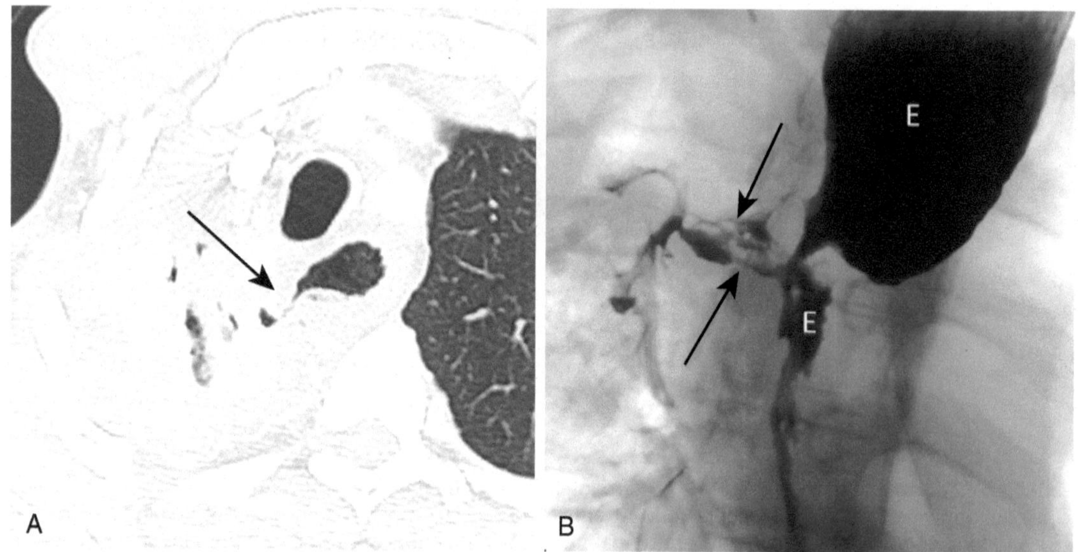

FIGURE 6.23 Esophagobronchial fistulas. Axial contrast-enhanced computed tomography image **(A)** and contrast esophagography **(B)** of a patient with lung cancer of the right upper lobe show multiple communications *(arrows)* between the esophagus *(E)* and bronchi in the right lung.

clinical symptoms such as chest pain and back pain are less common. A wide variety of imaging modalities may be used to make the diagnosis, including CT, aortography, bronchoscopy, and transesophageal echocardiography.

Bronchiectasis

Bronchiectasis refers to permanent irreversible dilation of the airways, specifically the bronchi, usually associated with inflammation of the airway wall. A wide variety of disease processes may result in bronchiectasis, the most common of which is infection. Respiratory syncytial virus (RSV) pneumonia is a frequent cause of bronchiectasis in children, and TB is a common cause of bronchiectasis affecting the upper lobes. Other causes include cystic fibrosis (CF); allergic bronchopulmonary aspergillosis (ABPA); chronic aspiration; and airway obstruction caused by airway neoplasm, foreign body, or extrinsic compression (see Table 6.3). Bronchiectasis can be described as diffuse or focal in distribution. Diffuse bronchiectasis may be caused by congenital abnormalities of the bronchi, systemic abnormalities of hose defense, abnormal mucus production, and abnormal ciliary clearance. In contrast, focal bronchiectasis tends to be the result of long-standing bronchial obstruction and is limited to one lung lobe or segment.

Various patterns of bronchiectasis are seen in specific disease processes. For instance, mucous plugging of the central airways may be seen in CF, ABPA, or Mounier-Kuhn syndrome and involvement of the upper lobes in CF, ABPA, and TB. In patients with CF, bronchiectasis is usually present in all lung lobes but is most pronounced within the upper lobes. Traction bronchiectasis is usually associated with radiation fibrosis caused by prior radiation therapy or diffuse lung diseases such as sarcoidosis, silicosis, or berylliosis. Because traction bronchiectasis reflects the sequela of adjacent interstitial fibrosis instead of intrinsic airway abnormality, airway wall thickening and mucous plugging are usually absent (Fig. 6.24). Although the underlying cause of bronchiectasis can often be determined by the pattern of imaging abnormalities or clinical history, the cause of bronchiectasis may not be identified in up to 50% of cases.

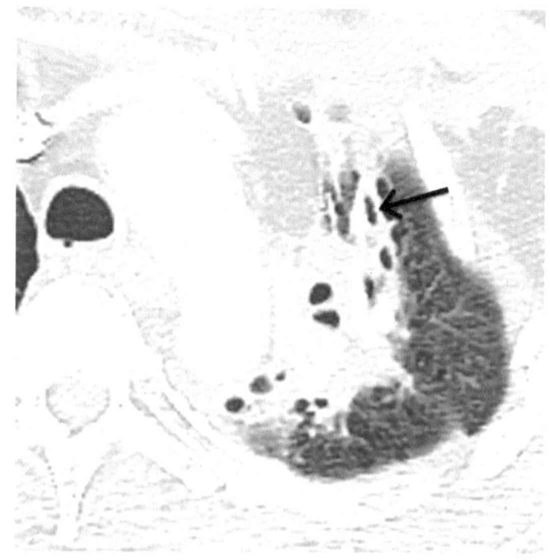

FIGURE 6.24 Traction bronchiectasis. Axial contrast-enhanced computed tomography image of a patient after radiation therapy shows left upper lobe opacity and volume loss. Regional bronchi are dilated but without bronchial wall thickening *(arrow)* consistent with traction bronchiectasis and adjacent fibrosis.

Three morphologic types of bronchiectasis have been described based on the morphology of the bronchi; the number of bronchial subdivisions that are present; and the appearance on MDCT: cylindrical, varicose, or cystic (Fig. 6.25). Cylindrical bronchiectasis is characterized by minimal dilation of the bronchi, which demonstrate a straight and regular outline and end squarely and abruptly. Varicose bronchiectasis refers to bronchi that are dilated but have sites of relative constriction and an overall bulbous appearance similar to that of varicose veins. Cystic bronchiectasis,

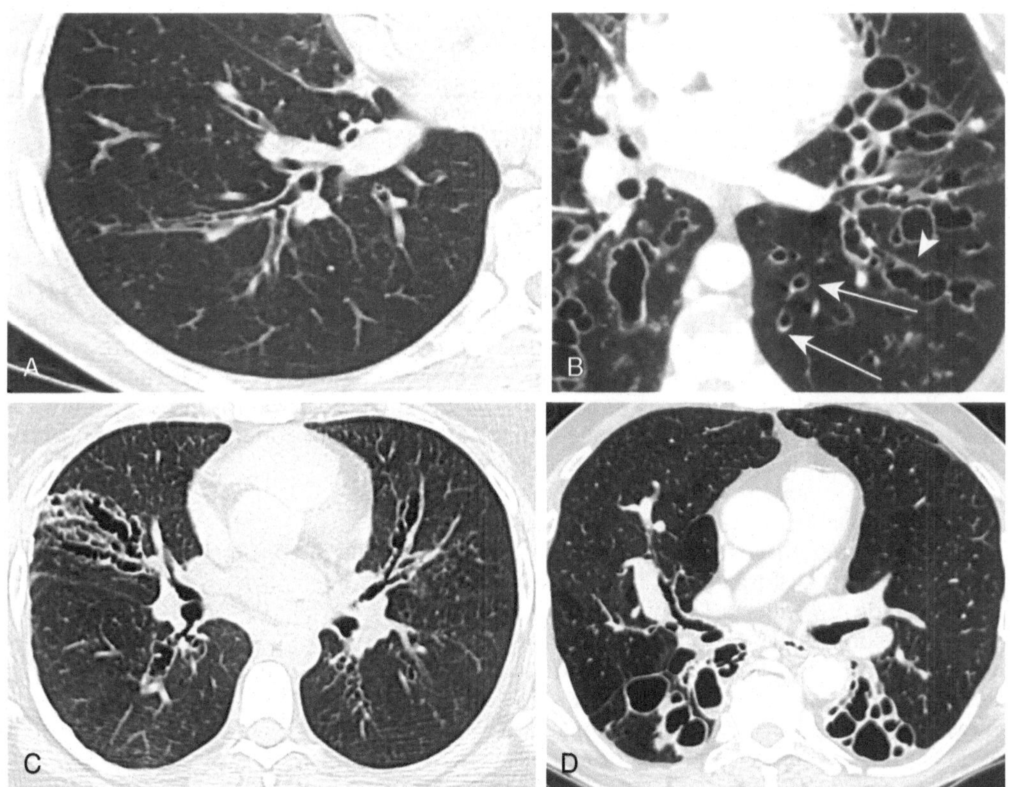

FIGURE 6.25 Three morphologic types of bronchiectasis. **A,** Axial computed tomography (CT) image of a patient with cystic fibrosis with bronchial wall thickening and mild smooth dilation of bronchi in the right lower lobe consistent with cylindrical bronchiectasis. **B,** Axial contrast-enhanced CT image of a patient with varicose bronchiectasis *(arrowhead)* and cystic bronchiectasis (lingula). Note the signet ring sign *(white arrows)* with the pulmonary artery seen adjacent to a dilated bronchus in cross section. **C,** Axial contrast-enhanced CT image of a patient with varicose bronchiectasis demonstrates bronchi that are dilated but have sites of relative constriction and an overall bulbous appearance similar to that of varicose veins. **D,** Axial contrast-enhanced CT image of a patient with cystic bronchiectasis, also known as saccular bronchiectasis, is characterized by ballooning of the bronchi, some of which contain secretions in the right lower lobe.

also known as saccular bronchiectasis, is characterized by ballooning of the bronchi.

Chest radiographs may be normal in the setting of mild bronchiectasis but become abnormal with greater severity of disease. When radiographic abnormalities are visible, linear or reticular opacities that follow the distribution of the bronchi, representing thickened airway walls, are the most common findings. A "tram-track" appearance is often seen in the setting of cylindrical bronchiectasis. Clusters of air-filled cysts may be present in cystic bronchiectasis. In the setting of superimposed infection, bronchial wall thickening increases and air–fluid levels develop within the cysts. Varying degrees of volume loss and atelectasis may be present in a lung lobe or segment in the setting of focal bronchiectasis.

Computed tomography is the imaging modality of choice for identifying and characterizing bronchiectasis, and both direct and indirect findings have been described. The characteristic direct finding is bronchial dilation with an increased bronchoarterial ratio. Whereas the normal bronchoarterial ratio is 0.65 to 1, the bronchoarterial ratio in bronchiectasis is greater than 1.5. A bronchoarterial ratio between 1 and 1.5 is nonspecific and can be encountered in situations such as patients older than 65 years and high altitudes. Additional direct findings include the lack of bronchial tapering, which is the earliest and most sensitive sign of bronchiectasis, and visualization of airways within 1 cm of the visceral pleura. Indirect findings include bronchial wall thickening, mucoid impaction or fluid-filled bronchi, centrilobular nodules or tree-in-bud opacities, and mosaic perfusion and air trapping caused by associated bronchiolitis.

Cylindrical bronchiectasis causes smooth dilation of the bronchi with lack of tapering, appearing as tram-track lines when the bronchus is in the plane of the scan and as a signet ring when seen in cross section. The "signet ring" sign refers to the appearance of a thickened and dilated bronchus associated with a smaller pulmonary artery branch identified in cross-section (Fig. 6.25, *D*). Varicose bronchiectasis demonstrates a beaded configuration when identified in the plane of the bronchus but may mimic cylindrical bronchiectasis in cross section. Cystic bronchiectasis appears as a string or cluster of cysts, and air–fluid levels may be seen in the setting of retained secretions.

Magnetic resonance imaging has been increasingly used for serial examinations of bronchiectasis in young patients because of the lack of ionizing radiation. T1- and T2-weighted turbo spin-echo sequences demonstrate the anatomy of the large airways, as well as potential abnormalities such as bronchial dilation, bronchial wall thickening, and mucous plugging. Hyperpolarized MRI with helium or xenon provides functional evaluation of air trapping.

Mucoid Impaction

Mucoid impaction, defined as airway filling by mucoid secretions, is associated with a wide variety of disease processes, resulting in bronchiectasis. Traditionally, the causes of mucoid impaction have been divided into obstructive versus nonobstructive or congenital versus acquired. A more recent approach uses a hybrid algorithm that is based on both the origin (congenital or acquired) and nature (inflammatory, infectious, or neoplastic) of the specific disease process.

When mucous and other secretions are retained in bronchioles and nondilated airways, the radiographic appearance typically is normal. In other cases, mucoid impaction may produce the so-called finger-in-glove sign caused by tubular or branching opacities that resemble fingers emanating from the central airways. CT effectively demonstrates mucoid impaction and enables differentiation from other abnormalities that may appear similarly on CXR such as arteriovenous malformation. Characteristic associated features include bronchiectasis, low-attenuation mucus inspissated in the bronchi, and connection with the central airways. In contrast, arteriovenous malformations demonstrate a nidus with efferent and afferent vessels on MDCT. IV contrast material may be administered to aid in the differentiation of unusual arteriovenous malformations from mucoid impactions.

Cystic Fibrosis

Cystic fibrosis is a multisystem disorder characterized by abnormalities of the exocrine glands in the airways, pancreas, colon, salivary glands, and sweat glands. It is the most common genetic disorder in whites, with a reported incidence of 1 in 2000 to 3500 live births, and is transmitted in an autosomal recessive inheritance pattern. The disease is characterized by a defect in the CF transmembrane regulator gene *(CFTR)* that results in abnormal transport of chloride across epithelial cells in mucous surfaces and production of thick secretions that impair mucociliary clearance. Elevated levels of sodium, chloride, and potassium are present in the sweat of affected patients. Patients typically present with recurrent respiratory infections and are susceptible to organisms such as *Staphylococcus aureus, Pseudomonas aeruginosa,* and *Haemophilus influenzae*. Associated abnormalities include exocrine pancreatic insufficiency, pansinusitis, infertility, bone demineralization, and biliary cirrhosis.

Computed tomography is the imaging modality of choice to evaluate CF and is more sensitive than radiography and PFTs in detecting early disease. Radiography is useful in evaluation of patients with new or exacerbation of symptoms because patients with CF are prone to develop complications such as infection and pneumothorax (Fig. 6.26). Bronchiectasis, which may be cylindrical, varicose, or cystic, is present within all lung lobes but is most pronounced in the upper lobes (Fig. 6.27). The presence of air-fluid levels in cystic bronchiectasis has been shown to correlate with acute exacerbation. Associated abnormalities resulting in

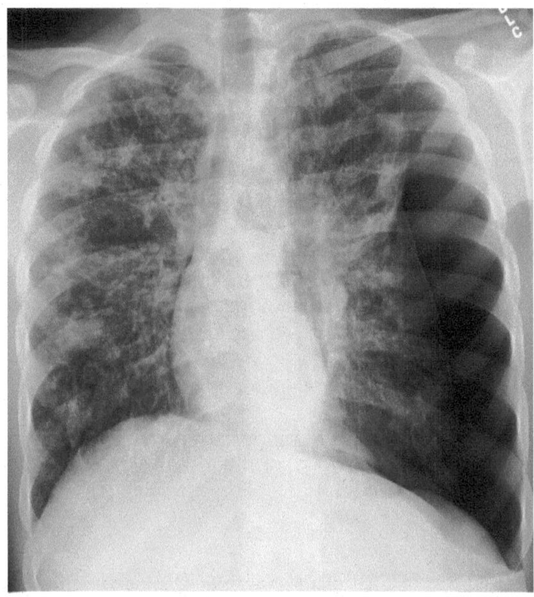

FIGURE 6.26 Cystic fibrosis. Posteroanterior chest radiograph shows large left pneumothorax with depression of the ipsilateral hemidiaphragm and contralateral shift of the mediastinum suggestive of tension. Note the bronchial wall thickening and tram tracking in the upper lobes.

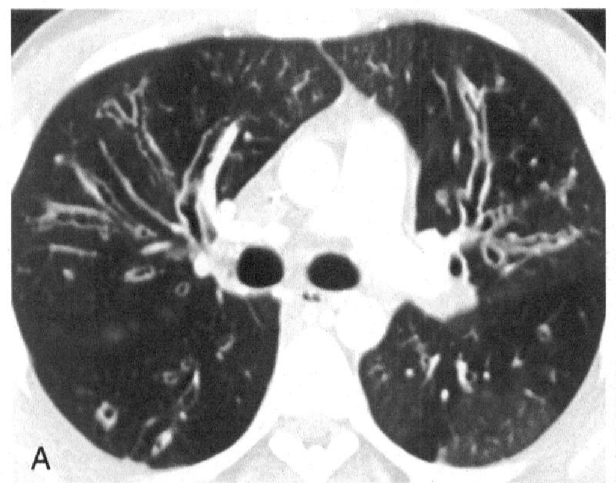

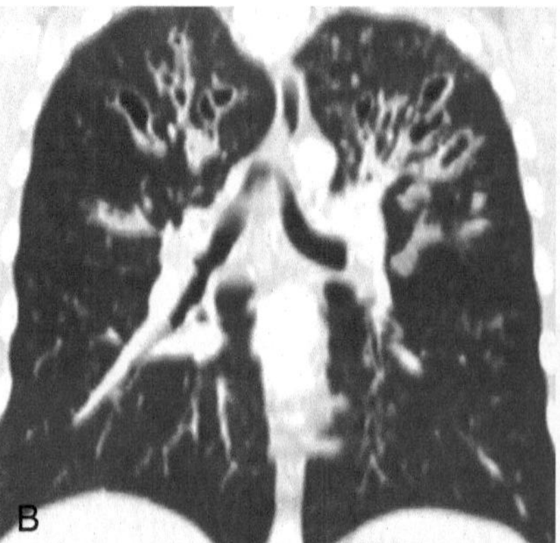

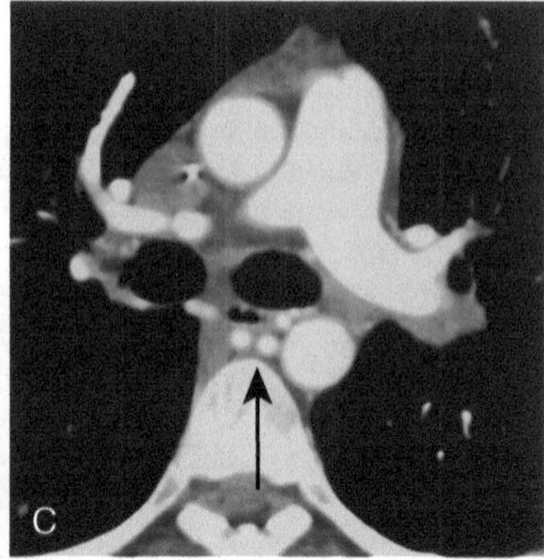

FIGURE 6.27 Cystic fibrosis. Axial **(A)** and coronal **(B)** contrast-enhanced computed tomography (CT) images show central and upper lobe predominant bronchiectasis, bronchial wall thickening, and mucous plugging. Axial contrast-enhanced CT in soft tissue windows of the same patient **(C)** demonstrates dilation of bronchial arteries *(arrow)*.

obstruction of small- and medium-sized airways include mucous plugging; V- or is -shaped tree-in-bud opacities or centrilobular nodules; and heterogeneous attenuation of the lungs caused by obstruction of small airways with resultant air trapping, referred to as "mosaic attenuation" (refer to Chapters 17 and 20), and expiratory air trapping may be present. Bronchial artery dilation can be observed (Fig. 6.27, *C*), possibly as a response to chronic inflammation and thrombosis of pulmonary vessels.

Magnetic resonance imaging may be used for monitoring of children with CF and readily demonstrates central bronchiectasis, bronchial wall thickening, and mucous plugging. High signal intensity on T2-weighted images and contrast enhancement of the bronchial walls may be seen in a setting of inflammation, and mucous plugging can manifest as intraluminal high signal intensity on T2-weighted images. Additional abnormalities such as air–fluid levels and pulmonary findings, including atelectasis and consolidation, may be identified. However, evaluation of the smaller, distal airways for bronchiectasis and other disease processes is limited. Hyperpolarized MRI using helium gas is sensitive for the detection of ventilatory defects, which correlate with PFTs and can be used to evaluate for treatment-related changes.

Patients are typically treated with a combination of chest physical therapy, mucolytics, bronchodilators, antibiotics, and pancreatic enzyme supplementation or replacement. Bronchial artery embolization is a treatment option for patients with hemoptysis. Lung transplantation may be performed in advanced lung disease.

Allergic Bronchopulmonary Aspergillosis

Allergic bronchopulmonary aspergillosis represents a hypersensitivity response to the presence of the *Aspergillus* fungus in the tracheobronchial tree. Affected patients typically have precipitating antibodies, skin sensitivity, elevated levels of IgE, and eosinophils in the airway walls and blood. Coexisting disorders such as asthma, atopy, and CF place the patient at risk for developing ABPA. The disease is characterized by repeated exacerbations that respond to the administration of oral corticosteroids.

Chest radiography typically demonstrates central branching, tubular opacities extending from the hila into the lungs along the distribution of the segmental and subsegmental bronchi, resulting in the finger-in-glove appearance. CT better demonstrates these abnormalities, as well as other findings such as mucoceles, which are dilated mucus-filled bronchi that may be of fluid density. The presence of a hyperattenuating mucous plug on CT, postulated to be caused by the presence of calcium and metal ions or desiccated mucus, is considered indicative of ABPA. When mucous plugs are cleared from the airways via expectoration, central, air-filled bronchiectatic airways may be identified. Lung findings such as atelectasis and consolidation (Fig. 6.28) may be present in acute exacerbation.

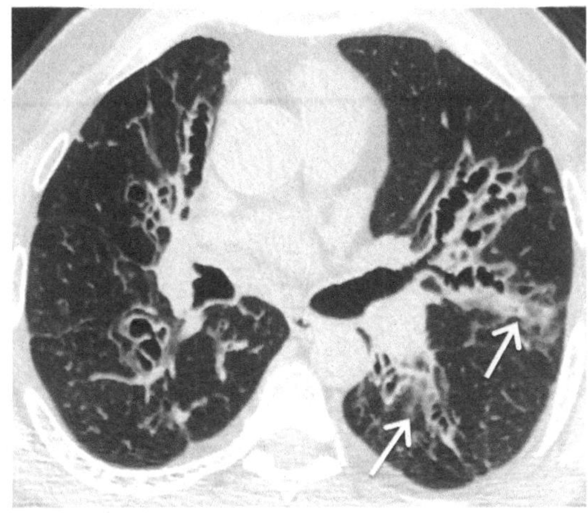

FIGURE 6.28 Allergic bronchopulmonary aspergillosis. Axial computed tomography image demonstrates bilateral central bronchiectasis and bronchial wall thickening. Peribronchial consolidative and ground-glass opacities *(arrows)* are suggestive of acute exacerbations.

Primary Ciliary Dyskinesia

Primary ciliary dyskinesia, also known as dyskinetic cilia syndrome, is a rare autosomal recessive genetic disorder characterized by a defect in ciliary structure and function. Because of resultant impaired mucus clearance, patients typically present with rhinitis, sinusitis, otitis media, and bronchiectasis, as well as reduced fertility because of impaired motility of spermatozoa. Approximately 50% of affected patients have situs inversus or heterotaxy. Kartagener syndrome represents a subset of patients with situs inversus, sinusitis, and bronchiectasis.

On CXR and MDCT, bilateral bronchiectasis is present and most pronounced in the lower lobes (Fig. 6.29). Associated findings include bronchial wall thickening, hyperinflation of the lungs, and regions of atelectasis or consolidation. Patients are treated with repeated courses of antibiotics and, in contrast to those with CF, have a normal life span.

Other Etiologies

A wide variety of rare diseases may result in bronchiectasis. Williams-Campbell syndrome is characterized by a congenital deficiency of cartilage associated with the subsegmental bronchi and results in dilation of the affected airways. Young syndrome, also known as obstructive azoospermia, is characterized by the clinical combination of sinopulmonary infections, infertility, and bronchiectasis. Yellow nail syndrome consists of the clinical triad of yellow nails, lymphedema, and pleural effusions.

Bronchiolitis

Bronchiolitis refers to diseases involving the small airways that lack cartilage and measure less than 2 mm and may be classified based on etiology and histologic features. The two primary forms of bronchiolitis include cellular or proliferative bronchiolitis and constrictive bronchiolitis (Table 6.4). The imaging findings associated with these various types of bronchiolitis are often nonspecific and may overlap, and various direct and indirect findings have been described. Whereas the direct findings are specifically related to the presence of fluid, cells, inflammation, and fibrosis associated with the bronchioles, indirect signs are related to obliteration of the airway lumen by fibrosis. The indirect signs include mosaic attenuation and air trapping and marked narrowing or obliteration of the airway lumen by fibrosis.

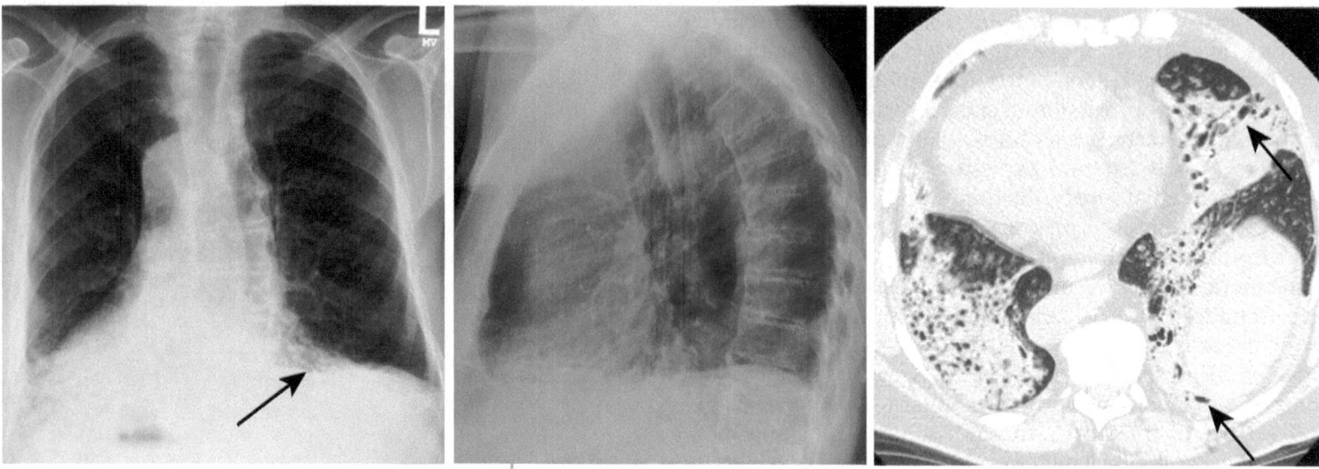

FIGURE 6.29 Primary ciliary dyskinesia. Posteroanterior **(A)** and lateral **(B)** chest radiographs show dextrocardia, hyperinflation, consolidations in the lower lobes, and a tram-track appearance (*arrow*, **A**) of the lower lobe airways. Axial contrast-enhanced computed tomography image **(C)** of the same patient demonstrates bronchiectasis *(arrows)* and patchy consolidation representing pneumonia.

TABLE 6.4 **Classification of Bronchiolitis**

Classification	Cause
Cellular (proliferative)	Acute infectious and noninfectious bronchiolitis Bronchiolitis associated with chronic large airway disease Subacute hypersensitivity pneumonitis Smoking-related respiratory bronchiolitis Follicular bronchiolitis Diffuse panbronchiolitis
Obliterative (constrictive)	Postinfectious conditions Lung and bone marrow transplantation Connective tissue disease Toxic fume inhalation Drugs Inflammatory bowel disease

Overview of Imaging Findings

Although chest radiographs are typically normal in cases of bronchiolitis, small, ill-defined nodules may occasionally be visible in the setting of acute infectious or noninfectious bronchiolitis, subacute hypersensitivity pneumonitis, or respiratory bronchiolitis (RB). Large pulmonary nodules, airspace opacities, and consolidation may be visible in cases of infection.

Air trapping, defined as an indirect finding of bronchiolitis, may be present on inspiratory and expiratory chest radiographs and fluoroscopy. Generalized air trapping may result in a decrease in diaphragmatic excursion, which typically changes to 1 to 2 cm from 3 to 4 cm in normal patients. Unilateral air trapping results in depression of the ipsilateral hemidiaphragm and contralateral shift of the mediastinum. Decubitus radiographs can be performed to evaluate for air trapping when patients cannot safely undergo inspiratory and expiratory imaging. In the setting of air trapping, the abnormal lung remains hyperinflated and lucent in the decubitus position, but the normal lung deflates.

Computed tomography is the imaging modality of choice to evaluate bronchiolitis because the ability to obtain high-quality multiplanar images and use expiratory technique for the investigation of air trapping is superior to CXR. During the inspiratory phase, direct findings of bronchiolitis include centrilobular nodules, tree-in-bud opacities, and mosaic attenuation. On expiratory CT, the normal lung decreases in volume and increases in attenuation. In regions of air trapping, the abnormal lung remains lower in attenuation, and the volume remains constant. The caliber of vessels within the region of air trapping may be diminished because of hypoxic vasoconstriction.

Infectious Bronchiolitis

Infectious bronchiolitis results from inflammation of the bronchioles caused by the presence of infectious organisms. A wide variety of causative agents have been identified, including childhood infections such as RSV, adenovirus, and *Mycoplasma pneumoniae*; fungal and viral diseases in immunocompromised patients; and other bacterial infections such as *Chlamydia* and typical and atypical mycobacteria. The clinical presentation in children is usually more severe than in adults and is characterized by symptoms of upper respiratory tract infection.

The most common manifestation of infectious bronchiolitis on CT is centrilobular nodules and tree-in-bud opacities (see Chapter 14).

Respiratory Bronchiolitis and Respiratory Bronchiolitis–Associated Interstitial Lung Disease

Respiratory bronchiolitis and respiratory bronchiolitis-associated interstitial lung disease (RB-ILD) are inflammatory diseases that affect smokers and, rarely, patients with collagen vascular diseases and mineral dust–induced diseases, and affect individuals 30 to 40 years of age. Patients with RB are asymptomatic, but those with RB-ILD present with clinical symptoms such as progressive shortness of breath and cough.

On CT, RB manifests as ill-defined centrilobular nodules that resemble those seen in hypersensitivity pneumonitis, and patchy ground-glass opacities, all of which typically

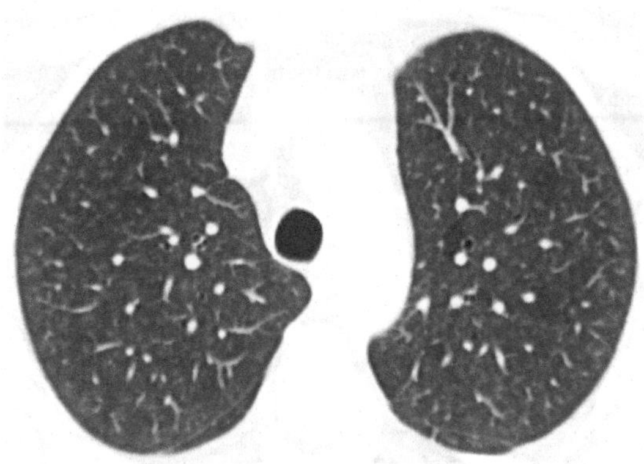

FIGURE 6.30 Respiratory bronchiolitis. Axial contrast-enhanced computed tomography image of an asymptomatic smoker demonstrates numerous ill-defined centrilobular ground-glass nodules in the upper lobes.

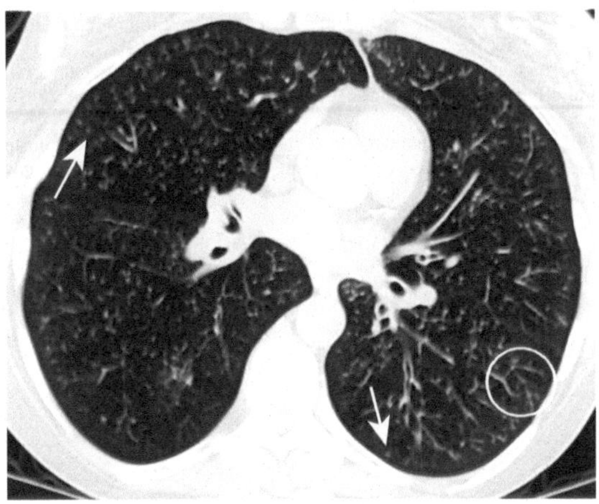

FIGURE 6.31 Follicular bronchiolitis. Axial contrast-enhanced maximum intensity projection computed tomography image shows numerous bilateral centrilobular nodules *(arrows)* and tree-in-bud opacities *(circle)*, which are typical abnormalities present in follicular bronchiolitis.

affect the upper lobes (Fig. 6.30). RB-ILD is characterized by centrilobular nodules in the upper lobes that are more pronounced than those seen in RB. Reticular opacities representing mild pulmonary fibrosis in the lower lobes and associated findings such as bronchial wall thickening and emphysema may also be present.

Smoking cessation is recommended for patients with RB and RB-ILD because the histologic abnormalities are reversible with cessation of smoking.

Follicular Bronchiolitis

Follicular bronchiolitis is a lymphoproliferative disorder characterized by proliferation of the lymphoid follicles in the walls of small airways and may be primary or secondary. Causes include connective tissue diseases such as rheumatoid arthritis and Sjögren syndrome, immunodeficiency, hypersensitivity reactions, and chronic airway infections.

Findings on chest radiographs, if present, include hyperinflation and small nodules and reticular or reticulonodular opacities. CT findings include centrilobular nodules and, less commonly, tree-in-bud opacities (Fig. 6.31). Additional findings include ground-glass opacities, bronchial dilation, and interlobular septal thickening. Corticosteroids are the mainstay of treatment for primary follicular bronchiolitis.

Diffuse Panbronchiolitis

Diffuse panbronchiolitis is an idiopathic disease characterized by inflammation of the respiratory bronchioles that is encountered in Asia, particularly Japan and Korea. However, cases have also been reported in America and Europe. Middle-aged men are typically affected, and there is no known association with smoking. Clinical symptoms include progressive cough, dyspnea, and severe pansinusitis.

Radiographic findings including small nodules and reticulonodular opacities are usually subtle. CT typically demonstrates a combination of bronchial wall thickening, centrilobular nodules, tree-in-bud opacities, bronchiectasis and bronchiolectasis, and air trapping.

Patients are typically treated with long-term low-dose erythromycin or other macrolides. Although an initial response is seen in 85% of patients, the long-term prognosis is poor, with progression of bronchiectasis typical.

Constrictive Bronchiolitis

Constrictive bronchiolitis is an irreversible disorder characterized histologically as concentric luminal narrowing of the membranous and respiratory bronchioles caused by inflammation and fibrosis. In contrast to other inflammatory bronchiolitis, direct signs of bronchiolitis such as bronchial wall thickening and peribronchiolar or tree-in-bud opacities are typically absent on radiograph and CT because of the small amount of abnormal tissue associated with airways. Mosaic attenuation, the most common finding, can be subtle on inspiratory CT. Expiratory CT is usually necessary to detect and confirm air trapping, which may be lobular, segmental, or lobar (see Chapter 20).

CONCLUSIONS

Airway diseases can have a variety of clinical presentations. Imaging is helpful in identifying the underlying anatomic abnormalities. CXR is often the initial imaging procedure, and radiologists should pay particular attention to the airways in patients with symptoms such as wheezing, stridor, and "adult-onset asthma." CT can delineate the size, location, distribution, and tissue characteristics of tracheobronchial abnormalities, which help narrow the differential diagnoses and guide further diagnostic procedures as needed.

SUGGESTED READING

Boiselle PM. Imaging of the large airways. *Clin Chest Med*. 2008;29:181-193.

Eichinger M, Heussel CP, Kauczor HU, et al. Computed tomography and magnetic resonance imaging in cystic fibrosis lung disease. *J Magn Reson Imaging*. 2010; 32(6):1370-1378.

Ferretti GR, Bithigoffer C, Righini CA, et al. Imaging of tumors of the trachea and central bronchi. *Thorac Surg Clin*. 2010;20:31-45.

Heidinger BH, Occhipinti M, Eisenberg RL, et al. Imaging of large airways disorders. *AJR Am J Roentgenol*. 2015;205(1):41-56.

Honings J, Gaissert HA, van der Heijden HF, et al. Clinical aspects and treatment of primary tracheal malignancies. *Acta Otolaryngol*. 2010;130:763-772.

Javidan-Nejad C. MDCT of trachea and main bronchi. *Radiol Clin North Am*. 2010;48:157-176.

Kang EY. Large airway diseases. *J Thorac Imaging*. 2011;26(4):249-262.

Kligerman SJ, Henry T, Lin CT, et al. Mosaic attenuation: etiology, methods of differentiation, and pitfalls. *Radiographics*. 2015;35(5):1360-1380.

Lee KS, Boiselle PM. Update on multidetector computed tomography imaging of the airways. *J Thorac Imaging*. 2010;25:112-124.
Martinez S, Heyneman LE, McAdams HP, et al. Mucoid impactions: finger-in-glove sign and other CT and radiographic features. *Radiographics*. 2008;28(5):1369-1382.
Milliron B, Henry TS, Veeraraghavan S, et al. Bronchiectasis: mechanisms and imaging clues of associated common and uncommon diseases. *Radiographics*. 2015;35(4):1011-1030.
Ngo AV, Walker CM, Chung JH, et al. Tumors and tumorlike conditions of the large airways. *AJR Am J Roentgenol*. 2013;201:301-313.
Park CM, Goo JM, Lee HJ, et al. Tumors in the tracheobronchial tree: CT and FDG PET features. *Radiographics*. 2009;29:55-71.
Pipavath SJ, Lynch DA, Cool C, et al. Radiologic and pathologic features of bronchiolitis. *AJR Am J Roentgenol*. 2005;185(2):354-363.
Wu CC, Shepard JA. Tracheal and airway neoplasms. *Semin Roentgenol*. 2013;48(4):354-364.

Chapter 7

The Pleura, Diaphragm, and Chest Wall

Lan Qian (Lancia) Guo and Jeanne B. Ackman

PLEURA

Anatomy and Physiology

The pleura is composed of two thin layers of mesothelium referred to as the visceral and parietal pleura. The visceral pleura covers the lung and fissural surfaces and the parietal pleura lines the mediastinum, ribs, and diaphragm. The visceral and parietal pleura differ in their arterial supply and their venous and lymphatic drainage. The visceral pleura is supplied by the pulmonary arterioles and capillaries and drains via the pulmonary veins, and the parietal pleura is supplied by systemic arterioles and capillaries, which drain into the systemic venous system via the azygous, hemiazygous, and internal mammary veins into the right atrium. The visceral and parietal pleura surround the hilum. Just below the hila, two layers of parietal pleura come together and extend inferiorly to the diaphragm to form a free edge known as the inferior pulmonary ligament, tethering the lower lung to the mediastinum.

The pleural space is a potential space and normally contains up to 10 mL of pleural fluid. Physiologic pleural fluid is constantly produced by the parietal pleura and absorbed by the lymphatics. Visceral pleural lymphatics drain centrally via the interlobular septae into the hila, and parietal pleural lymphatics drain into the thoracic duct.

Pleural Effusions

Abnormal accumulation of pleural fluid occurs when the rate of pleural fluid production outpaces the rate of absorption. There are two main types of pleural effusions: transudates and exudates. Transudates are usually caused by increased local capillary hydrostatic pressure and decreased oncotic pressure, as in the setting of hypoalbuminemia, congestive heart failure, hepatic cirrhosis, and renal failure with volume overload. In contrast, exudates result from infectious, inflammatory, and neoplastic processes with secondarily increased permeability of the microvascular circulation. Common causes of exudates include pneumonia, pleural tumors, and inflammatory conditions such as lupus and rheumatoid arthritis.

Specific Types of Pleural Effusions and Their Imaging Features

Freely Layering Pleural Effusion

A freely layering pleural effusion is more commonly transudative than exudative. On an upright chest radiograph (CXR), it manifests as blunting of the costophrenic angles, with an associated concave-upward interface known as the "meniscus sign" (Fig. 7.1). CXR projections differ in their sensitivity for detection of pleural effusions. The upright

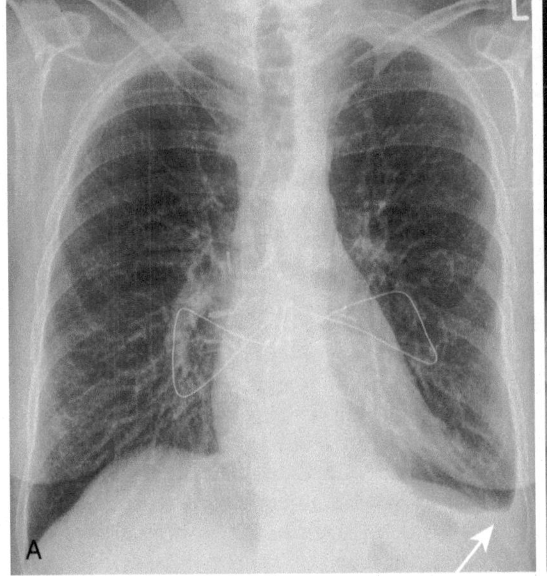

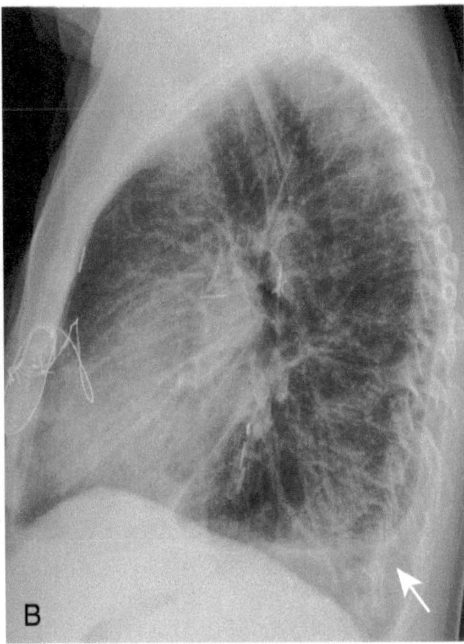

FIGURE 7.1 Meniscus sign. Posteroanterior **(A)** and lateral **(B)** chest radiographs show a small meniscus *(arrows)* in the left costophrenic angle in this woman after clamshell sternotomy and double-lung transplantation, representing a small left pleural effusion.

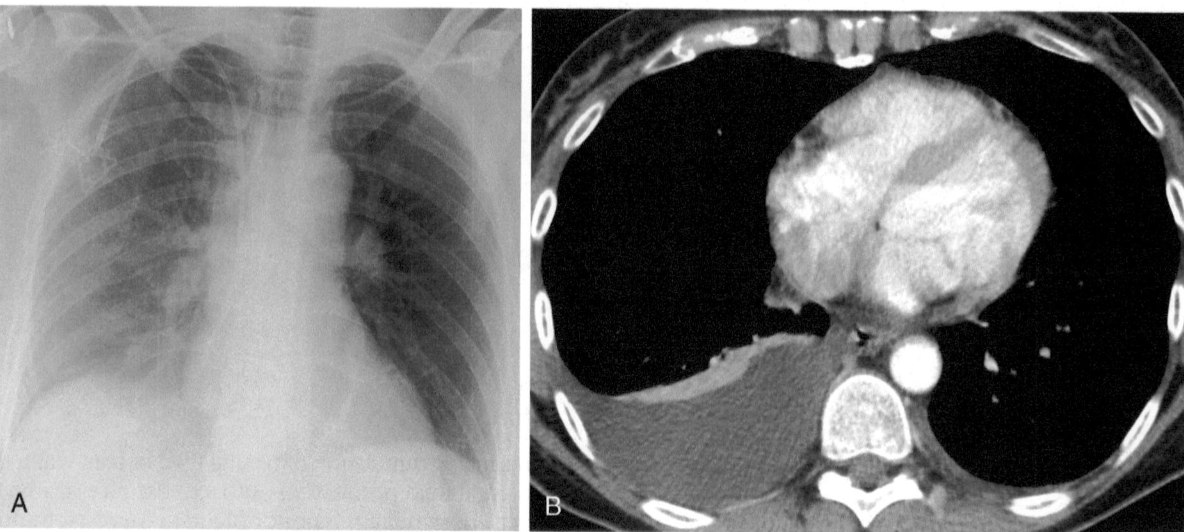

FIGURE 7.2 Freely layering right pleural effusion in a supine patient. **A,** Anteroposterior supine portable radiograph reveals graduated hazy attenuation from right apex to base caused by a small-to-moderate, layering right pleural effusion. An infusion port catheter terminates in the upper right atrium. **B,** Chest computed tomography (CT) scan with intravenous contrast shows the correlative water attenuation, layering right pleural effusion, with associated homogeneously enhancing and somewhat crescentic, mild right lower lobe relaxation atelectasis.

lateral projection is more sensitive than an upright frontal radiograph in the detection of very small pleural effusions, demonstrating as little as 50 to 75 mL of pleural fluid in the posterior costophrenic angles, the most dependent part of the thorax. Typically, closer to 200 mL of fluid is necessary to blunt the lateral costophrenic angles on a frontal CXR. On a supine CXR, a pleural effusion layers posteriorly, giving rise to hazy opacity overlying the lung, through which the pulmonary vessels can often still be visualized, with the extent of opacification depending on the size of the pleural effusion (Fig. 7.2). Pleural fluid may also track into the fissures (Fig. 7.3) and around the lung apex, producing an "apical cap."

When massive, pleural effusions may yield complete or near complete opacification of the ipsilateral hemithorax, with contralateral displacement of the mediastinum (Fig. 7.4). This contralateral shift can help distinguish complete hemithoracic opacification caused by a large pleural effusion from atelectasis alone; in the latter case, the mediastinum would be expected to shift ipsilaterally. Often, both pleural fluid and atelectasis are present, however, and their relative preponderance will dictate the degree of cardiomediastinal shift.

On chest computed tomography (CT), free-flowing pleural fluid produces a sickle-shaped water-attenuation opacity in the dependent aspect of the thorax. Compared with CXR, cross-sectional imaging by CT and magnetic resonance imaging (MRI) are more sensitive and specific in the detection of very small amounts of pleural fluid. Ultrasonography can also be used to image pleural fluid, provided there is an ample acoustic window.

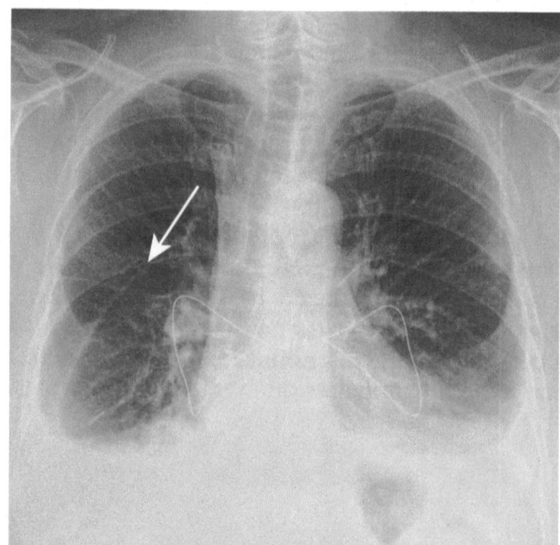

FIGURE 7.3 Bilateral pleural effusions with right major fissural extension *(arrow)*. Posteroanterior radiograph reveals small to moderate bilateral pleural effusions, right of which extends into and outlines the right major fissure in this woman status post clamshell sternotomy and double-lung transplantation.

Subpulmonic Pleural Effusion

Occasionally, free-flowing pleural fluid may accumulate in a subpulmonic position—that is, between the inferior surface of the lung and the hemidiaphragmatic pleura. In this situation, the lateral costophrenic angle may remain sharp until a large amount of fluid has accumulated and eventually spills into it. On a frontal CXR, a subpulmonic pleural effusion mimics elevation of the ipsilateral hemidiaphragm, yielding a "pseudo-diaphragm" appearance. However, closer scrutiny will reveal flattening of the medial aspect of the apparent hemidiaphragm with displacement of the peak of the apparent hemidiaphragm laterally (Fig. 7.5). On the left, increased distance between the apparent surface of the left hemidiaphragm and the underlying gastric bubble may also indicate the presence of a subpulmonic pleural effusion.

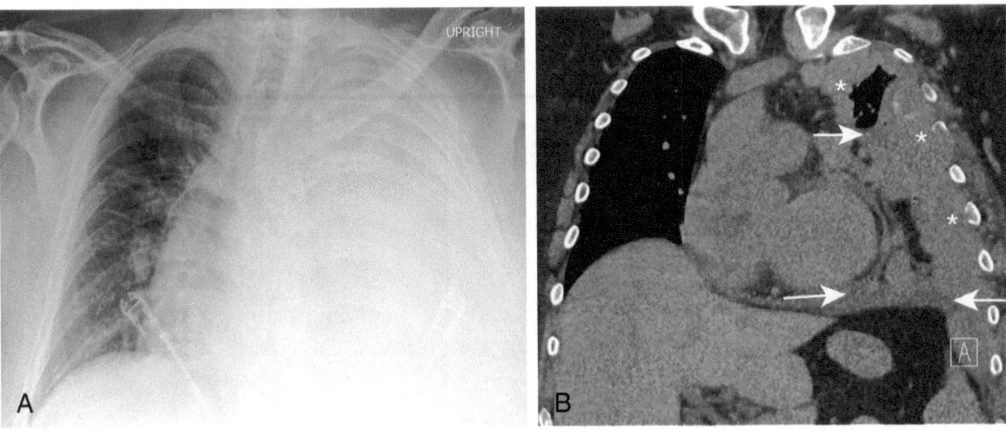

FIGURE 7.4 Extensive unilateral pleural disease with contralateral mediastinal shift in man with metastatic renal cell carcinoma. Posteroanterior chest radiograph **(A)** and corresponding coronal computed tomography (CT) scan **(B)** show near-complete left hemithoracic opacification with rightward cardiomediastinal shift, revealed by CT to be secondary to diffuse, nearly circumferential pleural thickening *(asterisks)*, pleural fluid *(arrows)*, and atelectasis (lung volume loss).

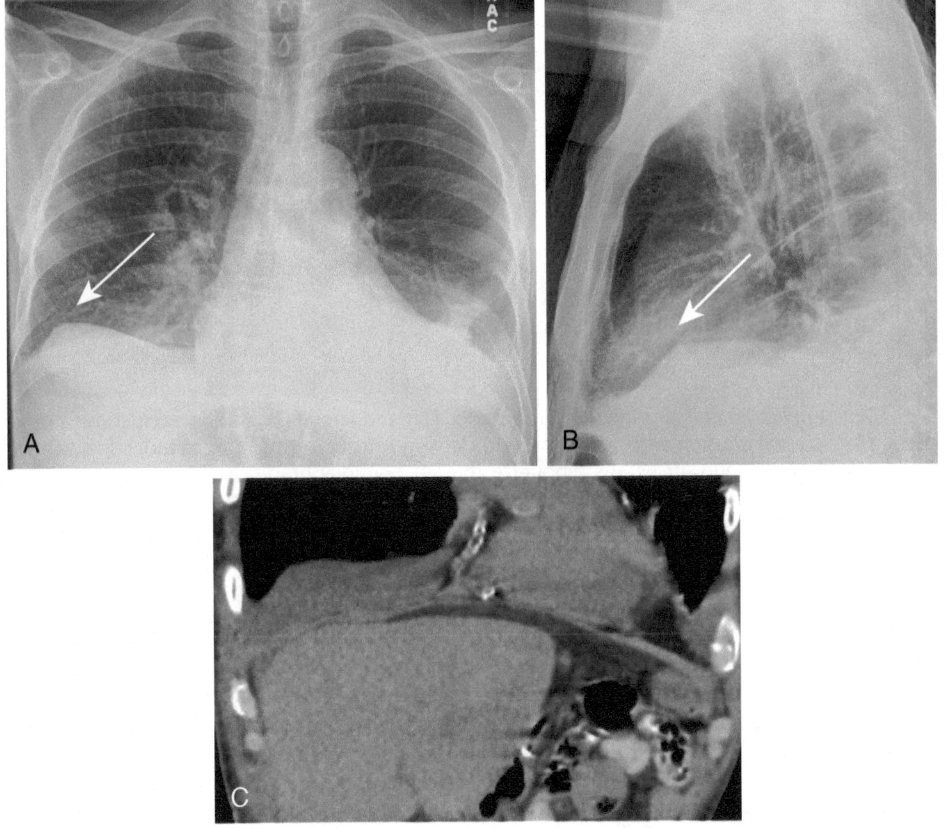

FIGURE 7.5 Subpulmonic pleural effusion. Posteroanterior **(A)** and lateral **(B)** chest radiographs demonstrate a right subpulmonic pleural effusion *(arrows)* simulating the right hemidiaphragm or creating a "pseudodiaphragm appearance" with its well-defined margin and a more lateral peak than would be expected for the right hemidiaphragm. A small left pleural effusion and bibasilar atelectatic changes are also present. **C,** Correlative coronal computed tomography scan without contrast showing the right subpulmonic pleural fluid and small left pleural effusion.

Loculated Pleural Effusion

Pleural fluid can become loculated when it no longer shifts freely in the pleural space, often because of adhesions between the visceral and parietal pleura. A loculated pleural effusion is usually exudative. If pleural adhesions are present and preexist the new pleural effusion, they may result in loculation of serous or transudative pleural fluid, which would otherwise layer. On CXR, CT, and MRI, a loculated pleural effusion does not behave according to the laws of

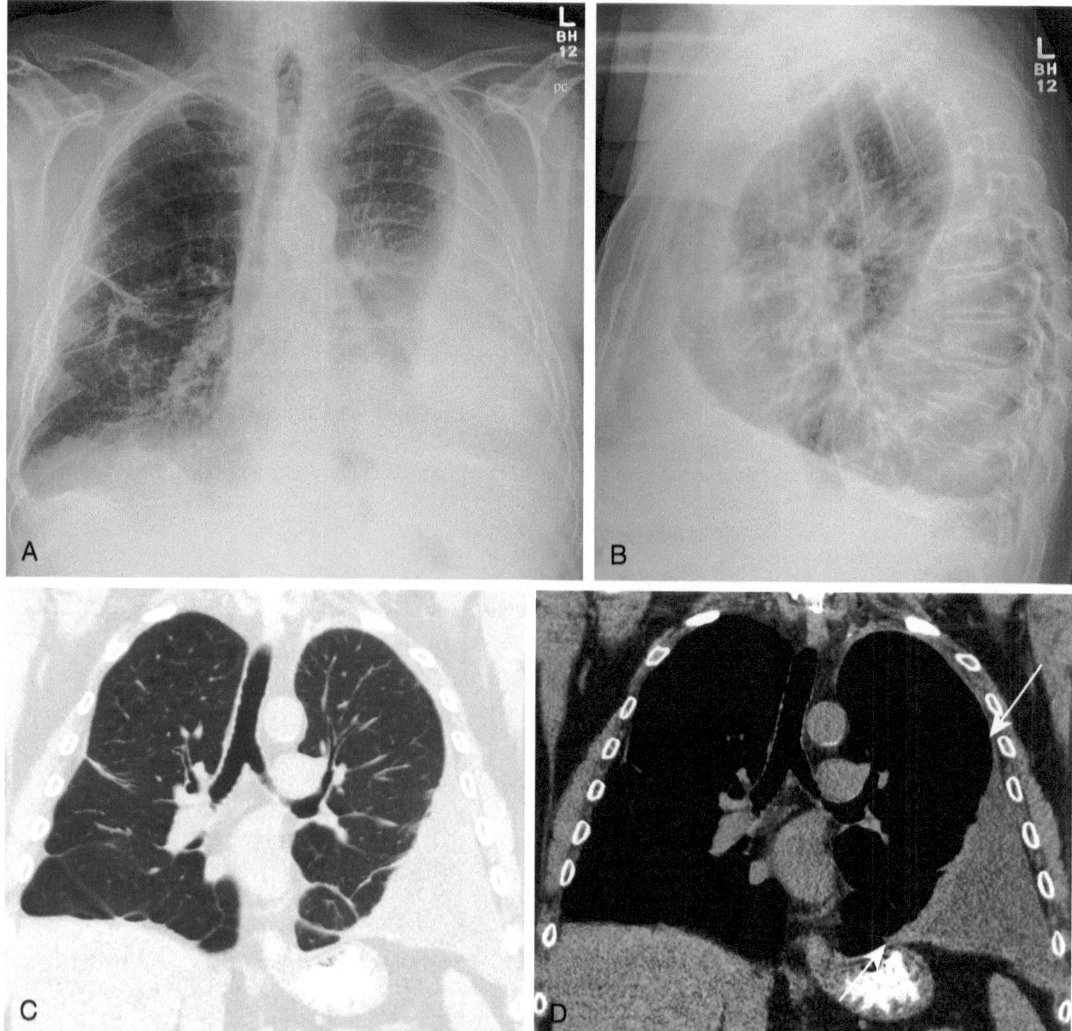

FIGURE 7.6 Loculated left pleural effusion. Posteroanterior **(A)** and lateral **(B)** radiographs show a moderate to large loculated left pleural effusion with wavy contour, defying gravity in this upright individual. The loculated pleural fluid and accompanying atelectasis silhouette the left hemidiaphragm and a portion of the left heart border. **C,** Corresponding coronal computed tomography (CT) lung window reveals parenchymal bands almost perpendicular to this loculated fluid that reflect traction of the lung by the diseased pleura. **D,** Corresponding coronal CT soft tissue window. Note the atelectasis along the diseased visceral pleura *(arrows)*.

gravity and manifests with fairly fixed morphology, despite change in patient position. It often exhibits an undulating, lobulated, or other gravity-defying contour, whether located dependently or nondependently within the thorax (Fig. 7.6). Occasionally, pleural fluid may accumulate within a fissure in such a manner that it mimics a mass or pseudotumor (Fig. 7.7). If necessary, right-side-down or left-side-down lateral decubitus views can be obtained to problem solve because free pleural fluid will shift and layer dependently on decubitus views, but loculated fluid will not. In general, however, when pleural fluid defies gravity, it is loculated, and no additional views are needed to make this determination. Ultrasonography at the bedside can be used to distinguish free-flowing from loculated pleural effusions and, similar to MRI, can better detect internal septations within an exudative pleural effusion than CXR and CT.

Hydropneumothorax

A hydropneumothorax is defined as the presence of air and fluid of any type in the pleural space. It often produces an air–fluid level in the pleural space on an upright CXR (Fig. 7.8). When an air–fluid level is present in the pleural space, its length classically varies on posteroanterior and lateral radiographs. Classically, a shorter air–fluid level may be seen on one view than the other. This feature helps to distinguish a hydropneumothorax or empyema from a lung abscess, in which the length of the air–fluid level is more apt to be equal on both views. Please see below for a further discussion of pneumothorax.

Empyema

An exudative pleural effusion with frank pus is referred to as an empyema. Most empyemas are caused by complications of bacterial pneumonia, an adjacent lung abscess, or both. They may also arise from chest trauma with introduced infection or superinfection, direct extension of a subphrenic abscess or vertebral osteomyelitis with phlegmon into the pleural space, and hematogenous spread of infection. The natural progression of an empyema consists of several phases: an exudative pleural

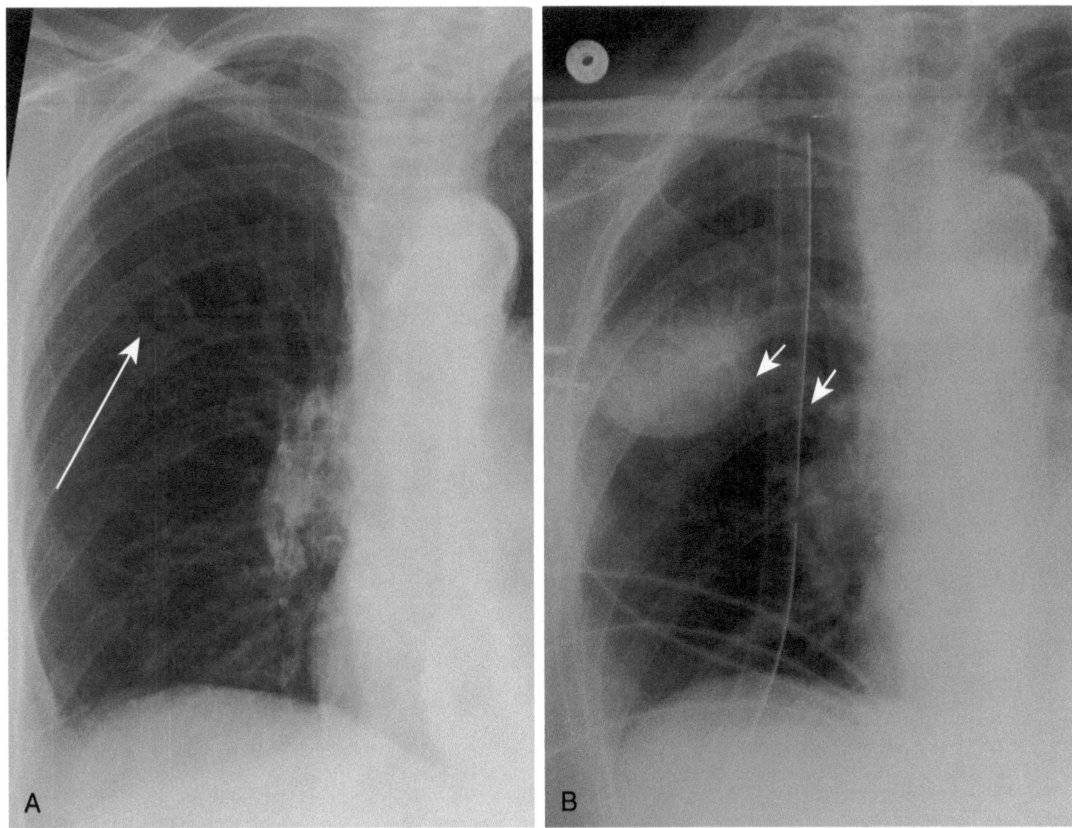

FIGURE 7.7 Pleural pseudotumor. **A,** Preoperative posteroanterior chest radiograph shows a small nodule in the right upper lung *(long arrow)*. **B,** Postoperative anteroposterior supine portable chest radiograph after wedge resection reveals a new oval, partially well-defined right midlung opacity at the level of the lateral aspect of the right major fissure. Its ill-defined upper border, representing an "incomplete border sign," indicates its pleural, rather than parenchymal, location and that this finding represents loculated pleural fluid in the fissure or a pleural pseudotumor rather than a pulmonary hematoma or other mass. The surgical staple line is largely medial to this loculated pleural fluid *(short arrows)*. A right chest tube is present.

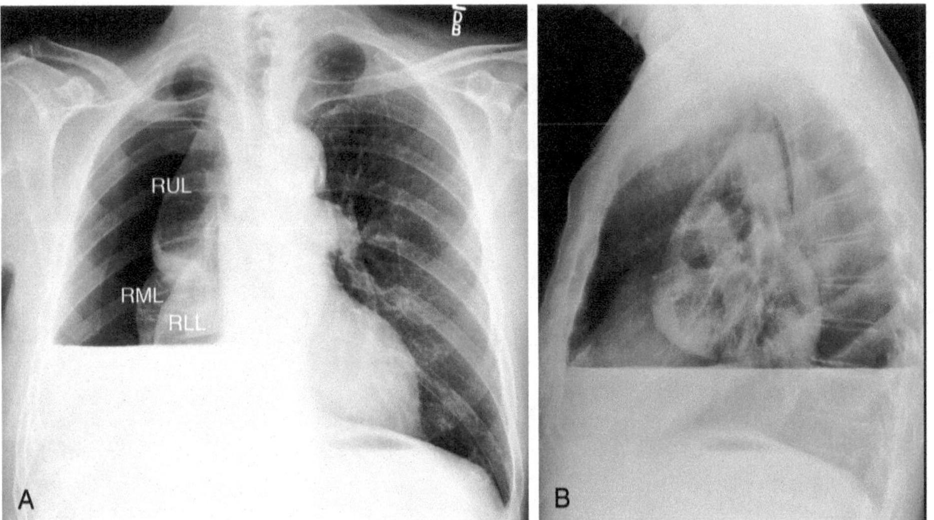

FIGURE 7.8 Hydropneumothorax. Posteroanterior (PA) **(A)** and lateral **(B)** chest radiographs show an air–fluid level (AFL) in the mid-to-lower hemithorax caused by pleural fluid interfacing with a large pneumothorax. The lung cancer–containing right lung is collapsed, with all three lobes identifiable as separate entities on the PA view. Note the discrepant length of the AFLs on the PA and lateral radiographs, another finding (besides the pneumothorax) indicative of the pleural, rather than parenchymal, location of this fluid. *RLL,* Right lower lobe; *RML,* right middle lobe; *RUL,* right upper lobe.

effusion acutely, then a fibrinopurulent phase, and later an organizing phase, when thickened pleura (termed a *fibrin peel*) develops. Early diagnosis and treatment of an empyema are of paramount importance to prevent potential complications, including bronchopleural fistula formation, recurrent empyema, and pleural thickening and fibrosis with trapped lung, the latter of which may require surgical decortication. When an empyema drains through an infection- or inflammation-created opening or sinus tract in the chest wall, it is referred to as empyema necessitans. Tuberculosis (TB), actinomycosis, and several fungal diseases are the most common precipitants of this finding (see Chapter 16).

On CXR, an empyema often manifests as a loculated pleural effusion. If an abnormal communication between the pleural space and the lung (bronchopleural fistula) develops, air accumulates in the pleural space, forming a hydropneumothorax.

The classic chest CT finding for empyema is the "split pleura sign," which manifests as enhancing, separated, and thickened leaves of visceral and parietal pleura encompassing a tense, bulging, lenticular collection of pleural fluid. When present, this finding is virtually diagnostic of an empyema (Fig. 7.9). MRI manifests similar findings; however, it is important to be aware that pleural enhancement is more readily apparent by MRI than CT

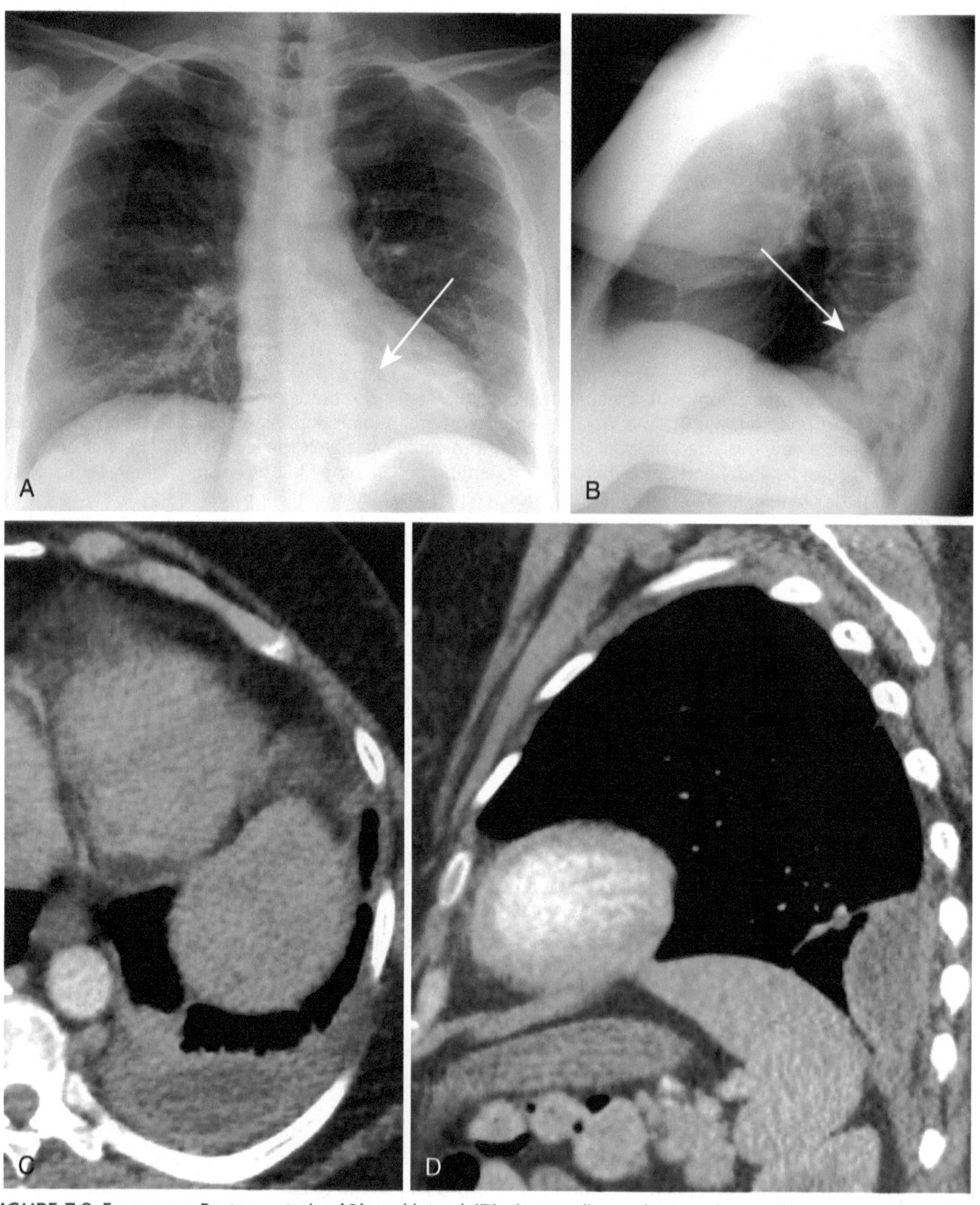

FIGURE 7.9 Empyema. Posteroanterior **(A)** and lateral **(B)** chest radiographs reveal a semilunar mass silhouetting the left paraspinal line and mimicking a left posterior mediastinal mass *(arrows)*. Axial **(C)** and sagittal **(D)** chest computed tomography scans with intravenous contrast reveal this radiographic finding to correspond to a loculated, lentiform left pleural effusion surrounded by thickened visceral and parietal pleura, the so-called split pleura sign of an empyema.

TABLE 7.1 Helpful Computed Tomography Features to Distinguish an Empyema From a Lung Abscess

Computed Tomography Features	Empyema	Lung Abscess
Shape	Lenticular	Round
Angle with pleura	Obtuse	Acute
Boundary with lung	Distinct; compresses adjacent lung	Less distinct boundary with the adjacent lung
Bronchovascular structures	Compressed and draped around an empyema	Terminate abruptly at the margins of a lung abscess
Split pleura sign	Present	Absent

because of MRI's higher soft tissue contrast and can be seen in other inflammatory and neoplastic processes besides empyema. As always, morphology and clinical context must be considered. Cross-sectional imaging is particularly helpful in distinguishing an empyema from a lung abscess (Table 7.1). Both CT and ultrasonography can be used to guide percutaneous diagnostic and therapeutic drainage of empyemas, particularly when composed of multiple loculations and septations.

Hemothorax

A hemothorax represents blood within the pleural space. Hemothoraces are most commonly caused by chest trauma, although hemorrhagic effusions may also occur in the setting of neoplasm, pulmonary infarction, infections such as TB, and coagulopathies. Chronic hemothoraces may result in chronic pleural thickening with tethering; multifocal parenchymal bands; and volume loss of the adjacent lung, otherwise known as a fibrothorax. If functionally limiting, this occurrence may warrant thoracotomy and decortication.

On CXR, a hemothorax may not be distinguishable from a free-flowing or loculated pleural effusion, although clinical history or findings compatible with acute chest trauma, such as pneumothorax and acute rib fractures, may suggest this entity. Recent pleural hemorrhage may be identified by the presence of hyperattenuating fluid on CT and T1 hyperintensity on MRI, as opposed to serous pleural fluid, which is of homogeneous water attenuation on CT and T1-hypointense and T2-hyperintense on MRI. A fluid-fluid level, sometimes referred to as a "hematocrit level," may be present because of dependent layering of the denser cellular elements and less dependent layering of the more serous elements of the blood (Fig. 7.10).

Chylothorax

Disruption of the major lymphatic channels, such as the thoracic duct, results in a chylothorax, with increased levels of triglycerides and cholesterol in the pleural fluid. Common causes of chylothorax include neoplasms (e.g., lymphoma), trauma (both surgical and nonsurgical), and infection (e.g., TB). Lymphangiomatosis is a rare cause (Fig. 7.11). A chylothorax is not readily distinguishable from a transudative pleural effusion on both CXR and CT. Despite the fat content, the CT attenuation is usually close to that of water. CT may be helpful in identifying the cause of chylothorax, such as lymphoma and chest trauma. MRI may be helpful in noninvasive confirmatory diagnosis of a chylothorax when the pleural fluid is T1-hyperintense (and hemorrhage is not a consideration) or when the fluid suppresses on opposed-phase chemical shift MRI secondary to the presence of microscopic fat and water in the same voxel.

Pneumothorax

Pneumothorax is defined as the abnormal presence of air or gas within the pleural space, or technically, the interpleural space. Air may enter the pleural space by several routes: via the lung, airways, esophagus, mediastinum (rarely, in the setting of pneumomediastinum), or the chest wall (in the setting of penetrating chest trauma).

Pneumothoraces may be spontaneous or secondary. Spontaneous pneumothoraces most commonly occur in otherwise healthy, tall, slender young men. They are caused by the rupture of small bullae or air pockets within the elastic fibers of the visceral pleura, most typically in the lung apices. Secondary causes of pneumothorax include a wide range of disease entities, such as chronic obstructive pulmonary disease, especially associated with apical bullae, cystic lung disease (e.g., cystic fibrosis, *Pneumocystis jiroveci* pneumonia, Langerhans cell histiocytosis, lymphangiomyomatosis), metastatic sarcoma (prototypically osteosarcoma), and rarely, pulmonary infarcts. Chest trauma, both open and closed or blunt, is a common cause of pneumothorax (see Chapter 13). Recent thoracic surgery, central line placement, thoracentesis, percutaneous biopsy of the lung and upper abdominal organs, and mechanical ventilation can result in iatrogenic pneumothorax (see Chapters 10 and 13). Catamenial pneumothorax is a rare manifestation of intrathoracic endometriosis and occurs in cyclic fashion, coincident with menses.

On CXR, a pneumothorax most commonly manifests as interpleural air—that is, air-filled lucency, devoid of vessels, located between the fine, smooth, thin visceral pleural line and the parietal pleura, generally along the chest wall but sometimes along the diaphragmatic parietal pleura, mediastinal pleura, or within a pulmonary fissure. A basic concept in imaging interpretation is that air rises. Therefore, on an upright CXR, a pneumothorax is most frequently, *but not always*, apical in location (Fig. 7.12). When the patient is supine, interpleural air typically collects anteriorly. Therefore, a pneumothorax may be more difficult to detect in a supine patient and may be anteromedial or basilar in location, for example. Anteromedial air in the pleural space may produce an abnormally sharp cardiomediastinal border. Air may also collect within the costophrenic sulcus, yielding a "deep sulcus sign" or within the cardiophrenic sulcus (see Chapter 10). Special maneuvers can help accentuate a small pneumothorax, including expiratory and decubitus views. An expiratory CXR may accentuate the size of the pneumothorax upon reduction in lung volume on expiration. Contralateral decubitus radiography can also be a problem-solving maneuver, with the interpleural air collecting nondependently.

Potential pitfalls in the diagnosis of pneumothorax on CXR include misinterpretation of skin folds (Fig. 7.13), overlying clothing, tubes and lines, an arching cortex of a rib, the bony contour of the superomedial scapula, the transverse process

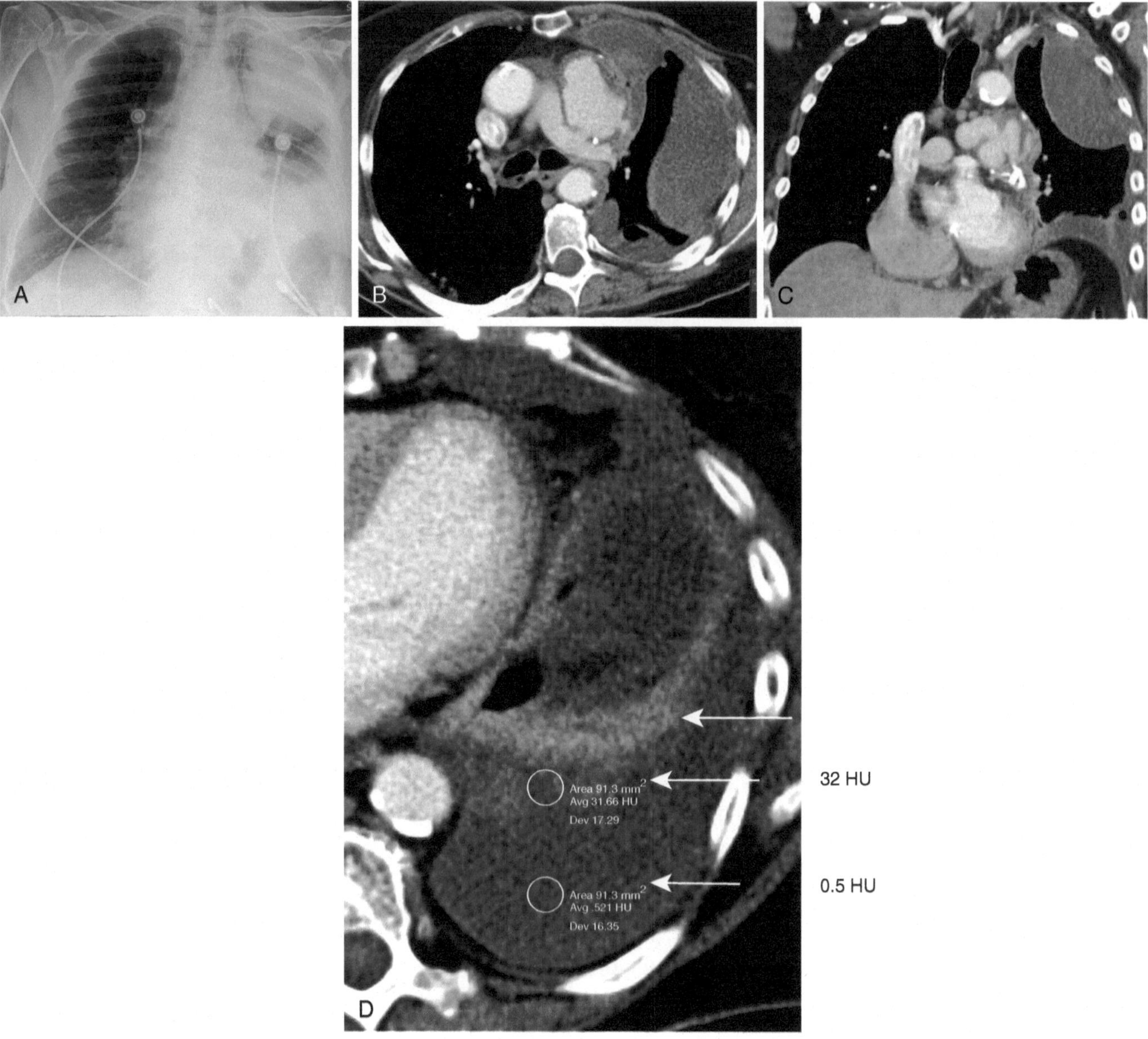

FIGURE 7.10 Hemothorax. **A,** Anteroposterior supine portable chest radiograph shows a multiloculated left pleural effusion or pleural masses (or both). **B** and **C,** Axial and coronal chest computed tomography (CT) scan with intravenous contrast shows correlative multiloculated pleural fluid collections. **D,** Axial CT more inferiorly reveals a fluid–fluid level composed of dependent, more serous hemorrhage of water attenuation—0.5 Hounsfield units *(bottom arrow)* and less dependent, more cellular hemorrhage measuring 32 Hounsfield units (HU) *(middle arrow)*, a so-called hematocrit level often characteristic of a subacute collection of blood. Homogeneously enhancing, crescentic relaxation atelectasis *(top arrow)* is present along the anterior aspect of this fluid.

of an upper thoracic vertebral body, and cavitary and cystic lung disease as a pneumothorax. With further scrutiny, a skin fold can be discerned from a pneumothorax because it becomes increasingly opaque up to its margin, with abrupt lucency along its outer border (it forms an edge, not a line). In contrast, the lung subjacent to a pneumothorax typically remains lucent against the visceral pleural line unless it is opacified by atelectasis or acute or chronic parenchymal disease. CT is much more sensitive and specific in the detection of pneumothorax than CXR. Unsuspected small pneumothoraces can be seen at the anteromedial and basal aspects of the thorax in a supine patient. Ultrasonography may also be used at the bedside in emergency and intensive care unit settings to detect a pneumothorax, but less reliably than CT. There is risk of missing a pneumothorax on MRI because the signal void of interpleural air is not that different from healthy, aerated, or nondiseased lung, particularly on pulse sequences that do not show the pulmonary vasculature. As with plain radiography, on MRI, one must look for absence of vascularity within the pneumothorax compared with the adjacent lung. Because MRI is more sensitive than CT in the detection of endometrial implants, MRI should be considered when a woman presents with chest pain during menses or when a catamenial pneumothorax is contemplated on CXR or CT. The most sensitive and specific MRI pulse sequence for the detection of endometrial implants is a non-contrast-enhanced ultrafast three-dimensional gradient echo fat-saturated T1-weighted sequence.

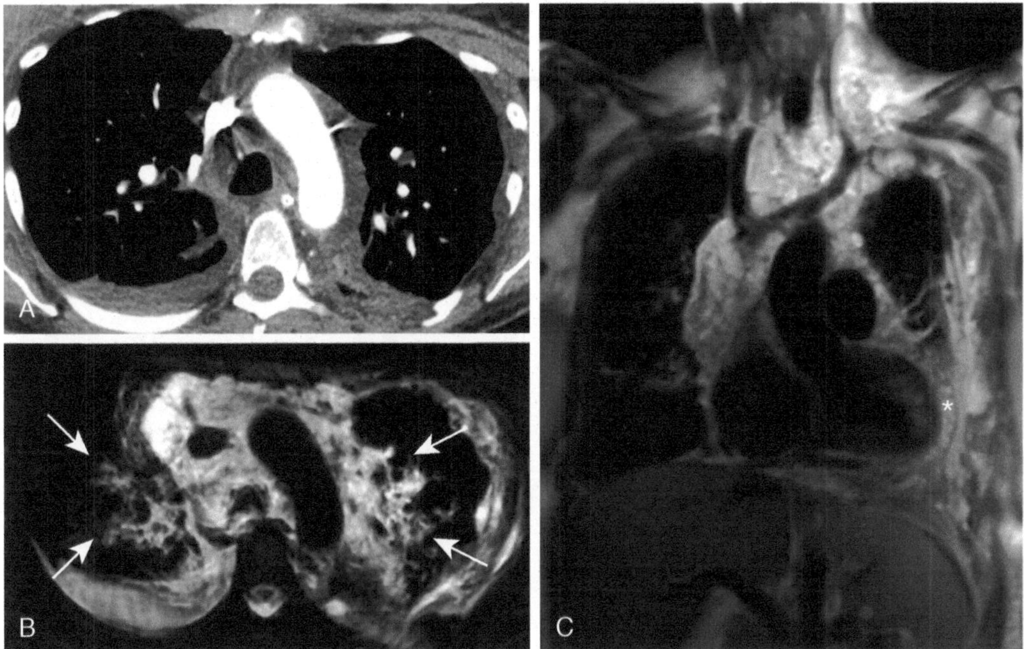

FIGURE 7.11 Chylothorax in the setting of lymphangiomatosis. **A,** Axial computed tomography (CT) scan shows low attenuation material in the mediastinum; tracking around and insinuating between the great vessels, trachea, and esophagus and essentially replacing all mediastinal fat. There is a small layering right pleural effusion. Indeterminate dependent material in the left posterior pleural–extrapleural space tracks partially around the left hemithorax. Axial **(B)** and coronal **(C)** fat-saturated T2-weighted magnetic resonance images acquired 2 weeks after the CT, revealing the indeterminate material throughout the mediastinum and left posterior pleural–extrapleural space to have increased over the short interval and to be composed of innumerable T2-hyperintense locules of fluid or cystic spaces, findings compatible with lymphangiomatosis. Note direct involvement of the peribronchovascular interstitium bilaterally *(arrows)* and direct involvement of the pericardial space *(asterisk)* through a defect created during remote resection of a mediastinal lymphangioma during childhood.

Tension Pneumothorax

A tension pneumothorax develops when the pleural pressure exceeds the alveolar pressure. It is often caused by a flap-like or ball-valve mechanism of the pleural defect, from which air that enters the pleural space cannot exit, resulting in a progressively expanded pleural space, with the ultimate potential for cardiovascular collapse because of impaired venous return and diminished cardiac output. Tension pneumothorax is a clinical diagnosis and medical emergency. On CXR, it classically manifests as collapse of the ipsilateral lung, contralateral shift of the mediastinum, ipsilateral hemidiaphragmatic depression, and widened and expanded ipsilateral intercostal spaces or lesser findings along this spectrum (Fig. 7.14).

Pneumothorax Ex Vacuo

When a pneumothorax arises upon drainage of pleural fluid in the setting of chronic pulmonary parenchymal disease, a malignant pleural effusion, or long-standing hepatic hydrothorax, for example, it may simply reflect the inability of the lung to reexpand fully rather than the presence of an air leak. In this circumstance, the pneumothorax is termed *pneumothorax ex vacuo* and may not warrant a chest tube (Fig. 7.15). A pneumothorax ex vacuo may resolve slowly or persist and has been associated with a poor prognosis.

Pneumonectomy Space

Pneumonectomy is defined as complete surgical removal of a lung. For pneumonectomy space dynamics, see Chapter 12.

It can be difficult to detect recurrent tumor amidst the chronic pneumonectomy rind and fluid by CT. MRI, with its higher soft tissue contrast and, in particular, dynamic contrast-enhanced MRI, may be more sensitive and specific in this regard (Fig. 7.16).

Asbestos-Related Pleural Disease (see Chapter 19)

Asbestos-related pleural disease may be benign or malignant and consists of pleural effusions, pleural thickening, pleural plaques, and mesothelioma. There is a latency period between asbestos exposure and radiographic manifestations. Asbestos-related pleural effusions may occur 10 to 20 years after exposure, can be asymptomatic, and typically resolve on their own. Pleural plaques are the most commonly recognized manifestation of prior asbestos exposure. They, too, are often asymptomatic and are incidentally discovered on imaging unless they are severe enough to cause a fibrothorax. They typically manifest as bilateral, multifocal, primarily parietal pleural thickening and may be calcified and/or noncalcified. On CXR and in tangent, pleural plaques display themselves as localized bandlike or nodular areas of pleural thickening. En face, pleural plaques may appear as irregular geometric opacities, sometimes giving rise to a "holly leaf appearance." Asbestos-related pleural plaques and pleural thickening relatively spare the lung apices, in contrast with pleural thickening by mesothelioma. Both may involve fissures. The presence of diaphragmatic pleural plaque is nearly

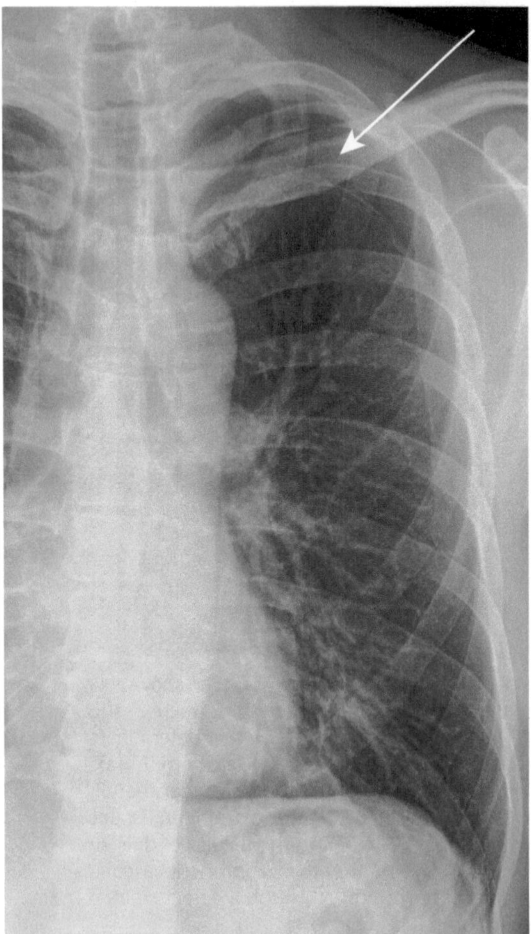

FIGURE 7.12 Pneumothorax. Posteroanterior chest radiograph reveals left apical lucency, through which no vessels pass, above a visceral pleural line *(arrow)*, representing a small left apical pneumothorax.

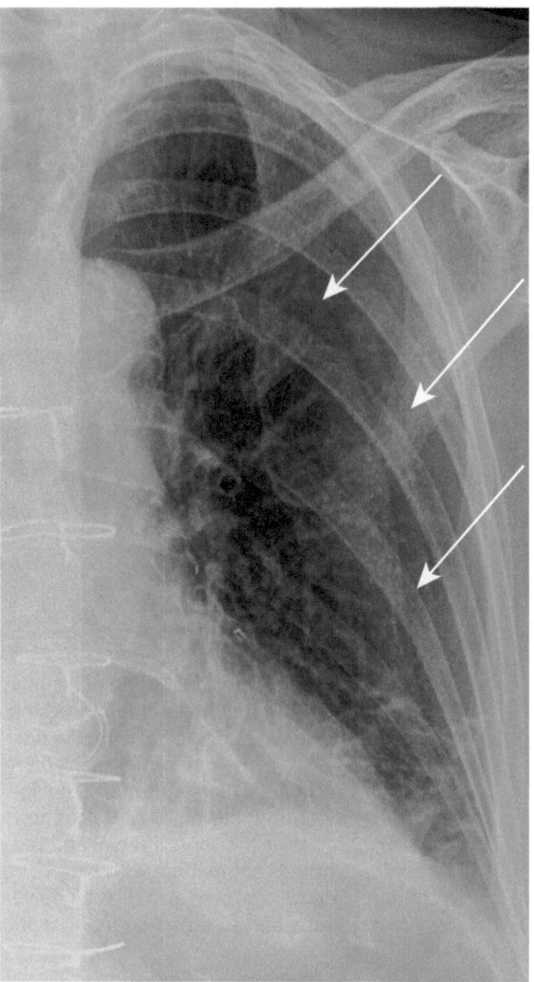

FIGURE 7.13 Skin folds. Anteroposterior supine portable chest radiograph reveals two adjacent skin folds *(arrows)* overlying the left hemithorax. Note the increasing attenuation, from medial to lateral, until the acute drop-off in attenuation at the edge of the skin fold, in contrast to the lucency found on either side of a pneumothorax (pulmonary parenchymal lucency on one side and interpleural lucency on the other). There has been a median sternotomy and coronary artery bypass graft with left internal mammary artery graft placement (the latter demarcated by surgical clips along the left cardiac margin).

pathognomonic for asbestos exposure. CT is more sensitive and specific than CXR in detecting pleural plaques (Fig. 7.17).

Non–Asbestos-Related Pleural Thickening

Non-asbestos-related pleural calcification and thickening may be caused by repeated pulmonary infection, prior empyema, prior surgery, radiation, or trauma, prior hemothorax, certain drugs such as methysergide, and rheumatoid arthritis. These non–asbestos-related forms of pleural thickening are more often unilateral and less multifocal.

Fibrothorax

A fibrothorax is defined as diffuse fibrosis and thickening of the pleura, with common causes including asbestos exposure, prior infection, empyema (classically from TB), chronic pleural inflammation (in the setting of rheumatoid arthritis or lupus), and hemothorax. When diffuse and extensive, it can limit the expansion of the lung, yielding a "trapped lung," and compromised respiration. Surgical decortication can be performed, if clinically warranted, to treat this entity. CT and MRI help differentiate benign diffuse pleural thickening from neoplastic pleural involvement. Benign fibrothorax rarely involves the mediastinal pleura and is seldom nodular and mass-like, unlike mesothelioma and pleural metastases. Follow-up imaging by CT or MRI can help distinguish between these entities if initial findings are indeterminate.

Thoracolithiasis

Thoracoliths are rare, calcified or noncalcified "rolling stones" within the pleural space that do not typically cause symptoms (Fig. 7.18).

Benign Pleural Tumors

Solitary Fibrous Tumor of the Pleura (Benign and Malignant)

Solitary fibrous tumors (SFTs) are rare mesenchymal neoplasms that most commonly arise from the pleura, although they may also occur in the mediastinum and elsewhere in the body. They account for less than 5% of all pleural tumors and are not associated with asbestos exposure. These tumors are slow growing. Patients can be asymptomatic or may present with local or systemic effects produced by the tumor. Hypertrophic osteoarthropathy has been reported, along with clubbing and episodic hypoglycemia. Histologically, the majority of SFTs arise from the visceral pleura. Most of these tumors are low-grade neoplasms of variable cellularity and collagen content. Myxoid change and collagen degeneration may occur. Approximately 20% to 30% of SFTs are malignant, based on histologic criteria including high cellularity, high mitotic activity, and pleomorphism. Nevertheless, even benign SFTs may behave in a malignant manner and recur years later; hence, benign histopathology at surgical resection is of limited reassurance.

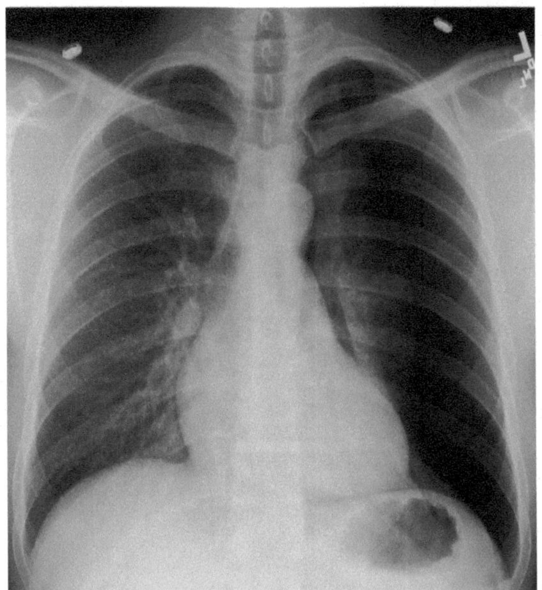

FIGURE 7.14 Tension pneumothorax. Posteroanterior chest radiograph demonstrates marked left hemithoracic lucency caused by a large left pneumothorax, with mild depression of the ipsilateral hemidiaphragm, widened left intercostal spaces, and rightward cardiomediastinal shift, compatible with an early tension pneumothorax.

On CXR, SFTs often manifest as well-circumscribed, rounded and/or mildly lobulated pleural masses, with or without pedunculation. When on a pedicle, they may shift in location between studies. These tumors may exhibit faded margins when viewed en face, referred to as an "incomplete border sign" typical of pleural and extrapleural lesions, in which the portion of the mass surrounded by air in the lung exhibits a sharp border and the portion contiguous with the pleura does not. On CT, most of these tumors are well-circumscribed and, when large, can form acute angles with the pleural surface. They may enhance heterogeneously on account of internal hemorrhage or cystic degeneration, particularly the larger, more malignant tumors. Calcifications may be present in up to 25% of cases.

On MRI, solitary fibrous tumors of the pleura (SFTPs) are often heterogeneous in signal; however, they often contain areas of very low T2 signal intensity when sufficiently fibrous, on account of the tightly bundled collagen (Fig. 7.19). When this low T2 signal is multifocal, the overall appearance has been referred to as the "chocolate chip cookie sign." These tumors have been observed to enhance gradually and strongly over several minutes on dynamic contrast-enhanced imaging. Malignant SFTs tend to be larger

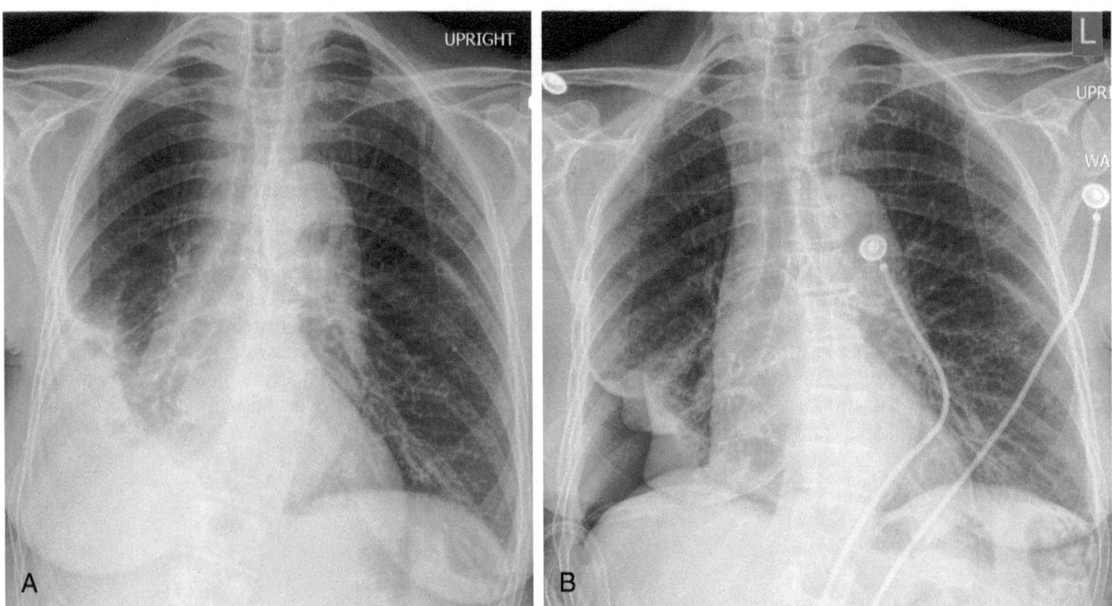

FIGURE 7.15 Pneumothorax *ex vacuo*. **A,** Upright anteroposterior (AP) chest radiograph before thoracentesis, revealing a loculated right pleural effusion containing a few locules of air that were iatrogenically introduced at the time of diagnostic thoracentesis. **B,** Upright AP chest radiograph after thoracentesis, revealing air at the site of previous loculated pleural fluid. The lung has not reexpanded into this space, hence the term *pneumothorax ex vacuo*.

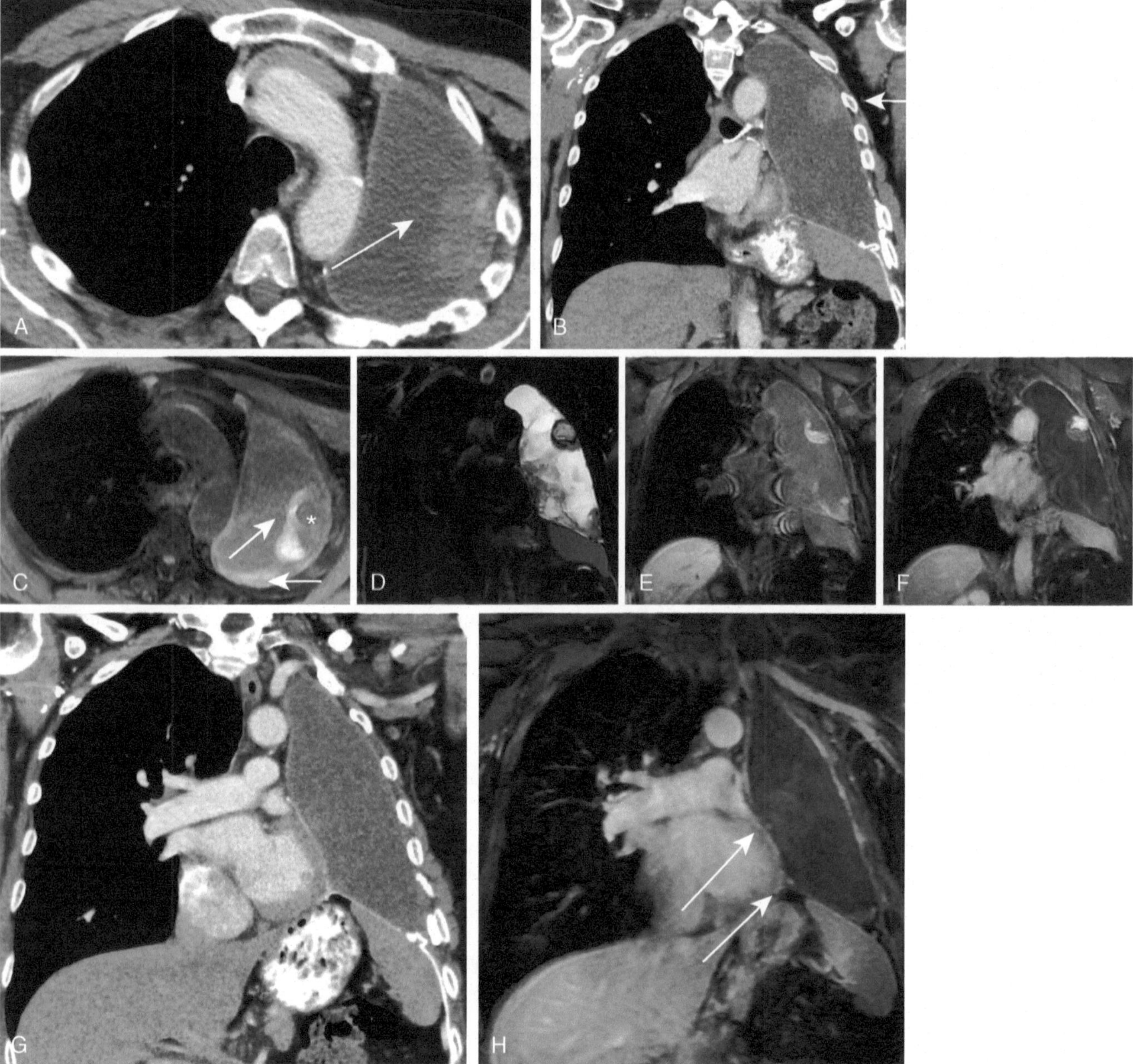

FIGURE 7.16 Recurrent mesothelioma in the pneumonectomy space. Axial **(A)** and coronal **(B)** computed tomography (CT) images with intravenous contrast show rounded, mixed attenuation mass-like opacity in the mid-to-upper lateral aspect of the left pneumonectomy space *(arrow)*. The composition of this finding is indeterminate by CT and may be hemorrhage or recurrent tumor. **C,** Axial fat-saturated precontrast T1-weighted image reveals T1-hyperintense material tracking around the round mass-like structure *(asterisk)* found on the CT and layering dependently *(arrows)*. Coronal T2-weighted **(D)**, coronal fat-saturated precontrast T1-weighted **(E)**, and coronal fat-saturated postcontrast T1-weighted images **(F)** showing the indeterminate mass on CT to be composed of solid, enhancing tumor surrounded by intrinsically T1-hyperintense hemorrhage. Matched coronal CT **(G)** and fat-saturated postcontrast magnetic resonance **(H)** images revealing tiny 3- to 4-mm enhancing nodules *(arrows)* in the inferomedial left pneumonectomy space, representing additional sites of recurrent (metastatic) mesothelioma that are invisible by CT.

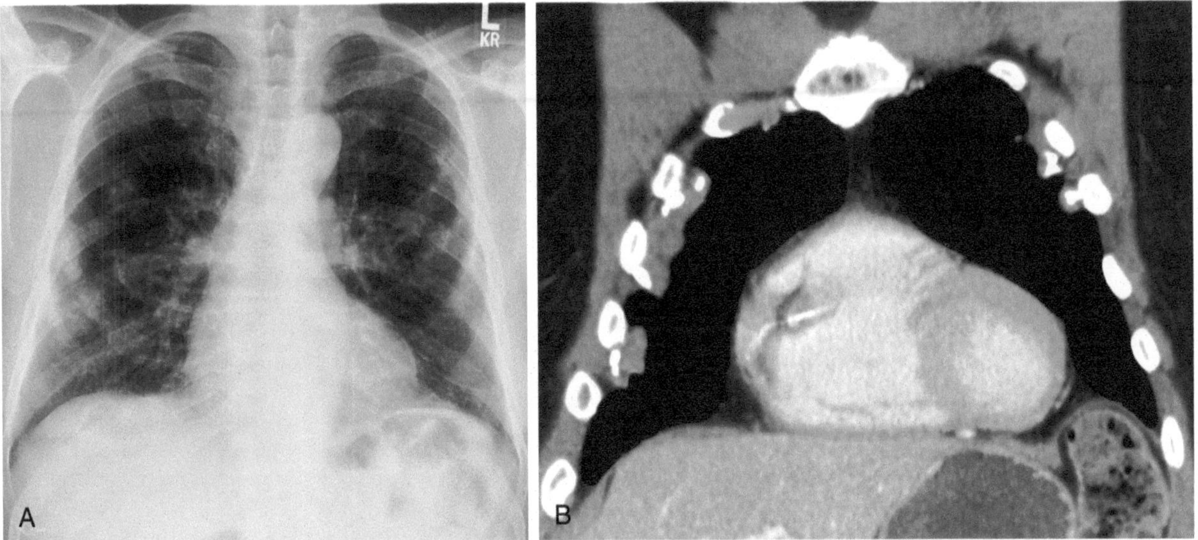

FIGURE 7.17 Asbestos-related pleural plaques. **A,** Posteroanterior chest radiograph reveals multiple bilateral calcified pleural plaques, many of which are en face. Some of these en face plaques resemble a holly leaf. **B,** Correlative coronal computed tomography scan showing multiple bilateral, partially calcified pleural plaques.

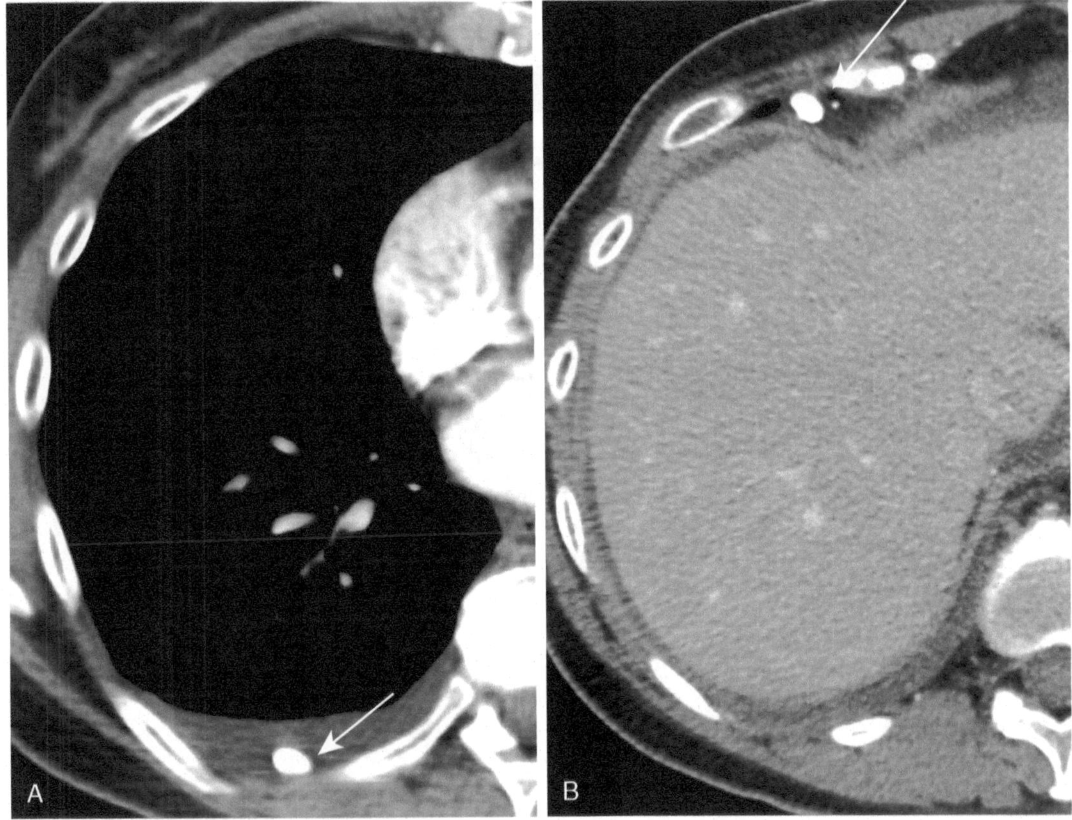

FIGURE 7.18 Thoracolith. **A,** Axial chest computed tomography (CT) scan revealing a small, ovoid, calcified nodule *(arrow)* located dependently within a small, layering right pleural effusion. **B,** Axial chest CT performed 3 weeks later showing interval movement of this thoracolith, now lodged in the right anterior costophrenic angle *(arrow)*, proving it to be a thoracolith, as opposed to a fixed, calcified parietal pleural nodule or plaque.

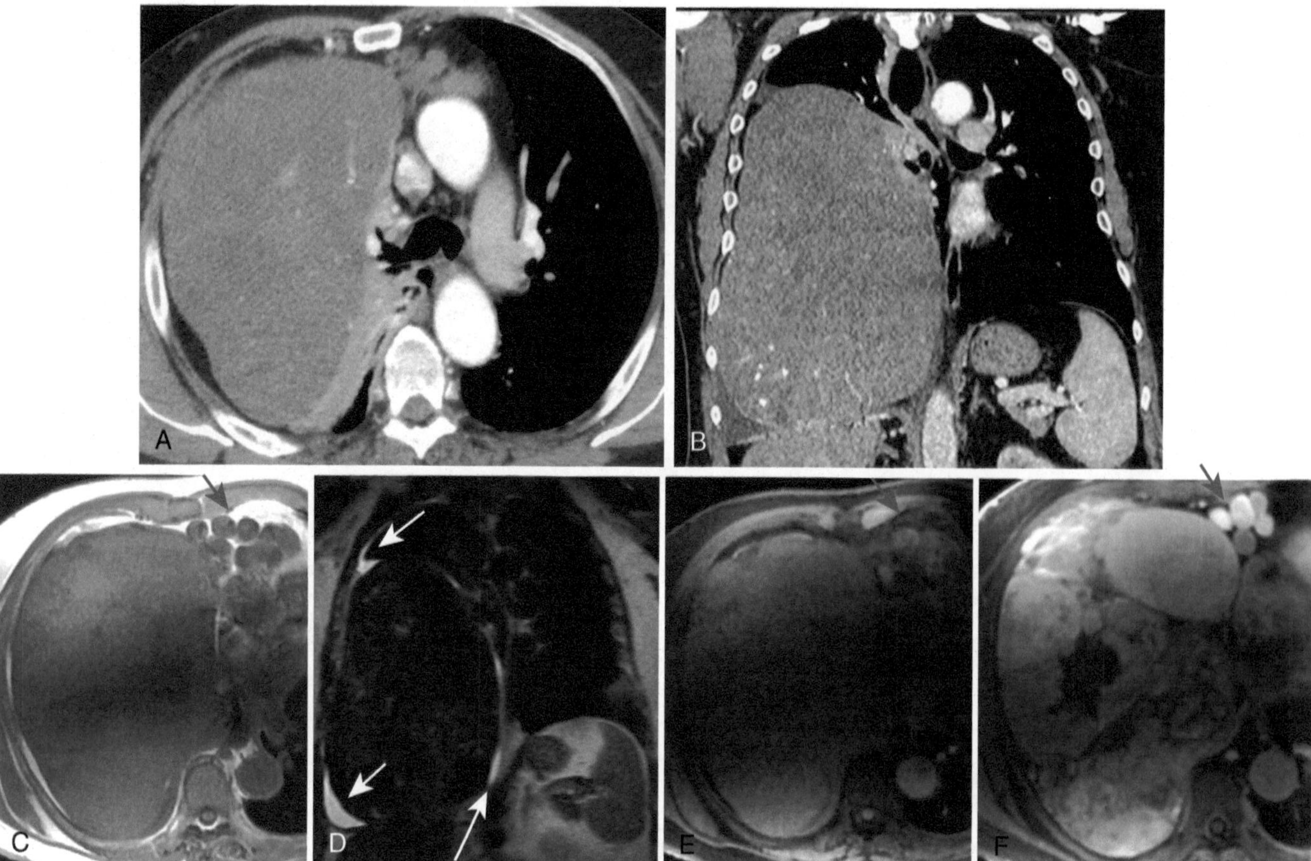

FIGURE 7.19 Solitary fibrous tumor (SFT), benign appearance. **A,** Axial computed tomography (CT) scan showing a large, well-circumscribed mass of slightly heterogeneous attenuation filling much of the right hemithoracic cavity, with extrapleural fat laterally and anteriorly and with compressive and relaxation atelectasis medially. There is leftward cardiomediastinal shift. **B,** Coronal CT scan shows this mass to depress and flatten the right hemidiaphragm. Axial T1-weighted **(C)**, coronal T2-weighted (**D**), and axial pre- **(E)** and postcontrast T1-weighted **(F)** magnetic resonance images reveal the mass to be of intermediate T1 signal and marked T2 hypointensity, with a partially circumferential T2-hyperintense pleural effusion *(white arrows)*. The mass enhances heterogeneously, along with the enhancing right pericardiophrenic varices *(gray arrow)* that have arisen as a result of venous compression by the mass. The marked T2 hypointensity of this mass, in conjunction with its solitary nature and location in the pleural space, confers a diagnosis of SFT of the pleura and excludes sarcoma, lymphoma, and a large lung cancer. These latter diagnoses would be T2-hyperintense on magnetic resonance imaging.

(>10 cm in diameter), more heterogeneous in CT attenuation and MR signal, and more T2-hyperintense (Fig. 7.20). These tumors may demonstrate aggressive features, including chest wall invasion. A small pleural effusion may accompany SFTPs. Hypertrophic osteoarthropathy, a periosteal reaction involving the diaphysis and metadiaphysis of the long bones of distal extremities, can occur not only in the setting of SFTP, but also in association with cardiovascular, hepatic, and gastrointestinal disorders. Clubbing of the fingers may be seen. When associated with a pulmonary condition, such as lung cancer, pulmonary metastatic disease, lung abscess, SFTP, and mesothelioma, it is termed *hypertrophic pulmonary osteoarthropathy* (HPOA).

Pleural Lipoma

Pleural lipomas are the most common benign tumor of the pleura. Most pleural lipomas are asymptomatic and discovered incidentally by imaging. CT and MRI are virtually diagnostic when the lesion is well-circumscribed and uniformly fatty—that is, isoattenuating or isointense to macroscopic fat on CT (Fig. 7.21) and MRI, respectively. However, the presence of an enhancing soft tissue component within an otherwise fatty pleural mass should heighten suspicion for liposarcoma and typically warrants resection.

Malignant Pleural Disease

Pleural Metastases

Pleural metastases account for the vast majority of malignant pleural disease. The most common malignancies to metastasize to the pleura include lung carcinoma, breast carcinoma, and gastrointestinal and genitourinary malignancies such as gastric and ovarian carcinomas. Pleural effusions are common in the setting of metastatic adenocarcinoma to the pleura. Pleural metastases may be asymptomatic, especially when limited, although patients may present with dyspnea, chest pain, and weight loss. Pleural metastases may also occur in the setting of invasive thymoma, although usually without a concurrent pleural effusion. In this scenario, they are sometimes referred to as "drop metastases" or "pleural seeding" (see Fig. 5.13 in Chapter 5).

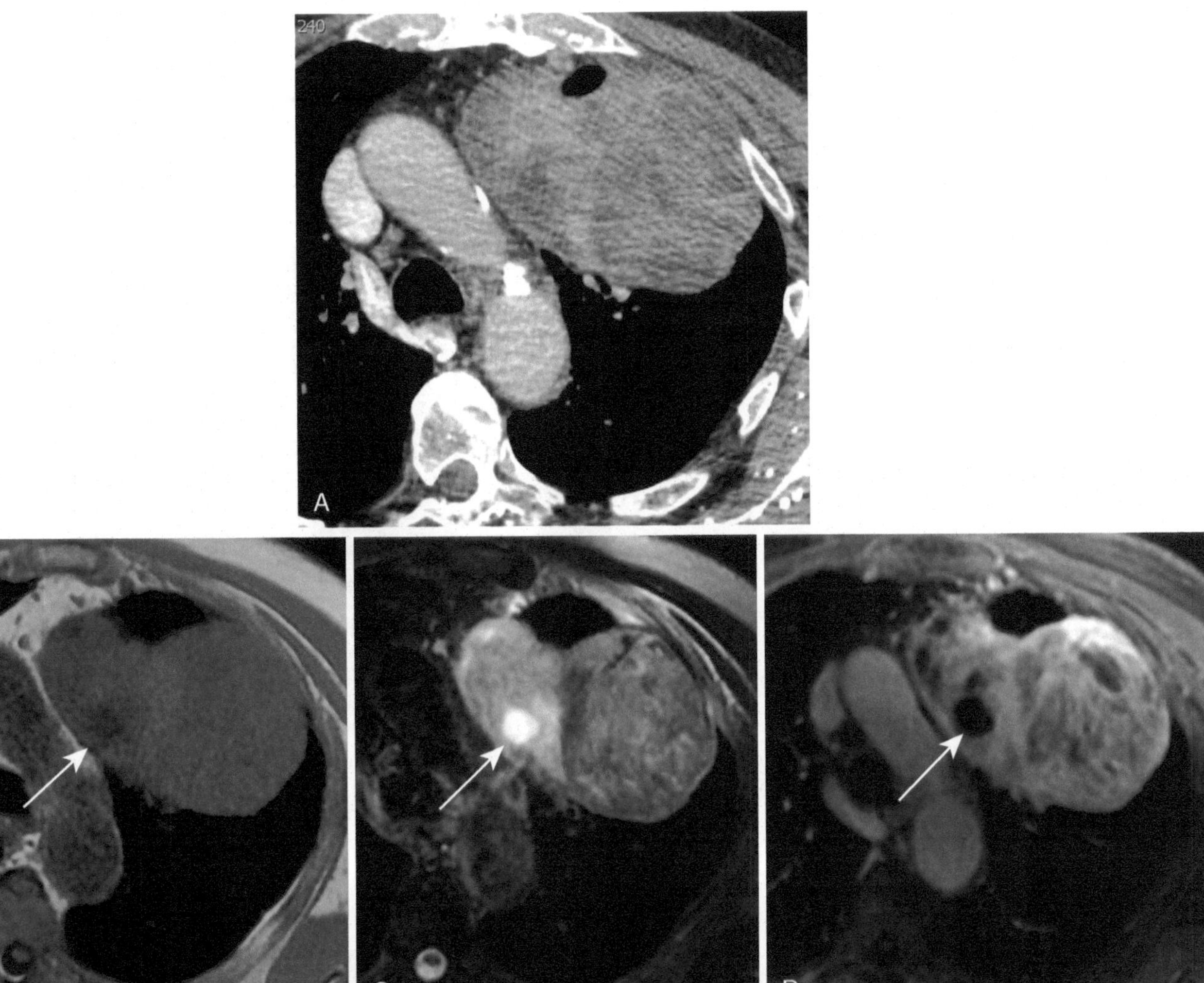

FIGURE 7.20 Solitary fibrous tumor of the pleura (SFTP), malignant appearance. **A,** Axial chest computed tomography (CT) scan with intravenous contrast shows a large, heterogeneously enhancing mass filling the anterior aspect of the left hemithoracic cavity with possible chest wall invasion. The intrathoracic compartment from which this mass arises is unclear by CT. The air pocket anteriorly represents normal aerated lung on the lung window (latter not shown). Axial T1-weighted **(B)**, axial T2-weighted **(C)**, and postcontrast fat-saturated axial T1-weighted **(D)** MR images reveal the mass to be very well circumscribed and pedunculated, displacing the anterior mediastinal fat pad to the right; it therefore likely arises from the pleural space. The mass is of heterogeneous but primarily intermediately-to-mildly hyperintense T1 signal and heterogeneous, primarily hyperintense T2 signal; it demonstrates heterogeneous and fairly intense enhancement. This MRI reveals no chest wall invasion. The nonenhancing, focal round area of T1-hypointense, T2-hyperintense signal *(arrow)* represents cystic change. There are scattered areas of focal, patchy low T2 signal within the mass representing fibrous tissue, sometimes referred to as the "chocolate chip cookie sign" of SFTs. The predominance of T2 hyperintensity, vigorous enhancement, and cystic change favor a malignant SFT over a benign SFT. The fibrous areas within the tumor favor SFT over a sarcoma.

On CXR, CT, and MRI, pleural metastatic disease may manifest as a layering or loculated pleural effusion, diffuse pleural thickening, or focal pleural nodules and masses. A malignant pleural effusion is the most common manifestation of metastatic pleural involvement by imaging. By CXR, however, it is often impossible to discern pleural thickening or masses from pleural fluid. CT more readily makes this distinction (Fig. 7.22), but it, too, can fall short in this regard. MRI is more sensitive and can virtually always distinguish pleural fluid from pleural thickening and is more capable than CT of showing the full extent of pleural disease (Figs. 7.23 and 7.24).

Mesothelioma

Mesothelioma is a rare primary pleural neoplasm strongly associated with asbestos exposure. There is usually a 20- to 40-year latency period between presentation and initial exposure. The amphibolic subtype of asbestos fiber has been shown to be the most carcinogenic. These tumors are most common in men between 50 and 70 years of age (male-to-female preponderance of 4:1). Most patients eventually become symptomatic, presenting with chest pain, dyspnea, and constitutional symptoms such as fever and weight loss. Histologically, mesothelioma can be divided

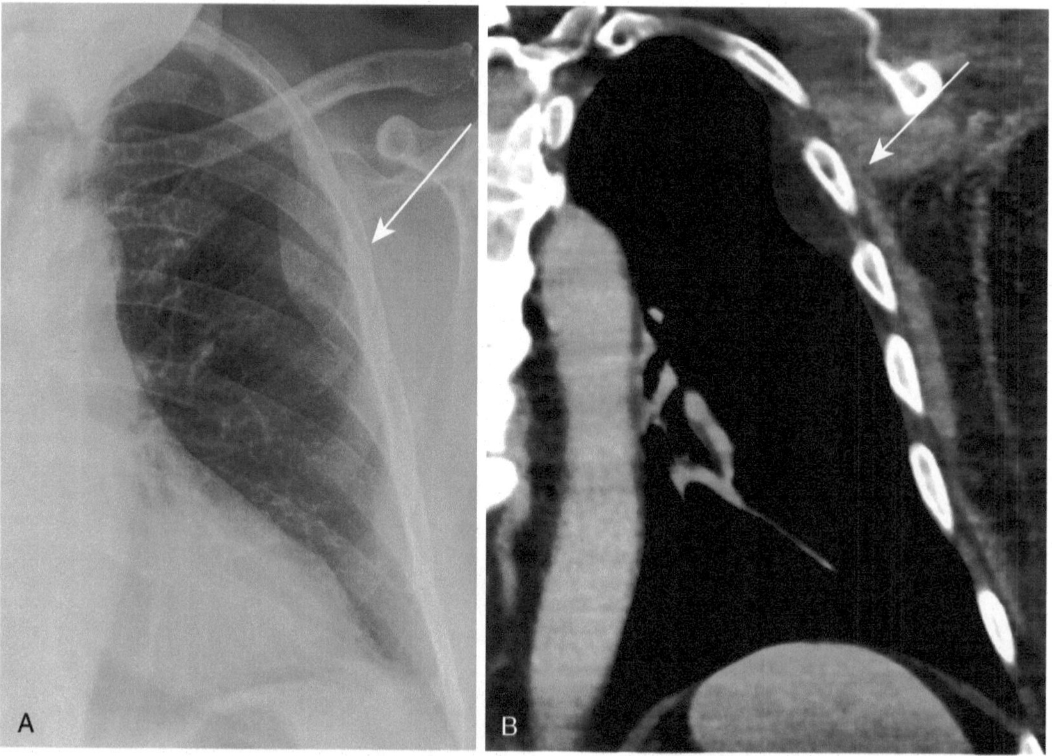

FIGURE 7.21 Pleural lipoma. **A,** Posteroanterior chest radiograph shows a peripheral left hemithoracic. Elongated mass *(arrow)* making obtuse angles with the lung and exhibiting an incomplete border sign, placing this lesion in the pleural or extrapleural space. **B,** Correlative coronal chest computed tomography scan reveals this mass *(arrow)* to be exclusively of fatty attenuation, proving it to represent a lipoma.

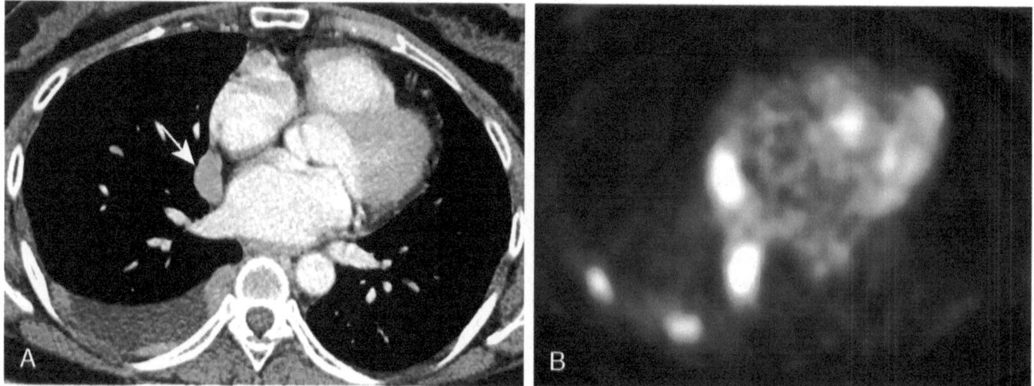

FIGURE 7.22 Pleural metastatic disease. **A,** Axial chest computed tomography scan with intravenous contrast shows multiple parietal pleural nodules amid a small, layering right pleural effusion, in addition to a paramediastinal pleural nodule *(arrow)*, representing metastatic adenocarcinoma to the pleura in this woman with breast cancer. **B,** Axial ^{18}FDG-PET (18-fluorodeoxyglucose positron emission tomography) scan reveals intense FDG-PET avidity of these metastatic pleural nodules.

into three major categories: epithelial, sarcomatoid, and mixed or biphasic, with all carrying a poor prognosis, although those with sarcomatoid features carry a worse prognosis. The epithelioid subtype is most common; the sarcomatoid subtype is less common and typically more aggressive.

Chest radiography can be nonspecific. Most patients present with diffuse pleural thickening and pleural effusion. The pleural thickening is usually lobulated and nodular. Mesothelioma is almost always unilateral. Coexistent calcified pleural plaques may be present and suggest prior asbestos exposure; however, their presence is not required for diagnosis of mesothelioma.

Computed tomography offers better delineation of tumor extent and distinction of pleural fluid from tumor than CXR (see Figs. 7.23 and 7.24). Mediastinal pleural involvement is more characteristic of malignant pleural tumors such as mesothelioma and pleural metastatic disease

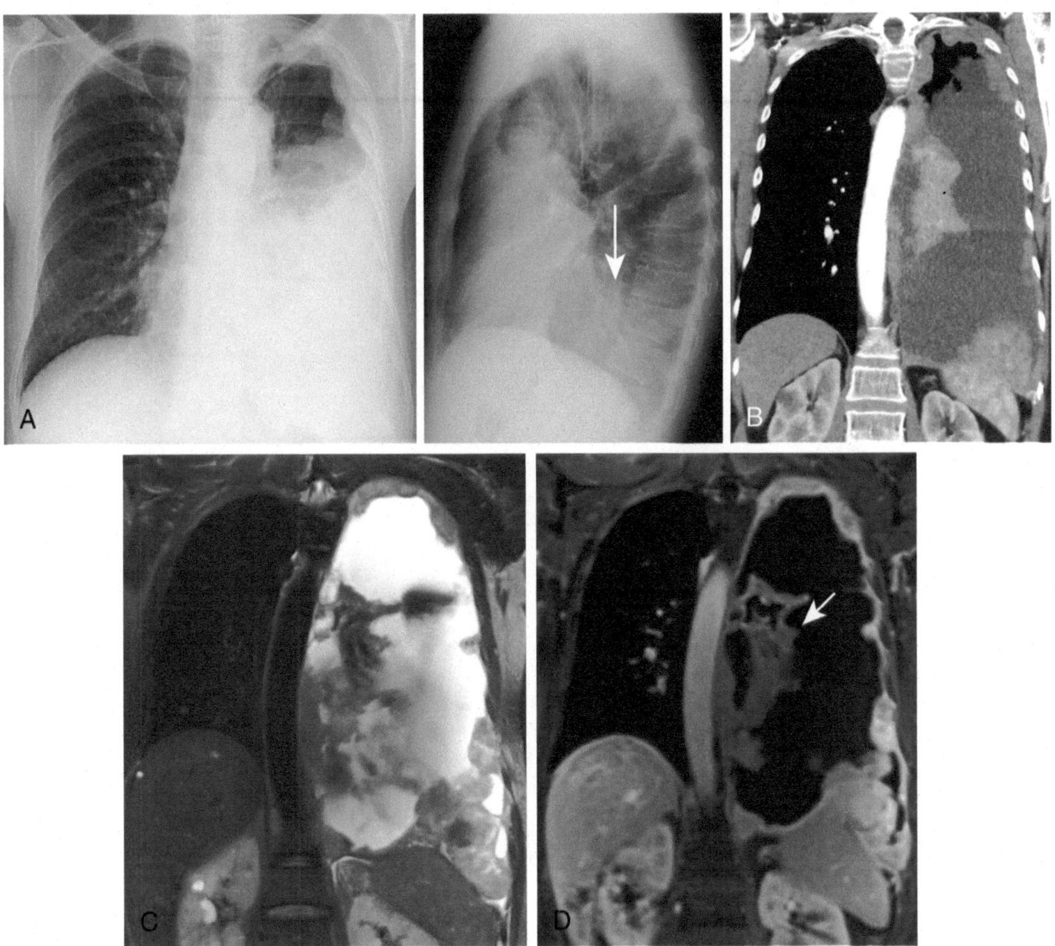

FIGURE 7.23 Mesothelioma. **A,** Posteroanterior and lateral chest radiographs show a partially circumferential, loculated left pleural effusion or pleural mass (or both), a suggestion of a layering component of this pleural effusion, given the meniscus on the upright lateral radiograph *(long arrow)*, and concurrent mid-to-lower pulmonary opacification. **B,** Coronal chest computed tomography (CT) scan with intravenous contrast shows the pleural opacification on chest radiography to be secondary to a combination of lobulated pleural thickening, pleural fluid, and atelectasis. Coronal T2-weighted **(C)** and coronal postcontrast **(D)** thoracic magnetic resonance images reveal the T2-hyperintense, enhancing solid pleural disease to be more extensive than shown by CT, involving the entire circumference of the left hemithorax. An associated large left pleural effusion and left lung atelectasis *(short arrow)* are again demonstrated.

than it is of benign asbestos-related pleural thickening or plaques. Common CT and MR findings of mesothelioma include diffuse and often circumferential pleural thickening, thickening of the interlobar fissures, and pleural effusion. Chest wall invasion (see Fig. 7.24), diaphragmatic invasion, and metastatic involvement of hilar and mediastinal lymph nodes can occur. Distant metastases are rare.

Multiplanar MRI offers superior delineation of extent of disease (see Figs. 7.23 and 7.24) and better demonstrates chest wall and diaphragmatic invasion than multiplanar CT secondary to its higher soft tissue contrast. Mesothelioma typically demonstrates iso- to mildly hyperintense T1-weighted signal, mild-to-moderate T2-hyperintensity to muscle, and vivid enhancement.

Mesothelioma is often intensely FDG-PET (18-fluorodeoxyglucose positron emission tomography) avid. Although FDG uptake in mesothelioma is higher than benign chronic pleural thickening, it can also be increased in inflammatory pleural disease. Greater FDG uptake in mesothelioma has been associated with a shorter survival time. FDG-PET imaging provides more accurate tumor staging and assessment of treatment response than CT, more readily detecting involved mediastinal lymph nodes and extrathoracic metastatic disease.

Pleural Lymphoma

Pleural lymphoma may be primary or secondary (spread from elsewhere), and of Hodgkin or non-Hodgkin type. It can mimic the appearance of mesothelioma (Fig. 7.25), with diffuse pleural thickening and a pleural effusion; however, it is more often associated with pronounced mediastinal lymphadenopathy than mesothelioma. Pleural lymphoma may alternatively present as a focal mass. Nonlymphomatous pleural effusions can arise in the setting of mediastinal lymphoma because of impaired lymphatic drainage by mediastinal lymphadenopathy.

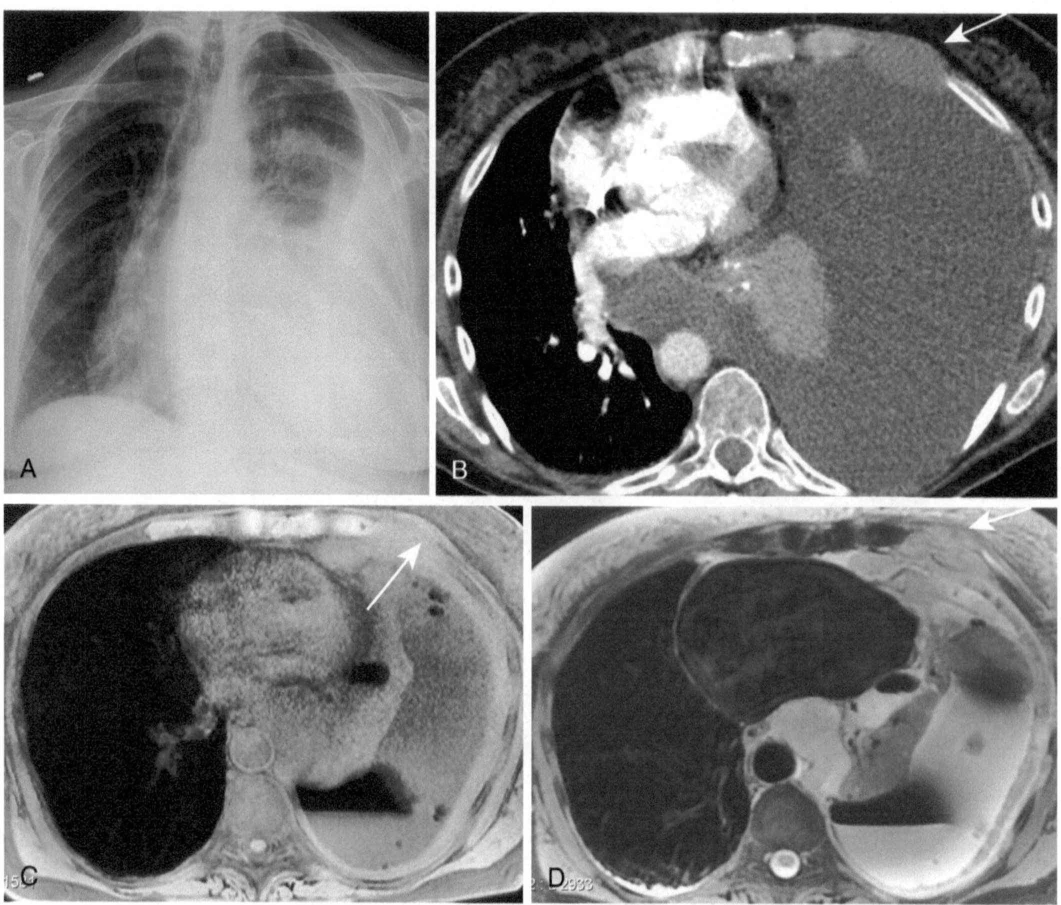

FIGURE 7.24 Mesothelioma invading the chest wall. **A,** Anteroposterior chest radiograph shows a moderate to large left pleural effusion, with associated atelectasis, obscuring much of left hemithorax, with rightward cardiomediastinal shift. **B,** Axial chest computed tomography (CT) scan reveals a large left pleural effusion yielding mass effect, with rightward cardiac displacement. There is complete left lung atelectasis. A left anterior intercostal chest wall mass is present *(arrow)*. Correlative axial T1- **(C)** and T2-weighted **(D)** MR images after thoracentesis reveal extensive, circumferential, intermediate T1 signal, T2-hyperintense, left hemithoracic pleural thickening and lobulation that are almost completely CT-occult. Left anterior intercostal chest wall invasion is again noted *(arrow)*.

DIAPHRAGM

Anatomy and Function

The diaphragm is the physical muscular barrier separating the thorax from the abdomen and serves as the primary muscle for ventilation. Dysfunction of the diaphragm can lead to dyspnea and respiratory failure. The two hemidiaphragmatic crura attach posteriorly to the upper lumbar vertebral bodies and intervertebral disks and are joined in the midline by the fibrous median arcuate ligament. The diaphragm is innervated by the right and left phrenic nerves, which originate from the third, fourth, and fifth cervical nerve roots. The diaphragm has a well-developed lymphatic drainage system, which explains the dissemination of neoplastic and infectious processes that can occur between the thorax and the abdomen. There are three main openings in the diaphragm that serve as major passageways for important structures between the thorax and abdomen: the inferior vena cava (IVC) hiatus, esophageal hiatus, and aortic hiatus. The IVC hiatus is at the T8 level and contains the IVC and branches of the right phrenic nerve. The esophageal hiatus is at the T10 level and contains the esophagus, vagus nerve, and sympathetic nerve branches. The aortic hiatus is at the T12 level and contains the aorta, azygous and hemiazygous veins, and thoracic duct. The cisterna chyli is also located at this level as well.

Diaphragmatic Eventration

An eventration of the diaphragm is a focal thinning of the diaphragmatic muscle, resulting in a focal bulge or superiorly convex contour of a portion of the hemidiaphragm. On CXR, there is a focal upward bulge of a portion of the affected hemidiaphragm, often better demonstrated on the lateral projection (Fig. 7.26).

Diaphragmatic Weakness and Paralysis

Diaphragmatic weakness (paresis) and paralysis may be caused by a wide range of disease entities, including cervical spinal trauma, cervical myelopathy, mediastinal tumors,

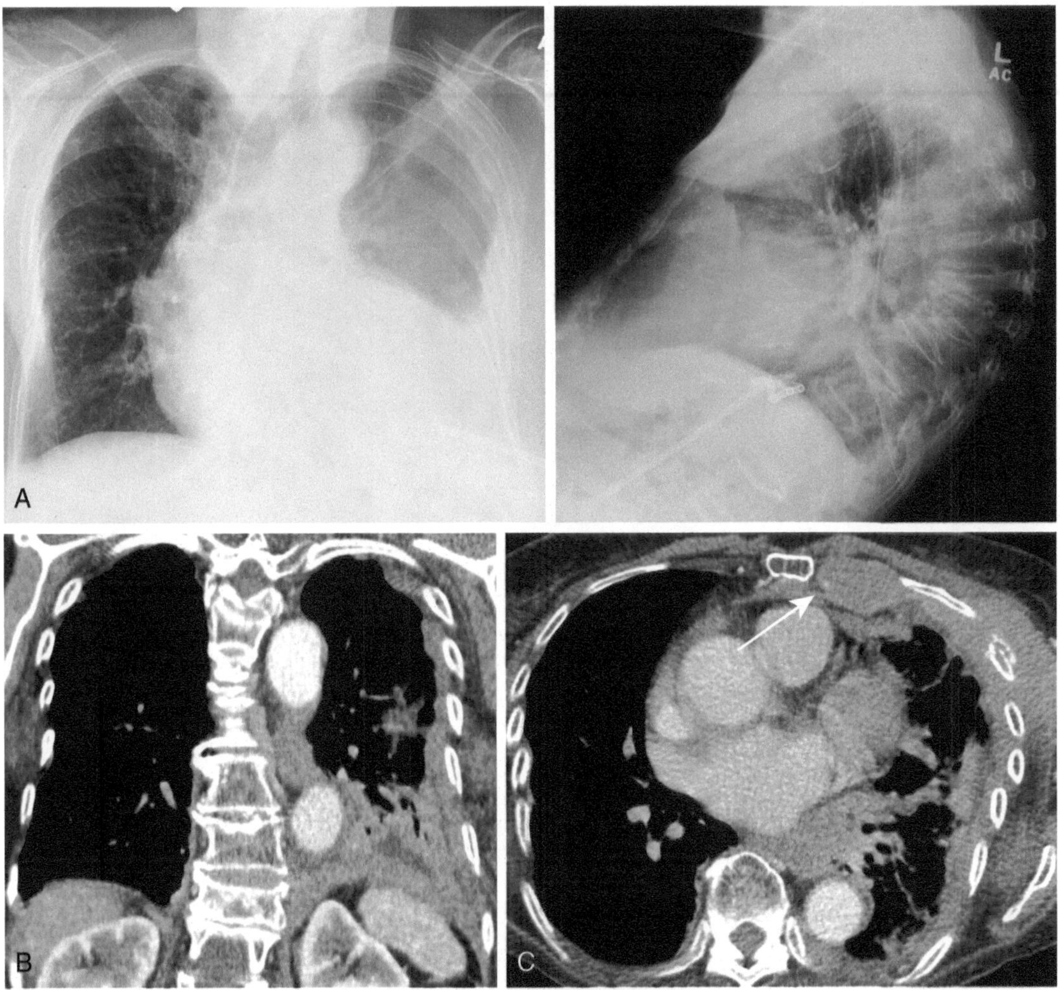

FIGURE 7.25 Pleural lymphoma. **A,** Posteroanterior and lateral chest radiographs show partially circumferential, loculated pleural fluid or lobulated pleural thickening, along with blunting of both posterior costophrenic angles. There is unrelated thoracic spinal kyphosis secondary to old, anteriorly wedged compression deformities. Coronal **(B)** and axial **(C)** computed tomography images confirm the presence of diffuse, nearly circumferential pleural thickening with left anterior intercostal chest wall invasion *(arrow)*. Atelectatic and interstitial changes were present in the lung, better demonstrated on lung windows that are not shown. The differential diagnosis for this appearance includes mesothelioma, metastatic adenocarcinoma to the pleura, and pleural lymphoma, the latter of which was proven at pathology.

neurodegenerative diseases such as amyotrophic lateral sclerosis, masses impinging on or involving the phrenic nerve, and phrenic nerve dysfunction of other etiology.

On CXR, CT, and MR, diaphragmatic weakness and paralysis manifest as elevation of the affected hemidiaphragm; however, it remains a diagnosis of exclusion, given many other causes of hemidiaphragmatic elevation, including other causes of lung volume loss, eventration, subphrenic collections and masses, and other abdominal pathology. There may also be hemidiaphragmatic pseudoelevation, for example, in the case of a subpulmonic pleural effusion. Review of prior chest imaging studies may help make this distinction. The fluoroscopic stiff test remains the imaging modality of choice for the diagnosis of diaphragmatic dysfunction, although sonographic evaluation of the diaphragm may be performed at the bedside if needed. It involves real-time observation of diaphragmatic motion during normal and deep inspiration and with sniffing. In normal individuals, both hemidiaphragms move inferiorly during inspiration. Decreased or delayed diaphragmatic excursion can be seen in the setting of diaphragmatic paresis. If there is hemidiaphragmatic paralysis, the affected hemidiaphragm demonstrates absent or even paradoxical movement, moving superiorly on inspiration. Sniffing more dramatically elicits the paradoxical motion of the hemidiaphragm that occurs with paralysis (Fig. 7.27). Although not yet widely used in clinical practice, dynamic MRI offers a real-time means of evaluating diaphragmatic function without ionizing radiation exposure. Coronal ultrafast balanced steady-state free precession (SSFP) gradient echo MRI can be used to acquire images of real-time diaphragmatic movement during free breathing and multiple sniffs (see Fig. 3.23 and associated video). Given MRI's greater cost than fluoroscopy, the MRI sniff test is best used during an already planned thoracic MRI in a patient with a mediastinal mass in the vicinity of the phrenic nerve (see Chapter 3).

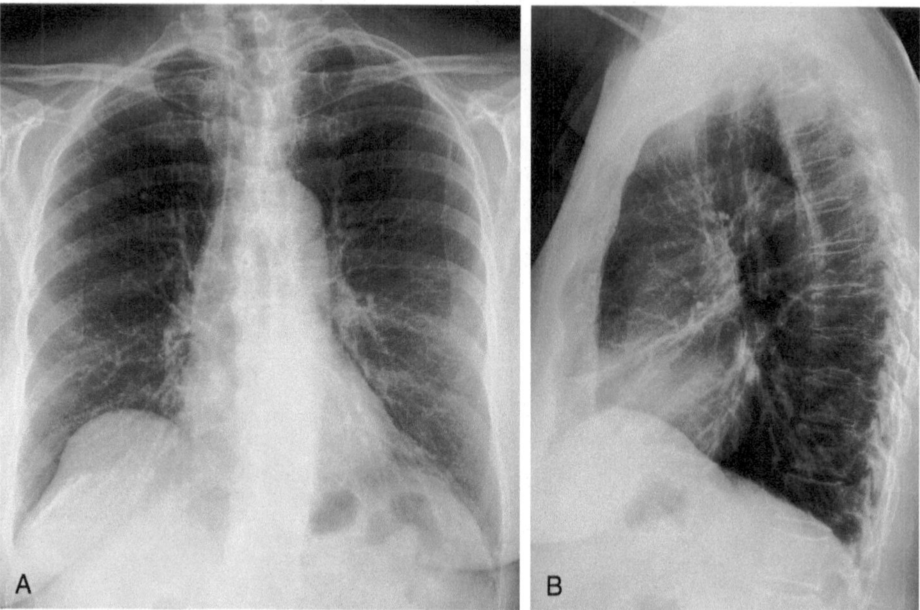

FIGURE 7.26 Diaphragmatic eventration. Posteroanterior **(A)** and lateral **(B)** chest radiographs reveal focal, convex-upward contour of the anteromedial aspect of the right hemidiaphragm, compatible with an eventration.

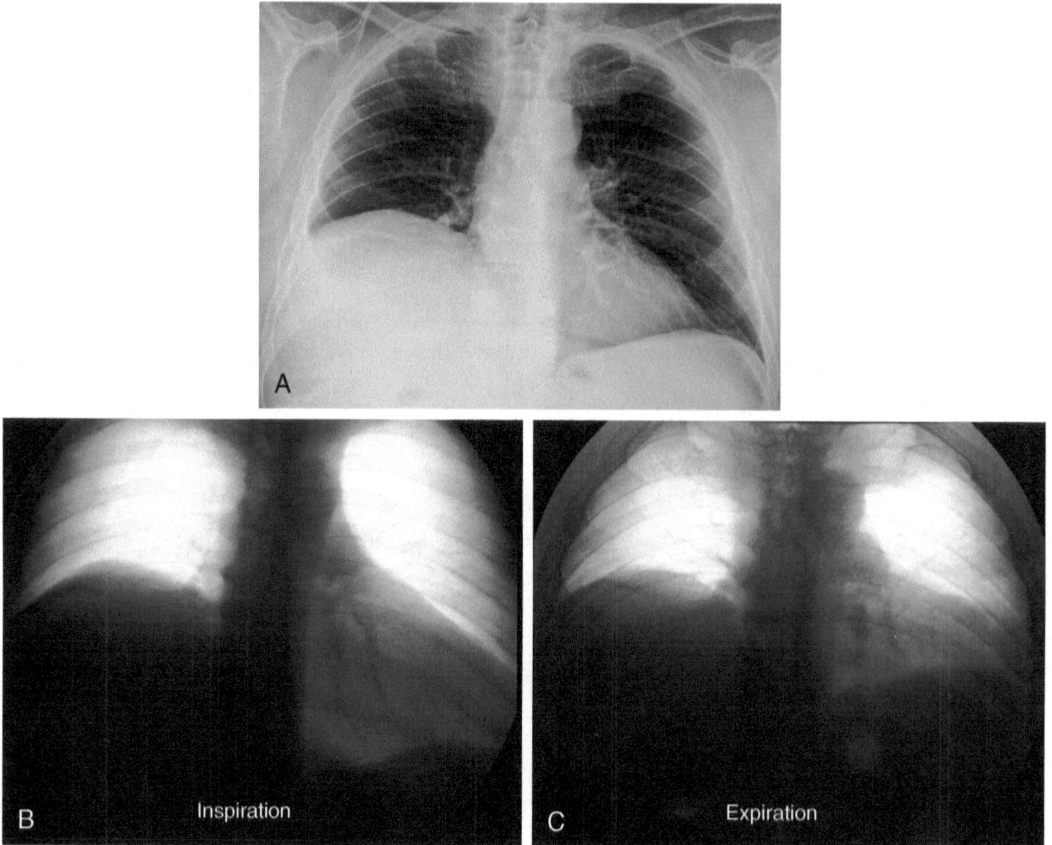

FIGURE 7.27 Right hemidiaphragmatic paralysis. **A,** Posteroanterior chest radiograph shows moderate to marked elevation of the right hemidiaphragm. Inspiratory **(B)** and expiratory **(C)** fluoroscopic spot radiographs of the diaphragm during a sniff test. There is near-complete lack of movement of the right hemidiaphragm upon inspiration and expiration, in contrast to the left hemidiaphragm, which demonstrates appropriate excursion, in terms of extent and direction. Sniff test confirmed paradoxical motion of the right hemidiaphragm.

Diaphragmatic Hernias

Hiatal Hernia (See Chapter 5)

Bochdalek Hernia

A Bochdalek hernia represents a developmental defect of the pleuroperitoneal folds or failure of fusion of the transverse septum with the intercostal muscle, resulting in herniation of abdominal contents through the posterior diaphragmatic foramen of Bochdalek into the thorax. It constitutes 90% of congenital diaphragmatic hernias and is more common on the left. It is usually small, containing only retroperitoneal fat; however, it may include the left kidney, the spleen, or both. It presents as a smooth upward bulge along the expected location of the posterior aspect of the left hemidiaphragm; the diaphragmatic defect can be confirmed by CT or MR (Fig. 7.28).

Morgagni Hernia

A Morgagni hernia represents herniation of abdominal contents into the thorax via the foramen of Morgagni, a congenital defect of fusion of the transverse septum of the diaphragm to the lateral body wall. It constitutes fewer than 10% of all congenital diaphragmatic hernias and most often occurs on the right. Contents of herniation may include the omentum, liver, and colon. On CXR, it commonly presents as a right cardiophrenic angle opacity (Fig. 7.29).

Traumatic Diaphragmatic Injury (see Chapter 13)

CHEST WALL

Congenital and Developmental Anomalies

Pectus Excavatum

Pectus excavatum is the most common congenital deformity of the chest wall. In this condition, the lower sternum is abnormally depressed, and the ribs on each side protrude anteriorly. The anteroposterior (AP) dimension of the thorax is reduced, resulting in leftward displacement and rotation

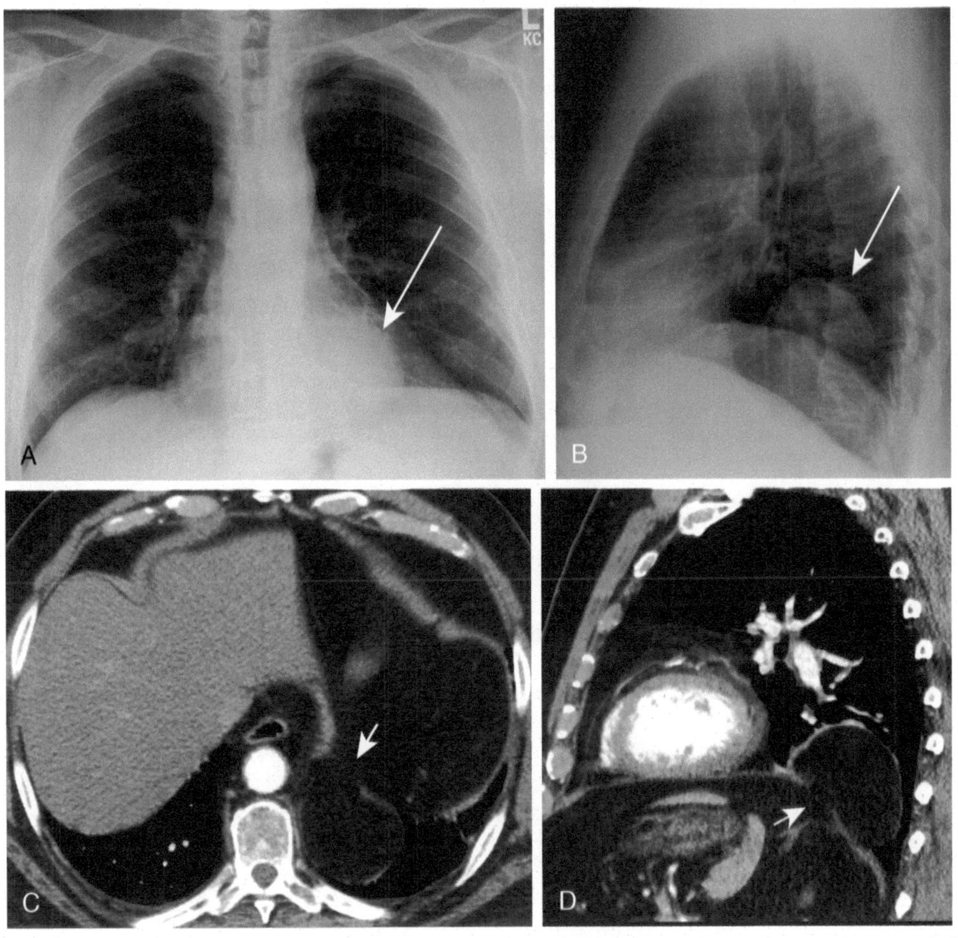

FIGURE 7.28 Bochdalek hernia. Posteroanterior **(A)** and lateral **(B)** chest radiographs reveal a rounded, well-circumscribed mass *(long arrows)* opacifying the inferoposteromedial aspect of the left hemithorax, whether due to a mediastinal mass or a Bochdalek hernia. Axial **(C)** and sagittal **(D)** chest computed tomography scans with intravenous contrast reveal the mass to be exclusively of fatty attenuation (aside from small traversing vessels), arising from the left subphrenic space and traversing a small defect *(short arrows)* in the posteromedial aspect of the left hemidiaphragm. Because there are no ancillary findings to suggest that this mass represents a fatty neoplasm and because of its passage through this characteristically located congenital-developmental diaphragmatic defect, this finding represents a fat-containing left Bochdalek hernia.

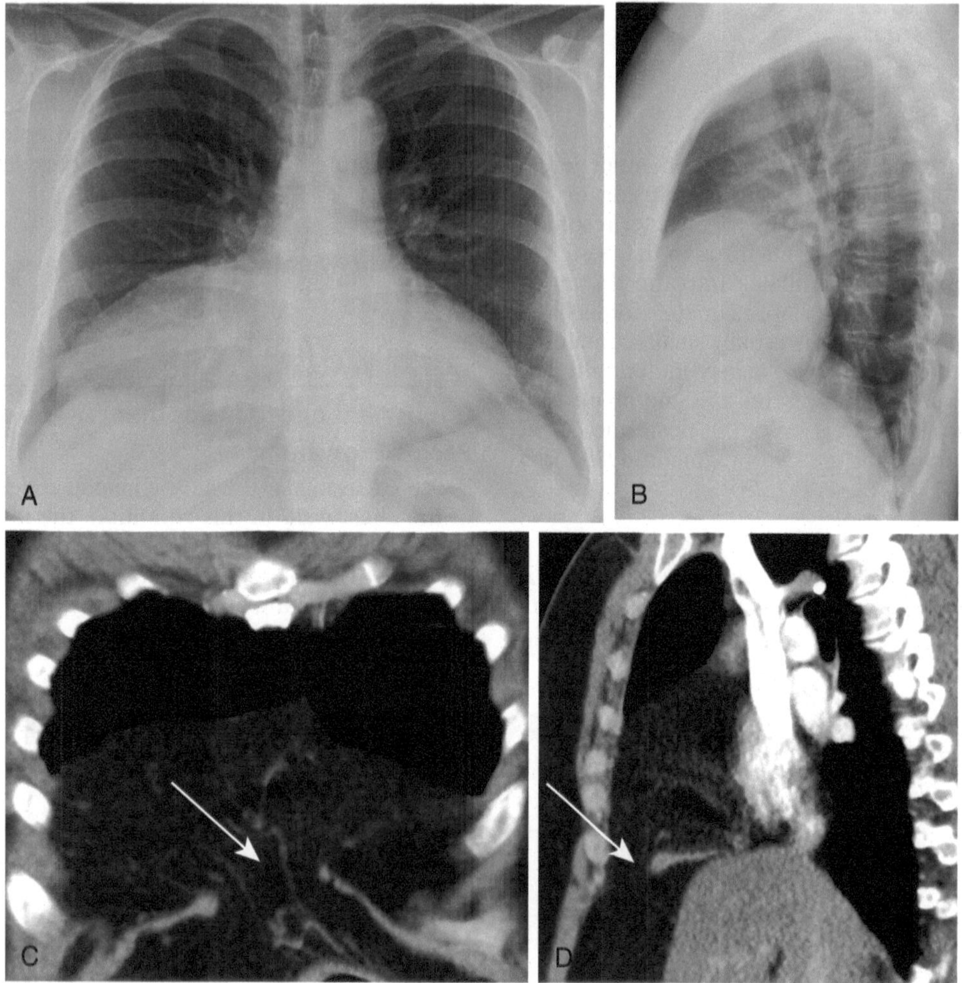

FIGURE 7.29 Morgagni hernia. Posteroanterior **(A)** and lateral **(B)** chest radiographs show a large, rounded, well-circumscribed mass filling much of the right anteroinferior hemithorax with sufficient lucency to allow pulmonary vessels to be visible through it, raising the likelihood of fatty consistency. Coronal **(C)** and sagittal **(D)** chest computed tomography scans with intravenous contrast show a large amount of fat- and vessel-containing subphrenic omentum passing through a right anteromedial diaphragmatic defect *(arrows)*, findings compatible with a Morgagni hernia.

of the heart and, in more severe cases, overt mass effect on the heart.

On frontal CXR, there is often increased opacity in the inferomedial aspect of the right hemithorax with apparent obscuration of the right heart border that can mimic right middle lobe pneumonia. However, the pectus deformity yielding this finding is easily discernable on the lateral projection. CT aids in quantification of the degree of deformity. The Haller index is calculated by dividing the inner transverse diameter of the thoracic cavity by the inner AP diameter on CT. A Haller index greater than 3.25 is often considered an indication for surgical correction (Fig. 7.30).

Pectus Carinatum

In pectus carinatum, the sternum protrudes anteriorly. It is much less common than pectus excavatum and is usually an isolated finding, although it is rarely associated with congenital heart disease (Fig. 7.31).

Poland Syndrome

Poland syndrome is a rare congenital anomaly in which there is unilateral congenital absence or hypoplasia of the pectoralis major and minor muscles. It can be associated with ipsilateral brachysyndactyly. On CXR, Poland syndrome classically manifests as a unilateral, hyperlucent hemithorax. Cross-sectional imaging by CT or MR can confirm this diagnosis (Fig. 7.32).

Neurofibromatosis Type 1–Related Changes

Neurofibromatosis type 1 is a multisystem neurocutaneous disorder and the most common phakomatosis. It is commonly associated with chest wall deformities such as kyphoscoliosis of the thoracic spine, dural ectasia, posterior element hypoplasia or scalloping, neural foraminal enlargement, rib notching, ribbon rib deformity, and cutaneous and subcutaneous neurofibromas arising from the peripheral nerves (Fig. 7.33).

Metabolic Conditions

Renal Osteodystrophy

Renal osteodystrophy is a constellation of skeletal findings that occurs in patients with chronic renal failure on account of secondary hyperparathyroidism and associated abnormal

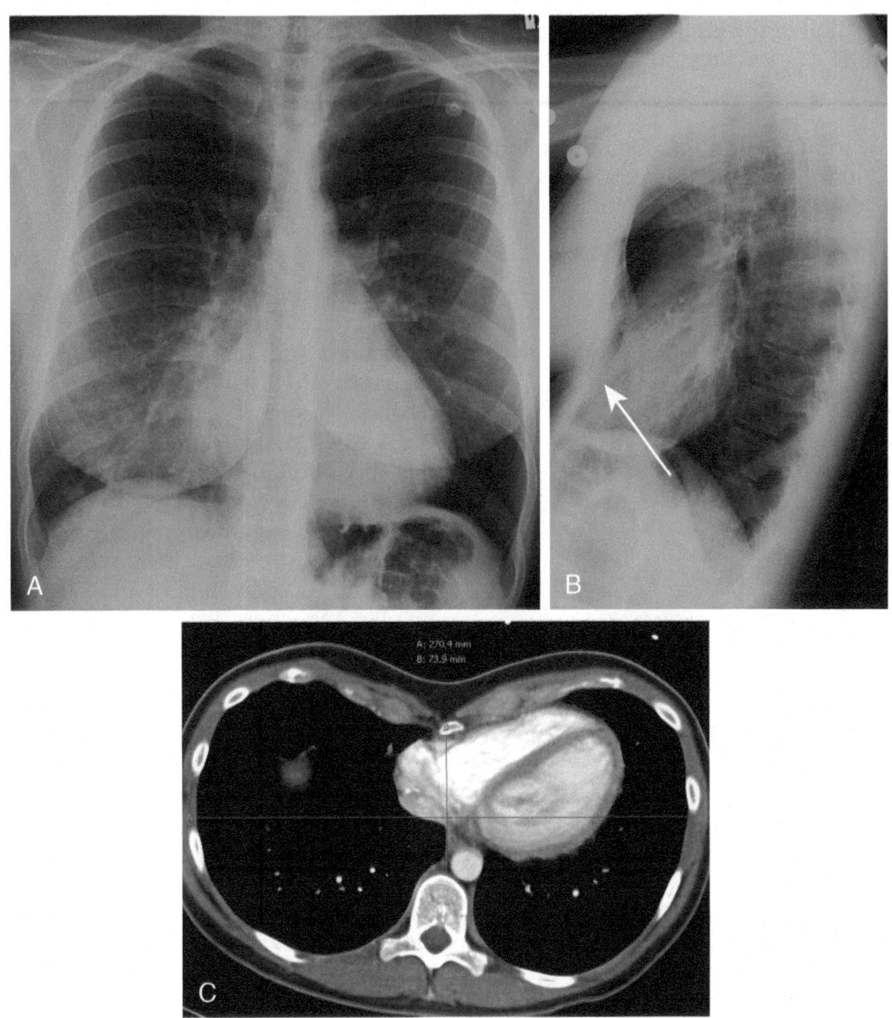

FIGURE 7.30 Pectus excavatum. Posteroanterior (PA) **(A)** and lateral **(B)** chest radiographs reveal concavity and depression of the lower sternum on the lateral radiograph *(arrow)*, causing some mass effect on the heart and, on the PA radiograph, a spread, less well-defined appearance of the right infrahilar vessels that partially silhouette the right heart border, mimicking right middle lobe (RML) pneumonia on the PA radiograph. There is no opacity overlying the heart on the lateral radiograph to confirm the presence of RML pneumonia, however. **C,** Axial chest computed tomography scan with intravenous contrast reveals a Haller index of 3.6, calculated by dividing the maximum transverse thoracic diameter of the thoracic cavity by the minimum anteroposterior diameter (in this case, 27.0 cm by 7.4 cm), with measurement endpoints along the *inner* chest wall.

calcium and vitamin D metabolism. In the thorax, osteopenia is a common early finding. Sclerosis of the endplates of multiple contiguous thoracic vertebral bodies, referred to as a "rugger-jersey spine," can also be seen (Fig. 7.34).

Sickle Cell Disease

In addition to pulmonary manifestations of acute chest syndrome and recurrent pneumonia caused by functional asplenia, sickle cell disease often leads to bone abnormalities in the thorax. Bone infarcts may involve the proximal humeri and endplates of thoracic vertebrae, with the latter resulting in "H-shaped vertebrae" or "fish vertebrae" (Fig. 7.35). Osteomyelitis is also a common complication.

Paget Disease

Within the thorax and adjacent proximal upper extremities, Paget disease can involve the spine, clavicle, humerus, and least frequently, the ribs. Typical manifestations of pagetoid bony involvement include bony expansion, cortical thickening, and coarsening of trabeculae (Fig. 7.36). Within the spine, the pagetoid thickening and sclerosis encasing the vertebral margins give rise to the so-called picture frame sign.

Inflammatory Conditions

Ankylosing Spondylitis

Ankylosing spondylitis is a form of seronegative spondyloarthropathy that frequently involves the spine. Early signs of spondylitis include small erosions with reactive sclerosis at the corners of vertebral bodies, giving rise to so-called shiny corners and vertebral body squaring. In the chronic stage, there is diffuse syndesmophyte formation caused by ossification of the annulus fibrosis of the intervertebral disks, leading to a "bamboo spine" appearance on lateral

CXR (Fig. 7.37). Ossification of the interspinous ligaments results in a "dagger spine" appearance on frontal CXR.

SAPHO Syndrome

SAPHO syndrome is a rare condition that includes a combination of synovitis, acne, pustulosis, hyperostosis, and osteitis. There may be a chronic osteomyelitic or infectious component to this entity. In the thorax, the anterior chest wall—in particular, the sternoclavicular joint—is the most common location of involvement, with osteitis, hyperostosis, cortical thickening, and often soft tissue swelling (Fig. 7.38).

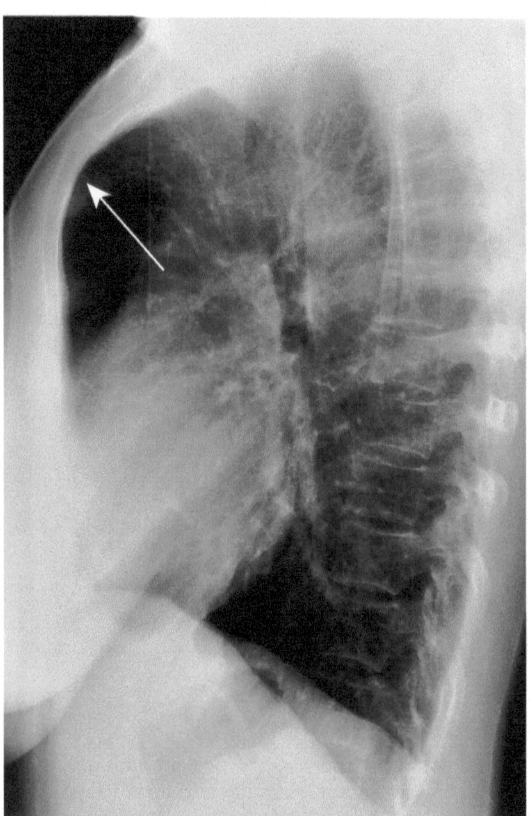

FIGURE 7.31 Pectus carinatum. Lateral chest radiograph demonstrates a marked outward convexity of the upper anterior chest wall *(arrow)*.

Infectious Diseases

Chest Wall Infections

Although primary infection of the chest wall is rare, it can occur spontaneously or in association with trauma, surgery (e.g., median sternotomy or thoracotomy), diabetes, or immunosuppression. Intravenous drug use is a well-recognized risk factor, with the sternoclavicular joint a frequent target of septic arthritis and osteomyelitis (Fig. 7.39). Chest wall infection also occurs secondary to contiguous spread of adjacent pulmonary or pleural infection.

Staphylococcus aureus and *Pseudomonas aeruginosa* are the most common causative organisms of pyogenic infection of the chest wall, which typically manifests as pyogenic osteomyelitis of the ribs and sternum. TB can involve the chest wall by either contiguous spread of pulmonary and pleural infection or by hematogenous seeding. When a pleural empyema extends out of the thoracic cavity into the adjacent chest wall and surrounding soft tissues, it is called empyema necessitans. Thoracic actinomycosis is an uncommon bacterial infection, caused by gram-positive *Actinomycetes* bacteria, which are a part of the normal oral flora. These bacteria can enter the lungs upon aspiration. Actinomycosis has the propensity to cross normal soft tissue planes because of its proteolytic enzymes and can directly invade the chest wall via the lungs and pleura. In immunocompromised hosts, fungal infections, including aspergillosis and mucormycosis, are also important considerations for chest wall infection; these infections may also invade the chest wall from the lung and pleura.

Chest radiography is insensitive in the detection of chest wall inflammation and infection until there is advanced soft tissue and bone destruction. Chest CT depicts loss of normal tissue planes, inferring the presence of soft tissue edema,

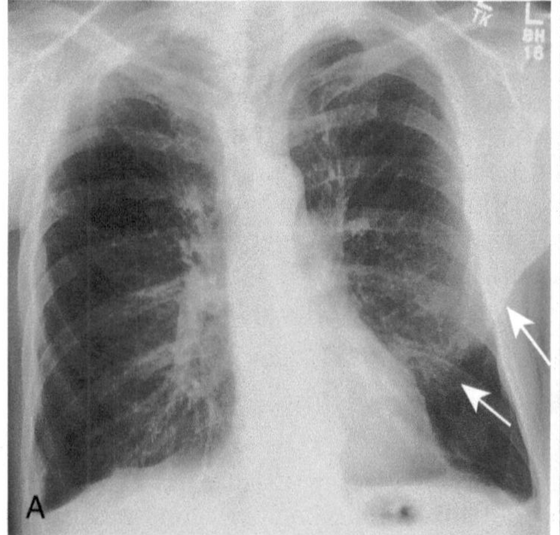

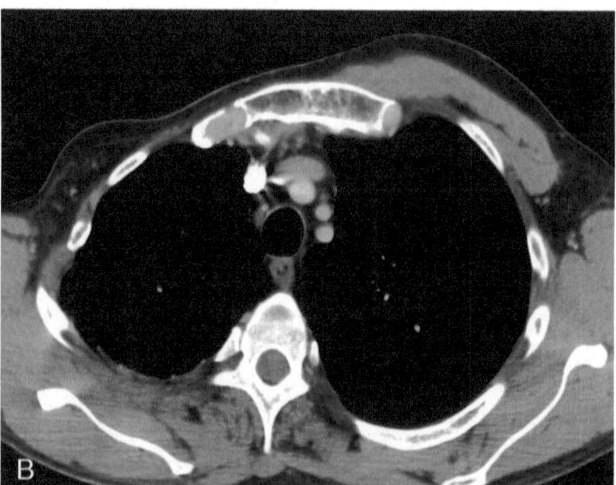

FIGURE 7.32 Poland syndrome. **A,** Posteroanterior chest radiograph revealing absence of the right pectoralis muscle shadow and a normal left pectoralis muscle shadow *(arrows)*. The absent right chest wall musculature creates the appearance of a "hyperlucent lung" on the right. Bilateral costophrenic blunting is present and unrelated. **B,** Chest computed tomography scan confirming congenital absence of the right pectoralis major and minor muscles. There is unrelated right apical pleural and parenchymal scarring and volume loss.

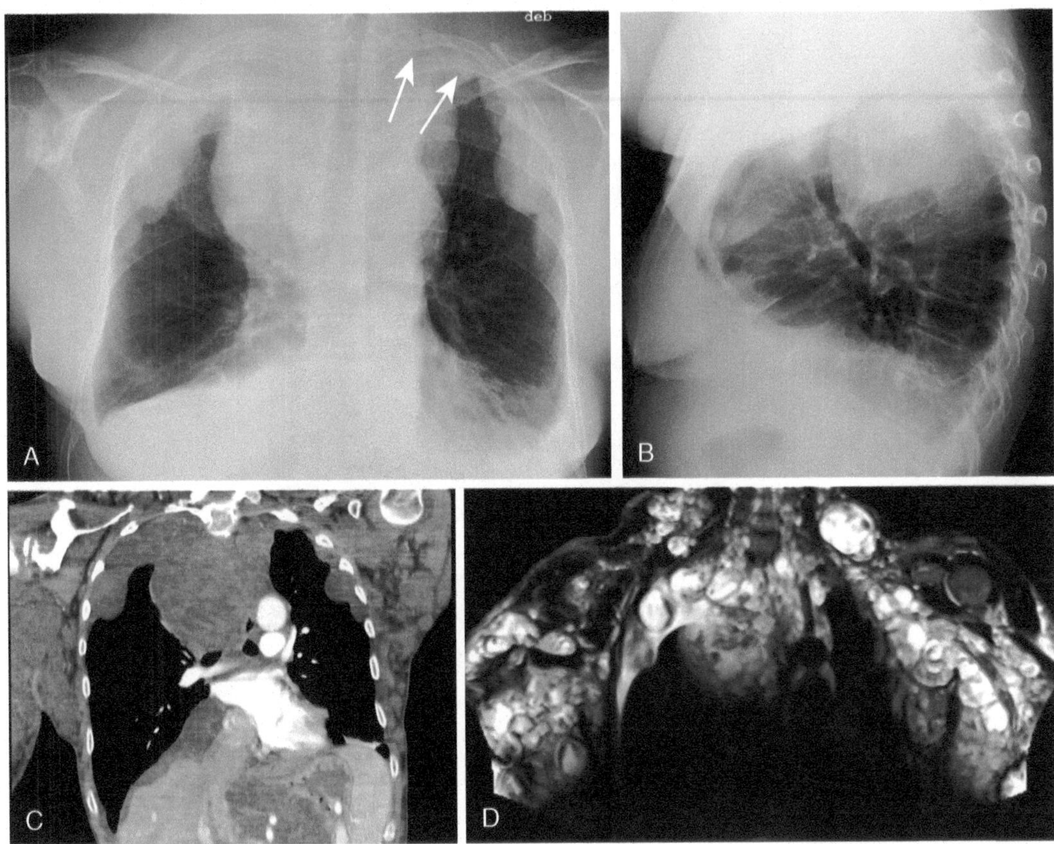

FIGURE 7.33 Neurofibromatosis involving the chest wall and mediastinum. Posteroanterior **(A)** and lateral **(B)** chest radiographs reveal a diffusely and irregularly thickened, relatively hyperattenuating chest wall in addition to extensive lobulated masses throughout much of the mediastinum and along upper pleural surfaces. Rib notching is most apparent within the left posterior second and third ribs *(arrows)*. **C,** Correlative coronal chest CT scan with intravenous contrast reveals innumerable soft tissue masses throughout the chest wall and mediastinum, along with contiguous involvement of the extrapleural space and upper extremities by neurofibromas. **D,** Corresponding segmented image from a coronal T2-weighted whole-body MR image shows these innumerable, well-circumscribed neurofibromas to exhibit heterogeneous T2-hyperintensity, with central and eccentric areas of relatively low T2 signal.

abscess, draining sinus tract, and osseous destruction. CT also facilitates evaluation of any concurrent pulmonary, pleural, and mediastinal pathology (Fig. 7.40). MRI and, in particular, short *tau* inversion recovery (STIR) and fat-saturated T2-weighted MRI sequences, are more sensitive than CT in the detection of chest wall and bone marrow edema and inflammation.

Diskitis-Osteomyelitis

Diskitis-osteomyelitis of the thoracic spine with associated paravertebral phlegmon or abscess can result in lateral displacement of the paraspinal lines, erosion and destruction of vertebral bodies on CXRs, and occasionally an empyema. Patients often present with back pain, fever, leukocytosis, and an elevated erythrocyte sedimentation rate (ESR). Compared with pyogenic infection, tuberculous spondylitis or Pott disease tends to spare the intervertebral disks in its earlier stage and more commonly involves multiple contiguous vertebral bodies on account of its spread along the underside of the anterior longitudinal ligament in the form of phlegmon or abscess, rather than via the disk spaces. Because of the more anterior predilection of involvement and the lesser initial disk involvement of TB, when compared with pyogenic infection, anteriorly wedged pathologic compression deformities are more apt to occur in tuberculous spondylitis than pyogenic spondylitis, with a resultant angular kyphosis or gibbus deformity. Although CT may better delineate cortical bone destruction, a later phase of osteomyelitis (see Fig. 7.40), MRI is more sensitive for detection of early bone involvement, spinal canal involvement, spinal cord compromise, and the presence of epidural abscess and phlegmon. MRI is therefore considered the test of choice for imaging of spinal infection (see Chapter 16 regarding Pott disease).

Benign Tumors and Tumor-like Conditions

Lipoma

Lipomas are the most common benign soft tissue neoplasm of the chest wall. These are often incidental findings and do not require treatment unless their growth over time appears unrelated to weight gain and raises the possibility of a low-grade liposarcoma. On CT, these lesions manifest as well-defined fatty masses with a thin, smooth, often

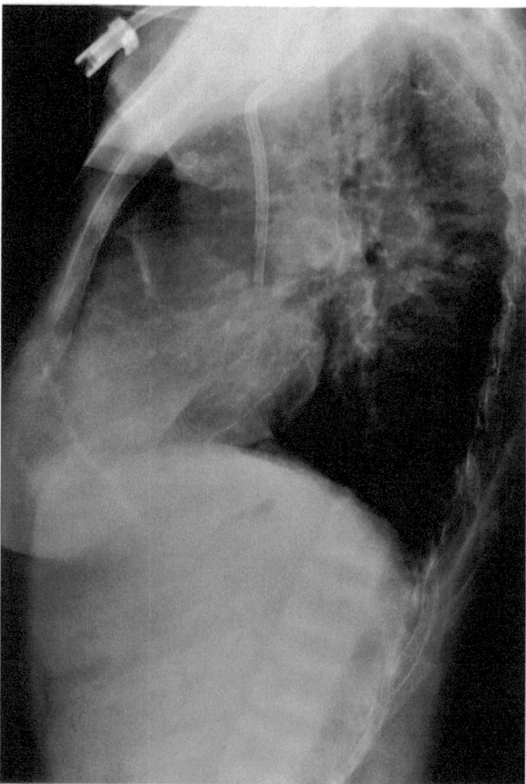

FIGURE 7.34 Rugger jersey spine of renal osteodystrophy. Lateral radiograph of chest and upper abdomen revealing band-like sclerosis along the superior and inferior endplates of every imaged vertebral body. A hemodialysis catheter terminates in the lower superior vena cava.

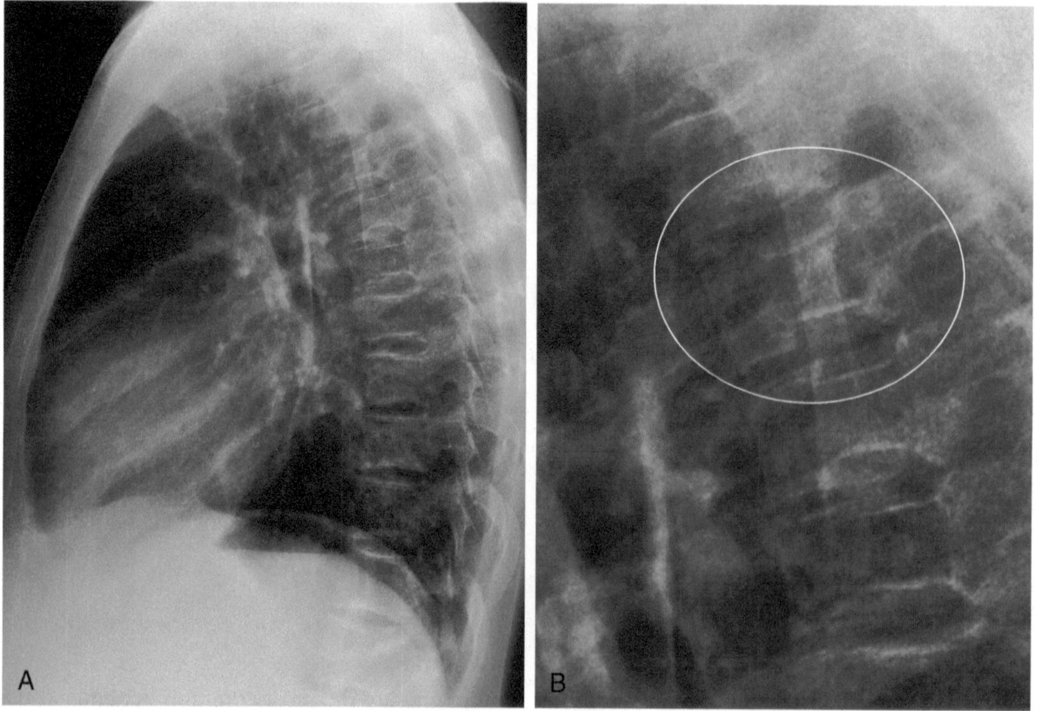

FIGURE 7.35 Sickle cell disease, H-shaped vertebrae. **A,** Lateral chest radiograph reveals multiple H-shaped vertebrae within the middle to upper thoracic spine secondary to sickle cell–induced endplate infarction and resultant endplate depression. **B,** Coned-down view of one of these H-shaped vertebrae *(circle)*.

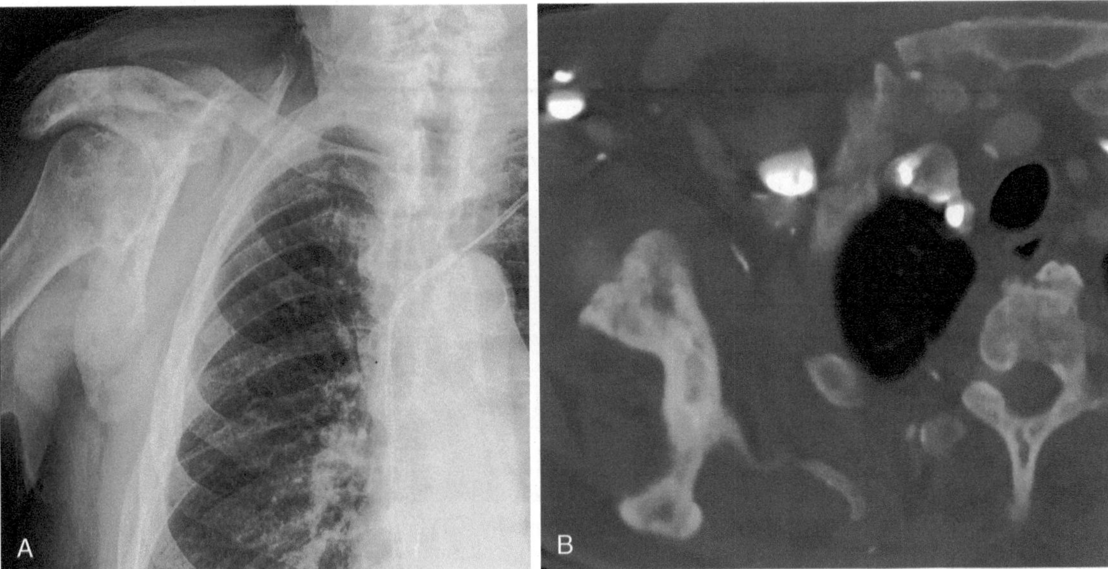

FIGURE 7.36 Paget disease. **A,** Posteroanterior chest radiograph shows a diffusely expansile, sclerotic appearance of the right scapula, with coarsened internal trabeculae. **B,** Correlative axial chest computed tomography bone window reveals the expanded right scapula with irregularly coarsened internal trabeculae and thickened cortex.

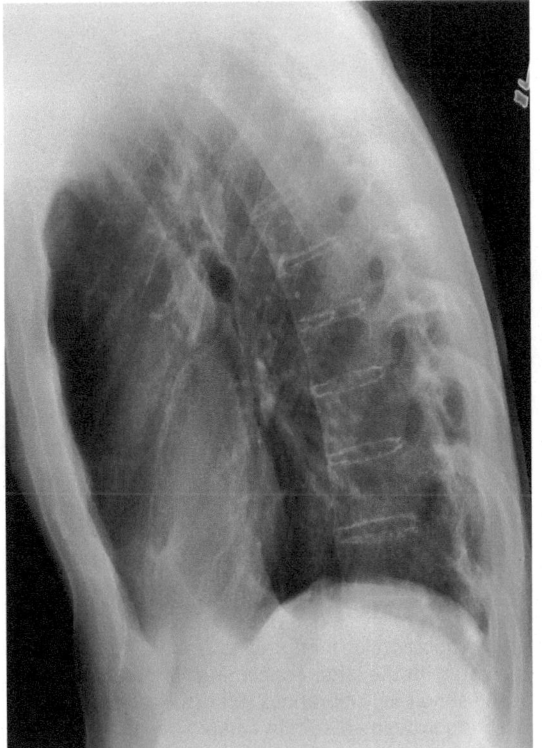

FIGURE 7.37 Ankylosing spondylitis. Lateral chest radiograph shows squaring of the vertebral bodies and fine, bridging syndesmophytes along all imaged thoracic vertebral bodies, resulting in a "bamboo spine" appearance.

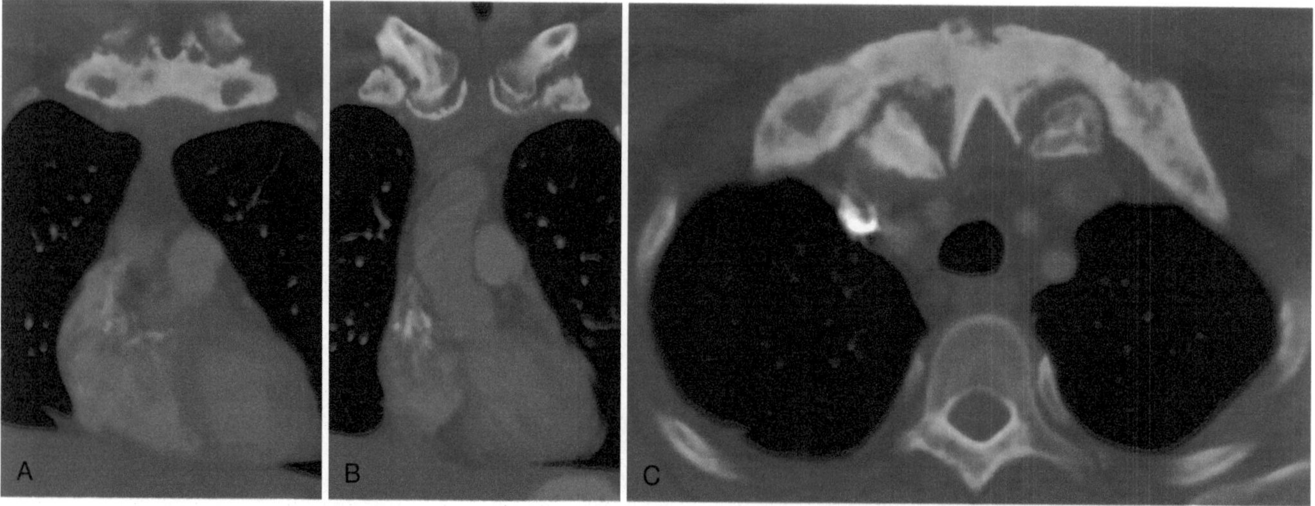

FIGURE 7.38 SAPHO syndrome. Coronal computed tomography (CT) bone windows of bilateral first costosternal joints **(A)** and bilateral sternoclavicular joints **(B)** showing bilaterally symmetric sclerosis or osteitis of the periarticular aspect of these bones, along with hypertrophic change of the medial clavicles. **C,** Correlative axial CT bone window showing dense sclerosis or osteitis of the manubrium, medial clavicles, and medial first ribs in addition to bony and cartilaginous hypertrophy and near-complete osseous fusion of the costomanubrial joints. This finding is not to be confused with blastic metastatic disease to bone.

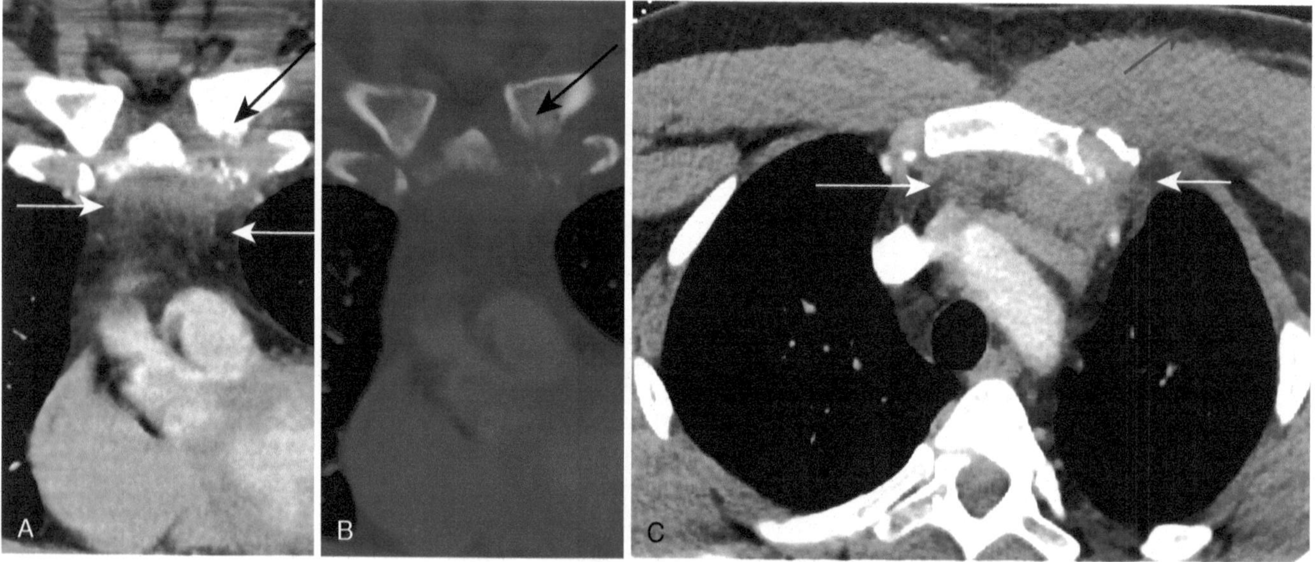

FIGURE 7.39 Sternoclavicular septic arthritis. **A,** Coronal chest computed tomography (CT) scan with intravenous contrast showing irregular lucency or erosive change of the inferomedial aspect of the left clavicular head *(black arrow)*, at the level of the left sternoclavicular joint and associated soft tissue stranding *(white arrows)* within the nearby anterior mediastinal fat, with the latter concerning for mediastinitis. **B,** Correlative coronal CT bone window. **C,** Axial CT scan showing abnormal, amorphous soft tissue attenuation material within the retromanubrial anterior mediastinal fat, representing acute mediastinitis *(white arrows)*. There is associated swelling of the medial left pectoralis musculature, which exhibits a less well-defined soft tissue plane with the adjacent subcutaneous fat, indicating secondary myositis and inflammation of the deep subcutaneous fat.

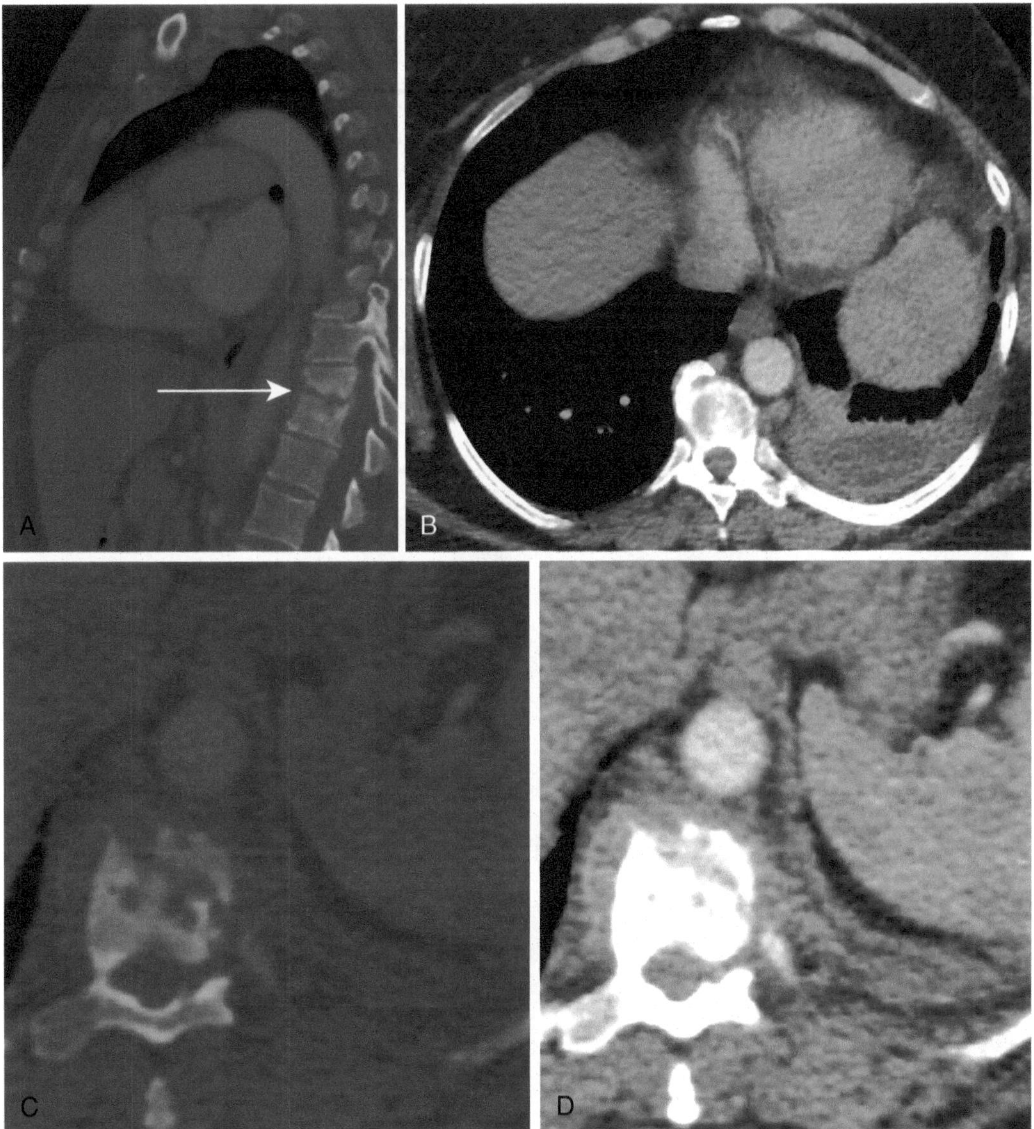

FIGURE 7.40 Thoracic spinal diskitis-osteomyelitis with empyema. **A,** Sagittal chest computed tomography (CT) bone window showing irregular intervertebral disk contour *(arrow)*, irregular endplate erosion and sclerosis, moderate pathologic compression deformity of T11, mild loss of height of T12, and a slight spinal kyphosis at this level *(arrow)*. **B,** Axial CT scan reveals a loculated left pleural effusion with the "split pleura sign" of an empyema and adjacent adherent atelectasis. **C,** Axial CT bone window reveals destructive erosive or lytic changes at the endplate. **D,** Corresponding axial CT soft tissue window shows abnormal bilateral paravertebral soft tissue attenuation material representing phlegmon. The presence of an epidural abscess cannot be excluded by CT but could be demonstrated by magnetic resonance imaging.

imperceptible capsule or pseudocapsule or no capsule (Fig. 7.41). Internal soft tissue attenuation components on CT or MRI within an otherwise fatty mass raise the possibility of a rare liposarcoma and warrant further diagnostic investigation or resection.

Neurogenic Tumors

Schwannomas and neurofibromas may involve the chest wall and can arise from intercostal nerves and more peripheral nerve branches (see Fig. 7.33). See Chapter 5 for additional information regarding the CT and MRI appearance of these lesions.

Hemangioma

Nonosseous chest wall hemangiomas are rare benign vascular neoplasms and can manifest as a soft tissue attenuation lesion, with or without phleboliths, within the chest wall on CXR. CT often demonstrates soft tissue attenuation masses with associated phleboliths and may show osseous remodeling. MRI provides superior delineation of the extent of the lesions. Nonosseous chest wall hemangiomas are characteristically markedly T2-hyperintense and exhibit early, intense enhancement. Vertebral body hemangiomas usually exhibit fatty attenuation and coarse internal trabeculation on CT and T1- and T2-hyperintensity on MR.

Enchondroma

Enchondromas are common benign medullary cartilaginous neoplasms. They most often occur in the tubular bones of the hands and feet, as well as long bones. On CXR, incidental enchondromas can be seen in the proximal humeri and, rarely, in the ribs. These are well-circumscribed lytic lesions within the medullary cavity, with a narrow zone of transition, typically containing rings and arcs calcification or chondroid matrix (Fig. 7.42). Multiple enchondromas, often unilateral, can be seen in Ollier disease. Ollier disease is more common than Maffucci syndrome, the latter of which manifests with multiple enchondromas and hemangiomas, lymphangiomas, or both. Maffucci syndrome carries an increased risk of malignancy, whether caused by sarcomatous degeneration of preexisting benign lesions (e.g., enchondroma into chondrosarcoma) or distinct central nervous system, gastrointestinal, and genitourinary malignancies.

Osteochondroma

Osteochondromas may be observed incidentally on CXR, arising from the bony thorax. These lesions can be sessile or pedunculated, with their medullary component continuous with the parent bone. They are capped by hyaline cartilage, which may be thin and difficult to identify or thick, with

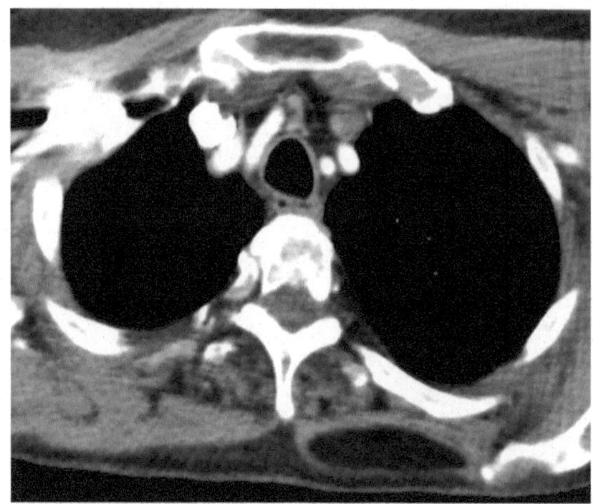

FIGURE 7.41 Chest wall lipoma. Axial chest computed tomography scan with intravenous contrast demonstrates a homogeneously fatty attenuation, well-circumscribed, oblong mass within the left trapezius muscle, representing an intramuscular lipoma.

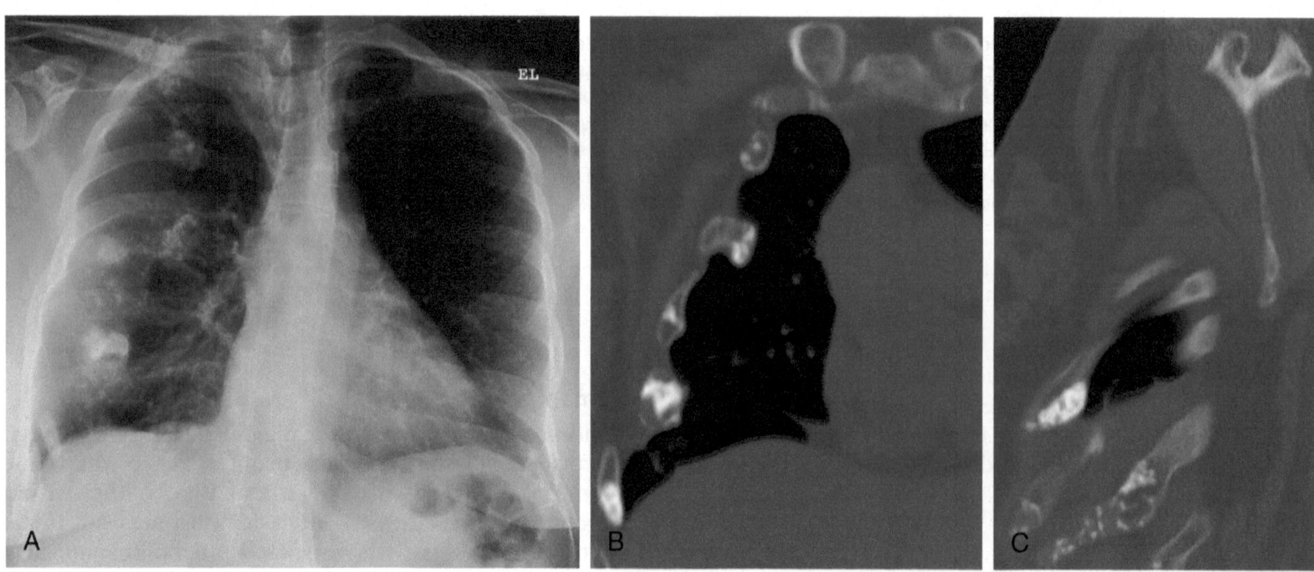

FIGURE 7.42 Enchondromatosis involving ribs. **A,** Posteroanterior radiograph demonstrates multiple expanded right anterior ribs with stippled and more confluent, calcified matrix. **B,** Correlative coronal chest computed tomography (CT) bone window. **C,** Sagittal chest CT scan showing stippled rings and arcs and more confluent calcifications within expanded segments of multiple anterolateral ribs. The stippled ring and arc calcification indicates cartilaginous matrix. Some of these enchondromas demonstrate lytic components.

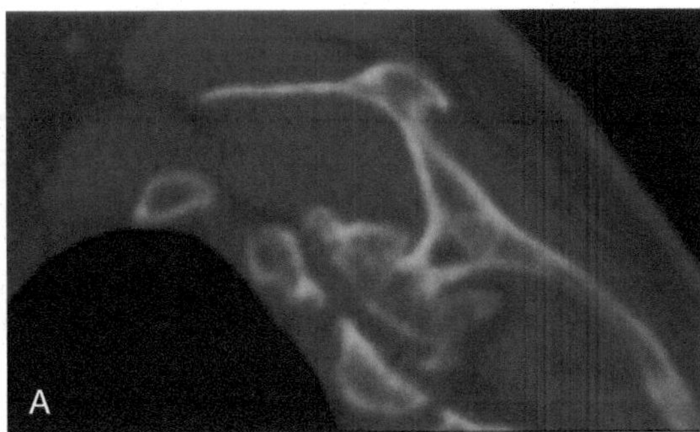
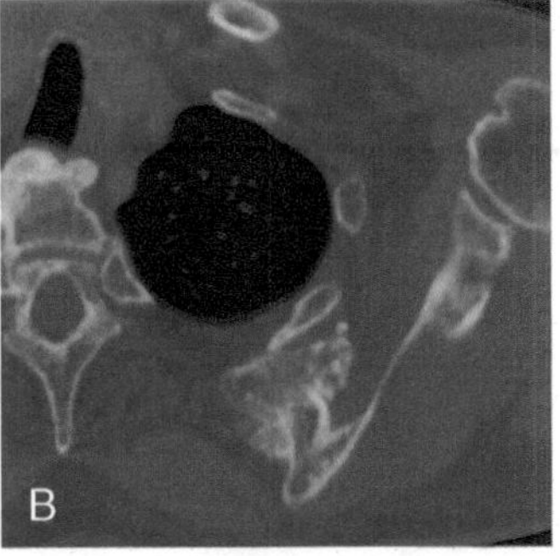

FIGURE 7.43 Osteochondroma arising from the scapula. Sagittal **(A)** and axial **(B)** computed tomography scan bone windows showing an exophytic, well-corticated bone lesion with partially cartilaginous cap (stippled calcified matrix) arising from the anteromedial aspect of the left scapula. Note the continuous marrow cavity between the scapula and this lesion.

rings and arcs calcification due to chondroid matrix (Fig. 7.43). Their cartilaginous cap can rarely degenerate into a chondrosarcoma.

Elastofibroma Dorsi

Elastofibroma dorsi is a soft tissue pseudotumor of the chest wall. It most commonly occurs in patients in their seventh decade, with a 4 to 1 female-to-male preponderance. These lesions are typically infrascapular in location, situated between the thoracic wall and the serratus anterior or latissimus dorsi muscles, and are often bilateral. Patients are often asymptomatic, although pain and a clicking or a snapping sensation with shoulder movement can occur. On CT, these lesions typically appear as poorly defined soft tissue masses with attenuation similar to that of the adjacent skeletal muscles and with interlaced fat (Fig. 7.44). On MRI, these masses demonstrate signal intensity similar to that of skeletal muscle, with a similar fascicular pattern that is intercalated with fat.

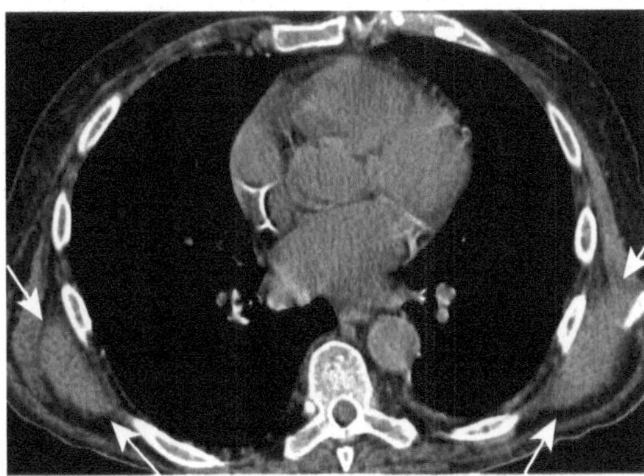

FIGURE 7.44 Bilateral elastofibroma dorsi. Axial chest computed tomography scan without contrast reveals bilateral, posterolateral, semilunar soft tissue attenuation masses *(arrows)*, partially subjacent to the inferior scapulae and serratus anterior muscles, resembling chest wall musculature and often missed or confused for chest wall musculature.

Fibrous Dysplasia

Fibrous dysplasia is the most common nonneoplastic, tumor-like condition of the ribs, but it can also occur in many other bones, including the proximal femur and humerus, tibia, pelvis, and craniofacial bones. Fibrous dysplasia can be monostotic or polyostotic. The monostotic form most commonly involves the ribs. It classically manifests as a well-circumscribed, expansile lesion with internal ground glass matrix (Fig. 7.45).

Malignant Tumors

Chest Wall Metastasis

The most common malignant chest wall tumors are osseous metastases and multiple myeloma, particularly in older adults. Bone metastases can be sclerotic or blastic (Fig. 7.46), lytic (Fig. 7.47), or mixed lytic and blastic. Metastatic disease can also involve the non-bony chest wall, particularly in melanoma, sarcoma, and advanced and often dedifferentiated or anaplastic adenocarcinoma.

Multiple Myeloma

Multiple myeloma typically yields well-defined or "punched out" lytic lesions, without sclerotic margins, and can involve the majority of the skeleton, including the bones of the thorax (Fig. 7.48). Radiographic skeletal series are therefore often used to screen for bony involvement by multiple myeloma. Pathologic rib fractures and compression deformities are frequent findings in the thorax in advanced disease.

Chondrosarcoma

The most common primary malignant osseous tumor of the chest wall is chondrosarcoma. Chondrosarcoma commonly arises from the costochondral junction and manifests as a large, multilobulated, lytic mass, with or without internal calcified chondroid matrix. They may also arise at the costovertebral junction. On CT, chondrosarcomas are typically of low attenuation and may contain chondroid matrix (stippled or rings and arcs calcification). Chondrosarcomas often demonstrate high signal intensity on T2-weighted MRI, reflecting their hyaline cartilage matrix, with internal signal voids because of calcifications. Peripheral and septal enhancement is often present, along with absent enhancement in cartilaginous and myxoid areas (Fig. 7.49). Other malignant tumors arising from the soft tissues of the chest wall in adults include fibrosarcoma and malignant fibrous histiocytoma.

Iatrogenic and Postsurgical Conditions

See Chapter 12.

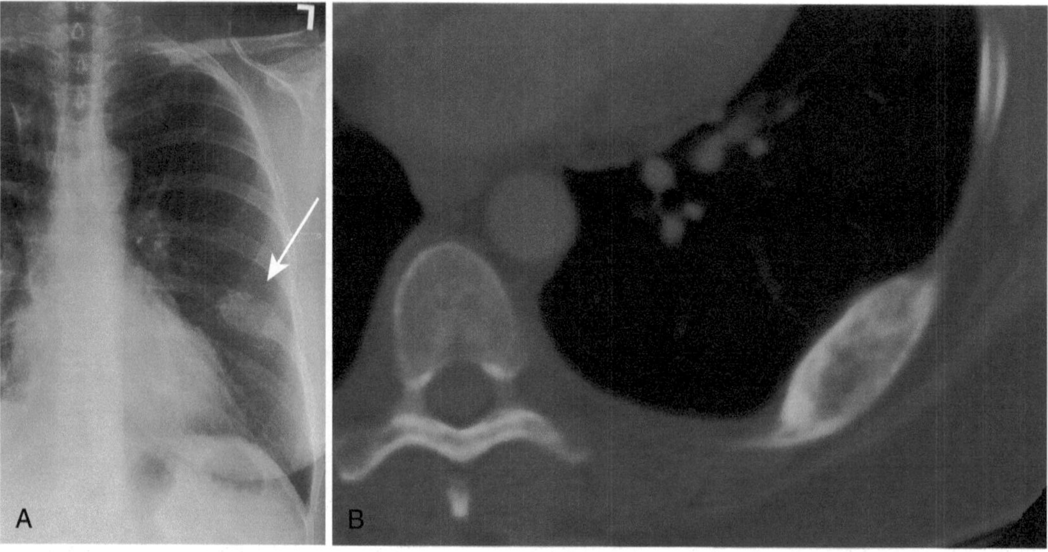

FIGURE 7.45 Fibrous dysplasia. **A,** Posteroanterior chest radiograph shows an expansile lesion with well-defined margins and hazy matrix within the left posterior eighth rib *(arrow)*. **B,** Correlative axial computed tomography bone window reveals this expansile rib lesion to exhibit an intact, albeit partially attenuated and partially thickened, sclerotic margin, ground-glass matrix, and some internal lucency.

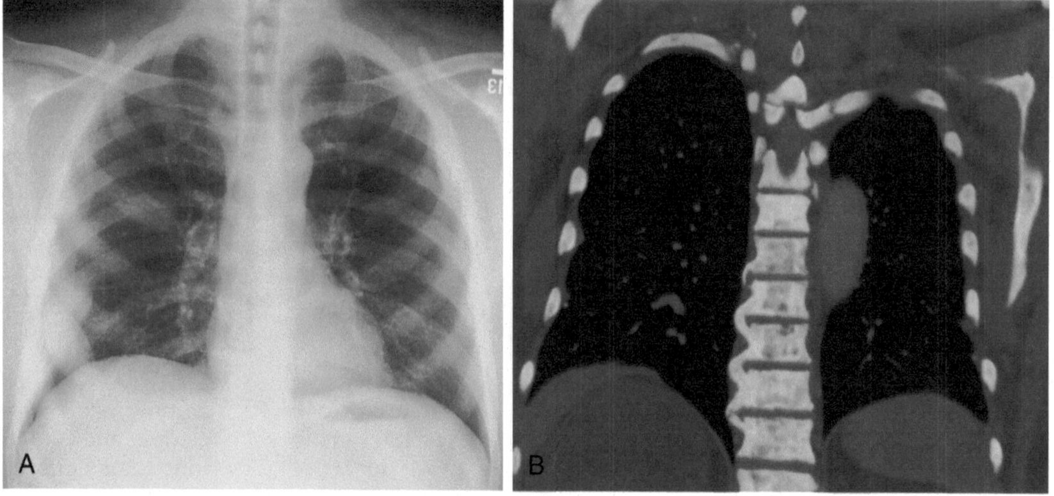

FIGURE 7.46 Diffuse blastic bony metastases. **A,** Posteroanterior chest radiograph demonstrating diffuse hyperattenuation of the ribs and spine secondary to diffuse blastic metastatic disease to bone in a woman with breast cancer, with occasional expansile blastic lesions (right anterior ribs 3 and 6, right posterolateral rib 8). **B,** Coronal chest computed tomography scan of a man with prostate cancer revealing diffuse blastic metastatic involvement of all bones of the thorax, including the spine, ribs, and scapulae.

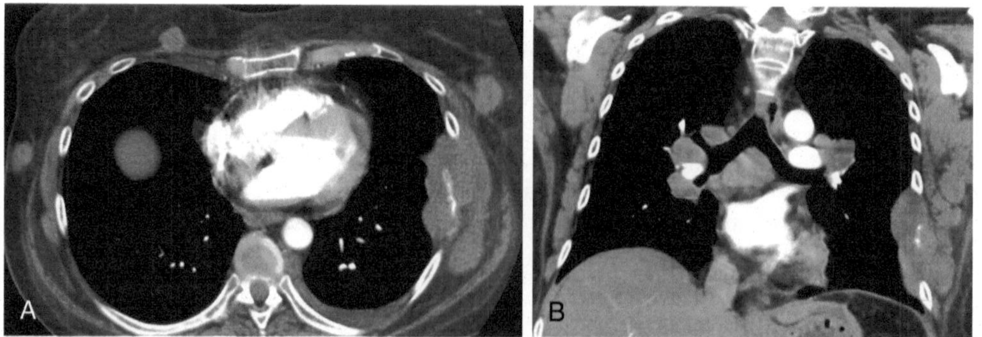

FIGURE 7.47 Chest wall metastases in a woman with melanoma. Axial **(A)** and coronal **(B)** computed tomography images showing multiple bilateral subcutaneous soft tissue nodules of varying size in addition to a destructive lytic rib lesion with cortical breakthrough and soft tissue mass extending into the thoracic cavity and outward, subjacent to the left serratus anterior muscle. A small layering left pleural effusion is present.

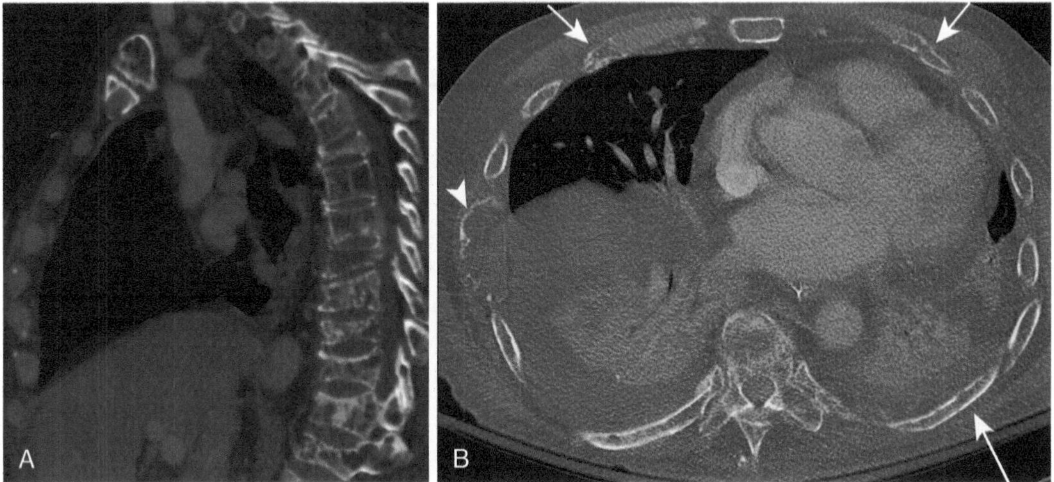

FIGURE 7.48 Multiple myeloma. **A,** Sagittal computed tomography (CT) bone window revealing diffuse pathologic compression deformities of the imaged portion of the thoracolumbar spine, with innumerable lytic lesions involving all bones of the imaged thorax. **B,** Axial CT bone window exhibiting innumerable lytic lesions within the ribs, sternum, and spine; multiple bilateral pathologic rib fractures *(long arrows)*; and a destructive, expansile, lytic lesion within a right lateral rib *(arrowhead.)*

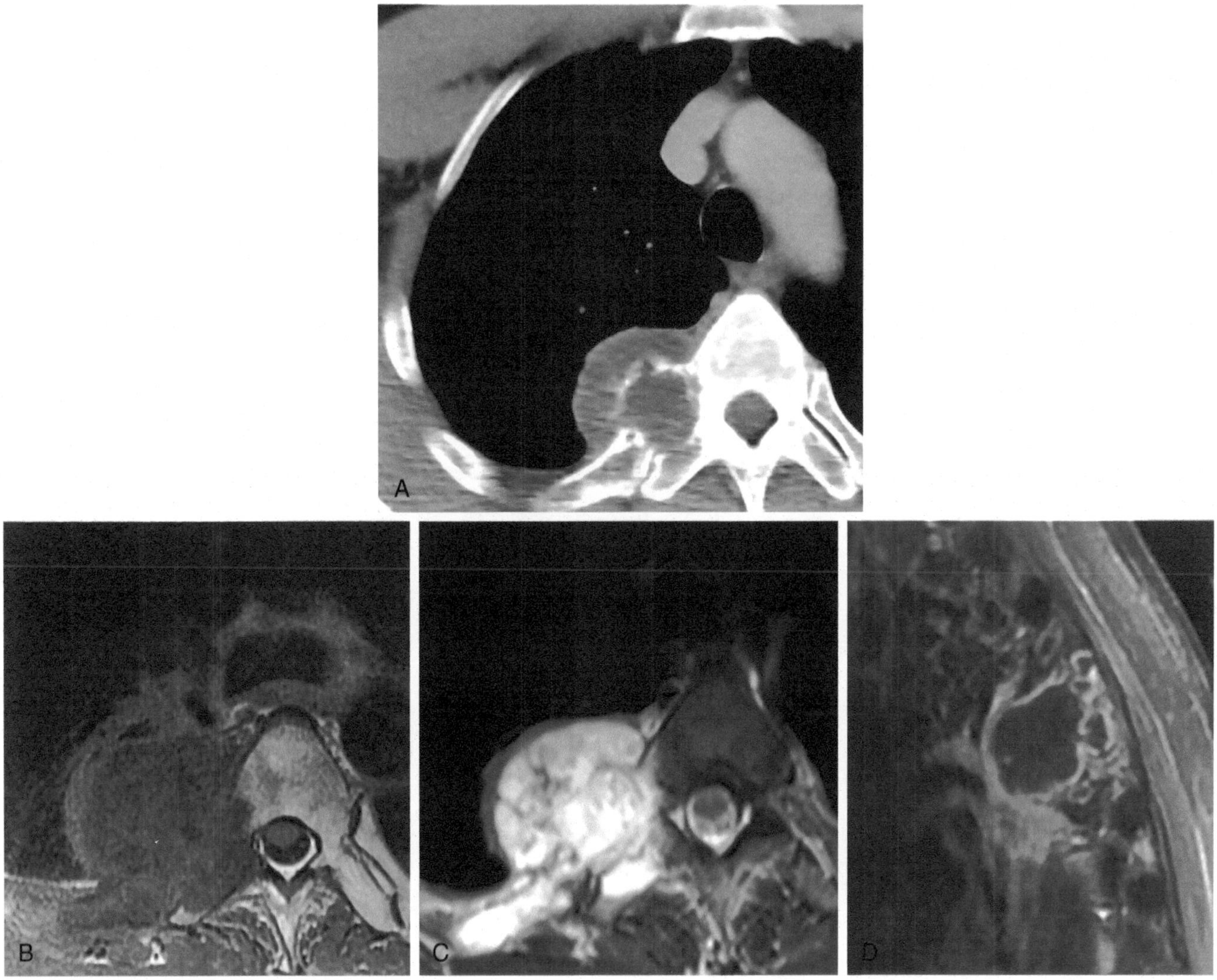

FIGURE 7.49 Chondrosarcoma arising at a costovertebral joint. **A,** Axial computed tomography (CT) scan with intravenous contrast shows an expansile lytic lesion with cortical breakthrough and soft tissue mass arising at a right costovertebral junction. Axial T1-weighted **(B)**, axial T2-weighted **(C)**, and sagittal fat-saturated postcontrast T1-weighted **(D)** MR images of this lesion reveal it to primarily rim-enhance, with a multicameral appearance composed of multiple nonenhancing locules of T1 hypointensity and T2 hyperintensity and surrounded by intermediate T1 and T2 signal septae, findings characteristic of cartilage. The extent of the lesion is more fully demonstrated by MRI, with involvement of the adjacent right rib, transverse process, and right lateral vertebral margin demonstrable by MRI but largely CT-occult.

SUGGESTED READINGS

Ginat DT, Bokhari A, Bhatt S, et al. Imaging features of solitary fibrous tumors. *AJR Am J Roentgenol.* 2011;196(3):487-495.

Hansell DM, Lynch DA, McAdams HP, et al. *Imaging of Diseases of the Chest.* St. Louis: Mosby-Elsevier; 2010.

Hussein-Jelen T, Bankier AA, Eisenberg RL. Solid pleural lesions. *AJR Am J Roentgenol.* 2012;198(6):W512-W520.

Jeung MY, Gangi A, Gasser B, et al. Imaging of chest wall disorders. *Radiographics.* 1999;19(3):617-637.

Levine BD, Motamedi K, Chow K, et al. CT of rib lesions. *AJR Am J Roentgenol.* 2009;193:5-13.

Light RW, Macgregor MI, Luchsinger PC, et al. Pleural effusions: the diagnostic separation of transudates and exudates. *Ann Intern Med.* 1972;77(4):507-513.

McDermott S, Levis DA, Arellano RS. Chest drainage. *Semin Intervent Radiol.* 2012;29(4):247-255.

Moskowitz H, Platt RT, Schachar R, et al. Roentgen visualization of minute pleural effusion. An experimental study to determine the minimum amount of pleural fluid visible on a radiograph. *Radiology.* 1973;109(1):33-35.

Nam SJ, Kim S, Lim BJ, et al. Imaging of primary chest wall tumors with radiologic-pathologic correlation. *Radiographics.* 2011;31(3):749-770.

Nason LK, Walker CM, McNeeley MF, et al. Imaging of the diaphragm: anatomy and function. *Radiographics.* 2012;32(2):E51-E70.

Ponrartana S, Laberge JM, Kerlan RK, et al. Management of patients with "ex vacuo" pneumothorax after thoracentesis. *Acad Radiol.* 2005;12(8):980-986.

Restrepo CS, Martinez S, Lemos DF, et al. Imaging appearances of the sternum and sternoclavicular joints. *Radiographics.* 2009;29(3):839-859.

Rosado-de-Christenson ML, Abbott GF, McAdams HP, et al. From the archives of the AFIP: localized fibrous tumor of the pleura. *Radiographics.* 2003;23(3):759-783.

Vix VA. Roentgenographic recognition of pleural effusion. *JAMA.* 1974;229:695-698.

Wang ZJ, Reddy GP, Gotway MB, et al. Malignant pleural mesothelioma: evaluation with CT, MR imaging, and PET. *Radiographics.* 2004;24(1):105-119.

Chapter 8

Congenital Thoracic Malformations

Justin Stowell, Matthew D. Gilman, and Christopher M. Walker

INTRODUCTION

Several congenital abnormalities of the thorax have been described, but most are rare. Classification of these anomalies is difficult because the embryologic basis often is not clearly understood. A classification based on anatomic structures uses the categories of trachea, bronchi, lung, and pulmonary vasculature. Although often described as separate entities, bronchopulmonary malformations are frequently interrelated, and features of different imaging and pathologic entities may coexist in the same lesion or separately in the same individual.

In children and adults, most congenital bronchopulmonary malformations (CBMs) can be diagnosed noninvasively with radiography, ultrasonography, computed tomography (CT), and magnetic resonance imaging (MRI). In this chapter, the more common congenital abnormalities encountered in adults are emphasized. Those more commonly identified in infancy are discussed in *Pediatric Radiology: The Requisites*. Congenital lesions of the heart, pericardium, and aorta are discussed in *Cardiac Radiology: The Requisites*.

TRACHEA

The most common congenital anomalies of the trachea include tracheomalacia, tracheal stenosis, tracheobronchomegaly, tracheoesophageal fistula (TEF), and tracheal bronchus. Tracheal agenesis and atresia are not discussed because they are associated with dismal prognosis, resulting in near-immediate postnatal death.

Tracheomalacia

Tracheomalacia refers to excessive pliability of tracheal cartilage, which leads to abnormal collapsibility of the trachea. It may be primary, associated with a localized absence or deficiency of the tracheal cartilage, or secondary, resulting from external compression by an extrinsic mass. Tracheomalacia may also occur in conjunction with other anomalies of the foregut, particularly TEF. Tracheomalacia must be differentiated from excessive dynamic airway collapse related to abnormal expiratory pressures. For example, collapse of a long segment of the intrathoracic trachea may occur in late expiration in patients with asthma, chronic bronchitis, and bronchiolitis caused by excessive anterior bowing of the posterior tracheal membrane rather than softening of tracheal cartilage.

Paired inspiratory and dynamic expiratory CT is excellent for evaluating tracheomalacia in adult patients. Anterior bowing of the posterior membrane and a greater than 70% cross-sectional area reduction of the trachea between inspiration and expiration are considered diagnostic. Other CT features of the tracheal lumen that are highly suggestive of tracheomalacia include a crescentic "frown" shape in expiration (Fig. 8.1) and a "lunate" morphology (coronal:sagittal ratio >1) in inspiration. The accuracy of these techniques is comparable with that of bronchoscopy, the gold standard for diagnosing tracheomalacia.

Congenital Tracheal Stenosis

Congenital tracheal stenosis is a rare condition characterized by fixed narrowing of the trachea. The three patterns of congenital tracheal stenosis (CTS) are (1) a diffuse or generalized hypoplasia, (2) a funnel-like stenosis (Fig. 8.2) often associated with an anomalous origin of the left pulmonary artery, and (3) segmental stenosis. The diffuse or funnel-like patterns may be associated with complete tracheal cartilage rings that replace the posterior membranous wall of the trachea. Patients with complete tracheal

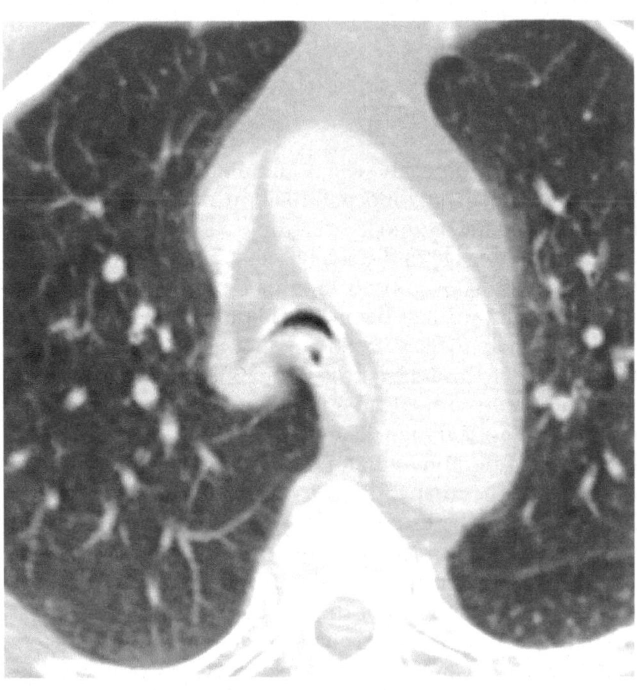

FIGURE 8.1 Tracheomalacia. Expiratory axial computed tomography image shows the "frown" sign with greater than 70% reduction in tracheal area from the inspiratory study (not shown).

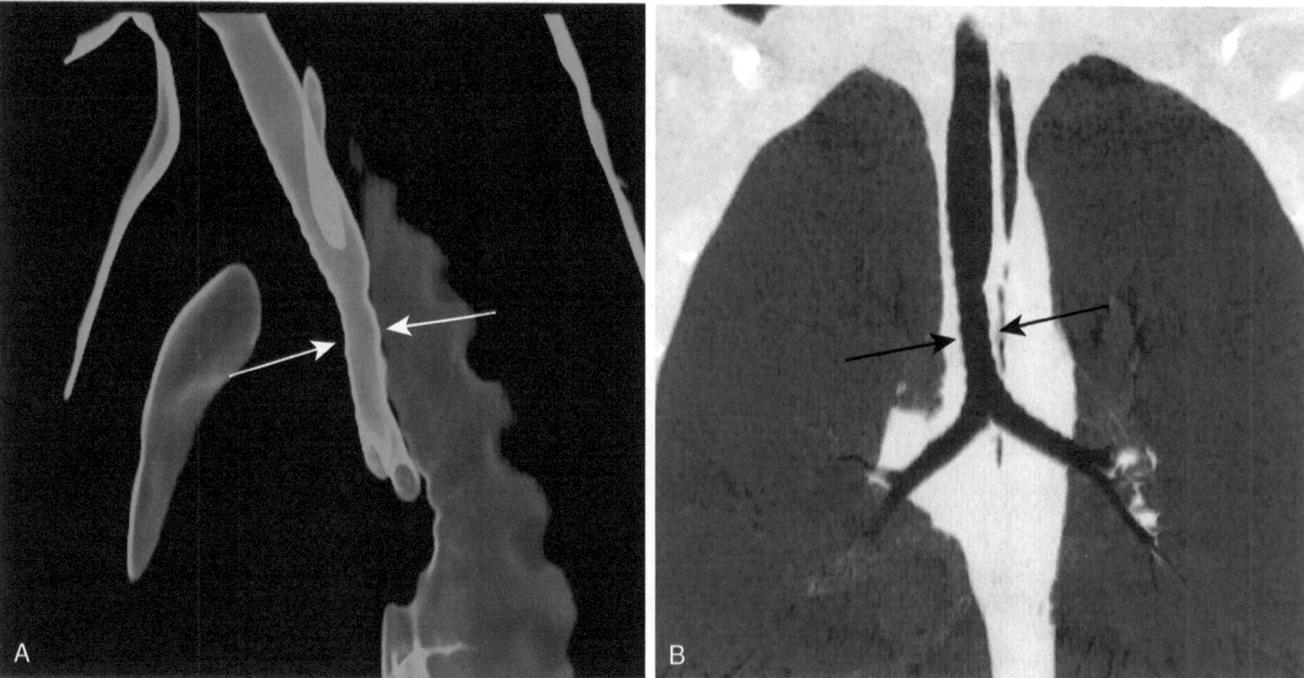

FIGURE 8.2 Congenital tracheal stenosis. External three-dimensional rendering **(A)** and coronal minimum intensity projection **(B)** of the trachea demonstrate smooth stenosis of the lower trachea *(arrows)*.

rings usually present with respiratory distress in the first few weeks of life, and this condition is associated with a high mortality rate. Rarely, the diagnosis is delayed until adulthood. Complete tracheal rings may be isolated events or may be associated with pulmonary vascular slings. CTS can be associated with abnormal bronchial branching patterns such as tracheal bronchus, bridging bronchus, and bronchial and lung agenesis. CTS has an association with other anomalies such as TEF, congenital heart disease, and skeletal abnormalities.

Congenital Tracheobronchomegaly

Tracheobronchomegaly (i.e., Mounier-Kuhn syndrome) is characterized by abnormal dilation of the trachea and bronchi thought secondary to atrophy of the elastic tissues and smooth muscle of the trachea and central bronchi. The disease is often diagnosed in adults, although symptoms of the condition may begin in childhood. In addition to tracheobronchomegaly, frequent outpouchings and possible diverticula of the intercartilaginous membranes are seen on radiography and CT, giving the trachea a characteristic corrugated appearance. The diagnosis can be established by chest radiography when the transverse diameter of the trachea is greater than 25 mm in men and 21 mm in women. Bronchomegaly is established when the diameters of the right and left main bronchi are greater than 21 and 18 mm in men and 20 and 17 mm in women. CT can confirm the increased diameter of the trachea in which a tracheal diameter greater than 3 cm and mainstem bronchi diameters greater than 2.4 cm are highly suggestive of Mounier-Kuhn syndrome (Fig. 8.3). Frequently, there is concomitant cystic bronchiectasis. Collapse of the trachea and central airways can be observed on expiratory imaging.

Tracheoesophageal Fistula

Congenital tracheoesophageal fistula (TEF) is invariably a pediatric disease. Most (70%–80%) occur in the presence of esophageal atresia with a distal TEF. However, about 4% of all TEFs occur with an otherwise normal esophagus (the so-called H-type fistula), and in these instances, patients may present in adult life with recurrent pneumonia. The esophagus communicates most often with the trachea (75%) and less frequently with the major bronchi. Congenital TEF carries a strong association with other congenital anomalies and is a component of the VACTERL association (vertebral anomalies, anal atresia, cardiac defects, TEF, renal anomalies, and limb defects). The chest radiograph may show evidence of bronchiectasis or an air-distended esophagus (Fig. 8.4). Esophagography can identify the fistulous communication between the tracheobronchial tree and pooling of oral contrast within the alveoli. See *Pediatrics: The Requisites* for more information about TEF.

Tracheal Bronchus

A tracheal bronchus is an abnormal bronchial branching pattern in which all or part of the upper lobe bronchial supply originates from the trachea. This usually occurs within 2 cm of the carina and most commonly on the right (Fig. 8.5). Although classically a tracheal bronchus is considered to arise from the trachea, the literature also refers to an anomalous bronchus originating from the proximal main bronchus above the carina as a tracheal bronchus. In a bronchus suis, or "pig bronchus," the entire upper lobe bronchial supply arises from the trachea. If all the segmental bronchi arise normally from the upper lobe bronchus (three segmental in the right upper lobe,

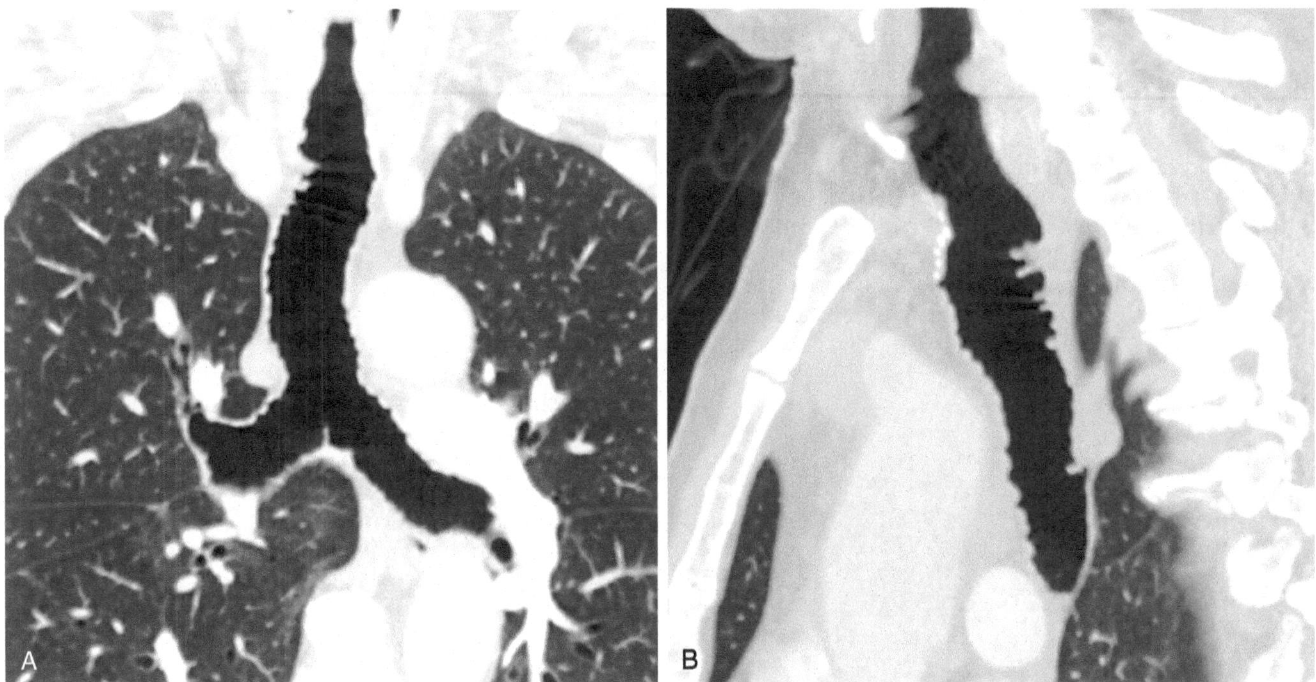

FIGURE 8.3 Congenital tracheobronchomegaly (Mounier-Kuhn syndrome). Coronal **(A)** and sagittal **(B)** chest computed tomography scans demonstrate tracheobronchomegaly. Saccular outpouchings between the cartilaginous rings give the trachea a corrugated appearance, best visualized on the sagittal reconstruction.

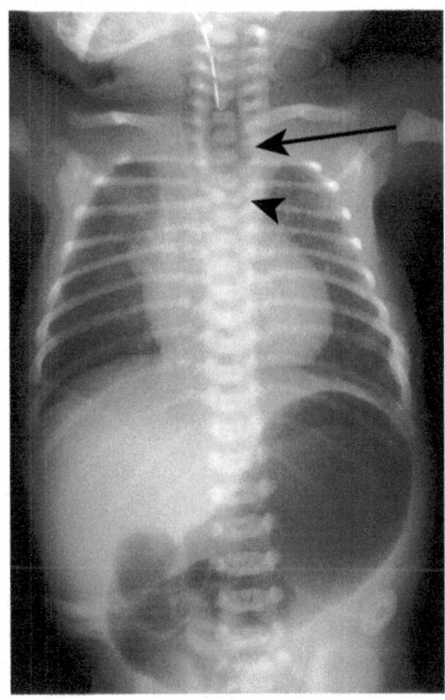

FIGURE 8.4 Congenital tracheoesophageal fistula. Frontal chest radiograph in a neonate with duodenal atresia and tracheoesophageal fistula (TEF). There are a mildly dilated, air-filled proximal esophagus *(arrow)* and T3 hemivertebra *(arrowhead)*. Findings are among the VACTERL complex (vertebral defects, imperforate anus, cardiac anomalies, TEF, and renal and limb anomalies). There is a double-bubble sign in the upper abdomen, indicating duodenal atresia.

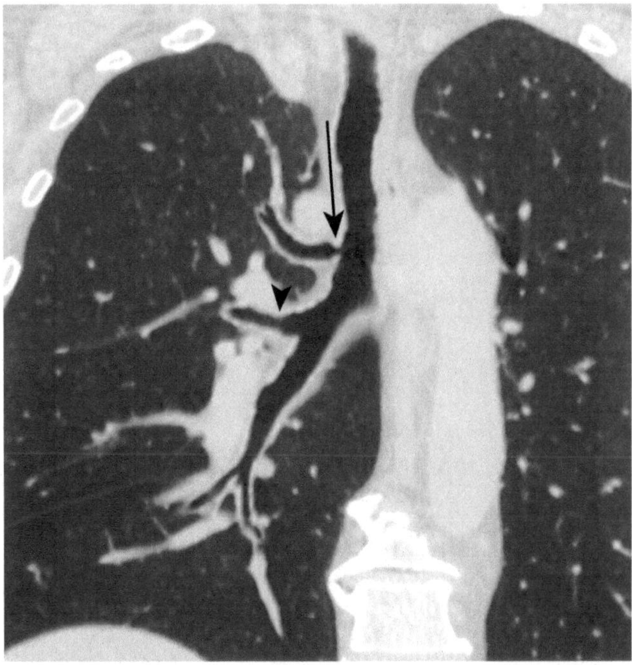

FIGURE 8.5 Tracheal bronchus. Coronal computed tomography scan shows a displaced apical segmental bronchus to the right upper lobe originating directly from the trachea *(arrow)*. In this case, the proximal lumen is stenotic, which is uncommon. The origins of the anterior and posterior right upper lobe segmental bronchi *(arrowhead)* were normal.

four segmental in the left upper lobe), the bronchus that arises from the trachea is referred to as supernumerary. If one or all of the normal upper lobe segmental bronchi are absent, the tracheal bronchus is referred to as displaced. Tracheal bronchi are usually of no clinical consequence. In a minority of patients, impaired drainage may result in air trapping, recurrent infections, or bronchiectasis. During endotracheal intubation, an endotracheal tube balloon cuff may inadvertently obstruct the aberrant bronchus, causing lobar or segmental atelectasis.

BRONCHI

Accessory Cardiac Bronchus

An accessory cardiac bronchus (ACB) is a supernumerary bronchus arising from the medial wall of the bronchus intermedius and extending toward the heart. ACB is uncommon, with a reported incidence of 0.07% to 0.5% but may be an incidental discovery on chest CT or bronchoscopy. Most are stumplike and blind ending (Fig. 8.6) and contain cartilage in their walls, distinguishing them from a diverticulum. Others may be more elongate, supplying a small lobule of underdeveloped pulmonary tissue referred to as a "cardiac lobe." ACB is often an incidental imaging or bronchoscopic finding in asymptomatic adults. Occasionally, an ACB may cause symptoms (e.g., hemoptysis) when associated with chronic inflammation or infection, retained secretions, foreign bodies, or rarely malignancy. Traumatic injury of ACB during bronchoscopy may lead to complications such as pneumothorax.

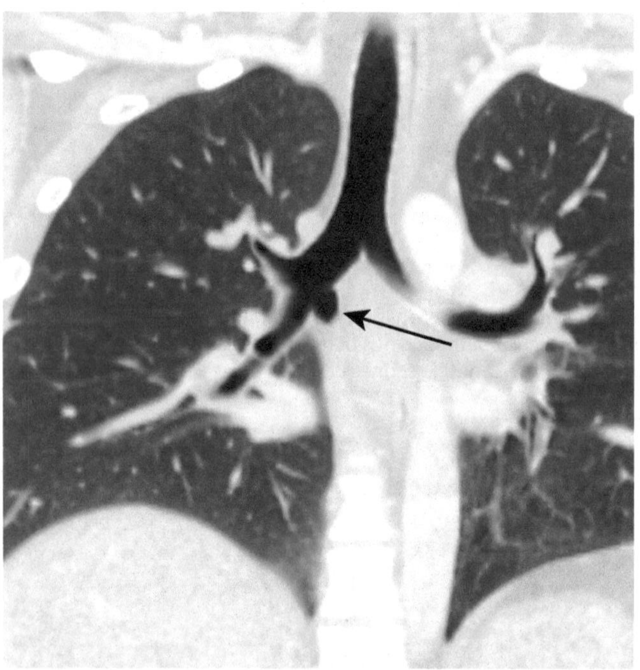

FIGURE 8.6 Accessory cardiac bronchus. Coronal contrast-enhanced computed tomography scan depicts a blind-ending accessory bronchus *(arrow)* extending from the medial wall of the bronchus intermedius.

Bronchial Isomerism

Bronchopulmonary isomerism refers to an identical pattern of bronchial branching and an equal number of lobes in each lung. Isomerism has a frequent association with abnormal left-to-right arrangement of the thoracic and abdominal organs, collectively known as heterotaxy syndrome. The most reliable imaging finding that defines right- or left-sided isomerism is the position of the mainstem bronchi in relation to the central pulmonary arteries. Bilateral eparterial bronchi (bronchus above the pulmonary artery in the hila) characterize the right bronchial isomerism type. Right-sided isomerism (bilateral right-sidedness) confers a poorer prognosis and frequent association with asplenia and severe congenital heart lesions. Bilateral hyparterial bronchi (bronchus below adjacent pulmonary arteries) define left isomerism (see Fig. 8.2). Left isomerism (bilateral left-sidedness) is associated with polysplenia.

Bronchial Atresia

In bronchial atresia, there is focal atresia of a lobar, segmental, or subsegmental bronchus with focal obliteration of the lumen. Distal to the point of atresia, the airways remain patent and accumulate a mucous plug or mucocele, one of the characteristic features on imaging. The most common site is the left upper lobe, particularly the apicoposterior segment. The right middle and right upper lobes are less common sites. The lobe or segment of the lung distal to the point of atresia is aerated by collateral air drift and

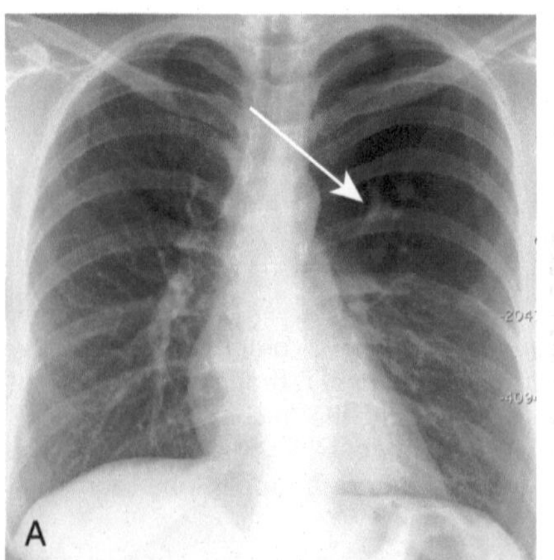

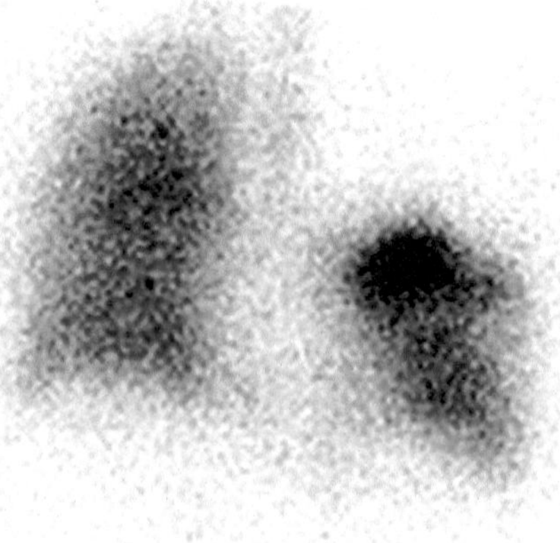

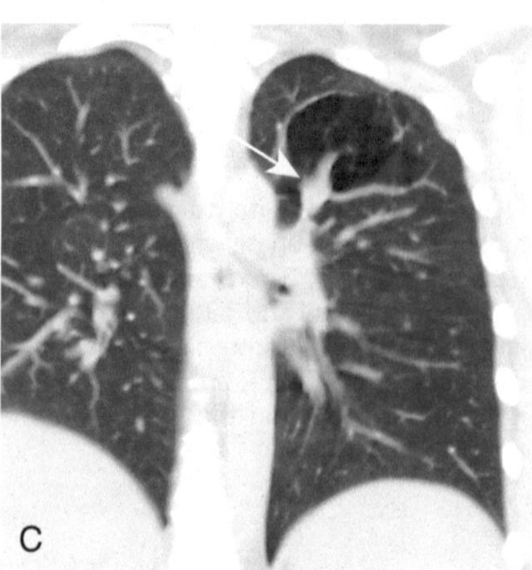

FIGURE 8.7 Bronchial atresia. **A,** Posteroanterior chest radiograph shows a hyperlucent left upper lobe with subtle rightward mediastinal shift. A left perihilar branching, tubular-shaped opacity *(arrow)* represents mucoid impaction distal to the atresia. **B,** Anterior projection ventilation scintigraphic image from a Tc-99m DTPA (technetium-99m-diethylene-triamine-pentaacetate) examination in the same patient shows lack of radiotracer distribution to the hyperlucent left upper lobe. **C,** Coronal computed tomography scan in a different patient shows a dilated mucus-filled bronchus *(arrow)* with distal hyperlucency caused by air trapping in the apicoposterior segment.

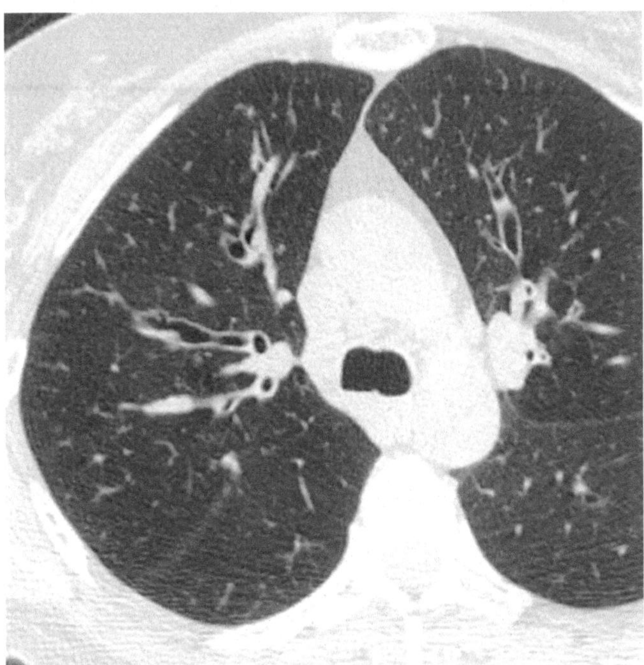

FIGURE 8.8 Williams-Campbell syndrome. Axial computed tomography scan demonstrates central cylindrical bronchiectasis and mild bronchial wall thickening affecting the fourth- through sixth-order bronchi. The trachea, distal bronchi, and bronchioles are of normal caliber.

becomes hyperinflated because of air trapping distal to the point of atresia. The chest radiograph may show an ovoid or branching nodule or mass that corresponds to the mucocele. Chest radiography may also show an area of hyperlucency in the affected segment(s) of the lung (Fig. 8.7). CT demonstrates a low-attenuation, nonenhancing, ovoid, or branching mass corresponding to the mucocele as well as characteristic hyperinflation in the lung distal to the mucocele (see Fig. 8.7). There may be an accompanying shift of the mediastinum and compression of the surrounding lung. It is important to consider and exclude an endobronchial mass (e.g., a carcinoid tumor) or a foreign body, which could have a similar appearance with a distal mucous plug and air trapping.

Congenital Bronchiectasis

Congenital bronchiectasis (i.e., Williams-Campbell syndrome) is rare. Williams-Campbell syndrome results from a congenital deficiency of bronchial cartilage affecting fourth- to sixth- order subsegmental bronchi. The cartilage deficiency leads to airway collapse, bronchiectasis, and pulmonary hyperinflation (Fig. 8.8). Acquired bronchiectasis (from chronic or recurrent infection) may also occur early in life as a result of other congenital, developmental, or genetic disorders. These conditions are listed in Box 8.1.

BOX 8.1 Developmental Disorders Associated With Bronchiectasis

Congenital cystic bronchiectasis
Primary hypogammaglobulinemia
Yellow nail syndrome
Cystic fibrosis
Immotile-cilia syndrome (Kartagener syndrome)

LUNGS

Pulmonary Underdevelopment

Pulmonary underdevelopment, also known as lung agenesis–hypoplasia complex, results from disordered in utero formation of the lungs and airways varying in severity from agenesis, to aplasia, to hypoplasia. In pulmonary agenesis, there is total absence of lung tissue, bronchi, and vasculature distal to the carina. This is distinguished from pulmonary aplasia in which a rudimentary bronchus ends in a blind pouch without lung tissue or pulmonary vasculature. In pulmonary hypoplasia, lung tissue and bronchi are present but are decreased in number or size. Pulmonary underdevelopment may be primary or secondary to an in utero pathologic process that prevents full development of the thoracic cavity. These conditions include decreased pulmonary vascular perfusion, oligohydramnios, or compression of the lung by a space-occupying mass (e.g., congenital diaphragmatic hernia). More than half of affected fetuses with pulmonary underdevelopment exhibit additional cardiovascular, gastrointestinal, or skeletal abnormalities.

The imaging appearance of agenesis–hypoplasia complex varies depending on the degree of pulmonary underdevelopment. In agenesis, chest radiography shows complete absence of an aerated lung in one hemithorax, pronounced decrease in volume of the affected hemithorax, and shift of the mediastinum to the affected side. There is usually compensatory overinflation of the contralateral normal lung that extends across the midline (Fig. 8.9). In pulmonary hypoplasia, the lung is decreased in size, and there may be similar signs of volume loss, but the appearance varies depending on the degree of pulmonary hypoplasia. In some cases, it may be difficult on radiography to distinguish severe pulmonary hypoplasia from aplasia or agenesis. In such instances, chest CT differentiates these entities by the presence or absence of a bronchus, pulmonary artery, and lung tissue. In pulmonary hypoplasia, a small pulmonary artery associated with transpleural collateral arteries may be seen in the affected lung.

Pulmonary hypoplasia must be differentiated from other conditions that can produce volume loss, including total atelectasis of the lung, severe bronchiectasis with collapse, and advanced fibrothorax caused by chronic pleural disease. CT is likely to be diagnostic in these cases.

Congenital Lobar Overinflation

Congenital lobar overinflation (CLO), also called congenital lobar hyperinflation, is characterized by progressive overdistention of a lobe thought secondary to bronchial obstruction and poststenotic air trapping related to a one-way ball-valve mechanism. The bronchial obstruction may be the result of an intrinsic cartilage deficiency or extraluminal compression by a vascular structure or mass (e.g., bronchogenic cyst). In some patients, lobar hyperinflation may be caused by an abnormal increase in alveoli (the so-called polyalveolar type). In CLO, the alveoli are overinflated, but there is

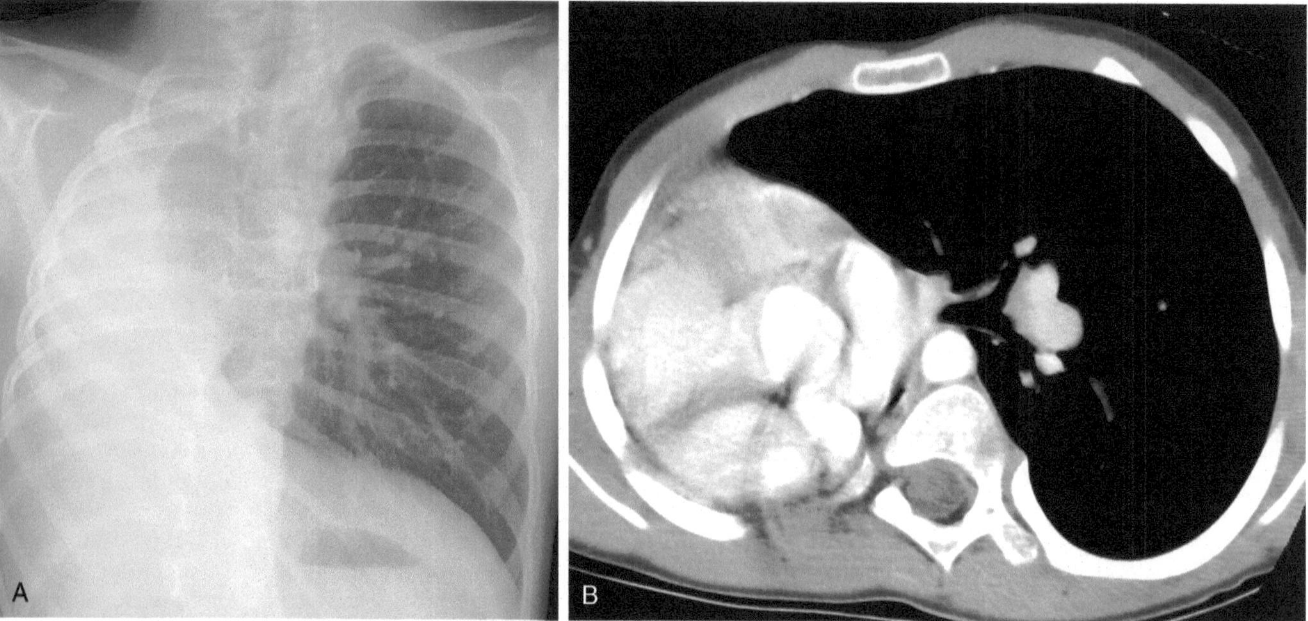

FIGURE 8.9 Pulmonary agenesis. **A,** Posteroanterior chest radiograph shows complete absence of the right lung, pronounced rightward mediastinal shift, and compensatory left lung hyperinflation. **B,** Axial contrast-enhanced chest computed tomography scan shows complete absence of pulmonary tissue, bronchi, and pulmonary vessels in the right hemithorax consistent with pulmonary agenesis.

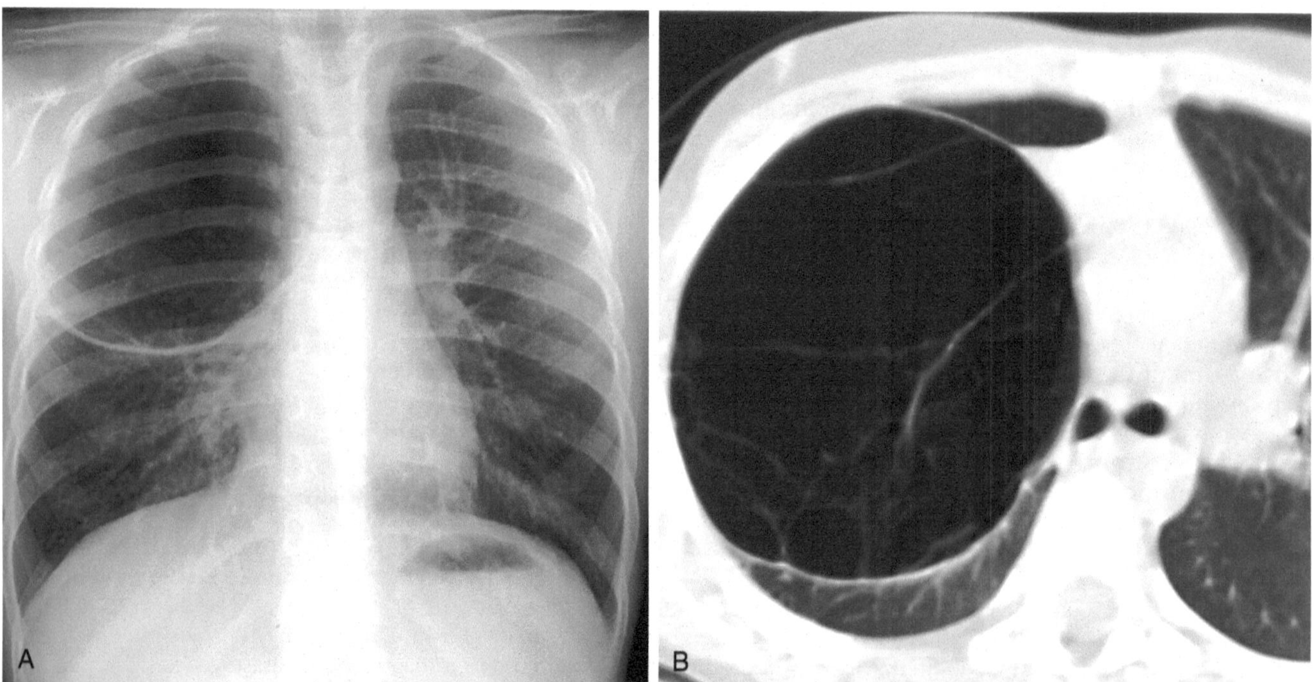

FIGURE 8.10 Congenital lobar overinflation (CLO). **A,** Chest radiograph shows asymmetric hyperlucency of the right upper lobe and mild left mediastinal shift. **B,** Axial image from chest computed tomography scan in lung window shows severe overinflation of the right upper lobe. CLO occurs most commonly in the left upper lobe but may be seen in any lobe.

no alveolar destruction. Therefore, the term *congenital lobar emphysema* is less accurate. CLO usually occurs in infants or young children, with boys being more frequently affected. The left upper lobe is most frequently involved followed by the right middle lobe.

The radiologic findings consist of hyperlucency and overinflation of the affected lobe with various degrees of mediastinal shift and atelectasis (Fig. 8.10). Occasionally in newborns, the lobe may appear opaque on radiography because of retained fetal lung fluid. The affected lung may then become progressively lucent as the fluid is absorbed by the pulmonary venolymphatic system. The differential diagnosis includes aspirated foreign body (older infants and toddlers); extraluminal compression of a bronchus by

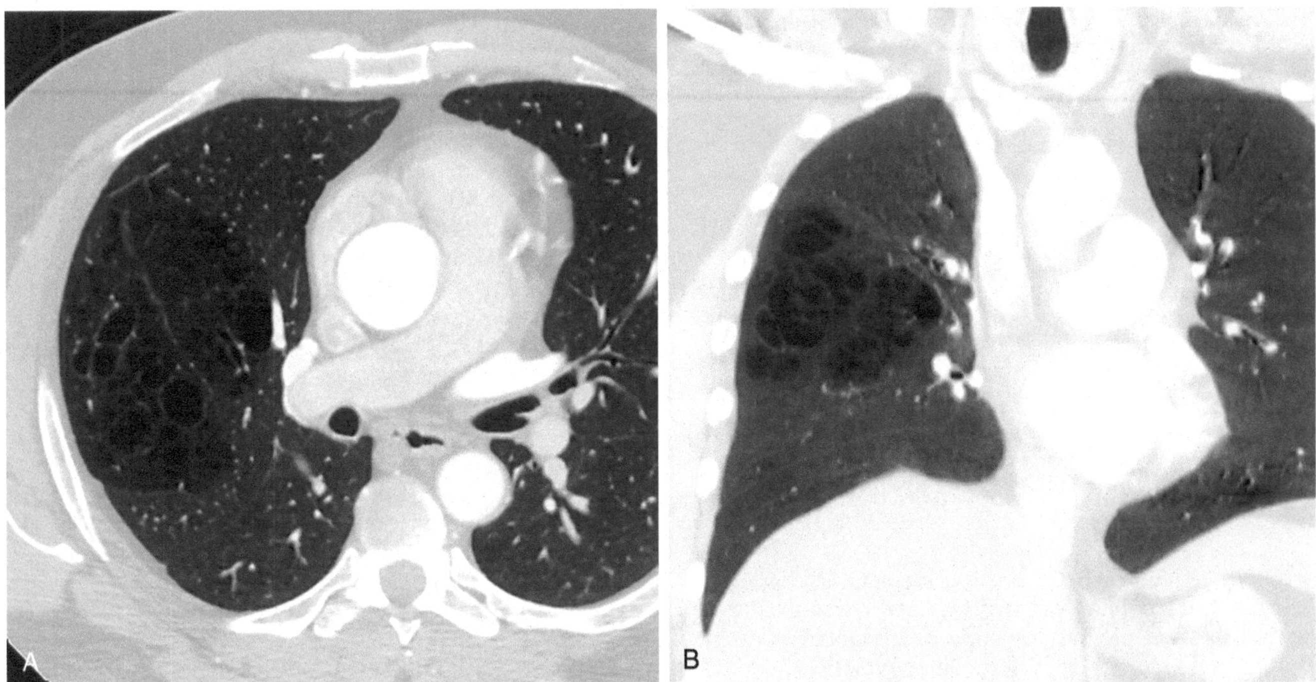

FIGURE 8.11 Congenital pulmonary airway malformation (CPAM), type I. Axial contrast-enhanced **(A)** and coronal minimum intensity projection **(B)** computed tomography scans show a right upper lobe multicystic mass containing large to medium-sized cysts. Type 1 CPAM is the most common subtype.

a bronchogenic cyst, teratoma, or other mass; bronchial atresia with overinflation; and a congenital lung cyst.

Cases of acute respiratory distress require surgical resection, particularly in the neonatal period. Supportive therapy may be considered, particularly for older children and children with milder symptoms because these lesions may regress. A few cases are asymptomatic and may not be diagnosed until adult life.

Congenital Pulmonary Airway Malformation

Congenital pulmonary airway malformations (CPAMs) are a heterogeneous group of congenital lung masses that result from disordered airway development. Originally described as congenital cystic adenomatoid malformation (CCAM), the name of this disorder has been changed to CPAM because not all of these lesions are cystic or adenomatoid pathologically. Patients usually present in infancy with respiratory distress caused by a space-occupying mass that compromises lung tissue. Roughly 80% of patients are younger than 6 months, although 17% of cases are reported in older children. Although controversial, rare cases have been reported in adults.

The most recent classification scheme consists of five types of CPAMs (types 0–4) based on cyst size and the histologic origin of the lesion in the tracheobronchial tree. Type I, the most common, is characterized by a single or multiple large cysts (2–10 cm) of bronchial or bronchiolar origin. Type II consists of single or multiple small cysts (≤2 cm) of bronchiolar origin. Type III is a predominantly solid lesion with small cysts, may contain adenomatous tissue, and is of bronchiolar-alveolar duct origin. Types 0 and IV CPAM are less common than types I to III. Type 0 CPAM represents acinar dysplasia or dysgenesis of large airways (trachea or bronchi) involving all lobes and is incompatible with life. Type IV CPAM originates from the acinus and consists of a large unlined cyst mimicking a type I lesion. Blood supply to most CPAMs is via pulmonary arteries and veins. However, hybrid lesions with features of extralobar sequestration may exhibit systemic blood supply.

The imaging findings vary with the lesion subtype. Chest radiography and chest CT of the type I lesion typically show unilateral, single, or multiple air-filled cysts (Fig. 8.11). In the neonatal period, the cyst may appear as a soft tissue mass that gradually becomes air filled as fetal lung fluid is cleared from the lesion. The cyst may be very large, occupying almost an entire hemithorax, producing mass effect, mediastinal shift, and compression of the remaining lung. A single dominant cyst may be surrounded by smaller cysts. Type II lesions typically manifest with multiple small uniform air-filled cysts. A type III lesion usually manifests as a solid intrathoracic mass or consolidation and may involve an entire lung. Although CPAM is most often unilateral, chest CT has found evidence of bilateral involvement in some cases.

In neonates with severe respiratory distress, this lesion may constitute a surgical emergency. The definitive treatment is surgical excision via lobectomy or segmentectomy. Although controversial, the association of recurrent infections and the small risk of malignancy with CPAMs represents the rationale for elective resection in asymptomatic patients.

The prognosis appears to be best for patients with type I lesions. If cysts are very large and interfere with normal pulmonary development, particularly if there is contralateral pulmonary hypoplasia, the prognosis is worse.

Pulmonary Sequestration

Pulmonary sequestration is a focal area of nonfunctioning lung tissue that lacks normal connection with the bronchial

TABLE 8.1 Differentiating Characteristics of Intralobar and Extralobar Sequestration

Intralobar	Extralobar
Arises within existing pulmonary visceral pleura	Contained within unique pleural envelope
Adult or adolescent	Infant or child
Recurrent infection	Infection rare
Variable appearance (mass or consolidation, cystic or multicystic, hyperlucent, mixed) but usually contains air	Homogeneous mass-like; rarely contains air
Pulmonary venous drainage (usually)	Systemic venous drainage (usually azygos or hemiazygos)

tree (i.e., sequestered) and receives systemic arterial supply. The sequestered lung tissue may be extralobar and contained within its own pleural envelope or intralobar contained within the visceral pleura of the affected lobe (Table 8.1). Extralobar sequestrations are generally considered to be congenital malformations. The origin of intralobar sequestration is more controversial, with some authors postulating that some intralobar sequestrations could be acquired lesions resulting from recurrent or chronic infection with bronchial obstruction and parasitization of systemic arterial supply from the aorta. Some cases of intralobar sequestration are identified on prenatal imaging and are considered congenital lesions. Some imaging and histologic features of bronchopulmonary sequestrations overlap with other bronchopulmonary malformations such as bronchial atresia, and other congenital lung abnormalities may coexist with a sequestration (so-called hybrid lesions).

Blood supply to the sequestered pulmonary tissue usually arises from the descending thoracic aorta, although the origin may be from the upper abdominal aorta or one of its major branches. The systemic arterial supply of pulmonary sequestrations may consist of one or more systemic arteries. The venous drainage pattern of intralobar and extralobar sequestration differs. Intralobar sequestration is usually drained by a branch of the inferior pulmonary vein to the left atrium, creating a left-to-left shunt. Extralobar sequestrations tend to drain to systemic veins, usually the azygous system.

Multiplanar and three-dimensional cross-sectional imaging with contrast-enhanced CT or MRI can further characterize these lesions and define their vascular supply and venous drainage. In equivocal cases, angiography may be used to demonstrate the anomalous vascular supply and drainage. The goals of imaging in pulmonary sequestration are to delineate the extent of the lesion, identify the systemic artery, identify if there are multiple systemic arteries, identify the venous drainage, evaluate for involvement below the diaphragm, and assess for complications such as superimposed infection.

Intralobar Sequestration

Intralobar sequestrations may manifest in adults as incidental radiographic abnormalities or in the context of recurrent pneumonias. They may appear as a mass or region of consolidation almost invariably in a posterior basal segment of the lower lobe. The mass or consolidation corresponding to the sequestration may contain air or air-fluid levels on chest radiography. They affect the left side twice as frequently as the right.

The chest CT appearance of intralobar sequestration varies depending on the degree of aeration and the presence or absence of associated infection. The lesion may appear as a solid mass, a water-density mass, an area of consolidation, a pure air-containing lesion, or a single cystic or multicystic lesion (Fig. 8.12). On CT, the cysts may contain air, fluid, or air–fluid levels. In intralobar sequestration, air gains entry into the sequestered lung from the normal surrounding lung by means of collateral ventilation or from fistulous communication to a normal airway as a result of infection. The presence of air–fluid levels or increased consolidation compared with prior examinations may raise the possibility of superimposed infection.

Extralobar Sequestration

Extralobar sequestration typically manifests in early infancy, occurring most frequently in the lower hemithorax between the lower lobe and the diaphragm (Fig. 8.13). Other locations include the mediastinum, within or below the diaphragm. Patients with extralobar sequestrations have a higher incidence of other malformations such as congenital diaphragmatic hernia, pulmonary aplasia–hypoplasia complex, and others. Extralobar sequestration in adults is usually diagnosed incidentally on imaging performed for other reasons. Rarely, an adult patient may be symptomatic and present with hemothorax, hemoptysis, infection, or infarction.

On chest radiography, the extralobar sequestration usually manifests as a single well-defined homogeneous mass in the lower thorax close to the posterior medial hemidiaphragm. An ectopic location is more commonly found with extralobar sequestration than intralobar and is a distinguishing feature. Ectopic locations include the mediastinum, pericardium, upper thorax, and upper abdomen. Because of their pleural covering, extralobar sequestrations characteristically do not to contain air. The presence of air within an extralobar sequestration may imply communication with the gastrointestinal tract, which could be evaluated with esophagography. On CT, extralobar sequestrations are usually homogeneous, well-defined, sometimes vascular masses of soft tissue attenuation. Occasionally, there may be perilesional hyperlucency or cystic change.

MEDIASTINUM

Foregut Duplication Cysts

Bronchogenic Cysts

Bronchogenic cysts are embryologic bronchopulmonary foregut malformations resulting from abnormal budding of the tracheobronchial tree. Bronchogenic cysts are lined by pseudostratified ciliated columnar epithelium and usually contain smooth muscle, mucous glands, and cartilage. Bronchogenic cysts may be filled with clear or mucoid material or contain layering milk of calcium. The features of bronchogenic cysts are covered in Chapter 5.

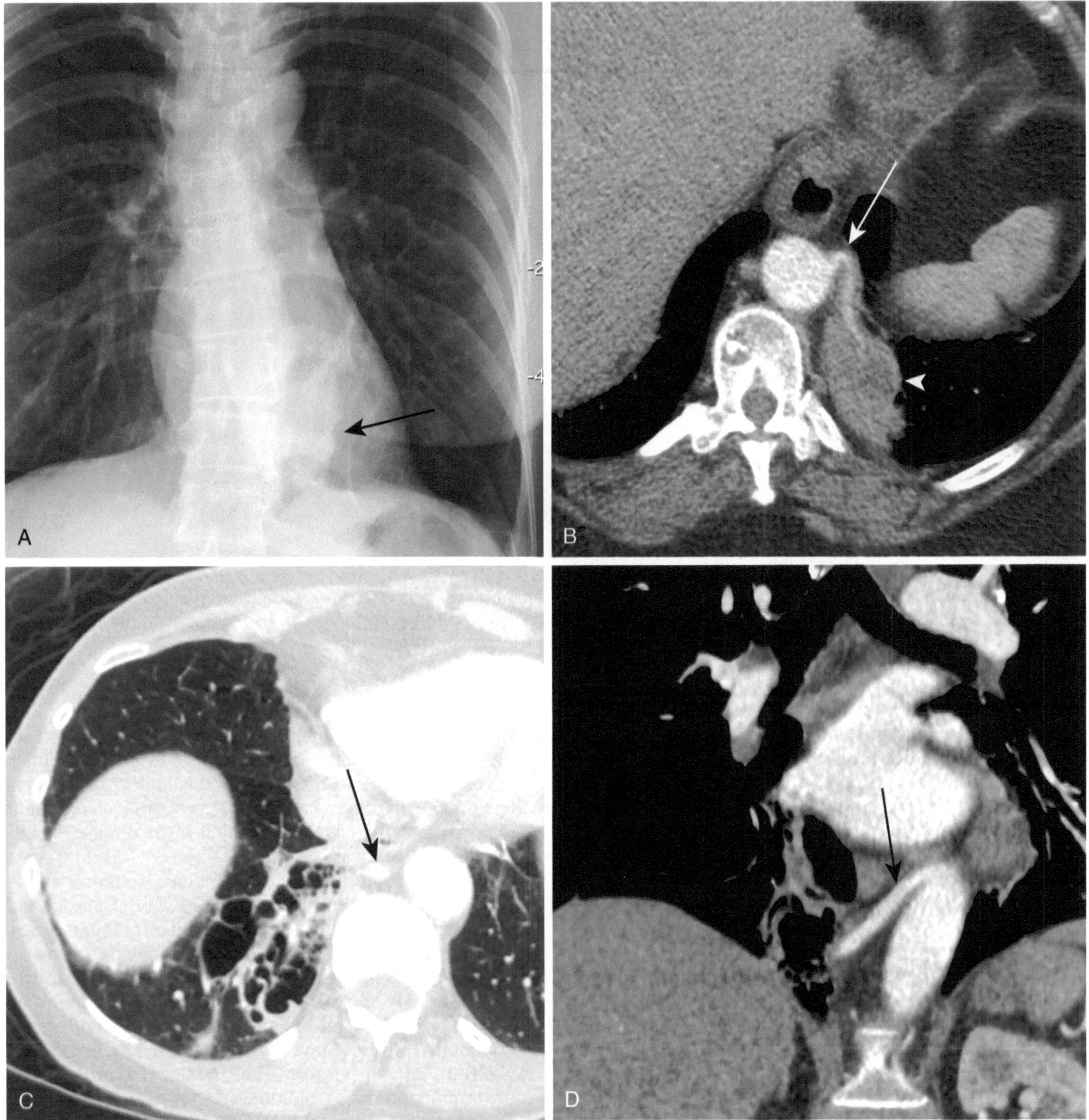

FIGURE 8.12 Intralobar sequestration. **A,** Chest radiograph shows a masslike lesion *(arrow)* in the left retrocardiac region, abutting the left hemidiaphragm. **B,** Axial contrast-enhanced computed tomography (CT) scan in the same patient demonstrates an aberrant systemic artery *(arrow)* arising from the descending thoracic aorta supplying the mass of sequestered lung tissue *(arrowhead)*. Axial **(C)** and coronal **(D)** contrast-enhanced CT from a different patient shows an aberrant artery *(arrows)* from the descending thoracic aorta supplying a medial right lower lobe mixed cystic and solid mass representing a sequestration.

Esophageal Duplication Cysts

Esophageal duplication cysts are similar to bronchogenic cysts yet remain histologically unique as they are lined with gastrointestinal mucosa instead of respiratory mucosa. Cysts containing gastric mucosa may lead to ulceration, hemorrhage, or perforation of the cyst. Two theories exist to explain their development including aberrant budding of the dorsal bud of the primitive foregut or abnormal recanalization of the foregut. The imaging features of esophageal duplication cysts are covered in Chapter 5.

Neurenteric Cysts

Neurenteric cysts are commonly discussed along with other foregut duplication cysts despite their unique embryologic

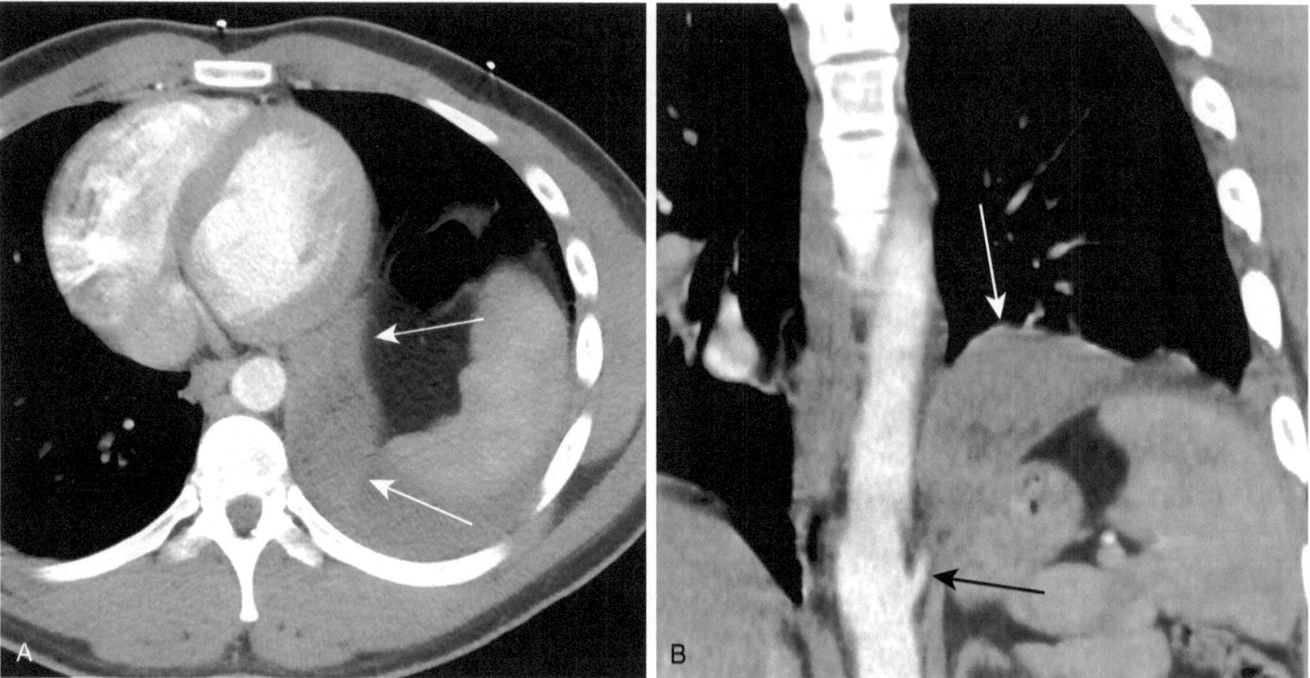

FIGURE 8.13 Extralobar sequestration with torsion. **A,** Axial contrast-enhanced computed tomography scan shows an extrapleural mass abutting the left hemidiaphragm *(white arrows)*. **B,** There is an abrupt cutoff of the aberrant artery from the descending thoracic aorta *(black arrow)*, suggesting torsion of the sequestration *(white arrow)*. A torsed and infarcted extralobar sequestration was confirmed on pathology.

origin and imaging features. They represent sequelae of incomplete separation of the notochord and endoderm manifesting in adult life as a paravertebral or extraaxial cyst. Vertebral ossification centers may fail to fuse as a consequence of persistent connection between the neurenteric cyst and the notochord, manifesting in the adult as bony anomalies of the spine. The imaging features of neurenteric cysts are covered in Chapter 5.

Thymic Cysts

Thymic cysts are rare and may be congenital or acquired. Congenital thymic cysts develop as a result of persistent patency of the thymopharyngeal duct. The imaging features of thymic cysts are covered in Chapter 5.

PULMONARY VESSELS

Congenital lung abnormalities involving pulmonary vessels range from purely vascular malformations with normal lung (e.g., pulmonary arteriovenous malformation [AVM]) to vascular malformations associated with abnormal lung development (e.g., hypogenetic lung syndrome, sequestration, interrupted pulmonary artery with lung agenesis or hypoplasia).

Anomalies of the Pulmonary Arteries

Proximal Interruption

Proximal interruption of the pulmonary artery is a rare congenital anomaly in which either the right or left pulmonary artery terminates usually within 1 cm of its origin. The term *proximal interruption* is preferred to congenital absence because the pulmonary arteries in the hilum and lung are typically intact but small in size. Proximal interruption of the right pulmonary artery is more common, and the interrupted pulmonary artery usually occurs opposite to the side of the aortic arch. Proximal interruption of the left pulmonary artery (with right aortic arch) has a higher incidence of associated congenital heart disease, such as tetralogy of Fallot.

Chest radiographic findings include reduced volume in the affected hemithorax with ipsilateral cardiac and mediastinal shift, absence of the hilar pulmonary arterial interface, elevated ipsilateral hemidiaphragm, and decreased number of pulmonary vessels in the affected lung (Figs. 8.14 and 8.15). Hyperinflation of the contralateral lung may occur with extension across the midline. Less commonly, rib notching may be seen in the presence of vigorous intercostal artery collaterals. Proximal absence or termination of the pulmonary artery can be confirmed by contrast-enhanced CT, which may also show enlarged bronchial, internal mammary, phrenic, or intercostal artery collaterals. Peripheral fine linear opacities and serrated pleural thickening from transpleural intercostal artery collaterals to the affected lung are common. The diagnosis can also be confirmed with spin-echo or steady-state free precession (SSFP) MRI. Proximal interruption must be distinguished from Swyer-James-Macleod syndrome, which shares many of the radiographic features. Unlike proximal interruption, Swyer-James-Macleod syndrome is associated with constrictive bronchiolitis and air trapping, which can be documented by expiratory CT. On chest radiography, proximal interruption of the right pulmonary artery may appear very similar to pulmonary venolobar syndrome but lacks the typical "scimitar vein" in the right lung base. Complications include bronchiectasis in the affected lung, recurrent infection, hemoptysis, and pulmonary

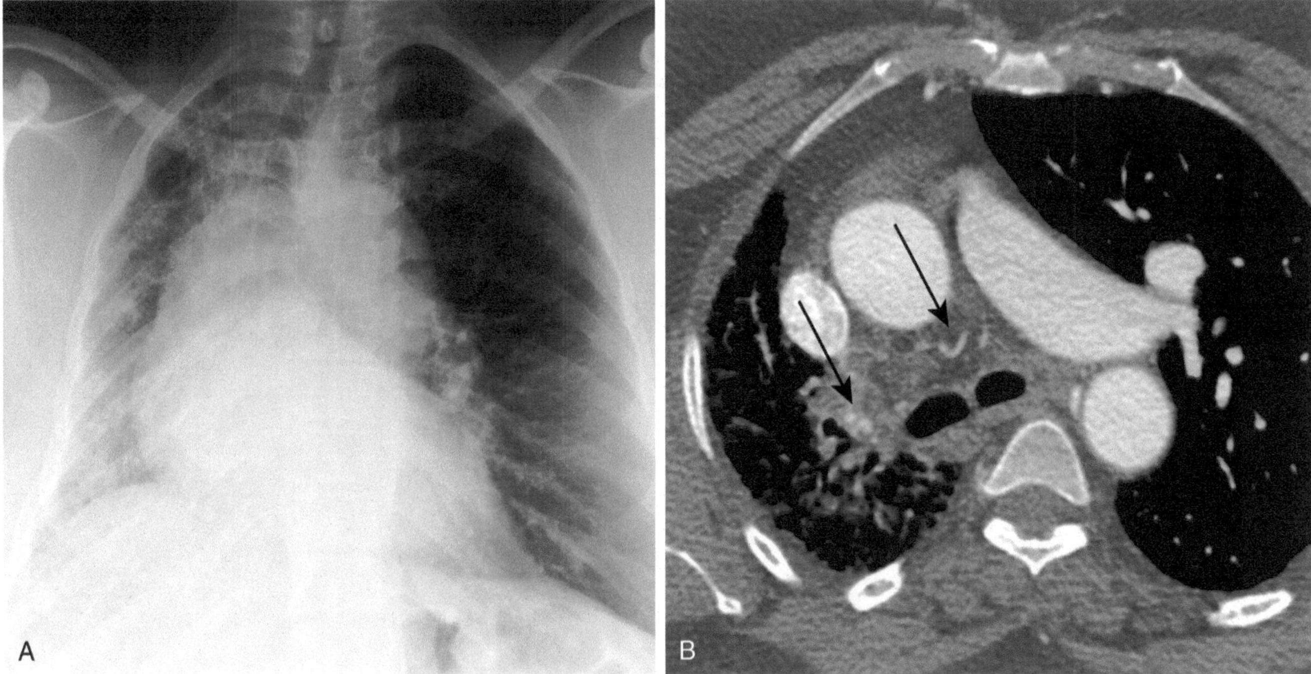

FIGURE 8.14 Proximal interruption of the right pulmonary artery. **A,** Posteroanterior chest radiograph depicts right hemithorax volume loss, rightward mediastinal shift, normal left-sided aortic arch and cardiomegaly. **B,** Axial contrast-enhanced computed tomography scan demonstrates absence of the right pulmonary artery with hypertrophied bronchial artery branches *(arrows)* supplying the right lung.

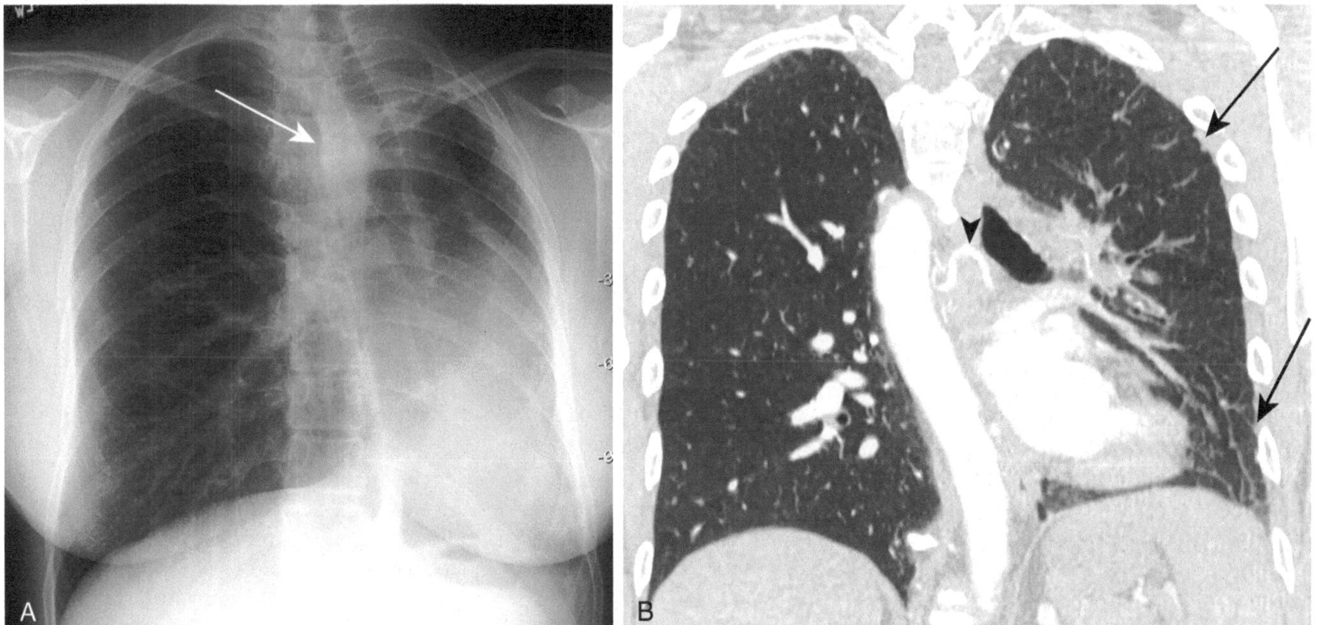

FIGURE 8.15 Proximal interruption of the left pulmonary artery. **A,** Posteroanterior chest radiograph exhibits similar but contralateral radiographic features to the patient in Fig. 8.14 and a right-sided aortic arch *(arrow)*. **B,** Coronal computed tomography lung window shows absence of the central left pulmonary artery, enlarged bronchial artery collaterals *(arrowhead)*, and reduced size of the left lung. Serrated pleural thickening and nodularity *(arrows)* are common in proximal interruption of the pulmonary artery and are associated with transpleural systemic collaterals from intercostal arteries. The interrupted pulmonary artery almost always occurs contralateral to the side of the aortic arch.

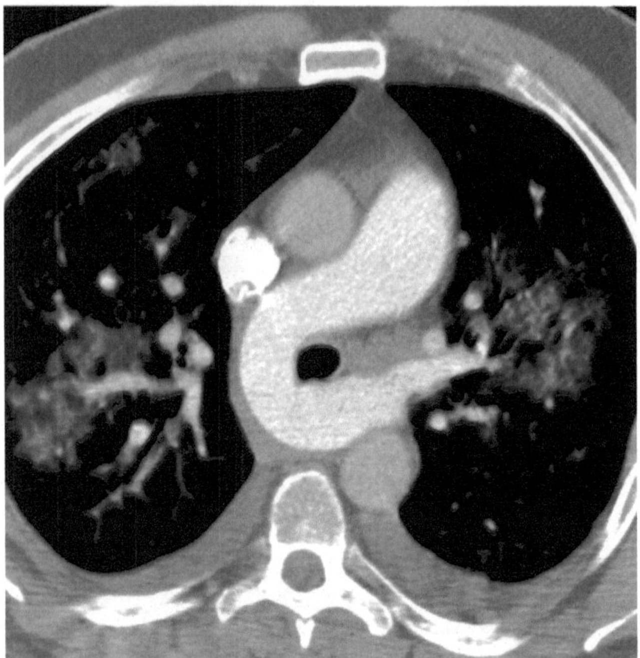

FIGURE 8.16 Pulmonary artery sling. Axial contrast-enhanced computed tomography scan shows the retrotracheal course of the left pulmonary artery, which mildly compresses the posterior wall of the trachea and compresses the esophagus. There are unrelated bilateral consolidation and small pleural effusions from pulmonary edema.

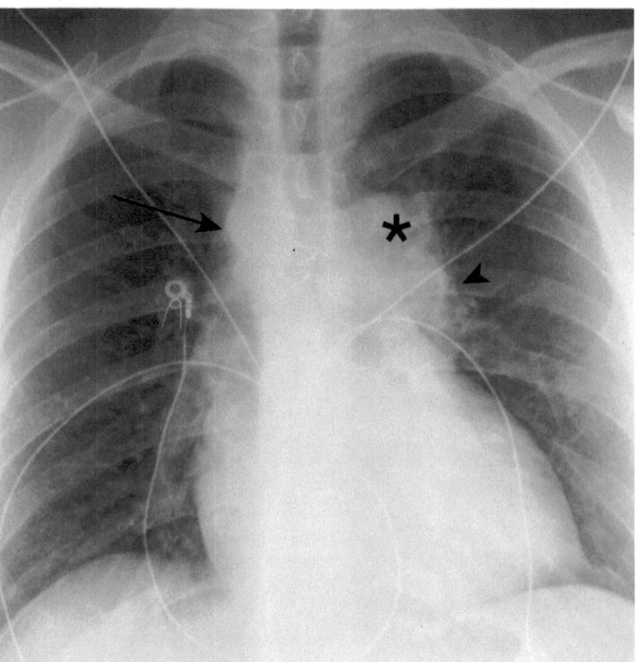

FIGURE 8.17 Pulmonary artery aneurysm. Posteroanterior chest radiograph in a patient with tetralogy of Fallot shows an enlarged main pulmonary artery *(asterisk)* and left pulmonary artery *(arrowhead)*. This represents a massive pulmonary artery aneurysm. There is a right aortic arch *(arrow)* seen in about 25% of patients with tetralogy of Fallot.

hypertension in up to 25%. Occasionally, patients may present with massive life-threatening hemoptysis.

Anomalous Origin of the Left Pulmonary Artery From the Right

Anomalous origin of the left pulmonary artery from the right (i.e., pulmonary artery sling) is an uncommon anomaly in which the left pulmonary artery arises from the posterior aspect of the right pulmonary artery. On its course to the left hilum, the anomalous artery passes between the esophagus and trachea. A "sling" is formed around the distal trachea and right main bronchus that may compress the right main bronchus and the trachea (Fig. 8.16). It may be an isolated finding or associated with cardiovascular anomalies or congenital tracheal stenosis, particularly the type caused by complete tracheal rings (the so-called ring-sling complex). Esophagram shows a focal impression on the anterior surface of the barium-filled esophagus in the region of the lower trachea. Ventilation-perfusion studies may show global hypoperfusion to the affected lung. Diagnosis can be easily established with contrast-enhanced CT or MRI.

Pulmonary Artery Stenosis or Coarctation

Pulmonary artery stenosis is a rare anomaly characterized by single or multiple coarctations of the pulmonary arteries, often with associated poststenotic dilation. Stenoses may be short- or long-segment, unilateral or bilateral, and may occur anywhere in the pulmonary arterial tree. This condition usually is associated with cardiac or other congenital anomalies.

The radiographic appearance varies depending on the location and number of stenoses. The pulmonary vasculature may appear normal, diminished, or increased. Main branch arterial stenosis may produce radiographic changes of diffuse oligemia to the supplied lung, as well as signs of pulmonary arterial hypertension and cor pulmonale.

Congenital Aneurysms of the Pulmonary Arteries

Congenital aneurysms of the pulmonary artery are rare and usually associated with other pulmonary abnormalities, such as arteriovenous fistulas or bronchopulmonary sequestration. Central pulmonary artery aneurysms are often the result of turbulent or increased flow associated with pulmonary valvular stenosis or patent ductus arteriosus (Fig. 8.17). See *Cardiac Radiology: The Requisites* for more information.

Anomalies of the Pulmonary Veins

Pulmonary Vein Stenosis and Unilateral Pulmonary Vein Atresia

Congenital pulmonary vein stenosis may occur in isolation or may be associated with other cardiac or venous anomalies (e.g., partial or total anomalous pulmonary venous connection). Pulmonary venous stenosis occurs on a spectrum of severity, involving long segments of the intraparenchymal pulmonary veins or localized stenosis at the junction of the left atrium and pulmonary vein. Stenosis or atresia is believed to occur from myofibroblastic proliferation in the walls of the pulmonary veins, leading to impaired return of oxygenated blood to the left atrium. Echocardiography and cardiac catheterization are frequently used in the diagnosis. Cardiac CT angiography (CTA) can also demonstrate pulmonary vein mural thickening, narrowing, or occlusion. Additional CT and radiographic findings may include pleural thickening, interlobular septal thickening, and reticulation in the lung drained by the affected pulmonary vein(s), representing

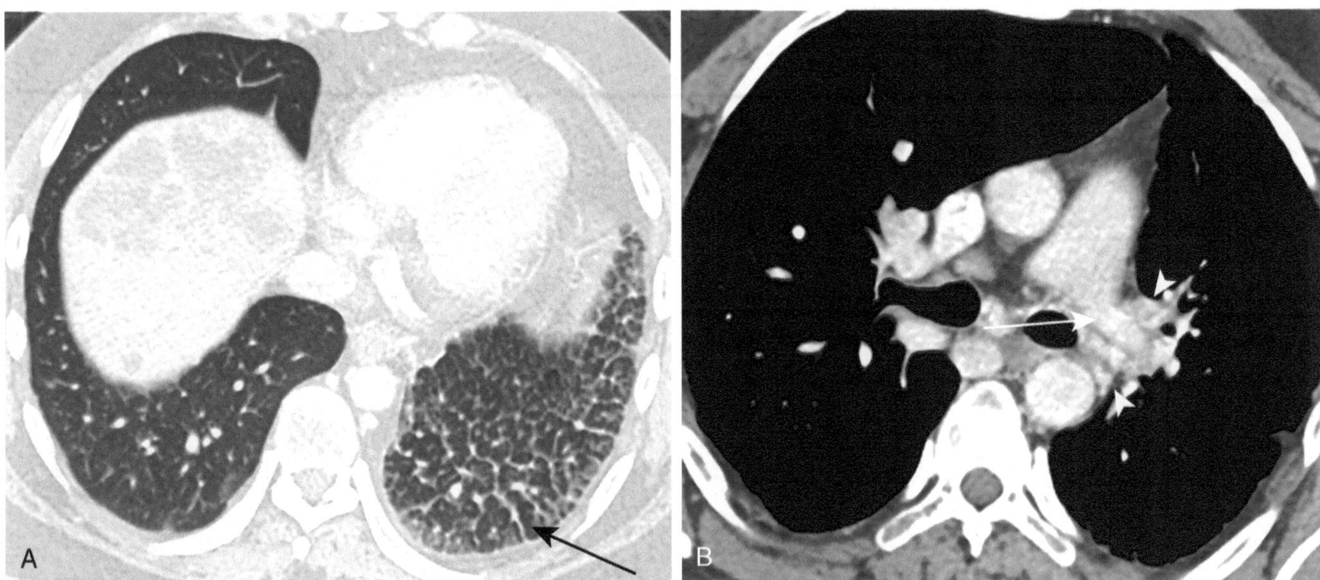

FIGURE 8.18 Pulmonary vein atresia. **A,** Axial chest computed tomography (CT) lung window shows left lung interlobular septal thickening *(arrow)* from chronic pulmonary edema caused by unilateral congenital atresia of the left pulmonary veins. **B,** Axial contrast-enhanced chest CT scan in the same patient shows a small left pulmonary artery *(arrow)* and numerous systemic venous collateral veins *(arrowhead)* connected to the pulmonary veins.

pulmonary edema and possibly fibrosis (Fig. 8.18). The ipsilateral pulmonary artery may be small in size.

Pulmonary Varix

A pulmonary varix is a rare localized enlargement of a segment of the pulmonary vein. It may be congenital or acquired. Acquired forms are caused by prolonged pulmonary venous hypertension, as seen in mitral valve disease. In the congenital variety, the varix occurs in a pulmonary vein that drains normally into the left atrium. Pulmonary varices are among the spectrum of features in Proteus syndrome. Although most patients with pulmonary varices are asymptomatic, there are rare cases of hemoptysis or dysphagia caused by pressure on the bronchi or esophagus, respectively.

Radiographically, pulmonary varices appear as smooth, rounded or lobulated masses of uniform density, frequently occurring in the lower lung zones, with the right greater than the left. A pulmonary varix may sometimes mimic a retrocardiac mass on chest radiograph. Contrast-enhanced CT or SSFP MRI can easily identify the vascular nature of the lesion, drainage into the left atrium, and characteristic venous phase peak enhancement (Fig. 8.19). The most important differential diagnosis is a pulmonary arteriovenous fistula. Contrast-enhanced CT should allow differentiation by demonstrating the absence of an enlarged feeding artery, enhancement during the venous phase, and drainage of the varix into the left atrium.

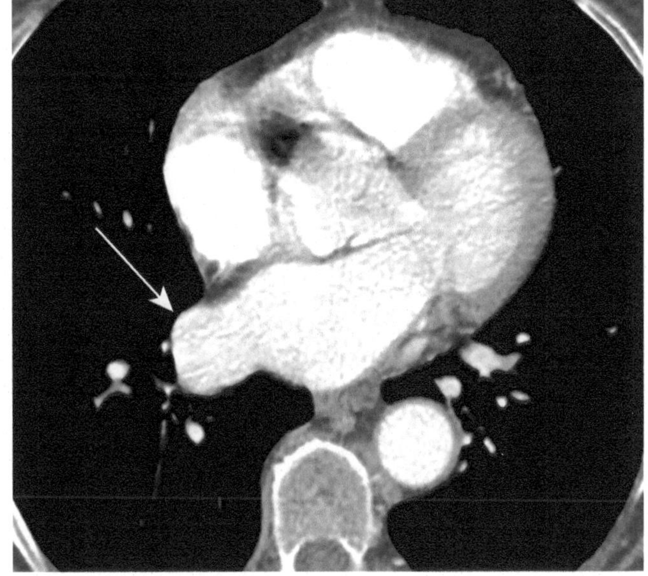

FIGURE 8.19 Pulmonary venous varix. Axial contrast-enhanced computed tomography scan shows an enlarged right inferior pulmonary vein *(arrow)* near the junction with the left atrium.

Meandering Pulmonary Vein

Rarely, pulmonary veins may take a variable course through the chest before draining normally into the left atrium. The abnormal course of the vein may have the radiographic appearance of anomalous pulmonary venous return; however, the vein ultimately connects to the left atrium. In such cases, the vein is referred to as a meandering pulmonary vein. Such vessels are usually discovered incidentally as isolated findings. Dilated meandering pulmonary veins may occasionally be detected on chest radiography as a solitary pulmonary nodule or prominent vessel with abnormal course but are best characterized by contrast-enhanced chest CT, which demonstrates the normal venoatrial connection of the meandering vein (Fig. 8.20).

Anomalous Pulmonary Venous Drainage

Anomalous pulmonary venous drainage is discussed in Chapter 9 of *Cardiac Radiology: The Requisites.*

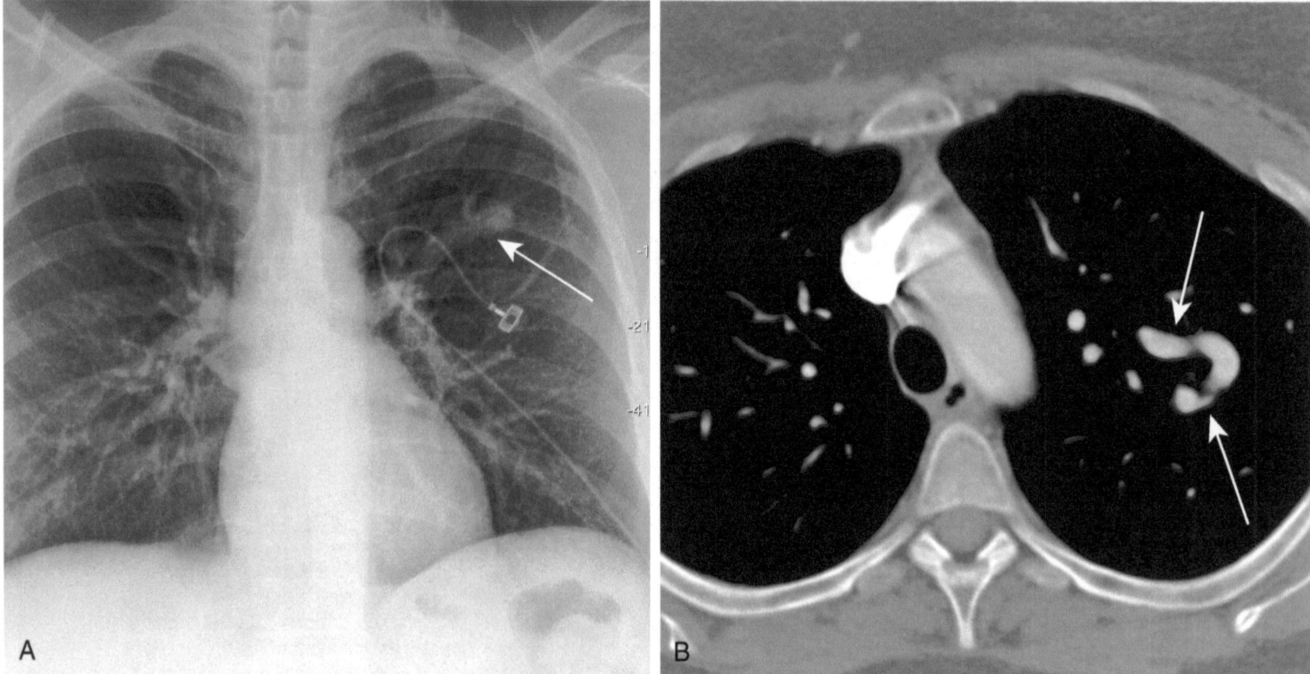

FIGURE 8.20 Meandering pulmonary vein. **A,** A tubular opacity *(arrow)* was detected in the left upper lobe on routine chest radiography. **B,** The patient underwent contrast-enhanced computed tomography scan, which confirmed the lesion to represent a dilated, tortuous left upper lobe pulmonary vein *(arrows)* that drained into the left superior pulmonary vein (not shown).

Anomalies Involving Arteries and Veins

Congenital Hypogenetic Lung Syndrome

Hypogenetic lung syndrome (also known as scimitar or congenital pulmonary venolobar syndrome) is a group of disorders of lung and vascular development that occur together. Although hypogenetic lung syndrome can occur on the left, it is almost exclusively a disorder of the right lung. The most consistent features of hypogenetic lung syndrome are anomalous pulmonary venous return of the right lung, which may be partial or complete, and pulmonary hypoplasia of the right lung, ranging from mild or severe. Hypogenetic lung syndrome is characterized by an anomalous pulmonary vein connecting the pulmonary veins of the right lung to the inferior vena cava (IVC), most commonly the infradiaphragmatic IVC just above the hepatic veins. The arterial supply to the right lung is often abnormal, with the right pulmonary artery reduced in size in 50% of cases and sometimes completely absent. Partial or complete systemic arterial supply of the right lung is common.

On chest radiography, the diagnostic feature is the identification of the anomalous vein coursing parallel to the right heart border that resembles a Turkish sword or scimitar (Fig. 8.21). The right lung is small in size, and there is cardiac dextroposition resulting from right lung hypoplasia. The degree to which the right lung is reduced in size and the degree of cardiac dextroposition depend on the severity of the pulmonary hypoplasia. There is decreased pulmonary vascularity in the right lung, and the unaffected left lung may become hyperinflated and extend across the midline anteriorly. Chest CTA clearly defines the anomalous pulmonary venous drainage, abnormalities of the central right pulmonary artery, and the systemic arterial supply to the right lung. Disorders of lobation and segmentation of the lung may be seen, including a bilateral left-sided bronchial branching pattern and a rare malformation referred to as "horseshoe lung." In horseshoe lung, the posterobasilar segments of the right and left lungs are fused across the midline by an isthmus of lung tissue crossing the mediastinum posterior to the pericardium and anterior to the aorta. There is an association of hypogenetic lung syndrome with pulmonary sequestration. Bronchial diverticula and stenosis may also be present and become a source for infection.

Systemic Arterial Supply to Normal Lung

Normal segments of lung may receive systemic arterial supply through anomalous systemic arteries (Fig. 8.22). Unlike pulmonary sequestration, the supplied pulmonary parenchyma and associated bronchi are morphologically normal. Furthermore, a normal capillary network develops around alveoli in this systemic arterial malformation, as opposed to the lack of an alveolar capillary network in pulmonary AVM, discussed subsequently. Venous drainage of the affected lung tissue is also normal. Systemic arterial supply to normal lung may represent a variant of the spectrum of pulmonary sequestration. Such congenital variants result in a left-to-left shunt, which rarely leads to congestive heart failure secondary to left ventricular overload and hypertrophy. Pulmonary arterial supply to the affected lung segments (typically the lower lobe) may remain intact or fail to develop. In patients who possess dual pulmonary and anomalous systemic arterial supply to the same lung segment, ligation or embolization of the anomalous vessel may be indicated to prevent hemorrhagic complications. Most individuals remain asymptomatic; however, life-threatening hemoptysis has been described.

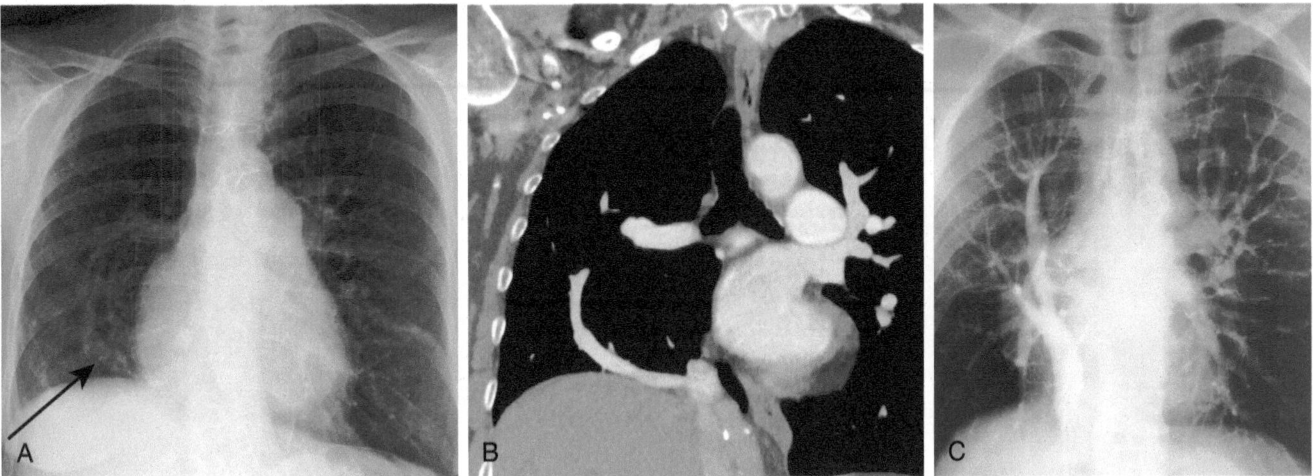

FIGURE 8.21 Hypogenetic lung (scimitar) syndrome. **A,** Posteroanterior chest radiograph shows an anomalous vessel *(arrow)* coursing toward the right hemidiaphragm. There is reduced volume in the right hemithorax associated with mild pulmonary hypoplasia. **B,** Oblique coronal contrast-enhanced computed tomography scan confirms venous drainage of the right lung by means of a single anomalous (scimitar) vein into the supradiaphragmatic inferior vena cava. **C,** Frontal image from a pulmonary angiogram in the pulmonary venous phase in a different patient shows anomalous pulmonary venous drainage of the right lung via the "scimitar vein" connecting to the inferior vena cava.

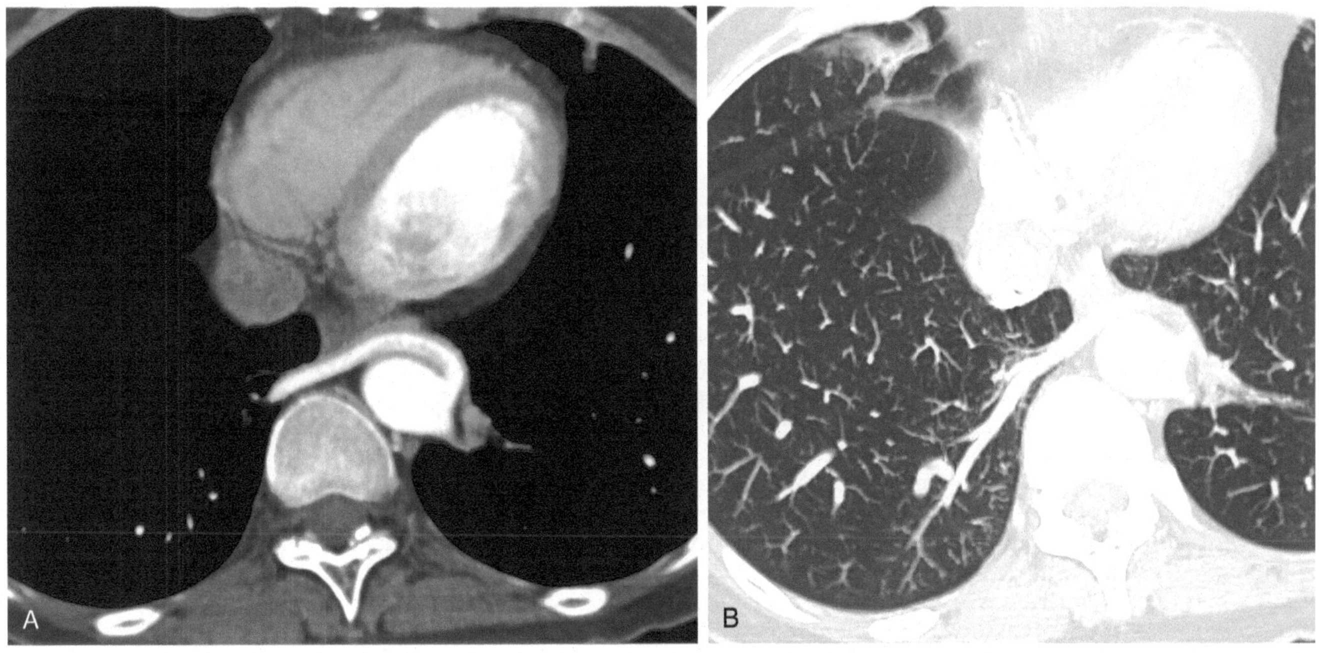

FIGURE 8.22 Systemic arterial supply to normal lung. **A,** Axial contrast-enhanced chest computed tomography scan shows a systemic artery arising from the descending thoracic aorta extending to the right lung. **B,** Axial maximum intensity projection image in lung window in the same patient shows the artery extending into normal right lower lobe lung parenchyma. This case is unusual in that the systemic artery arose from the contralateral aspect of the aorta and crossed the midline before supplying the right lower lobe.

Pulmonary Arteriovenous Malformation

A pulmonary AVM (arteriovenous fistula) is a direct communication between a pulmonary artery and pulmonary vein without an intervening capillary network. This direct communication between the pulmonary artery and vein results in a right-to-left shunt. Congenital pulmonary AVMs are thought secondary to a developmental defect in capillary formation. AVMs may also be acquired in patients with prior congenital heart disease, chronic liver disease, or certain infections such as tuberculosis or actinomycosis. Congenital pulmonary AVMs may be single or multiple (30%) or may be multisystem. Between 40% and 60% of patients with pulmonary arteriovenous fistulae have the inherited disorder known as hereditary hemorrhagic telangiectasia (Osler-Weber-Rendu disease), characterized by cutaneous and mucosal telangiectasias and occasionally arteriovenous fistulae in other organs. AVMs are classified as simple (80%)

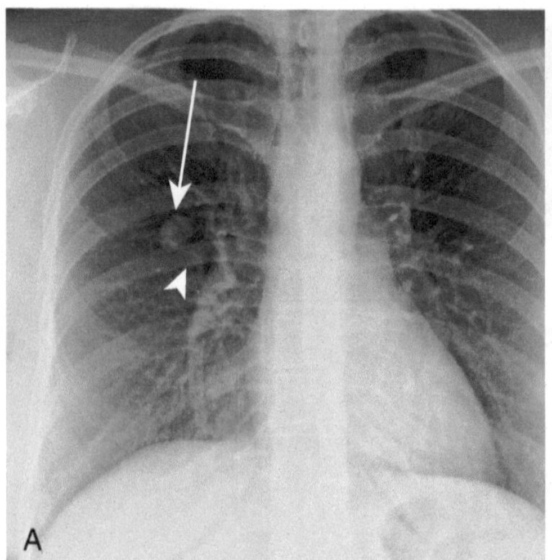

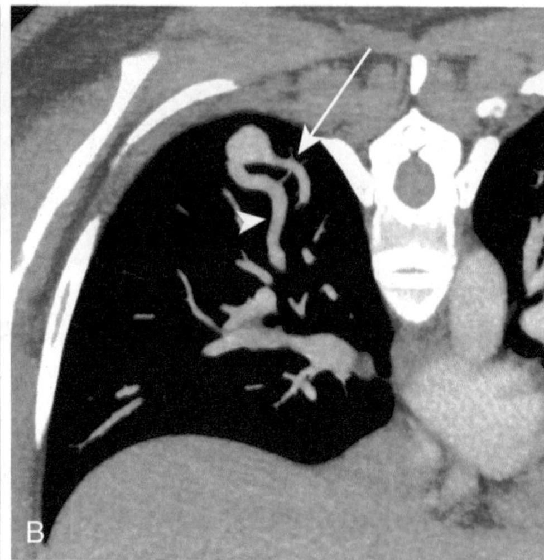

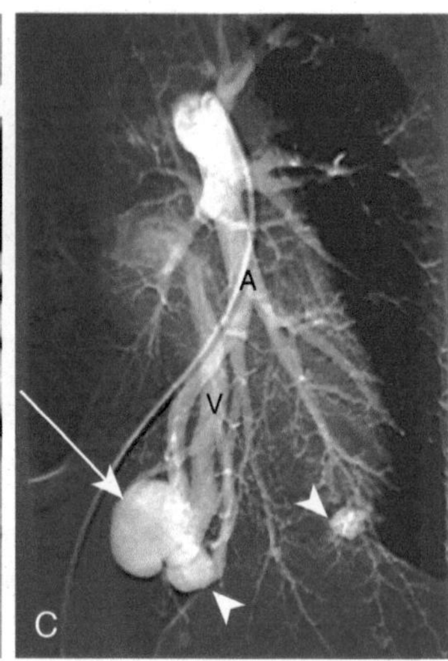

FIGURE 8.23 Pulmonary arteriovenous malformation (AVM). **A,** Pulmonary AVM is included in the differential diagnosis of a solitary pulmonary nodule *(arrow)* detected on chest radiography. Occasionally, a feeding vessel may be suggested on chest radiography *(arrowhead)*. **B,** Oblique coronal contrast-enhanced computed tomography scan clearly characterizes the feeding artery *(arrow)*, AVM, and draining vein *(arrowhead)*. **C,** Pulmonary angiogram in a different patient with hereditary hemorrhagic telangiectasia clearly depicts the arterial supply (labeled "A") and venous drainage (labeled "V") from a large left lower lobe AVM *(arrow)*. Note multiple smaller AVMs *(arrowheads)*. Angiography is not always required for diagnosis but may be used for therapeutic embolization of an AVM.

if there is a single feeding artery and a single draining vein; they are complex if there are two or more feeding arteries or two or more draining veins.

Most patients are asymptomatic, but cyanosis, dyspnea, and digital clubbing are the most common symptoms in the presence of significant right-to-left shunting. Central nervous system complications such as stroke and brain abscess may occur as a result of a paradoxical embolus through an AVM. Hemoptysis occurs in 7% of cases.

Chest radiography may depict single or multiple well-defined or lobulated nodules, representing the vascular nidus, typically in the medial or lower thirds of the lung. The feeding artery appears as a dilated vessel originating in the hilum, and the vein drains into the left atrium.

The classic morphology of pulmonary AVM (feeding artery, nidus, and draining vein) allows characterization by CT with or without contrast (Fig. 8.23). Pulmonary angiography historically has been the method of choice for the identification of the size, number, and architecture of pulmonary AVMs. However, multidetector CT with three-dimensional reconstruction is equivalent to angiography in the detection of small AVMs and in the delineation of the angioarchitecture before therapeutic embolization.

Congenital Anomalies of the Lymphatics

Four major types of developmental disorders affect the thoracic lymphatics: (1) pulmonary lymphangiectasis, characterized by rapidly fatal congenital anomalous dilation of the pulmonary lymph vessels; (2) localized lymphangioma, a multicystic lesion often occurring in the neck and mediastinum; (3) diffuse lymphangiomatosis, a proliferation of lymphatic vascular spaces in which visceral and skeletal involvement are common; and (4) lymphangioleiomyomatosis, a diffuse infiltrative lung disease characterized by haphazard proliferation of smooth muscle in the lungs and dilation of lymphatic spaces (see Chapter 18).

Lymphangiectasis

Because of the rapid fatality associated with pulmonary lymphangiectasis, affected neonates are seldom imaged, so it will not be discussed in detail here.

Lymphangioma

Lymphangiomas are focal masslike proliferations of lymphatic tissue characterized into three histologic subtypes: capillary, cavernous, or cystic. Lymphangiomas are discussed in Chapter 5.

Lymphangiomatosis

Lymphangiomatosis represents a more widespread, often multisystemic disorder with proliferation of infiltrating lymphangiomas, with a predilection for thoracic, neck and osseous (75%) involvement. In contrast to lymphangiectasis in which the lymphatics are dilated but normal in number, the primary abnormality in lymphangiomatosis is an increase in the number of lymphatics. Patients with lymphangiomatosis typically present later in life (late childhood) owing to a longer length of time and the hormonal changes required to produce growth and symptoms.

When confined to the thorax, the condition is referred to as diffuse pulmonary lymphangiomatosis (DPL). DPL manifests on imaging with diffuse, bilateral smooth thickening of the interlobular septa and peribronchovascular interstitium (Fig. 8.24). Diffusely increased CT attenuation of mediastinal fat is a frequent finding. Chylothorax, chylopericardium, and lytic osseous lesions are frequently found in association. On histology, there is proliferation of anastomosing lymphatic vessels in the pleural, interlobular septal, and peribronchovascular connective tissues. These lesions tend to exhibit progressive growth with compression of adjacent

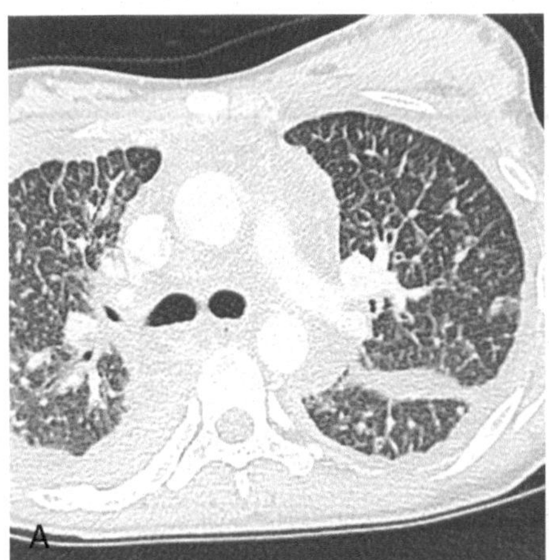

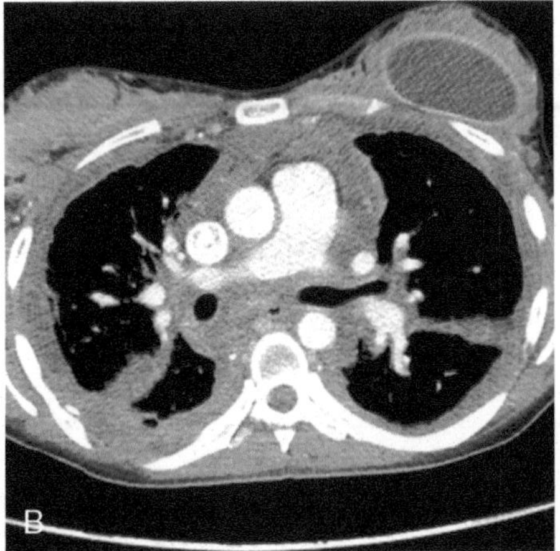

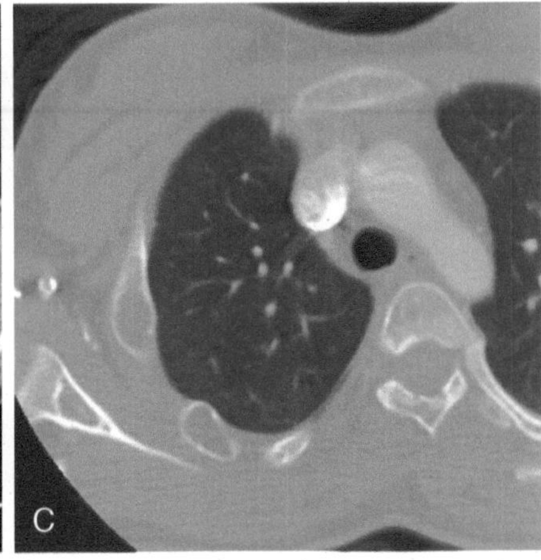

FIGURE 8.24 Diffuse lymphangiomatosis. Axial computed tomography (CT) scan in lung **(A)** and mediastinal **(B)** windows shows diffuse smooth interlobular and peribronchovascular interstitial thickening, pleural thickening and effusions, and mediastinal lymphatic infiltration in diffuse pulmonary lymphangiomatosis. **C,** Axial chest CT scan in a different patient shows expansile lytic lesions throughout the osseous structures, representing skeletal involvement of diffuse lymphangiomatosis.

structures. Complete surgical excision is seldom achievable, and lesions often recur. Other therapeutic options include percutaneous sclerotherapy. Cross-sectional imaging with CT or MR assists in defining the extent of the lesion as well as success of therapy. Lymphoscintigraphy may guide therapy and define lymphatic flow.

SUGGESTED READINGS

Barreiro TJ, Gemmel D. Accessory cardiac bronchus. *Lung*. 2014;192:821-822.

Biyyam D, Chapman T, Ferguson M, et al. Congenital lung abnormalities: embryologic features, prenatal diagnosis, and postnatal radiologic-pathologic correlation. *Radiographics*. 2010;30:1721-1738.

Boiselle PM, Ernst A. Tracheal morphology in patients with tracheomalacia: prevalence of inspiratory lunate and expiratory "frown" shapes. *J Thorac Imaging*. 2006;21(3):190-196.

Castaner E, Gallardo X, Rimola J, et al. Congenital and acquired pulmonary artery anomalies in the adult: radiologic overview. *Radiographics*. 2006;26:349-371.

Desir A, Ghaye B. Congenital abnormalities of intrathoracic airways. *Radiol Clin North Am*. 2009;47:203-225.

Dyer KT, Hlavacek AM, Meinel FG, et al. Imaging in congenital pulmonary vein anomalies: the role of computed tomography. *Pediatr Radiol*. 2014;44:1158-1168.

Eber E. Antenatal diagnosis of congenital thoracic malformations: early surgery, late surgery, or no surgery? *Semin Respir Crit Care Med*. 2007;28:35-366.

Ghaye B, Szapiro D, Fanchamps JM, et al. Congenital bronchial abnormalities revisited. *Radiographics*. 2001;21:105-119.

Gossage JR, Kanj G. Pulmonary arteriovenous malformations. A state of the art review. *Am J Respir Crit Care Med*. 1998;158(2):643-661.

Konen E, Raviv-Zilka L, Cohen RA, et al. Congenital pulmonary venolobar syndrome: spectrum of helical CT findings with emphasis on computerized reformatting. *Radiographics*. 2003;23(5):1175-1184.

Kothari NA, Kramer SS. Bronchial diseases and lung aeration in children. *J Thorac Imaging*. 2001;16(4):207-223.

Lee EY, Boiselle PM, Cleveland RH. Multidetector CT evaluation of congenital lung anomalies. *Radiology*. 2008;247:632-648.

Lee EY, Dorkin H, Vargas SO. Congenital pulmonary malformations in pediatric patients: review and update on etiology, classification, and imaging findings. *Radiol Clin North Am*. 2011;49(5):921-948.

Lee KS, Sun MR, Ernst A, et al. Comparison of dynamic expiratory CT with bronchoscopy for diagnosing airway malacia: a pilot evaluation. *Chest*. 2007;131:758-764.

Newman B. Congenital bronchopulmonary foregut malformations: concepts and controversies. *Pediatr Radiol*. 2006;36:773-791.

Porres DV, Morenza OP, Pallisa E, et al. Learning from the pulmonary veins. *Radiographics*. 2013;33:999-1022.

Raman SP, Pipavath SN, Raghu G, et al. Imaging of thoracic lymphatic diseases. *AJR Am J Roentgenol*. 2009;193(6):1504-1513.

Sandu K, Monnier P. Congenital tracheal anomalies. *Otolaryngol Clin North Am*. 2007;40:193-217.

Scalzetti EM, Heitzman ER, Groskin SA, et al. Developmental lymphatic disorders of the thorax. *Radiographics*. 1991;11:1069-1085.

Tsitouridis I, Tsinoglou K, Morichovitou A, et al. Scimitar syndrome versus meandering pulmonary vein: evaluation with three-dimensional computed tomography. *Acta Radiol*. 2006;47:927-932.

Walker CM, Wu CC, Gilman MD, et al. The imaging spectrum of bronchopulmonary sequestration. *Curr Probl Diagn Radiol*. 2014;43:100-114.

Woodring JH, Howard TA, Kanga JF. Congenital pulmonary venolobar syndrome revisited. *Radiographics*. 1994;14:349-369.

Woodring JH, Howard RS, Rehm SR. Congenital tracheobronchomegaly (Mounier-Kuhn syndrome): a report of 10 cases and review of the literature. *J Thorac Imaging*. 1991;6:1-10.

Yedururi S, Guillerman RP, Chung T, et al. Multimodality imaging of tracheobronchial disorders in children. *Radiographics*. 2008;28(3):e29.

Zylak CJ, Eyler WR, Spizarny DL, et al. Developmental lung anomalies in the adult: radiologic-pathologic correlation. *Radiographics*. 2002;22:S25-S43.

Chapter 9

Thoracic Lines and Tubes

Matthew D. Gilman

INTRODUCTION

Chest radiography serves a vital role in the management of critical care patients. Most patients in the intensive care unit (ICU) have at least one and frequently more than one device for central venous access, mechanical ventilation, hemodynamic monitoring, hemodynamic support, pleural drainage, or nutrition. The chest radiograph is an essential tool to assess these devices for proper position, to ensure proper function, and to avoid harm from malpositioned lines and tubes. Prompt recognition and reporting of malpositioning and complications are important to reduce morbidity related to thoracic lines and tubes. This chapter describes the use, proper placement, malpositions, and complications of the more common ICU monitoring and support devices.

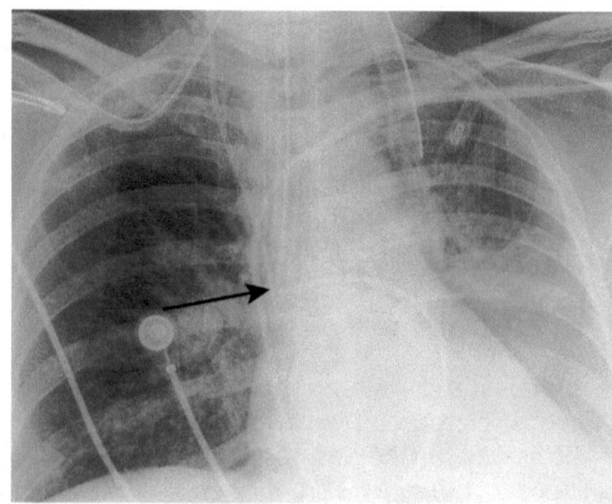

FIGURE 9.1 Right mainstem intubation. Anteroposterior chest radiograph shows the tip of the endotracheal tube *(arrow)* beyond the carina in the distal right mainstem bronchus. There is associated atelectasis of the left lower lobe.

AIRWAY TUBES

Endotracheal Tube

Endotracheal intubation is performed in patients who require airway protection, are hypoxemic, or are unable to sustain the work of breathing. The position of the endotracheal tube (ETT) is determined by measuring the distance from the tip of the ETT to the carina. In adult patients, the ideal position of the ETT is 3 to 7 cm from the carina with the neck in the neutral position. On each radiograph, assessment of ETT position is important because the ETT can move with changes in head position and with patient movement. The ETT can move up to 2 cm with changes in head position, and given the average length of the adult trachea is approximately 12 cm from the vocal cords to the carina, this potentially constitutes one third or more of the length of the trachea. In general, the "hose goes with the nose," meaning the ETT distal tip moves toward the carina with neck flexion and away from the carina with neck extension. Occasionally, on portable chest radiographs, it can be readily seen that the neck is in full flexion with the chin overlying the superior mediastinum. This information can be used to refine the interpretation of ETT position.

Complications of low ETT placement include bronchial intubation, most often right mainstem intubation because of the more vertical course of the right main bronchus relative to the left (Fig. 9.1). Bronchial intubation may lead to lobar or complete atelectasis of the nonintubated lung. Complications of high ETT placement include risk of extubation, injury to the vocal cords by the ETT cuff balloon, ineffective ventilation, and aspiration (Fig. 9.2). General complications of positive-pressure ventilation include barotrauma such as pneumothorax, pneumomediastinum, subcutaneous emphysema, and pulmonary interstitial emphysema (see Chapter 10). Tracheomalacia and tracheal stenosis may occur as delayed complications of endotracheal intubation.

Rare complications of traumatic endotracheal intubation include tracheal perforation, especially of the posterior membranous wall of the trachea. Perforation of the posterior membranous wall can also be associated with esophageal injury and mediastinitis. Rarely, hypopharyngeal perforation and tracheal rupture may occur (Fig. 9.3). Aspiration may occur at the time of intubation or when the ETT balloon cuff is deflated, at which time secretions may be released from above the cuff balloon into the lower airways. Rarely, aspirated foreign bodies such as teeth or dental work may be seen in the airways, esophagus, or stomach, particularly in difficult or traumatic intubations. Esophageal intubation is rare and manifests as an ETT to the left of the trachea rather than overlying the trachea. Air distention of the esophagus and stomach may also be seen due to esophageal insufflation by air (Fig. 9.4). Esophageal intubation can also result in esophageal perforation and manifest with pneumomediastinum. Today, esophageal intubation is rarely seen on postintubation radiographs because it is usually detected by auscultation or capnography, and it is usually corrected before the postintubation radiograph is obtained.

In addition to evaluating the ETT distal tip for proper positioning, it is also important to evaluate the size of the ETT cuff balloon. The ETT cuff balloon should fill the

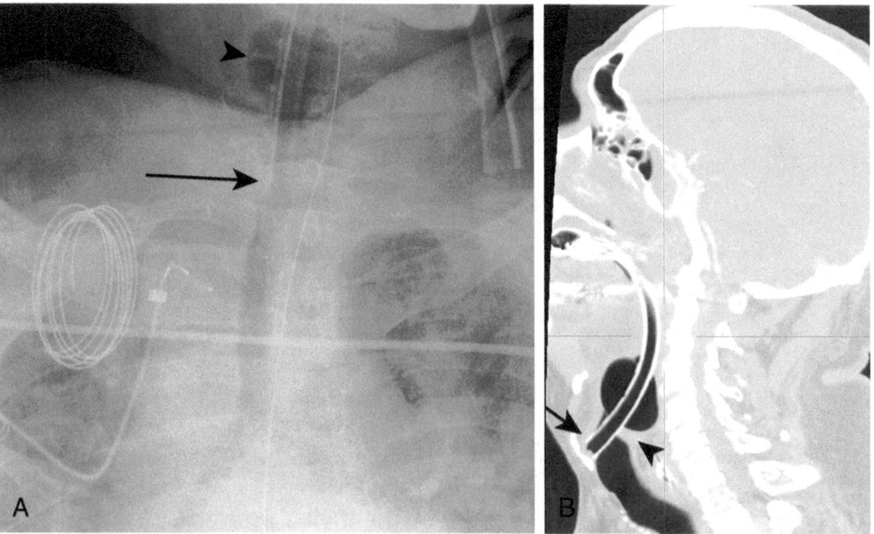

FIGURE 9.2 High endotracheal tube. **A,** Anteroposterior chest radiograph shows the tip of the endotracheal tube (ETT) *(arrow)* at the level of T1 measuring 11.5 cm above the carina. The ETT balloon cuff is overinflated *(arrowhead)*. **B,** Sagittal reconstruction from concurrent neck computed tomography scan in the same patient shows the ETT tip *(arrow)* just below the vocal cords *(arrowhead)*. The ETT cuff balloon is overdistended in the hypopharynx and is above the vocal cords.

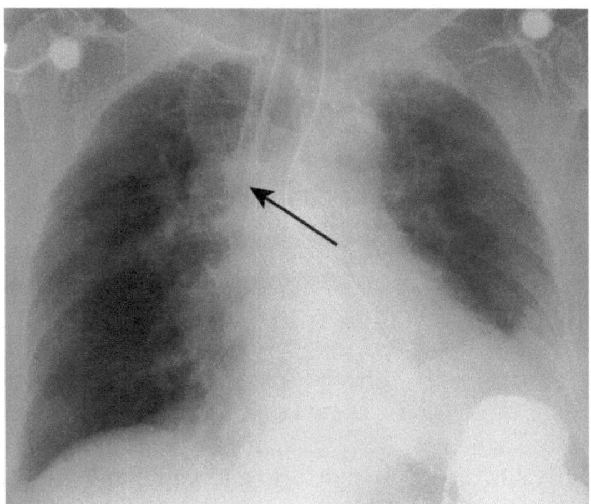

FIGURE 9.3 Tracheal rupture. Anteroposterior chest radiograph illustrates the radiographic findings of tracheal rupture, including overdistention of the endotracheal tube (ETT) cuff balloon, shortening of the distance from the balloon cuff to the distal tip *(arrow)*, and deviation of the ETT to the right. The ETT has perforated the wall of the trachea, and the distal ETT and cuff balloon reside in the right superior mediastinum. The distended cuff occluded the perforation of the trachea. When the ETT was removed, pneumomediastinum developed (not shown).

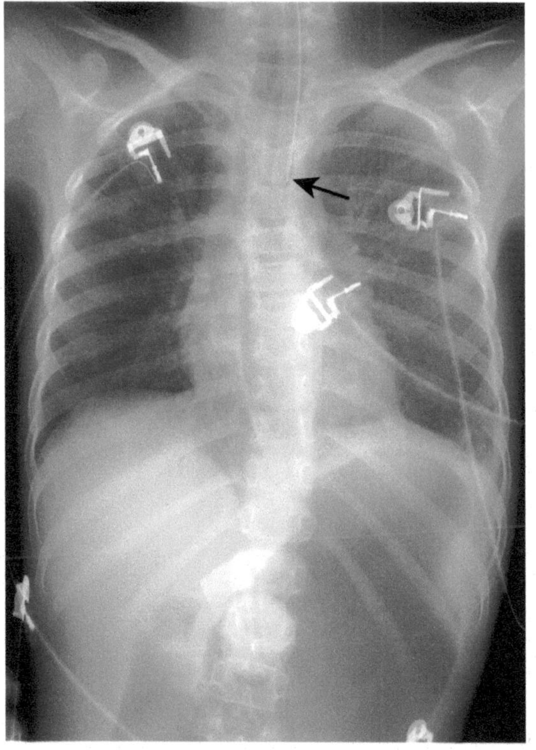

FIGURE 9.4 Esophageal intubation. Anteroposterior chest radiograph shows the endotracheal tube *(arrow)* external and to the left of the trachea with air distention of the esophagus and stomach.

lumen but not distend the tracheal wall. Overdistention of the trachea by the cuff balloon may cause ischemia in the tracheal wall, which could lead to tracheomalacia, tracheal rupture, or tracheal stenosis weeks to months after extubation. It has been reported in the thoracic surgical literature that when the ratio of the diameter of the tracheal cuff balloon to the diameter of the trachea is greater than 1.5, there is an increased risk of tracheal injury (Fig. 9.5).

Occasionally, a double-lumen ETT will be used for mechanical ventilation in cases requiring anatomic lung isolation. Such instances include controlled ventilation of one lung during thoracic surgery, unilateral lung lavage (e.g., alveolar proteinosis), in pulmonary hemorrhage, or in cases of severe infection to avoid spillage to the contralateral lung. For double-lumen ETTs, one lumen is placed in the lower trachea and the other lumen in the right or left main bronchus (Fig. 9.6). One ETT balloon cuff will be present in the trachea above the tracheal lumen orifice, and a second ETT balloon cuff will be in the intubated right

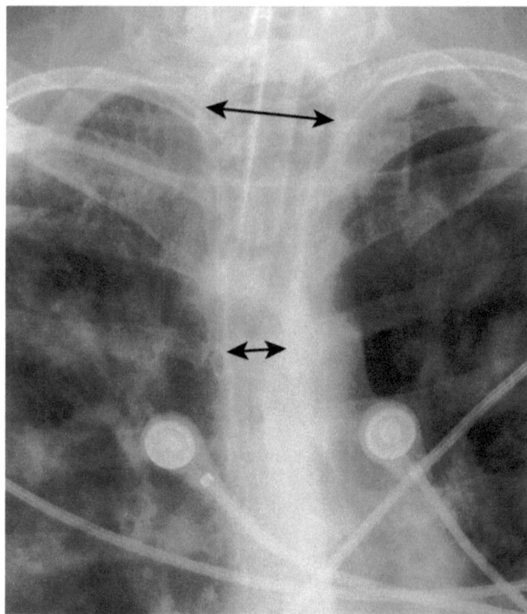

FIGURE 9.5 Overdistended endotracheal tube (ETT) balloon cuff. Anteroposterior chest radiograph shows the ETT cuff balloon diameter *(upper arrow)* exceeds twice the diameter of the normal trachea *(lower arrow)*. When the ratio of the width of the ETT balloon cuff to the width of the trachea exceeds 1.5, tracheal injury is more likely.

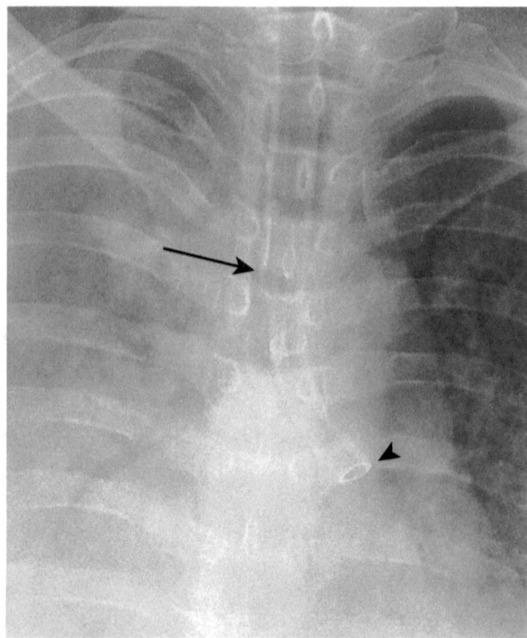

FIGURE 9.6 Double-lumen endotracheal tube (ETT). Anteroposterior chest radiograph shows a double-lumen ETT with right lung ventilation port in the trachea *(arrow)* and left lung ventilation port in the distal left mainstem bronchus *(arrowhead)*.

or left main bronchus. This isolates the lungs to separate respiratory circuits.

Tracheostomy Tube

Tracheostomy tubes are placed when patients require long-term mechanical ventilation. Unlike the ETT, the position of a properly secured tracheostomy tube is usually not affected by neck flexion or extension. Thus, a range of accepted distances of the tracheostomy tube distal tip to the carina is not usually used. An appropriately placed tracheostomy tube will be approximately one half to one third the distance from the stoma to the carina. A tracheostomy tube can move out if not properly secured, and this may be visible on chest radiographs. At the time of tracheostomy tube placement, a small amount of pneumomediastinum may be seen. A larger amount of pneumomediastinum at the time of tracheostomy tube placement raises the possibility of a tracheal leak or a tracheal or esophageal injury. Uncommonly, tracheostomy tube placement may result in pneumothorax. After a tracheostomy tube is removed, granulation tissue may result in tracheal stenosis at the cannulation site. Rarely, tracheostomy tubes can perforate the trachea or erode into an adjacent structure such as the innominate artery, leading to massive hemoptysis.

VASCULAR LINES

Central Venous Catheters

Central venous catheters (CVCs) are commonly used to provide central venous access for intravenous (IV) fluids, medications, nutrition, hemodialysis, and measurement of central venous pressure. There are four broad categories of CVCs: peripherally inserted central catheters (PICCs), temporary (nontunneled) CVCs, permanent (tunneled) CVCs, and implantable ports. The PICC is usually inserted by a forearm vein; the other central catheters are usually inserted via the internal jugular or subclavian vein.

The proper position of the distal tip of a CVC is in the superior vena cava (SVC) or at the junction of the SVC and right atrium (the cava atrial junction). Occasionally, a catheter tip is intentionally positioned in the superior right atrium for improved blood flow, particularly the dialysis catheters. In these cases, right atrial placement should be viewed with caution because of the potential for arrhythmias, cardiac injury, and valvular vegetations if the catheter is placed too low in the right atrium. Precise determination of catheter position on portable chest radiography is often challenging because catheter position is not fixed in location, and the catheter tip can move several centimeters with changes in patient position, arm position, phase of respiration, and radiographic technique.

Radiographic assessment of CVC position is important to ensure proper function of the catheter and to avoid catheter-related complications. Radiographs immediately after central line placement show malpositioned CVCs in about 30% of cases. Detection of catheter malposition requires detailed knowledge of the anatomy of the large and small thoracic veins, as well as variants in venous anatomy. Figure 9.7 shows the anatomy of the large central veins, with the line of demarcation between the axillary and subclavian vein at the lateral margin of the first rib. The small thoracic veins depicted in Fig. 9.7 are potential sites for catheter malposition, with the most common malpositions involving the azygous, internal mammary, and left superior intercostal veins.

Radiographic landmarks have been proposed to identify the cranial and caudal aspects of the SVC, although they are controversial and not always anatomically precise.

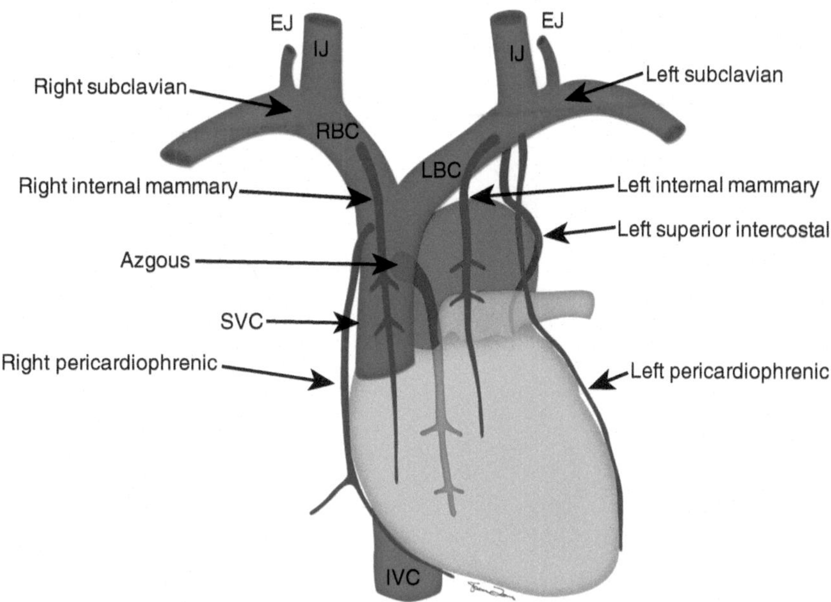

FIGURE 9.7 Thoracic venous anatomy. The lateral margin of the first rib is the demarcation between the axillary vein (extrathoracic) and the subclavian vein (intrathoracic). The subclavian veins join with the internal jugular (IJ) veins to form the brachiocephalic veins (left and right BCV). The brachiocephalic veins join to form the superior vena cava (SVC). The small thoracic veins that flow into the BCVs are illustrated, including the internal thoracic (internal mammary) veins, left superior intercostal vein, and pericardiophrenic veins. The azygous vein ascends into the mediastinum and extends over the right mainstem bronchus to insert into the posterior aspect of the superior vena cava. *EJ,* external jugular vein; *LBC,* left brachiocephalic vein; *RBC,* right brachiocephalic vein.

The use of specific anatomic landmarks is often limited by visibility, differences in patient positioning, rotation, and low lung volume technique. In most patients, the right first anterior intercostal space approximates the confluence of the brachiocephalic veins to form the cranial aspect of the SVC. However, a smaller number of patients have a very short SVC with a relatively low confluence of the brachiocephalic veins. For these patients, the right tracheobronchial angle may be a more accurate landmark (with the tracheobronchial angle defined as the junction of the right main bronchus and trachea). The junction of the SVC and right atrium (the cava atrial junction) can be approximated where the lower border of the bronchus intermedius crosses the right heart border. However, this landmark may not be anatomically precise in every case and is not visible on some portable chest radiographs. Although determination of the cranial and caudal aspects of the SVC may be imprecise on chest radiography, a catheter tip between the right tracheobronchial angle and 3 cm below the right tracheobronchial angle is almost always in the SVC.

One of the more common CVC malpositions is a catheter tip in the right atrium (Fig. 9.8). Subclavian catheters and PICCs can extend cephalad into the ipsilateral internal jugular vein. Catheters can also extend across midline and extend peripherally into the contralateral brachiocephalic or subclavian vein. Such catheter malpositions in the larger thoracic veins could lead to catheter malfunction, a less desirable location for infusion of substances requiring high flow, venous thrombosis, and delayed venous stenosis resulting from venous inflammation caused by the catheter tip or substances requiring higher venous flow to avoid venous irritation.

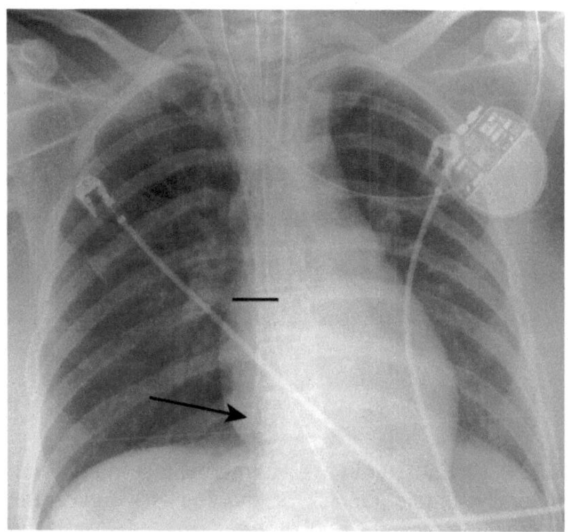

FIGURE 9.8 Central line in the right atrium. Anteroposterior chest radiograph shows a right central venous catheter extending beyond the superior cavoatrial junction (demarcated by a *horizontal line*) with its distal tip in the inferior right atrium *(arrow)*.

Central venous catheters can also extend into the small thoracic veins, including the azygous, internal mammary, and superior intercostal veins (Figs. 9.9 to 9.12). Catheters in small thoracic veins carry the risk of perforation, thrombosis, ineffective infusion, and ineffective venous blood return. Placement of a CVC in an artery is an urgent finding requiring prompt recognition and communication because of the potential for significant morbidity. Complications include bleeding, air or thrombotic embolus resulting in

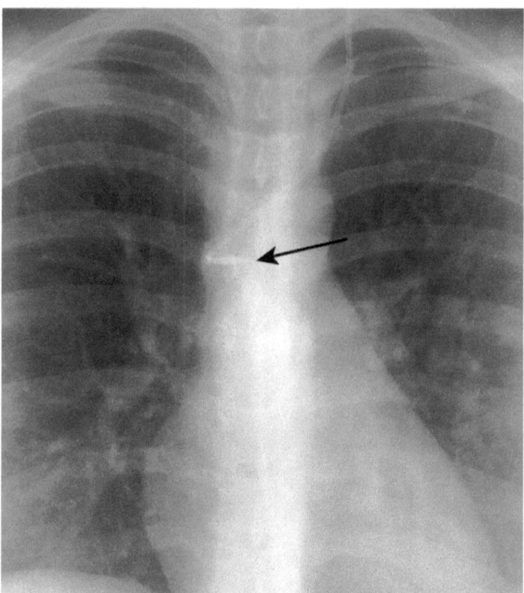

FIGURE 9.9 Catheter in the azygous vein. Anteroposterior chest radiograph shows the left internal jugular catheter tip is curved into the azygous vein *(arrow)*. The catheter extends from the superior vena cava into the azygous vein and extends posteriorly into the azygous arch.

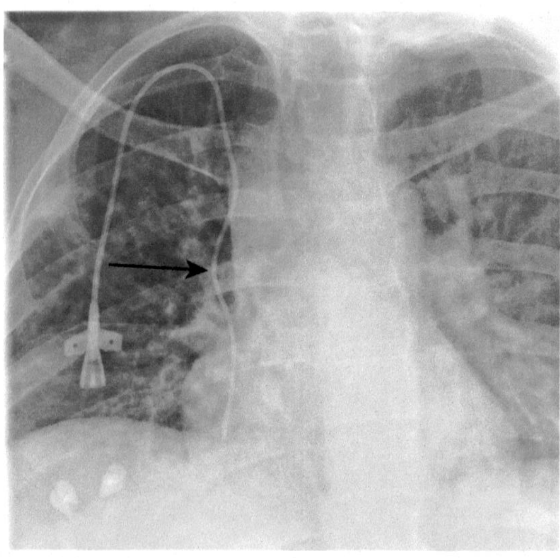

FIGURE 9.11 Catheter in the right internal mammary vein. Anteroposterior chest radiograph shows that the right-sided central venous catheter (CVC) is focally curved *(arrow)* at the level of the superior vena cava (SVC) and lies lateral to the SVC (extracaval). Normally, CVCs overlie the SVC and are not focally curved at this location. The focal curve and extracaval course have been termed the "extracaval shepherd's crook sign" and is a characteristic radiographic sign of right internal mammary vein catheter placement.

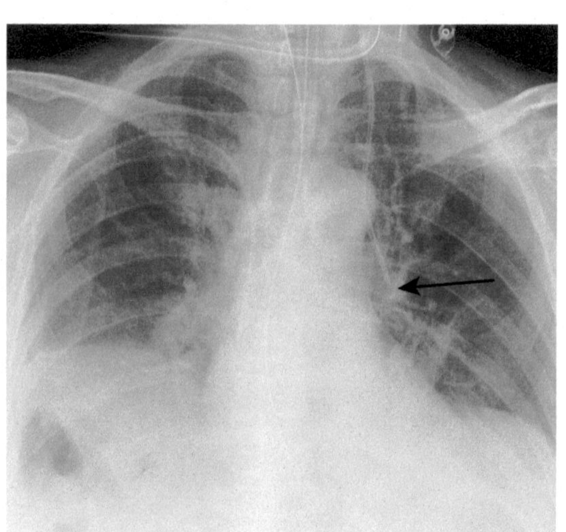

FIGURE 9.10 Catheter in the left internal mammary vein. Anteroposterior chest radiograph shows that the left-sided central venous catheter fails to cross the midline and terminates over the left hilum *(arrow)*. The appearance is consistent with placement in the left internal mammary vein, which was confirmed on chest computed tomography (not shown).

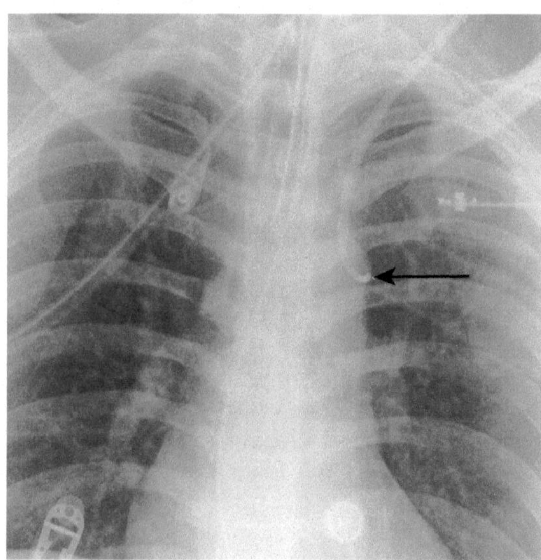

FIGURE 9.12 Catheter in the left superior intercostal vein. Anteroposterior chest radiograph shows that the left central venous catheter is curved lateral to the aortic arch *(arrow)* in the left superior intercostal vein.

stroke, and infusion of inappropriate substances directly to the brain (e.g., pressors or total parenteral nutrition). Arterial placement is sometimes but not always clinically suspected because of pulsatile flow through the catheter. Arterial placement is recognized on chest radiography by the course of a catheter that follows the anatomy of major arterial vessels rather than veins (Figs. 9.13 and 9.14).

Additional complications of CVC placement may include pneumothorax (up to 6% of lines), mediastinal hematoma, thrombosis, catheter fragmentation, catheter embolus, infection with line sepsis, endocarditis, and septic emboli (Fig. 9.15). An extravascular catheter or perforation of a vessel may manifest by mediastinal widening, development of an apical cap, or increasing pleural effusion caused by hemorrhage or infusion of IV fluid into the mediastinum or pleural space (Figs. 9.16 and 9.17). Left-sided catheters with a distal tip perpendicular and against the lateral wall of the SVC at the confluence of the innominate veins may place the patient at theoretical risk for venous perforation. Catheter narrowing or fragmentation may occur from compression between the first rib and clavicle, which has been termed the *pinch-off syndrome* (Fig. 9.18).

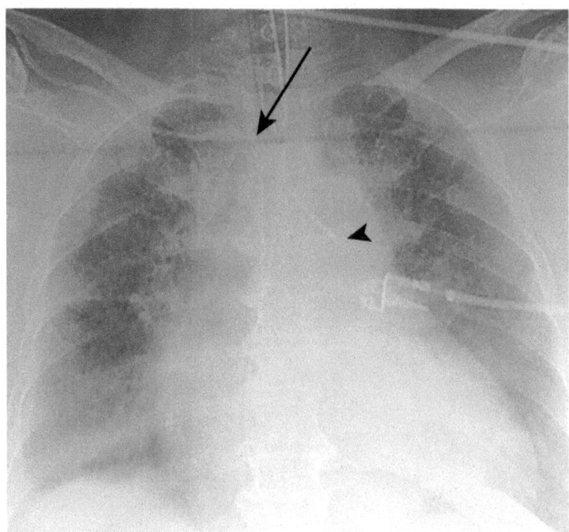

FIGURE 9.13 Arterial placement of right central venous catheter (CVC). Anteroposterior chest radiograph shows the right subclavian CVC courses superiorly away from the medial right first rib *(arrow)* and crosses the midline with the distal tip over the aortic arch *(arrowhead)*. The catheter follows the arterial course of the right subclavian artery and right brachiocephalic artery to the aorta.

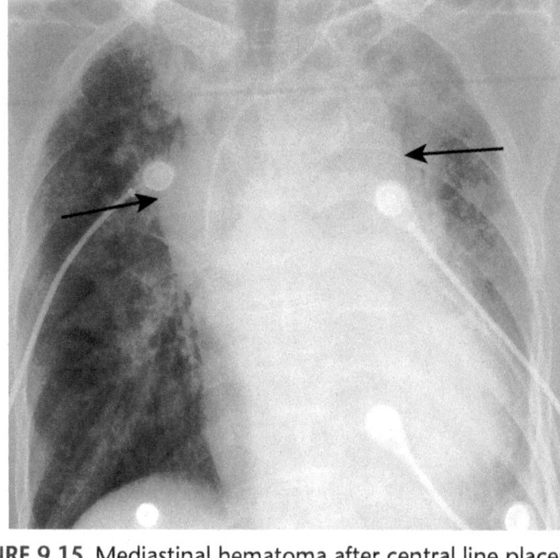

FIGURE 9.15 Mediastinal hematoma after central line placement. After difficult insertion of the left central venous catheter, an anteroposterior chest radiograph shows acute mediastinal widening *(arrows)* consistent with a mediastinal hematoma confirmed on computed tomography (not shown).

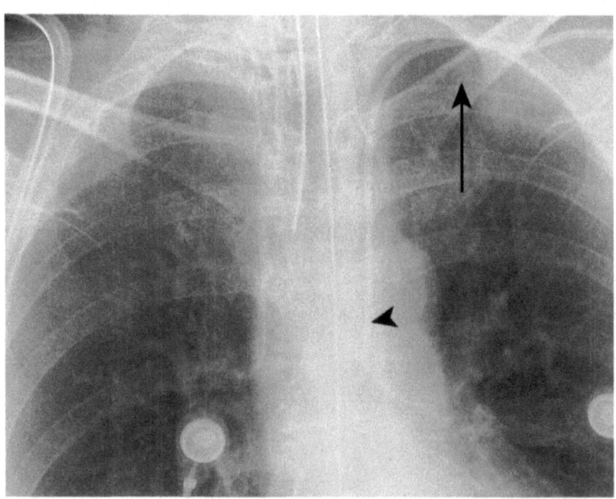

FIGURE 9.14 Arterial placement of left central venous catheter (CVC). Anteroposterior chest radiograph shows that the left subclavian CVC extends above the left clavicle *(arrow)*, descends overlying the left subclavian artery, fails to cross the midline, and terminates over the aorta *(arrowhead)*. The catheter is in the left subclavian artery and aorta.

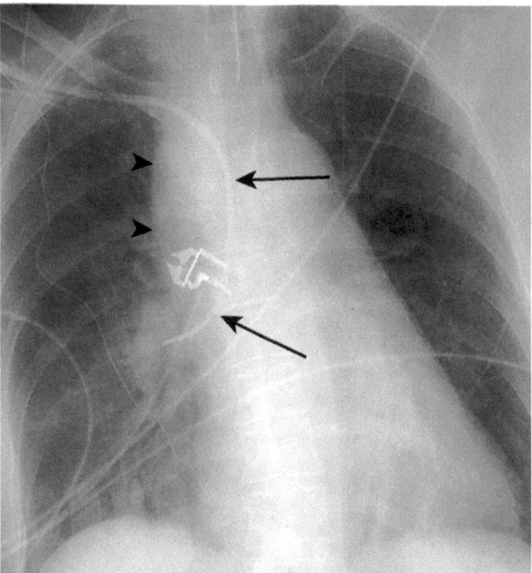

FIGURE 9.16 Extravascular catheter. Anteroposterior chest radiograph shows the right subclavian central venous catheter has a bizarre course *(arrows)* that does not conform to thoracic venous or arterial anatomy. There are acute thickening and increased density of the right paratracheal stripe consistent with hematoma *(arrowheads)*. The findings are consistent with an extravascular catheter with associated right paratracheal hematoma.

Pulmonary Artery Catheter

The pulmonary artery catheter (PAC) is a balloon-tipped catheter that allows measurement of pulmonary arterial, central venous, and pulmonary capillary wedge pressures. Cardiac output and systemic vascular resistance can also be calculated. This information can be used to monitor intravascular volume status and assess the cause of hypotension (e.g., hypovolemia, cardiac failure, or sepsis). With the balloon uninflated, the ideal location of the distal PAC tip is beyond the pulmonic valve and within the right or left main pulmonary arteries but no farther than the proximal interlobar or proximal left descending pulmonary artery. When the PAC balloon is inflated, the catheter tip and balloon will migrate forward to its wedge position.

Pulmonary artery catheters that are too proximal may be curled in the right atrium or right ventricle or extend into the IVC or hepatic veins (Fig. 9.19). Catheters located in the right heart will not be able to obtain proper pressure measurements and can cause atrial and ventricular arrhythmias. Pulmonary artery occlusion and pulmonary infarct can occur if the catheter is occlusive in a small pulmonary artery, if there is persistent inflation of the balloon, or if thrombus forms near the distal tip of the catheter (Fig. 9.20). Catheters that are located too distal can also result in pulmonary artery perforation, pulmonary artery rupture, or

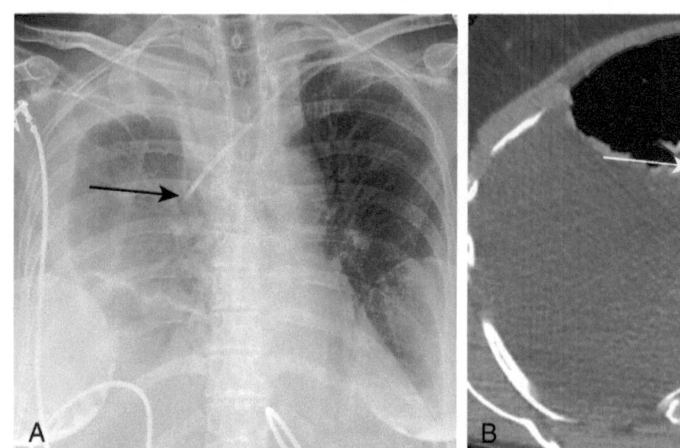

FIGURE 9.17 Catheter perforation of the superior vena cava (SVC) and infusothorax. **A,** Anteroposterior chest radiograph shows a left subclavian central venous catheter with distal tip lateral to the margin of the SVC *(arrow)*. There is a large right pleural effusion that increased in size after intravenous (IV) fluid infusion. **B,** Axial image from contrast-enhanced chest computed tomography shows the distal tip of the catheter external to the SVC *(arrow)* and a large low-density right pleural effusion from infusion of IV fluid into the pleural space (infusothorax).

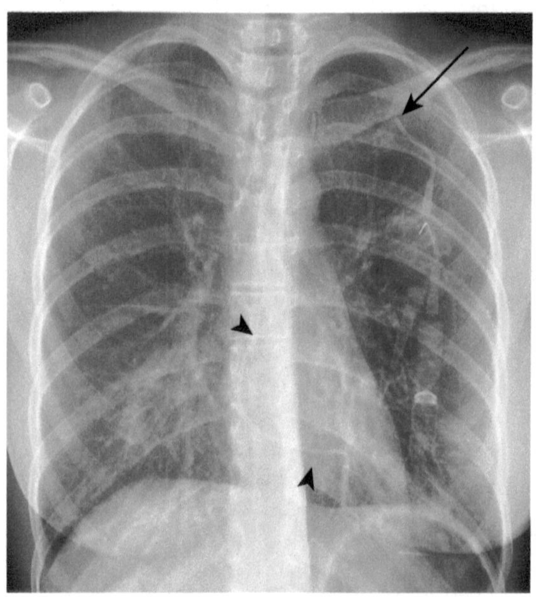

FIGURE 9.18 Catheter fracture with catheter fragment in the right heart. Posteroanterior chest radiograph shows fracture of the left-sided port catheter between the left first rib and clavicle *(arrow)* and a catheter fragment in the right heart *(arrowheads)*. The catheter fracture is likely the result of compression of the catheter between the first rib and clavicle, the catheter "pinch-off syndrome."

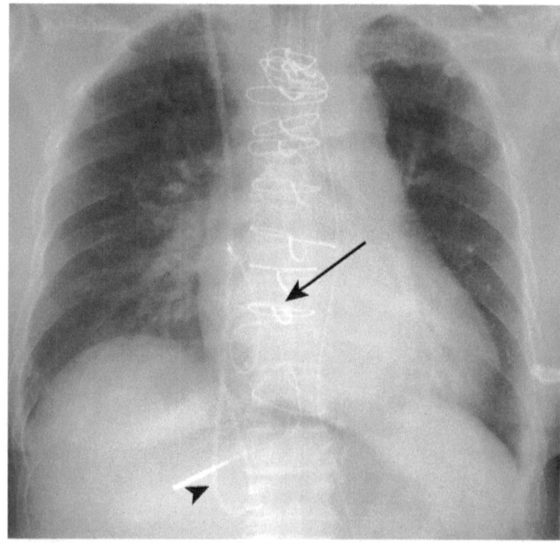

FIGURE 9.19 Pulmonary artery catheter (PAC) looped into the inferior vena cava (IVC). Anteroposterior chest radiograph shows the PAC distal tip in the right atrium *(arrow)* with a retrograde loop of the PAC extending into the IVC *(arrowhead)*.

pulmonary artery pseudoaneurysm (Fig. 9.21). Rarely, PACs can result in looping, knots, or cardiopleural perforation.

PLEURAL AND ENTERIC TUBES

Chest Tubes

Chest tubes are commonly used for evacuation of pneumothorax, pleural effusion, empyema, and hemothorax. The proper position of the pleural tube is determined by whether the tube is intended to evacuate fluid or air. In general, chest tubes placed for evacuation of pneumothorax are directed anterior and to the apex. Tubes placed for evacuation of fluid are placed posterior and in the base. Tubes placed for drainage of loculated collections are placed in the specific location of the collection, often under image guidance. In general, if the tube fails to drain the targeted collection, malposition is suspected, and additional imaging (such as CT) may be indicated.

For surgical chest tubes, the proximal side hole of the tube is located on the radiopaque line within the tube. The side hole is identified on radiography as a focal discontinuity in this radiopaque line. The proximal side hole should be within the confines of the pleural space. A proximal port outside the pleural space can be a source for air leak or extravasation of lytic or sclerosing agents into the soft tissues of the chest wall (Fig. 9.22). Chest tubes that are located within the fissure can be suggested by the lack of a gentle curve at the insertion site, horizontal course, oblique course, and a course directly at the hilum (Fig.

9.23). Because of its location within the fissure, a fissural chest tube has the potential for ineffective drainage. Rarely, intrafissural tubes may result in herniation of the lung into the lumen of the tube, resulting in infarction at the tube end hole or proximal side hole. Extrapleural placement of a chest tube into the chest wall or placement below the diaphragm may be suspected when the chest tube fails to adhere to the anatomic confines of the pleural space or when the tube fails to drain. Subdiaphragmatic chest tube placement could result in injury to abdominal organs, including the liver, spleen, and bowel (Fig. 9.24). Rarely, chest tubes may be placed within the lung parenchyma, resulting in pulmonary laceration, hematoma, hemothorax, infarct, hemorrhage, and bronchopleural fistula. Rarely, a chest tube may be placed into the mediastinum, with the potential for injury to the heart, esophagus, or great vessels (Fig. 9.25).

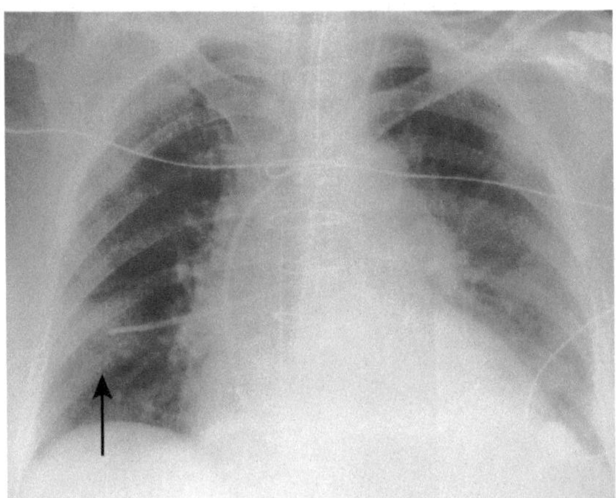

FIGURE 9.20 Peripheral pulmonary artery catheter (PAC) and pulmonary infarct. Anteroposterior chest radiograph shows a PAC extending well beyond the proximal interlobar pulmonary artery, likely in a small subsegmental pulmonary artery. There is a wedge-shaped consolidation distal to the catheter caused by a pulmonary infarct *(arrow)*.

Another cause of ineffective drainage includes kinking of the chest tube. This occurs more often with the smaller pigtail catheters but can also happen with the larger surgical chest tubes.

Nasogastric and Orogastric Tube and Feeding Tube

Nasogastric tubes (NGT) and orogastric tubes (OGTs) are frequently placed for administration of medication, nutritional support, or suction of gastric contents. Enteric tubes may be placed through the nose (NGT) or directly in the mouth (OGT). The proper position of an NGT or

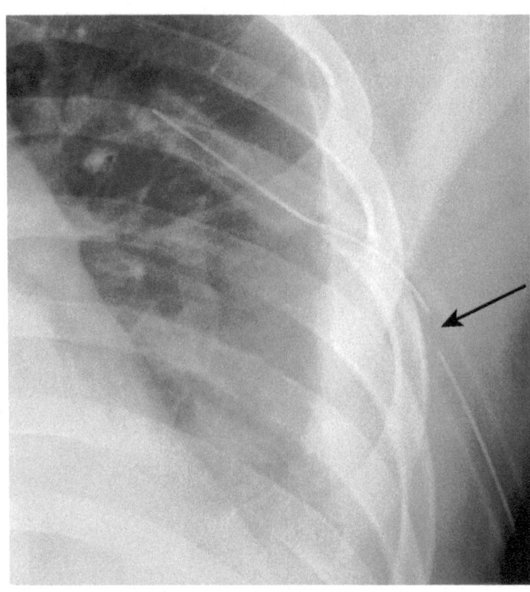

FIGURE 9.22 Chest tube proximal port external to the pleural space. Anteroposterior chest radiograph in a patient with a postoperative chest tube. The chest tube proximal port (side hole) is in the soft tissues of the left chest wall external to the pleural space *(arrow)*.

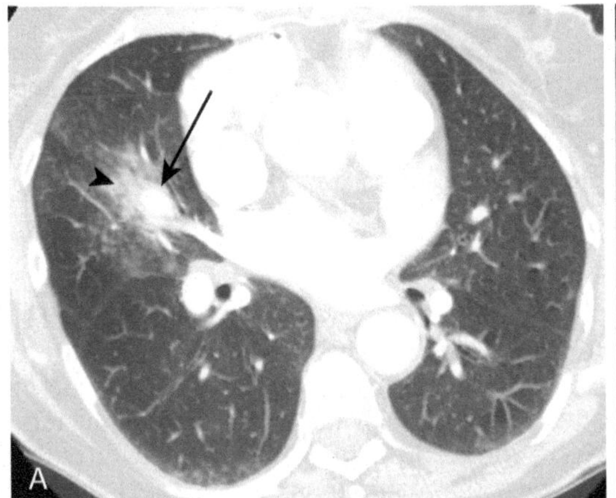

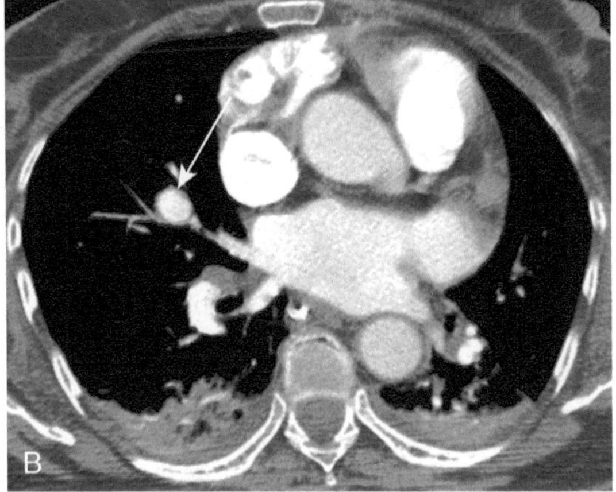

FIGURE 9.21 Pulmonary artery pseudoaneurysm from pulmonary artery catheter (PAC). **A,** Axial image in lung windows from contrast-enhanced chest computed tomography (CT) scan in a patient with a PAC in place and subsequent hemoptysis. CT shows pulmonary hemorrhage *(arrowhead)* adjacent to a pulmonary artery pseudoaneurysm *(arrow)*. **B,** Axial image from the same patient 1 day later shows the enhancing pseudoaneurysm adjacent to the distal aspect of the lateral segmental pulmonary artery in the right middle lobe *(arrow)*. The patient subsequently underwent catheter pulmonary angiography and coil embolization.

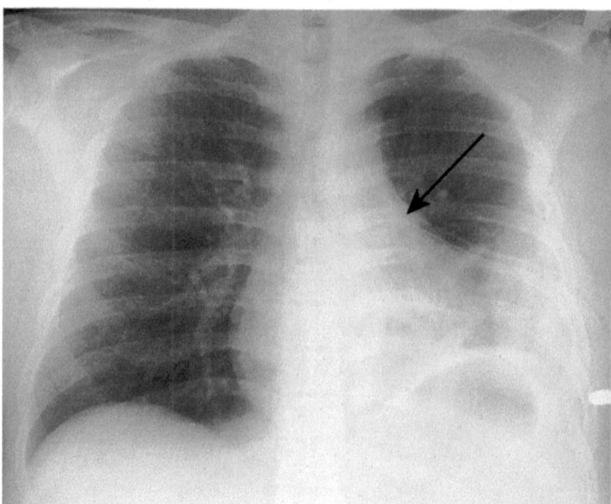

FIGURE 9.23 Fissural chest tube. Anteroposterior chest radiograph in a patient with chest tube placed for drainage of hemothorax. The chest tube is relatively straight, directed at the hilum *(arrow)*, and there was ineffective drainage of the left hemothorax. There is a bullet in the left chest wall.

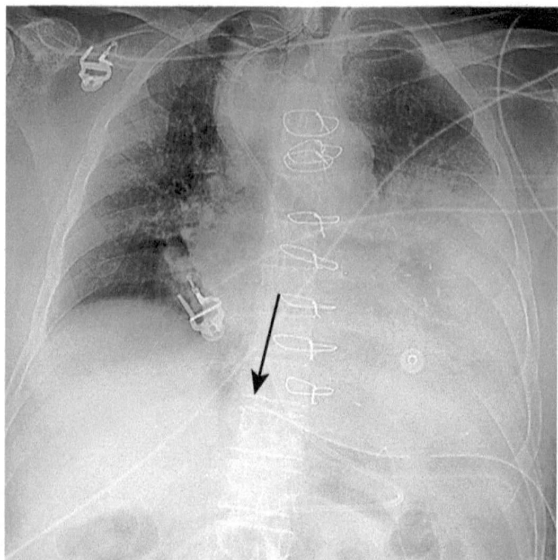

FIGURE 9.24 Subdiaphragmatic chest tube. Anteroposterior chest radiograph in a patient with left chest tube placed for parapneumonic effusion. The left chest tube is quite inferior in location and crosses the midline *(arrow)*, suggesting the tube is subdiaphragmatic. Clinically, there was no output from the chest tube, and the chest tube was confirmed to be intraabdominal on an abdominal computed tomography scan performed to evaluate for abdominal organ injury.

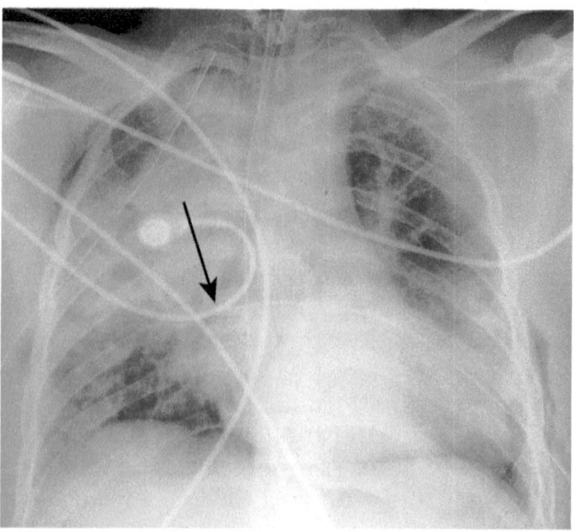

FIGURE 9.25 Mediastinal chest tube. Anteroposterior chest radiograph performed after tube and line placement in a patient after a motor vehicle accident. The left chest tube extends across the midline with the distal tip over the right heart border *(arrow)*. The tube was confirmed to extend from the left pleural space and across the mediastinum and to terminate in the right pleural space.

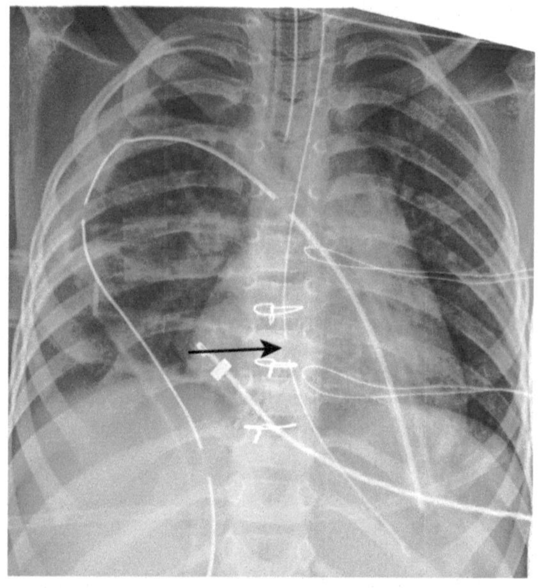

FIGURE 9.26 Nasogastric tube (NGT) proximal port in the distal esophagus. Anteroposterior chest radiograph shows the proximal port *(arrow)* of the NGT to be in the distal esophagus. Both the distal tip and proximal port should be below the gastroesophageal junction.

OGT is within the stomach with both the distal tip and proximal side hole beyond the gastroesophageal junction. When present, the proximal side hole is visible as a focal discontinuity in the radiopaque line of the enteric tube. If the side hole is present in the distal esophagus, it could be a source for aspiration or ineffective gastric suction.

The feeding tube is a smaller, flexible catheter often with a weighted tip. During placement, many feeding tubes require a wire stiffener, which is removed after insertion. The ideal position of the feeding tube distal tip is postpyloric in the second portion of the duodenum to minimize gastric residuals and risk of aspiration. However, location in the gastric antrum or other parts of the duodenum is often accepted.

One of the more common malpositions of the NGT and feeding tubes is placement of the distal tip or proximal side hole in the esophagus, which can be corrected by advancing the tube farther into the stomach (Fig. 9.26). NGTs and feeding tubes may be inadvertently placed into the tracheobronchial tree. In some cases, the NGT or feeding tube could extend into the bronchi (Fig. 9.27) or even the pleural space, with the feeding tubes at greatest risk for pleural perforation (Fig. 9.28). After removal of any pleural or parenchymal enteric tube, a chest radiograph should immediately be obtained because of the increased likelihood of resulting pneumothorax. Occasionally, NGT

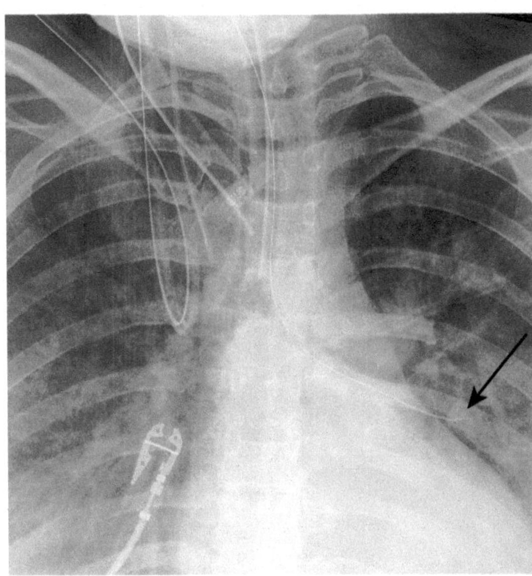

FIGURE 9.27 Nasogastric tube (NGT) in the left lower lobe bronchus. Anteroposterior chest radiograph shows the NGT in the trachea adjacent to the endotracheal tube, extending into the left main bronchus with the distal tip in the left lower lobe bronchus *(arrow)*.

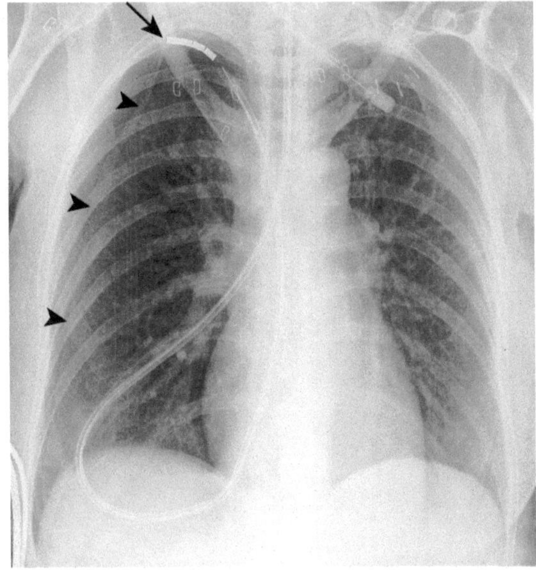

FIGURE 9.28 Feeding tube in the right pleural space. Anteroposterior chest radiograph shows a weighted feeding tube extending from the trachea, into the airways of the right lung, extending through the visceral pleura, with the weighted tip residing in the pleural space in the right apex *(arrow)*. There is an associated right pneumothorax *(arrowheads)*.

or feeding tubes may become coiled in the oropharynx or esophagus. Rarely, pharyngeal, esophageal, or gastric perforation may occur. Clues to such complications include development of pleural effusion after tube placement, pneumomediastinum, or pneumoperitoneum. Caution must be taken when considering placement of enteric tubes in patients who have undergone recent esophageal, gastric, or otolaryngologic surgery.

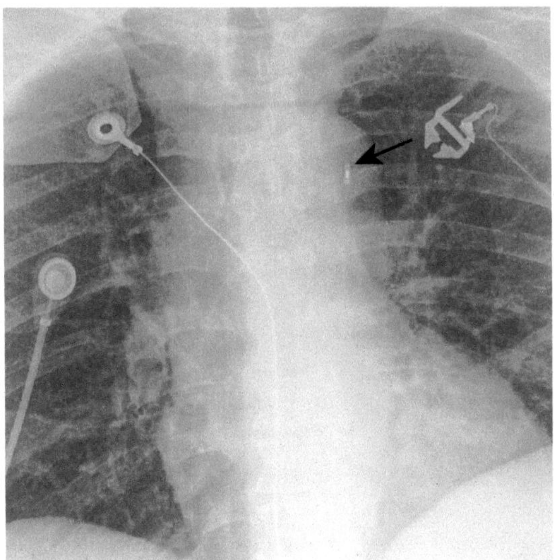

FIGURE 9.29 Intraaortic balloon pump (IABP). Anteroposterior chest radiograph showing appropriate positioning of the IABP with distal tip overlying the center of the aortic arch 1.9 cm below the superior aspect of the aortic arch *(arrow)*.

RESPIRATORY AND HEMODYNAMIC SUPPORT DEVICES

Intraaortic Balloon Pump

An intraaortic balloon pump (IABP) is a circulatory assist device that provides circulatory support to patients with cardiogenic shock and augments coronary perfusion. The IABP provides cardiac counterpulsation in which the balloon inflates during diastole and deflates during systole. Diastolic inflation of the IABP increases diastolic pressure in the ascending aorta, augmenting coronary perfusion, increasing the oxygenation of the myocardium, and thereby increasing cardiac output. Systolic deflation of the IABP decreases cardiac afterload, decreases left ventricular work, and decreases myocardial oxygen demand. The catheter is usually placed from the femoral artery retrograde into the descending thoracic aorta, where a balloon approximately 26 cm in length resides in the descending thoracic aorta. The superior position of the catheter is determined by a metallic tip visible on chest radiography. The proper position of the IABP distal tip is in the descending thoracic aorta distal to the origin of the left subclavian artery or approximately 2 cm below the superior aspect of the aortic arch on chest radiograph (Fig. 9.29). High catheter placement risks injury to the aortic arch, including dissection or pseudoaneurysm. Extension into the left subclavian artery or left carotid artery can also occur, resulting in intermittent occlusion, vascular injury, or emboli within the left common carotid, left vertebral, or left subclavian artery (Fig. 9.30). Low placement of the IABP may result in ineffective counterpulsation or intermittent occlusion of major abdominal aortic branches, including the superior mesenteric artery or renal arteries (Fig. 9.31). Aortic dissection is a rare complication and may be suspected if there is placement of the IABP along the lateral margin of the aorta, loss of definition of the descending aorta, or enlargement of the descending thoracic aorta (Fig. 9.32).

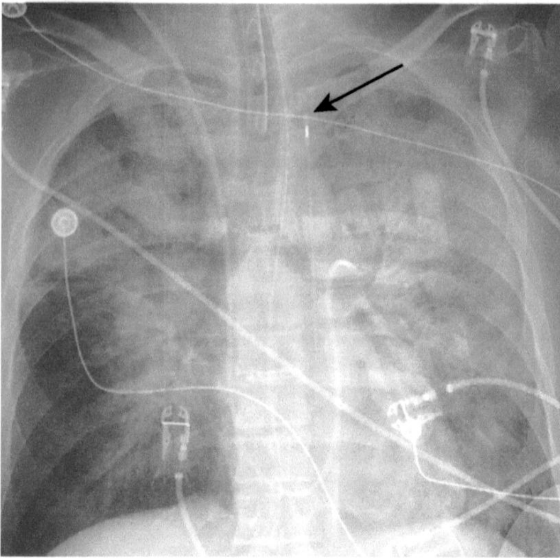

FIGURE 9.30 Intraaortic balloon pump (IABP) too high. Anteroposterior chest radiograph shows the distal tip of the IABP several centimeters superior to the aortic arch within the left subclavian artery *(arrow)*.

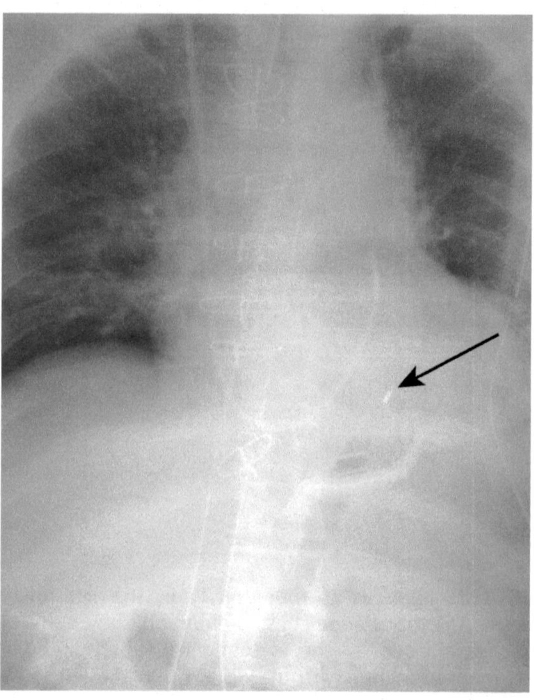

FIGURE 9.31 Intraaortic balloon pump (IABP) too low. Anteroposterior chest radiograph shows the distal tip of the IABP is too low, overlying the descending aorta at the level of the left hemidiaphragm *(arrow)*. Note that the IABP is inflated on this image. In this location in the lower thoracic aorta, there will be ineffective counterpulsation and intermittent occlusion of the superior mesenteric artery, renal arteries, and possibly inferior mesenteric artery.

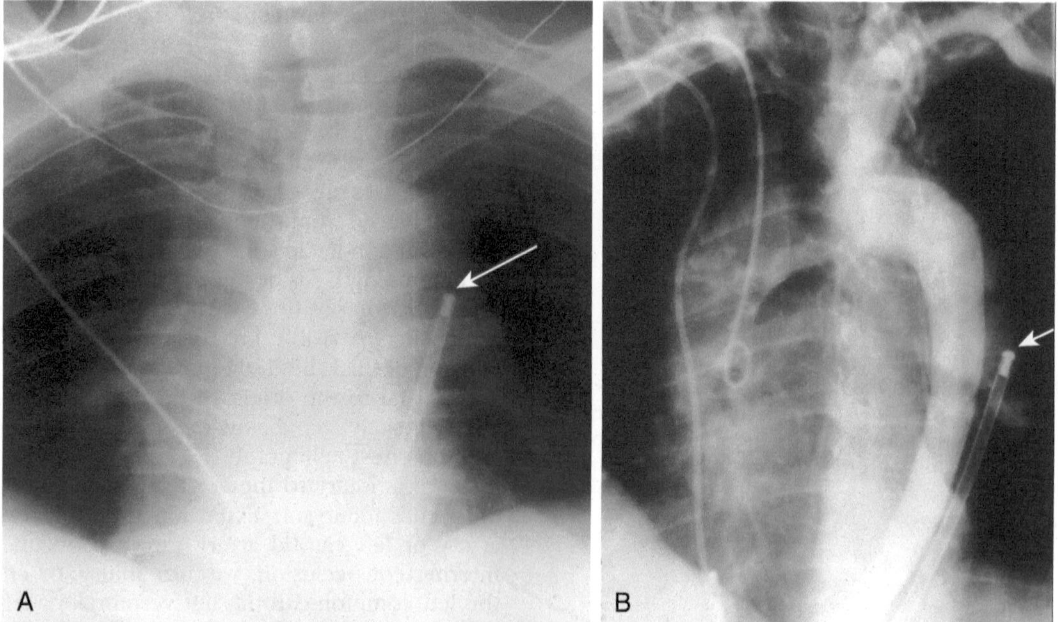

FIGURE 9.32 Aortic dissection caused by an intraaortic balloon pump (IABP). **A,** Anteroposterior chest radiograph shows an IABP overlying the descending aorta. The IABP is relatively inferior in location and overlies the lateral margin of the aorta *(arrow)*. **B,** Image from catheter angiography shows a contrast-enhanced true lumen and the IABP in the non–contrast-enhanced false lumen of an aortic dissection *(arrow)*.

Extracorporeal Membrane Oxygenation

Extracorporeal membrane oxygenation (ECMO) is increasingly being used in adult patients to sustain life in severe respiratory failure, cardiogenic shock, and failure to wean from cardiopulmonary bypass (CPB). The two most common forms of ECMO are venovenous and venoarterial ECMO.

Venovenous ECMO

Venovenous ECMO (VV ECMO) is used for patients with respiratory failure such as acute respiratory distress syndrome, severe interstitial lung disease, and lung transplants with severe graft dysfunction. VV ECMO may be used as a bridge to lung transplant or during recovery from acute lung injury. Several possible VV ECMO configurations may be used. In a femorojugular VV ECMO configuration, deoxygenated blood is withdrawn from a drainage cannula introduced into the femoral vein with distal tip in the IVC just below the IVC right atrial junction. The deoxygenated blood is sent to the oxygenator, and the oxygenated blood is returned by a return cannula introduced into the internal jugular vein with the distal tip at the SVC–right atrial junction (Fig. 9.33). Femorofemoral VV ECMO is less commonly seen, in which a drainage cannula is placed into the femoral vein with the distal tip in the lower IVC above the bifurcation of the iliac veins. The return cannula is placed in the ipsilateral or contralateral femoral vein with the distal tip in the right atrium.

Bicaval dual-lumen VV ECMO cannulas are also available, in which deoxygenated blood is withdrawn and oxygenated blood returned via one cannula containing two lumens (one lumen for drainage and one lumen for return). In these dual-lumen VV ECMO cannulas, the cannula enters the right internal jugular vein and extends through the right brachiocephalic vein, through the SVC, and through the right atrium, with the distal tip residing in the IVC (Fig. 9.34). Deoxygenated blood is withdrawn from side holes positioned in the SVC and IVC (i.e., bicaval). Oxygenated blood is returned through a return side port positioned in the right atrium and directed toward the tricuspid valve. Less commonly, a bicaval dual-lumen ECMO cannula may be placed from below through the IVC, through the right atrium, with the distal tip in the SVC. In VV ECMO, the drainage and return of blood are entirely right sided, and aortic blood flow is normal (anterograde).

Venoarterial Extracorporeal Membrane Oxygenation

Venoarterial ECMO (VA ECMO) is used for patients with severe cardiac failure and cardiogenic shock. Whereas VV ECMO provides only respiratory support, VA ECMO provides both hemodynamic and respiratory support. In VA ECMO, the withdrawal of deoxygenated blood is from the right side (venous), and the return of oxygenated blood is to the left side (arterial).

In central VA ECMO, cannulas are placed directly into the right atrium (drainage cannula) and ascending aorta (return cannula) through an open sternum at the time of

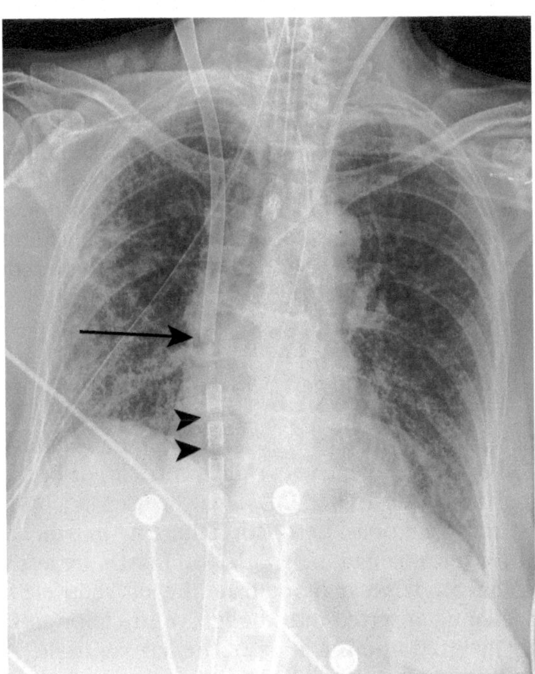

FIGURE 9.33 Misplaced venovenous extracorporeal membrane oxygenation (ECMO) access cannula. Anteroposterior chest radiograph shows the return cannula for oxygenated blood terminating in the lower superior vena cava *(arrow)*. The drainage cannula for withdrawal of deoxygenated blood has its distal tip and side holes in the right atrium *(arrowheads)*. For venovenous ECMO, the access cannula would ideally be in the inferior vena cava (IVC) just below the IVC right atrial junction. In this case, positioning of the access cannula in the right atrium below the return cannula allows recirculation of oxygenated blood through the ECMO circuit.

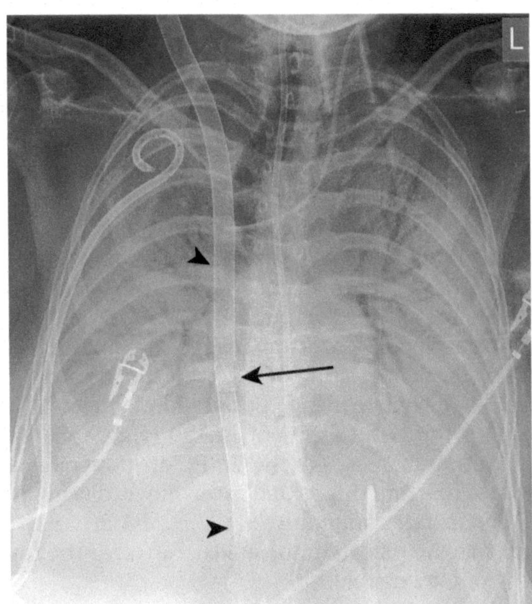

FIGURE 9.34 Bicaval dual-lumen venovenous extracorporeal membrane oxygenation (ECMO) cannula. Anteroposterior chest radiograph in a patient with severe acute respiratory distress syndrome. A bicaval dual-lumen ECMO cannula extends through the right internal jugular vein, brachiocephalic vein, superior vena cava (SVC), and right atrium with distal tip in the inferior vena cava (IVC). Side holes in the SVC and IVC *(arrowheads)* serve as the access holes through which deoxygenated blood is withdrawn and sent to the oxygenator. The return port for oxygenated blood is positioned in the right atrium directed toward the tricuspid valve *(arrow)*.

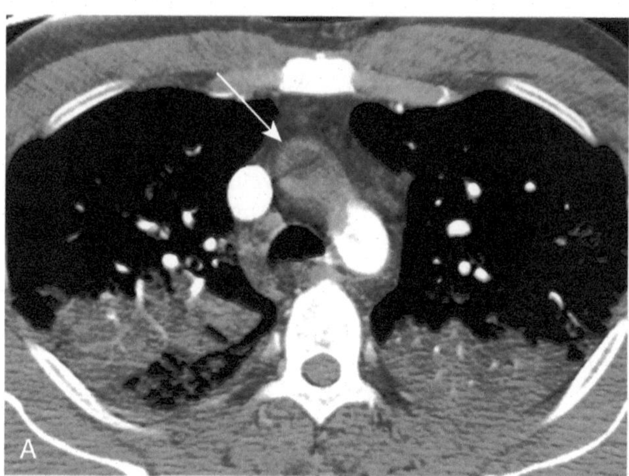

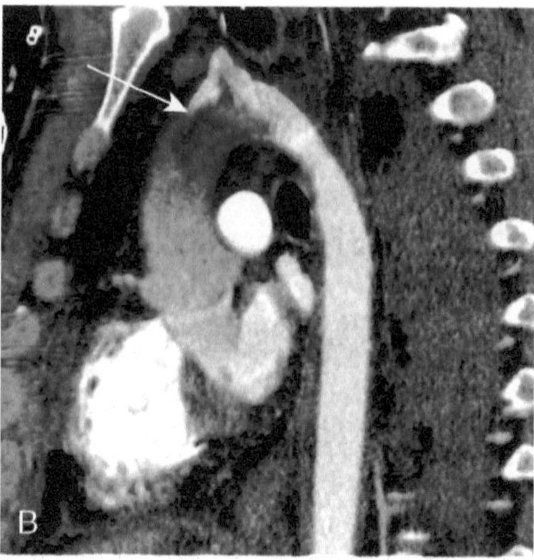

FIGURE 9.35 Flow artifact associated with venoarterial extracorporeal membrane oxygenation (VA ECMO). **A,** Axial contrast-enhanced computed tomography (CT) image from CT pulmonary angiography in a patient on VA ECMO. There are dense contrast in the superior vena cava from right internal jugular injection of contrast, contrast in the pulmonary arteries, and contrast in the distal aortic arch from retrograde flow up the aorta from a VA ECMO return catheter in the common iliac artery (not shown). There is low attenuation in the ascending aorta *(arrow)* in this early phase of imaging. **B,** Sagittal CT image of the aorta from the same patient shows heterogeneous low attenuation in the ascending aorta *(arrow)*, which could be intraaortic thrombus or mixing artifact associated with VA ECMO. In this case, no intraaortic thrombus was found at the time of surgery for pulmonary artery thromboendarterectomy for pulmonary embolism (not shown), confirming this finding represented mixing artifact associated with VA ECMO.

cardiac surgery. Central VA ECMO is typically seen in the context of failure to wean from CPB after cardiac surgery.

In peripheral VA ECMO, withdrawal of deoxygenated blood (drainage cannula) is often by a cannula placed into the femoral vein extending through the IVC, through the right atrium, with the distal tip at the junction of the SVC and right atrium. Blood is sent to the oxygenator, and the oxygenated blood is returned by an arterial return cannula typically entering the femoral artery and terminating in the common iliac artery or distal aorta. This oxygenated blood flows retrograde up the aorta, providing oxygenated blood and hemodynamic support to the aortic arch and ascending aorta. If cardiac output is minimal and the patient is on full VA ECMO support, oxygenated blood can be pumped retrograde all the way to the aortic valve. If there is increased cardiac output or if VA ECMO support (flow rate) is decreased, a "mixing cloud" can occur in the ascending aorta consisting of deoxygenated blood ejected from the left ventricle and retrograde oxygenated blood flowing up the aorta from VA ECMO (Fig. 9.35). As the cardiac output increases or the VA ECMO flow rate further decreases, this "mixing cloud" can move distally in the aorta. Much less commonly, a VA ECMO arterial return cannula may be placed in the axillary artery if the femoral artery is not accessible.

Extracorporeal Membrane Oxygenation Complications

Complications of peripheral ECMO cannulas are similar to those of other central venous and arterial catheters. Cannula malposition, pneumothorax, hemothorax, hematoma, and cardiac injuries may occur. On serial radiographs, care should be taken to assess for any change in ECMO catheter position that could suggest cannula migration.

Venoarterial ECMO has implications for CT imaging because patients on VA ECMO may have inconsistent aortic contrast mixing that varies depending on cardiac output, flow rate of the oxygenator, and bolus timing. When patients on VA ECMO are imaged with chest CT early after initiation of contrast injection, flow artifacts can occur that mimic aortic dissection or intraaortic thrombus. The addition of a delayed imaging series after contrast injection may be helpful in patients on VA ECMO to confirm resolution of such filling defects and to avoid this imaging pitfall. Patients on VA ECMO who require CT pulmonary angiography for assessment of pulmonary embolism may have difficulty achieving adequate pulmonary artery contrast enhancement because of siphoning of blood by the drainage cannula in the right atrium. ECMO flow rates may need to be reduced or temporarily withheld to allow sufficient pulmonary artery contrast bolus enhancement.

Ventricular Assist Devices

Ventricular assist devices (VADs) replace or augment the function of the left ventricle, right ventricle, or both. Left ventricular assist devices (LVADs) may be used as a bridge to cardiac transplant or as "destination therapy" in patients not eligible for transplantation. A variety of LVADs are available. Most LVAD models take blood from the left ventricle by an inflow cannula inserted into the left ventricle or an LVAD directly inserted into the apex of the left ventricle. Blood is then pumped from the LVAD to the aorta by an outflow cannula anastomosed to the ascending or descending aorta (Fig. 9.36). Some LVADs reside entirely within the left ventricle via a catheter crossing the aortic valve (Impella, Abiomed) with blood pumped from the left ventricular chamber across the aortic valve into the ascending aorta, thereby augmenting cardiac output.

Complications of VADs include pneumothorax, postoperative hemothorax, hemopericardium, mediastinal hemorrhage, thrombus formation with thromboembolism, inflow/

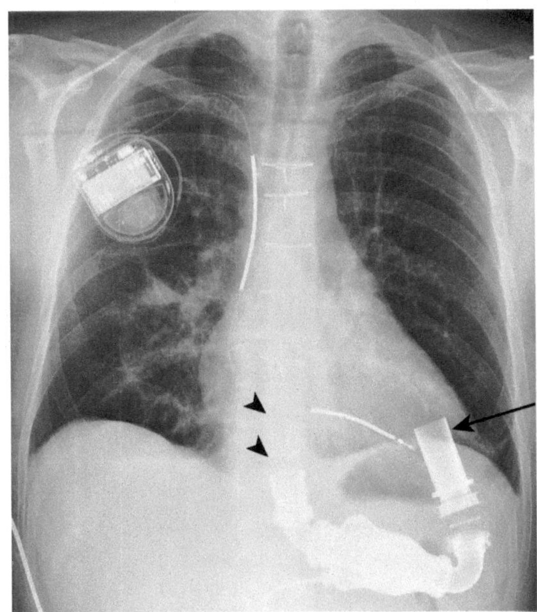

FIGURE 9.36 Left ventricular assist device (LVAD) and implantable cardioverter defibrillator (ICD). Anteroposterior view of the chest shows a left ventricular assist device over the upper abdomen. The inflow cannula overlies the apex of the left ventricle *(arrow)*. The majority of the outflow cannula connecting to the ascending aorta is radiolucent *(arrowheads)* and not visible on chest radiography but can be visualized on computed tomography (not shown). This patient also has an ICD device in place with shock coil in the right ventricle and in the superior vena cava.

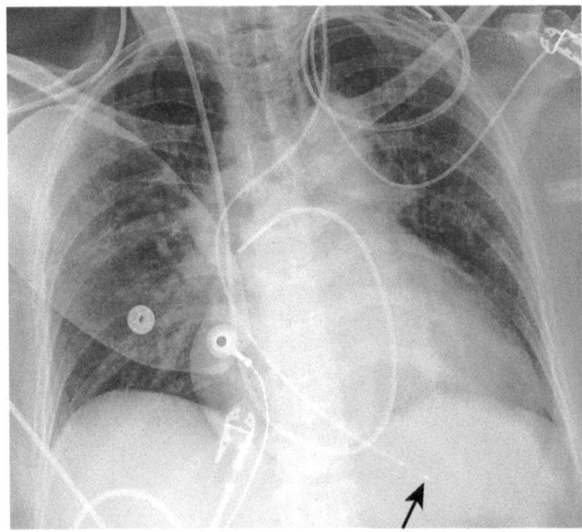

FIGURE 9.37 Temporary transvenous pacing lead. Anteroposterior chest radiograph shows a left internal jugular temporary transvenous pacing lead with distal tip in the inferior right ventricle *(arrow)*.

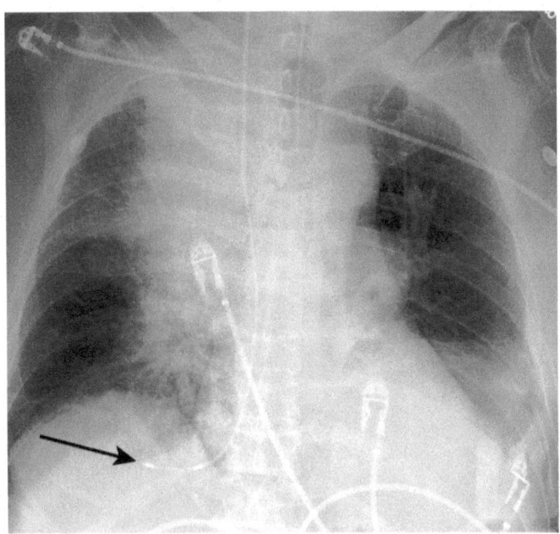

FIGURE 9.38 Malpositioned transvenous pacing lead in the hepatic vein. Anteroposterior chest radiograph shows a right internal jugular transvenous pacing lead overlying the liver in a hepatic vein *(arrow)*.

outflow cannula obstruction, aortic dissection, and infection. These findings may manifest on chest CT as kinking of the outflow cannula; anastomotic tearing of the cannula; thrombus in the cannula; left ventricular thrombus; and hemorrhage in the mediastinum, pleura, or pericardium. Air and fluid collections around the pump, power or drive line, and cannulas may indicate the presence of VAD infection.

CARDIAC CONDUCTION DEVICES

Cardiac Pacemakers

Temporary and permanent cardiac pacemakers are used to treat various cardiac conduction system abnormalities, including sinus node dysfunction, heart block, severe bradycardias, and arrhythmias. Chest radiography is an important modality to assess the placement and structural integrity of the pacing device.

Temporary pacing leads are commonly placed in the ICU setting via the internal jugular, subclavian, or femoral veins. The transvenous temporary lead is usually placed within the trabecula of the right ventricle in the region of the apex of the right ventricle (Fig. 9.37).

Permanent pacemakers are commonly seen on chest radiography and may be placed into the heart by a transvenous, epicardial, or subxiphoid approach. Transvenous placement is the most common in which the leads are placed via the subclavian, internal jugular, or cephalic veins. In single-lead pacers, a right ventricular lead is wedged into the trabecula of the right ventricle and contacts the endocardium of the right ventricle, often near the apex of the right ventricle. In dual-lead pacemakers, one lead is placed into the right ventricle and a second lead into the right atrium. This right atrial lead is most often placed into the right atrial appendage and shows an upward curve of the lead when properly wedged into the right atrial appendage.

A biventricular pacemaker may be placed to synchronize the contraction of the right and left ventricles. A biventricular pacemaker requires an additional lead to directly pace the epicardium of the left ventricle. This is accomplished by placing an additional lead through the right atrium; into the coronary sinus or great cardiac vein; and ultimately into a cardiac vein side branch, where the distal tip contacts and paces the left ventricular epicardium.

Immediate complications of pacemaker placement may include pneumothorax, hemothorax, hematoma, lead malpositioning, and cardiac perforation or tamponade (Figs. 9.38 and 9.39). In the early period before the leads are fibrosed in place, the leads may become dislodged. One of the more common leads to dislodge is the right atrial appendage lead.

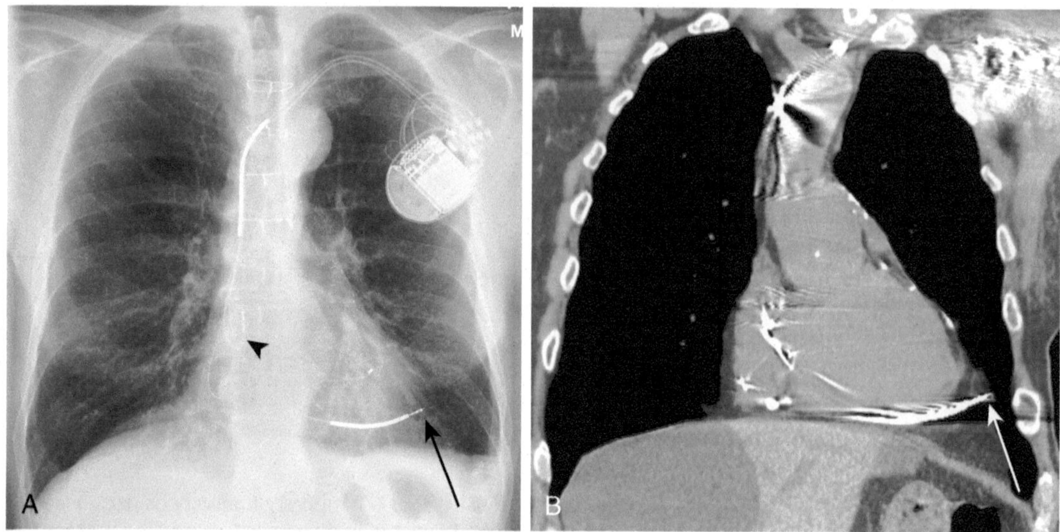

FIGURE 9.39 Right ventricular pacing lead perforation of the right ventricle. **A,** Posteroanterior (PA) chest radiograph shows an implantable cardioverter defibrillator (ICD) biventricular pacing device with right atrial, right ventricular, and left ventricular leads. The tip of the right ventricular lead appeared more lateral than on prior radiographs *(arrow)*, prompting computed tomography (CT) to evaluate lead location. Note the normal upward turn of the right atrial pacing lead *(arrowhead)*. **B,** Coronal image from non–contrast-enhanced chest CT shows the right ventricular lead has perforated through the wall of the right ventricle and the pericardium and resides in the pericardial fat external to the heart *(arrow)*.

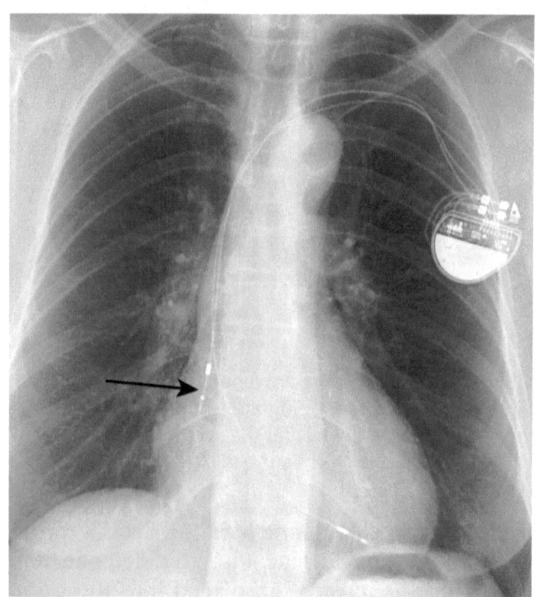

FIGURE 9.40 Right atrial pacing lead dislodged from the right atrial appendage. Posteroanterior view of the chest shows the right atrial lead vertically suspended in the right atrium *(arrow)*. Previously, this lead had a normal upward turn similar to the right atrial lead in Fig. 9.39. The lead has become dislodged from the atrial appendage, is suspended vertically in the right atrium, and will not reliably capture for atrial pacing.

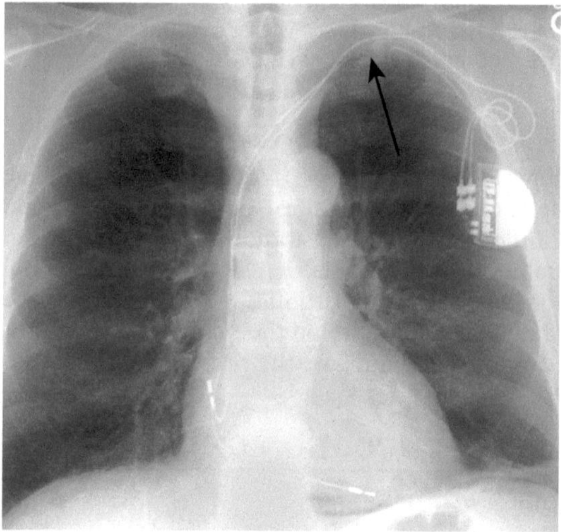

FIGURE 9.41 Fractured right atrial pacer wire. Posteroanterior chest radiograph shows the right atrial pacing lead is fractured and discontinuous between the left first rib and clavicle *(arrow)*. This is the so-called subclavian crush syndrome.

Radiographically, a right atrial lead that initially showed a normal upward curve may become vertically suspended in the right atrium, dislodged from the right atrial appendage (Fig. 9.40). The dislodged lead will not reliably contact the right atrial wall and therefore may not capture. Such leads are usually removed and replaced into the atrial appendage to ensure proper lead capture. Leads may also become dislodged when PACs pass through the heart. Coronary sinus leads have no screws or tines to hold them in place and may be at greatest risk for dislodgment by PACs.

A long-term complication of cardiac pacing leads is lead fracture between the first rib and clavicle, the so-called subclavian crush syndrome (Fig. 9.41). The other more common locations that pacing leads can fracture are at the pulse generator and near the lead tip. Leads may become disconnected from the pulse generator, allowing the generator to rotate in the chest wall. Traction on the pacing leads and lead dislodgment can also occur if the patient repeatedly manipulates the generator, called the "twiddler syndrome." Myocardial perforation by a pacing lead may be suggested by a changed or unusual course of the lead or distal tip. Uncommonly, pacemakers may become infected in the generator pocket or along the leads, requiring removal of the pacemaker generator and externalization of the leads.

Implantable Cardioverter Defibrillator

Implantable cardioverter defibrillators (ICDs) can be combined with cardiac pacemakers to provide cardioversion or defibrillation for the potentially fatal arrhythmias of ventricular tachycardia and ventricular fibrillation. ICDs have a characteristic thick shock coil in the right ventricle and often a second coil in the SVC or brachiocephalic veins. The complications of ICDs are similar to those of cardiac pacemakers. Lead extrusion is a rare complication and is a potential cause of inappropriate ICD shocks or lead failure. In lead extrusion, the sheath of the ICD lead becomes torn, and a lead segment protrudes through the tear, creating a loop in the lead that is external to the ICD lead sheath (referred to as "externalization"). This occurs most often at sites of lead curving and bending.

SUGGESTED READINGS

Aslamy Z, Dewald CL, Heffner JE. MRI of central venous anatomy: implications for central venous catheter insertion. *Chest.* 1998;114(3):820-826.

Carr CM, Jacob J, Park SJ, et al. CT of left ventricular assist devices. *Radiographics.* 2010;30(2):429-444.

Conrardy PA, Goodman LR, Lainge F, et al. Alteration of endotracheal tube position. Flexion and extension of the neck. *Crit Care Med.* 1976;4(1):8-12.

Costelloe CM, Murphy WA Jr, Gladish GW, et al. Radiography of pacemakers and implantable cardioverter defibrillators. *AJR Am J Roentgenol.* 2012;199(6):1252-1258.

Funaki B. Central venous access: a primer for the diagnostic radiologist. *AJR Am J Roentgenol.* 2002;179(2):309-318.

Godoy MC, Leitman BS, de Groot PM, et al. Chest radiography in the ICU: Part 1, Evaluation of airway, enteric, and pleural tubes. *AJR Am J Roentgenol.* 2012;198(3):563-571.

Godoy MC, Leitman BS, de Groot PM, et al. Chest radiography in the ICU: Part 2, Evaluation of cardiovascular lines and other devices. *AJR Am J Roentgenol.* 2012;198(3):572-581.

Goodman LR, Conrardy PA, Laing F, et al. Radiographic evaluation of endotracheal tube position. *AJR Am J Roentgenol.* 1976;127(3):433-434.

Hurwitz LM, Goodman PC. Intraaortic balloon pump location and aortic dissection. *AJR Am J Roentgenol.* 2005;184(4):1245-1246.

Jain VR, White CS, Pierson RN 3rd, et al. Imaging of left ventricular assist devices. *J Thorac Imaging.* 2005;20(1):32-40.

Knisely BL, Collins J, Jahania SA, et al. Imaging of ventricular assist devices and their complications. *AJR Am J Roentgenol.* 1997;169(2):385-391.

Ridge CA, Litmanovich D, Molinari F, et al. Radiographic evaluation of central venous catheter position: anatomic correlation using gated coronary computed tomographic angiography. *J Thorac Imaging.* 2013;28(2):129-133.

Rollins RJ, Tocino I. Early radiographic signs of tracheal rupture. *AJR Am J Roentgenol.* 1987;148(4):695-698.

Rubinowitz AN, Siegel MD, Tocino I. Thoracic imaging in the ICU. *Crit Care Clin.* 2007;23(3):539-573.

Vesely TM. Central venous catheter tip position: a continuing controversy. *J Vasc Interv Radiol.* 2003;14(5):527-534.

Chapter 10

Acute Thoracic Conditions in the Intensive Care Unit

Susan E. Gutschow and Christopher M. Walker

INTRODUCTION

Thoracic imaging plays a vital role in the management of intensive care unit (ICU) patients. The chest radiograph provides critical information regarding placement of life support devices, complications such as barotrauma, intravascular volume status, and a wide spectrum of underlying diseases. A systematic review of the life-support devices, lungs, pleura, mediastinum, bones, and extrathoracic soft tissues ensures that all important observations are made. To ensure radiographic interpretation is accurate, it is important to have as much clinical information as possible and to use the benefit of prior radiographs. Additional studies may be used to clarify a radiographic abnormality, including decubitus views, bedside ultrasonography, or computed tomography (CT).

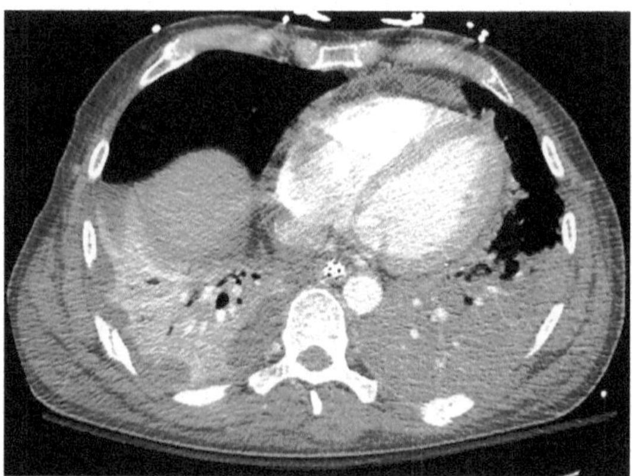

FIGURE 10.1 Right lower lobe atelectasis and left lower lobe pneumonia. Axial contrast-enhanced computed tomography shows hypoenhancing left lower lobe lung parenchyma indicating the presence of pneumonia. There is decreased volume and hyperenhancement of the right lower lobe consistent with atelectasis adjacent to pleural effusion.

PULMONARY DISEASE

Atelectasis

Atelectasis, a common finding in critically ill patients, represents areas of nonaerated lung that in the acute setting is often due to obstructive mucous plugging or nonobstructive relaxation atelectasis. The extent may vary from linear bands of subsegmental atelectasis to more extensive patchy opacification to lobar collapse. Radiographically, the appearance may be indistinguishable from pneumonia because both can demonstrate air bronchograms or manifest clinically with fever. However, atelectasis is usually basal and tends to have a left lower lobe predominance, particularly after cardiac surgery. Typically, atelectasis appears and resolves more rapidly than pneumonia and is associated with signs of volume loss, including fissural displacement, bronchovascular crowding, or hemidiaphragm elevation, among others. On contrast-enhanced CT, atelectasis may be differentiated from pneumonia as atelectasis manifests with intense enhancement owing to crowding of the vascular structures (Fig. 10.1).

Aspiration

Patients with an altered level of consciousness are at risk for aspiration. The clinical and radiographic appearance is determined by the volume and nature of the aspirate and by the position of the patient. Aspiration occurs in the dependent regions of the lung; with the patient in a supine position, it involves the posterior segments of the upper lobes and the superior and posterior basal segments of the lower lobes (Fig. 10.2). Importantly, aspiration is a common phenomenon in intubated patients, often occurring despite the presence of an inflated endotracheal balloon.

Three types of aspirates have been described with different radiologic outcomes. The aspiration of acidic gastric contents produces a chemical pneumonitis (Mendelson syndrome), resembling noncardiogenic pulmonary edema. The onset of symptoms occurs within minutes, and there may be associated bronchospasm, hypotension, or hypoxemia. Fever and leukocytosis are common. Clinical and radiographic resolution usually occurs within a couple of days, although some patients may progress to severe acute respiratory distress syndrome (ARDS). The aspiration of innocuous fluids such as blood or water is rarely clinically significant unless the fluid volume is large. The radiograph is typically normal, but the aspiration of food or oral pathogens may result in pneumonia with the typical appearance of persistent consolidation in the dependent regions of the lung.

Pneumonia

Pneumonia may be divided broadly into infection acquired in the community and infection acquired in hospital or nursing home patients, with the latter more often caused

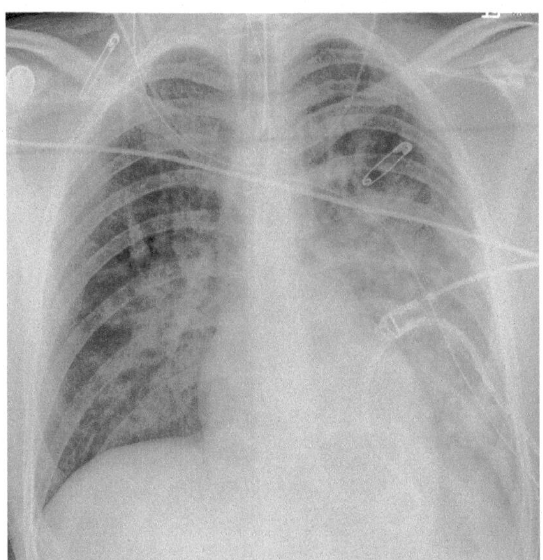

FIGURE 10.2 Aspiration. Frontal chest radiograph shows left greater than right mid and lower lung zone predominant consolidation in a patient with witnessed massive aspiration. The heart borders are sharp, indicating the consolidation is in the lower lobes. Radiographs earlier that day were normal (not shown).

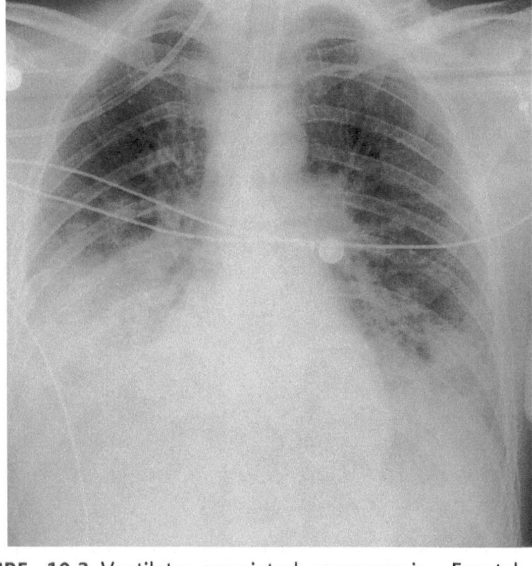

FIGURE 10.3 Ventilator-associated pneumonia. Frontal chest radiograph shows right greater than left mid and lower lung zone consolidation, which developed 3 days after endotracheal tube intubation. There are likely small associated pleural effusions. *Haemophilus influenzae* was recovered from bronchoalveolar lavage fluid.

by multidrug-resistant bacteria. Health care–associated pneumonia (HCAP) is defined as pneumonia developing in a patient receiving health care services, including recent hospitalization, nursing home care, wound care, or dialysis. Hospital-acquired pneumonia (HAP) is defined as pneumonia manifesting 48 hours or later after hospital admission. HAP is typically caused by bacterial pathogens and is associated with high morbidity and mortality rates. It is the second leading cause of nosocomial infection, trailing only urinary tract infections. Ventilator-associated pneumonia (VAP) is defined as pneumonia manifesting at least 48 to 72 hours after endotracheal tube (ETT) intubation (Fig. 10.3). VAP complicates the clinical course of up to 30% of ventilated patients, with a mortality rate as high as 80%.

The diagnosis of pneumonia is sometimes difficult in ICU patients but is defined by the presence of a new or progressive airspace opacity on the chest radiograph that is associated with purulent sputum, fever, or leukocytosis. However, fever and leukocytosis may be absent, or the white blood cell count may be elevated from a number of other causes. The radiographic appearance may be similar to that of atelectasis, pulmonary edema, pulmonary hemorrhage, or pulmonary infarct. Asymmetric pulmonary edema caused by underlying emphysema or asymmetric clearing of edema can also mimic pneumonia. In the presence of ARDS, the airspace opacification of diffuse alveolar damage may mask the appearance of pneumonia. The presence of positive sputum cultures may be misleading, reflecting colonization rather than infection. Colonization of the oropharyngeal tube and ETT by pathogenic bacteria occurs early, usually within 24 hours of intubation. The reliability of cultures from aspirated or expectorated tracheal sections is low, and protected brush catheter specimens obtained through bronchoscopy provide a more accurate diagnosis of a lower respiratory tract infection. Compared with radiography, the diagnosis of pneumonia is easier to make on contrast-enhanced CT, with pneumonia manifesting as areas of hypoattenuating and hypoenhancing lung parenchyma in contrast to densely enhancing lung in atelectasis (see Fig. 10.1). Other CT features helpful in the diagnosis of pneumonia include airspace nodules, tree-in-bud opacities, and nondependent consolidation. Complications of pneumonia include abscess and empyema and are more likely to occur with hospital or HCAP compared with community-acquired pneumonia.

Septic pulmonary emboli can originate from multiple extrapulmonary sources, including infective endocarditis, infected intravenous catheters, or thrombophlebitis. The classic appearance of septic emboli consists of peripheral, poorly marginated nodular or wedge-shaped opacities with or without cavitation, which may increase in number or change appearance from one day to the next. The nodules may manifest the *feeding vessel sign*. They may be seen on chest radiography but are best demonstrated on CT (Fig. 10.4). When large, tricuspid or pulmonic valvular vegetations may be visible on CT.

Pulmonary Embolism

Critically ill patients are likely to have risk factors for venous thromboembolism. In a study of medical intensive care patients, 33% developed deep venous thrombosis (DVT) despite prophylaxis, and most cases occurred within the first week. Approximately 10% of patients with DVT will develop pulmonary emboli, and 10% of these are fatal. Many thromboembolic episodes, however, are unrecognized. Autopsy studies of hospitalized patients report a prevalence ranging from 9% to 28%.

Pulmonary CT angiography has proved invaluable in the assessment of the dyspneic intensive care patient. CT angiography provides an accurate, noninvasive assessment of the pulmonary arteries by demonstrating even small

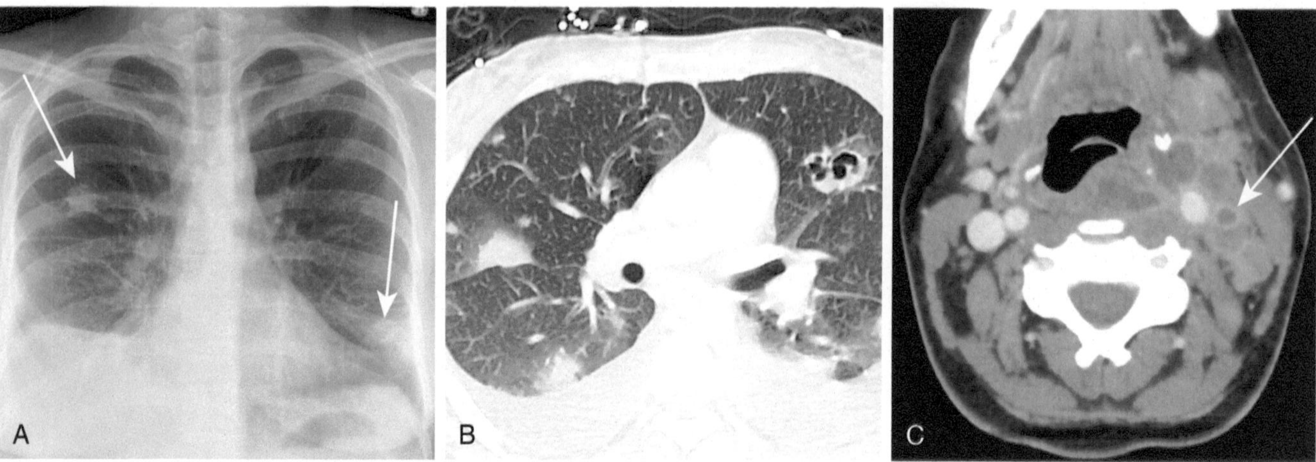

FIGURE 10.4 Septic emboli. **A,** Frontal chest radiograph demonstrates bilateral nodules *(arrows)*. **B,** Contrast-enhanced computed tomography (CECT) confirms peripheral pulmonary nodules of various sizes, including a left upper lobe cavitary nodule. **C,** CECT of the neck identifies the source of the septic emboli, thrombophlebitis of the left internal jugular vein (Lemierre syndrome) *(arrow)* with surrounding abscess and effacement of the airway. The cause of the abscess was *Fusobacterium necrophorum*.

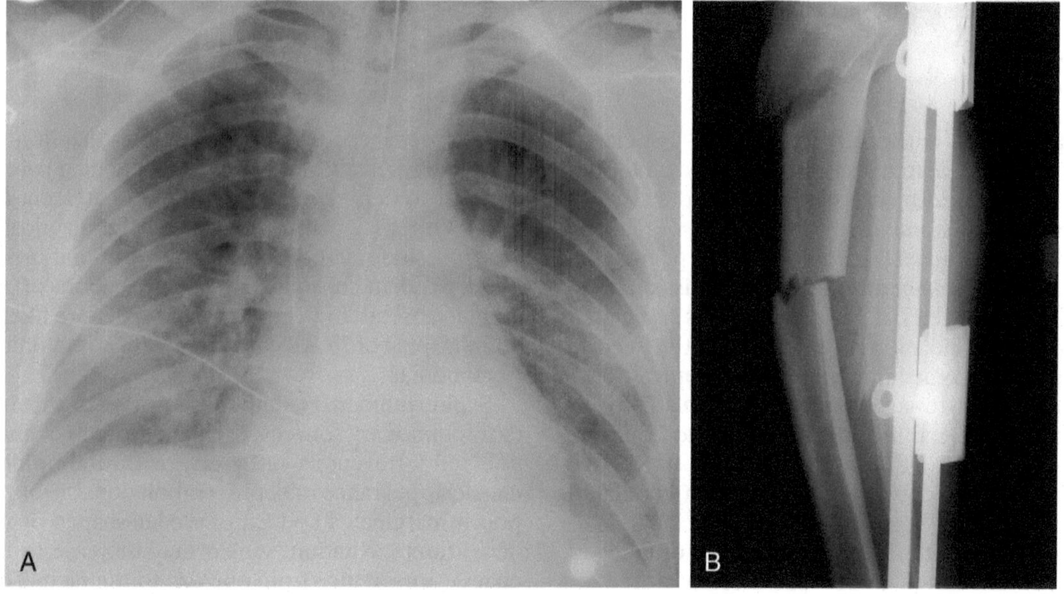

FIGURE 10.5 Fat emboli. **A,** Frontal chest radiograph obtained 4 days after significant trauma demonstrates patchy bilateral airspace opacities. In contrast to pulmonary contusion, which usually manifests as airspace disease within 24 hours of the inciting trauma, fat embolism syndrome has a lag in the radiographic appearance of opacities. Note absent pleural effusions, which helps differentiate from cardiogenic pulmonary edema. **B,** Lower extremity radiograph confirms comminuted fractures involving the tibia and fibula.

peripheral emboli and allows identification of nonembolic causes of respiratory distress. Studies have shown that up to two thirds of patients with an initial suspicion of pulmonary embolism have an alternate diagnosis. The radiographic, scintigraphic, CT, and conventional pulmonary angiographic features of pulmonary thromboembolism are discussed in Chapter 11.

Fat embolism is a rare complication of long bone fracture. Most patients are asymptomatic and may have normal radiographs, but a percentage go on to develop fat embolism syndrome (FES). FES is a symptom triad of lung, skin, and cerebral involvement that develops within 1 to 3 days of injury. The mechanism of injury is believed to be primarily due to an endothelial inflammatory reaction incited by the production of free fatty acids rather than mechanical vessel obstruction. Clinically, FES can be diagnosed by identifying fat in the urine. CT rarely demonstrates endoluminal fat filling defects but instead resembles diffuse alveolar damage of ARDS, including focal or diffuse consolidation, ground-glass opacity, and small (<10 mm) pulmonary nodules (Fig. 10.5). The lag in appearance of radiographic abnormalities helps differentiate FES from pulmonary contusion, with the latter diagnosis typically manifesting as geographic airspace consolidation or ground-glass opacities within 24 hours of the inciting trauma. Unlike cardiogenic pulmonary edema, pleural effusions are often absent in FES.

Amniotic fluid embolism (AFE) is a rare pregnancy complication with a reported maternal mortality rate of 80%. Most cases begin during early labor but can develop up to 48 hours after delivery and result from uterine contractions forcing amniotic fluid into the bloodstream through small uterine vein tears. Other cases may occur during surgical or traumatic placenta disruption, including cesarean delivery, curettage abortion, and amniocentesis. Similar to FES, the pathophysiology of AFE is thought to be due to an inflammatory and anaphylactic reaction rather than mechanical vessel obstruction. Radiographic findings consist of diffuse bilateral heterogeneous opacities resembling pulmonary edema or diffuse alveolar damage.

Air embolism can be classified into two types: venous air embolism and arterial air embolism. Venous air embolism occurs when air is introduced into systemic veins and travels to the right ventricle and pulmonary arteries. Arterial air embolism occurs when air enters the pulmonary veins, left ventricle, and systemic arterial circulation. Air embolism is discussed in more detail in Chapter 11.

Pulmonary Edema

Pulmonary edema is an abnormal accumulation of fluid in the extravascular compartments of the lung and is broadly divided into cardiogenic and noncardiogenic edema. Cardiogenic edema is caused by increased pulmonary capillary hydrostatic pressure, typically caused by left heart failure or fluid overload. In theory, when the pulmonary capillary wedge pressure (PCWP) rises to 12 to 18 mm Hg, pulmonary venous hypertension develops and results in pulmonary vascular engorgement. In chronic pulmonary venous hypertension, vascular redistribution may be seen on true upright chest radiographs where the upper lung zone pulmonary veins become larger than the lower lung zone pulmonary veins. As the PCWP increases to 18 to 24 mm Hg, interstitial edema develops and on radiography is characterized by vascular indistinctness or perihilar haze, peribronchial cuffing (Fig. 10.6), subpleural edema, and septal thickening. Accumulation of fluid within the interlobular septa is seen as fine linear horizontal opacities extending to the pleural surface (Kerley B lines) (Fig. 10.7) or as perihilar linear opacities that are longer and central (Kerley A lines). Further increases in the PCWP result in alveolar edema and may appear as the *bat-wing pattern* with bilateral perihilar opacities (Fig. 10.8) or as diffuse consolidation. Although in theory a patient should progress from pulmonary venous hypertension to interstitial edema and eventually alveolar edema, the reality is that this sequence is often unpredictable. Pulmonary edema may also be asymmetric because of patient positioning or preferentially affect the right upper lung zone because of acute mitral insufficiency from papillary muscle rupture or severe mitral regurgitation of any cause (Fig. 10.9). An atypical pattern and distribution of pulmonary edema may also be seen in emphysema or pulmonary fibrosis in which

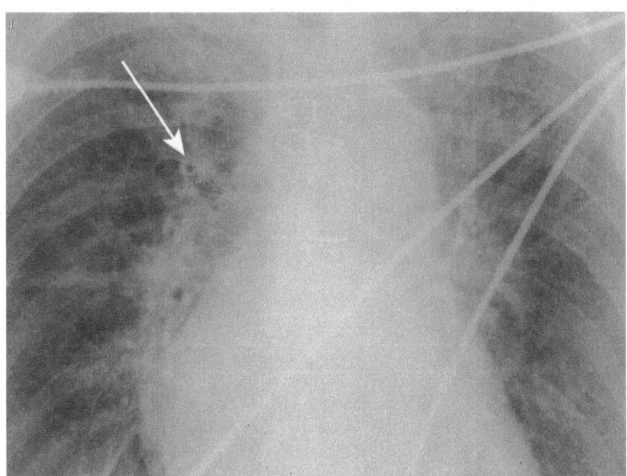

FIGURE 10.6 Cardiogenic interstitial pulmonary edema. Coned frontal radiograph reveals peribronchial cuffing *(arrow)* and indistinct perihilar vessels in a patient with interstitial pulmonary edema.

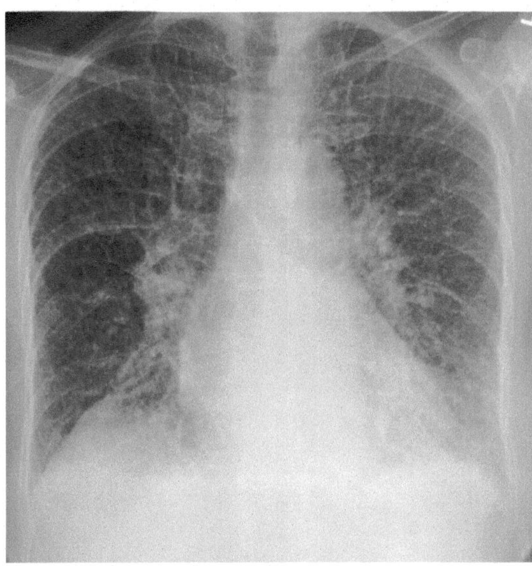

FIGURE 10.7 Cardiogenic interstitial pulmonary edema. Frontal radiograph demonstrates short peripheral lines perpendicular to the pleura (Kerley B lines) in a patient with interstitial pulmonary edema. Kerley B lines represent interstitial edema within thickened interlobular septa.

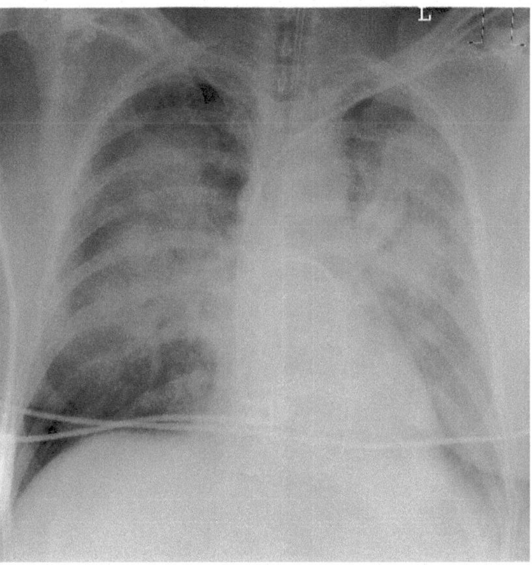

FIGURE 10.8 Cardiogenic alveolar pulmonary edema. Frontal radiograph demonstrates a bat-wing pattern of perihilar consolidation surrounded by a radiolucent peripheral zone of normal lung in keeping with alveolar pulmonary edema in a patient with acute myocardial infarction.

the pulmonary edema manifests in areas not destroyed by underlying lung disease (Fig. 10.10). Associated findings in cardiogenic pulmonary edema include cardiomegaly, pleural effusions, and a widened vascular pedicle.

The vascular pedicle is the width of the superior mediastinum as measured from the right lateral border of the superior vena cava at the point at which it crosses the right main bronchus to the left lateral margin of the left subclavian artery as it arises from the aortic arch. A serial change in the width of the vascular pedicle reflects circulating blood volume and provides a useful assessment of the patient's intravascular volume status. In 95% of normal individuals, the vascular pedicle is between 38 and 58 mm wide. Because of the wide normal range, comparison of serial radiographs for an individual patient is more useful than an absolute measurement. However, similar radiographic positioning is required for accurate comparison, and portable supine radiographs are rarely directly comparable. With fluid overload, the vascular pedicle typically widens (Fig. 10.11), but in cases of pulmonary edema from left heart failure, only half of patients have a widened vascular pedicle. Patients with permeability pulmonary edema have a normal vascular pedicle.

The posttherapeutic lag phase describes the discrepancy between the improving PCWP and the lack of radiographic

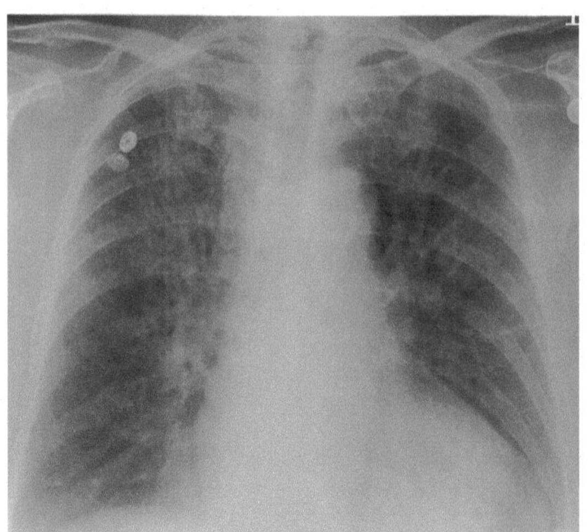

FIGURE 10.9 Asymmetric pulmonary edema. Frontal radiograph shows focal right upper lobe consolidation representing asymmetric pulmonary edema in a patient with severe mitral regurgitation.

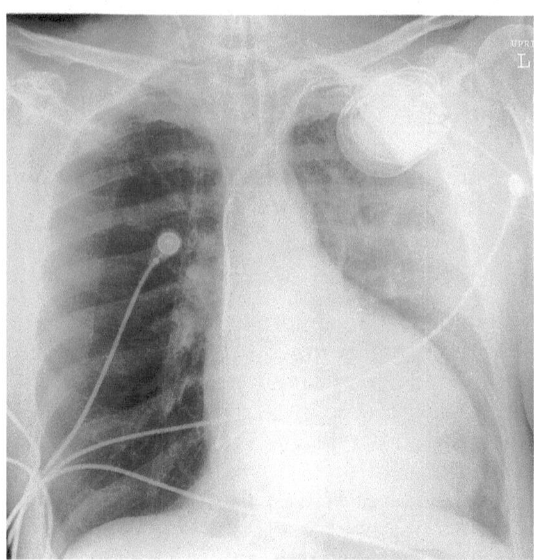

FIGURE 10.10 Asymmetric pulmonary edema. Frontal chest radiograph demonstrates hyperlucency of the right lung caused by severe emphysema, with asymmetric pulmonary edema in the less affected left lung.

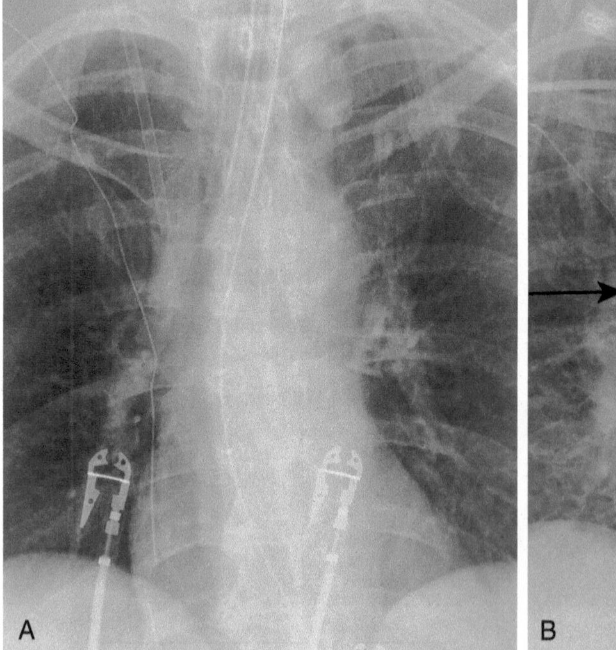

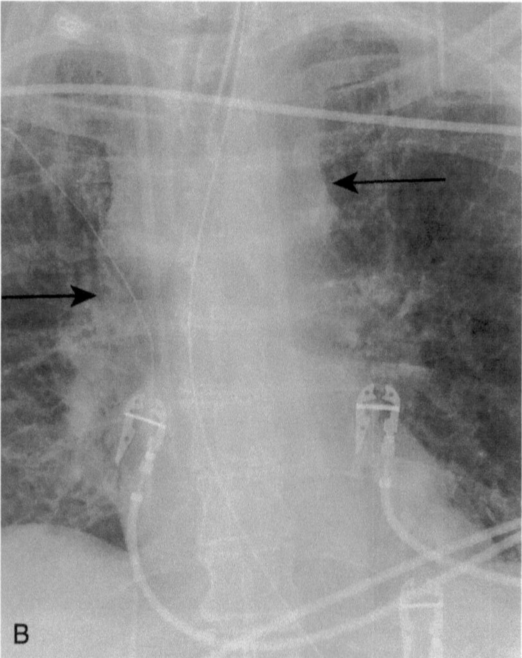

FIGURE 10.11 Fluid overload and pulmonary edema. Composite image with frontal chest radiograph before **(A)** and after **(B)** the administration of 12 L of intravenous fluids shows widening of the vascular pedicle *(arrows)*, enlargement of the azygous vein, and diffuse interstitial edema.

resolution of edema. Even after the wedge measurements have returned to normal and the patient's symptoms have improved, it may still take hours or days for the reabsorption of large amounts of extracellular fluid and therefore clearing of the radiographic abnormality. This phenomenon is frequently seen in patients with left-sided heart failure.

Noncardiogenic edema is caused by increased capillary permeability or decreased plasma oncotic pressure and can be seen in multiple settings, including central nervous system injury, near drowning, high-altitude pulmonary edema, renal impairment, drug use, lung reexpansion, blood transfusion, postpneumonectomy, and diffuse alveolar damage. The radiographic appearance may be indistinguishable from cardiogenic edema, although cardiomegaly and pleural effusions are less common in noncardiogenic causes of edema. Diffuse alveolar damage (DAD) results from injury to the alveolar capillaries and epithelium. DAD is absent in some cases of noncardiogenic edema caused by drugs (e.g., heroin) but may be severe in other cases. The degree of DAD influences the time course of the radiographic abnormality: When DAD is absent, the radiographic findings are likely to be transient, but severe DAD may result in permanent lung damage.

Acute respiratory distress syndrome is a clinical diagnosis of acute respiratory failure characterized by profound hypoxia associated with a chest radiograph demonstrating widespread pulmonary opacification with air bronchograms (Fig. 10.12). The risk factors for developing ARDS include multiple trauma, fat emboli, sepsis, severe pneumonia, aspiration of gastric contents, and multiple transfusions. Patients often have more than one risk factor. The initiating event may occur hours or days before, as with sepsis or fat emboli, or ARDS may develop acutely, as after gastric aspiration. The resultant DAD causes a generalized permeability defect that produces noncardiogenic pulmonary edema. Acute lung injury (ALI) is on the same spectrum as ARDS. Both involve acute onset, bilateral radiographic abnormalities, and absence of left atrial hypertension, but they differ in the degree of hypoxemia, with ARDS being the most severe form of disease. Although ALI has a ratio of arterial oxygen to the fraction of inspired oxygen (PaO_2/FiO_2) of 300 mm Hg or less, ARDS is defined by a ratio of 200 mm Hg or less.

Acute respiratory distress syndrome is traditionally divided into three phases: exudative, proliferative, and fibrotic. The exudative phase involves the leaking of circulating fluid into the interstitium and alveolar space. Initial imaging may be normal, with eventual development of interstitial and subsequent alveolar edema. Typically, in acute exudative-stage ARDS, the supine radiograph demonstrates extensive airspace opacification, which appears to symmetrically involve both lungs, preferentially involving the lung periphery (Fig. 10.13, *A*). CT reveals the lung involvement as heterogeneous, with a mixture of ground-glass opacity and normal aerated lung anteriorly and areas of dense consolidation dependently. In addition to the ventral-dorsal gradient, the abnormal density of the lung increases in a cephalocaudal direction (Fig. 10.13, *B*). The parenchymal pattern represents the generalized capillary leak (i.e., ground-glass opacification), the local lung injury (i.e., consolidation), and the dependent atelectasis from a prolonged supine position. Dense, asymmetric consolidation predominates in patients with direct injury to the lung, such as pneumonia or aspiration (see Fig. 10.12), and ground-glass opacification (i.e., permeability edema) is the predominant finding in patients with alveolar damage from an extrapulmonary insult such as sepsis or hypotension. The "crazy paving" pattern of ground-glass opacities and interlobular septal thickening may also be seen on CT, although this is not specific for ARDS. In contrast to cardiogenic and hypervolemic edema, the vascular pedicle is not widened, the heart is not enlarged, pleural effusions are small or absent, and there is no upper lobe vascular redistribution. When visualized, the upper lobe vessels are constricted rather than dilated. The lung volumes are

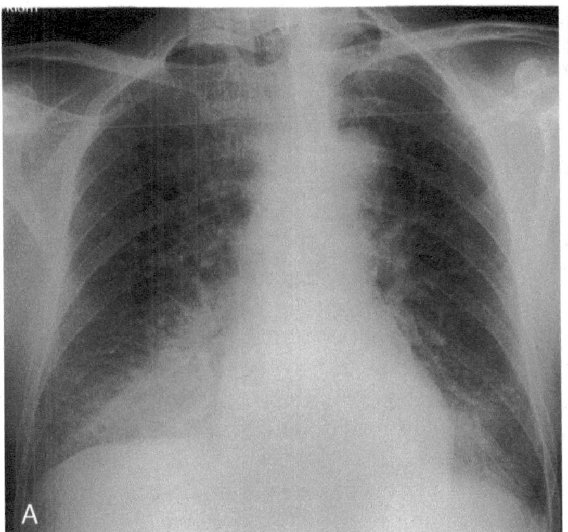

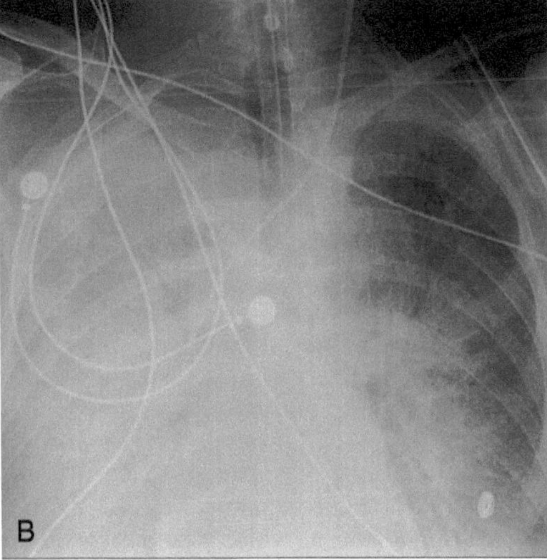

FIGURE 10.12 Diffuse alveolar damage (DAD) and acute respiratory distress syndrome (ARDS). **A,** Frontal radiograph shows right greater than left lower lobe consolidation compatible with pneumonia. **B,** Frontal radiograph performed 6 hours later shows interval endotracheal intubation and marked progression of diffuse right greater than left consolidation typical of DAD with ARDS. Whereas asymmetric opacities with DAD typically occur with pulmonary causes, symmetric opacities are more typical of nonpulmonary causes of diffuse alveolar damage.

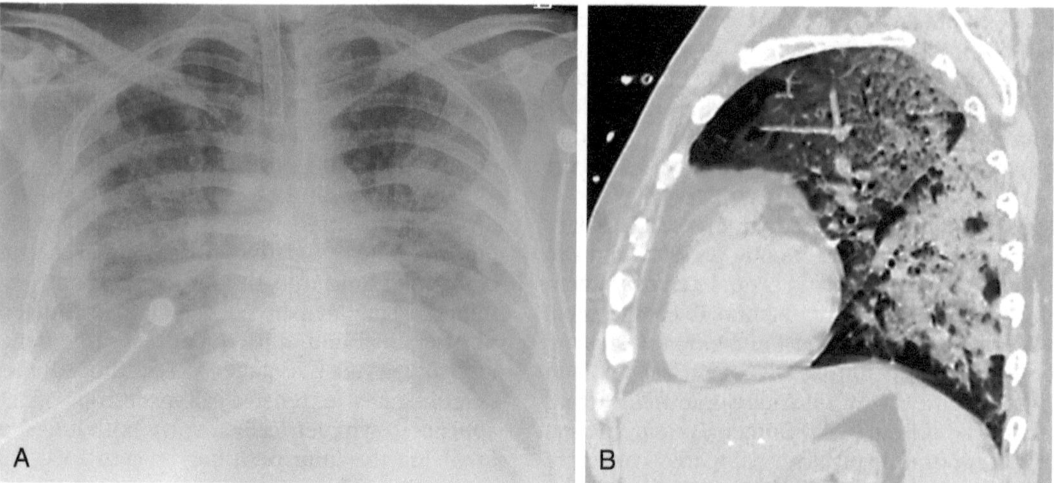

FIGURE 10.13 Acute exudative phase of diffuse alveolar damage (DAD) and acute respiratory distress syndrome (ARDS). **A,** Frontal radiograph demonstrates bilateral consolidation with a peripheral distribution typical of DAD with ARDS, in this case caused by the H1N1 influenza strain. **B,** Sagittal contrast-enhanced computed tomography scan from a different patient shows characteristic ventral-dorsal and cephalocaudal gradient of ground-glass opacity and consolidation.

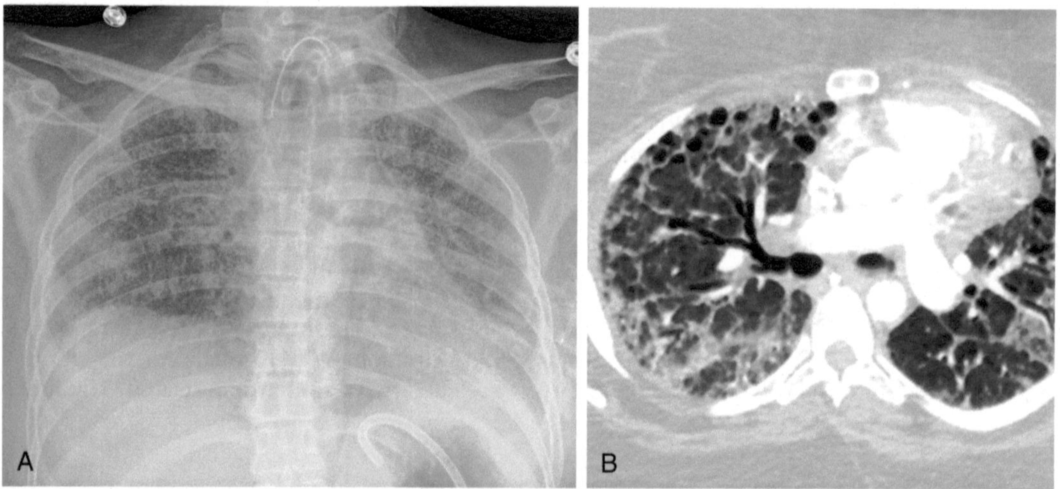

FIGURE 10.14 Chronic or fibrotic phase of diffuse alveolar damage (DAD). **A,** Frontal radiograph shows diffuse coarse reticular opacities and diminished lung volumes. **B,** Axial contrast-enhanced computed tomography scan from a different patient demonstrates anterior lung predominance of fibrosis and cysts associated with reticular and ground-glass opacities typical of the chronic phase of DAD.

reduced, but because of mechanical ventilation, this may not be apparent.

The second, proliferative, phase of ARDS occurs on days 3 to 10 after the initial insult and involves the migration of fibroblasts and type II pneumocytes, which secrete proteins such as collagen. The continuation of this process eventually leads to more collagen production with fibrosis and destruction of alveolar spaces, the so-called fibrotic stage (Fig. 10.14, *A*). In patients who survive ARDS, some have no long-term sequelae, but others have a residual pulmonary function deficit and variable amounts of lung fibrosis. Chronic CT findings that may be seen include cysts of varying sizes that occur in both dependent and nondependent lung (Fig. 10.14, *A*). Ground-glass and reticular opacities may also be seen preferentially involving the anterior nondependent lung. This nondependent distribution suggests that the major contributor to lung fibrosis may be ventilator-induced lung injury rather than alveolar damage because the dependent consolidated lung is protected from the ventilator and oxygen therapy.

Bacterial pneumonia is a common and frequently missed complication of ARDS. The diffuse airspace opacification of ARDS often obscures the radiographic findings of pneumonia. However, the CT finding of dense, nondependent consolidation should raise the suspicion of coexistent infection.

Most patients with ARDS require mechanical ventilation for survival, often for prolonged periods and with high peak end-expiratory pressure. Barotrauma is a well-recognized complication associated with a high mortality rate. The most common manifestation is the development of extraalveolar air collections, particularly pneumothorax and pneumatocele formation.

Acute Exacerbation of Interstitial Lung Disease

Patients with interstitial lung disease (ILD) may experience acute exacerbation of their disease, which is characterized by clinical worsening of dyspnea and new imaging opacities. This may occur in usual interstitial pneumonitis (UIP), hypersensitivity pneumonitis, or connective tissue disease–associated ILD. The imaging differential diagnosis for new diffuse opacities in a patient with underlying ILD includes infection (including pneumocystis), pulmonary edema, pulmonary hemorrhage, and an acute exacerbation of underlying ILD. Histologically, acute exacerbation of UIP generally falls into three patterns: diffuse alveolar damage, organizing pneumonia, or fibroblastic foci superimposed on underlying fibrosis. Imaging findings may be indistinguishable from ARDS, infection, or edema and include variable amounts of ground-glass opacity and consolidation, which may be diffuse, peripheral, or multifocal (Fig. 10.15). The distribution of the CT findings correlates with prognosis: Patients with diffuse or multifocal type have higher mortality rates than those with peripheral disease. Often echocardiography and bronchoscopy are needed to exclude heart failure and coexistent infection, respectively.

Pulmonary Hemorrhage

Pulmonary hemorrhage can be localized or diffuse and can result from a number of causes, including infection, tumors, bronchiectasis, lung biopsy, trauma, pulmonary infarction, vasculitis, or connective tissue disorders. Diffuse pulmonary hemorrhage (DPH) is a syndrome defined by a triad of clinical and radiographic findings, including hemoptysis, iron deficiency anemia, and a chest radiograph showing bilateral consolidation with apical sparing. The differential diagnosis and diagnostic and therapeutic approaches depend on whether the patient is immunocompetent or immunocompromised. DPH in immunocompetent hosts includes causes such as Goodpasture syndrome, systemic lupus erythematosus, granulomatosis with polyangiitis (formerly Wegener granulomatosis), and idiopathic pulmonary hemosiderosis. In immunocompromised hosts, DPH is caused by thrombocytopenia or coagulopathy and frequently coexists with other abnormalities such as infection or chemotherapy- or radiation-induced lung injury.

Radiographic differentiation of pulmonary hemorrhage from pneumonia or edema may be difficult because all can produce diffuse consolidation. Although the presence of hemoptysis and a dropping hematocrit should suggest the diagnosis of DPH, hemoptysis is not always present. Other clinical and laboratory data are frequently needed, including absence of fever, absence of elevated white blood cell count, elevated carbon monoxide–diffusing capacity, and presence of hemosiderin-laden macrophages in sputum or bronchoalveolar lavage fluid. In contrast to pneumonia, a rapid radiographic improvement is common with pulmonary hemorrhage. Within several days, the consolidation resolves leaving reticular opacities, with interlobular septal thickening developing as the blood products are absorbed and carried away via lymphatics. Complete radiographic resolution occurs within 2 weeks.

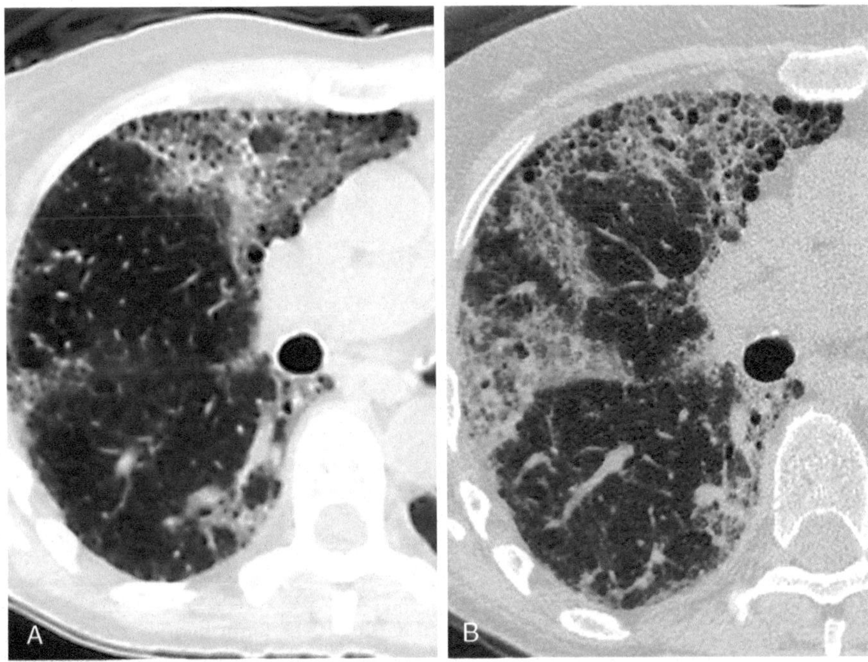

FIGURE 10.15 Acute interstitial lung disease exacerbation. Composite image of a patient with usual interstitial pneumonia in the setting of rheumatoid arthritis. **A,** Baseline computed tomography shows a mixture of ground-glass opacity and honeycombing. **B,** During an episode of acute exacerbation, there is a sudden increase in ground-glass opacity, which was accompanied clinically by worsening dyspnea.

ABNORMAL AIR COLLECTIONS

Subcutaneous Air

Barotrauma from prolonged or high-pressure ventilation may result in subcutaneous air, pulmonary interstitial emphysema (PIE), pneumomediastinum, and pneumothorax. Subcutaneous air confined to the cervical region suggests possible injury to the upper airway or esophagus during intubation. Subcutaneous air in the chest wall should alert the radiologist to the presence of a pneumothorax, with the lateralization indicated by the distribution of the air. A continuous increase in the volume of subcutaneous air adjacent to a chest tube indicates a malfunctioning tube or improper wound dressing.

Pneumothorax

On an upright radiograph, the pneumothorax is identified as a thin white line (i.e., visceral pleural line) with an absence of vessels superiorly and laterally. On a radiograph obtained with the patient supine, pleural air preferentially collects anteriorly and may outline mediastinal structures. A classic manifestation of pneumothorax in the supine patient is *the deep sulcus sign,* with sharp delineation of the anterior costophrenic sulcus and adjacent diaphragmatic and cardiac contours (Fig. 10.16). A large supine pneumothorax may result in hyperlucency of the affected hemithorax compared with the opposite lung. Decubitus views with the side of interest up can confirm the diagnosis.

A subpulmonic pneumothorax appears as a hyperlucent upper quadrant of the abdomen and sharp margination of the adjacent hemidiaphragm (Fig. 10.17). This may be associated with a *deep sulcus sign*. The anterior and posterior diaphragmatic surfaces may be visualized, a finding known as the *double-diaphragm sign*. Loculated pneumothoraces can be difficult to identify in supine patients, and in selected patients, a CT scan is indicated for diagnosis and drainage.

Tension pneumothorax occurs when intrapleural air accumulates progressively, allowing the pleural pressure in the affected hemithorax to exceed the atmospheric pressure. This is caused by a valve effect, which allows gas to enter the pleural space during inspiration but blocks the escape of gas during expiration. Radiographic findings of a pneumothorax under tension include contralateral mediastinal shift, ipsilateral widening of the intercostal spaces, and flattening of the ipsilateral hemidiaphragm (Fig. 10.18). These radiographic signs should alert the radiologist to the possibility of tension physiology, although ultimately it is a clinical diagnosis requiring the presence of hypotension. Tension pneumothorax is a medical emergency, usually treated with emergent needle thoracostomy followed by conventional tube thoracostomy.

Pulmonary Interstitial Emphysema

Pulmonary interstitial emphysema represents air dissecting around the bronchovascular sheath and lymphatics (Fig. 10.19). Air from alveolar rupture may dissect along the axial interstitium centrally (Macklin effect), resulting in pneumomediastinum, or peripherally resulting in pneumothorax. Radiographically, PIE is recognized as lucent streaks radiating from the hilum in a nonbranching, disorganized pattern that is most readily seen against a background of consolidation (e.g., ARDS). Larger radiolucencies seen in a perihilar or subpleural distribution represent air cysts or pneumatoceles. Subpleural cysts increase the risk of pneumothorax.

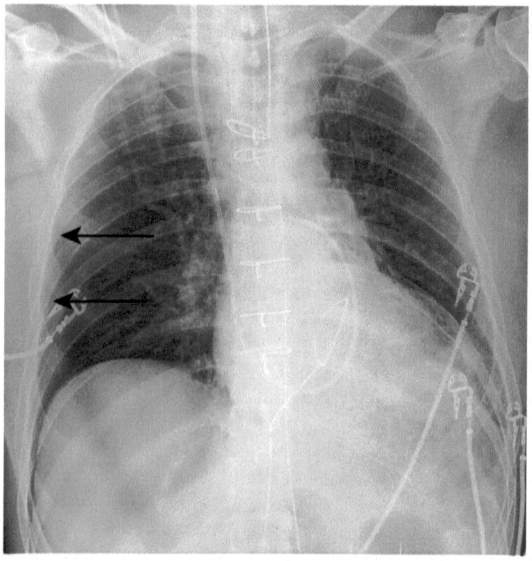

FIGURE 10.16 Pneumothorax. Frontal radiograph shows a right deep sulcus sign as well as lucency overlying the liver in keeping with right basilar pneumothorax in this supine patient. The visceral pleural line is faintly visualized laterally *(arrows)*.

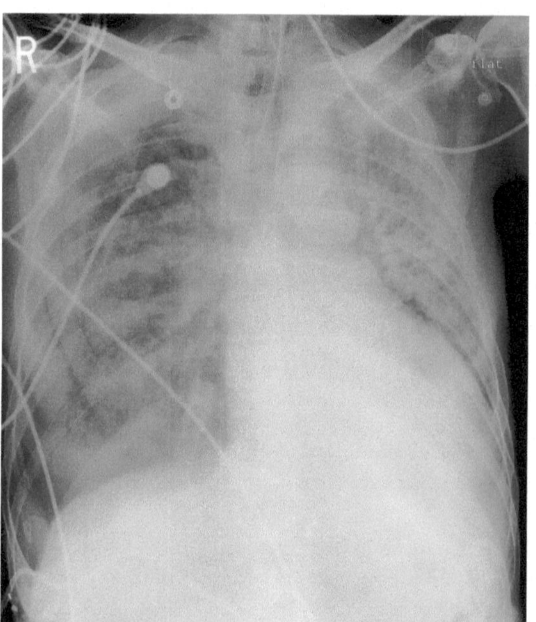

FIGURE 10.17 Right hydropneumothorax. Frontal radiograph in a supine patient with a right-sided hydropneumothorax. Note the right costophrenic angle is hyperlucent, there is absence of vascularity in the right base, and the radiopaque pleural effusion tracks to the apex. No air–fluid level is seen because the patient is in the supine position.

Pneumomediastinum

Pneumomediastinum is the presence of extraluminal air within the mediastinum, and it may be spontaneous due to alveolar rupture with dissection of air via the Macklin effect or traumatic due to tracheobronchial or esophageal rupture. Radiographically, pneumomediastinum is seen as vertically oriented air lucencies outlining the contours of the mediastinal structures, such as the medial border of the superior vena cava, the great vessels of the arch, around the pulmonary arteries, and along the thoracic aorta (Fig. 10.20). Air may also extend superiorly into the neck subcutaneous tissues or rarely inferiorly into the retroperitoneum. The superior aspect of the central diaphragm is normally not visible inferior to the heart extending across midline, but it can be seen in patients with pneumomediastinum or pneumopericardium and is referred to as the *continuous diaphragm sign*.

Pneumomediastinum is usually more apparent on lateral radiographs, but CT is the most sensitive for detection and can also help evaluate for coexistent tracheobronchial or

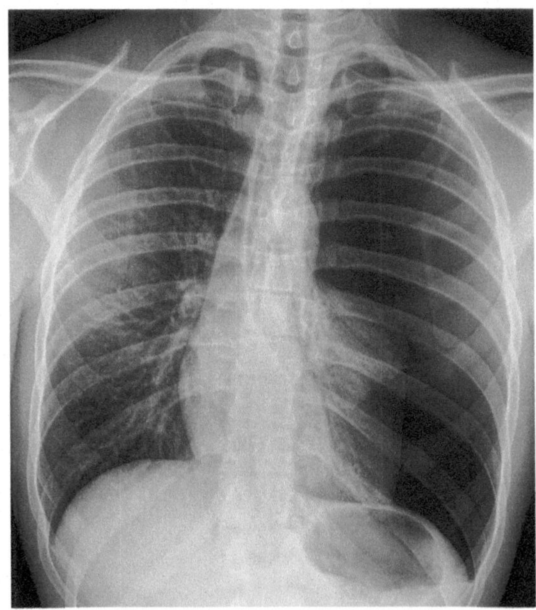

FIGURE 10.18 Tension pneumothorax. Frontal radiograph reveals a large left pneumothorax with contralateral mediastinal and tracheal shift. Note left rib interspace widening and flattening of the left hemidiaphragm, findings that raise the possibility of tension physiology, which was confirmed clinically.

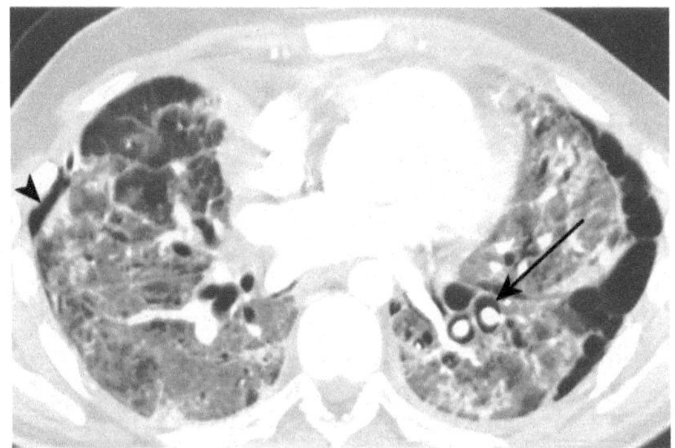

FIGURE 10.19 Pulmonary interstitial emphysema and pneumothorax from barotrauma. Axial contrast-enhanced computed tomography scan demonstrates air surrounding vessels in the left lower lobe *(arrow)* compatible with pulmonary interstitial emphysema. Note the small right-sided pneumothorax *(arrowhead)* with chest tube in this patient with chronic phase of diffuse alveolar damage.

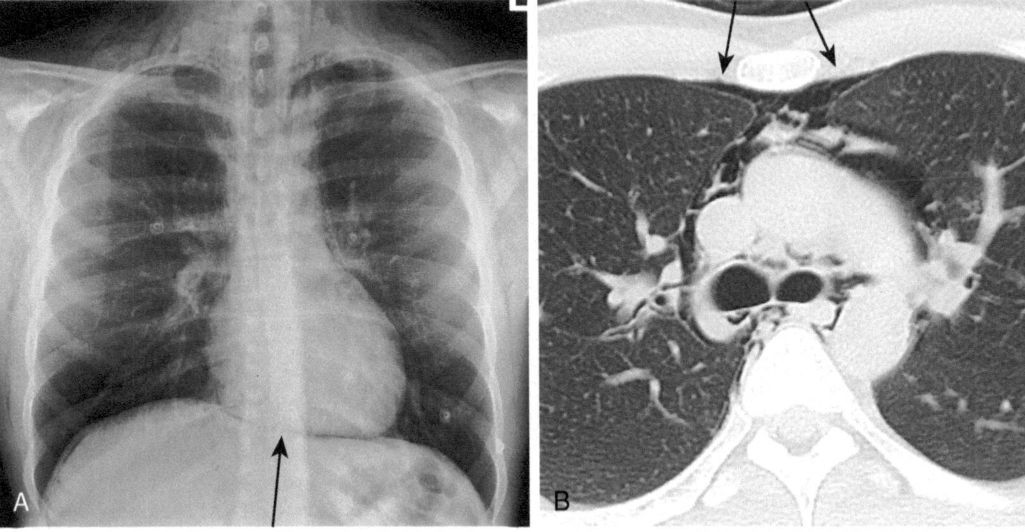

FIGURE 10.20 Pneumomediastinum. **A,** Frontal radiograph depicts lucency from pneumomediastinum outlining the heart, aorta, and trachea with air extending into the neck. Note the presence of the *continuous diaphragm sign (arrow)* as mediastinal air outlines the superior diaphragmatic surface beneath the heart. This surface is normally obscured by contact with the cardiac silhouette. **B,** Axial computed tomography scan demonstrates lucency outlining the main bronchi and great vessels, compatible with pneumomediastinum. Occasionally, the extrapleural air may create a pseudopneumothorax *(arrows)* because of the displacement of the parietal pleura from the chest wall. Decubitus imaging may be useful to differentiate pseudopneumothorax from true pneumothorax because the air collection in the latter shifts location with changes in positioning.

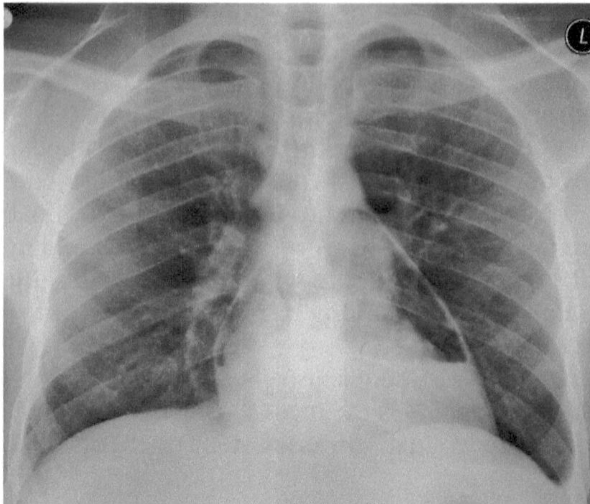

FIGURE 10.21 Hydropneumopericardium. Frontal radiograph demonstrates air surrounding the left ventricle, left atrium, and right atrium, which is confined to the pericardial space. Air–fluid level indicates the presence of hydropneumopericardium.

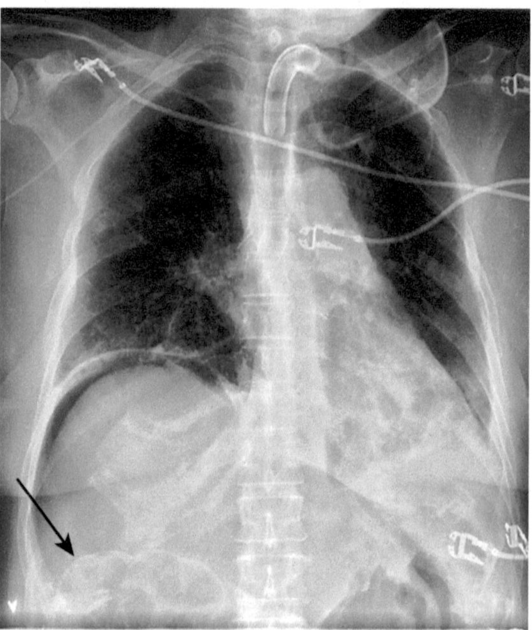

FIGURE 10.22 Pneumoperitoneum. Upright frontal radiograph depicts a large amount of subdiaphragmatic intraperitoneal air. Note the Rigler sign in the right upper abdomen *(arrow),* which results when intraluminal and free air outlines the bowel wall. The large oval radiolucency overlying the abdomen represents the football sign of pneumoperitoneum.

esophageal rupture. Medial pneumothorax or pneumopericardium can be difficult to differentiate from pneumomediastinum on portable chest radiography, and decubitus views may help make this distinction. The configuration of pneumomediastinum remains unaltered on decubitus imaging, but air in the pleural space or pericardium will rise to the highest nondependent location.

Pneumopericardium

Pneumopericardium is air within the confines of the pericardial space and is usually caused by intrapericardial thoracic or cardiac surgery or penetrating trauma (Fig. 10.21). Hemopericardium or pericardial fluid may also be present. Tamponade physiology is rare but possible, particularly in cases of trauma, and is termed *tension pneumopericardium*. Signs of pericardial tamponade on CT include compression of the right heart chambers, flattening or inversion of the right ventricular wall, inverted interventricular septum, and enlargement of the superior vena cava and inferior vena cava.

Pneumoperitoneum

Pneumoperitoneum is air within the peritoneal cavity, frequently caused by recent surgery, peritoneal dialysis, or perforated hollow viscus. The radiographic appearance of pneumoperitoneum on portable chest radiography is variable, and numerous signs have been described. Subdiaphragmatic air is the most common finding on upright views (Fig. 10.22). Supine radiographs may demonstrate the *cupola sign*, *Rigler sign*, *football sign*, or *falciform ligament sign*, among others. The *cupola sign* occurs when air accumulates under the central tendon of the diaphragm (Fig. 10.23). Whereas the *continuous diaphragm sign* in pneumomediastinum tends to be straight, the *cupola sign* in pneumoperitoneum tends to be curved. The *Rigler sign* is visualized when intraluminal air and intraperitoneal free air outline the inner and outer bowel walls, respectively.

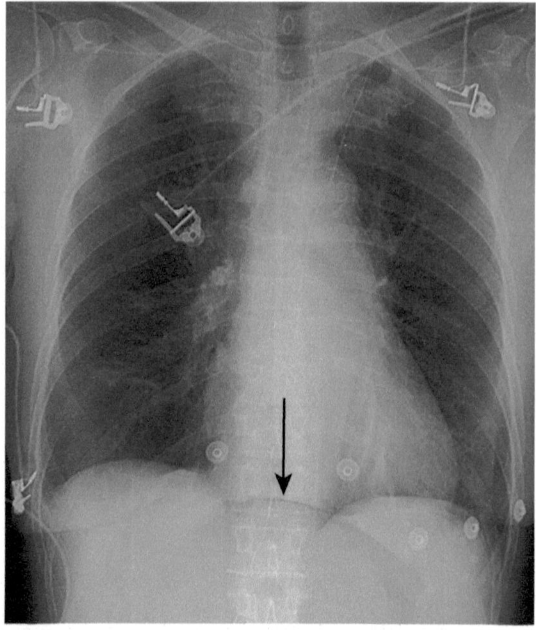

FIGURE 10.23 Pneumoperitoneum. Semi-upright frontal radiograph demonstrates the cupola sign from air that has accumulated under the central tendon of the diaphragm *(arrow)*. This air creates a convex interface, in contrast to the lucency in the *continuous diaphragm sign* of pneumomediastinum, which tends to be more horizontal.

The *football sign* is seen in cases of massive pneumoperitoneum, frequently in children with necrotizing enterocolitis, and may coexist with *the falciform ligament sign* in which air outlines the anterior abdominal wall extending to the liver.

FLUID COLLECTIONS

Pleural Effusions

Most pleural effusions in intensive care patients are small and uncomplicated, and they occur postoperatively. Chest radiography, sometimes supplemented by decubitus views, is usually sufficient to document a pleural effusion. Large unilocular effusions, multilocular parapneumonic effusions, empyemas, and hemothoraces may require tube drainage.

Percutaneous image-guided catheter drainage has become the procedure of choice. Sonography may be used for diagnostic thoracentesis and for bedside catheter drainage of free-flowing pleural effusions. CT is particularly valuable in the evaluation of complex pleural-pulmonary disease. CT accurately depicts the size of a collection and the presence of loculation. CT also enables identification of associated complications, such as lung abscess or bronchopleural fistula. A more in-depth discussion of pleural effusion is provided in Chapter 7.

Pericardial Effusion

Pericardial effusion is caused by fluid accumulating in the potential space between the serous visceral and serous parietal pericardium. A small amount of fluid (up to 50 cc) is normal, and even small to moderate effusions may be radiographically occult. On ICU radiographs, pericardial fluid is rarely distinctly visible and instead results in diffuse enlargement of the cardiopericardial silhouette, resulting in a globular or "water bottle" appearance. Changes in cardiopericardial size may be evident on serial radiographs (Fig. 10.24). When larger, in the retrosternal region on the lateral view, there may be a *fat pad sign* (sometimes termed the *Oreo cookie* or *sandwich sign)* in which a vertical stripe of pericardial fluid is outlined anteriorly by mediastinal fat and posteriorly by subepicardial fat. Rapid accumulation of fluid may result in cardiac tamponade, which can cause hemodynamic collapse and ultimately death if left untreated. CT findings of tamponade are discussed earlier under Pneumopericardium.

Infusothorax

A rare complication of central venous catheter placement is the catheter-related pleural effusion, or infusothorax. Infusothorax is estimated to occur in 0.5% of adults with catheters and is secondary to catheter penetration through a vessel wall with subsequent extraluminal infusion of fluid. Radiologists should have a high level of suspicion for infusothorax or other catheter-related problem when a patient with a central venous catheter has a rapidly enlarging pleural effusion.

Hemothorax, Empyema, and Chylothorax

Please see the sections on trauma, pleura, and postoperative complications for descriptions of hemothorax, empyema, and chylothorax.

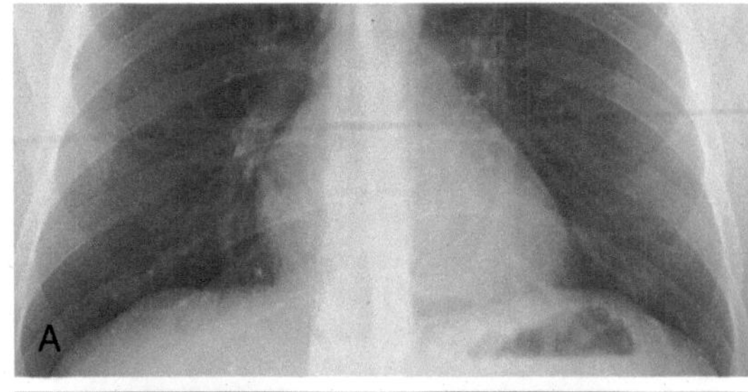

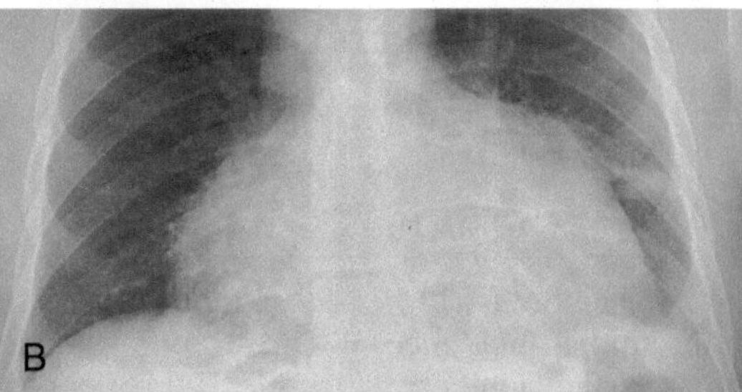

FIGURE 10.24 Pericardial effusion. Composite image with normal cardiac silhouette **(A)** and marked enlargement of the cardiac silhouette **(B)** with a globular contour indicating the presence of a large pericardial effusion.

SUGGESTED READINGS

Akira M, et al. Computed tomography findings in acute exacerbation of idiopathic pulmonary fibrosis. *Am J Respir Crit Care Med*. 2008;178(4):372-378.

Bentz MR, Primack SL. Intensive care unit imaging. *Clin Chest Med*. 2015;36:219-234.

Cabrera-Benitez NE, et al. Mechanical ventilation-associated lung fibrosis in acute respiratory distress syndrome: a significant contributor to poor outcome. *Anesthesiology*. 2014;121:189-198.

Cascade ON, Kazerooni EA. Aspects of chest imaging in the intensive care unit. *Crit Care Clin*. 1995;10(2):247-263.

Desai SR, Wells AU, Suntharalingam G, et al. Acute respiratory distress syndrome caused by pulmonary and extra pulmonary injury: a comparative computed tomographic study. *Radiology*. 2001;218:689-693.

Goodman LR, Fumagalli R, Tagliabue P, et al. Adult respiratory distress syndrome due to pulmonary and extra pulmonary causes: CT, clinical, and functional correlations. *Radiology*. 1999;213:545-552.

Han D, et al. Thrombotic and nonthrombotic pulmonary arterial embolism: spectrum of imaging findings. *Radiographics*. 2003;23(6):1521-1539.

Hirsch DR, Ingenito EP, Goldhaber SZ. Prevalence of deep venous thrombosis among patients in medical intensive care. *JAMA*. 1995;274:335-337.

Khashper A, et al. Nonthrombotic pulmonary emboli. *AJR Am J Roentgenol*. 2012;198:W152-W159.

Kuhlman HE, Singha NK. Complex disease of the pleural space: radiographic and CT evaluation. *Radiographics*. 1997;17:63-79.

Mattison LE, Coppage L, Alderman DF, et al. Pleural effusions in the medical ICU: prevalence, causes, and clinical implications. *Chest*. 1997;111:1018-1023.

Marik PE. Aspiration pneumonitis and aspiration pneumonia. *N Engl J Med*. 2001; 344(9):665-671.

Primack SL, Miller RR, Muller NL. Diffuse pulmonary hemorrhage: clinical, pathologic, and imaging features. *AJR Am J Roentgenol*. 1995;164:295-300.

Rossi SE, Goodman PC, Franquet T. Nonthrombotic pulmonary emboli. *AJR Am J Roentgenol*. 2000;174:1499-1508.

Chapter 11

Pulmonary Embolus and Pulmonary Vascular Diseases

Shaunagh McDermott and Matthew D. Gilman

PULMONARY EMBOLUS

Pulmonary embolus (PE) is a common clinical problem with an annual incidence of 4 to 21 per 10,000 people per year, rising significantly to 1 in 100 patients after 80 years of age. Autopsy studies have shown that PE is the second leading cause of sudden, unexpected, nontraumatic death in outpatients, and it is not diagnosed premortem in most cases. The all-cause, 30-day mortality rate after diagnosed PE is about 8%. The mortality rate of untreated PE has been estimated to be 30%. Although the prompt and accurate diagnosis of PE is important, imaging can lead to undesirable consequences such as increased cost, ionizing radiation exposure, and potential overdiagnosis. Another potential consequence of initial computed tomography (CT) for PE is that additional CT follow-up examinations may be performed. One study that followed 300 patients initially evaluated in the emergency department for PE using CT pulmonary angiography (CTPA) found that over the next 4 years, 900 subsequent CT studies were performed in patients with a mean cumulative dose estimate of 31 mSv (range, 7-297 mSv).

Although imaging has a key role in the diagnosis of PE and in risk stratification, clinical assessment of the patient is the first and most crucial step. The symptoms and signs of acute PE include dyspnea, pleuritic chest pain, tachypnea, tachycardia, and hemoptysis. When PE is suspected, the utilization of clinical decision support improves the outcome for patients and reduces unnecessary imaging. Validated scoring systems, such as the Wells, simplified Wells, and modified Geneva scores, are recommended. Based on these scores, when PE is deemed likely, the clinician should proceed to imaging; in low likelihood patients, a D-dimer test can be performed to help exclude the diagnosis of PE, and imaging should only be obtained if the D-dimer test result is positive.

Imaging of Pulmonary Embolus

Chest Radiography

Although the majority of chest radiographs of patients with acute PE show an abnormality, the radiographic findings are nonspecific. A major role of the chest radiograph is to exclude other diagnoses that might mimic a PE, such as pneumothorax, pneumonia, or rib fractures, and to provide information that helps in interpreting the scintigram.

Radiographic signs of a PE without infarction include atelectasis, oligemia of the lung beyond the occluded vessel (Westermark sign) (Fig. 11.1), or a large central pulmonary artery caused by central thrombus (Fleischner sign) (Fig. 11.2) with abrupt tapering of the occluded pulmonary artery distally, creating the "knuckle sign." Radiographic signs of PE with infarction include peripheral wedge-shaped consolidation abutting the pleura (i.e., Hampton hump)

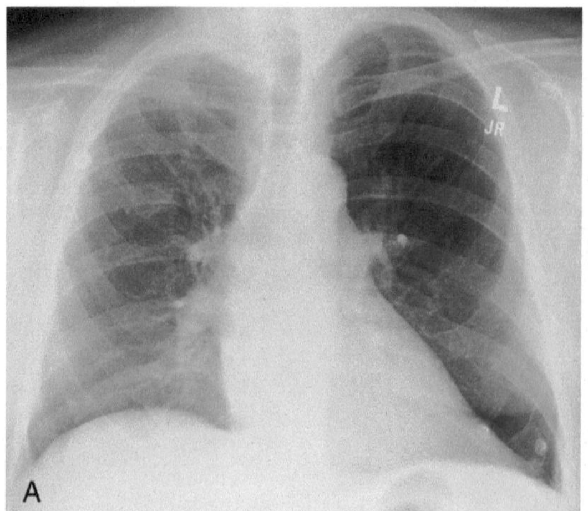

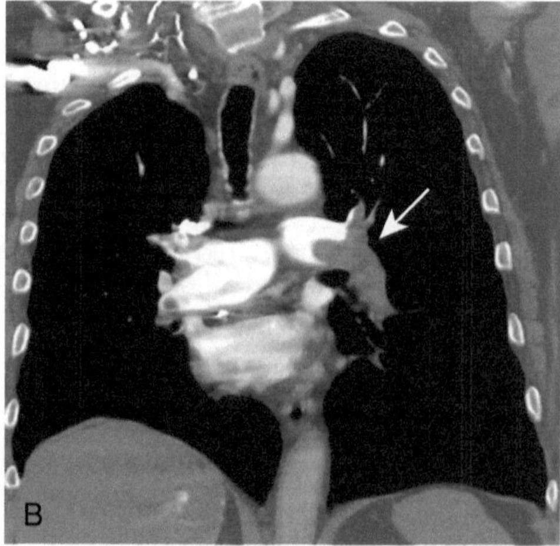

FIGURE 11.1 Westermark sign. **A,** A frontal chest radiograph shows increased lucency (oligemia) of the left lung (Westermark sign). **B,** Coronal image from computed tomography pulmonary angiography shows a pulmonary embolus in the distal left main pulmonary artery extending into and completely occluding the left upper and left lower lobe pulmonary arteries *(arrow)*.

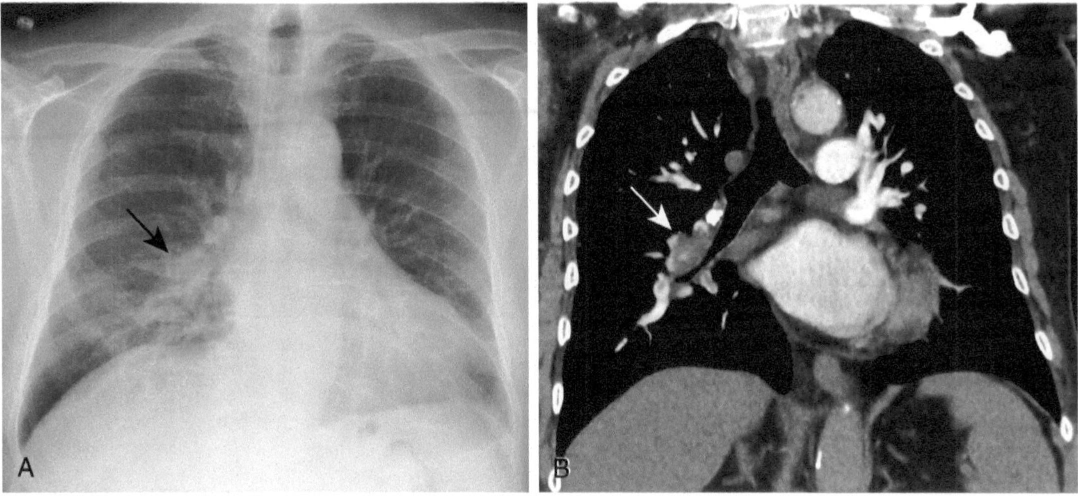

FIGURE 11.2 Fleischner sign. **A,** Frontal chest radiograph demonstrating enlargement of the right lower lobe pulmonary artery (Fleischner sign) *(arrow)*. **B,** Coronal image from computed tomography pulmonary angiography demonstrates a filling defect in a distended right lower lobe pulmonary artery *(arrow)*.

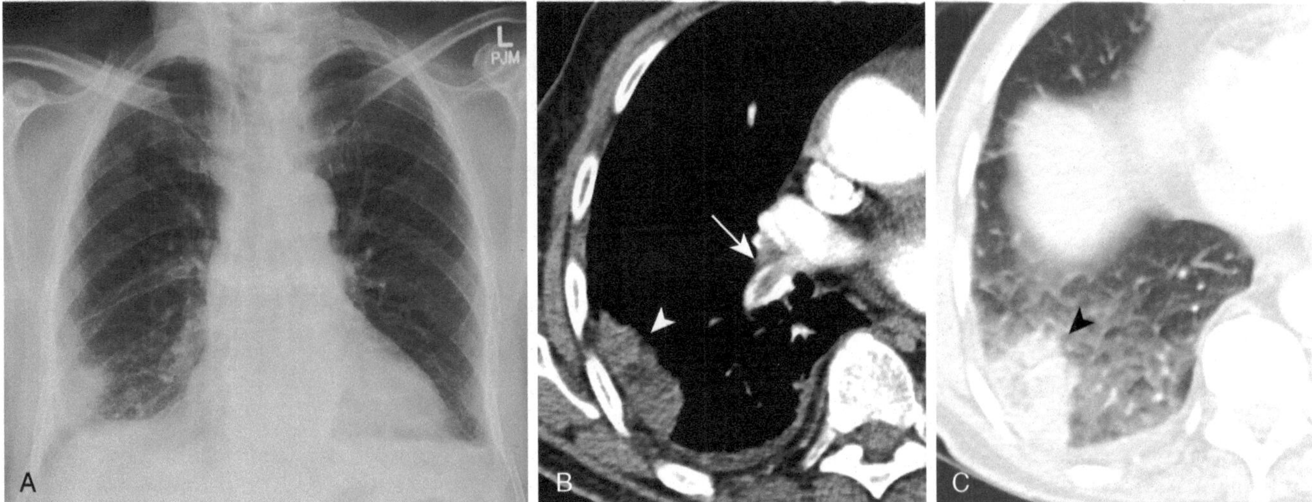

FIGURE 11.3 Pulmonary infarct and Hampton hump. **A,** Frontal chest radiograph demonstrates a wedge-shaped opacity in the right lower lung near the costophrenic sulcus, abutting the pleura (Hampton hump). **B,** Axial computed tomography (CT) image on mediastinal windows demonstrates a filling defect in the right lower lobe pulmonary artery *(arrow)* and a wedge-shaped area of consolidation abutting the pleura *(arrowhead)*. **C,** Axial CT image on lung windows shows a wedge-shaped area of consolidation abutting the pleura *(arrowhead)* consistent with an infarct. A small right pleural effusion is noted.

(Fig. 11.3), atelectasis, elevated hemidiaphragm, and pleural effusion. The Prospective Investigation of Pulmonary Embolus Diagnosis (PIOPED) demonstrated that these radiographic signs do not provide sufficient information to accurately establish or exclude the diagnosis of PE.

Ventilation/Perfusion Scintigraphy

The scintigram relies on indirect radiologic signs for the diagnosis of PE. Xenon 133 and technetium-99m (^{99m}Tc) diethylenetriamine-pentaacetic acid are the usual inhaled ventilation agents, and ^{99m}Tc macroaggregated human albumin is the perfusion agent that is injected intravenously. To make the diagnosis of PE, the perfusion scan must show two or more apex-central, wedge-shaped defects in a segmental or larger vascular distribution, together with evidence of normal ventilation in the same lung segments (ventilation/perfusion [V/Q] mismatch) (Fig. 11.4). When interpreting the scintigram, it is important to evaluate a current chest radiograph.

Based on the PIOPED II criteria, V/Q scans are reported according to the likelihood of a PE being present as one of the following: normal, very low probability for PE (<10%), low probability for PE (10%–19%), intermediate probability for PE (20%–79%), or high probability for PE (>80%). Diagnostic accuracy is greatest when the V/Q scan is combined with clinical probability. An in-depth discussion about scintigraphy can be found in *Nuclear Medicine: The Requisites*.

Evaluation of the Leg Veins

Lower extremity venous ultrasonography has a role to play in patients with nondiagnostic pulmonary vascular imaging

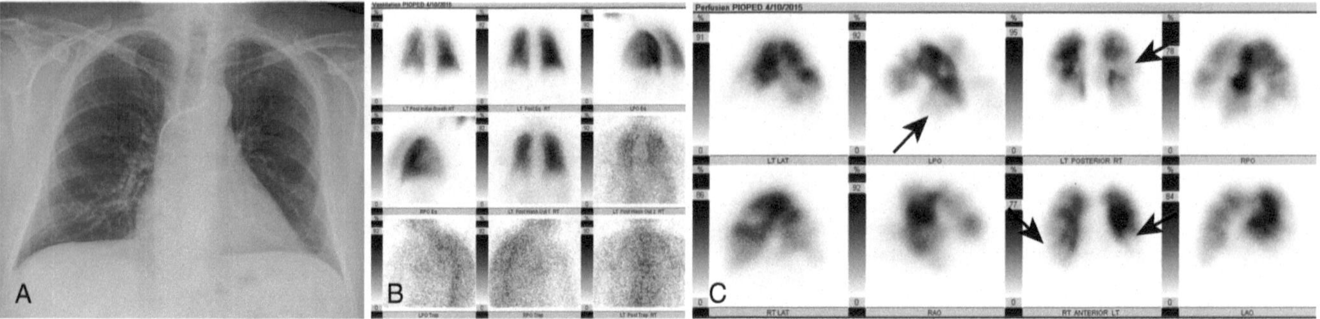

FIGURE 11.4 Pulmonary embolism on ventilation/perfusion scan. **A,** Frontal chest radiograph in a patient presenting with shortness of breath after heart transplantation demonstrates clear lungs. Incidental note is made of a retained implantable cardioverter defibrillator (ICD) lead fragment. **B,** Ventilation images appear normal. **C,** Perfusion images demonstrate several bilateral moderate and large perfusion defects *(arrows)* with no matching defects on the ventilation images or on the recent chest radiograph, consistent with a high probability of pulmonary embolism.

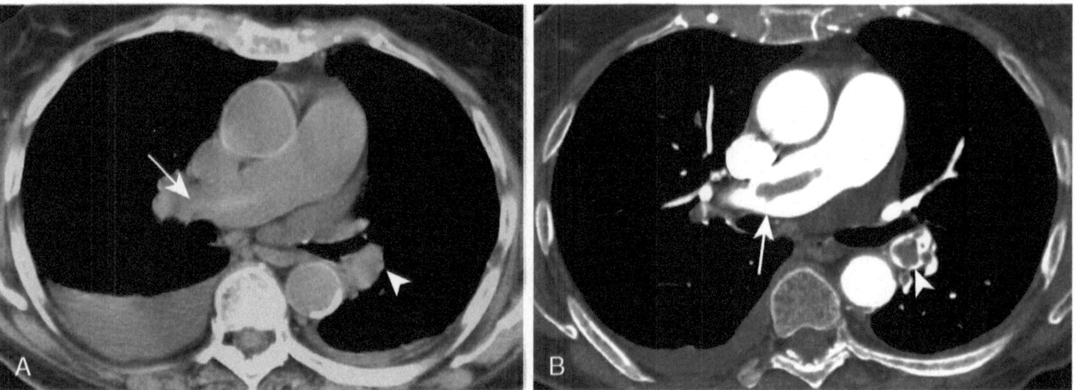

FIGURE 11.5 Pulmonary embolism on noncontrast and contrast-enhanced chest computed tomography (CT) scan. **A,** Axial noncontrast CT image demonstrates a hyperattenuating filling defects in the right main *(arrow)* and left lower lobe *(arrowhead)* pulmonary arteries. **B,** These were confirmed to be pulmonary emboli on CT pulmonary angiography. Small pleural effusions are noted bilaterally.

and in patients who cannot or do not want to undergo a CT scan because diagnosing a deep venous thrombus (DVT) is tantamount to diagnosing a PE from the standpoint of anticoagulation. Studies have shown that ultrasonography of the legs is positive for DVT in 10% to 20% of patients with suspected PE but without leg symptoms or signs, and it is positive in approximately 50% of patients with proven embolism. However, all patients with suspected PE in whom the ultrasonography negative for DVT require pulmonary vascular imaging.

Multidetector CT (MDCT) venography of the pelvis and lower extremities is simple and accurate and when combined with CTPA provides a fast and comprehensive analysis of thromboembolic disease. It can be performed with the same contrast bolus used for the chest CT. However, because of radiation dose concerns, this method should not be used routinely in all patients. According to the Fleischner Society's guidelines, CT venography should only be considered when an expeditious complete vascular examination is desired clinically.

Computed Tomography

On noncontrast chest CT scans, an incidental PE can be identified as a hyperattenuating filling defect (Fig. 11.5). For the evaluation of suspected PE, CTPA has become the modality of choice because of technical advances, its immediate and widespread availability, and its ability to identify alternative diagnoses for the patient's symptoms such as pneumonia, pleural disease (including pneumothorax, pleural effusion, and pleuritis), pericarditis, aortic dissection, and esophagitis. MDCT can acquire contrast-enhanced images of the entire chest with a reconstructed slice thickness of 1 mm in 8 seconds or less. Multidetector scanners allow improved vascular resolution because of narrow slice thickness and less motion artifact because of faster scan times. Diagnostic accuracy for PE detection is constantly increasing, with sensitivity and specificity of recently developed CT scanners reaching up to 94% to 96% and 94% to 100%, respectively.

The fundamental goals of CTPA acquisition is to provide high-contrast opacification of the pulmonary arterial circulation using the lowest possible volume of contrast material, keeping the acquisition time as short as possible to mitigate motion artifacts, and minimizing radiation dose while maintaining acceptable levels of image noise. Contrast bolus timing can be determined either by using a test bolus or by using bolus tracking with the region of interest (ROI) placed in the right ventricle or main pulmonary artery. The appropriate window width and level settings are important to identify small emboli, webs, or flaps. Excessively bright vessel contrast can obscure subtle emboli. Some suggest using PE-specific settings with a window width and level

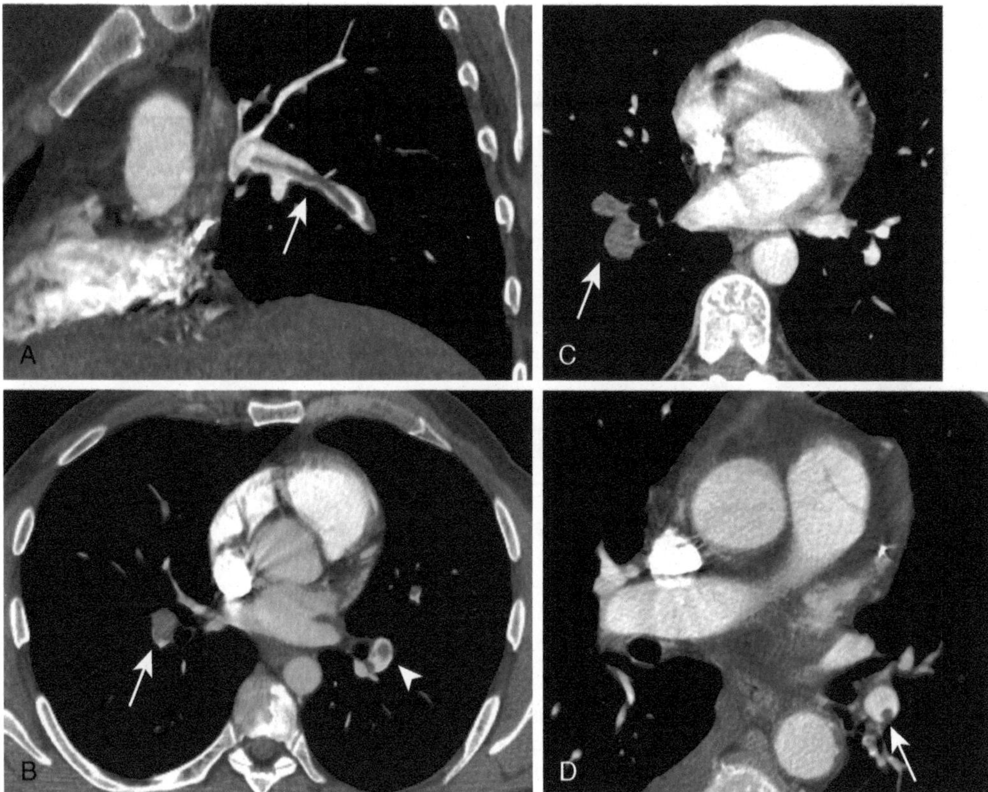

FIGURE 11.6 Computed tomography findings of acute pulmonary embolus. **A,** There is a central filling defect surrounded by contrast within a right lower lobe segmental pulmonary artery *(arrow)* (railway track sign). **B,** There are complete occlusion of the right lower lobe pulmonary artery *(arrow)* and a central filling defect surrounded by contrast (polo mint sign) in the left lower lobe pulmonary artery *(arrowhead)*. **C,** There are completely occluded segmental right lower lobe segmental pulmonary arteries *(arrow)*, which are distended compared with the corresponding left lower lobe segmental pulmonary arteries. **D,** There is an eccentric filling defect in the left lower lobe pulmonary artery *(arrow)*, which forms an acute angle with the pulmonary arterial wall.

of 700 and 100 HU, respectively. Others have suggested a window width equal to the mean attenuation of the enhanced main pulmonary artery plus two standard deviations and a window level equal to half of this value.

Findings of an acute PE on CTPA include complete arterial occlusion, partial filling defects surrounded by contrast, or a peripheral filling defect that makes an acute angle with the arterial wall (Fig. 11.6). Pulmonary infarcts, when present, are peripheral and extend to the pleural surface (Fig. 11.7). Pulmonary infarcts may appear as consolidation or ground-glass opacities and may contain bubbly lucencies. They generally have a wedge-shaped configuration but may become nodular as they resolve. The diagnostic criteria for acute PE are outlined in Table 11.1.

Dual-energy CT (DECT) pulmonary angiography provides several potential advantages over single-energy scans. The ability to reconstruct virtual monoenergetic images at varying energy levels allows the radiologist to retrospectively select the kV that provides the best compromise between vascular attenuation (with increased vascular attenuation at lower kV levels) and acceptable image noise. DECT may help salvage a CTPA study that would be considered nondiagnostic because of suboptimal contrast opacification on a single energy scanner. It can also allow prospective reduction in the required contrast volume. Another advantage of dual-energy CTPA is the ability to superimpose an iodine map overlay on the standard images to create a dual-energy perfusion map of the lungs. These are static images that indirectly display blood volume rather than time-resolved dynamic CT perfusion imaging. These perfusion maps display the iodine-perfused lung tissue, analogous to scintigraphy, and allow visualization of parenchymal perfusion defects distal to vessels affected by PE (Figs. 11.8 and 11.9). This may enhance the detection of smaller, peripheral emboli compared with single-energy CTPA, which does not provide such perfusion maps.

Computed tomography pulmonary angiography also has a role to play in assessing the severity of hemodynamic compromise from acute PE and to identify patients at increased risk for fatal or nonfatal adverse events, thus guiding clinical management toward more aggressive therapy. The main methods used to categorize the hemodynamic relevance and severity of PE are imaging signs of right heart strain, methods for clot burden quantification, and lung perfusion measurements. Imaging markers of right heart strain include a right ventricle–left ventricle ratio of greater than 1 (Fig. 11.10), reflux of contrast into the hepatic veins, dilated main pulmonary artery, and straightening or leftward bowing of the interventricular septum (Box 11.1). To calculate the right ventricle–left ventricle ratio, the ventricular chambers are measured in the axial plane at their widest points between the inner surface of the free wall and the surface of the interventricular septum, which may be at slightly different axial images. The right ventricle–left ventricle ratio has the

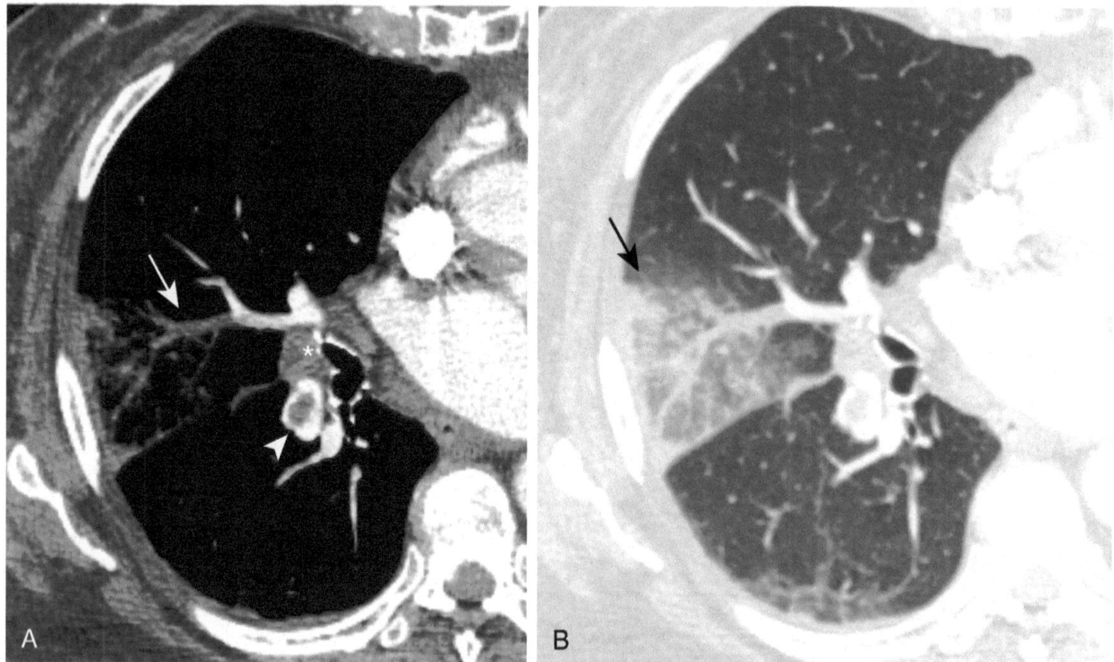

FIGURE 11.7 Pulmonary infarct. **A,** Axial computed tomography image on mediastinal windows demonstrates complete occlusion of a subsegmental right middle lobe pulmonary artery *(arrow)* and a central filling defect in the right lower lobe pulmonary artery (polo mint sign) *(arrowhead)*. Note is made of a right hilar lymph node *(asterisk)*. **B,** Corresponding axial image on lung windows demonstrates a wedge-shaped ground-glass opacity distal to the occluded right middle lobe pulmonary artery, consistent with a pulmonary infarct *(arrow)*.

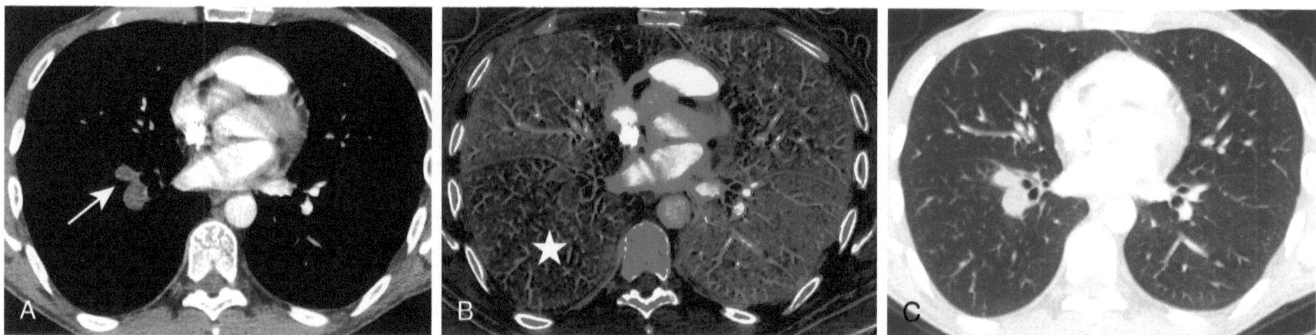

FIGURE 11.8 Pulmonary embolism on dual-energy computed tomography. **A,** Axial image on mediastinal windows depicting filling defects and complete occlusion of two right lower lobe pulmonary arteries *(arrows)*. **B,** Perfusion map demonstrates decreased perfusion of the right lower lobe *(star)* compared with the remainder of the lungs. **C,** There is no corresponding abnormality of the lung parenchyma on lung windows.

TABLE 11.1 Computed Tomography Findings of Acute and Chronic Pulmonary Embolus

	Acute Embolus	Chronic Embolus
Filling defect	Complete filling defect Central filling defect surrounded by contrast • Polo mint sign (in cross section) • Railway track sign (in long axis) Eccentric filling defect with acute angle with pulmonary artery wall	Complete filling defect Peripheral, crescent-shaped defect with obtuse angle with pulmonary artery wall Web or flap (linear filling defect) Contrast flowing through thickened, often constricted, artery caused by recanalization of chronic thrombus Calcification of the thrombus
Vessel size	Normal or dilated	Normal or smaller than adjacent patent vessels (constricted)
Ancillary findings	Peripheral, wedge-shaped opacities (infarcts) Perfusion defect (dual energy) Imaging markers of right heart strain	Extensive bronchial or other systemic collateral vessels Mosaic perfusion pattern in the lungs CT findings of pulmonary hypertension

CT, Computed tomography.

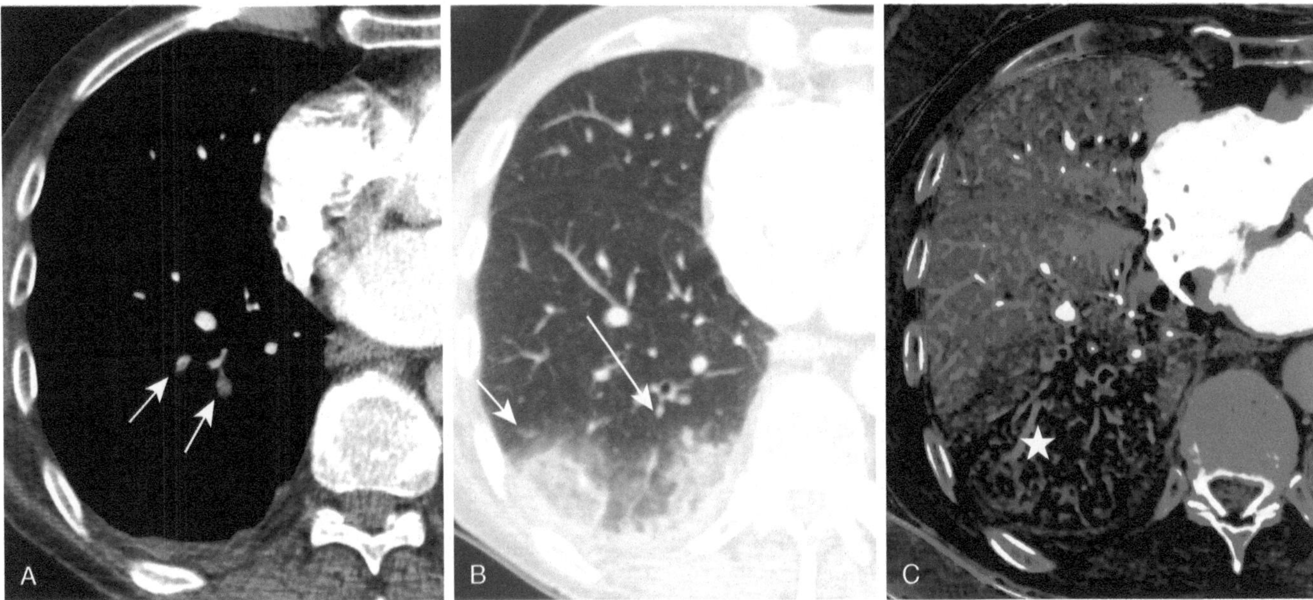

FIGURE 11.9 Pulmonary embolism and infarct on dual-energy computed tomography (CT). **A,** Axial image shows filling defects in two right lower lobe pulmonary arteries *(arrows)*. **B,** Axial image demonstrates two peripheral wedge-shaped ground-glass opacities (infarcts) *(arrows)*. **C,** The perfusion map demonstrates decreased perfusion in the right lower lobe *(star)*, which involves a larger area of the lung parenchyma than the ground-glass opacity associated with the infarcts, representing a mismatch. An area of decreased perfusion on the perfusion map that is larger than the CT opacity is a typical finding in pulmonary embolism with infarct. In cases of pneumonia, the area of decreased perfusion on dual-energy CT is of similar size to the area of consolidation.

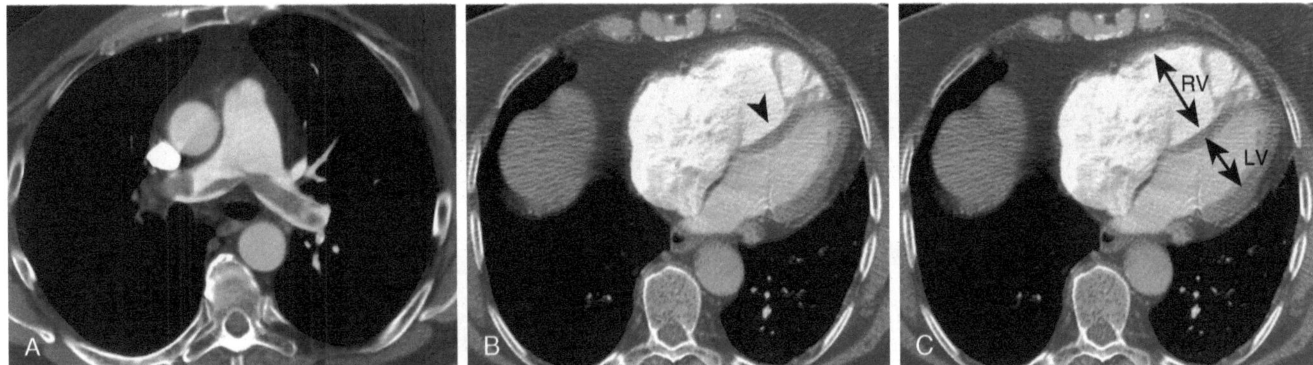

FIGURE 11.10 Saddle embolus and right heart strain. **A,** Axial image depicts a saddle embolus. **B,** Axial image through the heart shows a right ventricle–left ventricle (RV/LV) ratio greater than 1. There is also bowing of the interventricular septum toward the left ventricle *(arrowhead)*. These findings are consistent with right heart strain. **C,** The same image as *B* shows the measurements used to calculate the RV/LV ratio, which is greater than 1 on this image. Sometimes the widest diameter from the interventricular septum to the inner surface of the ventricular free wall may be different on different images at different levels.

BOX 11.1 Imaging Markers of Right Heart Strain

Right ventricle–left ventricular ratio greater than 1
Reflux of contrast into the hepatic veins
Dilated main pulmonary artery
Straightening or leftward bowing of the interventricular septum

strongest predictive value and most robust evidence base for adverse clinical outcomes in patients with acute PE. Clot burden assessments, such as the Mastora and Qanadli scores, are cumbersome and not routinely used in clinical practice. Dual-energy perfusion maps may have prognostic value because a correlation between the extent of perfusion defects on the perfusion maps and adverse clinical outcome has been shown.

Although CTPA has been shown to be highly sensitive and specific when pretest clinical decision support is used, it is surprisingly inaccurate in patients with low pretest probability, with false-positive rates as high as 42%. One study found that PEs diagnosed on CTPA were frequently overdiagnosed (26% of cases) when compared with the consensus opinion of a panel of expert chest radiologists. Discordance occurred more often when the original reported PE was solitary (46% of reported solitary PEs were considered negative on retrospective review) and located in a segmental or subsegmental pulmonary artery (27% of segmental and 59% of subsegmental PE diagnoses were considered negative on retrospective review).

There are pitfalls in the interpretation of CTPA that can result in the misdiagnosis of PE (Fig. 11.11). These include patient-related factors such as respiratory motion, image noise, and flow-related artifact. Motion artifacts are best appreciated on lung window settings and can create the "seagull" sign or can be identified by a rapid change in the position of vessels on contiguous images. Image noise increases as patient size increases and can make the evaluation of segmental and subsegmental vessels difficult, resulting in indeterminate readings or misdiagnosis of PE. Flow-related artifacts, caused by mixing of unopacified blood and contrast material, can result in a transient interruption of contrast enhancement. This transient interruption of contrast enhancement is likely related to deep inspiration, resulting in a wave of unenhanced blood from the inferior vena cava entering the right atrium, right ventricle, and pulmonary arteries just before image acquisition. Flow-related artifacts can usually be identified by ill-defined margins or attenuation level above 78 HU. Another artifact that can limit the interpretation of CTPA is a streak or beam-hardening artifact from dense contrast within the superior vena cava, which can overlie the right pulmonary artery and medial upper lobe pulmonary arteries. In areas of consolidation or atelectasis, an unenhanced or poorly opacified vessel may result because of focally increased vascular resistance with slow flow. This can also result in a misdiagnosis of PE. Recognition of this phenomenon is important because the unenhanced vessel may be normal, containing no PE, or the poor contrast enhancement may obscure a true embolus. A false diagnosis of PE can also be made if a poorly opacified pulmonary vein or a mucus-plugged bronchus is misidentified as a pulmonary artery.

After the diagnosis of PE is made, patients should receive appropriate treatment without delay. The treatment should be tailored to the individual patient and his or her clinical condition. Treatment options include anticoagulation, placement of an inferior vena cava filter, systemic thrombolysis, pulmonary artery catheter-directed

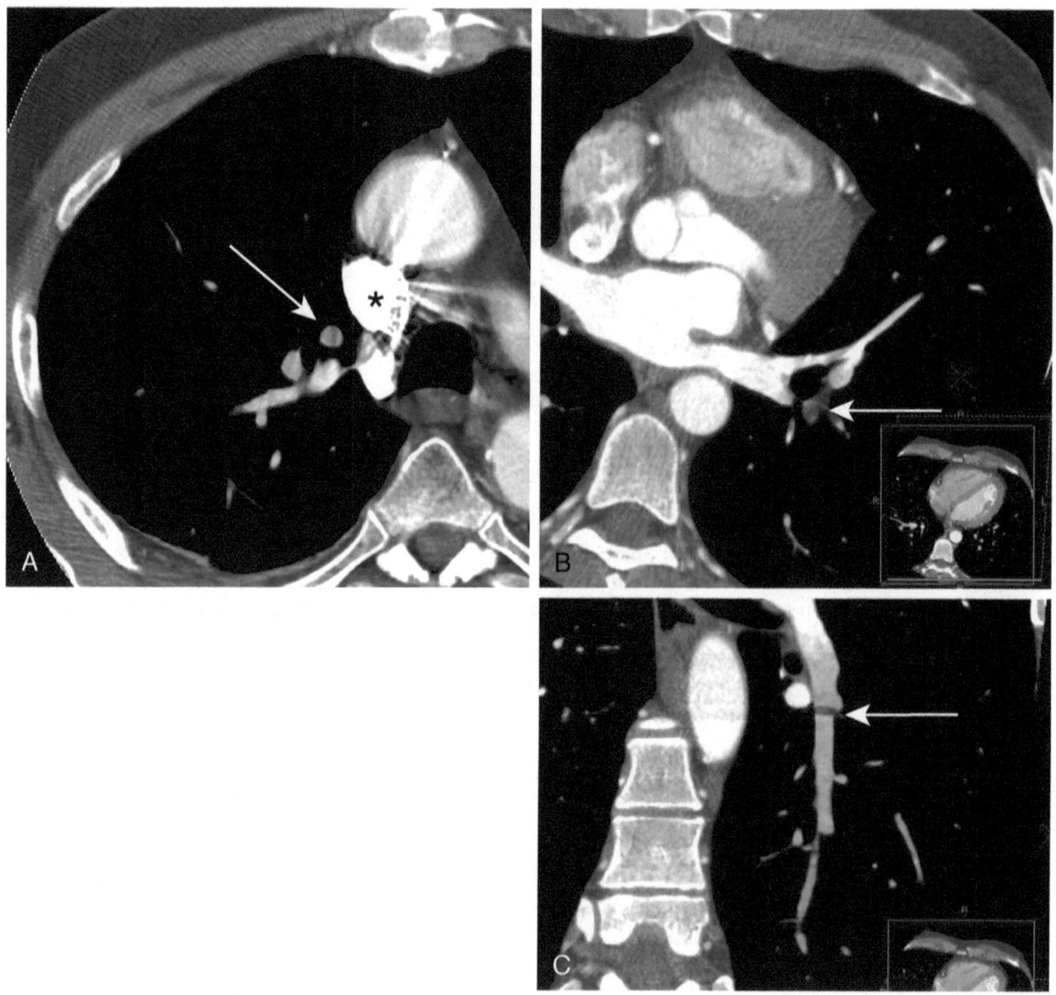

FIGURE 11.11 Pitfalls in the interpretation of computed tomography pulmonary angiography. **A,** Apparent filling defect in a right upper lobe pulmonary artery *(arrow)* is caused by a streak or beam-hardening artifact from dense contrast within the superior vena cava *(asterisk)*. **B,** Apparent filling defect of a left lower lobe pulmonary artery on axial image *(arrow)* is confirmed to be secondary to slab or misalignment artifact on the corresponding coronal multiplanar reformation **(C)** *(arrow)*. Apparent filling defects perpendicular to the pulmonary artery on corresponding multiplanar reformations are typically artifacts.

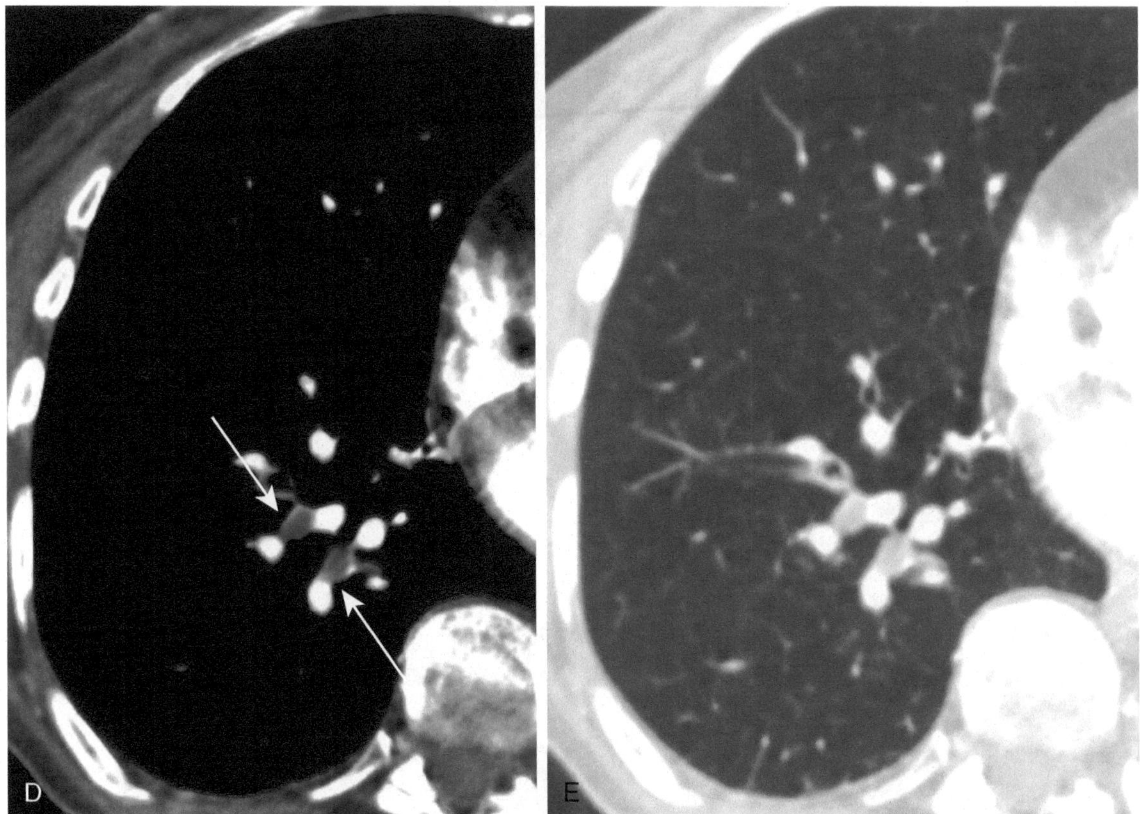

FIGURE 11.11, cont'd D, Low-attenuation tubular structures *(arrows)* in the right lower lobe could be misidentified as filling defects in the pulmonary arteries, but the pulmonary arteries can be seen posterior and lateral to these structures. The tubular low-attenuation structures are mucous plugs within right lower lobe segmental bronchi. **E,** Mucous plugging is confirmed on the corresponding axial image in lung windows.

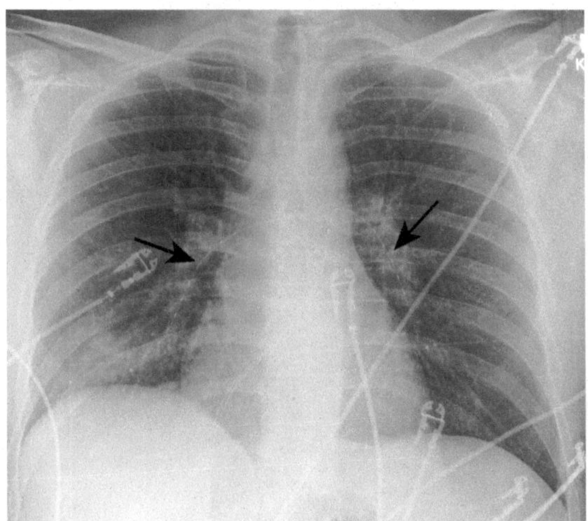

FIGURE 11.12 Pulmonary artery thrombolysis catheters. Frontal chest radiograph demonstrating pulmonary artery thrombolysis catheters in the main pulmonary artery extending into both lower lobe pulmonary arteries *(arrows)*.

pharmacologic thrombolysis (Fig. 11.12), percutaneous mechanical thrombolysis, and surgical embolectomy. Readers are referred to another volume in this book series, *Vascular & Interventional Radiology: The Requisites*, for a complete description of percutaneous procedures for the management of acute PE.

Most pulmonary emboli resolve without sequelae. However, in a small percentage of patients, particularly those with large or recurrent emboli, incomplete resolution of the thrombi may occur. Findings on CTPA of a chronic PE include complete occlusion of a vessel that is smaller than adjacent patent vessels, a web or flap within a contrast-filled artery, a crescent-shaped filling defect that forms obtuse angles with the pulmonary arterial wall, or contrast flowing through thickened pulmonary arteries because of recanalization (Fig. 11.13). There are secondary signs of chronic PE, including extensive bronchial or other systemic collateral vessels, mosaic attenuation of the lungs, or CT changes caused by pulmonary hypertension (Fig. 11.14). The diagnostic criteria for chronic PE are outlined in Table 11.1.

Angiography

Pulmonary angiography involves percutaneous advancement of a catheter through a peripheral vein through the right atrium and right ventricle to the pulmonary arteries under fluoroscopic guidance. After the injection of intravascular contrast, images are acquired at a rapid rate. The angiographic signs of PE include a partial filling defect within a contrast-filled vessel and complete occlusion of the vessel, producing an abrupt vascular cutoff (Fig. 11.15). Although pulmonary angiography had been considered the gold standard for the diagnosis of PE, it has become almost entirely supplanted by CTPA. Currently, the main clinical utility of conventional pulmonary angiography is for

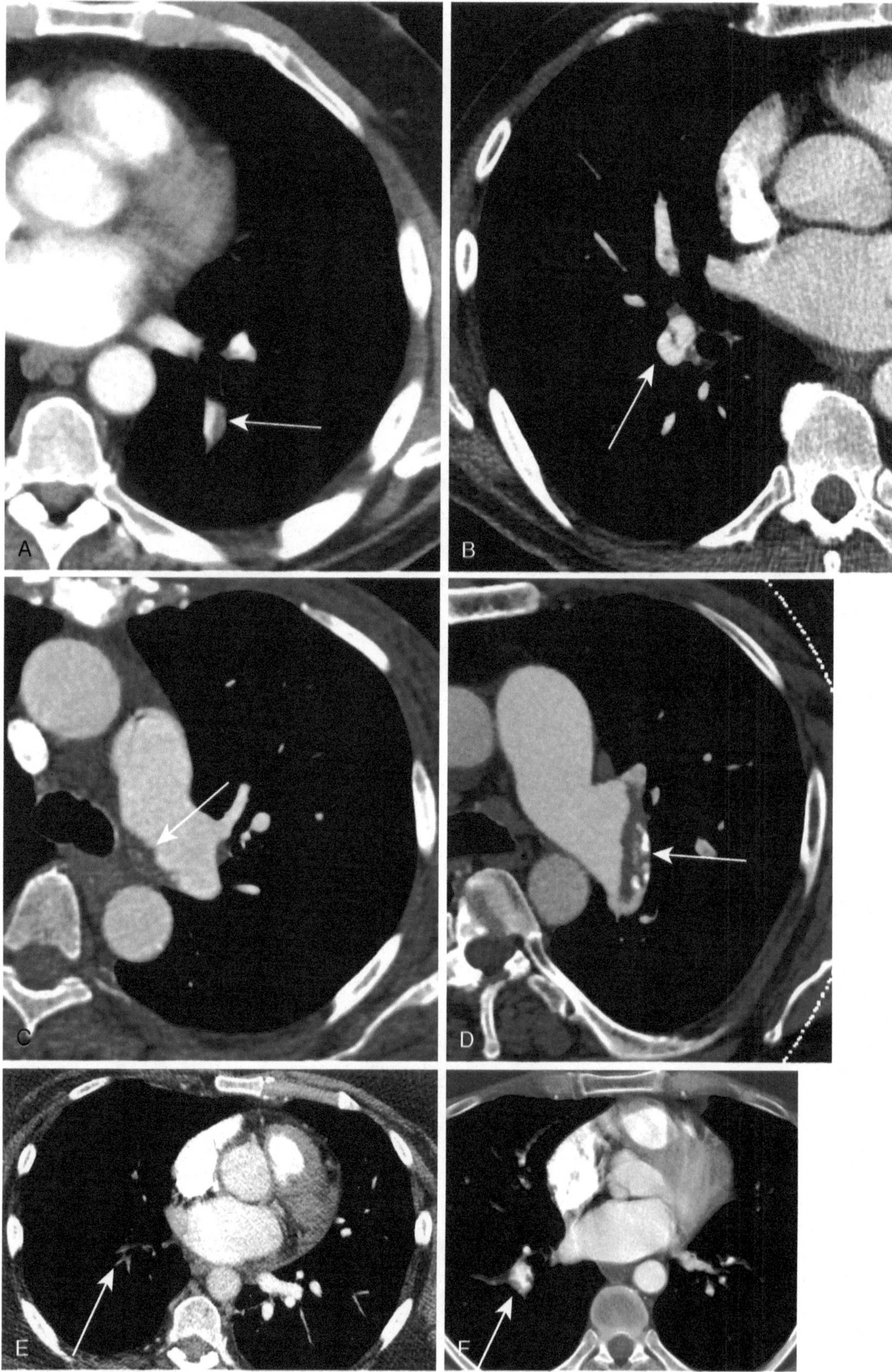

FIGURE 11.13 Computed tomography (CT) findings of chronic pulmonary embolus. Multiple axial CT images with intravenous contrast. **A,** There is a peripheral filling defect in a left lower lobe pulmonary artery, which forms an obtuse angle with the pulmonary artery wall *(arrow)*. **B,** There is a web within a contrast-filled right lower lobe pulmonary artery *(arrow)*. **C,** There is a peripheral filling defect in the left main pulmonary artery with obtuse angles with the pulmonary artery wall *(arrow)*. **D,** A peripheral filling defect in the left main pulmonary artery with foci of calcification *(arrow)*. **E,** Complete occlusion of right lower lobe segmental pulmonary arteries *(arrow)*, which are constricted compared with the corresponding left lower lobe pulmonary arteries. **F,** There is contrast flowing through a right lower lobe pulmonary artery, which has irregularly thickened walls secondary to recanalization of the vessel *(arrow)*.

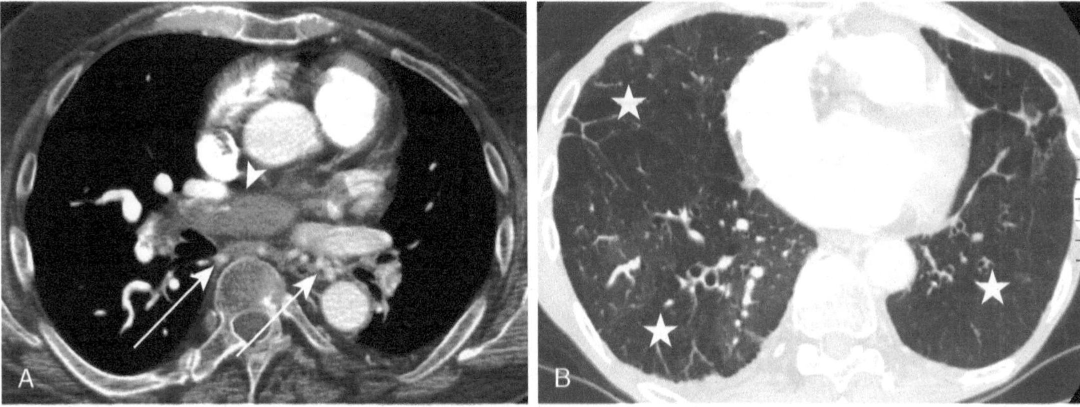

FIGURE 11.14 Secondary signs of chronic pulmonary embolism (PE). **A,** Axial computed tomography in mediastinal window shows multiple enlarged bronchial arteries *(arrows)* secondary to an occluding chronic PE in the right main pulmonary artery *(arrowhead)*. **B,** Axial image in lung windows depicts sharply demarcated regions of hypoattenuation in both lungs, with reduced vessel size *(stars)* interspersed with adjacent areas of normal attenuation or relative hyperattenuation consistent with mosaic attenuation. Note the marked constriction of the pulmonary arteries in areas of hypoattenuation.

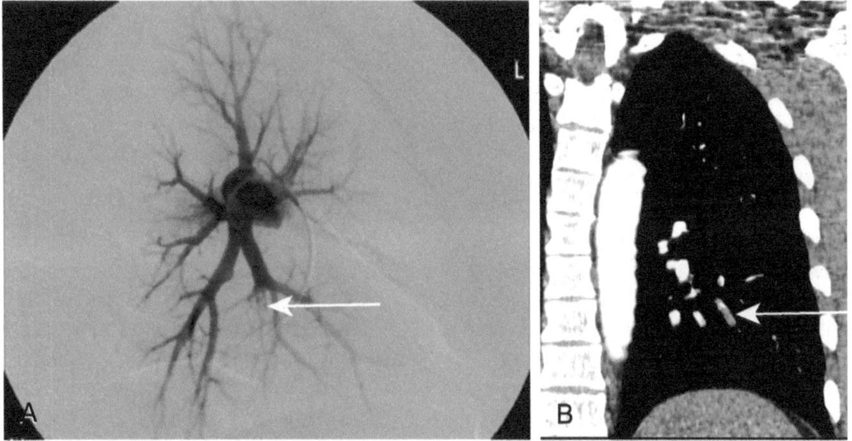

FIGURE 11.15 Pulmonary embolism on pulmonary angiogram. **A,** Digital subtraction angiogram demonstrates a filling defect and abrupt cutoff of a left lower lobe pulmonary artery *(arrow)*. **B,** Coronal computed tomography pulmonary angiography image shows the corresponding filling defect *(arrow)*.

therapeutic intervention and, in selected cases, preoperative evaluation of the pulmonary arteries.

Magnetic Resonance Angiography

With recent improvements in technology, magnetic resonance angiography (MRA) shows promise for the detection of PE. MRA has the advantage of using neither ionizing radiation nor iodinated contrast. These advantages allow the use of multiphasic acquisitions and the potential for repeated contrast injections, resulting in improved technical success rates when the initial acquisition is compromised by poor bolus timing or patient motion. Disadvantages of MRA compared with CTPA include longer acquisition times, limiting the suitability of long MRI protocols in dyspneic patients, and lower spatial resolution, which likely contributes to the lower sensitivity for the detection of subsegmental emboli. There is also concern about nephrogenic systemic fibrosis, which occurs rarely in patients with poor renal function who receive gadolinium-containing contrast material. Furthermore, the relative lack of familiarity with MRA for evaluation of PE may contribute to technical inconsistency, the primary reason for the underperformance of MRA for the detection of subsegmental emboli in the PIOPED III study.

The pulmonary arteries are evaluated in a segment-by-segment method, similar to the evaluation of CTPA images. Although the criteria for the diagnosis of PE are similar for MRA and CTPA, an important difference is the fact that completely occlusive emboli can appear as abrupt vessel cutoffs on MRA, analogous to cutoff vessels seen in conventional angiography. This may make the identification of occlusive emboli more difficult on MRA than on CTPA because an absent vessel may be more challenging to identify. The PIOPED III study concluded that technically adequate MRA had a sensitivity of 92% and a specificity of 99%, but 25% of patients had technically inadequate images.

Unenhanced MRA techniques can also be used for patients with suspected PE. These include balanced steady-state free precession techniques, three-dimensional (3D) fresh blood imaging using 3D fast spin-echo-based sequences, and arterial spin-labeling techniques.

NONTHROMBOTIC PULMONARY EMBOLUS

Nonthrombotic PE is an uncommon condition. It usually involves particles that are so small that they do not present as intraarterial filling defects. Possible causes include droplets of fat, bubbles of air or nitrogen, amniotic fluid, tumors, and foreign bodies such as talc or cement.

Septic Embolus

Septic emboli can occur when fragments of thrombus include microorganisms, typically bacterial; however, fungi or parasites can also be involved. Please refer to Chapter 14 for more details.

Fat Embolus

This is a rare complication of a long bone fracture. Other rarer causes include hemoglobinopathy, major burns, pancreatitis, overwhelming infection, tumors, blood transfusion, and liposuction. Please refer to Chapter 10 for more details.

Air Embolus

Air embolism can be classified into two types: venous air embolism and arterial air embolism. Venous air embolism occurs when air is introduced into systemic veins and travels to the right ventricle and pulmonary arteries. Causes of venous air embolism to the right ventricle and pulmonary arteries include peripheral intravenous (IV) placement, radiologic IV contrast administration, central line placement or removal, dialysis, pacemaker placement, trauma, and certain surgical procedures (otolaryngologic, orthopedic, obstetrics and gynecology, and especially neurosurgical procedures). Venous air embolism is reported in 12% to 23% of patients undergoing contrast-enhanced CT, but venous air emboli are typically of no clinical significance when small in volume. Moderate amounts of venous air embolism may result in a noncardiogenic pulmonary edema pattern. Large venous air embolism may show hyperlucency in the heart, pulmonary arteries, or hepatic veins and can be fatal.

Arterial air embolism occurs when air enters the pulmonary veins, left ventricle, and systemic arterial circulation. Arterial air embolism may occur by direct entry of air into the pulmonary veins during lung biopsy, radiofrequency or microwave lung ablation, thoracic or cardiac surgery, or penetrating trauma. Paradoxical embolism of a venous air embolism can occur when there is a right-to-left communication through a septal defect, patent foramen ovale, or pulmonary AVMs.

Either venous or arterial air embolism can result from decompression sickness (divers), barotrauma associated with positive pressure ventilation, and penetrating and rarely blunt chest trauma.

The pathologic effects of air embolism occur through vascular obstruction "air block" or vasoconstriction. Air emboli can also cause vascular inflammation and endothelial injury. Arterial air embolism is typically a more serious event and can be morbid even with a small arterial air embolism. The heart and brain are the most vulnerable end organs in arterial air embolism, potentially resulting in stroke, seizure, or myocardial infarction.

Amniotic Fluid Embolus

This is a rare but highly fatal complication of pregnancy. It occurs when amniotic fluid is forced into the bloodstream through small tears in the uterine veins during normal labor or when the placenta is disrupted by surgery or trauma. Please refer to Chapter 10 for more details.

Tumor Embolus

Intravascular pulmonary metastases are seen in up to a quarter of autopsies but are much less frequently identified before death. Common extrapulmonary malignancies that cause tumor emboli include hepatocellular, breast, renal, gastric and prostate carcinoma, and choriocarcinoma. The majority involve subsegmental pulmonary arteries and arterioles. However, right atrial myxomas and renal cell carcinoma tend to embolize to the large central and segmental pulmonary arteries. CT findings depend on the size of the involved pulmonary arteries, with large emboli in the main or lobar pulmonary arteries causing filling defects that mimic acute PE. Tumor emboli that affect the segmental and subsegmental pulmonary arteries produce multifocal dilation or beading of the pulmonary artery, and those affecting secondary pulmonary lobule arterioles have a tree-in-bud appearance. Although tumor emboli may occur suddenly and mimic thrombotic emboli, they often demonstrate growth on serial scans (Fig. 11.16).

Foreign Body Embolus

Talc and cellulose emboli are common among drug addicts. These materials are used as fillers in tablets taken orally but are insoluble and when injected become trapped in the pulmonary vasculature, causing thrombosis, inflammation, and eventually giant cell reaction. Findings on chest radiographs progress from initial widespread small nodules to large areas of increased opacity that resemble the progressive massive fibrosis seen in patients with silicosis. There may also be evidence of pulmonary hypertension. On CT, tree-in-bud opacities can be identified.

Cement (polymethacrylate) embolus is a potential complication of percutaneous vertebroplasty. Both radiography and CT may demonstrate tubular areas of high-attenuation cement outlining the pulmonary arteries (Fig. 11.17). Catheter embolus can also occur and may happen when the introducer needle tears off a fragment of a catheter as the introducer needle is being removed. Chest radiography shows the fragment in an unusual location, such as the heart or pulmonary artery, which can be confirmed on CT. Another substance that can cause a nonthrombotic embolus is iodinated oil, used for lymphangiography or for transcatheter oil chemoembolization for treatment of hepatocellular carcinoma. Embolization of brachytherapy seeds used for the treatment of prostate cancer has also been described.

PULMONARY HYPERTENSION

Pulmonary hypertension is a hemodynamic and pathophysiologic condition defined as an increase in mean pulmonary arterial pressure of 25 mm Hg or more at rest as assessed by right heart catheterization. The current classification

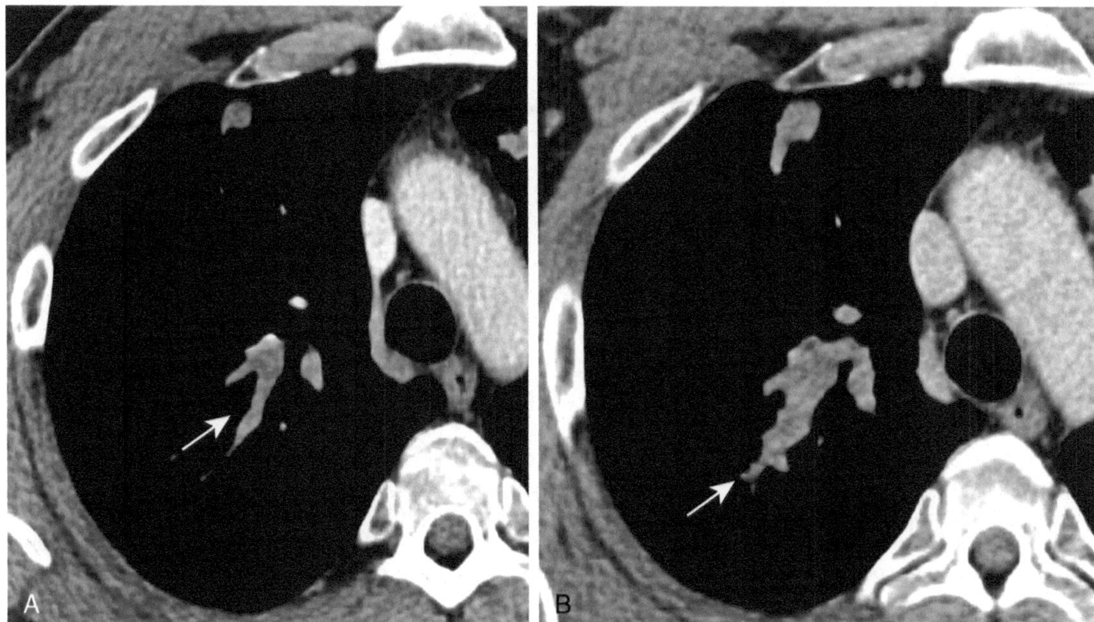

FIGURE 11.16 Tumor embolus. **A,** Axial computed tomography image in a 67-year-old man with hepatocellular carcinoma depicts a branching structure in the right upper lobe *(arrow),* which is in the distribution of a pulmonary artery. **B,** Follow-up imaging 6 months later shows that this lesion *(arrow)* has increased in size and has a beaded appearance consistent with enlargement of a tumor embolus. Note an additional smaller tumor embolus anteriorly.

of pulmonary hypertension is clinically based and groups diseases with similar pathophysiologic features and therapeutic approaches (Box 11.2). A diagnosis of pulmonary arterial hypertension (PAH) is made only in the absence of other causes of pulmonary hypertension. The presenting symptoms are initially those of exertional dyspnea, but patients may have reduced exercise tolerance, fatigue, exertional chest pain, and syncope as right ventricular function becomes compromised. Because of these nonspecific symptoms, the diagnosis is usually delayed by an average of 2 years. Imaging plays an important role in the detection, characterization, and monitoring of pulmonary hypertension.

Imaging of Pulmonary Hypertension

Chest Radiography

The features of pulmonary hypertension on a chest radiograph include cardiomegaly, right atrial and right ventricular dilation, and enlarged central pulmonary arteries (Fig. 11.18). In PAH, the pulmonary vessels are typically dilated centrally and attenuated peripherally (pruned). On chest radiographs, enlargement of the main pulmonary artery results in a prominent convex contour. On posteroanterior, erect chest radiographs, the normal transverse diameter of the right interlobar artery as it descends adjacent to the bronchus intermedius is less than or equal to 16 mm. The left pulmonary artery is seen better on the lateral projection and should measure no more than 18 mm from the posterior margin of the artery to the upper limit of the left upper lobe bronchus. In the setting of long-standing, severe PAH, the enlarged central pulmonary arteries may develop peripheral, atherosclerotic calcification. This is an unusual finding and is most frequently seen in patients with PAH secondary to Eisenmenger syndrome, a condition characterized by a reversal in the direction of a long-standing, severe left-to-right shunt. On the lateral view, there may be reduced retrosternal air space as a result of right ventricular dilation.

Chest radiography may also depict features that are indicative of the underlying cause of pulmonary hypertension, such as interstitial lung disease, emphysema, chest wall deformities, and left-sided heart disease.

Ventilation/Perfusion Scintigraphy

In the setting of the evaluation of pulmonary hypertension, V/Q scintigraphy is mainly performed to identify potentially surgically treatable chronic thromboembolic pulmonary hypertension (CTEPH) and to differentiate it from other causes of pulmonary hypertension. In CTEPH, there are typically multiple segmental perfusion defects with maintenance of normal ventilation, resulting in a mismatch of perfusion and ventilation in the affected bronchopulmonary segment (Fig. 11.19). This differs from nonthrombotic causes of pulmonary hypertension, in which the V/Q scan may be normal or may demonstrate mismatched nonsegmental defects in the perfusion, giving a moth-eaten appearance. V/Q has a very high sensitivity and specificity in differentiating CTEPH from idiopathic PAH and is more sensitive for evaluation of CTEPH than CT.

Computed Tomography

Pulmonary arterial hypertension can be reliably predicted when (1) the diameter of the distal main pulmonary artery is greater than or equal to 29 mm and the segmental artery-to-bronchus ratio is greater than 1:1 in three of four pulmonary lobes or (2) the ratio of the distal main

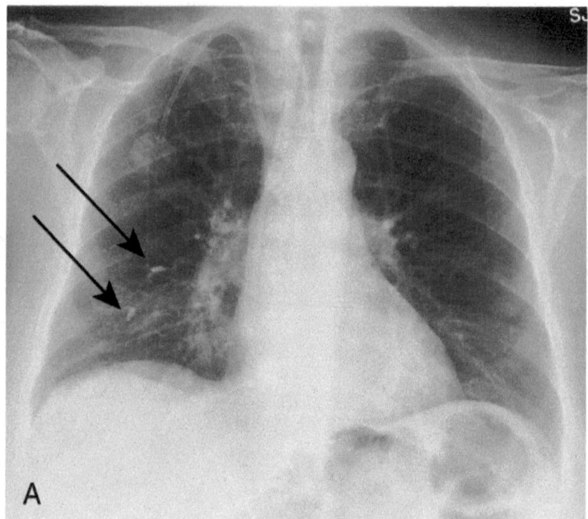

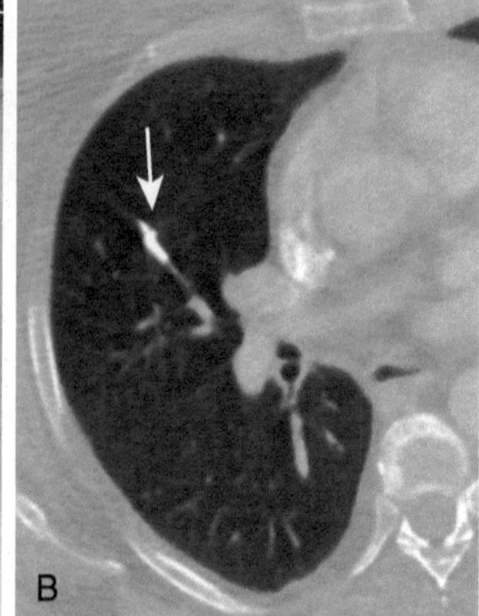

FIGURE 11.17 Cement embolism. **A,** Frontal chest radiograph in a 78-year-old man who had previously undergone lumbar vertebroplasty, depicting two foci of tubular high attenuation in the right lower lung *(arrows)*. **B,** Axial computed tomography image confirming high-attenuation material within a right middle lobe subsegmental pulmonary artery consistent with a cement embolus *(arrow)*.

BOX 11.2 Clinical Classification of Pulmonary Hypertension (Nice, 2013)

1 Pulmonary arterial hypertension (PAH)
- 1.1 Idiopathic PAH
- 1.2 Heritable
  - 1.2.1 BMPR2
  - 1.2.2 ALK-1, endoglin, SMAD9, CAV1, KCNK3
  - 1.2.3 Unknown
- 1.3 Drug-induced and toxin-induced
- 1.4 Associated with
  - 1.4.1 Connective tissue diseases
  - 1.4.2 HIV infection
  - 1.4.3 Portal hypertension
  - 1.4.4 Congenital heart disease
  - 1.4.5 Schistosomiasis

1′ Pulmonary veno-occlusive disease and/or pulmonary capillary hemangiomatosis

1″ Persistent pulmonary hypertension of the newborn

2 Pulmonary hypertension owing to left heart disease
- 2.1 Left ventricular systolic dysfunction
- 2.2 Left ventricular diastolic dysfunction
- 2.3 Valvular disease
- 2.4 Congenital/acquired left heart inflow/outflow tract obstruction and congenital cardiomyopathies

3 Pulmonary hypertension owing to lung disease and/or hypoxia
- 3.1 Chronic obstructive pulmonary disease
- 3.2 Interstitial lung disease
- 3.3 Other pulmonary disease with mixed restrictive and obstructive pattern
- 3.4 Sleep-disordered breathing
- 3.5 Alveolar hypoventilation disorders
- 3.6 Chronic exposures to high altitudes
- 3.7 Developmental abnormalities

4 Chronic thromboembolic pulmonary hypertension (CTEPH)

5 Pulmonary hypertension with unclear multifactorial mechanisms
- 5.1 Hematologic disorders: chronic hemolytic anemia, myeloproliferative disorders, splenectomy
- 5.2 Systemic disorders: sarcoidosis, pulmonary Langerhans cell histiocytosis, lymphangiomyomatosis, neurofibromatosis, vasculitis
- 5.3 Metabolic disorders: glycogen storage disease, Gaucher disease, thyroid disorders
- 5.4 Others: tumorous obstruction, fibrosing mediastinitis, chronic renal failure, segmental pulmonary hypertension

ALK-1, Activin receptor-like kinase type 1; *BMPR2,* bone morphogenetic protein receptor type 2; *CAV1,* caveolin 1; *KCNK3,* potassium channel superfamily K member-3; *SMAD9,* mothers against decapentaplegic 9.

pulmonary artery diameter to the ascending aortic diameter is greater than 1:1, particularly in patients younger than 50 years. In patients with fibrotic lung disease, the ratio of the pulmonary artery diameter to the ascending aortic diameter is a more reliable indicator of pulmonary hypertension than the absolute main pulmonary artery diameter. The CT diameter of the main pulmonary artery is measured in the scanning plane of its bifurcation at a right angle to its long axis and just lateral to the ascending aorta. Complications of sustained PAH that can be seen on CT include central pulmonary artery thrombosis, atherosclerosis of the pulmonary arteries (Fig. 11.20), and pulmonary artery dissection. Cardiac features of pulmonary hypertension include right ventricular hypertrophy (defined as a wall thickness of more than 4 mm), straightening or leftward bowing of the interventricular septum, right ventricular dilation (right ventricle diameter–left ventricle diameter ratio greater than 1), dilation of the inferior vena cava and hepatic veins, and pericardial effusion.

In cases of CTEPH, CT also demonstrates signs of chronic pulmonary thromboembolism as described previously. The increased bronchial artery blood flow secondary to chronic obstruction of the pulmonary arteries results in dilated bronchial arteries (≥1.5 mm in diameter) and nonbronchial systemic collaterals such as inferior phrenic, intercostal, and internal mammary arteries, which are seen in 73% of patients with CTEPH compared with only 14% of patients with IPAH. Mosaic perfusion is characterized by sharply demarcated

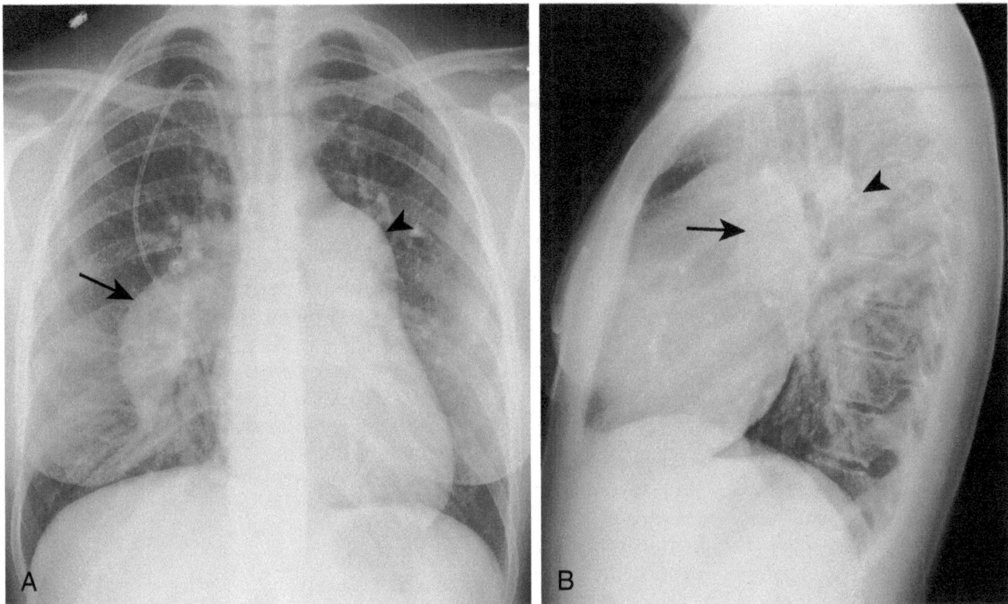

FIGURE 11.18 Pulmonary hypertension. **A,** Posteroanterior chest radiograph shows enlargement of the main pulmonary artery *(arrowhead)* and interlobar pulmonary artery *(arrow)*. Note is also made of a Port-A-Cath. **B,** Lateral chest radiograph shows enlargement of the right pulmonary artery *(arrow)* and left pulmonary artery *(arrowhead)*.

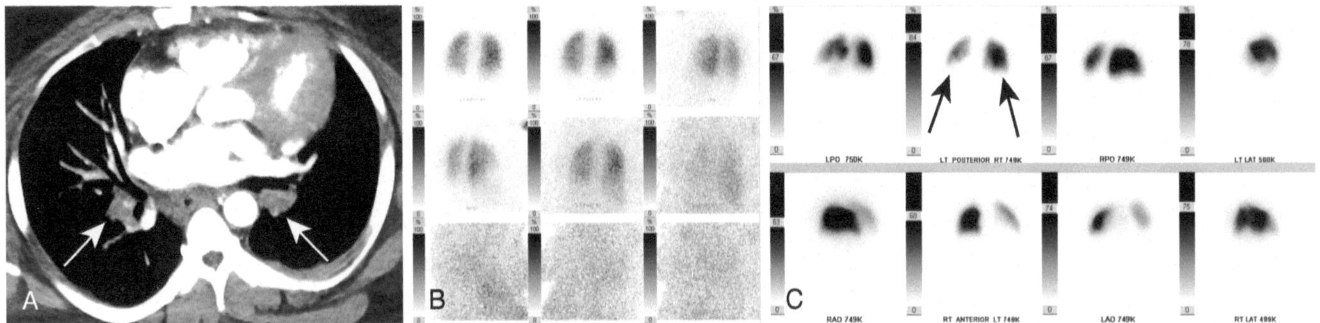

FIGURE 11.19 Chronic thromboembolic pulmonary hypertension. **A,** Axial chest computed tomography image demonstrating complete occlusion of bilateral lower lobe pulmonary arteries *(arrows)*. **B,** Ventilation scan demonstrates normal ventilation. **C,** Perfusion imaging demonstrates large perfusion defects in the lower lobes bilaterally *(arrows)*. These findings were unchanged from a prior study and are consistent with chronic thromboembolic pulmonary hypertension.

regions of lung hypoattenuation with reduced vessel size and without air trapping, interspersed with adjacent areas of normal lung attenuation or relative hyperattenuation (see Fig. 11.14) and is seen more often in patients with pulmonary hypertension caused by chronic PE than in those with pulmonary hypertension secondary to cardiac or lung disease. Other parenchymal findings frequently seen in CTEPH include peripheral opacities caused by prior infarction and cylindrical bronchial dilation. Bronchial dilation usually occurs at the segmental or subsegmental level in areas of severely stenosed or completely occluded pulmonary arteries. CT may also be used to see if patients will benefit from surgery. Patients are considered for thromboendarterectomy if disease is present in the main, lobar, or segmental arteries. Patients with distal disease usually undergo medical treatment.

Computed tomography findings of pulmonary venoocclusive disease (PVOD) include dilated central pulmonary arteries; widespread, smoothly thickened interlobular septa; and ground-glass opacities in a diffuse, geographic, mosaic, perihilar, patchy, or centrilobular pattern. Septal lines and poorly defined centrilobular ground-glass opacities are helpful findings in distinguishing between PVOD and idiopathic PAH. In cases of pulmonary capillary hemangiomatosis, main pulmonary arterial enlargement and widespread ill-defined centrilobular ground-glass nodules are seen on CT (Fig. 11.21).

Magnetic Resonance Imaging

Cardiac MR imaging (MRI) can be used to assess morphologic changes of pulmonary hypertension, including right ventricular dilation and hypertrophy, right atrial enlargement, flattening or leftward bowing of the interventricular septum, and tricuspid regurgitation. A delayed pattern of contrast enhancement with a midwall distribution at the

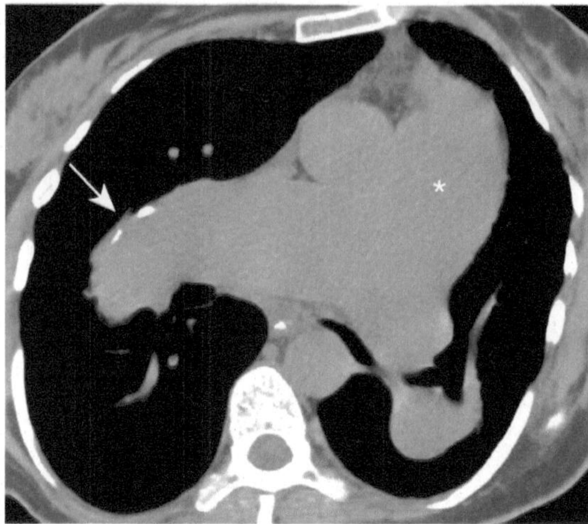

FIGURE 11.20 Eisenmenger syndrome with pulmonary hypertension and pulmonary arterial calcification. Axial unenhanced computed tomography image demonstrating enlarged main pulmonary artery *(asterisk)*, right main pulmonary artery, interlobar pulmonary artery, and left main pulmonary artery. There is associated calcification of the wall of the interlobar pulmonary artery *(arrow)*.

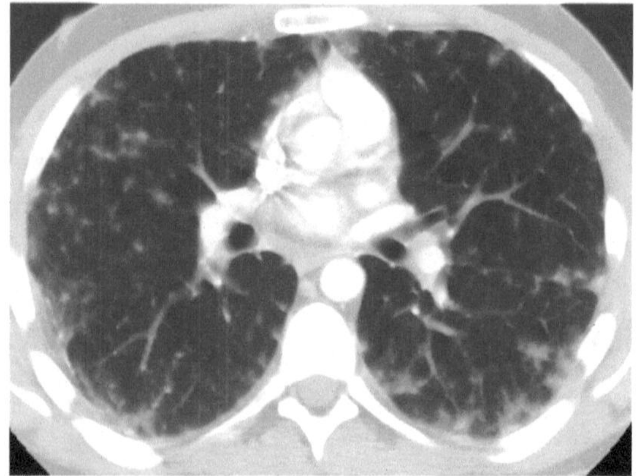

FIGURE 11.21 Pulmonary capillary hemangiomatosis. Axial image from contrast-enhanced computed tomography in lung window shows multiple patchy ground-glass nodules in this patient with pulmonary capillary hemangiomatosis.

right ventricular septal insertion has been described in patients with chronic pulmonary hypertension.

PULMONARY VASCULITIS

Vasculitis is an inflammatory process affecting blood vessels. Pulmonary vasculitis may constitute a primary (most cases are idiopathic) disorder or may be secondary to other conditions. Underlying conditions in the secondary vasculitides include infectious diseases, connective tissue disorders, malignancies, and hypersensitivity disorders. Vasculitis can be broadly classified depending on the size of the predominantly affected vessel into small-, medium-, and large-vessel vasculitis (Box 11.3). Lung involvement can present via three major pathologic mechanisms:

- Necrosis of pulmonary parenchyma with inflammatory cell infiltration
- Stenosis of the tracheobronchial tree secondary to inflammation
- Diffuse alveolar hemorrhage secondary to pulmonary capillaritis

BOX 11.3 Classification of Vasculitides

- Large-vessel vasculitis
  - Takayasu arteritis
  - Giant cell arteritis
- Medium-vessel vasculitis
  - Polyarteritis nodosa
  - Kawasaki disease
- Small-vessel vasculitis
  - Antineutrophil cytoplasmic antibody–associated vasculitis
    - Granulomatosis with polyangiitis
    - Eosinophilic granulomatosis with polyangiitis
    - Microscopic polyangiitis
  - Immune complex small-vessel vasculitis
    - Antiglomerular basement membrane disease
    - Cryoglobinemic vasculitis
    - Immunoglobulin A vasculitis
    - Hypocomplementemic urticarial vasculitis
- Variable vessel vasculitis
  - Behçet disease
  - Cogan syndrome
- Vasculitis associated with systemic disease
  - Lupus vasculitis
  - Rheumatoid vasculitis
  - Sarcoid vasculitis
- Vasculitis associated with probable etiology
  - Hepatitis C virus–associated cryoglobinemic vasculitis
  - Hepatitis B virus–associated vasculitis
  - Syphilis-associated aortitis
  - Drug-associated immune complex vasculitis
  - Drug-associated antineutrophil cytoplasmic antibody–associated vasculitis
  - Cancer-associated vasculitis
  - Other

Large-Vessel Vasculitis

The two main diseases involving the large vessels are *Takayasu arteritis* and *giant cell arteritis*. They predominantly affect the aorta and its largest branches, such as the major arteries to the extremities and to the head and neck. However, pulmonary artery involvement occurs in 50% to 80% of patients with Takayasu arteritis, predominantly as a late manifestation of the disease. Stenosis or occlusion of the segmental and subsegmental arteries and less commonly of the lobar or main pulmonary artery are the most characteristic findings. CT manifestations of pulmonary artery involvement include wall thickening (Fig. 11.22) and enhancement in the early phases and mural calcification and luminal stenosis or occlusion in the chronic phase. In chronic cases, collaterals can develop depending on the site and severity of the stenosis. MRI can also demonstrate the smooth wall thickening of the involved vessels, which may show enhancement. The presence of mural enhancement is suggestive of active disease. MRI is preferred over CT because it avoids radiation in this young population. Positron emission tomography (PET) with 18-fluorodeoxyglucose (^{18}FDG) can show FDG uptake in acutely inflamed vessels and can also be helpful in monitoring these patients as the intensity of FDG accumulation decreases in response

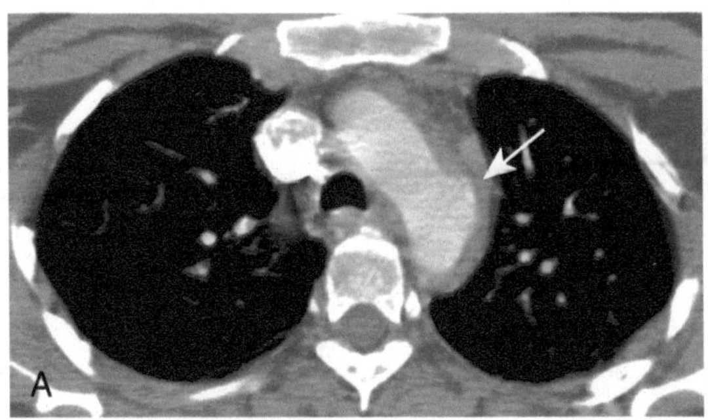

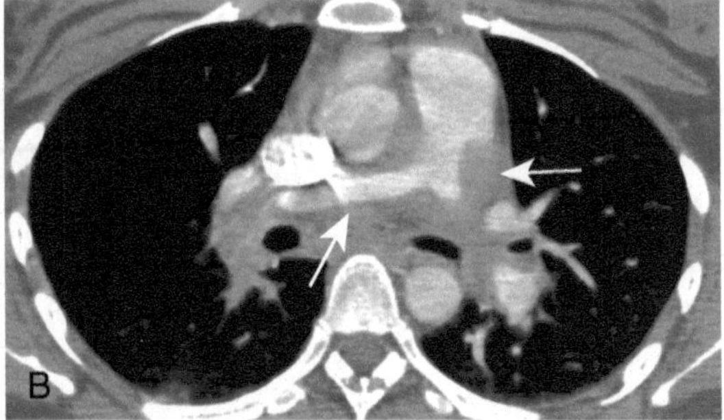

FIGURE 11.22 Takayasu arteritis. Axial images from chest computed tomography with intravenous contrast demonstrates **(A)** thickening of the aorta and a focal aneurysm of the aortic arch *(arrow)*. **B,** Thickening and narrowing of the main pulmonary arteries bilaterally *(arrows)* in a patient with Takayasu arteritis

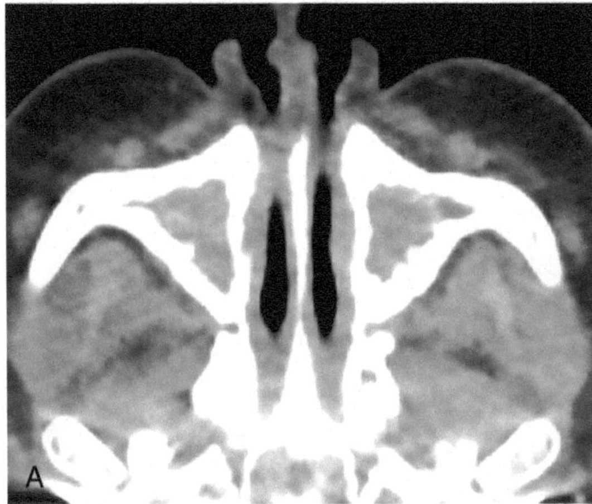

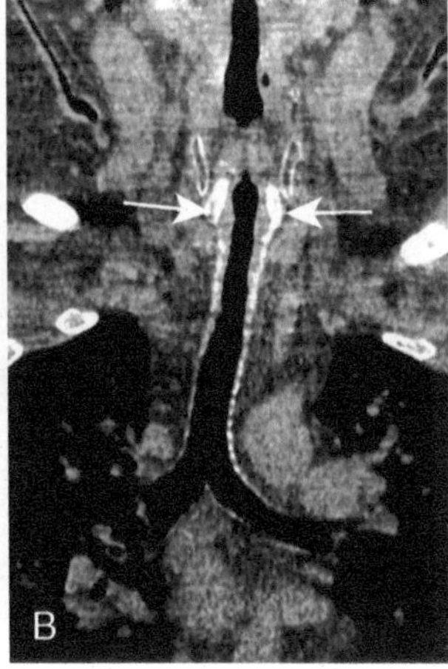

FIGURE 11.23 Granulomatosis with polyangiitis. **A,** Axial image of the sinuses demonstrates complete opacification of the maxillary sinuses bilaterally. **B,** Reconstructed coronal image shows diffuse thickening of the subglottic trachea *(arrows)*. The patient was confirmed to have granulomatosis with polyangiitis on serologic testing.

to treatment. Pulmonary artery involvement is much less common with giant cell arteritis than with Takayasu arteritis.

Medium-Vessel Vasculitis

Medium-vessel vasculitis predominantly affects the medium arteries, such as the main visceral arteries and their branches. The two major forms are *polyarteritis nodosa* and *Kawasaki disease*. Lung involvement is extremely rare in polyarteritis nodosa, and its presence argues against this entity. Kawasaki disease usually occurs in children younger than 5 years. The coronary arteries are often involved, and the aorta and large arteries may be involved.

Small-Vessel Vasculitis

Small-vessel vasculitis is defined as vasculitis that affects vessels smaller than arteries, such as arterioles, venules, and capillaries; however, small-vessel vasculitis may also affect arteries, thus overlapping with medium- and large-vessel vasculitides. It is subdivided into antineutrophil cytoplasm antibody (ANCA)-associated vasculitis (AAV) and immune complex small-vessel vasculitis.

Antineutrophil Cytoplasm Antibody–Associated Vasculitis

Antineutrophil cytoplasm antibody-associated vasculitides are the most common primary systemic small-vessel vasculitides in adults and include three major diseases: granulomatosis with polyangiitis, eosinophilic granulomatosis with polyangiitis, and microscopic polyangiitis.

Granulomatosis With Polyangiitis. Formerly referred to as Wegener granulomatosis, granulomatosis with polyangiitis (GPA) is the most common AAV. The classic triad includes upper airway disease (including otitis; sinusitis; epistaxis; rhinorrhea; ulceration; and subglottic, tracheal, and bronchial stenosis) (Fig. 11.23), lung involvement (clinically presenting as hemoptysis, chest pain, dyspnea, and cough), and glomerulonephritis (presenting as hematuria and azotemia), although patients may not have all these symptoms at initial presentation. The upper respiratory tract is affected in almost all patients, and the lungs and kidneys are involved in 90% and 80% of patients, respectively.

The most common chest radiographic and CT abnormalities of GPA are pulmonary nodules and masses, seen at presentation in up to 90% of patients with pulmonary disease (Fig. 11.24). The nodules and masses are usually multiple and bilateral and tend to involve mainly the subpleural regions or less commonly the peribronchovascular regions. They have no predilection for the upper or lower lung zones. The nodules can coalesce into larger masses greater than 10 cm in diameter. Larger nodules, greater than 2 cm, frequently cavitate. The cavities are usually thick walled with an irregular inner margin, but they may become thin walled and decrease in size with treatment. On contrast-enhanced CT scans, most noncavitated nodules

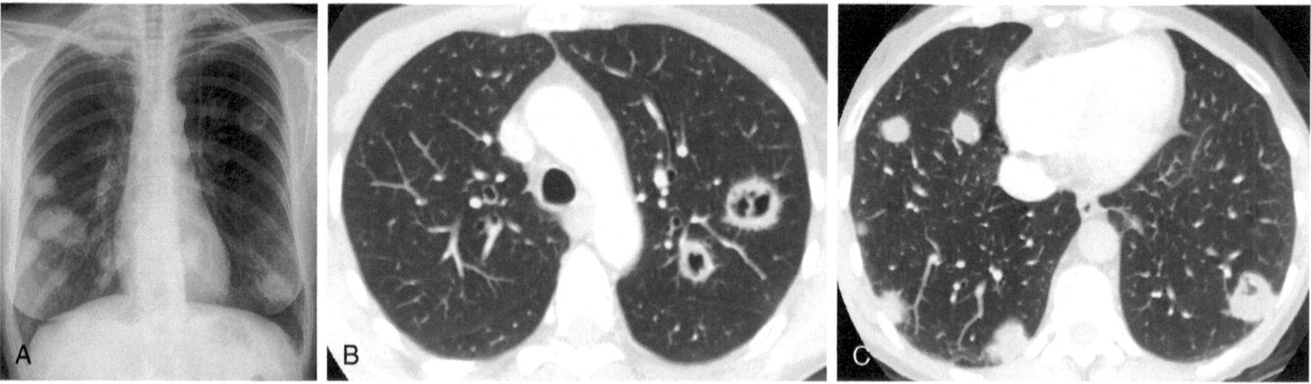

FIGURE 11.24 Granulomatosis with polyangiitis. **A,** Frontal chest radiograph demonstrating bilateral nodules and masses, some of which demonstrate cavitation. **B,** Axial computed tomography (CT) image at the level of the aortic arch shows cavitary nodules in the left upper lobe. Note that the nodules have thick walls. **C,** Axial CT image at the level of the lung bases shows bilateral pulmonary nodules. This was confirmed to be granulomatosis with polyangiitis on biopsy.

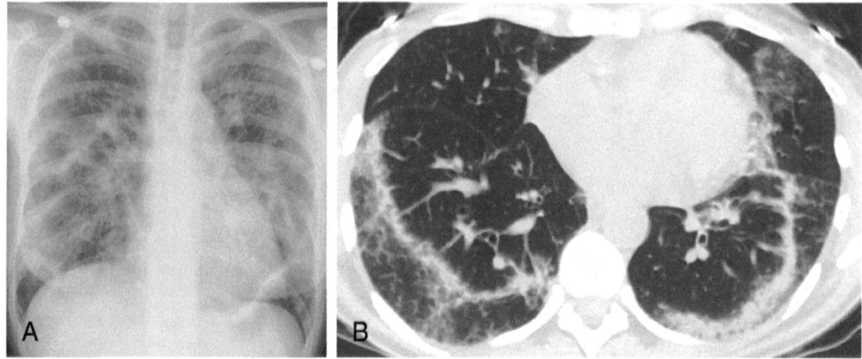

FIGURE 11.25 Eosinophilic granulomatosis with polyangiitis. **A,** Frontal chest radiograph demonstrates diffuse lung disease with bilateral lower lung zone–predominant bandlike pulmonary opacities. **B,** Axial chest computed tomography scan shows a strongly peripheral pattern of consolidation and ground-glass opacities in this patient with eosinophilic granulomatosis with polyangiitis.

or masses demonstrate central low attenuation, which may reflect necrosis, with or without peripheral enhancement. A rim of ground-glass opacity surrounding the pulmonary lesion (the CT halo sign) is seen in up to 15% of cases. A reverse halo appearance may also be seen, likely reflecting an organizing pneumonia reaction in the periphery of focal hemorrhage. There may be evidence of an artery, leading into a nodule or mass, known as the feeding vessel sign.

Consolidation and ground-glass opacities are the second most common radiographic manifestation and can be seen in 25% to 50% of patients. The opacities can be patchy or diffuse and reflect either vasculitic pulmonary disease in the form of pneumonitis or alveolar hemorrhage. Airway abnormalities are also common with GPA, with segmental or subsegmental bronchial wall thickening seen in 40% to 70% of patients. Larger airways are involved in 30% of patients. Concentric wall thickening caused by inflammation leading to airway stenosis is seen in 15% of patients. Involvement of the subglottic trachea is most typical, with variable involvement of the vocal cords, distal trachea, and proximal mainstem bronchi. The main differential diagnosis for GPA (typically subpleural nodules and masses) includes infection such as septic emboli and abscess; neoplasm, including hematogenous metastases and lymphoma; and when peribronchovascular lesions predominate, organizing pneumonia and Kaposi sarcoma.

Eosinophilic Granulomatosis With Polyangiitis. Formerly called Churg-Strauss syndrome, it consists of a triad of eosinophilia, asthma, and necrotizing vasculitis. Virtually all patients have asthma. Pulmonary hemorrhage and glomerulonephritis are less commonly seen in EGPA than in other types of AAV. Involvement of other organs, such as the skin, kidneys, cardiac, gastrointestinal system, and neurologic system, is common.

Abnormal chest radiographic findings are seen in more than 70% of patients with EGPA. The most common radiographic manifestation consists of bilateral, nonsegmental areas of consolidation without a predilection for any lung zone. The areas of consolidation can be transient, resembling Loeffler syndrome, or predominantly peripheral, resembling chronic eosinophilic pneumonia or organizing pneumonia (Fig. 11.25). Pleural effusions are seen in approximately one third of patients. The most common abnormality on CT, seen in up to 90% of patients, is bilateral areas of ground-glass opacity or consolidation. The pulmonary opacities are usually lower lobe predominant and peripheral in distribution, although peribronchial and random distributions can also be seen. Interlobular septal thickening is another

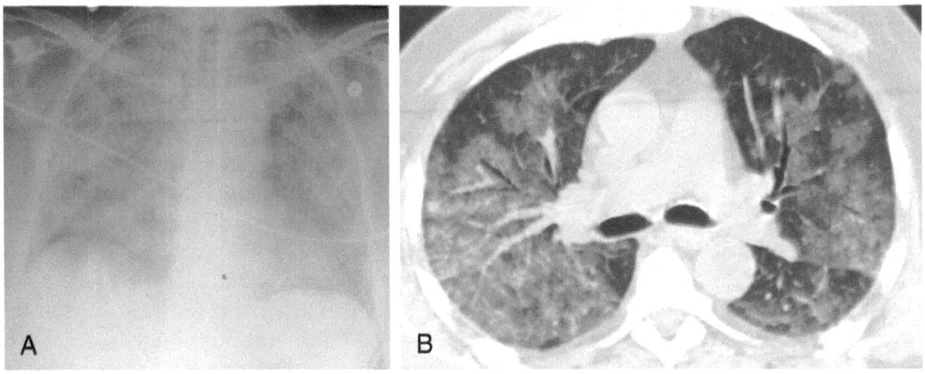

FIGURE 11.26 Diffuse alveolar hemorrhage associated with small-vessel vasculitis. **A,** Frontal chest radiograph demonstrates bilateral, diffuse airspace opacities. **B,** Axial computed tomography scan demonstrates diffuse ground-glass opacities in this patient with diffuse alveolar hemorrhage caused by small-vessel vasculitis.

relatively common finding, seen in approximately 50% of patients. This thickening may be secondary to pulmonary edema secondary to cardiac involvement, eosinophilic infiltration of the septa, or mild fibrosis. Less common manifestations include a diffuse reticular pattern or small and large nodular opacities that seldom cavitate. Unilateral or bilateral pleural effusions are seen on CT in up to 50% of patients and may be caused by left heart failure secondary to cardiomyopathy or by eosinophilic pleuritis. Airway involvement presents as small centrilobular nodules and tree-in-bud opacities, bronchial dilation, and bronchial and bronchiolar wall thickening.

Microscopic Polyangiitis. Characterized by the coexistence of pulmonary hemorrhage and glomerulonephritis, microscopic polyangiitis is the most common cause of pulmonary-renal syndrome. Pulmonary involvement is less common than renal manifestations and is seen in 30% of patients. Radiologically, it manifests as diffuse alveolar hemorrhage secondary to pulmonary capillaritis. The radiographic features consist of patchy or diffuse bilateral airspace opacities. CT is more definitive in the assessment of lung involvement, demonstrating patchy or diffuse ground-glass opacities and consolidation (Fig. 11.26). The findings are usually widespread but may be more prominent in the perihilar regions, with relative sparing of the lung apices and the costophrenic regions. Ill-defined centrilobular nodules may be the predominant pattern in some patients. The presence of dense consolidation represents complete filling of the alveoli with blood.

Within days of an acute episode of hemorrhage, interlobular septal thickening can be seen in association with the ground-glass opacity (crazy-paving pattern) as hemosiderin-laden macrophages accumulate in the interstitium. Complete clearing of airspace and interstitial opacities usually occurs within 10 to 14 days if no further hemorrhage occurs. Repeated episodes of pulmonary hemorrhage may result in a persistent reticular pattern with areas of honeycombing and traction bronchiectasis. This reflects interstitial hemosiderin deposition and mild lung fibrosis.

Immune Complex Small-Vessel Vasculitides

The immune complex small-vessel vasculitides include antiglomerular basement membrane disease, immunoglobulin A vasculitis, hypocomplementemic urticarial vasculitis, and cryoglobulinemic vasculitis.

Antiglomerular Basement Membrane Disease. *Goodpasture disease* is a term used for patients with glomerulonephritis and pulmonary hemorrhage with antiglomerular basement membrane (anti-GBM) antibodies. Pulmonary involvement occurs in 40% to 60% of patients, with the typical imaging features of diffuse alveolar hemorrhage being seen.

Immunoglobulin A Vasculitis. Formerly known as Henoch-Schönlein purpura, pulmonary involvement is rare in children but more common in adults. Deposition of anti-GBM IgA leads to alveolitis and capillaritis, and imaging features related to diffuse alveolar hemorrhage are seen. Pleural effusions can also be seen. Interstitial fibrosis with the usual interstitial pneumonia pattern has also been reported.

Hypocomplementemic Urticarial Vasculitis. Pulmonary involvement is reported in 20% of patients, with the most common manifestations being chronic obstructive pulmonary disease and asthma. Panacinar emphysema with a basilar predominance is commonly seen. Pleural effusions have also been reported.

Cryoglobulinemic Vasculitis. Pulmonary involvement is rare, occurring in only 2% of cases. The imaging features are related to diffuse alveolar hemorrhage.

Variable Vessel Vasculitis

Behçet disease can affect vessels of any size and type. Behçet disease is a chronic multisystemic vasculitis characterized by recurrent oral and genital ulcerations, with associated inflammatory skin, articular, ocular, gastrointestinal, or central nervous system lesions. Thoracic involvement has been reported in up to 8% of patients. Behçet disease is the most common cause of pulmonary artery aneurysms (Fig. 11.27). Typically, these pulmonary artery aneurysms are fusiform or saccular, commonly multiple and bilateral, and located in the main or lower lobe pulmonary arteries. Frequently, these pulmonary artery aneurysms are partially or totally thrombosed. On a chest radiograph, the presence of a pulmonary artery aneurysm may be suggested by hilar enlargement or a round perihilar area of increased opacity. CT findings include thickening of the wall of the aorta or superior vena cava caused by vasculitis, superior vena cava obstruction, thromboembolism, and pulmonary infarction. Intracardiac thrombi and endomyocardial fibrosis can occur, which are better appreciated on MRI. Small-vessel involvement by Behçet disease can cause mosaic attenuation on CT. Pleural effusions can also be seen secondary to either superior vena cava obstruction or pulmonary infarction.

Other Causes of Vasculitis

Vasculitis can also be associated with or caused by a systemic disease. Common associations include collagen vascular disease such as rheumatoid arthritis, systemic lupus erythematosus, systemic sclerosis, sarcoidosis, and relapsing polychondritis. In these cases of secondary vasculitis, the small vessels are typically involved with evidence of capillaritis.

Drugs such as propylthiouracil, gemcitabine, transretinoic acid, and crack cocaine may also cause pulmonary capillaritis. Imaging studies usually depict the findings of diffuse alveolar hemorrhage (Fig. 11.28). Foreign materials such as talc, starch, cellulose, and maltose, which are used as filler for tablets and capsules, when injected in suspension by drug abusers can cause a foreign body granulomatous reaction that is centered on arterioles. Radiographic findings include small pulmonary nodules. CT findings include centrilobular small nodules or vascular tree-in-bud opacities within the secondary pulmonary lobule.

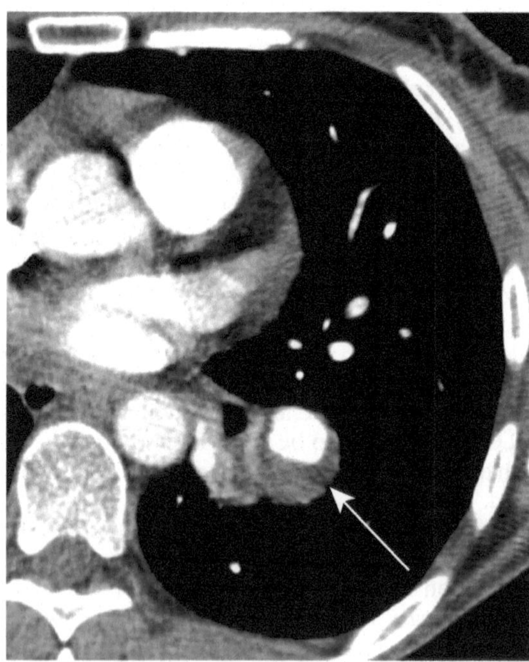

FIGURE 11.27 Behçet disease. Axial image from contrast-enhanced chest computed tomography scan shows a fusiform aneurysm with peripheral thrombus in the left lower lobe pulmonary artery *(arrow)*. The patient was confirmed to have Behçet disease on biopsy of the pulmonary artery.

PULMONARY ARTERY PSEUDOANEURYSM

Pulmonary artery pseudoaneurysms are rare and may be idiopathic or may be related to infection, primary or secondary lung neoplasm, pulmonary hypertension, or vasculitis. Trauma is another cause, most commonly as a result of pulmonary artery perforation caused by improper placement of a pulmonary artery catheter or a penetrating injury and very rarely as a result of blunt injury. In the appropriate clinical setting, a pulmonary artery aneurysm or pseudoaneurysm should be considered in patients who present with hemoptysis or when chest a radiograph demonstrates hilar enlargement or a new focal lung mass that is stable or has increased in size over subsequent radiographs. CTPA is thc noninvasive imaging modality of choice for the workup of patients with suspected PAP (Fig. 11.29). One study found that PAPs are usually solitary except in cases caused by endocarditis or metastatic disease, and they show a strong predilection for peripheral pulmonary artery branches. Those associated with endocarditis may not occur at the site of a consolidation or cavitary lesion, and those secondary to neoplasms most often occur at sites where tumor nodules or masses encase the pulmonary arteries. A ground-glass halo or a hemothorax is unusual in the absence of trauma. A high index of suspicion and awareness of the imaging findings are required because this entity is often underreported. Percutaneous endovascular treatment with direct coil embolization, stenting, or embolization

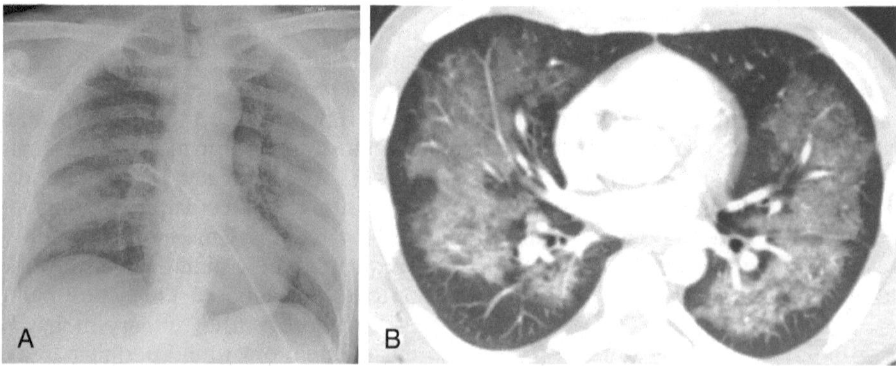

FIGURE 11.28 Diffuse alveolar hemorrhage associated with cocaine use. **A,** Frontal chest radiograph demonstrates bilateral airspace opacities. **B,** Axial chest computed tomography scan demonstrates diffuse bilateral ground-glass opacities with subpleural sparing. This patient had diffuse alveolar hemorrhage secondary to pulmonary capillaritis associated with a cocaine overdose.

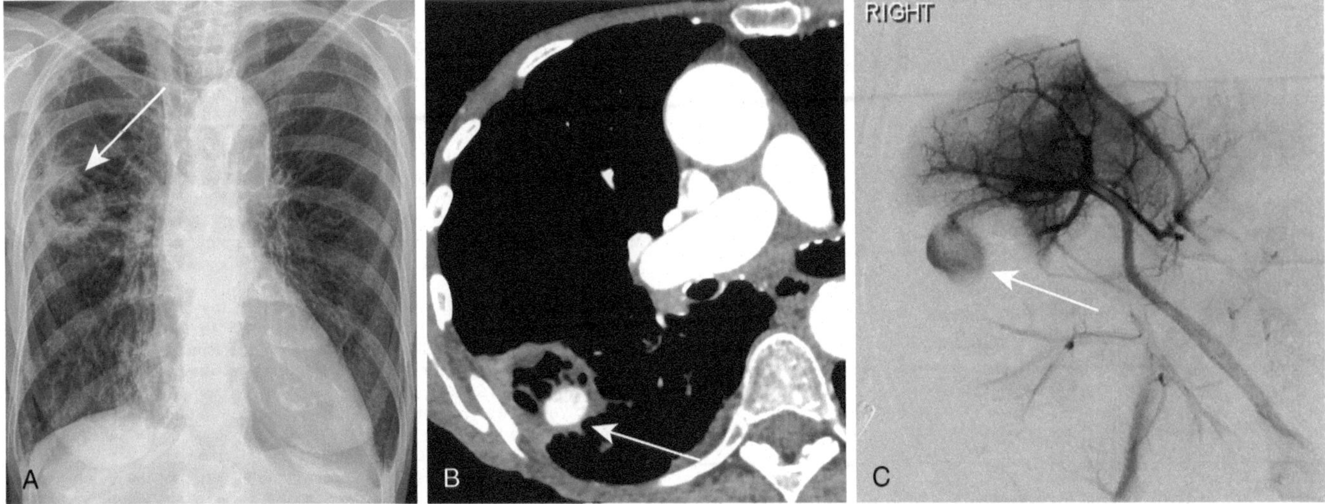

FIGURE 11.29 Pulmonary artery pseudoaneurysm caused by atypical mycobacterial infection. **A,** Frontal chest radiograph demonstrates a cavitary nodule with a thick wall in the right upper lung *(arrow)*. **B,** On the contrast-enhanced axial computed tomography image there is an avidly enhancing nodule within the wall of the cavity *(arrow)* consistent with a pulmonary artery pseudoaneurysm. **C,** This was confirmed on pulmonary artery angiography and was successfully treated by percutaneous coil embolization.

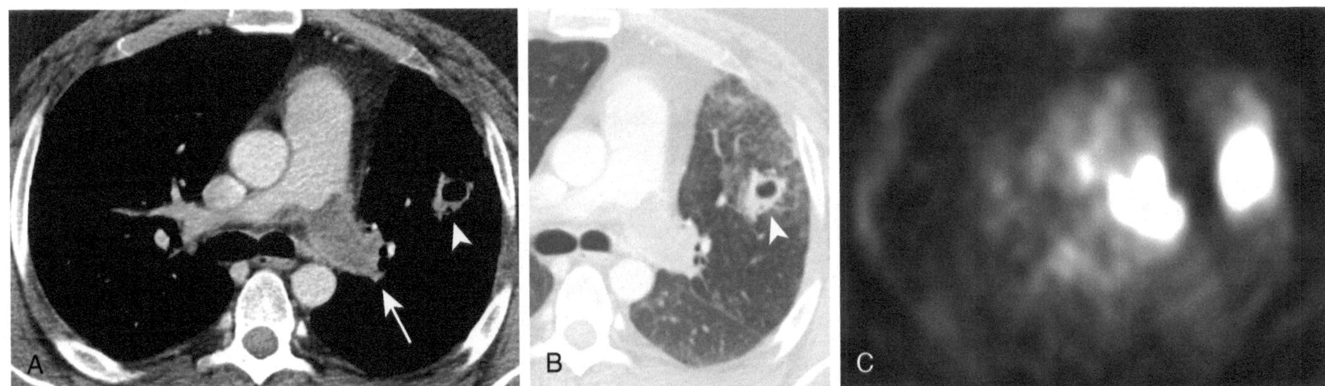

FIGURE 11.30 Pulmonary artery angiosarcoma. **A,** Axial contrast-enhanced computed tomography scan demonstrates a complete filling defect occluding the left main pulmonary artery *(arrow)*. **B,** Corresponding image on lung window shows a cavitary nodule in the left upper lobe *(arrowhead)*. **C,** Both the filling defect and the cavitary nodule demonstrate intense uptake on 18-fluorodeoxyglucose positron emission tomography. This was confirmed to be a pulmonary artery angiosarcoma on biopsy. The cavitary nodule represented a lung metastasis.

of the feeding vessel are effective and safe therapeutic options.

PULMONARY ARTERIOVENOUS MALFORMATION

Pulmonary arteriovenous malformations are abnormal communications between pulmonary arteries and veins. They tend to occur in the lower lobes and can be single or multiple. Commonly, pulmonary AVMs are congenital with a strong association with hereditary hemorrhagic telangiectasia (Rendu-Osler-Weber disease). Other causes are outlined in Box 11.4. Please refer to Chapter 8

PRIMARY PULMONARY ARTERY SARCOMA

Primary pulmonary artery sarcoma (PA sarcoma), although rare, is the most frequent sarcoma of the great arteries. It usually affects middle-aged people, favoring women slightly. Common presenting symptoms are similar to those of PE, including progressive dyspnea, cough, and chest pain; however, symptom onset is usually more gradual. Imaging is often as confounding as the clinical presentations, with many similarities between PA sarcoma and PE. Chest radiographs may demonstrate a hilar mass, prominent pulmonary artery, or decreased peripheral pulmonary vessels. On CT, PA sarcoma is usually unilateral, most commonly originates in the main pulmonary artery, and may demonstrate retrograde growth into the right ventricle. Imaging features may mimic a pulmonary embolus, but the filling defects tend to be more nodular and can demonstrate enhancement on CT or MRI. PA sarcoma can also demonstrate uptake of ^{18}FDG on PET (Fig. 11.30). Another differentiating feature of PA sarcoma from a PE is extension of the mass into the lung parenchyma or mediastinum.

BOX 11.4 Causes of Pulmonary Arteriovenous Malformation

Hereditary hemorrhagic telangiectasia
Hepatic cirrhosis
Penetrating chest trauma
Mitral stenosis
Schistosomiasis
Actinomycosis
Fanconi syndrome
Metastatic thyroid carcinoma
After surgery for congenital heart disease
Idiopathic

SUGGESTED READINGS

Albrecht MH, Bickford MW, Nance JW Jr, et al. State-of-the-art pulmonary CT angiography for acute pulmonary embolism. *AJR Am J Roentgenol.* 2017;208(3):495-504.

Bendel EC, Maleszewski JJ, Araoz PA. Imaging sarcomas of the great vessels and heart. *Semin Ultrasound CT MR.* 2011;32(5):377-404.

Castaner E, Alguersuari A, Gallardo X, et al. When to suspect pulmonary vasculitis: radiologic and clinical clues. *Radiographics.* 2010;30(1):33-53.

Chen Y, Gilman MD, Humphrey KL, et al. Pulmonary artery pseudoaneurysms: clinical features and CT findings. *AJR Am J Roentgenol.* 2017;208(1):84-91.

Chung MP, Yi CA, Lee HY, et al. Imaging of pulmonary vasculitis. *Radiology.* 2010;255(2):322-341.

Devaraj A, Sayer C, Sheard S, et al. Diagnosing acute pulmonary embolism with computed tomography: imaging update. *J Thorac Imaging.* 2015;30(3):176-192.

Frazier AA, Franks TJ, Mohammed TL, et al. From the archives of the AFIP: pulmonary veno-occlusive disease and pulmonary capillary hemangiomatosis. *Radiographics.* 2007;27(3):867-882.

Grosse C, Grosse A. CT findings in diseases associated with pulmonary hypertension: a current review. *Radiographics.* 2010;30(7):1753-1777.

Han D, Lee KS, Franquet T, et al. Thrombotic and nonthrombotic pulmonary arterial embolism: spectrum of imaging findings. *Radiographics.* 2003;23(6):1521-1539.

Mahmoud S, Ghosh S, Farver C, et al. Pulmonary vasculitis: spectrum of imaging appearances. *Radiol Clin North Am.* 2016;54(6):1097-1118.

McCann C, Gopalan D, Sheares K, et al. Imaging in pulmonary hypertension, part 1: clinical perspectives, classification, imaging techniques and imaging algorithm. *Postgrad Med J.* 2012;88(1039):271-279.

Metter D, Tulchinsky M, Freeman LM. Current status of ventilation-perfusion scintigraphy for suspected pulmonary embolism. *AJR Am J Roentgenol.* 2017;1-6.

Nagle SK, Schiebler ML, Repplinger MD, et al. Contrast enhanced pulmonary magnetic resonance angiography for pulmonary embolism: building a successful program. *Eur J Radiol.* 2016;85(3):553-563.

Ohno Y, Yoshikawa T, Kishida Y, et al. Unenhanced and contrast-enhanced MR angiography and perfusion imaging for suspected pulmonary thromboembolism. *AJR Am J Roentgenol.* 2017;1-14.

Pena E, Dennie C, Veinot J, et al. Pulmonary hypertension: how the radiologist can help. *Radiographics.* 2012;32(1):9-32.

Saad N. Aggressive management of pulmonary embolism. *Semin Intervent Radiol.* 2012;29(1):52-56.

Simonneau G, Gatzoulis MA, Adatia I, et al. Updated clinical classification of pulmonary hypertension. *J Am Coll Cardiol.* 2013;62(25 suppl):D34-D41.

Stein PD, Chenevert TL, Fowler SE, et al. Gadolinium-enhanced magnetic resonance angiography for pulmonary embolism: a multicenter prospective study (PIOPED III). *Ann Intern Med.* 2010;152(7):434-443, W142-W143.

Wittram C, Maher MM, Yoo AJ, et al. CT angiography of pulmonary embolism: diagnostic criteria and causes of misdiagnosis. *Radiographics.* 2004;24(5):1219-1238.

Chapter 12

The Postoperative Chest

Bojan Kovacina, Jo-Anne O. Shepard, and Subba R. Digumarthy

INTRODUCTION

For optimal interpretation of imaging studies done after thoracic surgery, it is essential to understand the surgical techniques and the possible complications. The common surgical procedures that are performed in the lung, pleura, mediastinum, and chest wall are discussed in this chapter.

LUNG SURGERIES

Open and Minimally Invasive

Almost all thoracic surgical procedures in the past have been performed via open lung approach, requiring either sternotomy or thoracotomy to gain access to intrathoracic structures. Sternotomy could be either partial or complete, depending on the procedure and the access required. Thoracotomy consists of division of one of major muscles groups in the chest wall and entering a hemithorax cavity through an intercostal space. Spreading of the intercostal space to gain a wider access window occasionally requires an additional partial rib resection or may cause rib fracture. Minimally invasive thoracic surgery, mainly referred to as video-assisted thoracoscopic surgery (VATS), has recently replaced the open lung approach for almost all indications, except lung transplant and pneumonectomy. VATS requires three to four entrance ports through which a videothorascope and trocars are introduced, thereby decreasing the risk for wound or incisional complications. Furthermore, VATS is better tolerated than open lung surgery because of reduced length of the hospital stay and marked decrease in the degree and duration of postoperative pain.

Wedge Resection

Wedge resection is a type of lung surgery during which a small nonanatomic portion of lung is excised. Pulmonary vessels, bronchus, and lymphatics in the affected segment are usually preserved. Common indications for this type of surgery are lung biopsy for diffuse lung disease, excisional biopsy of indeterminate lesions, and resection of single or multiple metastases. More rarely, wedge resection is used as a salvage procedure for primary lung carcinoma in patients who cannot tolerate larger anatomic lung resection. As well, sublobar resection may sometimes be the preferred resection for peripheral small minimally invasive cancer. A dense linear opacity representing a surgical staple line is typically visualized at the site of resection on postoperative radiographs. An associated small parenchymal hematoma usually develops during the early postoperative period and is characterized as a focal airspace opacity surrounding the staple line (Fig. 12.1) that gradually resolves in the following days or weeks. Small amounts of adjacent atelectatic lung and mild parenchymal distortion can additionally be present and are best appreciated on computed tomography (CT).

Bullectomy and Blebectomy

Blebectomy consists of resection of apical blebs. This procedure is usually performed in the context of recurrent pneumothorax and sometimes may be followed by mechanical pleurodesis. Bullectomy, or excision of a single bulla or multiple large bullae, is performed when bullae are causing atelectasis of adjacent lung parenchyma. The resection of these bullae favors reexpansion of the atelectatic lung and improvement in the patient's respiratory function. The radiologic findings after bullectomy and blebectomy are subtle. In fact, if normal lung parenchyma fully reexpands after the surgery, signs of these surgical procedures may only be the absence of bullae or blebs that were documented on preoperative imaging and possibly surgical staple lines (Fig. 12.2).

Volume Reduction Surgery

Lung volume reduction surgery has traditionally been used for treatment of severe emphysema. Nonanatomic resection of lung parenchyma most severely affected by emphysema has been shown to improve patients' respiratory status and quality of life, particularly if upper lobes are diseased. This type of surgery is often considered when medical therapy fails to improve symptoms. Volume reduction surgery may also be performed in the context of lung transplant in which donor lungs are reduced in size to fit in the recipient's chest. Long surgical staple lines are typically the only findings appreciated on radiographs. CT scan additionally demonstrates adjacent parenchymal distortion and smaller-than-usual size of the lobe that underwent reduction.

Segmentectomy

Segmentectomy is a type of anatomic lung surgery defined by the resection of one or several segments of a pulmonary lobe. Examples of surgeries involving resection of more than one segment are basal segmentectomy (all basal segments of a lower lobe, sparing the superior segment), lingulectomy (lingular inferior and superior segments), and upper division left upper lobectomy (LUL) (anterior and apicoposterior segments of LUL, sparing lingular segments). Accompanying draining lymph nodes are dissected with the segment(s) as

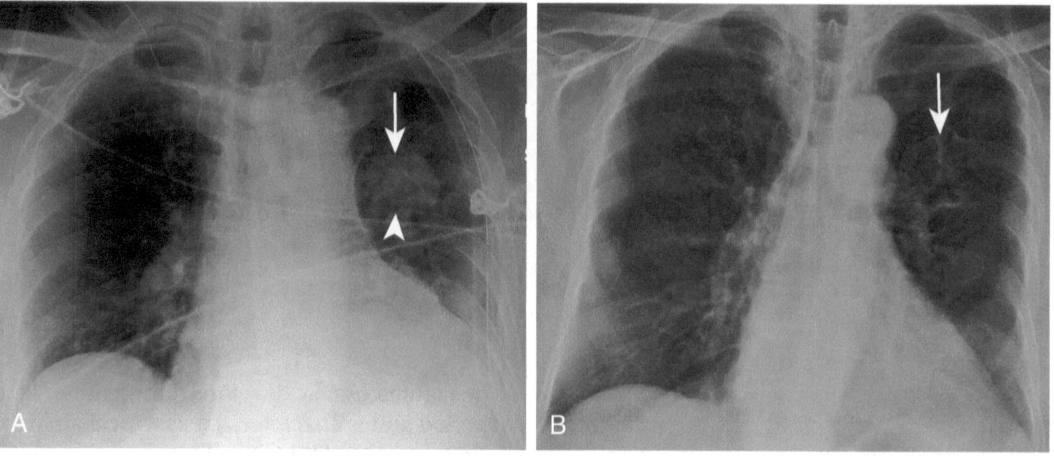

FIGURE 12.1 Images after left upper lobe wedge resection with associated parenchymal hematoma. **A,** Supine chest radiograph 3 days after surgery demonstrates surgical staple line *(arrow)* and associated parenchymal hematoma *(arrowhead)*. **B,** Posteroanterior chest radiograph 5 months later reveals complete resolution of a hematoma. Note the staple line *(arrow)*.

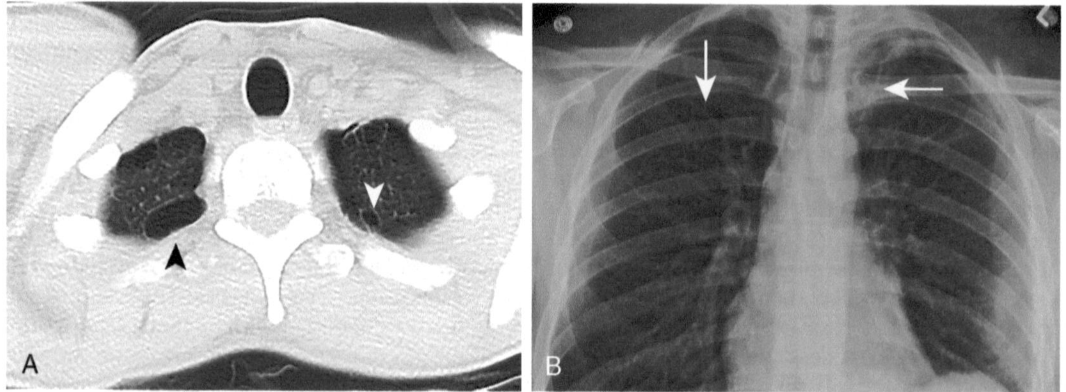

FIGURE 12.2 Apical blebectomy. **A,** Axial chest computed tomography image in a patient with a history of recurrent pneumothorax demonstrates biapical blebs *(arrowheads)*. **B,** Posteroanterior chest radiograph of the same patient 1 month postoperatively demonstrates apical surgical staple lines *(arrows)*.

well. This surgery can be used for resection of lung cancers if lobectomy cannot be tolerated by a patient because of poor lung function. Additional indications include excision of metastasis, benign tumors, and focal parenchymal processes (e.g., bronchiectasis). The postoperative appearance is characterized by a smaller-than-expected size of the affected lobe. The lobar bronchus remains patent, but the segmental bronchus is resected. A surgical staple line may or may not be visualized, depending on whether staples or sutures were used during surgery.

Lobectomy

Lobectomy is considered as a definitive surgical procedure for most lung cancers. It implies resection of one (or more) lobes along with regional lymph nodes. In addition to lung cancers, some benign processes (e.g., severe bronchiectasis) and congenital anomalies (e.g., congenital pulmonary airway malformation) are indications for a lobectomy. Sleeve lobectomy is a type of lobectomy during which a diseased lobe, corresponding lobar bronchus, and segment of the mainstem bronchus are resected en bloc. The remaining lobar bronchus is subsequently connected to the residual portion of the main bronchus in end-to-end fashion. This surgery is usually performed as a lung-sparing procedure for central lung cancers invading the main bronchus as an alternative to pneumonectomy. Radiographic findings of lobectomy are similar to those of total lobar collapse. In both processes, there are volume loss of the affected lung, displacement of the hila, shift of the mediastinal structures, and elevation of the ipsilateral hemidiaphragm. Some findings, however, are characteristic of lobectomy. In particular, the presence of surgical clips in the hilar region and postthoracotomy changes (if open lung surgery was performed) confirm prior surgical resection (Fig. 12.3). The absence of the fissure in the left lung and characteristic reorientation of fissures in the right lung after lobectomy is another finding differentiating lobectomy from lobar collapse and is easily seen on CT. Occasionally, a surgeon may decide to use an additional vascularized tissue to reinforce the bronchial stump and prompt its healing. This usually is achieved by additional blood supply to the stump from muscle flaps (intercostal, latissimus dorsi, or

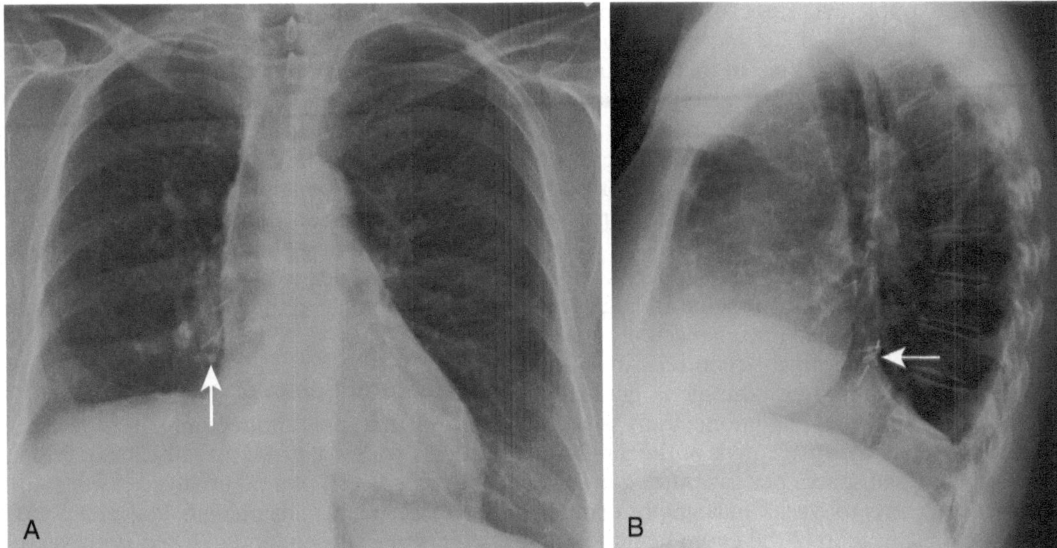

FIGURE 12.3 Images after right lower lobectomy. Posteroanterior **(A)** and lateral **(B)** chest radiographs 1 year after surgery demonstrate volume loss of the right lung, elevation of the right hemidiaphragm, and surgical clips in the right infrahilar region *(arrows)*.

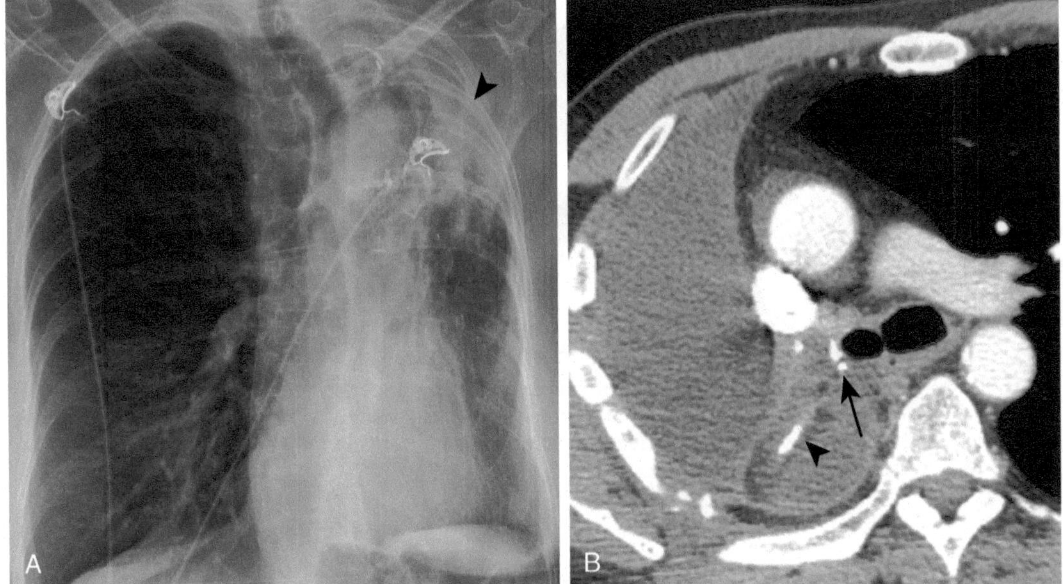

FIGURE 12.4 Intercostal muscle flap used for bronchial stump reinforcement **A,** Anteroposterior chest radiograph after left upper lobectomy demonstrates volume loss of the left lung and opacity in the left upper hemithorax extending from the left hilum to the chest wall *(arrowhead)*. **B,** Axial chest computed tomography scan in a different patient after right pneumonectomy reveals hilar surgical clips *(arrow)* and muscle flap *(arrowhead)*.

pectoralis) or fat flaps (omentum, pericardial fat pad). On postoperative radiographs, the ipsilateral hilum appears larger than expected. Additionally, a large triangular opacity extending from the hilum to the chest wall can be seen if a muscle flap was used (Fig. 12.4). CT scans demonstrate soft tissue and fat density material in the region of bronchial stump tracking to the chest wall. It should be noted that these radiologic findings are present from the first postoperative radiograph and usually do not subsequently change in appearance. In contrast, progressive enlargement of the ipsilateral hilum and formation of new soft tissue density in the region of the stump in a later postoperative stage should raise a strong suspicion of local tumor recurrence.

Pneumonectomy

Surgical removal of an entire lung is indicated for lung cancers that invade central structures, such as the mainstem bronchus and main pulmonary artery, and those that extend through fissures. Given its higher rate of morbidity and mortality than lesser anatomic resections, a pneumonectomy is usually performed as a last resort. It is the only surgical lung resection that is not routinely performed with VATS. There are three types of pneumonectomies: classic, intrapericardial, and extrapleural. The classic pneumonectomy consists of resection of a lung and corresponding hilar lymph nodes. Tumor invasion of pericardium or intrapericardial portions of pulmonary artery or veins is an indication for intrapericardial pneumonectomy. This type of pneumonectomy implies resection or ligation of intrapericardial portions of pulmonary artery, vein, or both in addition to excision of affected lung. When a partial resection of pericardium is performed, it is followed by pericardial reconstruction with a mesh (Fig. 12.5). After pneumonectomy, the earliest postoperative radiographs demonstrate predominantly air-filled pneumonectomy space with midline position of mediastinal structures. After the chest tube is clamped or removed, the air is gradually reabsorbed, and fluid fills the pneumonectomy space. This is manifested by cranial displacement of the air–fluid level, usually two intercostal spaces per day. After the air is entirely reabsorbed over days to weeks, radiographs demonstrate characteristic opacification of the entire hemithorax, which is typically attributable to a combination of fluid and shifted mediastinal structures (Fig. 12.6). Eventually, some of the fluid gets reabsorbed as well, causing mediastinal structures to shift even more into ipsilateral hemithorax. The amount and rate of fluid reabsorption are variable and may take weeks to months. More often than not, some fluid chronically persists within the pneumonectomy space with a smooth peripheral margin and concave margin toward the hilum, best appreciated on CT scan (see Fig. 12.4). High-density mesh (either bovine or polytetrafluoroethylene in nature) can be appreciated at the site of pericardial and diaphragmatic reconstruction if resection was performed during the surgery. In the immediate postoperative period, pulmonary edema may be seen in the residual lung, more commonly in the left lung after right pneumonectomy (Fig. 12.7).

Extrapleural Pneumonectomy

Extrapleural pneumonectomy is performed in selected patients with malignant mesothelioma. It requires resection of lung, parietal pleura, involved portions of pericardium, and ipsilateral hemidiaphragm. Pericardial and diaphragmatic defects are subsequently closed with synthetic graft and mesh. Findings on postoperative radiographs are similar to those after classic pneumonectomy. CT additionally demonstrates a curvilinear hyperdensity extending from the chest wall medially toward the midline and a round or oval

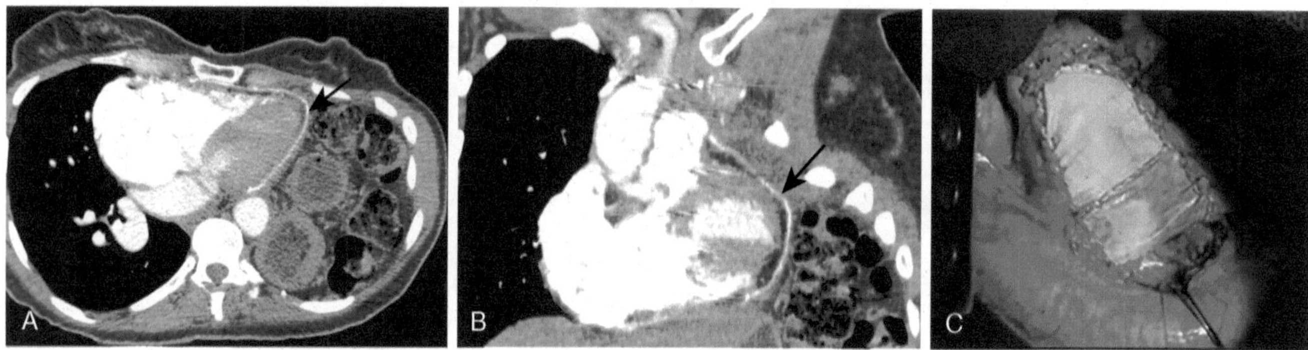

FIGURE 12.5 Images after left intrapericardial pneumonectomy and pericardial defect reconstruction Axial **(A)** and coronal **(B)** images of chest computed tomography scans 2 years after surgery demonstrate hyperdense pericardial patch *(straight arrows)*. **C,** Intraoperative image of a pericardial synthetic patch. (Courtesy of Michael Lanuti, MD, Boston, MA.)

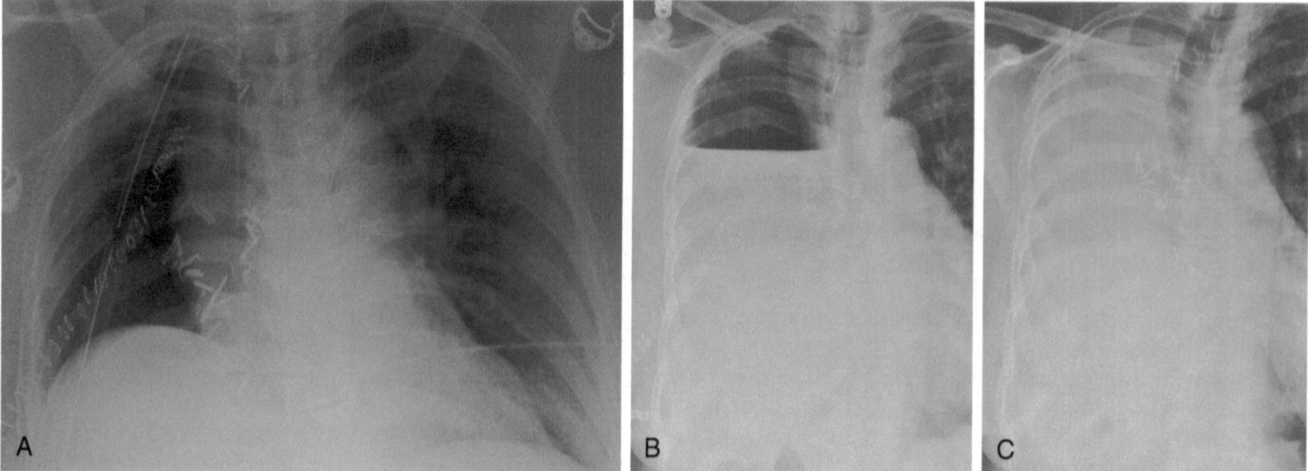

FIGURE 12.6 Post right pneumonectomy. **A** to **C,** Serial postoperative chest radiographs demonstrate gradual resorption of air and filling of right postpneumonectomy space with fluid. Note also the gradual shift of the mediastinum to the right.

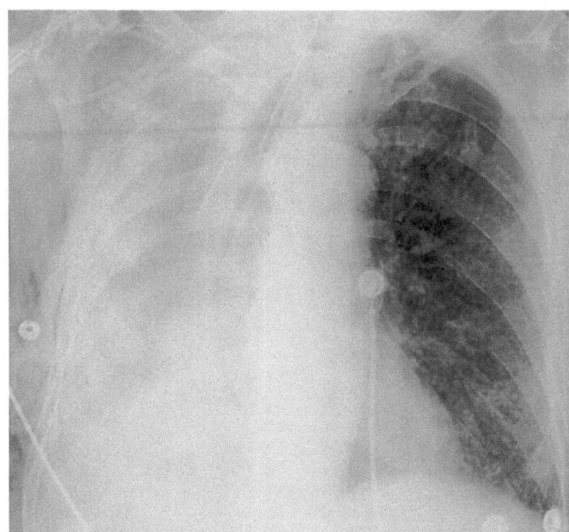

FIGURE 12.7 Postpneumonectomy pulmonary edema. Anteroposterior chest radiograph in the immediate postoperative period after right pneumonectomy demonstrates vascular indistinctness and perihilar fullness consistent with pulmonary edema in the left lung.

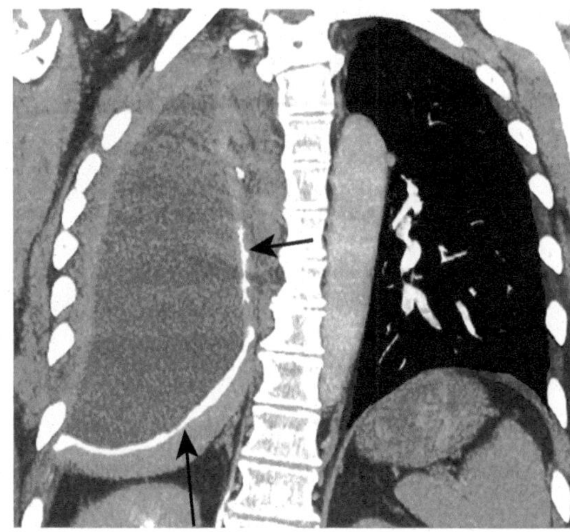

FIGURE 12.8 Post right extrapleural pneumonectomy. Coronal chest computed tomography image in a patient 2 years after right extrapleural pneumonectomy. Note the hyperdense diaphragmatic and pericardial patches *(arrows)* as well as chronic fluid within the postpneumonectomy space.

hyperdensity overlying the heart, representing reconstructed hemidiaphragm and pericardial mesh, respectively (Fig. 12.8). Almost all complications after classic pneumonectomy may also happen after extrapleural pneumonectomy.

Complications

Air Leak

Small pneumothorax is an expected early finding after a lung resection. It invariably resolves with an indwelling chest tube inserted at the time of the surgery. Pneumothorax that persists despite a chest tube for longer than 7 to 10 days suggests an air leak.

Bronchopleural Fistula

Connection between the pleural space and larger bronchus is defined as bronchopleural fistula (BPF). The incidence of this complication ranges from 0.4% to 3%. Central BPF is commonly caused by dehiscence of sutures and staples or necrosis at the level of the bronchial stump. After pneumonectomy, this commonly occurs in the early postoperative period (within the first 2 weeks). The risk factors for the development of BPF include preoperative infection, radiation, right pneumonectomy, residual tumor at the stump, a long stump, extensive mediastinal or hilar lymph node dissection, diabetes, and steroid use. Surgical reclosure is a preferred treatment in the absence of pleural infection because it minimizes the risk of possible complications, such as empyema, acute respiratory distress syndrome (ARDS), and aspiration of the pleural fluid into the contralateral lung. If not already performed at the time of initial resection, a vascularized flap is used to cover the stump to promote adequate vascular supply and promote healing. The radiographic appearance of BPF varies depending on the size of the fistula. New or an increasing amount of air in the ipsilateral pleural space is a typical presentation (Fig. 12.9). If a large amount of air develops in the pleural space in the context of large BPF, it can sporadically result in a tension pneumothorax. Characteristic radiographic findings of BPF after pneumonectomy consist of increased air in the pneumonectomy space with caudal drop of more than 2 cm of preexisting air-fluid level, failure of fluid to fill the pneumonectomy space, reoccurrence of air in the previously opacified hemithorax, and contralateral shift of the mediastinal structures. In addition to these radiographic findings, CT scans may directly demonstrate a connection between the pleural space and the airway.

Lobar Torsion

Postoperative lobar torsion is a rare complication after thoracic surgery. It is most frequently seen after lobectomy, although it can occur after sublobar resection, severance of pleural adhesions, and parietal pleurectomy. Although any lobe can be affected, torsion of the right middle lobe is the most commonly seen, usually after right upper lobectomy. Lobar torsion can be partial or complete, depending on the degree of rotation of its vascular pedicle. Predisposing factors include the presence of complete fissures, long slender hilar pedicle, absence of postoperative adhesions, and complete division of the inferior pulmonary ligament during upper lobectomy. Urgent surgical reduction of torsion is required to prevent venous congestion, occlusion of the arterial supply, infarction, and gangrene of the affected lobe. Radiographic findings of a lobar torsion are subtle and nonspecific. Consolidated lobe in an unusual position and change in position of an opacified lobe on serial radiographs may be seen on early postoperative radiographs. CT is much more sensitive in detection of an ongoing lobar torsion, particularly given its ability to create multiplanar reformats. The CT appearance of the torsed lung parenchyma depends on the duration and degree of torsion. It typically consists of a combination of ground-glass opacity; interlobular septal thickening in early stages; and lack of enhancement, consolidation, and necrosis as it progresses (Fig. 12.10). Moreover, CT may additionally demonstrate bronchial cut-off, tapered occlusion or distortion of the proximal pulmonary artery and vein, and abnormal orientation of the fissures.

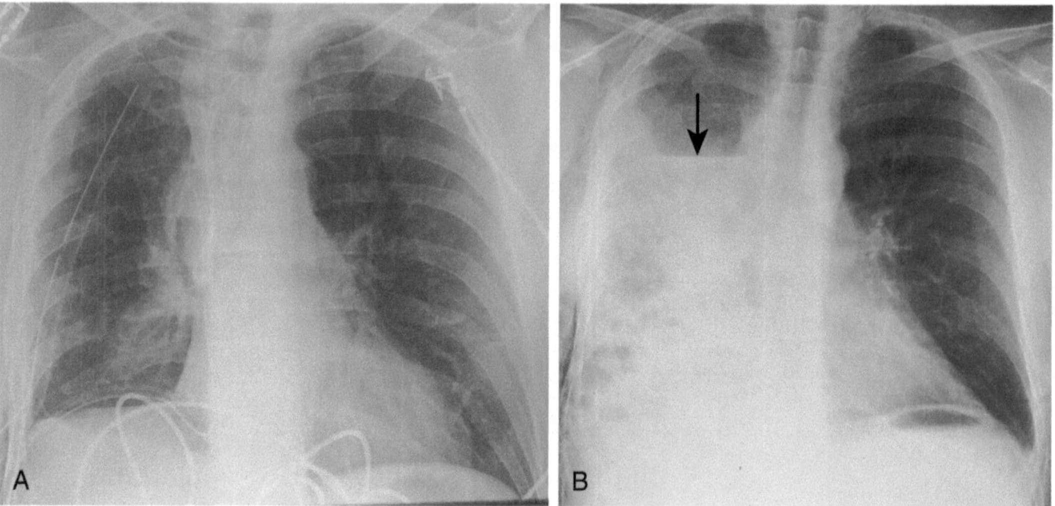

FIGURE 12.9 Bronchopleural fistula (BPF) after right upper lobectomy. **A,** Anteroposterior chest radiograph 3 days after surgery shows volume loss of the right lung and indwelling chest tubes without pneumothorax. **B,** Posteroanterior chest radiograph 10 days later demonstrates BPF, manifested by new right hydropneumothorax with air–fluid level *(arrow)*.

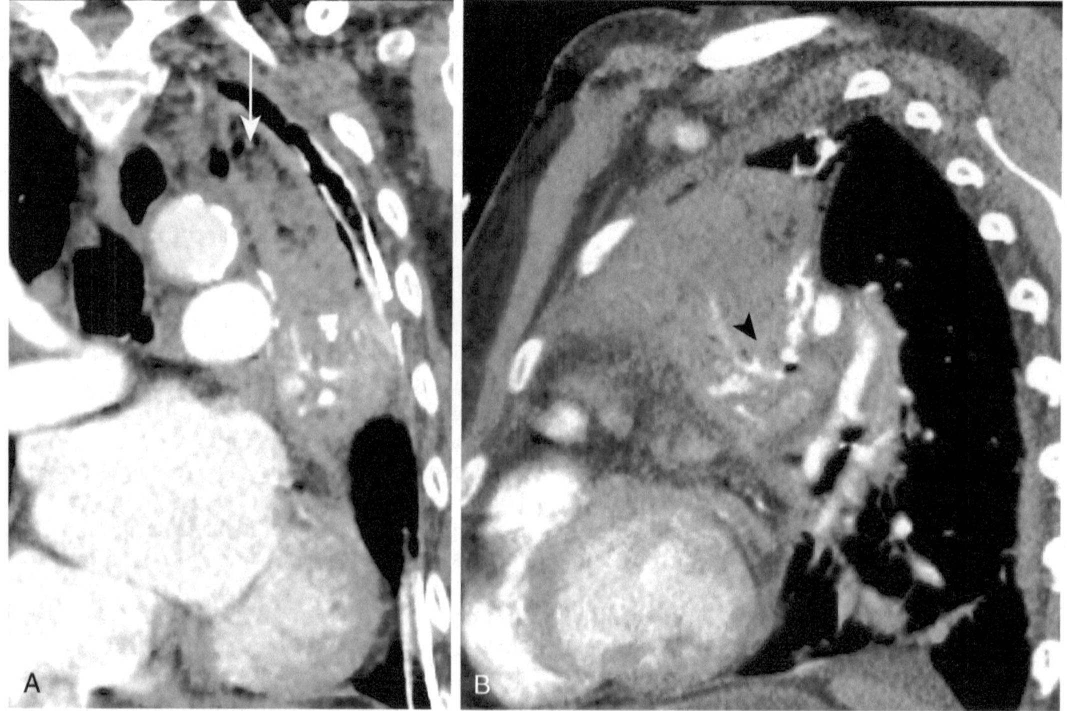

FIGURE 12.10 Lingular torsion after lingula-sparing left upper lobectomy. Coronal **(A)** and sagittal **(B)** chest computed tomography images days after surgery demonstrate a collapsed lingula in the upper and anterior left hemithorax. Note the absence of normal enhancement and the presence of gas in the necrotic portion of the lobe *(arrow)* and abnormal orientation of hilar vessels *(arrowhead)*.

Venous Infarct

Pulmonary venous infarct is a rare complication after thoracic surgery, predominantly seen after lobectomy. It happens because of pulmonary vein thrombosis, compression, or unintended ligation during surgery. Hemoptysis is a common presenting symptom. Timely diagnosis is essential to preserve the viability of the rest of the lung parenchyma. Therapeutic options consist of antibiotics, angioplasty, stent insertion, and resection of the affected lobe. Radiologic findings depend on the stage of venous infarct: early hemorrhagic and late fibrotic stages. Radiographic findings of the hemorrhagic stage initially are manifestations of increased pressure in pulmonary veins and capillaries, which are radiographically manifested by reticular opacities with or without enlarged pulmonary veins in the portion of the lung drained by the affected veins. Afterward, patchy irregular opacities predominate, which are signs of parenchymal

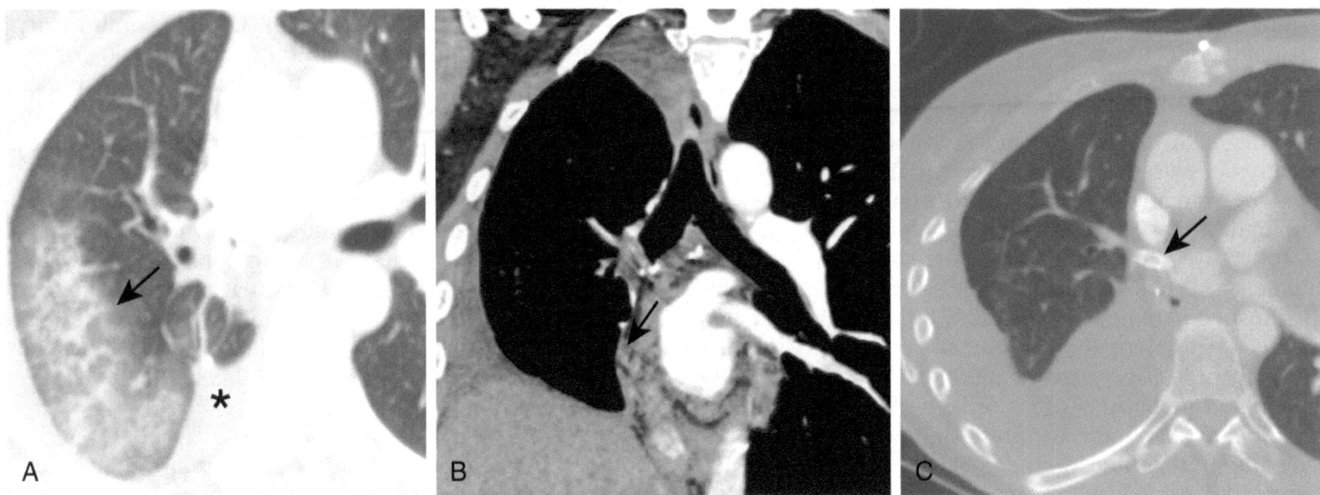

FIGURE 12.11 Venous infarct. Axial **(A)** and coronal **(B)** chest computed tomography (CT) images in lung and mediastinal windows 3 weeks after right middle and lower bilobectomy demonstrate right pleural effusion *(asterisk)*, occluded right superior pulmonary vein *(arrowhead)*, and peripheral ground-glass opacity with septal thickening in the RUL *(arrow)* consistent with venous infarction. **C,** Axial chest CT image after right superior pulmonary vein stent insertion *(arrow)* reveals resolution of previously seen parenchymal infarct and persistent right pleural effusion.

hemorrhage. On CT, a venous infarct typically demonstrates interlobular septal thickening, ground-glass opacities located septally near venules, and scattered airspace opacities, consistent with areas of hemorrhage and infarct (Fig. 12.11). Furthermore, visceral pleura of the implicated lung may be thickened because of venous collaterals. Late fibrotic phase demonstrates characteristic findings of parenchymal fibrosis, consisting of intralobular and interlobular septal thickening, honeycombing, and parenchymal distortion. By demonstrating the exact level of venous occlusion, CT, magnetic resonance imaging, and pulmonary angiography with delayed venous phase are useful for confirmation of diagnosis and for treatment planning.

Cardiac Herniation or Torsion

Cardiac herniation through a surgically made pericardial defect is a potential complication of intrapericardial pneumonectomy. This complication always appears on the side of the resection and is more common after a right intrapericardial pneumonectomy. Because a cardiac volvulus or torsion may develop depending on the amount of herniated heart, an emergent surgical reduction and pericardial defect repair are performed. Predisposing factors for the development of cardiac herniation include failure to repair a pericardial defect, rapid intraoperative repositioning of the patient with the pneumonectomy side placed dependently, positive-pressure ventilation, connection of a chest tube to high suction, and sudden increase of intrathoracic pressure from coughing. Presenting clinical signs and symptoms depend on the side on which herniation occurs. Cardiac herniation into the right postpneumonectomy space causes kinking of the superior vena cava and counterclockwise rotation of the heart around the axis of the vena cava, which results in decreased venous return, tachycardia, and hypotension. Cardiac herniation into the left pneumonectomy space is associated with myocardial strangulation by the pericardial sac and usually manifests with decreased cardiac output, ventricular arrhythmias, and

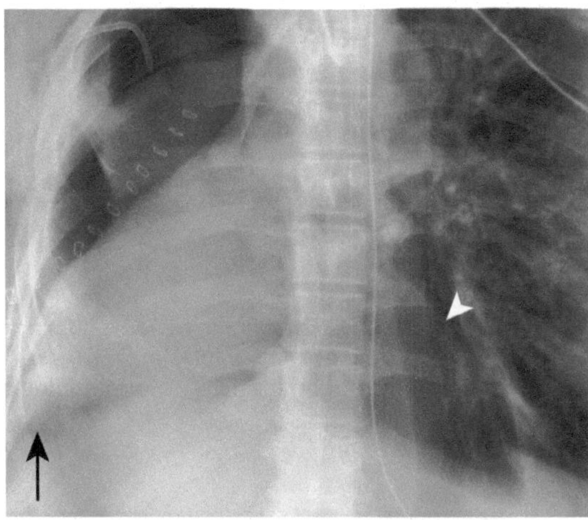

FIGURE 12.12 Cardiac herniation after right intrapericardial pneumonectomy. Anteroposterior chest radiograph obtained immediately postoperative demonstrates rotation and displacement of the cardiac silhouette into the right postpneumonectomy space consistent with cardiac herniation or torsion. Note the cardiac apex in the right costophrenic sulcus *(straight arrow)* and gas in the empty pericardial sac *(arrowhead)*.

myocardial infarction. Cardiac herniation has characteristic features on radiography; thus, CT is virtually never needed or performed for diagnosis. Early partial herniation presents with the "snow cone sign" in which a small portion of the heart protrudes through the pericardial defect. Air within the empty pericardial sac with the cardiac silhouette positioned in the pneumonectomy space is a diagnostic feature of cardiac herniation or torsion on early postoperative radiographs (Fig. 12.12). Cardiac apex in right lateral or posterior costophrenic angle, clockwise rotation of a pulmonary artery catheter, and marked kinking of a central venous line are additional signs of this complication after right pneumonectomy. A convex hemispheric left heart contour and a prominent notch between the great vessels and more lateral herniating cardiac margin are seen after left pneumonectomy.

Diaphragmatic Dehiscence

Diaphragmatic graft dehiscence is a specific but rare complication of extrapleural pneumonectomy, with a reported incidence ranging from 1.7% to 8.1% and most often seen within the first week after surgery. Tight diaphragmatic graft, postoperative ileus, and increased pressure in the abdomen augment the risk of this complication. On radiographs, the most common manifestation of a diaphragmatic patch dehiscence is herniation of intraabdominal organs into the empty postoperative hemithorax. Because the liver has limited mobility because of its partial fixation to the peritoneum, diaphragmatic graft failure or rupture may be radiographically subtle on the right side. The presence of a herniated gastric air bubble or air-filled bowel loops into the postoperative left hemithorax strongly suggests dehiscence of a left hemidiaphragmatic patch. CT is a confirmatory test, usually demonstrating intrathoracic herniation of the abdominal organs secondary to detachment of a diaphragmatic graft from one of its attachment points or caused by a focal defect within the graft itself (Fig. 12.13).

Other Early Complications

Aspiration, parenchymal hemorrhage, pneumonia, lung abscess (Fig. 12.14), atelectasis, hemothorax, and empyema are additional early complications that may be seen after lung surgeries. The radiologic findings of these processes in the postoperative setting do not differ from their general appearance described elsewhere in this book.

Tumor Recurrence

Tumor can reoccur at the bronchial stump after lobectomy or pneumonectomy or along a surgical staple line in the context of sublobar lung resection. Tumor may also

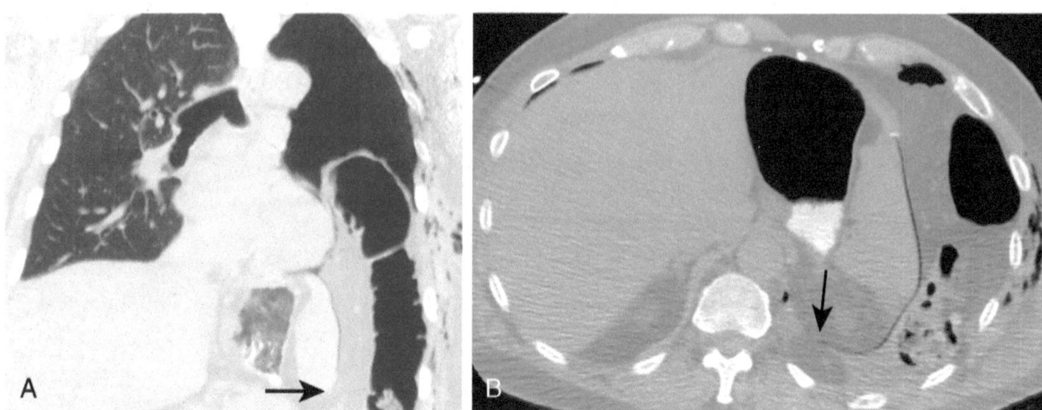

FIGURE 12.13 Diaphragmatic patch dehiscence after left extrapleural pneumonectomy. Coronal **(A)** and axial **(B)** chest computed tomography images 1 week after left extrapleural pneumonectomy show herniation of bowel loops and intraabdominal fat into postpneumonectomy space caused by left diaphragmatic patch dehiscence *(straight arrows)*.

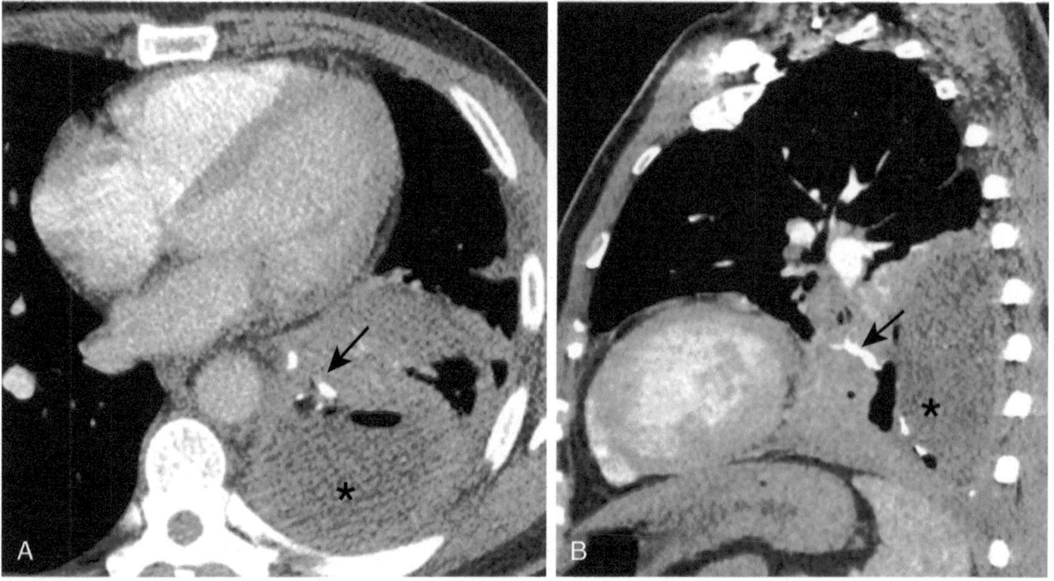

FIGURE 12.14 Lung abscess at the staple line. Axial **(A)** and sagittal **(B)** chest computed tomography images after wedge resection of a left lower lobe nodule demonstrate an abscess with air–fluid level *(asterisk)* posterior to the surgical staple line *(arrow)*.

recur in parietal pleura and mediastinal lymph nodes. This complication usually happens within the first 2 years after resection. Radiographically, recurrent tumors may not be visible, especially if they are small in size. The larger tumors may present as increasing masslike opacities in the surgical bed or cause return of the mediastinal structures to their preoperative position in the context of previous pneumonectomy. A growing mass at the level of lung resection on serial CT scans strongly suggests tumor recurrence (Fig. 12.15). Positron emission tomography (PET) is usually helpful in confirming the diagnosis or differentiating the recurrent tumor from postoperative fibrosis (Fig. 12.16).

Postpneumonectomy Syndrome

Postpneumonectomy syndrome usually happens in the first 2 years after the lung resection and is predominantly seen in children and young adults. It clinically presents with dyspnea, inspiratory stridor, and recurrent pneumonias. The syndrome implies excessive displacement of the heart and other mediastinal structures into the pneumonectomy space, which causes rotation of the mediastinum and compression of the contralateral mainstem bronchus in between the pulmonary artery anteriorly and spine and aorta posteriorly. Treatment consists of surgical repositioning of the mediastinum more centrally in the thorax. The suggestive radiographic findings include a smaller than usual pneumonectomy space and marked hyperinflation of the contralateral lung. CT scan allows adequate assessment of the postpneumonectomy space and demonstrates the location of narrowing or compression of the mainstem bronchus by mediastinal vessels and the spine.

LUNG TRANSPLANTATION

Technique

Lung transplant implies transplantation of bilateral lower lobes, single lung, or both lungs. In bilateral lobar transplantation, the lobes are procured from two living donors. Lung transplant may occasionally be combined with heart transplantation. The major indications for lung transplantation are chronic obstructive pulmonary disease, idiopathic pulmonary fibrosis, cystic fibrosis, and idiopathic pulmonary hypertension. Whereas transplantation of a single

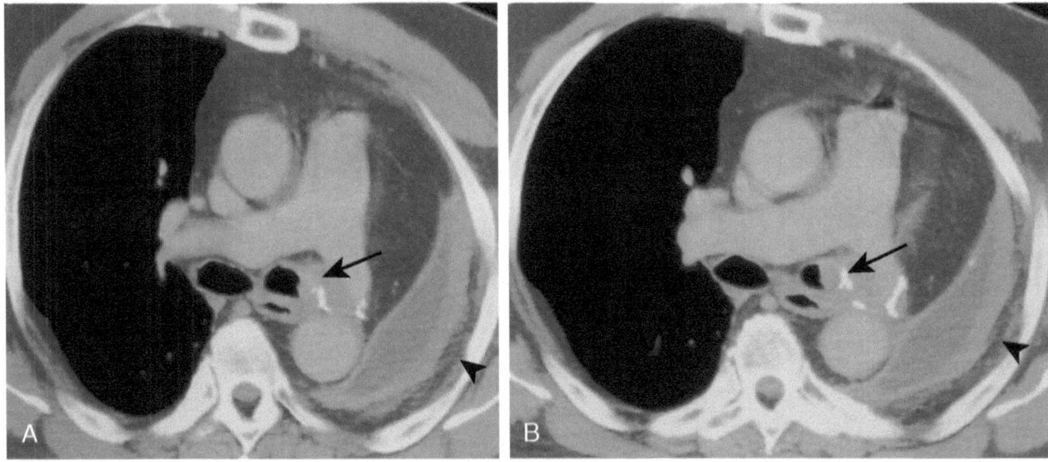

FIGURE 12.15 Tumor recurrence after left pneumonectomy. **A** and **B,** Axial chest computed tomography images obtained 6 months and 17 months after surgery demonstrate increasing soft tissue mass at the level of bronchial stump *(arrow)* representing local tumor recurrence. Note chronic residual fluid in the left postpneumonectomy space *(arrowhead).*

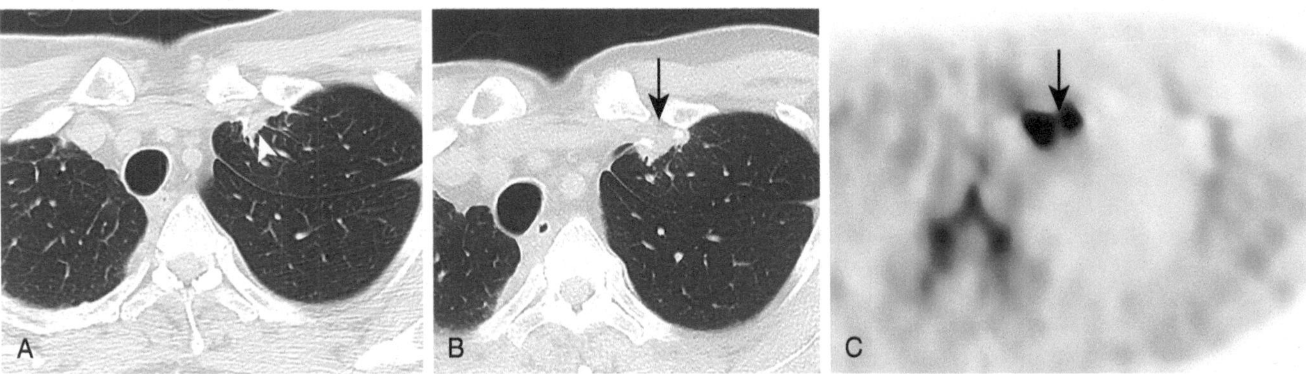

FIGURE 12.16 Tumor recurrence after left upper lobe anterior segmentectomy. **A,** Axial chest computed tomography (CT) image 2 years after surgery. Note the expected minimal scar adjacent to the surgical staple line *(arrowhead).* Axial chest CT image **(B)** and corresponding positron emission tomography image **(C)** 2 years later reveal enlarged soft tissue opacity adjacent to the surgical staple line *(arrow)* with associated increased fluorodeoxyglucose uptake *(arrow),* consistent with recurrent cancer.

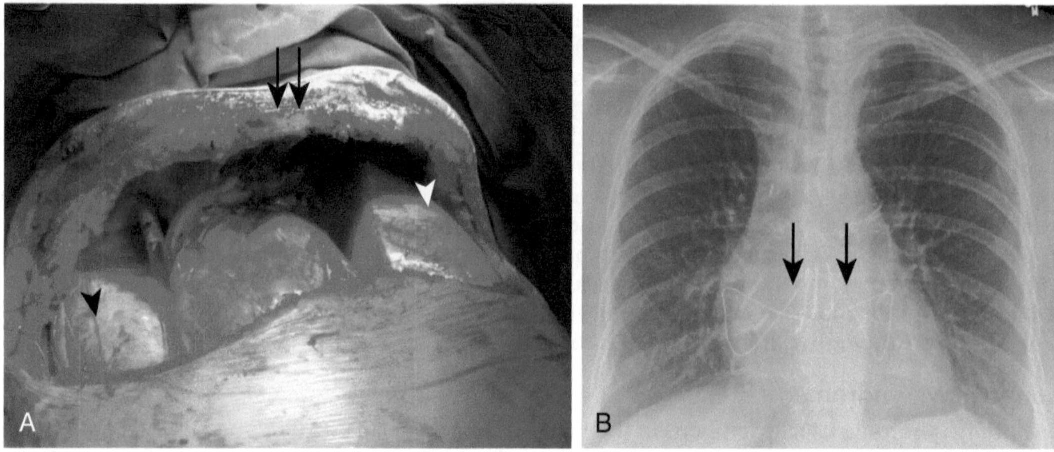

FIGURE 12.17 Transverse (clamshell) sternotomy for double-lung transplant. **A,** Transverse splitting of the lower sternum *(arrows)* to gain access for double-lung transplant *(arrowheads)*. **B,** Posteroanterior chest radiograph showing clamshell sternotomy wires *(arrows)*. (*A* courtesy of John Wain, MD, Boston, MA.)

lung usually is performed through posterior thoracotomy, transverse thoracosternotomy (clamshell incision) is required for double-lung transplantation (Fig. 12.17). The airway connection is achieved with an end-to-end anastomosis between the donor and recipient mainstem bronchi. If these bronchi are of different size, a telescope technique may be used, during which the smaller bronchus is telescoped and inserted into the larger bronchus. Expected postoperative radiographic findings depend on the type of lung transplantation. After sequential double-lung transplant, typical findings consist of characteristic transverse thoracosternotomy (clamshell) wires and surgical clips in hilar regions (see Fig. 12.17). Surgical staple lines may be seen in upper lung zones if additional volume reduction of donor lungs was performed. After single-lung transplantation, radiographs usually demonstrate an asymmetric size and appearance of the lungs with the normal donor lung and abnormal native lung (Fig. 12.18). Vascular and airway anastomosis are more readily seen by CT.

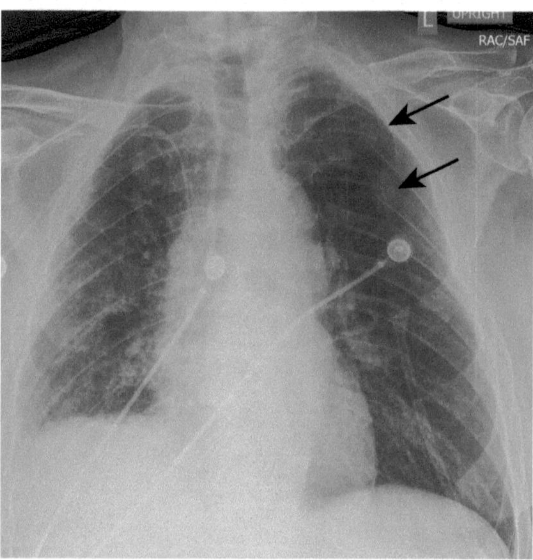

FIGURE 12.18 Post left lung transplant for idiopathic pulmonary fibrosis. Anteroposterior chest radiograph 1 month postoperative demonstrates asymmetric appearance of lungs, with decreased volume and diffuse reticular opacities in the native right lung with pulmonary fibrosis. Note the clear slightly hyperinflated transplanted left lung and postthoracotomy changes in the left posterior fourth and fifth ribs *(arrows)*.

Complications

Reperfusion Edema

Reperfusion edema is a form of noncardiogenic edema and characteristically occurs within the first 24 hours after a lung transplant, peaks in severity on postoperative day 4 to 5, and usually improves by the end of the first week, although it may persist for several months. Reperfusion edema is caused by increased capillary permeability resulting from multiple factors, including interruption of lymphatic flow, decreased surfactant production, donor lung denervation, and ischemia. Other causes of respiratory distress in the early posttransplant period, including acute lung rejection and infection, need to be excluded before the diagnosis of reperfusion edema is made. The chest radiograph typically demonstrates peribronchial cuffing, subpleural septal lines, and an indistinctness of the pulmonary vessels (Fig. 12.19). Enlarged cardiac silhouette and pleural effusions, typically seen with cardiogenic edema, are usually absent in the context of reperfusion edema. Moreover, a patchy peripheral distribution of opacities is relatively specific to noncardiogenic edema, which if severe, can have a radiographic appearance similar to that of ARDS. CT is infrequently used to evaluate reperfusion edema; if performed, its purpose usually is to exclude other causes of acute respiratory dysfunction.

Anastomotic Dehiscence

Anastomotic dehiscence is a serious complication, with the reported incidence ranging from 1% to 10% after lung transplant. It usually occurs within the first month after surgery. Interruption of the native bronchial circulation, long donor bronchial stump, and excessive peribronchial resection during harvesting are associated with an increased risk of donor bronchus ischemia, which is the main factor in the development of posttransplant anastomotic dehiscence.

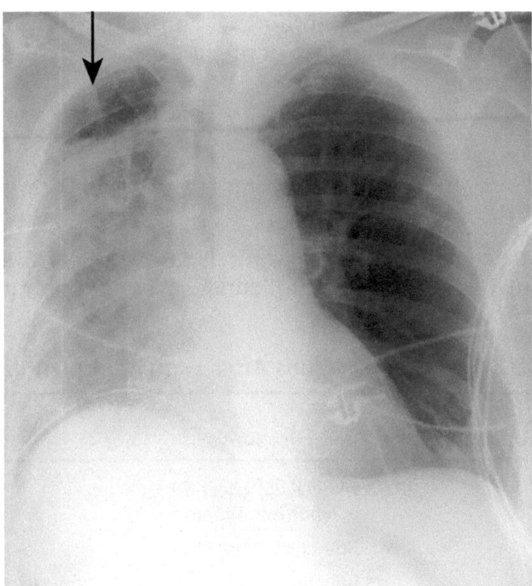

FIGURE 12.19 Reperfusion edema. Anteroposterior chest radiograph 5 days after right lung transplant demonstrates opacification of the right lung caused by reperfusion edema. There are a right basilar chest tube and a small right apical pneumothorax *(arrow)*. Note hyperinflation of the left lung caused by emphysema.

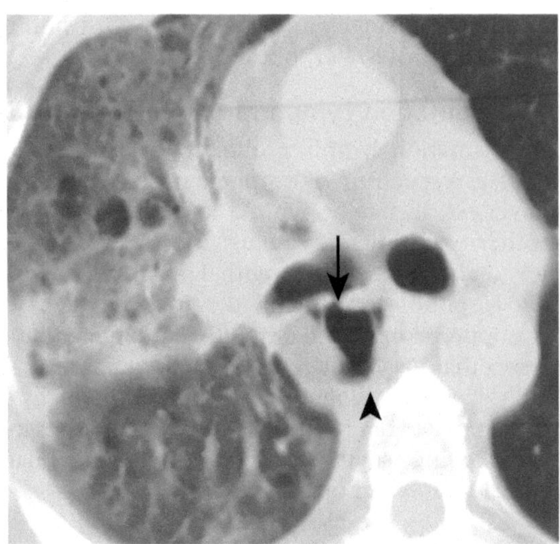

FIGURE 12.20 Bronchial anastomotic dehiscence after right lung transplant. Axial chest computed tomography image 2 weeks after surgery demonstrates anastomotic dehiscence *(arrow)* with posterior extraluminal air collection *(arrowhead)*. Note the hypoinflated right lung with additional underlying reperfusion edema.

Other risk factors for this complication include prolonged donor mechanical ventilation time, acute rejection, and preoperative and postoperative pulmonary infections. Morbidity and mortality rates of an anastomotic dehiscence increase with the presence of concurrent infection or BPF. Partial dehiscence can be treated conservatively with close surveillance and antibiotics. Severe cases of dehiscence may necessitate temporary endobronchial stent insertion and open surgical repair. Radiographic findings of anastomotic dehiscence are signs of air leak or decreased lung expansion, such as new or persistent pneumothorax, pneumomediastinum, and atelectasis of the lung or lobe. Although perianastomotic mucosal ischemia, which represents the earliest sign of dehiscence, is typically detected only by bronchoscopy, CT can reliably diagnose dehiscence by directly demonstrating a focal anastomotic wall defect (Fig. 12.20). Additional CT findings include irregular or narrowed airway and perianastomotic extraluminal air collection.

Anastomotic Stricture

Although stenosis is the most common anastomotic complication after lung transplant, it rarely occurs in the immediate postoperative period. It is usually seen 3 to 4 months after the surgery. The reported incidence of this complication ranges from 5% to 10%. Early postoperative airway stenosis may be caused by surgically created anastomotic narrowing or bronchial mucosal edema. Late stenosis is caused by granulation tissue secondary to bronchial ischemia, healing of a dehiscence, and perianastomotic infection. Flexible bronchoscopy is considered the gold standard for the diagnosis. Multiple endoscopic and surgical treatment options are available, including balloon bronchoplasty, cryotherapy, laser photoresection, stent insertion, and bronchial anastomotic reconstruction. Chest radiographs have a limited role in diagnosing airway stenosis. In contrast, CT with multiplanar reformats is reported to have high accuracy in detecting anastomotic stenosis in transplant recipients, typically manifested by endobronchial luminal narrowing. Moreover, dynamic or expiratory CT can be used to investigate for possible bronchomalacia.

Rejection

Transplant rejection is categorized into hyperacute, acute, and chronic rejection. Hyperacute rejection happens immediately after the surgery and is caused by preformed antibodies to donor-specific antigens. The process is usually fulminant and rapidly evolving. Radiologically, it is manifested by diffuse relatively homogeneous opacification of donor lung(s). Acute rejection is cell-mediated process usually occurring within the first 3 weeks after transplantation. Patients may be asymptomatic or may present with dyspnea, fever, and impaired pulmonary function test (PFT) results. Clinically and radiologically, an acute rejection may be difficult to differentiate from reperfusion edema and infection; thus, transbronchial biopsy usually is required for definite diagnosis. Radiography and CT demonstrate mid to lower lobe opacities, interlobular septal thickening, and pleural effusions. CT also shows patchy or diffuse ground-glass opacities, whose extent depends on the severity of rejection (Fig. 12.21). Chronic rejection is usually manifested by bronchiolitis obliterans. It is a principal factor responsible for limited long-term survival of allografts, shown to affect more than 50% of patients. Prior episodes of acute rejection, viral infections, and gastroesophageal reflux are major risk factors for this complication. Patients generally present with worsening respiratory status documented by obstructive pattern on PFTs. Radiologically, chronic rejection demonstrates typical findings of bronchiolitis obliterans, such as mosaic attenuation of lung parenchyma, air trapping on expiratory CT, bronchiectasis, and bronchial cuffing or bronchial wall thickening. Rarely, a chronic rejection may manifest by development of upper lobe fibrosis, characterized radiologically by usual interstitial pneumonitis pattern of parenchymal changes in upper lobes with minimal if any involvement of lower lobes (Fig. 12.22).

Posttransplantation Lymphoproliferative Disorder

Posttransplantation lymphoproliferative disorder (PTLD) encompasses a spectrum of lymphoid neoplasms of variable aggressiveness. It may be limited to lungs or additionally affect other extrathoracic organs. This rare complication is believed to be associated with Epstein-Barr virus and typically responds to antiviral therapy and decrease in immunosuppression. Single or multiple pulmonary nodules and masses that may contain air bronchograms are characteristically seen on radiographs. CT may additionally show a surrounding halo of ground-glass opacity and interlobular septal thickening, small pleural effusions, and hilar and mediastinal lymphadenopathy (Fig. 12.23).

Other Complications

Several other complications may be seen after lung transplant, whose radiologic manifestations are not different from their general appearance described elsewhere in this book (Table 12.1). These consist of infection, pneumothorax, pleural effusions, hemothorax, empyema, organizing pneumonia, and recurrence of primary disease (particularly sarcoidosis).

PLEURAL PROCEDURES

Pleurodesis

The main objective of pleurodesis is obliteration of the potential space within a pleural cavity by promoting

TABLE 12.1 Complications After Lung Transplantation

Weeks Since Transplant	Complications
0–2	Hyperacute rejection, ischemia-reperfusion injury
0–4	Bronchial dehiscence
>0	Infections (bacterial, viral, and fungal)
>1	Acute rejection
>4	Viral and community-acquired pneumonia
>12	Chronic rejection and posttransplantation lymphoproliferative disorder

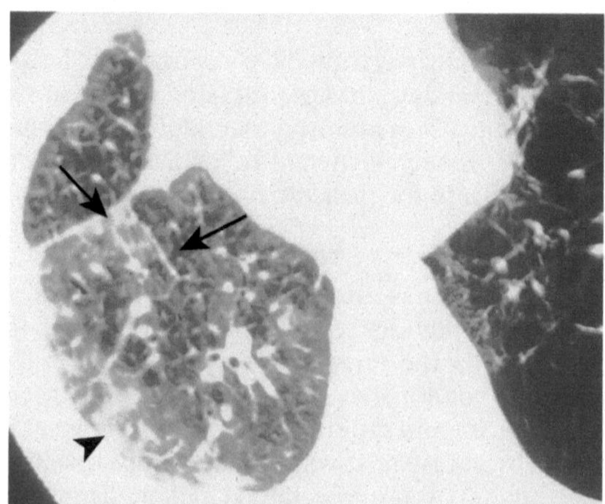

FIGURE 12.21 Acute rejection after single-lung transplant for emphysema. Axial chest computed tomography image demonstrates diffuse ground-glass opacification with thickening of the interlobular septa *(arrow)* and nodular foci of consolidation *(arrowhead).*

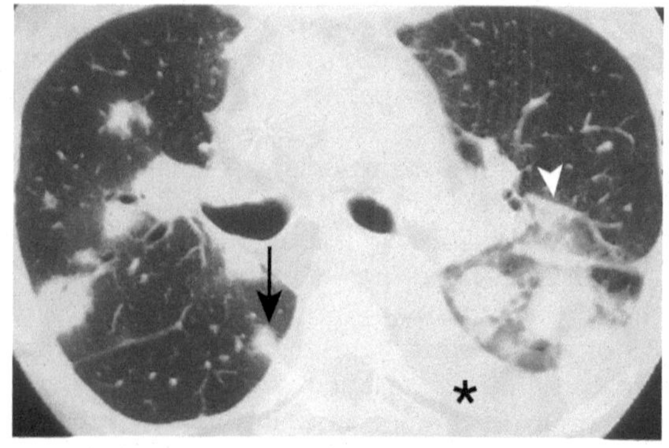

FIGURE 12.23 Posttransplant lymphoproliferative disease (PTLD) after double-lung transplant. Axial chest computed tomography image demonstrates nodules *(arrow)*, consolidation *(arrowhead)*, and pleural effusions *(asterisk)*.

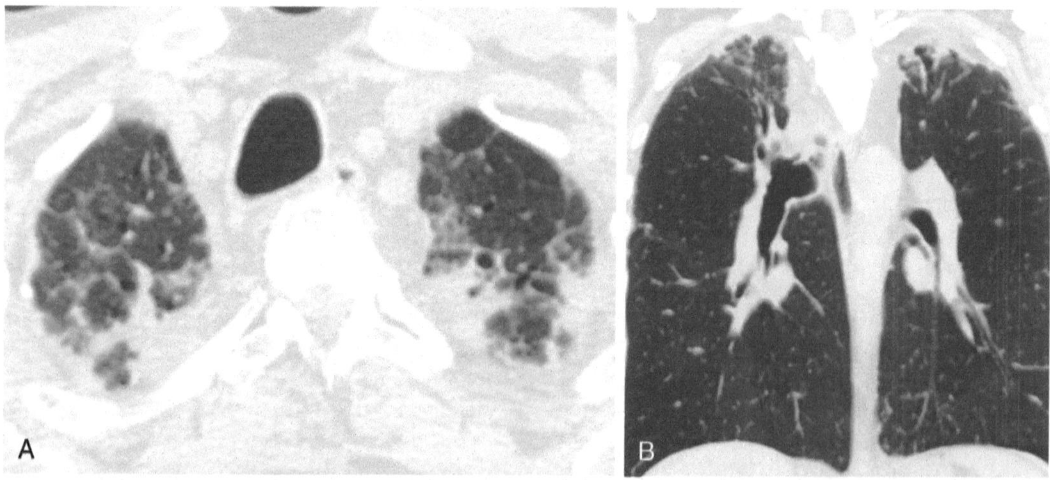

FIGURE 12.22 Chronic rejection. Axial **(A)** and coronal **(B)** chest computed tomography images after bilateral lung transplant demonstrate biapical pleuroparenchymal opacities with architectural distortion and fibrosis.

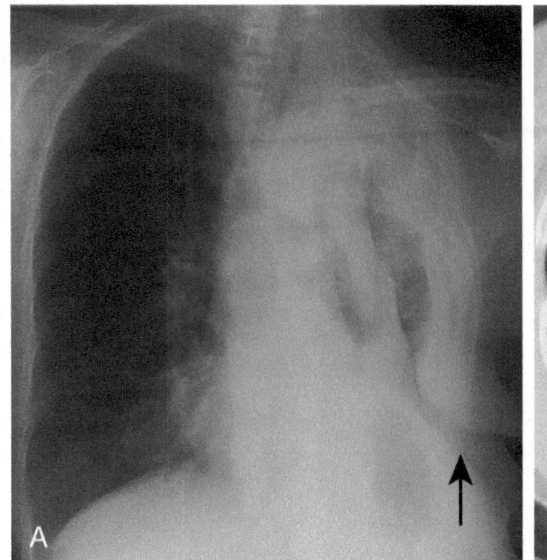

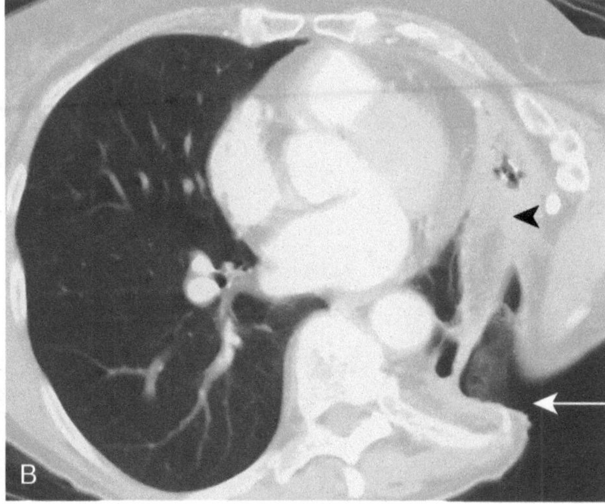

FIGURE 12.24 Post Eloesser flap for chronic left empyema. **A,** Posteroanterior chest radiograph 1 month postoperative demonstrates deformity of the left chest wall, resection of left lateral ribs, and characteristic crescent-shape lucency *(arrow)*. **B,** Axial chest computed tomography image of the same patient reveals communication between the pleural space and the skin defect *(arrow)* and near-complete obliteration of the pleural space *(arrowhead)*.

adhesive pleuritis. This procedure is indicated for recurrent pneumothorax and pleural effusions, particularly those that are malignant in nature. The pleuritis is obtained by either mechanical or chemical irritation of the pleura. Mechanical pleurodesis may be achieved via thoracotomy or VATS and consists of pleural abrasion with scratch pads. It usually is preferred in younger patients for benign causes. Chemical pleurodesis is accomplished by insertion of sclerosant (talc, bleomycin, tetracycline) or cytostatic (cisplatin) agents into pleural space. Talc particles are seen as hyperdense foci or linear opacities in a pleural space on radiographs and CT scans and may be associated with an increased FDG (fluorodeoxyglucose) uptake on PET scan. Other types of pleurodesis do not have specific radiologic findings and may only demonstrate residual pleural thickening and/or resolution of previously seen pleural effusion or pneumothorax.

Decortication and Pleurectomy

Pleurectomy is defined as resection of parietal (partial) or parietal and visceral (complete) pleura. It is performed in selected patients with mesothelioma or in patients with organized hemothorax, fibrothorax, and empyema. Decortication consists of surgical removal of thick fibrous material deposited in pleural space and along pleurae. It is usually performed after a failed attempt of percutaneous drainage of empyema or organized hemothorax. Both of these procedures are now commonly performed by VATS. The clinical history of a prior pleurectomy or decortication is necessary for adequate interpretation of postprocedural studies, given the lack of specific radiologic findings.

Open Pleural Drainage

Open pleural drainage involves the surgical creation of a fistula between the skin and pleural space through the chest wall. An Eloesser flap or window is the most common type of such drainage and consists of a U-shaped incision through the skin and chest wall muscles with additional resection of two or three underlying ribs. The skin or muscle flap is folded inward into the pleural space and fixed to the parietal pleura. This allows creation of an opening in the chest wall communicating with the pleural space. Historically, this procedure was performed for tuberculous empyema. The procedure is now uncommon and is mainly indicated for chronic empyema in patients who failed initial conservative treatment and who would not tolerate more extensive surgical treatment (e.g., decortication or pleurectomy). Radiologic findings of Eloesser flaps consist of a characteristic chest wall defect from the flap creation. A crescent-shaped lucency is commonly seen projecting over the soft tissues on radiographs, which is related to the original skin or muscle incision. Connection between the pleural space and the skin can readily be seen on CT scans (Fig. 12.24). Depending on the stage of empyema drainage, the pleural space may be completely or partially obliterated.

MEDIASTINAL SURGERIES

Esophagectomy

Esophagectomy is resection of a part of the esophagus and is indicated for tumors (both benign and malignant) and several other nontumoral processes, such as achalasia, strictures, corrosive injury, and esophageal perforation. There are many different surgical techniques for esophagectomy, broadly categorized into transthoracic and transhiatal approaches. Similar to lung surgeries, minimally invasive surgical techniques have gained much popularity in recent years. During esophagectomy, the resected portion of the esophagus is replaced by a conduit that is anastomosed to the residual esophagus. This conduit may be formed by either stomach or bowel graft (colon or jejunum). If the stomach is used, the conduit is first mobilized and then pulled up and placed within the chest, in a paravertebral, right paratracheal, or retrosternal position. If a bowel conduit is used, the graft is resected, and an enteroenteric (or enterocolonic) anastomosis is created. The graft is subsequently transposed into the chest and connected cranially to the residual esophagus and caudally to the stomach. The major difference between transthoracic and

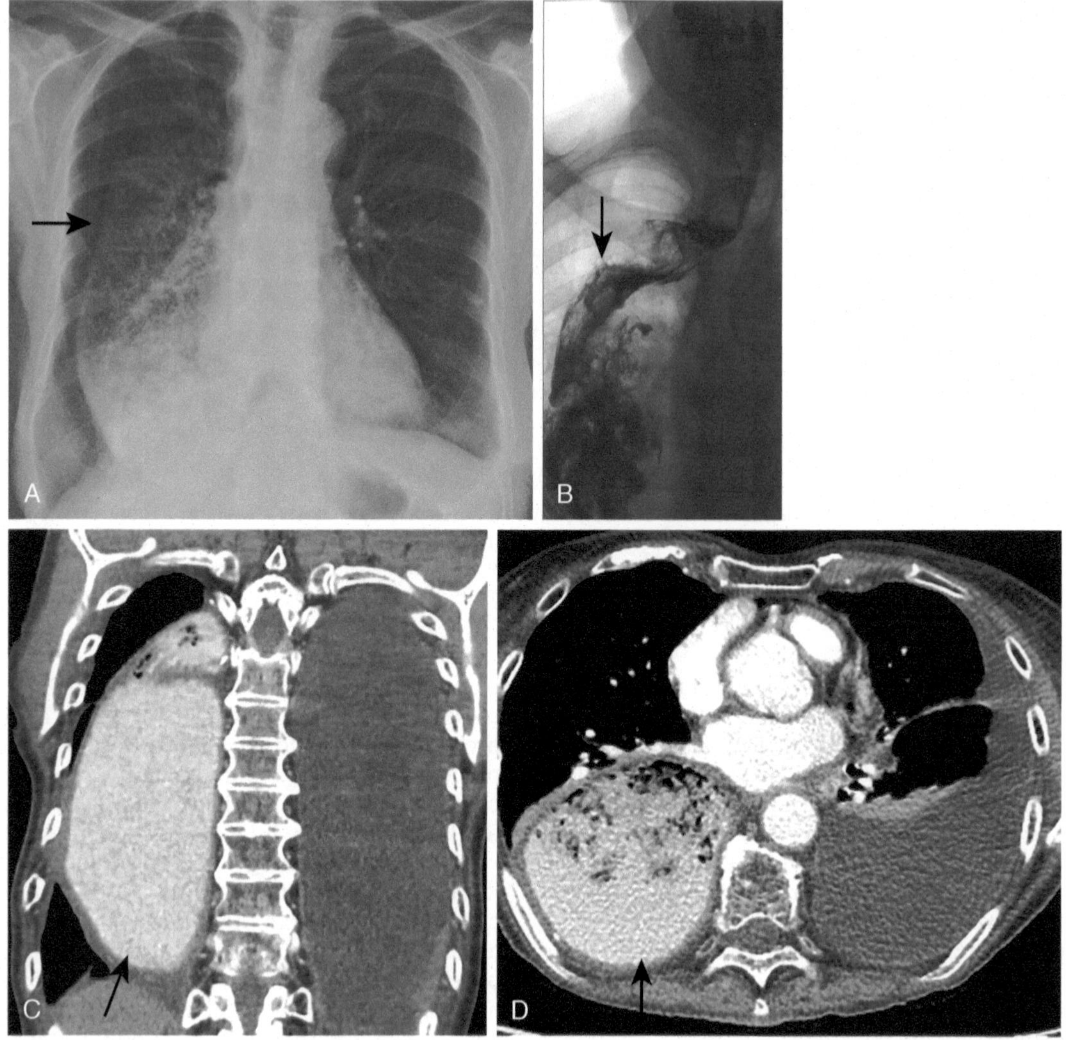

FIGURE 12.25 Post Ivor Lewis esophagectomy. **A,** Posteroanterior chest radiograph 10 weeks postoperative demonstrates heterogeneous tubular structure in the right hemithorax consistent with gastric pull-through *(arrow)*. **B,** Esophagogram performed on the same day demonstrates oral contrast filling the gastric pull-through *(arrow)* without signs of anastomotic stenosis or leak. Coronal **(C)** and axial **(D)** chest computed tomography images 1 week later reveal contrast-filled gastric pull-through in the posterior right hemithorax *(arrows)*. Note moderate left pleural effusion.

transhiatal esophagectomies is a need for thoracotomy in the transthoracic approach. Transhiatal esophagectomy is performed through laparotomy and a left cervical incision. It requires an additional challenging step of blunt dissection and mobilization of the mid mediastinal esophagus by the surgeon's hand through the esophageal hiatus. Normal postoperative appearance on radiographs, esophagograms, and CT scans varies depending on the surgical approach and conduit used. For adequate interpretation of such studies, it is essential to know the type of esophagectomy performed, location of the anastomosis, type of conduit, and position of the conduit within the intrathoracic cavity. Radiographically, a widened mediastinum with abnormal contours is almost always seen. Gas bubbles within the conduit may or may not be seen and, if present, could be difficult to differentiate from potential complications, such as anastomotic leak or mediastinal abscess. Postthoracotomy changes may or may not be present, depending on the surgical approach. Esophagography is routinely performed on postoperative day 7 to 10 and together with CT scan may be used to define the anatomy of the conduit and detect complications (Fig. 12.25).

Mediastinal Tumor Resection

Multiple surgical approaches exist for resection of nonesophageal mediastinal tumors. These all imply some degree of sternotomy or thoracotomy, although there has been recent interest in minimally invasive surgical procedures or VATS. Complete median sternotomy and clamshell sternotomy are preferred for resection of large mediastinal tumors because these offer wider exposure to the mediastinum than other less extensive approaches. Clamshell sternotomy, which implies inframammary horizontal incision with transverse sternotomy at the fourth intercostal space level, is most commonly used if tumor extends into both hemithoraces.

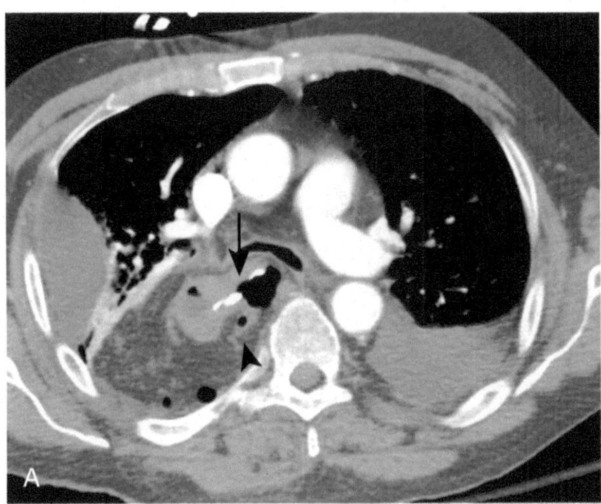

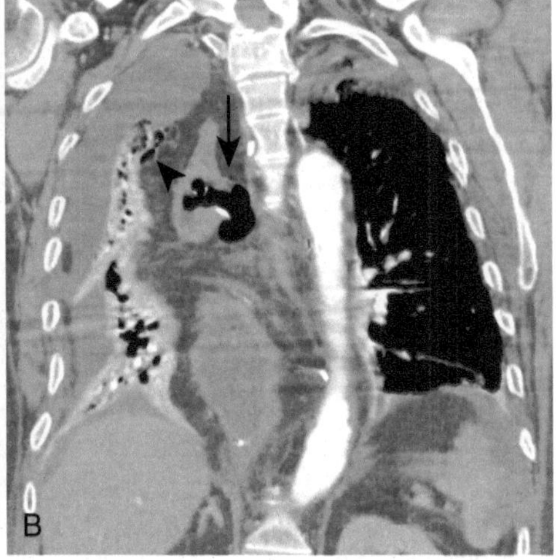

FIGURE 12.26 Esophageal anastomotic dehiscence after Ivor Lewis esophagectomy. Axial **(A)** and coronal **(B)** chest computed tomography images 8 days after surgery demonstrate dehiscence of esophagogastric anastomosis at the suture line *(arrow)*. Note the extraluminal gas bubbles tracking posteriorly and into the omentum *(arrowhead)*.

Postoperative imaging depends on the surgical procedure and approach. Median sternotomy wires and clamshell sternotomy wires have characteristic radiographic distribution: five or six wires in horizontal orientation and vertical distribution for the former and two parallel wires in vertical orientation at the fourth or fifth interspace for the latter. Additional partial rib resection or healed rib fracture may be present if a thoracotomy was required during tumor resection. Widening of the mediastinum and presence of surgical clips usually are the only nonosseous signs of surgery on radiographs. In addition to the radiographic findings, CT may further demonstrate mediastinal fat stranding, tissue distortion, mediastinal gas bubbles, and small postoperative fluid collections or seromas in the surgical bed. Postoperative air and fluid should resolve by 1 month.

Complications

Anastomotic Leak

Anastomotic leak is a recognized complication of esophagectomies, occurring in 10% to 44% of cases. It is more common following esophagectomy using gastric conduit than those using bowel grafts. Predisposing factors for anastomotic leak include arterial and venous ischemia of the perianastomotic tissue, excessive or inadequate tension on the anastomosis, postoperative conduit gaseous distention, infection, technical errors, and extrinsic compression of the anastomosis by chest tube or thoracic inlet structures. Anastomotic leaks have a reported mortality rate of 2% and commonly occur within the first 10 days after surgery. Clinical manifestations and treatment depend on the severity of the leak. Sepsis, septic shock, and drainage of gastrointestinal content from chest tubes may be seen in the setting of a large anastomotic dehiscence. Smaller leaks may present with fever and leukocytosis. The majority of small leaks are, however, subclinical and are first detected on a routine postoperative esophagography. Subclinical leaks are usually small and contained by adjacent tissues and frequently resolve with a conservative management consisting of nasogastric tube decompression, nutritional support, and antibiotics. If leakage progresses or an abscess forms close to the trachea and aorta, percutaneous or surgical drainage may be required. Large leaks are usually treated with an urgent thoracotomy and an anastomotic revision with reinforcement. The initial esophagography is usually performed with water-soluble contrast agents to detect the presence of large anastomotic leaks or obstruction. If large leaks are absent and the study appears normal, additional images are obtained with thin barium to assess for subtle smaller leaks. Contrast agent extraluminal extravasation at the level of anastomosis is diagnostic of a leak. Anastomotic dehiscence is commonly occult on postoperative radiographs. Larger leaks may demonstrate new gas bubbles and air-fluid levels within the mediastinum, with or without mediastinal widening or pleural effusions. CT scan performed after oral contrast administration is more sensitive than radiographs in detecting anastomotic dehiscence and is particularly useful in unstable patients (Fig. 12.26). Additionally, CT scan may demonstrate associated complications such as abscess or empyema.

Esophagopleural Fistula

Esophagopleural fistula (EPF) usually is seen in the context of anastomotic esophageal leak. This complication may also occur after lung resection such as lobectomy and pneumonectomy if the esophagus is injured during resection of a tumor or mediastinal lymph nodes. Drainage of food particles or gastric contents through a pleural drainage catheter or skin incision is a typical clinical sign of this complication. Postoperative esophagopleural fistula is associated with a high mortality rate and requires a prompt intervention. Antibiotics, feeding jejunostomy, and drainage of the pleural cavity with chest tube are the first lines of treatment. However, a surgical intervention is frequently required. Extension of the oral contrast into the pleural space during esophagography is a diagnostic finding of EPF. Postoperative radiographs typically demonstrate increasing pleural effusion or new air-fluid levels in the pleural space.

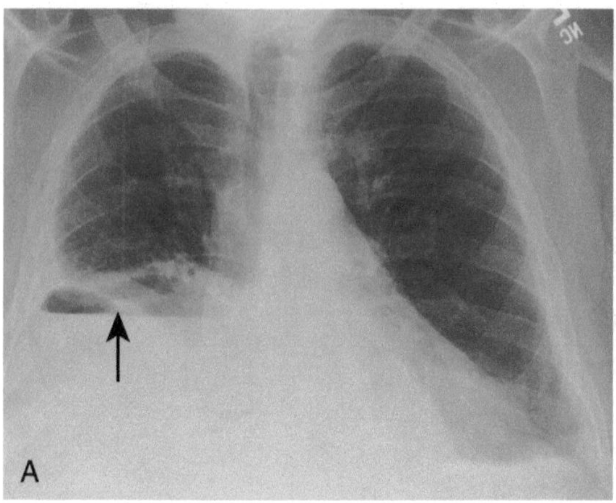

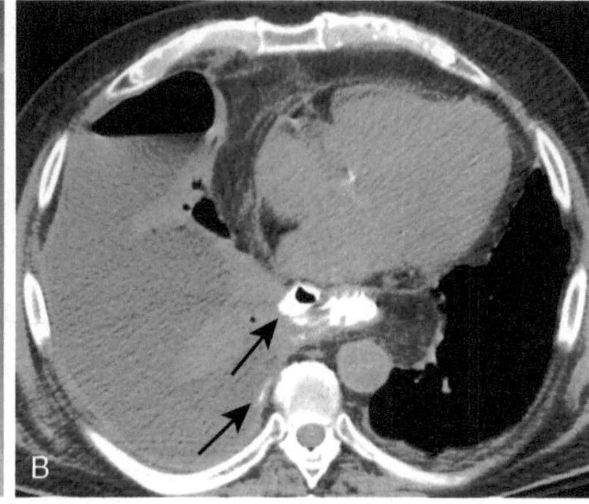

FIGURE 12.27 Esophagopleural fistula after Ivor Lewis esophagectomy. **A,** Posteroanterior chest radiograph 14 days postoperative demonstrates moderate right hydropneumothorax. Note intrapleural air–fluid level *(straight arrow)*. **B,** Axial computed tomography image reveals a small amount of extravasated oral contrast in the right pleural space *(arrows)*.

On CT scan, a diagnosis is obtained by visualization of extravasated oral contrast in the pleural space and direct esophagopleural communication (Fig. 12.27). CT is also useful in excluding potential associated empyema and abscess.

Anastomotic Stricture

Esophagogastric or esophagocolonic anastomotic stricture is usually caused by technical complications or wound healing in the early postoperative period. Delayed anastomotic stricture is typically caused by prior anastomotic leak or local tumor recurrence. Dysphagia is a common presenting symptom. This complication is radiologically diagnosed with demonstration of proximal esophageal dilation with the transition point at the level of anastomosis on esophagography or CT scan. Initially, it is treated with endoscopic balloon dilatation.

Chylothorax

Postoperative chylothorax most commonly develops because of disruption of the thoracic duct or one of its major tributaries. Lymph accumulates in the posterior mediastinum until it ruptures the mediastinal pleura and extends into a pleural space. Chylothorax commonly forms on the right side if an injury or transection occurred below the T6 level. If an injury to the duct occurred more cranially, a chylothorax is usually seen on the left side. Although chylothorax is a recognized complication of esophagectomy, this entity can also be seen after pneumonectomy, mediastinal tumor resection, aggressive mediastinal nodal dissection, and cervical and abdominal surgeries. A triglyceride concentration greater than 110 mg/dL in the pleural fluid is diagnostic of chylothorax. Persistent chylothorax is frequently treated with thoracic duct ligation to prevent metabolic and nutritional deficiencies, which may develop if chylous leak persists. Other treatment options include creation of a pleuroperitoneal shunt or a pleurovenous shunt and percutaneous embolization and sclerosis of a thoracic duct. Radiographically, a chylothorax presents as pleural fluid that quickly increases in amount or persists despite an indwelling chest tube. This condition has a nonspecific appearance on CT scan and may be indistinguishable from simple pleural effusion. If needed on rare occasion, a lymphangiography may be used to demonstrate extravasation of dense contrast into the mediastinum and pleural cavity, confirming the diagnosis of chylothorax (Fig. 12.28).

Nerve Injury

Recurrent laryngeal nerve injury can happen during cervical esophageal mobilization and creation of cervical anastomosis. This may predispose a patient to aspiration and pneumonia. Another nerve that may potentially be injured in the context of esophagectomy is a phrenic nerve. Although rarer than with lung surgeries, an injury of a phrenic nerve usually presents itself with persistently elevated ipsilateral hemidiaphragm on postoperative radiographs. This complication may be temporary or permanent. Paradoxical motion of the abnormal hemidiaphragm at the "sniff test," during which a patient is asked to vigorously and swiftly take a breath through the nose while the motion of the hemidiaphragm is monitored by ultrasonography or chest fluoroscopy, is diagnostic of diaphragmatic paralysis caused by phrenic nerve injury (see Chapter 7).

Mediastinal Hematoma

A small mediastinal hematoma is a common finding after thoracic surgery and usually does not require any further intervention. Clinically significant mediastinal hemorrhage is rare, with a reported incidence of 2.5%. Mediastinal hematoma may be caused by inadequate hemostasis of mediastinal and chest wall arteries, injury to mediastinal veins, inappropriate intraoperative insertion of vascular lines, and disruption of vascular anastomosis with or without infection. When large, hematoma may cause mass effect on adjacent structures, particularly on the trachea and the superior vena cava. Radiographic findings of a large mediastinal hematoma include mediastinal widening, obscuration of the aortic arch, deviation of the trachea, displacement of a nasogastric tube, left apical pleural cap, and widened right paratracheal stripe. CT confirms the diagnosis of hematoma by demonstrating a dense collection of 50 to 90 Hounsfield units (HU) that does not enhance after intravenous contrast administration. A contrast-enhanced CT scan may be used to assess the integrity of vascular structures

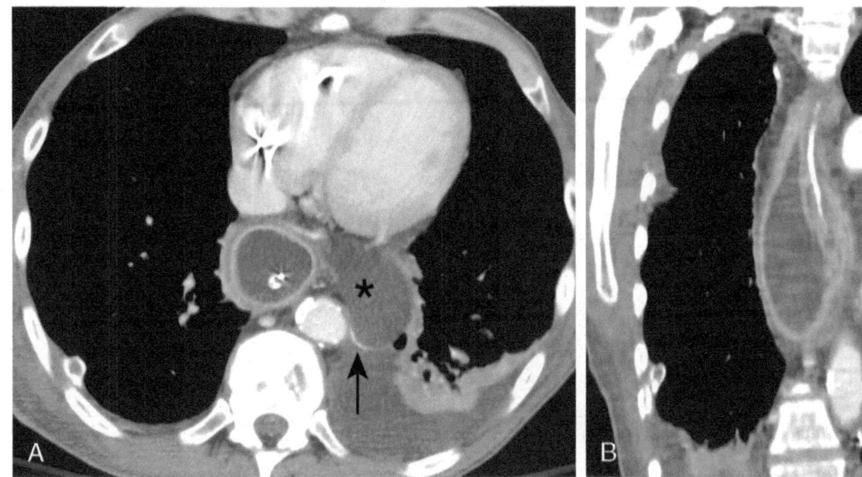

FIGURE 12.28 Chylothorax after McKeown procedure. Axial **(A)** and coronal **(B)** chest computed tomography images after a lymphangiography demonstrate left pleural effusion and left mediastinal collection *(asterisk)* with a small amount of extravasated contrast *(straight arrow)* from disrupted lymphatic channels or thoracic duct. Note the nasogastric tube in the gastric pull-through.

and to exclude other causes of mediastinal widening on radiographs.

Sternal Dehiscence and Osteomyelitis

Sternal dehiscence and osteomyelitis are uncommon complications after thoracosternotomy and sternotomy (median or clamshell). Seen in up to 89% of dehiscence cases, specific signs of sternal dehiscence on chest radiographs are rotation and unraveling of the sternal wires, as well as characteristic displacement of the wires named "wandering wires," in which wires pull out or cut through the sternum rather than break. CT may demonstrate separation of the sternal incision and features of osteomyelitis such as demineralization of the bone, osteolysis, periostitis, adjacent inflammation, and fluid collection (Fig. 12.29).

CHEST WALL SURGERIES

Types and Techniques

Numerous different surgical techniques are used for chest wall tumor resection, congenital deformity correction, and defect reconstruction. Common entities and their radiographic appearance are discussed in this section.

Resection of superior sulcus tumor (Pancoast tumor) is a special case and requires a different approach from regular upper lobectomy. Although the tumor originates in the lung parenchyma, it commonly extends extrapleurally and potentially invades the brachial plexus, subclavian vessels, first rib, vertebrae, and lower cervical muscles. Given the location of tumor and adjacent vital structures, excision of all neoplastic tissue is considered a challenging task. In addition to upper lobectomy, resection may include the clavicle, first or second ribs (or both), subclavian vessels, adjacent muscles, and even a portion of the brachial plexus and part of the vertebrae, depending on cancer extension. The postoperative imaging appearance depends on the extent of surgical resection. The loss of volume of the involved hemithorax, absence of upper ribs, and deformity of the structures in the ipsilateral apical region are typical radiologic findings. Focal lung herniation into the chest wall can occur at the site of rib resection (Fig. 12.30).

The Nuss procedure is a surgical procedure used for correction of severe sternum excavatum. It is indicated in symptomatic patients with Haller index larger than 3 (ratio of maximal transverse diameter of intrathoracic cavity over the smallest distance between the posterior sternum and anterior cortex of vertebral body, measured on axial CT images; see Chapter 7). The surgical procedure requires insertion of a stainless steel bar through the retrosternal space in transverse orientation and its fixation to the chest wall. The inserted bar displaces the sternum outward and corrects the initial deformity. The bar is left in place for 2 to 5 years and is eventually removed. Radiographs demonstrate a characteristic appearance consisting of a horizontal bar in the lower chest on a frontal view that is easily localized in the retrosternal space on a lateral view (Fig. 12.31).

RETAINED SURGICAL FOREIGN BODIES

Retained surgical instruments and surgical material, such as sponges, is rare but an important complication of thoracic surgical procedures. Recognition of these foreign bodies in intraoperative and in the immediate postoperative imaging can be challenging but is critical to avoid surgical reexploration and complications. If there is suspicion of a retained surgical foreign body or discrepancy in the instrument count in the operating room, the radiologic interpretation can be improved by the following steps: (1) communication with the surgical team to clarify the nature, shape, and size of the missing surgical foreign body; (2) ensuring a technically adequate radiologic study and, if required, repeating the study and additional views and extending the field of view; (3) direct communication with the surgeon to resolve the validity of suspicious findings; and finally (4) comparing with a dedicated radiograph of the missing foreign body when in doubt. The commonly encountered foreign bodies are retained needles, guidewires, and sponges (Fig. 12.32).

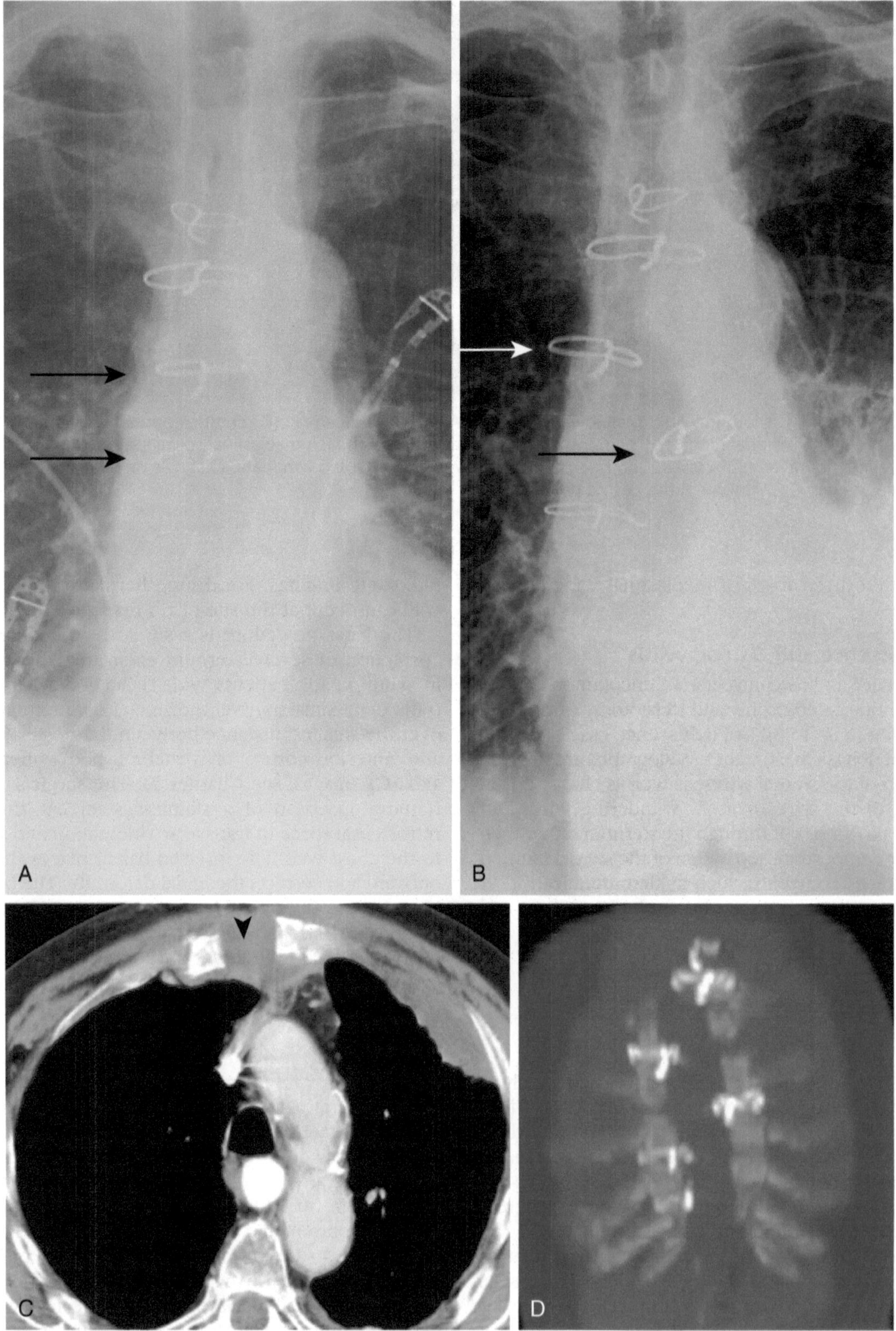

FIGURE 12.29 Sternal dehiscence and osteomyelitis **A,** Chest radiograph obtained 7 days after surgery shows normal alignment of sternal wires. **B,** Chest radiograph obtained 11 days later shows wandering wires with leftward or rightward displacement of the sternal wires in relation to their initial position *(arrows)*. **C,** Axial chest computed tomography (CT) image demonstrates separation of sternal wires with associated rim-enhancing fluid collection *(arrowhead)*. **D,** Maximum intensity projection reformatted coronal CT image demonstrates sternal dehiscence with "wandering wires."

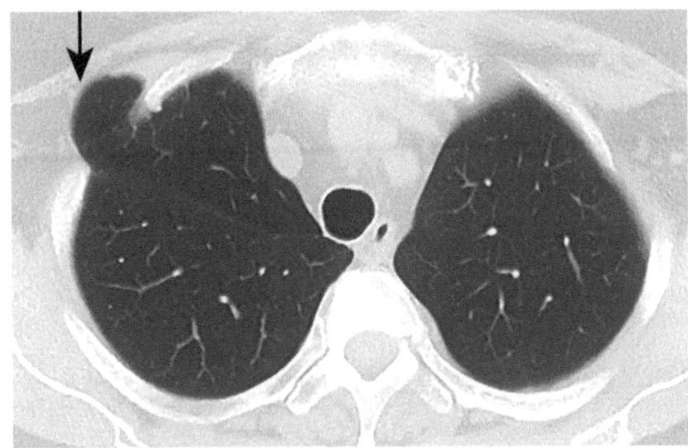

FIGURE 12.30 Lung herniation after right upper lobectomy. Axial chest computed tomography image 5 years after surgery demonstrates focal lung herniation through thoracotomy defect *(arrow)*.

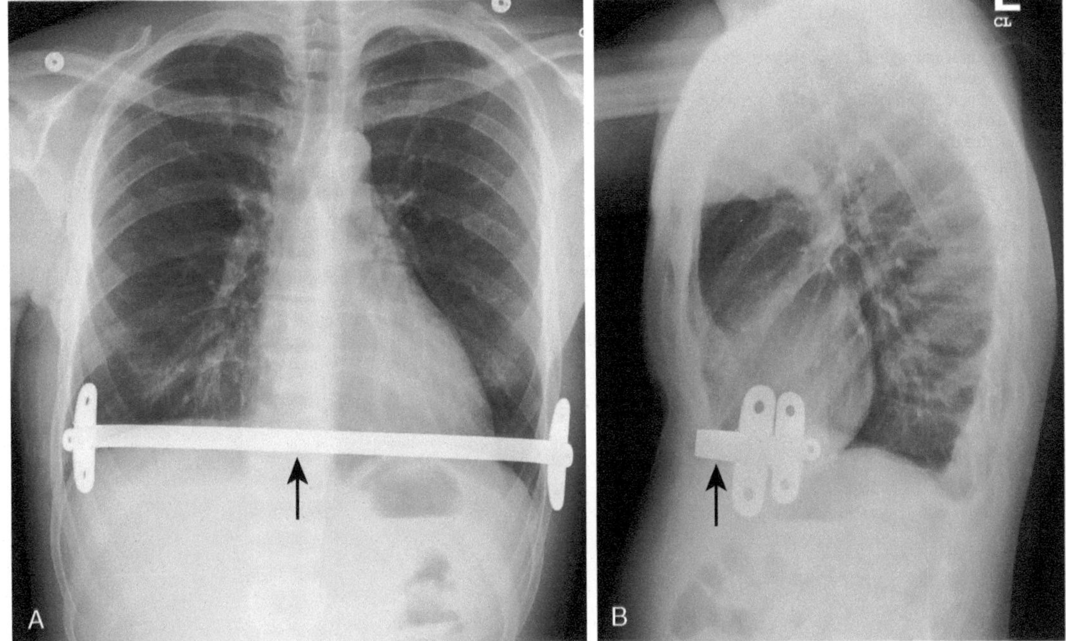

FIGURE 12.31 Post–Nuss bar procedure for pectus excavatum. Posteroanterior **(A)** and lateral **(B)** chest radiographs 6 months after surgery demonstrate a characteristic stainless steel bar in the retrosternal space *(arrow)* inserted during the surgery.

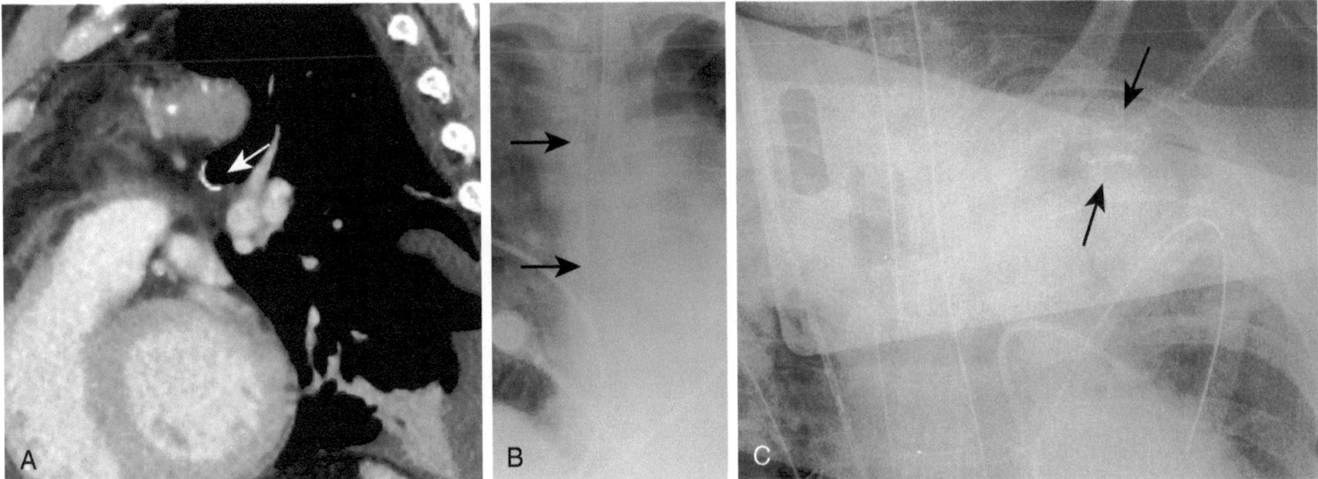

FIGURE 12.32 Retained surgical foreign bodies. **A,** Sagittal chest computed tomography image after mediastinal surgery shows a retained surgical needle *(arrow)* in the aortopulmonary window. **B,** Supine chest radiograph after venogram shows a retained guidewire in the heart and superior vena cava *(arrows)*. **C,** Intraoperative radiograph shows a retained surgical sponge in the left upper chest *(arrows)*.

SUGGESTED READINGS

Arndt RD, Frank CG, Schmitz AL, et al. Cardiac herniation with volvulus after pneumonectomy. *AJR Am J Roentgenol*. 1978;130:155-156.

Asrani A, Kaewlai R, Digumarthy S, et al. Urgent findings on portable chest radiography: what the radiologist should know-review. *AJR Am J Roentgenol*. 2011;196:S45-S61.

Brady MB, Brogdon BG. Cardiac herniation and volvulus: radiographic findings. *Radiology*. 1986;161:657-658.

Boiselle PM, Mansilla AV, Fisher MS, et al. Wandering wires: frequency of sternal wire abnormalities in patients with sternal dehiscence. *AJR Am J Roentgenol*. 1999;173:777-780.

Chae EJ, Seo JB, Kim SYK. Radiographic and CT findings of thoracic complications after pneumonectomy. *Radiograobics*. 2006;26:1449-1467.

Chang MY, Sugarbaker DJ. Extrapleural pneumonectomy for diffuse malignant pleural mesothelioma: techniques and complications. *Thorac Surg Clin*. 2004;14:523-530.

Felson B. Lung torsion: radiographic findings in nine cases. *Radiology*. 1987;162: 631-638.

Flanagan JC, Batz R, Saboo SS. Esophagectomy and gastric pull-through procedures: surgical techniques, imaging features and potential complications. *Radiographics*. 2015;36:107-121.

Friedman PJ, Hellekani CAG. Radiologic recognition of bronchopleural fistula. *Radiology*. 1977;124:289-295.

Goodman LR. Postoperative chest radiograph. II. Alterations after major intrathoracic surgery. *AJR Am J Roentgenol*. 1980;134:803-813.

Gurney JW, Arnold S, Goodman LR. Impeding cardiac herniation: the snow cone sign. *Radiology*. 1986;161:653-655.

Hansell DM, Lynch DA, McAdams HP, et al. Pleura and pleural disorders. In: Hansell DM, eds. *Imaging of Diseases of the Chest*. London: Mosby Elsevier; 2010:1003-1064.

Hobert JM, Libshitz HI, Chasen MH, et al. The postlobectomy chest: anatomic consideration. *Radiographics*. 1987;7:889-911.

Liu PS, Levine MS, Torigian DA. Esophagopleural fistula secondary to esophageal wall ballooning and thinning after pneumonectomy: findings on chest CT and esophagography. *AJR Am J Roentgenol*. 2006;186:1627-1629.

LoCicero J. Segmentectomy and lesser pulmonary resection. In: Shields TW, eds. *General Thoracic Surgery*. Philadelphia: Lippincott Williams & Wilkins; 2005:496-502.

Kim EA, Lee KS, Shim YM, et al. Radiographic and CT findings in complications following pulmonary resection. *Radiographics*. 2002;22:67-86.

Kim TF, Lee KH, Kim YH, et al. Postoperative imaging of esophageal cancer: what chest radiologists need to know. *Radiographics*. 2007;27:409-429.

Krishnam MS, Suh RD, Tomasian A, et al. Postoperative complications of lung transplantation: radiologic findings along a time continuum. *Radiographics*. 2007;27:957-974.

Kuhlman JE, Singha NK. Complex disease of the pleural space: radiographic and CT evaluation. *Radiographics*. 1997;17:63-79.

Massard G, Wihlm JM. Early complications. Esophagopleural fistula. *Chest Surg Clin N Am*. 1999;9:617-631.

McKenna RJ Jr, Houck W, Fuller CB. Video-assisted thoracic surgery lobectomy: experience with 1100 cases. *Ann Thorac Surg*. 2006;81:421-426.

Nachiappan A, Digumarthy S, Sharma A, et al. An overview of lung surgeries: postoperative CT findings and complications. *Internet Journal of Radiology*. 2009;12:1-7.

Ng YL, Paul N, Patsios D, et al. Imaging of lung transplantation: review. *AJR Am J Roentgenol*. 2009;192:S1-S13.

Parissis H, Young V. Treatment of pnacoas tumors from surgeons prospective: re-appraisal of the anterior-manubrial sternal approach. *J Cardiothorac Surg*. 2010;5:102.

Pinstein ML, Winer-Muram H, Eastridge C, et al. Middle lobe torsion following right upper lobectomy. *Radiology*. 1985;155:580.

Semenkovich JW, Glazer HS, Anderson DC, et al. Bronchial dehiscence in lung transplantation: CT evaluation. *Radiology*. 1995;194:205-208.

Shapiro MP, Gale ME, Daily BDT. Eloesser window thoracostomy for treatment of empyema: radiographic appearance. *AJR Am J Roentgenol*. 1988;150:549-552.

Stark DD, Federle MP, Goodman PC, et al. Differentiating lung abscess and empyema: radiography and computed tomography. *AJR Am J Roentgenolà*. 1983;141:163-167.

Stirling GR, Babidge WJ, Peacock MJ, et al. Lung volume reduction surgery in emphysema: a systematic review. *Ann Thorac Surg*. 2001;72:641-648.

Waldhausen JA, Pierce WS. Segmental resection. In: Waldhausen JA, Pierce WS, eds. *Johnson's Surgery of the Chest*. Chicago: Year Book Medical Publishers; 1985:143-165.

Williamson WA, Tronic BS, Levitan N, et al. Pulmonary venous infarction. *Chest*. 1992;102:937-940.

Wright CD, Wain JC, Mathisen DJ, et al. Postpneumonectomy bronchopleural fistula after sutured bronchial closure: incidence, risk factors, and management. *J Thorac Cardiovasc Surg*. 1996;112:1367-1371.

Chapter 13
Thoracic Trauma

Efren J. Flores, Laura L. Avery, and Jeanne B. Ackman

INTRODUCTION

In the United States, 25% of trauma-related deaths are secondary to thoracic injuries, which can result from either penetrating trauma or blunt trauma. Penetrating chest trauma is less frequent but deadlier than blunt chest trauma and commonly results from gunshot and stabbing. Surgery is more frequently required for penetrating thoracic injury than blunt injury. The most common causes of blunt trauma are motor vehicle collisions and falls. Increased morbidity and mortality are associated with multiple rib fractures, increased age, and a higher Injury Severity Score (ISS). The ISS is an anatomic scoring system that provides an overall assessment of the severity of multiple injuries, dividing the body into six regions (Box 13.1): head and neck, face, chest, abdomen, extremities, and external (skin).

Each body region receives an Abbreviated Injury Score (AIS) from 1 to 6 (Table 13.1) based on the severity of injury, with a score of 6 non-survivable. The three most severely injured regions have their score squared and added together to generate the overall ISS score. The ISS overall score values range from 0 to 75. In cases in which a body region gets an AIS of 6, the ISS is automatically assigned a value of 75.

Supine anteroposterior portable chest radiographs (AP portable CXRs) are the first line of imaging evaluation for chest trauma patients because they can be obtained at the bedside. CXRs demonstrate placement of central lines and tubes, in addition to injuries such as tension pneumothorax, displaced fractures, and hemothorax. Other injuries, such as traumatic aortic injury (TAI), lung lacerations and contusions, tracheobronchial injuries, cardiac injuries, and thoracic spine injuries, are better depicted by cross-sectional imaging and most commonly by multidetector computed tomography (MDCT). MDCT with intravenous (IV) contrast provides better anatomic detail and more accurate characterization of thoracic injuries, allowing for more precise assessment and patient management than CXR. Dual-energy CT (DECT) provides additional information beyond standard MDCT and may provide more accurate diagnosis. For example, virtual noncontrast postprocessing of DECT images can be used to differentiate active hemorrhage, with extravasation of high-attenuation IV contrast, from calcifications and can also be used to demonstrate decreased organ perfusion.

BOX 13.1 Injury Severity Score (ISS) Body Regions

- Head and neck
- Face
- Chest
- Abdomen
- Extremity
- External (skin)

PULMONARY, PLEURAL, AND DIAPHRAGMATIC INJURIES

Lung Contusions and Lacerations

Lung contusions occur when the energy from a chest wall injury is transmitted to the lung parenchyma. This energy disrupts the alveolar capillary network, resulting in hemorrhage in the alveoli and pulmonary interstitium. Contusions manifest as hazy opacity and consolidation on CXR (Fig. 13.1). They may not be evident on initial radiographs, materializing 6 to 12 or more hours later. Contusion on CT manifests as one or more areas of ground-glass attenuation or consolidation in the geographic distribution of injury. Contusions do not respect anatomic boundaries, unlike typical pneumonias. Lung contusions often resolve, or at least improve, within 48 hours of their appearance. If consolidation worsens beyond this time frame, then other causes for the consolidation, such as aspiration, other pneumonia, and acute respiratory distress syndrome, should be considered.

Lung lacerations are tears of the lung parenchyma that may fill with air (pneumatocele), blood (hematocele), or both (air–fluid level). They are typically spherical because the elastic recoil of the lung parenchyma retracts the laceration in all directions within the disrupted region. Lung lacerations are often difficult to identify on CXR because of adjacent lung contusion. Cross-sectional imaging by CT provides clear visualization and better characterization of lung laceration (see Fig. 13.1), which can occur in several ways (Table 13.2). Lung lacerations usually take weeks to heal and typically leave a parenchymal scar. Pulmonary

TABLE 13.1 Abbreviated Injury Score (AIS)

AIS Score	Injury
1	Minor
2	Moderate
3	Serious
4	Severe
5	Critical
6	Non-survivable

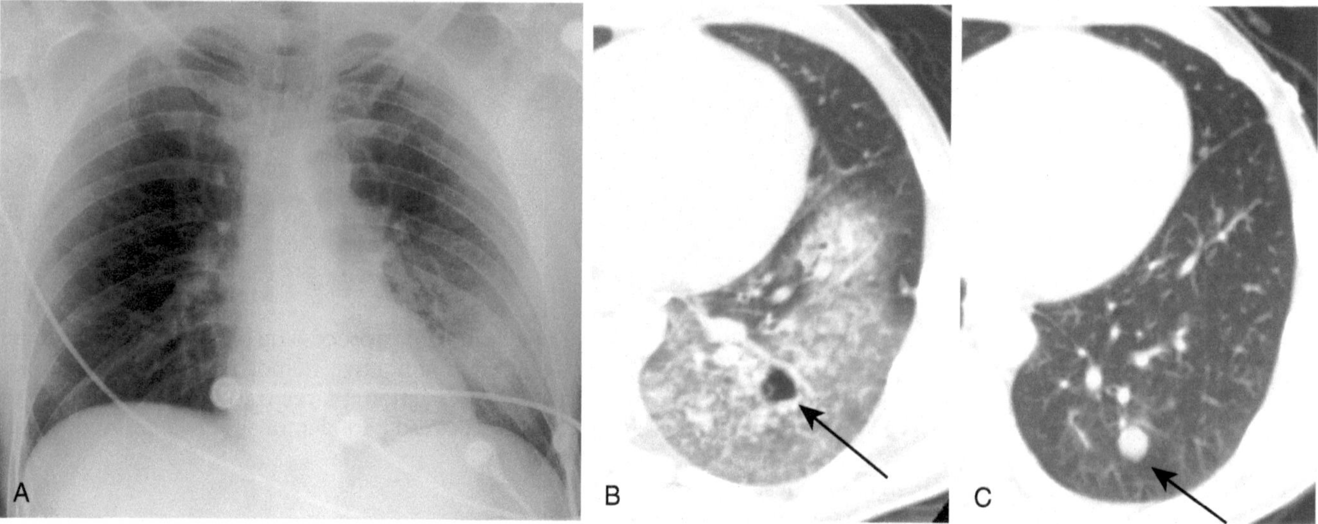

FIGURE 13.1 Left lung contusion, laceration, and hematoma. Portable anteroposterior chest radiograph **(A)** demonstrates hazy opacities in the middle to lower left lung. Axial computed tomography (CT) image **(B)** demonstrates a lung laceration in the left lower lobe *(arrow)* with surrounding ground glass, consistent with surrounding contusion and hemorrhage. Follow-up chest CT performed 4 weeks later **(C)** demonstrates interval resolution of lung contusion and healing of lung laceration, with residual small lung nodule representing a hematoma *(arrow)*.

TABLE 13.2 **Lung Laceration Types**

	Laceration Type	Description
Type 1	Compression rupture laceration	Lung parenchymal rupture caused by sudden compression of chest wall
Type 2	Compression shear laceration	Shear injury against an adjacent vertebral body, usually in posterior lower lobes
Type 3	Rib penetration tear	Puncture injury from adjacent rib fracture penetrating pleural space and injuring lung parenchyma
Type 4	Adhesion tear	Preexisting pleural-parenchymal adhesions causing a tear from chest wall trauma

hematomas can take months to resolve and can be mistaken for neoplasm.

Tracheobronchial Injuries

Tears and fractures of the tracheobronchial tree are rare. Often their diagnosis is delayed secondary to lack of recognition on initial imaging studies. The vast majority of these injuries occurs within 2 cm of the carina and affects the left and right mainstem bronchi with equal frequency. The most common radiographic findings are pneumomediastinum, pneumothorax, and subcutaneous emphysema. Tracheal lacerations are usually longitudinal and located at the junction of the cartilaginous and membranous portions of the trachea. In patients with tracheobronchial transection, the associated pneumothorax is the result of a traumatic tear of the mediastinal pleura. This continuous leakage of air from the tracheobronchial tear into the pleural space results in a persistent pneumothorax that does not resolve despite chest tube placement on continuous wall suction. With complete transection of the mainstem bronchus, the affected lung may rarely fall into the dependent aspect of the thoracic cavity, resulting in the "fallen lung sign" on CXR or CT. The imaging findings of tracheobronchial injury (Box 13.2) are better assessed by CT. These findings include a sharply angulated bronchus, bronchial narrowing with periluminal air, and bronchial discontinuity (Fig. 13.2). Incomplete tears may not cause a pneumothorax and may therefore be underrecognized. The resultant delayed diagnosis can lead to stenosis of the affected bronchus, sometimes presenting as atelectasis.

BOX 13.2 Computed Tomography Imaging Findings of Tracheobronchial Injury

- Sharply angulated bronchus
- Tracheobronchial narrowing with periluminal air
- Discontinuity of the tracheobronchial tree
- Bronchial stenosis with atelectasis (delayed presentation)

Injuries of the Pleural Space

Pneumothorax

Injuries to the pleural space are most commonly the result of a chest wall injury associated with rib fractures that cause air to enter the pleural space (Fig. 13.3). Because air rises, one would expect the air in pneumothoraces to collect at the lung apices of an upright patient and anteriorly in a supine patient; however, there are many exceptions. For example, if there are pleural adhesions, air may not be able to migrate freely to the expected location. Rarely, air in the pleural cavity may solely collect inferolaterally, even in an upright patient. A "deep sulcus" sign can develop on a supine radiograph when a moderate to large

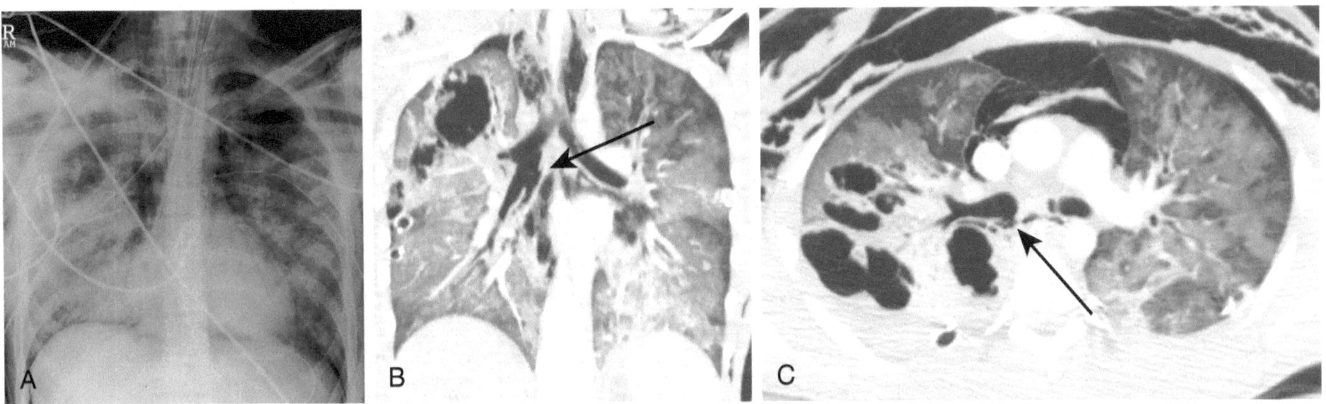

FIGURE 13.2 Posttraumatic laceration of bronchus intermedius. Portable anteroposterior chest radiograph **(A)** demonstrates an endotracheal tube and bilateral chest tubes, extensive subcutaneous emphysema, pneumomediastinum, and bilateral pneumothoraces. Coronal **(B)** and axial **(C)** computed tomography images demonstrate focal discontinuity *(arrow)* and peribronchial air *(arrow)* from laceration of the bronchus intermedius and associated pneumothorax and pneumomediastinum. Note the surrounding extensive right lung lacerations and bilateral contusions.

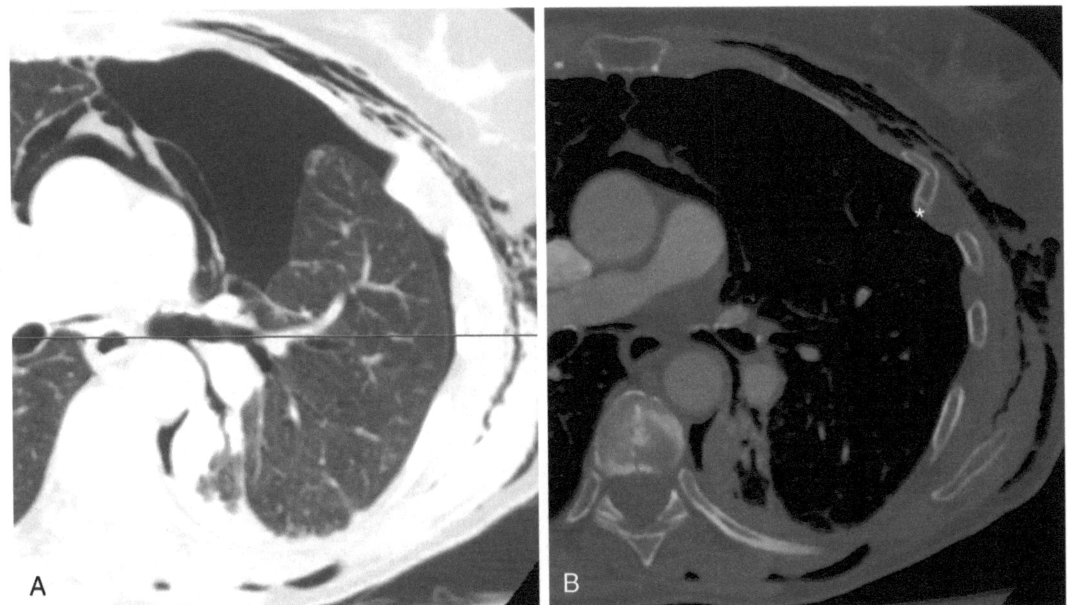

FIGURE 13.3 Left rib fracture and pneumothorax. Axial computed tomography images in lung **(A)** and bone **(B)** windows demonstrate a displaced and angulated left rib fracture *(arrow)*, with associated moderate left pneumothorax, partial collapse of the left lung, and pneumomediastinum.

pneumothorax extends inferiorly into and expands the costophrenic angle along the ipsilateral hemidiaphragm. An unusually sharp delineation of the cardiomediastinal border by lucency on a supine radiograph is a sign of a medial pneumothorax. Air may also collect in the subpulmonic space in a supine patient (a basilar pneumothorax) and even in an upright patient if there are pleural adhesions. A tension pneumothorax is a life-threatening condition that occurs when increasing intrapleural pressure compresses and contralaterally displaces cardiomediastinal structures, yielding hemodynamic instability on account of decreased central venous return. The key imaging findings for tension pneumothorax are the presence of a large pneumothorax, with contralateral shift of the mediastinum, ipsilateral widening of the intercostal spaces, and depression of the ipsilateral hemidiaphragm (Box 13.3). See Chapter 7 for additional information regarding pneumothoraces.

BOX 13.3 Key Radiographic Findings for Tension Pneumothorax

- Contralateral shift of mediastinal structures
- Ipsilateral widening of intercostal spaces ("flaring" of ribs)
- Depression of ipsilateral hemidiaphragm

Hemothorax

A hemothorax typically results from traumatic injury to an intercostal vessel, with blood dissecting into the

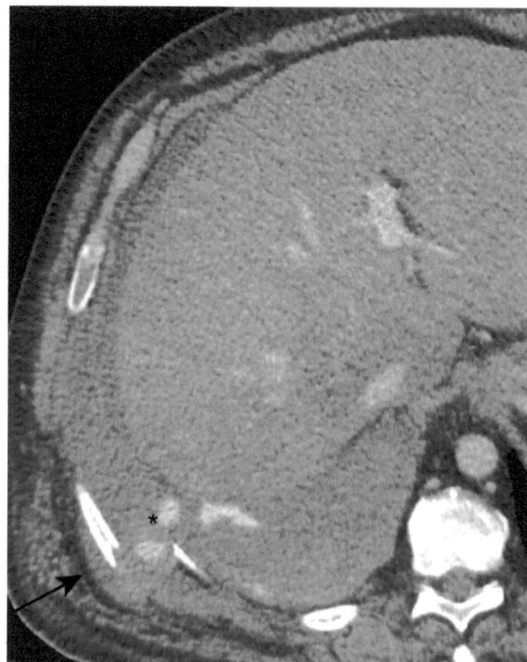

FIGURE 13.4 Rib fracture with hemothorax. Axial contrast-enhanced computed tomography demonstrates a displaced right rib fracture *(arrow)*, with an associated hemothorax and active contrast extravasation *(arrowheads)* from a lacerated intercostal artery.

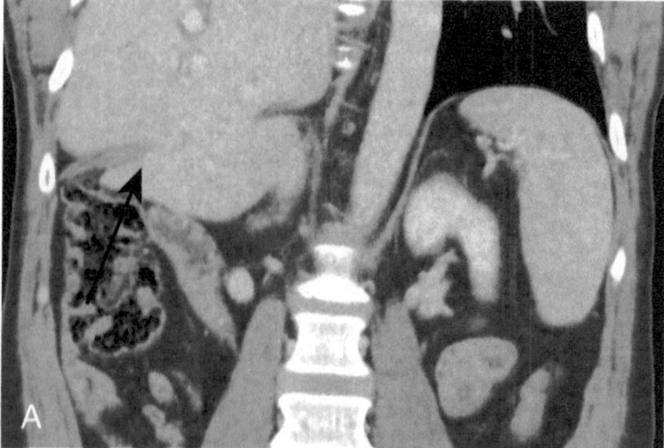

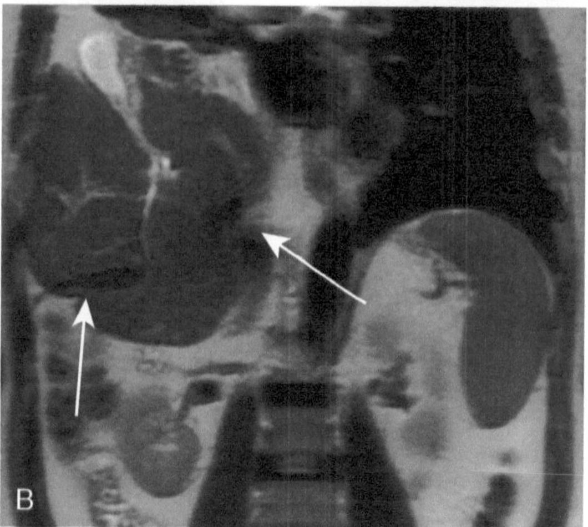

FIGURE 13.5 Right hemidiaphragmatic injury with liver herniation. Coronal computed tomography image **(A)** demonstrates focal discontinuity of the right hemidiaphragm *(arrow)*, consistent with a tear that results in herniation of the liver. Coronal T2-weighted magnetic resonance image **(B)** delineates the focal discontinuity of the right hemidiaphragm, with herniation of the liver into the thorax and resultant "collar sign" *(arrows)*.

pleural space. Radiographs cannot differentiate between a pleural effusion composed of simple fluid (hydrothorax) and a pleural effusion composed of blood (hemothorax). However, CT can differentiate between these two entities. On CT, a hydrothorax demonstrates an attenuation of 0 to 20 Hounsfield units (HU); an acute hemothorax will more commonly demonstrate an attenuation of 35 to 60 HU (Fig. 13.4).

Diaphragmatic Injuries

Traumatic diaphragmatic tears and ruptures result from a combination of increased abdominal pressure from blunt trauma and shear injury of the diaphragm. Diaphragmatic ruptures have high clinical impact caused by impaired ventilation of the lung on the affected side, on account of reduced diaphragmatic function. Abdominal visceral herniation into the thoracic cavity through the diaphragmatic defect can result in organ incarceration and ischemia, in addition to a further reduction in diaphragmatic function and lung volume. Early diagnosis with imaging is the key to early detection and management of this type of injury. Right hemidiaphragmatic injury (Fig. 13.5) is less common than left-sided injury (3:1) because of the protective effect of the liver under the right hemidiaphragm. Diaphragmatic injuries sometimes are difficult to diagnose because of the variable appearance of the diaphragm, especially in older patients. Chest radiographs may demonstrate intrathoracic herniation of abdominal viscera through the diaphragmatic defect (Fig. 13.6). On cross-sectional imaging, a "collar sign" has been described in cases in which an abdominal structure such as liver or bowel demonstrates a focal narrowing from diaphragmatic constriction as it passes through the diaphragmatic defect. Prompt recognition of this sign is key to management of these patients because this constriction can result in vascular compromise and ischemia of the abdominal organ. Another classic sign on cross-sectional imaging described with diaphragmatic tears is the "dependent viscera sign," which occurs when the herniated abdominal viscera lies dependently against the chest wall, because the diaphragm no longer supports it.

Computed tomography provides a more precise assessment of diaphragmatic injuries and the involved abdominal viscera than CXR because of its intrinsic high anatomic resolution and additional benefits from coronal and sagittal reformations. Cross-sectional imaging modalities allow detection of small injuries that are missed by radiographs, in addition to visualization of the diaphragmatic defect, abdominal viscera at risk for ischemia, with a "collar sign," and other associated findings such as hemothorax, hemoperitoneum, and liver and splenic lacerations that suggest acute injury. When the presence of diaphragmatic injury is inconclusive by CT, MRI can make this diagnosis. The normal diaphragmatic muscle is smooth, curvilinear, continuous, and T2-hypointense. A diaphragmatic defect disrupts these normal MRI features (Fig. 13.7).

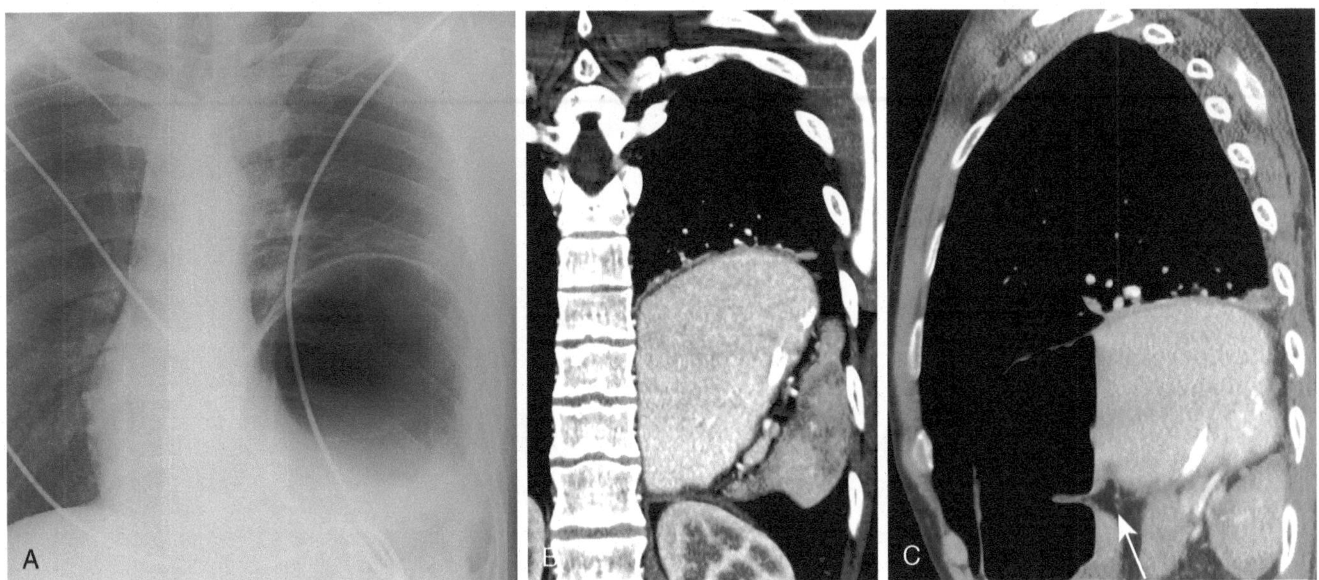

FIGURE 13.6 Left hemidiaphragmatic injury with organoaxial gastric volvulus. **(A)** Frontal chest radiograph demonstrates a nasogastric tube above the left hemidiaphragm within a herniated stomach. **(B)** Coronal computed tomography (CT) image confirms the herniation of the stomach through a posttraumatic left diaphragmatic injury. **(C)** Sagittal CT image demonstrates the greater curvature of the stomach to be cranial to the lesser curvature *(arrow)*, indicating an organoaxial volvulus.

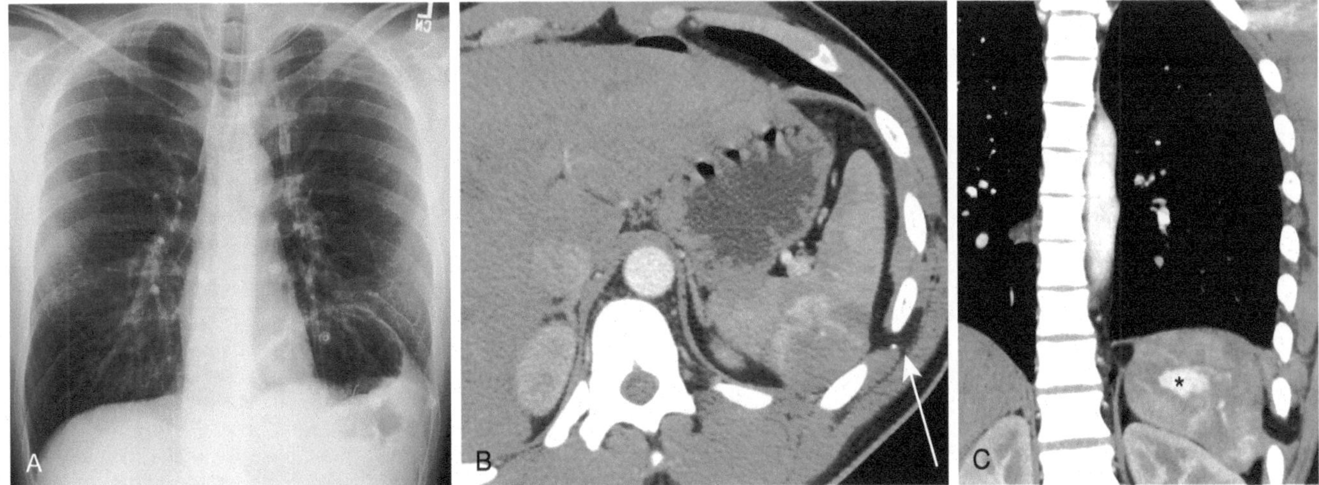

FIGURE 13.7 Left hemidiaphragmatic stabbing injury and splenic laceration. Frontal chest radiograph **(A)** demonstrates an elevated left hemidiaphragm. Axial contrast-enhanced computed tomography (CT) image **(B)** demonstrates a splenic laceration, with evidence of active contrast extravasation and a left hemidiaphragmatic laceration secondary to a stabbing injury, with intercostal herniation of peritoneal fat *(long arrow)*. Coronal CT image **(C)** demonstrates a posttraumatic splenic pseudoaneurysm *(asterisk)* and herniation of peritoneal fat through the diaphragmatic laceration and intercostal space.

MEDIASTINAL INJURIES

Traumatic Aortic and Great Vessel Injuries

Traumatic aortic injuries (TAI) from blunt trauma have a 70% fatality rate at the scene of the accident. The most common sites of thoracic aortic injury are those in which the aorta is relatively fixed and include the aortic root, the aortic isthmus, and the distal descending aorta as it passes through the diaphragmatic hiatus. The majority of patients who survive the initial injury and are transported to the hospital demonstrate an injury at the aortic isthmus, which is the part of the aorta just distal to the left subclavian artery at the level of the ligamentum arteriosum. Rapid deceleration injury results in vascular shear because of differential deceleration of the mobile aortic arch compared with the relatively fixed descending aorta at the location of the ligamentum arteriosum. Injuries involving the aortic root (Fig. 13.8) are associated with critical cardiovascular complications, including coronary arterial injury and hemopericardium, which may result in cardiac tamponade.

Radiographic findings suggesting TAI (Box 13.4) include mediastinal widening at the level of the aortic arch, loss of the aortic arch contour and descending aortic contour,

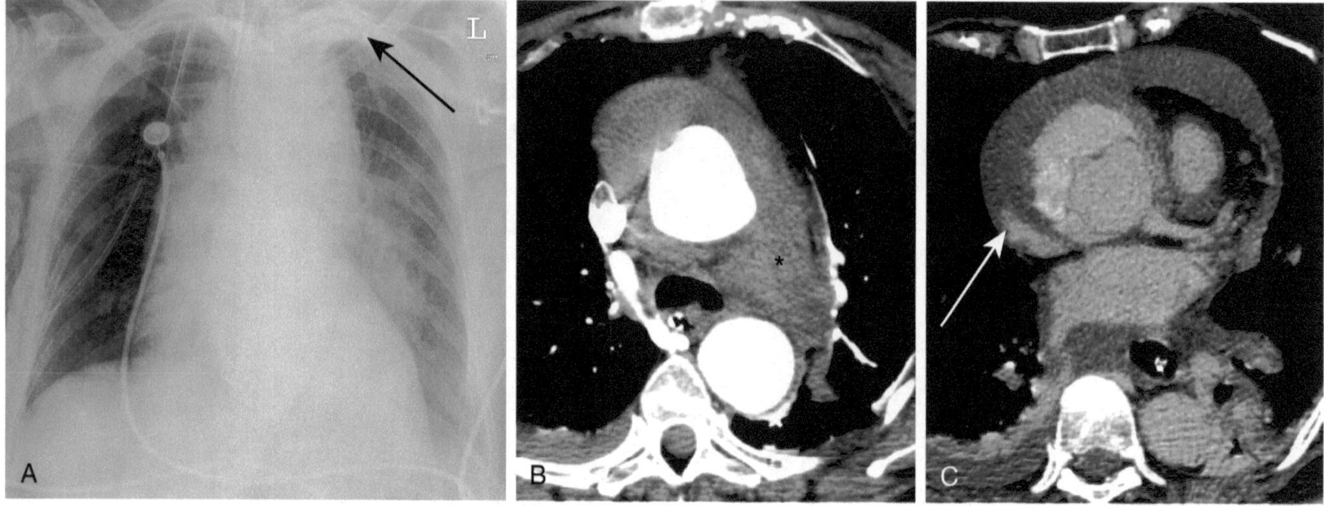

FIGURE 13.8 Aortic root tear and hemopericardium. Portable anteroposterior chest radiograph **(A)** demonstrates mediastinal widening, loss of the aortic contour, left apical cap *(arrow)*, and displacement of the trachea and nasogastric tube to the right. Axial contrast-enhanced computed tomography angiography (CTA) of the chest **(B)** demonstrates hemomediastinum *(asterisk)*. In addition to traumatic dissection of the ascending aorta *(long arrow)*, delayed axial CTA **(C)** images demonstrate active extravasation *(arrow)* of contrast at the aortic root, representing an aortic tear.

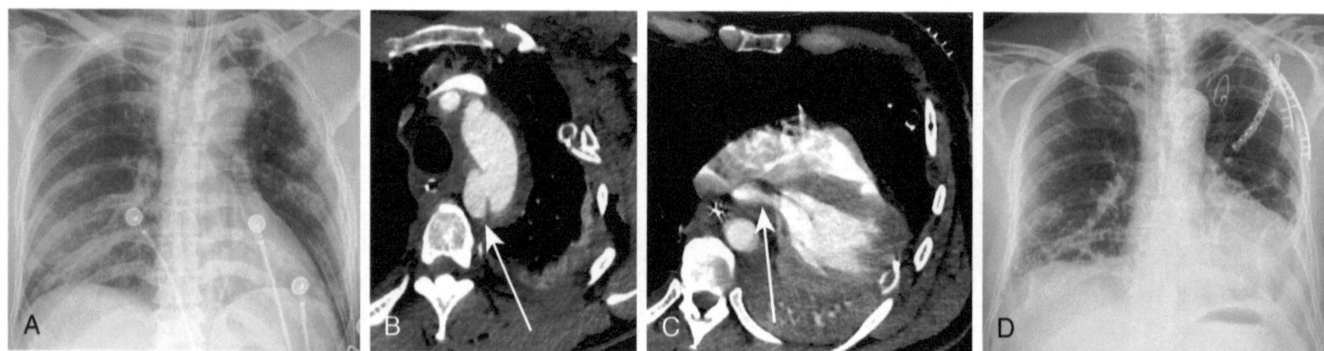

FIGURE 13.9 Traumatic aortic injury with pseudoaneurysm and cardiac herniation. Portable anteroposterior chest radiograph (CXR) **(A)** demonstrates multiple left-sided rib fractures and loss of the normal aortic contour. Axial computed tomography angiography images of the chest **(B)** demonstrate a posttraumatic aortic pseudoaneurysm *(arrow)*, with associated mediastinal hematoma **(C)**, posterior displacement and rotation of the heart, and severe narrowing of the left atrium *(arrow)*, consistent with posterior cardiac herniation. Frontal CXR **(D)** demonstrates postoperative changes from open reduction and internal fixation of multiple rib fractures and aortic graft repair.

BOX 13.4 Radiographic Findings Associated With Traumatic Aortic Injury

- Mediastinal widening
- Loss of aortic contour
- Left apical cap
- Rightward displacement of nasogastric tube

displacement of the nasogastric tube, and a left apical cap (the latter caused by hemorrhage tracking around the apical pleural or extrapleural space).

Computed tomography angiography (CTA) is the most appropriate study for evaluation of TAI, given its rapid, high-resolution depiction of the injury and associated findings, with a sensitivity and specificity of more than 90% for detection of TAI. CT imaging findings of TAI include an intimal flap or aortic dissection, pseudoaneurysm, acute contrast extravasation, abrupt contour irregularity or narrowing of the aorta, mediastinal hematoma, and hemopericardium. One of the most common types of TAIs is a traumatic pseudoaneurysm (Fig. 13.9) caused by disruption of the aorta, resulting in a focal saccular outpouching of the aorta that is contained by adventitia. It is usually associated with mediastinal hemorrhage. TAI is usually treated with endovascular graft repair. Prompt diagnosis of this type of injury is critical to decrease morbidity and mortality in these patients. An important mimic of aortic pseudoaneurysm is an enlarged ductus diverticulum; however, without injury, the adjacent mediastinal fat should be "clean" and without evidence of mediastinal hemorrhage.

Esophageal Injuries

The majority of esophageal injuries result from penetrating trauma. Esophageal injuries resulting from blunt trauma are uncommon because of the protective effect of adjacent mediastinal structures and the chest wall. Blunt trauma most commonly affects the cervical esophagus and the gastroesophageal junction because these areas are less protected than the intrathoracic esophagus. The most common types of esophageal injuries caused by blunt trauma are partial or complete rupture of the esophagus and intramural hematoma. Various proposed mechanisms of blunt esophageal injury include increased intraluminal pressure with a closed glottis, ischemia, and perforation resulting from disruption of the esophageal vascularity and injury against the thoracic spine. The most common radiographic findings are mediastinal widening, pneumomediastinum, and pleural effusion. CT findings may include pneumomediastinum, mediastinitis, extraluminal oral contrast in the mediastinum and pleural space, pleural effusion, esophageal wall thickening, and esophageal wall defect. Further assessment of the specific site of esophageal rupture is usually performed with water-soluble contrast esophagography. Recent literature supports that the use of CT with water-soluble oral contrast, administered while the patient is on the scanner table, can be as effective in determining the site of esophageal perforation in many cases. MRI can demonstrate an intramural hematoma of the esophagus because of its high soft tissue contrast, but it is not typically used in the acute setting (see Chapter 5 for additional information regarding esophageal injury).

Cardiac and Pericardial Injuries

Cardiac and pericardial injuries typically result from penetrating trauma, but they can also occur as a result of high-energy blunt trauma in association with a sternal fracture. Patients with cardiac injuries have an abnormal electrocardiogram and elevated cardiac enzymes resulting from injury to the myocardium. Types of injuries include cardiac contusion, myocardial and valvular rupture, and hemopericardium, with or without cardiac tamponade. The radiographic findings are nonspecific and include an acutely enlarged cardiac silhouette and pulmonary edema from compromised cardiac function. Both CT and echocardiography provide more precise evaluation of cardiac injuries than CXR. Although MRI can illustrate these findings and can also evaluate cardiac function, it is not typically used in the acute clinical setting.

THORACIC SKELETAL INJURIES

Rib Fractures

The presence of chest wall fracture may indicate a serious internal injury. Fractures of the scapula, the sternum, or the first and second ribs are often indicative of high-energy trauma. Unless the trauma is quite forceful, injury to the first and second ribs is resisted by the stronger chest wall architecture in this area, girded by the scapula and clavicle. These fractures are most conspicuous on CXR when they are displaced. When nondisplaced, they may be difficult to detect. An overlying trauma board on the radiograph can obscure some of these structures and pose an additional challenge when evaluating for subtle injury. Further evaluation by CT is helpful and often required to assess for additional injuries.

Upper rib fractures are strongly associated with injuries to the aorta and great vessels. Displaced fractures of the lower ribs are associated with injuries to the diaphragm, liver, and spleen. A flail chest occurs in cases in which three or more contiguous segmental rib fractures (fractures in two or more places) are present (Fig. 13.10). Prompt recognition of a flail chest is important because it results in inadequate ventilation to the affected lung caused by altered chest wall respiratory mechanics. Failure to recognize and treat this entity hinders patient recovery. There is increasing evidence that patients with flail chest pathology will have a shorter recovery when they undergo open reduction and internal plate fixation (ORIF) of rib fractures. Traumatic lung herniation is a rare surgical emergency that occurs in patients with a large traumatic chest wall defect and

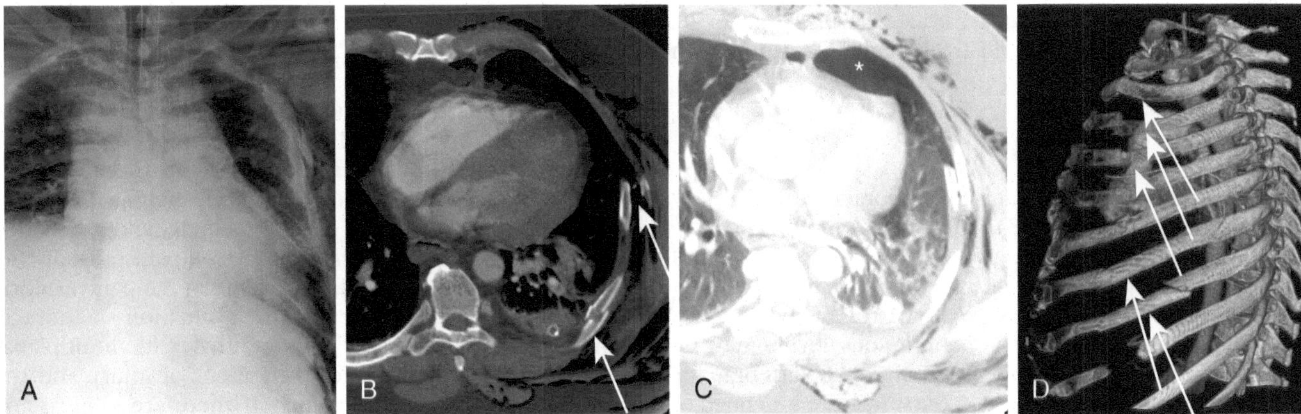

FIGURE 13.10 Flail chest. Portable anteroposterior chest radiograph **(A)** demonstrates multiple left-sided segmental rib fractures, a left pneumothorax with a deep sulcus sign, and subcutaneous emphysema. Axial computed tomography images in bone **(B)** and lung windows **(C)** demonstrate multiple displaced left rib fractures *(arrow)* and a pneumothorax *(asterisk)*. Preoperative planning three-dimensional image of the chest **(D)** demonstrates multiple consecutive segmental rib fractures *(arrows)* compatible with a flail chest.

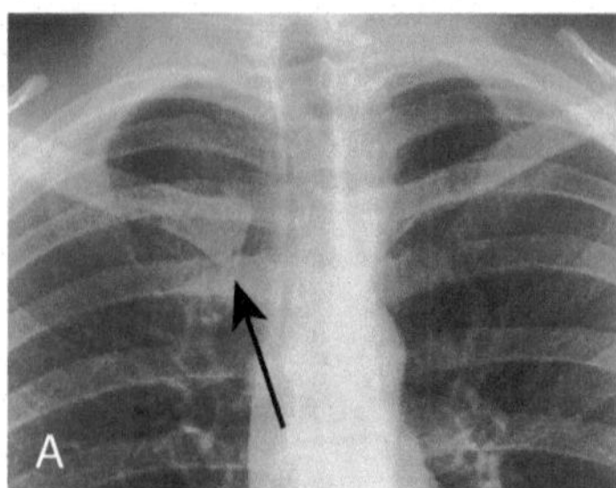

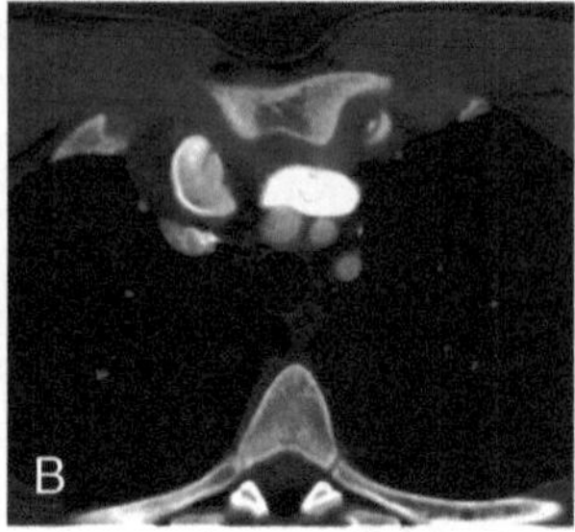

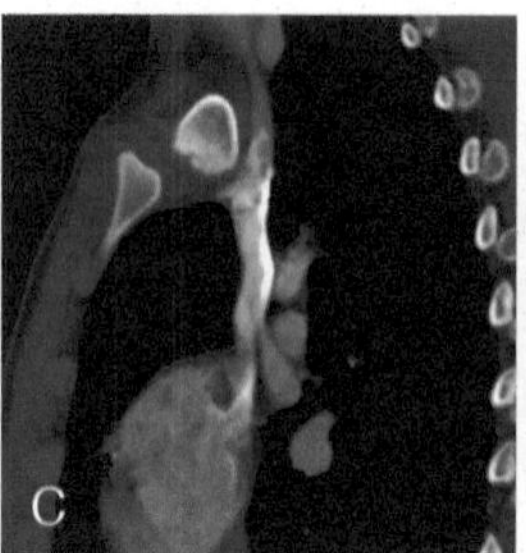

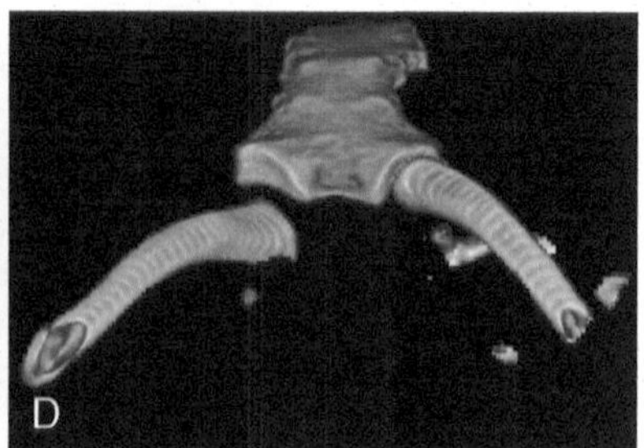

FIGURE 13.11 Posterior dislocation of the right sternoclavicular joint. Coned-down frontal chest radiograph **(A)** demonstrates asymmetric widening of the right sternoclavicular joint, compared with the left, with a small fracture of the right clavicular head *(arrow)*. Axial **(B)** and sagittal **(C)** computed tomography images demonstrate posterior dislocation of the right clavicular head. Three-dimensional **(D)** image used for preoperative planning clearly depicts the misaligned right clavicle with respect to the sternum.

can result in lung incarceration and ischemia. CT is the modality of choice for further assessment of patients with rib fractures, given their association with other internal injuries that can substantially change clinical management.

Sternal and Clavicular Injuries

Clavicle fracture and sternoclavicular dislocation are usually the result of direct blunt impact and can cause life-threatening injury to the adjacent great vessels, the trachea, and the esophagus. Posterior sternoclavicular dislocation (Fig. 13.11) carries higher morbidity and mortality than anterior sternoclavicular dislocation. Although clavicle fractures are readily visualized on radiographs, sternoclavicular dislocations are not, unless they are cranially or caudally displaced. CT is the modality of choice to assess these fractures and associated injuries.

Sternal fractures result from direct high-energy blunt trauma and are associated with cardiac and aortic injury. Unfortunately, chest radiography seldom identifies nondisplaced sternal fractures. Displaced sternal fractures are more identifiable on lateral chest radiographs or on dedicated sternal radiographs. By contrast, CT provides clear visualization of sternal fractures (Fig. 13.12) and associated injuries. Continuous monitoring of patients with sternal fracture by telemetry and serial cardiac enzymes is generally performed because of the relatively high association with cardiac injury.

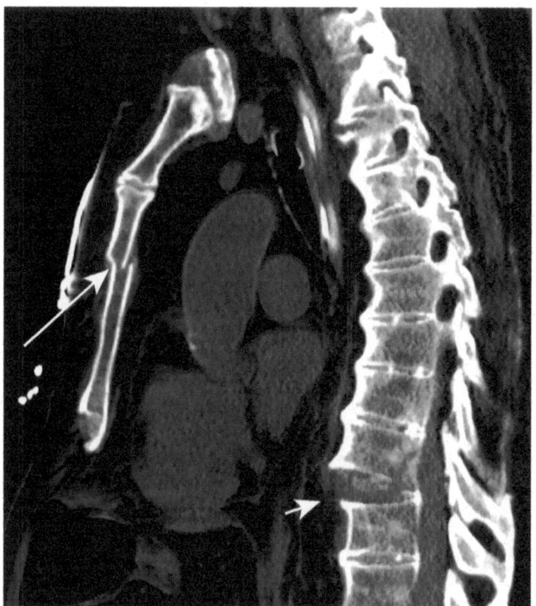

FIGURE 13.12 Sternal fracture and extension fracture of the thoracic spine. Sagittal computed tomography image of the chest demonstrates a sternal fracture *(long arrow)* and associated extension fracture *(short arrow)* of the thoracic spine.

Thoracic Spine Injuries

The most frequent mechanism of thoracic spinal injury is hyperflexion (Fig. 13.13). The most common thoracic vertebral injuries are wedge compression fractures and burst fractures, particularly near the thoracolumbar junction (T9–T12). Multiple fractures are often present and, in cases of axial loading, multiple noncontiguous levels may be affected. Therefore, careful assessment of all vertebrae for additional fractures is required. A burst fracture is defined as a compression fracture of the vertebral body, with associated disruption of the anterior and middle columns. Burst fractures are strongly associated with spinal cord injury because the posteriorly displaced fracture fragments may directly traumatize the spinal cord (Fig. 13.14). A high percentage of patients with thoracic spine fracture-dislocation (Fig. 13.15) have neurologic deficits related to partial or complete cord transection or spinal cord hematoma.

Radiographic findings in patients with thoracic spine injuries include loss of vertebral body height, increased interpedicular distance, a missing pedicle, and a widened paravertebral stripe or laterally displaced paraspinal line(s), with the latter caused by hemorrhage in the paravertebral space. CT provides more precise evaluation of thoracic spine injuries than chest radiography, with multiplanar reconstructions that depict the extent of injury and the potential for spinal cord injury. If there are clinical and imaging findings that suggest injury to the spinal cord, MRI is the modality of choice for more definitive and comprehensive assessment of spinal cord integrity and ligamentous and osseous injuries on account of its higher soft tissue contrast.

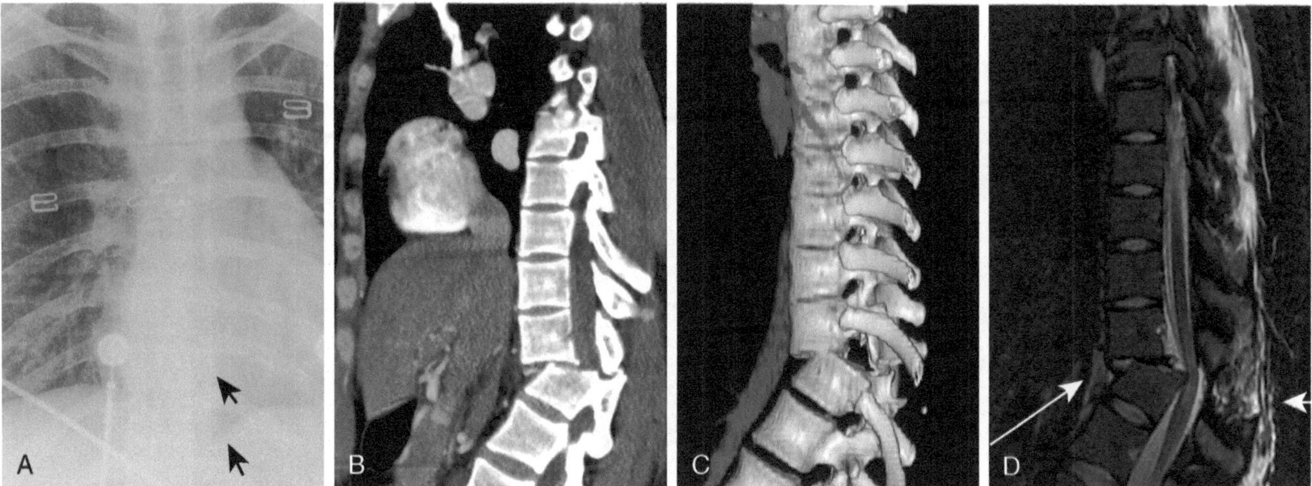

FIGURE 13.13 Fracture dislocation of the thoracic spine with acute cord compression. Portable anteroposterior chest radiograph **(A)** demonstrates thickening of the left paraspinal stripe *(arrows)*. Sagittal computed tomography **(B)** and three-dimensional reformatted images **(C)** demonstrate a three-column fracture-dislocation of the thoracic spine secondary to a hyperflexion injury. There is severe stenosis of the spinal canal. Sagittal fat-saturated T2-weighted magnetic resonance image **(D)** demonstrates severe spinal canal stenosis and a posteriorly displaced vertebral body impinging on the spinal cord. Please note prevertebral hematoma *(long arrow)* and hemorrhage in the posterior soft tissues *(short arrow)*, consistent with ligamentous injury.

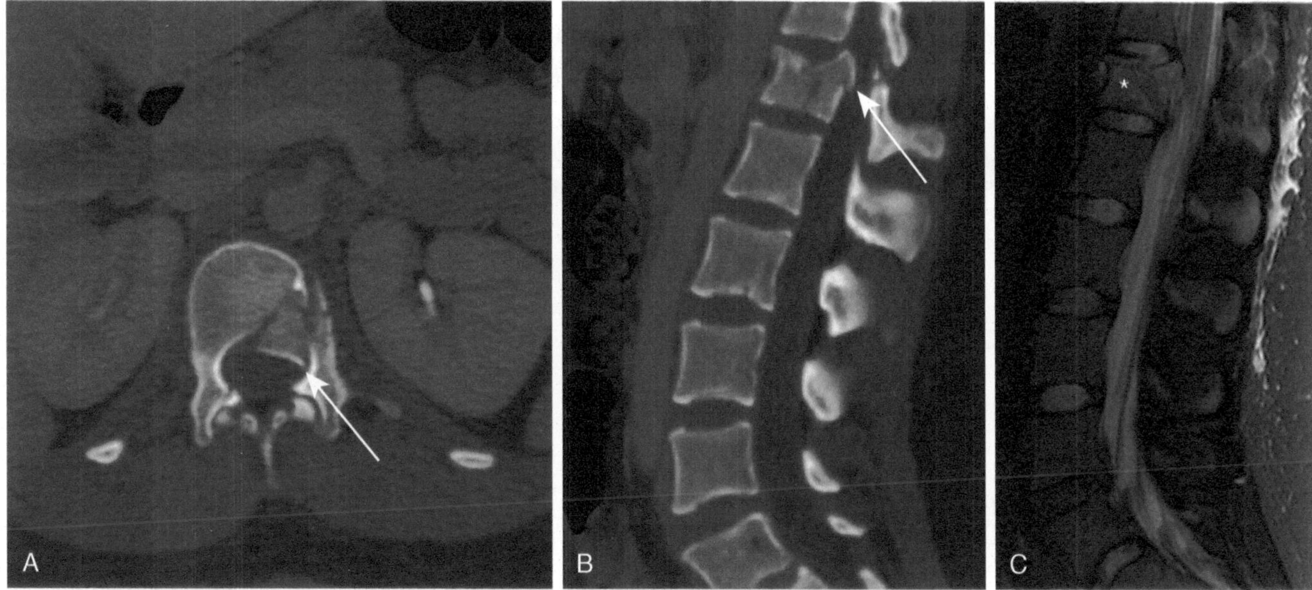

FIGURE 13.14 T12 burst fracture. Axial **(A)** and sagittal **(B)** computed tomography images demonstrate a burst fracture of the T12 vertebral body, with posterior displacement of a fracture fragment into the spinal canal *(arrows)*. Sagittal fat-saturated T2-weighted magnetic resonance image **(C)** demonstrates bone marrow edema and hemorrhage within the T12 vertebral body secondary to acute burst fracture *(asterisk)*, with retropulsion and resultant moderate stenosis of the spinal canal at this level.

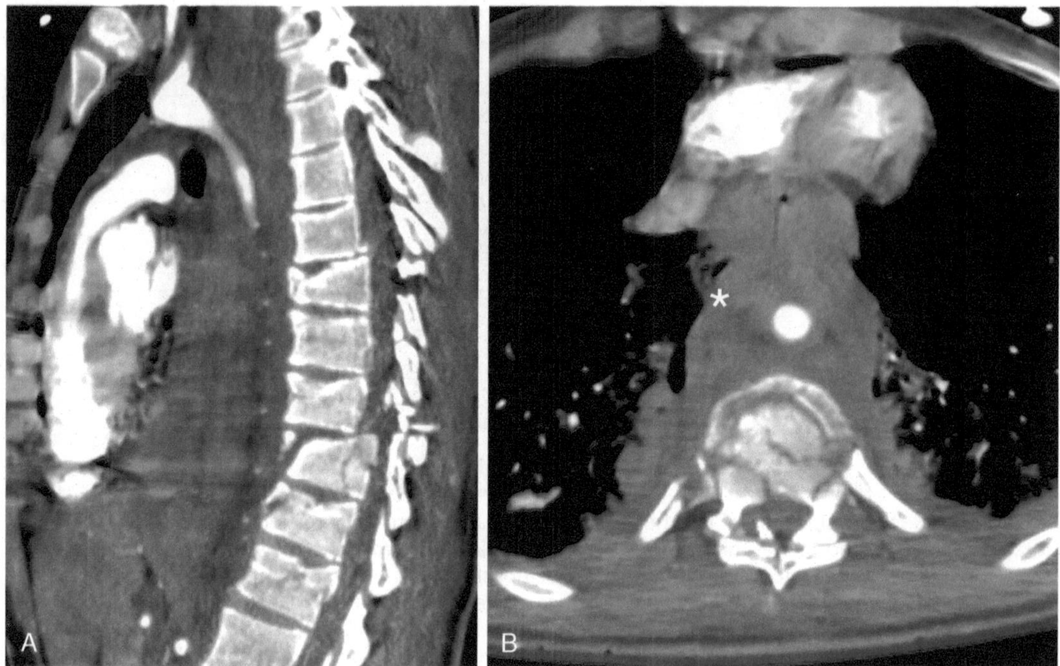

FIGURE 13.15 Extensive thoracic spine fracture-dislocation: Sagittal **(A)** and axial **(B)** computed tomography images of the chest demonstrate extensive, multilevel fracture-dislocation of the thoracic spine, resulting in severe spinal stenosis and spinal cord injury. Bilateral paravertebral hematoma, extending into the visceral mediastinum *(asterisk)*, displaces the mediastinal structures anteriorly, including the aorta, esophagus, and heart.

SUGGESTED READINGS

Aran S, Shaqdan KW, Abujudeh HH. Dual-energy computed tomography (DECT) in emergency radiology: basic principles, techniques, and limitations. *Emerg Radiol*. 2014;21:391-405.

Battle CE, Hutchings H, Evans PA. Risk factors that predict mortality in patients with blunt chest wall trauma: a systematic review and meta-analysis. *Injury*. 2012;43:8-17.

Chung JS, Cox CW, Mohammed TLH, et al. ACR appropriateness criteria. Blunt chest trauma. *J Am Coll Radiol*. 2014;11:345-351.

Demehri S, Rybicki F, Desjardins B, et al. ACR Appropriateness Criteria: blunt chest trauma-suspected aortic injury. *Emerg Radiol*. 2012;19:287-292.

Dreizin D, Munera F. Multidetector CT for penetrating torso trauma: state of the art. *Radiology*. 2015;227:338-355.

Iochum S, Ludig T, Walter F, et al. Imaging of diaphragmatic injury: a diagnostic challenge? *Radiographics*. 2002;22:103-118.

Ketai L, Brandt MM, Schermer C. Nonaortic mediastinal injuries from blunt chest trauma. *J Thorac Imaging*. 2000;15:120-127.

Zinck SE, Primack SL. Radiographic and CT findings in blunt chest trauma. *J Thorac Imaging*. 2000;15:87-96.

Chapter 14

Community-Acquired Pneumonia

John W. Nance

INTRODUCTION

Pneumonia is an important cause of morbidity and mortality, with tremendous variability in its clinical and imaging manifestations, treatment, and outcomes. Many individuals with mild pneumonias never come to medical attention, but other patients ultimately succumb to infections that cause extensive local and systemic damage. Likewise, pneumonia on imaging studies may manifest with minimal findings or demonstrate extensive tissue necrosis. This heterogeneity poses a challenge for both referring clinicians and radiologists.

Nearly any parenchymal opacity can represent pneumonia, and a wide variety of noninfectious diseases can simulate infection. Frustrations are compounded by the relative lack of specific imaging features to suggest a particular organism when infection is diagnosed. Even though empiric treatment paradigms have become more common, optimal therapy remains pathogen driven, and diagnosticians naturally wish to provide the most specific information possible.

Despite these challenges, imaging is extremely important throughout the care cycle of pneumonia. Chest radiographs remain an important tool in making the initial diagnosis, scoring disease severity, assessing resolution, and identifying complications; furthermore, certain radiographic patterns can suggest broad categories of organisms.

Chest computed tomography (CT) has excellent sensitivity to detect infection and its complications and search for causes of slow resolution and may have greater utility in narrowing the list of potential causative organisms. After the diagnosis is established, both chest radiography and CT play important roles in following the response to treatment and monitoring for the development of complications.

MECHANISMS AND PATTERNS OF INFECTION

Overall, most community-acquired pneumonias result from inhalation of infected droplets, particularly those between 0.5 and 5 μm. Smaller droplets tend to be exhaled and larger droplets deposited in the upper airways. The second most common route of infection is aspiration of nasopharyngeal organisms. More rare causes include hematogenous spread from extrathoracic sources of infection (most commonly tricuspid endocarditis), direct extension from a localized site of infection (e.g., mediastinal or transdiaphragmatic spread), and inoculation from a penetrating wound. The development of pneumonia and the resulting imaging features depend on the interplay between the size of the inoculum, virulence of the organism, and host response.

Inhalational Pneumonia

Ideally, pneumonia is classified according to the responsible pathogen; however, the causative organism is not detected in approximately half of the patients hospitalized for community-acquired pneumonia in the United States. Therefore, clinical and pathogenetic classification schemes are commonly used to guide management. There are three forms of inhalational pneumonia with distinct pathologic and radiographic features: lobar pneumonia, bronchopneumonia, and interstitial pneumonia. Although there is some overlap in their imaging appearance, particularly depending on the chronicity of infection and host response, categorization into one of these three forms can suggest a range of likely organisms and potentially guide management decisions.

Lobar Pneumonia

The most common pattern seen in community-acquired pneumonia, lobar pneumonia, develops when organisms reach the distal airspaces, usually in the subpleural lung. Although the term *lobar* is traditionally and commonly used, sublobar distributions are more commonly seen, and airspace consolidation of any size can manifest as a radiographic "lobar pneumonia" pattern. The organisms involved in lobar pneumonia characteristically cause a rapid, profuse edematous exudate that extends directly into adjacent acini via terminal airways and communicating channels (the pores of Kohn). Fluid and organisms expand in a confluent rather than nodular pattern, leading to the typical consolidative appearance at radiography (Fig. 14.1). Air bronchograms are often preserved and, when present, argue against a central obstructing lesion as a contributing factor to the pneumonia. Volume loss is usually minimal, and there may even be expansion of the affected lobe caused by extensive edema, resulting in the *bulging fissure sign* (Fig. 14.2). Expansion is classically described in *Klebsiella* infection but is possible with any organism causing lobar pneumonia. Lobar pneumonia is most commonly unifocal but may be multifocal; the latter situation portends a worse prognosis. Another radiographically distinct form of lobar pneumonia is spherical or "round" pneumonia, which is more commonly seen in childhood and results in a rounded consolidation with or without air bronchograms (Fig. 14.3). There is little clinical significance in making the distinction of round pneumonia; it is thought to simply represent a specific pattern of spread caused by poorly developed collateral air circulation, especially in younger patients.

Particular care must be taken when interpreting cases in patients with emphysema or other structural lung disease. Infectious involvement within the abnormal lung parenchyma is variable, which can lead to bizarre patterns that can simulate necrosis, chronic cavitary disease (e.g., tuberculosis), or cancer. Differentiation of infectious consolidation and lung cancer can be difficult even in patients with normal lung parenchyma, highlighting the importance of follow-up imaging. Whereas persistent or slowly enlarging consolidations or masses should raise suspicion for cancer (Fig. 14.4), rapid changes are much more characteristic for infections (see Fig. 14.3).

Streptococcus pneumoniae is the most common cause of lobar pneumonia, but other typical bacteria (most commonly *Klebsiella pneumoniae* and *Legionella pneumophila*), atypical bacteria (*Mycoplasma pneumoniae*), and fungi can result in lobar consolidation. Radiography is not able to further distinguish among these organisms; therefore, clinical, demographic, and epidemiologic factors must be used in conjunction with the radiographic pattern to rank the likelihood of various pathogens.

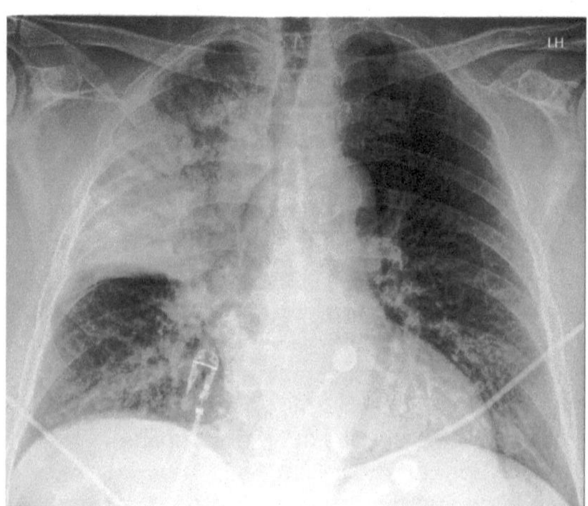

FIGURE 14.1 Lobar pneumonia pattern. Anteroposterior chest radiograph demonstrates airspace consolidation throughout the right upper lobe with central air bronchograms, compatible with lobar pneumonia.

Bronchopneumonia

The bronchopneumonia pattern is seen when organisms initially infect the bronchial and bronchiolar mucosa. In contrast to lobar pneumonia, there is a rapid suppurative response with relatively little fluid production. The process spreads through the airways into the peribronchiolar alveoli, which become filled with edema and pus, resulting in the early radiographic appearance of multiple, ill-defined centrilobular nodular opacities, usually ranging from 5 to 10 mm. Nodules may be ground glass, consolidative, or both depending on the degree of alveolar filling. The intense initial host response can serve to limit initial spread, resulting in a patchy pattern. Continued infection results in spread through airways into adjacent pulmonary lobules, and eventually there may be a confluent consolidation indistinguishable from lobar pneumonia. The pattern may be recognized on both radiography and CT; the latter can better distinguish the nodular opacities and may be able to suggest confluent bronchopneumonia rather than lobar pneumonia when centrilobular nodules are seen surrounding regions of consolidation (Fig. 14.5). Because of the association with the small airways, there tends to be a component of

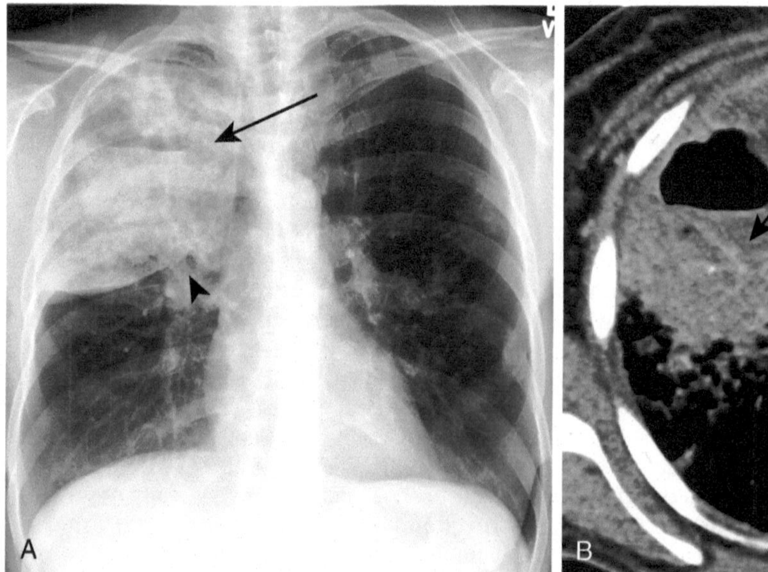

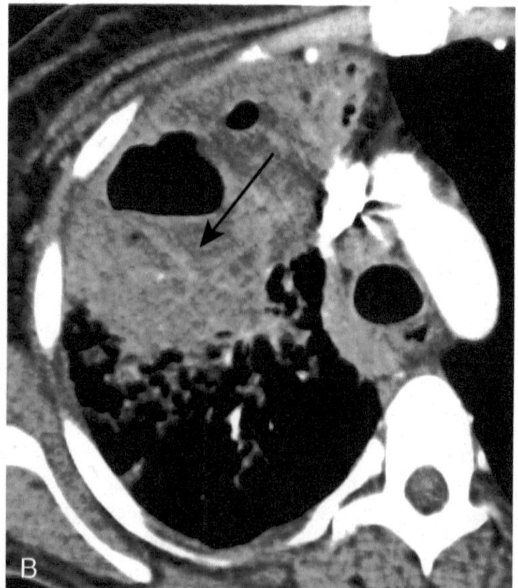

FIGURE 14.2 Lobar pneumonia with abscess and bulging fissure. **A,** Posteroanterior chest radiograph demonstrates consolidation throughout the right upper lobe with an air–fluid level *(arrow)* and mild convexity of the right minor fissure (*bulging fissure sign; arrowhead*). **B,** Axial computed tomography demonstrates the consolidation, central abscess, and the *CT angiogram sign (arrow)*, which can be seen in any process causing parenchymal consolidation, including lung cancer, pulmonary lymphoma, and pneumonia. Methicillin-resistant *Staphylococcus aureus* was isolated.

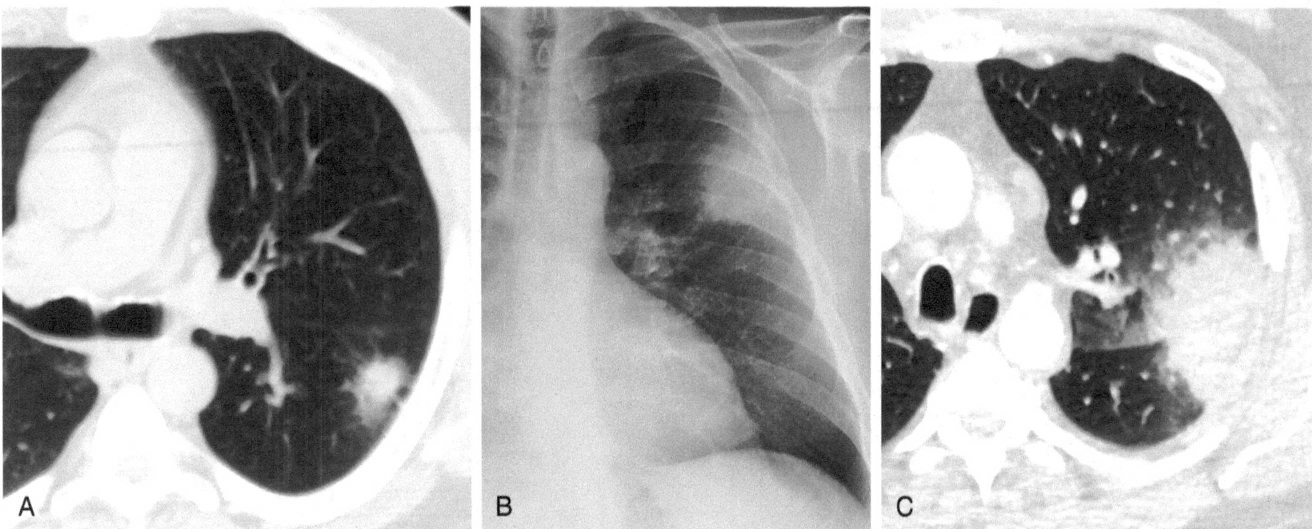

FIGURE 14.3 Rapidly growing "round" pneumonia. **A,** Axial computed tomography (CT) image demonstrates a nodule in the superior segment of the left lower lobe. Note the surrounding ground-glass halo, which can be seen in a variety of infections in addition to classic angioinvasive aspergillosis. **B,** Posteroanterior chest radiograph obtained 2 weeks later shows interval enlargement of the nodule, which is now masslike. **C,** Axial CT image further demonstrates the masslike consolidation, which is now crossing the left major fissure. *Streptococcus anginosis* and *Enterobacter aerogenes* were isolated, implicating aspiration as the mechanism of infection.

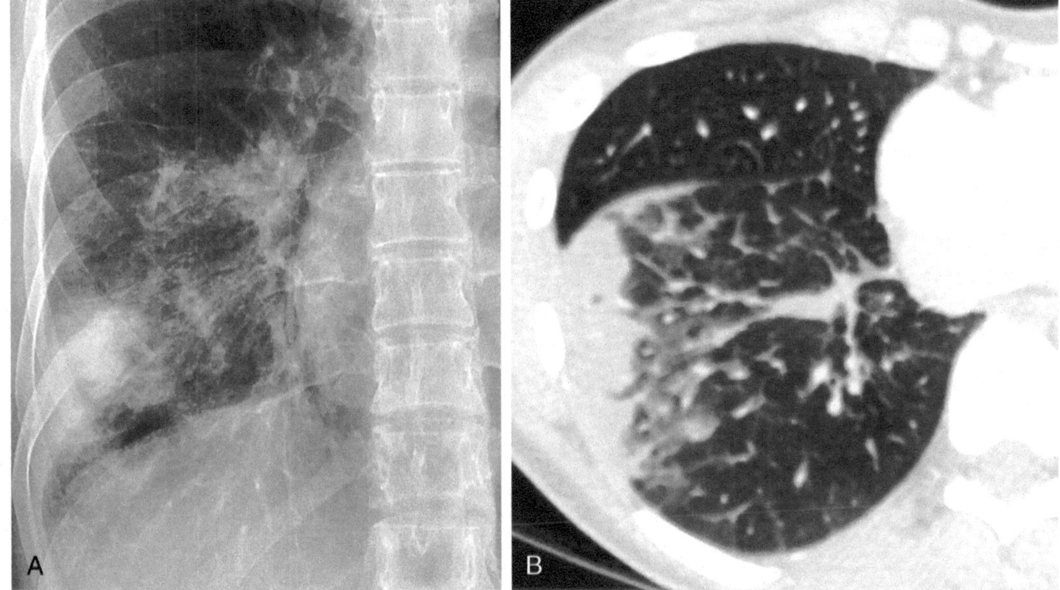

FIGURE 14.4 Adenocarcinoma mimicking pneumonia. **A,** Coned posteroanterior chest radiograph demonstrates an airspace consolidation in the right lower lung, initially thought to represent pneumonia in a patient presenting with cough. **B,** Axial image from later computed tomography, acquired because of delayed resolution of the suspected pneumonia, demonstrates the consolidation with surrounding ground-glass and interlobular septal thickening. Subsequent biopsy revealed adenocarcinoma.

volume loss. In addition, multifocal and bilateral disease is more commonly seen in bronchopneumonia compared with lobar pneumonia.

Typical bacterial organisms are the most common cause of nonmycobacterial community-acquired bronchopneumonia, including *Staphylococcus aureus*, gram-negative organisms, anaerobic bacteria, and *L. pneumophila*. Note that these tend to be more virulent organisms; accordingly, there is a tendency for greater tissue destruction, which can lead to cavitation or necrosis, abscess formation, and residual scarring.

Interstitial Pneumonia

Mononuclear cell infiltration around the bronchial and bronchiolar walls with extension into the interstitium of alveolar walls typifies interstitial pneumonias, most commonly caused by viral organisms and *Mycoplasma pneumoniae*. There are two predominant histopathologic

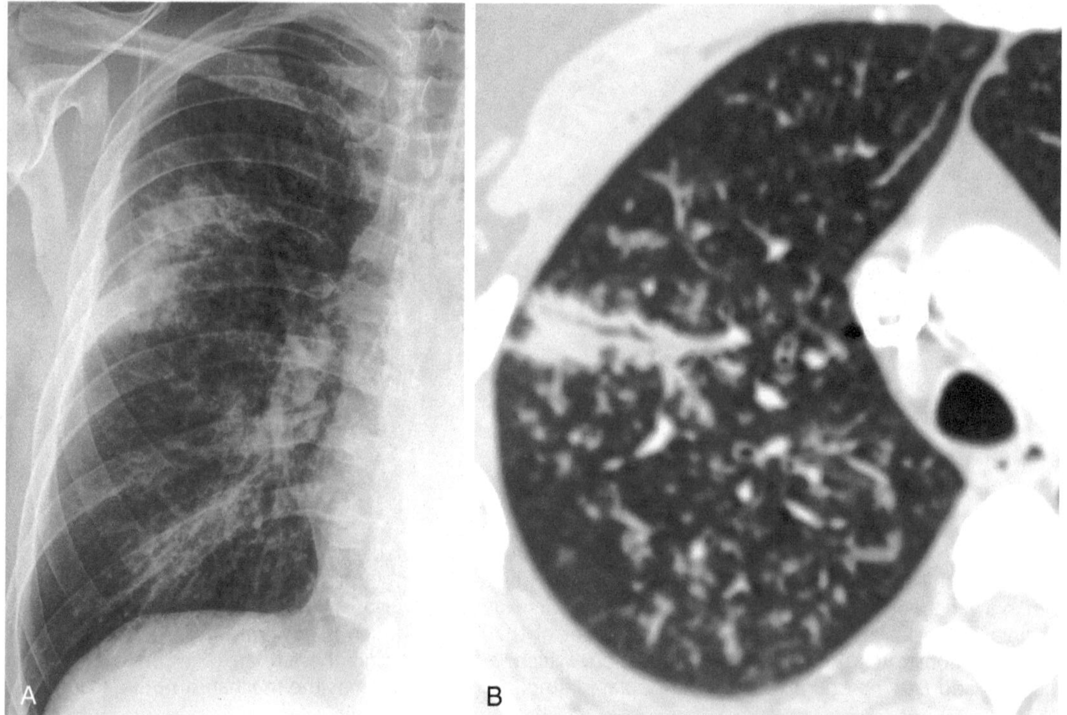

FIGURE 14.5 Bronchopneumonia pattern. **A,** Posteroanterior chest radiograph demonstrates an airspace consolidation in the right upper lobe with surrounding nodular opacities throughout the right lung. **B,** Computed tomography shows a right upper lobe consolidation containing an air bronchogram and surrounding tree-in-bud and centrilobular nodules, compatible with bronchopneumonia. The mixed consolidative and nodular morphology demonstrated in this case is commonly seen in bronchopneumonia.

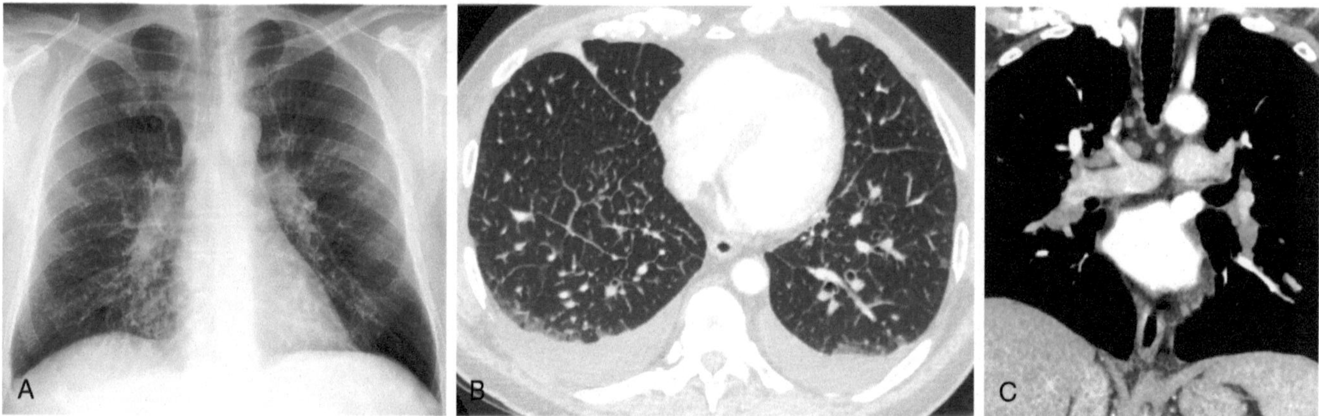

FIGURE 14.6 Interstitial pattern, pleural effusions, and lymphadenopathy. **A,** Posteroanterior chest radiograph demonstrates an interstitial pattern, with diffuse reticular opacities, and prominent hila suggestive of mild lymphadenopathy. **B,** Axial image from subsequent chest computed tomography (CT) more clearly reveals interlobular septal thickening and small bilateral pleural effusions. **C,** Coronal CT reconstruction demonstrates mildly enlarged mediastinal and hilar lymph nodes. The patient was subsequently diagnosed with babesiosis, a relatively rare malaria-like disease caused by the *Babesia* blood parasite.

manifestations with corresponding radiographic features; however, it is important to note that these two forms represent the ends of a spectrum, and most cases show features of both. The more chronic insidious form is characterized by a pure interstitial mononuclear cell infiltrate. Accordingly, radiographs may show bronchial or bronchiolar thickening (or both), manifesting as tram tracks and ring shadows, or ill-defined reticular or reticulonodular opacities. Likewise, CT can show bronchial or bronchiolar wall thickening (or both), interlobular septal thickening (Fig. 14.6), or ground-glass opacities caused by intralobular septal thickening. The distribution can be patchy (Fig. 14.7) or diffuse. Because there is airway involvement, patchy segmental or subsegmental atelectasis is often present.

The more acute form of interstitial pneumonia can result in the histopathologic pattern of diffuse alveolar damage

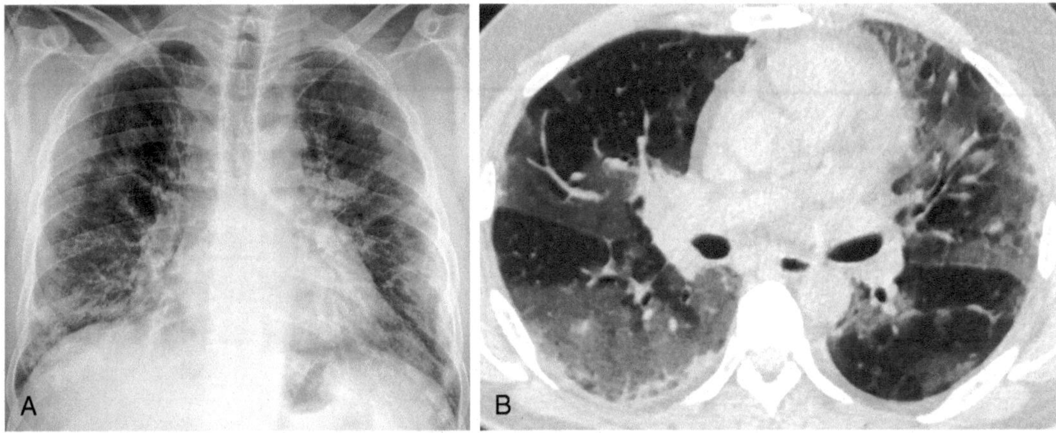

FIGURE 14.7 Influenza. **A,** Posteroanterior chest radiograph demonstrates diffuse hazy and patchy opacities. **B,** Contemporaneously acquired computed tomography demonstrates patchy, ground-glass opacities. The patient tested positive for influenza A virus, H1N1 subtype.

(see Chapter 10). In addition to interstitial thickening, proteinaceous exudate extends into the alveolar spaces, forming characteristic hyaline membranes. Radiographically, this manifests as a more consolidative process that mimics bronchopneumonia, although the extent is usually more diffuse.

Aspiration Pneumonia

Aspiration is a common process with varying clinical manifestations and levels of severity. For example, it is estimated that approximately half of all healthy adults silently aspirate without clinical consequence. Risk factors for aspiration play a large role in the pathogenesis and include altered levels of consciousness, alcoholism, drug addiction, esophageal disease, periodontal and gingival disease, seizure disorders, and nasogastric tubes.

The chronicity, volume, and contents of aspiration dictate the clinical syndrome. Isolated bland aspiration is clinically silent in most cases. Chronic aspiration or aspiration of irritants, most commonly gastric acid, can result in a sterile bronchiolitis or pneumonitis. Imaging manifestations can include bronchial or bronchiolar wall thickening, tree-in-bud nodules, and ground-glass or consolidative centrilobular nodules. Distribution is largely dependent on patient positioning at the time of aspiration: The basilar and posterior lung segments are most commonly involved in upright, semiupright, or supine patients, but the "axillary" (i.e., lateral) subsegments of the right upper lobe anterior and posterior segments are most commonly affected in patients who aspirate while in the right lateral decubitus position, often while sleeping. Noninfectious aspiration is usually characterized by fairly rapid clearance in less than a week. Mendelson syndrome is a specific form of aspiration that results from large-volume aspiration of gastric acid, causing chemical pneumonitis and acute lung injury, including acute respiratory distress syndrome (ARDS). The radiographic manifestations simulate pulmonary edema, usually in a diffuse distribution. Lipoid pneumonia is another distinct form of noninfectious aspiration and is usually caused by chronic ingestion of exogenous lipoid material, such as mineral oil for chronic constipation. On radiographs, lipoid pneumonia appears as a chronic consolidation or mass, which can simulate lung cancer. The consolidations demonstrate low attenuation on CT, attesting to the lipoid contents (Fig. 14.8).

Aspiration pneumonia usually results from aspiration of oropharyngeal organisms. In healthy adults, the majority of the oropharyngeal colonizers are of low virulence, but some can cause pulmonary infection. Chronically ill or hospitalized patients tend to have more virulent colonizers. Infections are most commonly caused by mixed gram-negative aerobic (*S. pneumoniae, S. aureus, Haemophilus influenzae,* and *L. pneumophila*) and anaerobic (*Bacteroides, Prevotella, Fusobacterium,* and *Peptostreptococcus* spp.) bacteria. Necrosis and abscess formation are common (Fig. 14.9).

Chronic aspiration, both infectious and sterile, can result in nonspecific fibrotic changes in affected areas, often at the lung bases, sometimes simulating interstitial lung disease in a patchy posterior- or basilar-predominant distribution.

Hematogenous and Direct Spread of Infection

Pneumonia of hematogenous origin is much less common than inhalational and aspiration pneumonia, particularly in immunocompetent individuals. The most common scenario is seeding of septic emboli, usually from tricuspid endocarditis and less commonly from systemic thrombophlebitis or venous line infection. Intravenous drug users and patients with long-standing indwelling catheters are most commonly affected. Both CT and radiography demonstrate irregular pulmonary nodules that are usually multiple and peripheral in distribution; they are often wedge shaped and abut the pleura (Fig. 14.10). There tends to be a basilar predominance in accordance with the apicobasilar gradient of pulmonary blood flow. The size of the nodules is variable, and cavitation is common but not uniform, particularly early in the disease process. CT sometimes demonstrates a vessel apparently abutting the nodule (*feeding vessel sign*).

Less commonly, septic bacterial infection can result in massive seeding of the lungs with a miliary (i.e., very small nodular) pattern; however, this is more commonly seen in hematogenous dissemination of granulomatous infections and in immunocompromised individuals (see Chapter 15).

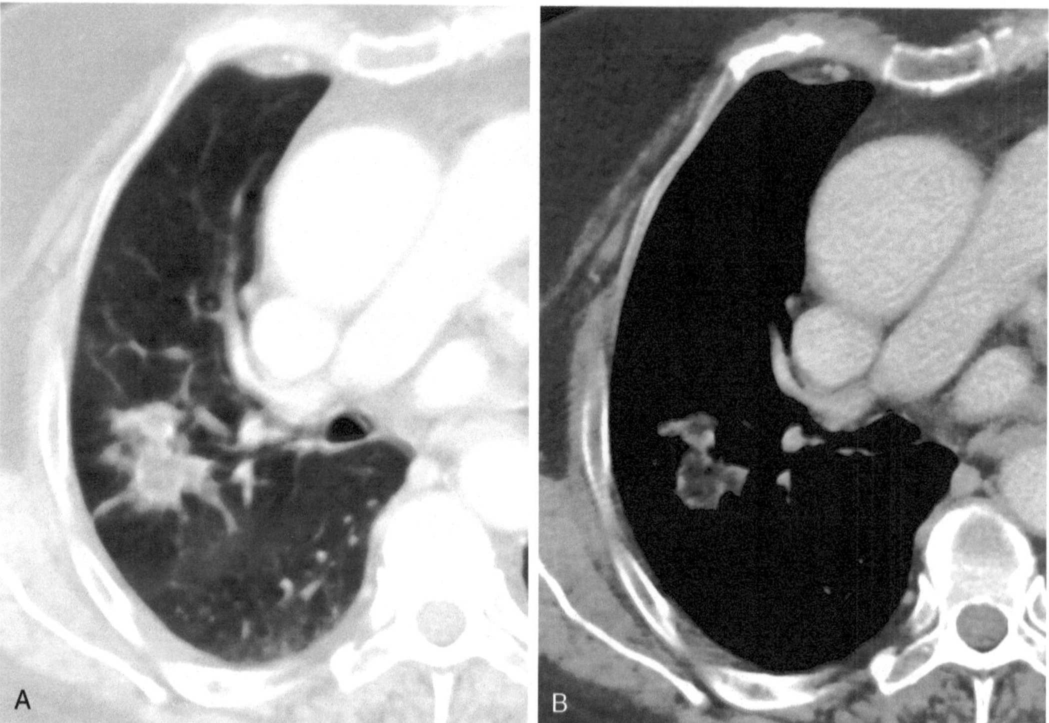

FIGURE 14.8 Lipoid pneumonia. **A,** Axial computed tomography image displayed with lung window and level shows a bilobed irregular nodule that was persistent on previously acquired serial radiographs. **B,** The same image displayed with soft tissue window and level demonstrates low attenuation within the nodule, similar to body wall fat. The patient reported a history of chronic mineral oil consumption.

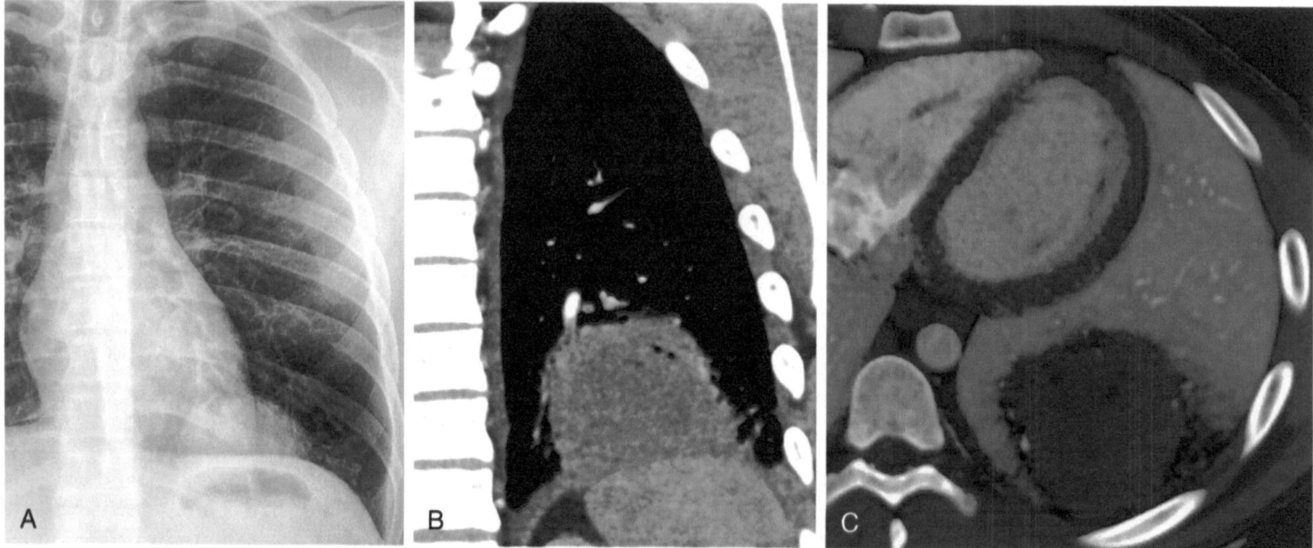

FIGURE 14.9 Aspiration pneumonia with abscess. **A,** Posteroanterior chest radiograph demonstrates a left lower lobe mass. **B,** Coronal computed tomography reconstruction demonstrates low attenuation within the mass. **C,** Lung perfusion blood volume reconstruction shows a perfusion defect associated with the mass. Subsequent percutaneous drainage demonstrated *Fusobacterium* spp., an anaerobic, gram-negative bacteria that is a pathologic colonizer of the oropharynx.

Direct spread of infection can result from penetrating wounds or subdiaphragmatic, chest wall, or mediastinal sources, such as liver abscess or esophageal rupture. There is often pleural involvement and localized consolidation adjacent to the source of the infection, and abscess formation is common.

Patterns of Host Response to Infection

The time to radiographic resolution, histopathologic response, and imaging sequelae depend on the pathogenetic type of infection, the extent of damage, and the host's immunologic response.

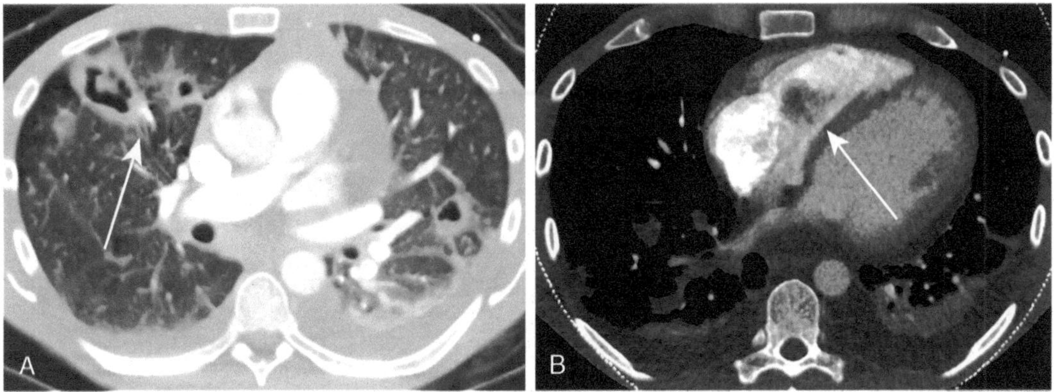

FIGURE 14.10 Septic emboli. **A,** Axial computed tomography (CT) image demonstrates multifocal cavitary nodules and masses, including one with a prominent *feeding vessel sign (arrow)*. **B,** A large tricuspid vegetation *(arrow)* can be seen on the non–electrocardiogram-gated chest CT image. The patient had a history of intravenous drug abuse.

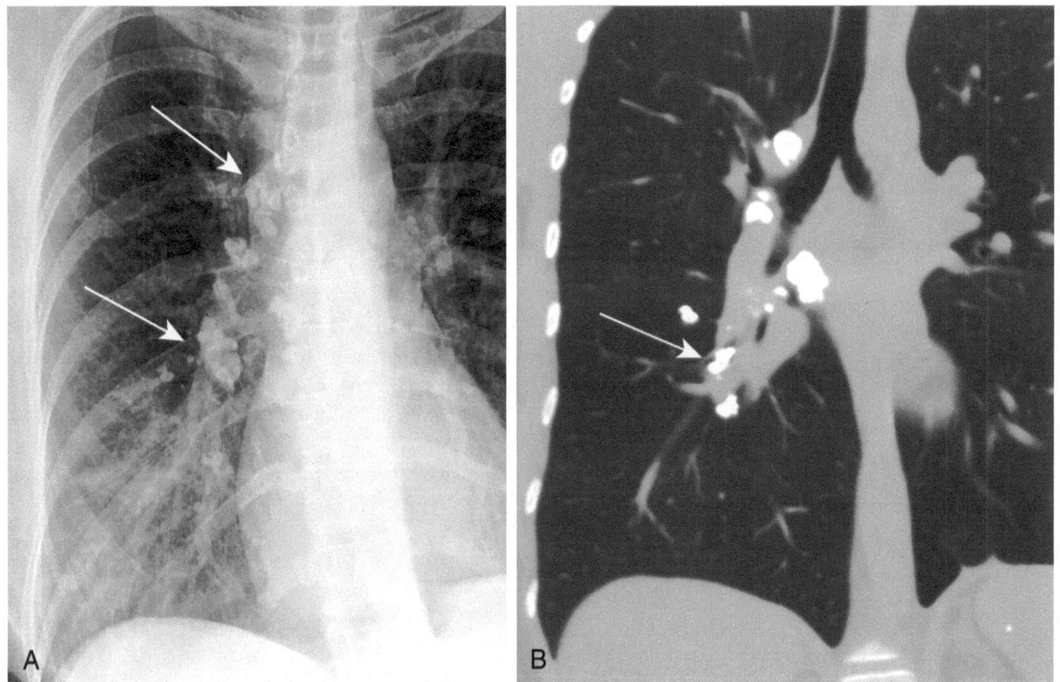

FIGURE 14.11 Recurrent pneumonia caused by a broncholith. **A,** Posteroanterior chest radiograph demonstrates a right lower lung consolidation and several calcified right hilar and mediastinal lymph nodes *(arrows)*. **B,** Coronal computed tomography reconstruction demonstrates the calcified mediastinal and hilar nodes, including an intrabronchial node extending into the right lower lobe bronchus *(arrow)*.

Although radiographic clearance notoriously lags behind clinical improvement, adequately treated healthy adults with uncomplicated lobar pneumonia should demonstrate near-complete imaging resolution in 6 to 8 weeks. Adequately treated older or chronically ill individuals may take 2 months or longer to demonstrate full radiographic resolution. In either case, the consolidation progressively decreases in size and attenuation and typically leaves no residual scarring, a frequent exception being patients with underlying parenchymal damage by emphysema. Cases that do not show clearance within 2 months should undergo further evaluation to exclude treatment failure, inaccurate initial diagnosis, or an underlying structural abnormality such as obstructing broncholith or neoplasm (Fig. 14.11 and Box 14.1).

Bronchopneumonia or interstitial pneumonia usually takes longer to clear, particularly if there is significant alveolar epithelial injury. In cases severe enough to cause damage to the alveolar basement membrane, organizing fibroblastic tissue (i.e., organizing pneumonia) is the usual histopathologic response. Often, consolidation begins to coalesce and coarsen around bronchovascular structures (Fig. 14.12). This process can become self-perpetuating in some patients, leading to a pathologic form of organizing pneumonia and necessitating a course of steroids. Varying degrees of fibrosis may occur in affected areas, manifesting as architectural distortion, volume loss, and bronchiectasis.

COMPLICATIONS

Cavitation and Abscess

Lung parenchymal necrosis with cavitation can occur in pneumonia, particularly that produced by virulent bacteria, including *S. aureus* (see Fig. 14.2), *S. pneumoniae,* gram-negative bacilli, and anaerobic bacteria. If the inflammatory process is localized, a lung abscess will form. It is usually rounded and focal, simulating a mass. With liquefaction of the central inflammatory process, a communication may develop with the bronchus; air enters the abscess, forming a cavity, which often contains an air-fluid level. The walls of the cavity may be smooth, but more often they are thick and irregular. Lung abscesses are treated medically with extended antibiotics and rarely with percutaneous drainage or surgery. They usually do not require more invasive intervention because drainage occurs spontaneously through the tracheobronchial tree.

Multiple small cavities or microabscesses may develop in necrotizing pneumonia, which on both CT and radiography appear as multiple lucent foci within a consolidation. This should not be confused with pneumonia superimposed on emphysema, which can have a similar appearance. If necrosis is extensive, arteritis and vascular thrombosis may occur in an area of intense inflammation, causing ischemic necrosis and death of a portion of lung. This particular complication, sometimes called "pulmonary gangrene," is most typical of *K. pneumoniae* and other pneumonias producing lobar enlargement. Radiography demonstrates multiple areas of cavitation, often with air-fluid levels (Fig. 14.13). Portions of dead lung may slough and form intracavitary masses.

BOX 14.1 Causes of Slowly Resolving or Recurrent Pneumonia

UNDERLYING STRUCTURAL ABNORMALITIES

- Central obstruction (e.g., lung cancer)
- Bronchiectasis
- Chronic obstructive pulmonary disease or emphysema
- Extensive fibrosis or scarring (e.g., sarcoidosis)
- Inadequate antimicrobial therapy

Systemic Disease

- Diabetes mellitus
- Congestive heart failure
- Alcoholism
- Advanced malignancy
- Chronic corticosteroid use

Incorrect Initial Diagnosis

- Adenocarcinoma
- Granulomatosis with polyangiitis
- Drug reaction

Pneumatocele Formation

Pneumatoceles form either from alveolar rupture or in an area of necrosis and cavitation in which the granulation tissue has become epithelialized. Airways leading to the air-filled sac become obstructed, and a ball-valve phenomenon leads to progressive enlargement; ultimately, the pneumatocele appears as a thin-walled cyst (see Fig. 14.12). As expected by the mechanism of formation, this complication is most commonly seen with pneumonia caused by virulent organisms; the classic offender is *S. aureus*. Pneumatoceles can be single or multiple and are variable in size. They may show rapid change in size and location on serial radiographs, and they can resolve over time.

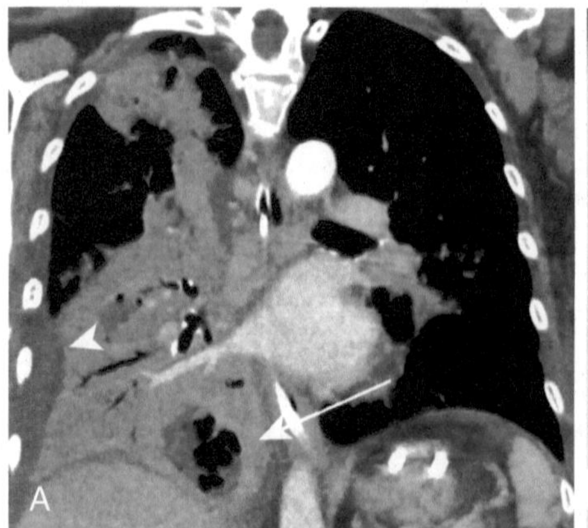

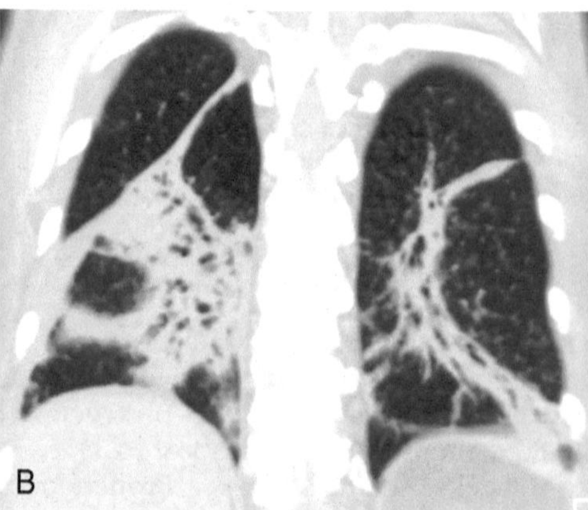

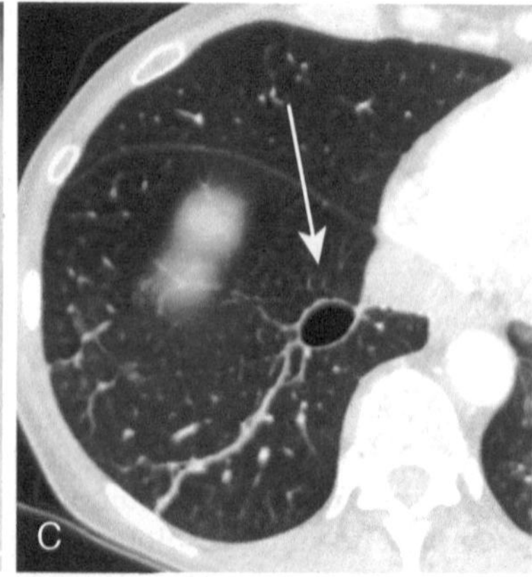

FIGURE 14.12 Complications of pneumonia. The patient initially presented with a flulike illness, which progressed to acute respiratory distress syndrome. **A,** Coronal computed tomography (CT) reconstruction 1 month after the initial presentation demonstrates a large right lung consolidation with a right lower lobe abscess *(arrow)* and parapneumonic pleural effusion *(arrowhead)*. Mixed organisms were isolated from sputum, including *Klebsiella* spp., *Stenotrophomonas maltophilia, Acinetobacter* spp., and *Escherichia coli*. **B,** Coronal CT reconstruction acquired 6 weeks later shows dense peribronchovascular consolidations, compatible with organizing pneumonia as a response to diffuse alveolar damage. **C,** Axial CT image 3 months later shows a pneumatocele and scarring in the right lower lobe at the site of the previous abscess *(arrow)*.

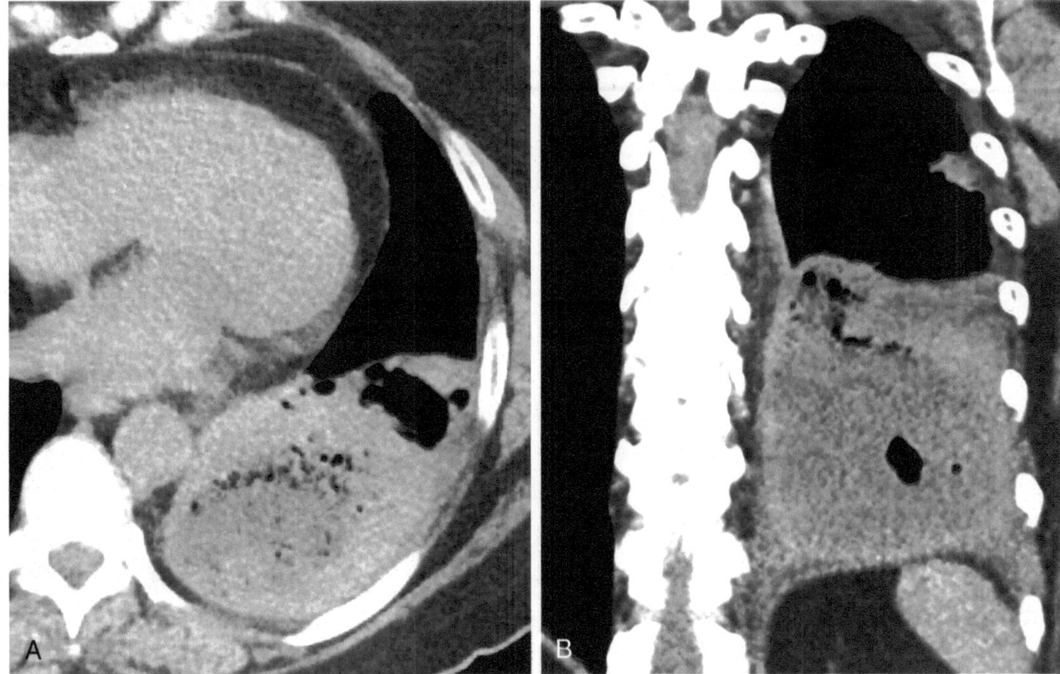

FIGURE 14.13 Pulmonary gangrene. Axial **(A)** and coronal **(B)** computed tomography reconstructions demonstrate left lower lobe consolidation with a central hypoattenuating component and numerous small bubbly lucencies. Subsequent left lower lobectomy demonstrated a necrotic lung. Culture from the resected specimen grew gram-positive rods, *Fusobacterium nucleatum,* anaerobic gram-negative rods, and actinomyces.

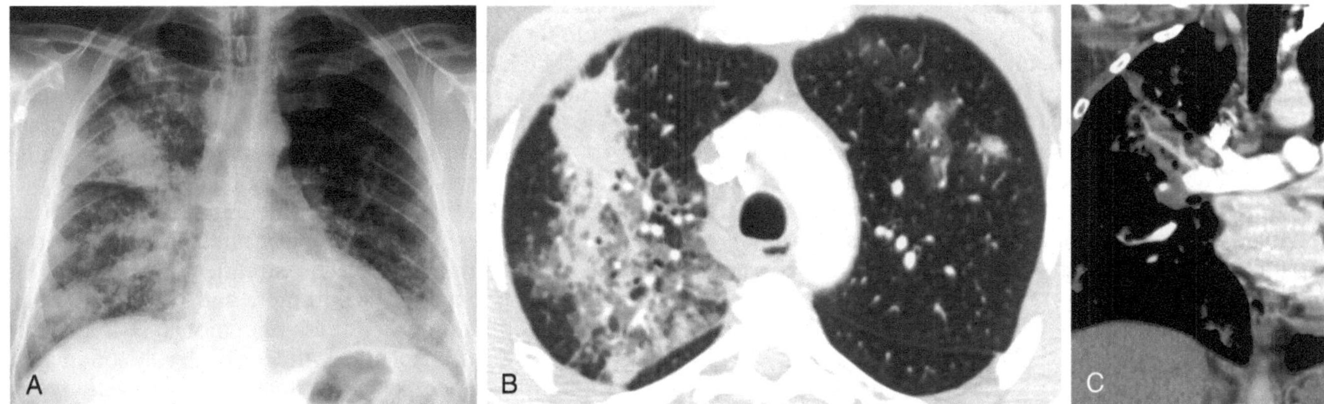

FIGURE 14.14 Masslike and consolidative coccidioidomycosis. **A,** Posteroanterior chest radiograph demonstrates patchy consolidative and masslike opacities throughout the right lung, with intervening reticulonodular opacities. **B,** Computed tomography (CT) shows the masslike consolidation, as well as patchy, heterogeneous ground-glass and nodular opacities. **C,** Coronal CT reconstruction reveals mild right hilar and mediastinal lymphadenopathy. Acute coccidioidomycosis was diagnosed in this patient who had recently returned from a horseback-riding trip to the southwestern United States.

Lymphadenopathy

Intrathoracic lymphadenopathy that can be recognized on standard radiographs is uncommon in most bacterial and viral infections; some notable exceptions include *Mycobacterium tuberculosis, Pasteurella tularensis,* and *Yersinia pestis*. Lymphadenopathy may be associated with fungal infections (Fig. 14.14) or bacterial infections that are long-standing or virulent, as in lung abscesses. CT may show slightly enlarged reactive nodes (>1 cm) in patients with common bacterial infections that are not visible on standard radiography.

Pleural Complications

Pleural effusion is a common complication of pneumonia, occurring in about 40% of cases. Most effusions are parapneumonic (i.e., reactive and sterile). Infection of the pleural space with empyema requiring drainage is a less common but important complication of some pneumonias. Imaging cannot reliably differentiate infected from noninfected pleural fluid; however, the development of loculations (particularly if they develop rapidly), pleural thickening and enhancement, and stranding of the extrapleural fat are suggestive of exudative rather than transudative effusions

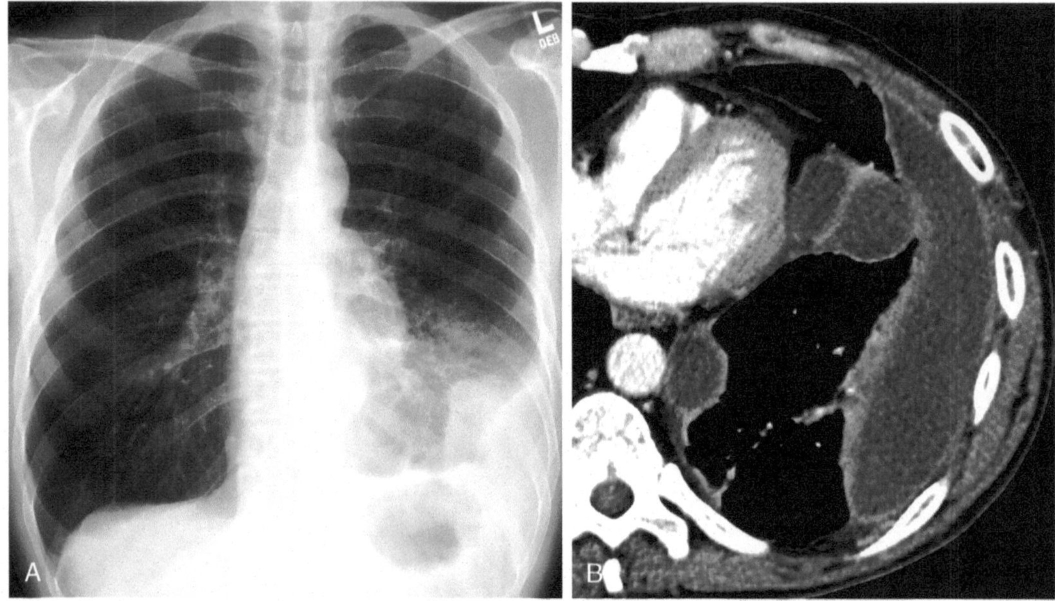

FIGURE 14.15 Empyema. **A,** Posteroanterior chest radiograph demonstrates left lower lung pneumonia and loculated pleural fluid. **B,** Chest computed tomography better defines a multiloculated left pleural effusion with associated pleural thickening and enhancement, the *split pleura sign*. Subsequent drainage revealed mixed organisms, likely secondary to aspiration.

(Fig. 14.15). These signs may warrant diagnostic thoracentesis, as empyemas, as opposed to lung abscesses, usually require percutaneous drainage to fully resolve. Large pleural effusions and empyema are more commonly seen with more virulent organisms, including *S. aureus, Streptococcus pyogenes,* gram-negative bacteria, and anaerobic bacteria.

Bronchopleural fistula is a related complication in which lung necrosis leads to a fistulous communication between the airways and the pleural space, resulting in an empyema with an air-fluid level. Although not always visible, the fistulous connection can sometimes be seen on CT and should be sought in suspected cases to help guide surgical management.

Other Complications

Rapidly progressive and fulminant bacterial or viral pneumonia may result in ARDS. In the preantibiotic era, bronchiectasis was an extremely common complication of bacterial pneumonia, but the incidence of postinfectious bronchiectasis has declined with the advent of antibiotics. Recurrent pneumonias are frequently found in patients with predisposing factors such as chronic obstructive lung disease, bronchiectasis, alcoholism, and diabetes (see Box 14.1). Although recurrent or persistent pneumonia in the same location raises the possibility of an obstructing endobronchial lesion caused by a foreign body or tumor, lung cancer accounts for fewer than 5% of such cases.

CLINICAL APPROACH TO PNEUMONIA

It is important to have a basic understanding of the clinical approach to the diagnosis and management of community-acquired pneumonia. Distinctions that should be made in a patient with pneumonia involve the setting in which the infection was acquired (i.e., community acquired vs healthcare associated) and the immune status of the patient. This chapter is focused on community-acquired pneumonia in immunocompetent patients. Infections in this setting can be further stratified based on the acuity, signs, and symptoms with which the patient presents. "Typical" and "atypical" pneumonia syndromes are most commonly encountered in the community, with differentiating clinical features (Table 14.1). Aspiration pneumonia has some distinguishing features, but the presentation and imaging overlap with typical pneumonia; likewise, chronic pneumonia has overlapping clinical features with the atypical pneumonia syndrome.

Patients cannot always be stratified into one of the described pneumonia syndromes, and the clinical diagnosis of community-acquired pneumonia is not always straightforward, explaining the critical role of imaging to confirm suspected cases. Some patients with typical pneumonia, especially older adults, do not present with cough, fever, or an elevated white blood cell count, and a significant number of patients hospitalized for pneumonia are ultimately found to have pulmonary edema, lung cancer, ARDS, pulmonary embolism, and so on. Nevertheless, given the potentially devastating consequences of inadequate treatment, the threshold for imaging and antimicrobial treatment is understandably low in patients presenting with a pneumonia-like syndrome.

BACTERIAL PNEUMONIA

In most clinical settings, bacteria are the most important pathogens involved in community-acquired pneumonia. Viral respiratory infections, although much more common, are less likely to progress to frank pneumonia and are usually limited to the upper respiratory tract. Bacteria can cause a typical pneumonia syndrome, an atypical pneumonia, or an aspiration pneumonia. Chronic bacterial infection can be seen in patients with structural abnormalities (e.g.,

TABLE 14.1 Clinical Pneumonia Syndromes

Pneumonia Syndrome	Clinical Features	Imaging Features	Common Organisms
Typical community-acquired pneumonia	• Acute presentation • Productive cough • Purulent sputum • Fever and chills • Leukocytosis • Chest pain • Absence of upper respiratory symptoms or initial upper respiratory infection followed by acute worsening (suggesting bacterial superinfection of initial viral infection) • Elevated procalcitonin (≥0.25 μg/L) • More vague symptoms are often present in older adults or debilitated patients (e.g., confusion, afebrile)	• Radiographs show new opacities: lobar, sublobar, or multifocal airspace consolidations; patchy or nodular opacities • Lobar or bronchopneumonia patterns are possible • Variable complications	• *Streptococcus pneumoniae* • *Haemophilus influenzae* • *Staphylococcus aureus* • *Klebsiella pneumoniae* • *Pseudomonas aeruginosa* • *Legionella pneumophila* • *Moraxella catarrhalis*
Atypical community-acquired pneumonia	• Subacute course without clinical deterioration • Nonproductive cough • Normal or mildly elevated WBC count • Systemic and extrapulmonary manifestations (headache, myalgias) • Variable fever • Clustered/epidemic outbreaks • Procalcitonin level ≤0.1 μg/L	• Radiographs demonstrate reticulonodular opacities, which are usually multifocal or diffuse • Patchy ground-glass or interstitial pattern on CT • Complications are less common unless typical bacterial superinfection or ARDS develops	• *Mycoplasma pneumoniae* • *Chlamydia* spp. • Viruses • *Coxiella burnetii*
Aspiration pneumonia	• Abrupt presentation in a hospitalized or predisposed individual • Events are sometimes witnessed in the health care setting • It is estimated that 5%–15% of community-acquired pneumonias are caused by aspiration	• Radiographs demonstrate new posterior and basilar opacities that can be nodular, patchy, or consolidative • Often difficult to distinguish from atelectasis, especially on portable radiographs • CT shows bronchopneumonia or lobar pneumonia patterns in posterior and basilar lung segments • Complications, including cavitation, are not uncommon • Debris in the central airways and bronchial or bronchiolar wall thickening and mucous plugging can be seen	• Mixed infections with the following: • Anaerobic oral flora • *Escherichia coli* • *S. aureus* • *S. pneumoniae* • *H. influenzae* • *P. aeruginosa*
Chronic pneumonia	• Chronic cough, low-grade fever, and flulike symptoms • Sometimes progressive to productive cough or hemoptysis • Variable weight loss, chest pain or pleurisy, and manifestations of chest wall involvement	• Highly variable but can initially be consolidative or nodular • Often progresses to a chronic necrotizing consolidative or nodular focus with variable involvement of surrounding pleura, mediastinum, and chest wall	• *Actinomyces* spp. • *Nocardia* spp. • Fungi

ARDS, Acute respiratory distress syndrome; *CT,* computed tomography; *WBC,* white blood cell.

bronchiectasis) and with certain organisms (e.g., *K. pneumoniae*). The most common pathogenetic patterns are lobar pneumonia and bronchopneumonia; nodular consolidations and ground-glass opacities are less frequent (Fig. 14.16). Again, these patterns are not organism specific, and any given bacterial pathogen can manifest in a variety of ways.

Table 14.2 describes the most common bacterial pathogens, associated risk factors, and clinical and radiographic characteristics. Note the wide overlap in both clinical and radiographic characteristics of the organisms. In most cases, imaging will be unable to specify an organism, but this lack of specificity has no bearing on patient management in most cases, such as those of uncomplicated pneumonia treated empirically. More important, the radiologist should be able to suggest the diagnosis of pneumonia, specify alternative diagnostic considerations where appropriate, describe the pathogenetic pattern and extent of disease, and identify any complications.

VIRAL PNEUMONIA

Although extremely common, viral respiratory infections come to clinical attention relatively infrequently in adults. The majority of cases that require hospitalization are attributed to influenza or bacterial superinfection. Most viruses, however, do have the potential to cause severe pneumonia that can rapidly progress to ARDS, and new viruses are constantly emerging with varying pathogenicity (e.g., Middle

East respiratory syndrome coronavirus). Viral pneumonias are more likely than bacterial to occur in clustered or epidemic outbreaks, emphasizing the importance of up-to-date epidemiologic data and a comprehensive patient travel history.

The classic pathogenetic and radiographic pattern associated with viral infection is interstitial pneumonia.

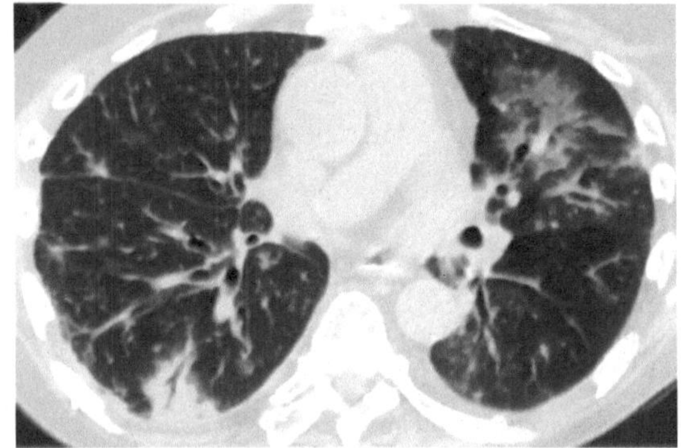

FIGURE 14.16 *Pseudomonas* pneumonia. Axial computed tomography image demonstrates patchy ground-glass opacities and nodular consolidation, which are less frequent imaging manifestations of bacterial pneumonias but can be seen with *Pseudomonas, Staphylococcus, and Legionella* spp.

Interstitial pneumonia represents a spectrum ranging from mild mononuclear cell infiltration and associated thickening of the interstitial spaces to diffuse alveolar damage with diffuse consolidation. Mild viral pneumonias can present with normal radiographs or demonstrate mild bronchial wall thickening or reticulonodular opacities. CT often demonstrates interstitial thickening, bronchial wall thickening, tree-in-bud opacities, and patchy ground-glass opacities. Distribution is often bilateral and multifocal (Fig. 14.17). Worsening infections result in increased disease extent and progressively confluent and consolidative opacities. Some viral pneumonias, such as varicella, may manifest as a nodular pattern. Others, such as Epstein-Barr pneumonia, often manifest with lymphadenopathy. Acute clinical worsening or a new focal consolidation suggests bacterial superinfection, particularly if there is associated necrosis or cavitation. Common viral pathogens and their features are described in Table 14.3.

FUNGAL PNEUMONIA

The most clinically important fungal pneumonias, such as invasive aspergillosis and candidiasis, are typically seen in immunocompromised patients (see Chapter 15). The endemic fungi, on the other hand, are quite common in healthy individuals but come to clinical attention relatively rarely. Actinomycosis and nocardiosis are caused by bacterial

TABLE 14.2 **Common Bacterial Infections**

Organism	Epidemiology and Risk Factors	Clinical Characteristics	Imaging Characteristics
	Gram-Positive Bacteria		
Streptococcus pneumoniae	• Most common community-acquired pneumonia • More common in adults • Occurs in healthy and debilitated individuals • Predisposition in patients with splenic disorders (sickle cell disease, splenectomy, hematologic malignancies)	• Typical pneumonia syndrome (see Table 14.1) in most patients: high fever, productive cough, shaking chills, and pleuritic chest pain • Manifestations may be atypical or overshadowed in older or debilitated patients	• Most commonly lobar or sublobar consolidation • Multifocal consolidation and bronchopneumonia pattern less common • Can present as "round" pneumonia • Can produce bulging fissure • Effusions in just under half of cases
Staphylococcus aureus	• Rare in healthy adults • More common in children and infants • Common nosocomial pathogen • Superinfectant after viral infection • Hematogenous spread (septic emboli) in IV drug abusers and patients with indwelling catheters	• Typical pneumonia syndrome; patients are often very ill • Clinical worsening after viral pneumonia • Occasional hemoptysis	• Inhalational form more often demonstrates a bronchopneumonia pattern, but lobar consolidation can also be seen • Typically bilateral; lower lobe predominant • Cavitation, empyema, and pneumatocele formation • Multiple septic emboli in hematogenous form
Streptococcus pyogenes	• Much less common than the other gram-positive bacteria • Predominantly occurs in very young and old patients • Occasionally epidemic • Can follow other bacterial or viral infections	• Typical pneumonia syndrome, sometimes with blood-streaked sputum	• Multifocal lobar consolidation or bronchopneumonia pattern can be seen • Lower lobe predominant • Often causes pleural effusions
Bacillus anthracis	• Spore-forming organism found in soil, ingested by animals, seen in agricultural areas • Used in terrorist attacks in the United States in October 2001	• Cutaneous, GI, and inhalational forms • Initial presentation similar to an upper respiratory tract infection, with rapid progression to respiratory failure, shock, and death	• Mediastinal widening on radiographs secondary to hemorrhagic lymphadenitis and mediastinitis; nodes are hyperattenuating on CT • Pleural effusions common • Peribronchovascular airspace opacities are disproportionately scant relative to lymphadenopathy

TABLE 14.2 Common Bacterial Infections—cont'd

Organism	Epidemiology and Risk Factors	Clinical Characteristics	Imaging Characteristics
		Gram-Negative Bacteria	
Klebsiella pneumoniae	• Usually in middle-aged or older patients • More common in those with chronic lung disease and in patients with alcoholism • Often aspirated	• Severe typical pneumonia syndrome, often with painful respiration and shortness of breath • Green or "currant jelly" sputum can be seen • Can become chronic, in which case it simulates TB	• Lobar consolidation, more commonly in the upper lobes • Bulging fissures, cavitation, effusions, and pulmonary gangrene can be seen • Occasional bronchopneumonia
Escherichia coli	• Typically hospitalized or chronically ill patients • Aspirated or direct extension across the diaphragm	• Typical pneumonia syndrome	• Lower and posterior lung bronchopneumonia • Commonly cavitary • Pleural effusions common
Pseudomonas aeruginosa	• Typically hospitalized or debilitated patients • Associated with bronchiectasis, particularly those taking glucocorticoids • Chronic colonizer in patients with cystic fibrosis	• Severe typical pneumonia syndrome • Occasional blood-streaked sputum	• Bronchopneumonia or consolidative patterns • Lower lobe predominant, often multifocal or bilateral • Cavitation and pleural effusions may occur
Haemophilus influenzae	• Most common in debilitated patients, young children, and older adults • Particularly common in patients with COPD	• Typical pneumonia syndrome on a background of chronic illness • Can cause bronchitis without bronchopneumonia in adults and epiglottitis in children or adults	• Bronchopneumonia • Lower lobe predominant • Cavitation and pleural effusion are rare
Legionella pneumophila (Legionnaires' disease; legionellosis)	• Usually affects older men with underlying chronic illness • Resides in water sources; airborne spread	• Wide range of clinical manifestations, from mild flulike illness (Pontiac fever) to ARDS and death • GI symptoms, particularly diarrhea, are common • Headache, encephalopathy, hematuria, and renal insufficiency more commonly seen than in other bacterial pneumonias • Usually diagnosed through urine serology	• Peripheral focal consolidation, usually in upper lobes initially, with rapid spread to other lobes • Cavitation is uncommon in immunocompetent patients • Relatively slow resolution
Moraxella catarrhalis	• Usually seen in patients with chronic illnesses or varying levels of immunosuppression, including patients on chronic corticosteroids	• Upper or lower respiratory infections are possible • Clinical disease is usually mild	• Nonspecific radiographic patterns • When the lower respiratory tract is involved, usually presents with a bronchopneumonia pattern
Chlamydophila pneumoniae	• Increasingly recognized cause of community-acquired pneumonia in adults • Seen in healthy and immunocompromised patients	• Often preceded by pharyngitis with progression to atypical pneumonia syndrome (see Table 14.1), with nonproductive cough and fever • Variable clinical severity	• Usually patchy or homogeneous middle or lower lobe consolidation • Can present with a diffuse reticulonodular pattern (interstitial pneumonia), similar to viruses
Chlamydophila psittaci (psittacosis)	• Inhalation of infected aerosolized material from any avian species	• Variable, ranging from asymptomatic to fulminant disease with multisystem failure • Atypical or typical pneumonia syndromes are possible • History (birds) is key to diagnosis	• Variable patterns, including patchy multifocal consolidations or extensive lower lung-predominant reticulations • Pleural effusions are common but usually small
Francisella tularensis (tularemia)	• Transmitted through handling or ingesting small animals or tick bites • Occasionally clustered outbreaks • Typhoidal form results from ingestion of infected meat or water and presents with GI symptoms • Ulceroglandular form occurs via direct inoculation	• Either of typhoidal or ulceroglandular forms can cause pneumonia • Pneumonic tularemia presents as a typical pneumonia syndrome, often severe	• Consolidation, usually solitary but occasionally multifocal • Pleural effusions, mediastinal and hilar lymphadenopathy are seen in ≈50% of patients
Coxiella burnetii (Q fever)	• Rickettsial disease most common in the western and southwestern United States • Transmitted through infected dust from animals	• Flulike illness, with fever, dry cough, myalgias, and headache • Pneumonia in less than half of infected patients	• Variable radiographic patterns, including unifocal or multifocal consolidations or interstitial pattern (reticulonodular) • Cavitation is rare • Occasional pleural effusions

Continued

TABLE 14.2 **Common Bacterial Infections—cont'd**

Organism	Epidemiology and Risk Factors	Clinical Characteristics	Imaging Characteristics
		Gram-Negative Bacteria	
Anaerobes: *Bacteroides, Fusobacterium, Peptococcus, Peptostreptococcus, Prevotella, Propionibacterium* spp.	• Typically aspirated; therefore, associated with risk factors for aspiration • More commonly seen in patients with poor dental hygiene	• Sudden typical pneumonia syndrome of varying severity • Often mixed with aerobic organisms	• Bronchopneumonia pattern is most common • Lower and posterior lung predominance • Cavitation is common
Other: *Mycoplasma pneumoniae*	• Technically not a bacteria but a bacterial-like organism • Accounts for up to 20% of cases of community-acquired pneumonia • Often seen in winter months in clustered outbreaks	• Classically presents with the atypical pneumonia syndrome, including insidious onset, low-grade fever, nonproductive cough • Extrapulmonary manifestations include otitis, nonexudative pharyngitis, and diarrhea	• Classically demonstrates the interstitial pattern, with reticulonodular opacities on radiographs and patchy ground-glass on CT • Can progress to patchy consolidative or nodular opacities (i.e., lobar or bronchopneumonia pattern, respectively)

ARDS, Acute respiratory distress syndrome; *COPD,* chronic obstructive pulmonary disease; *CT,* computed tomography; *GI,* gastrointestinal; *IV,* intravenous; *TB,* tuberculosis.

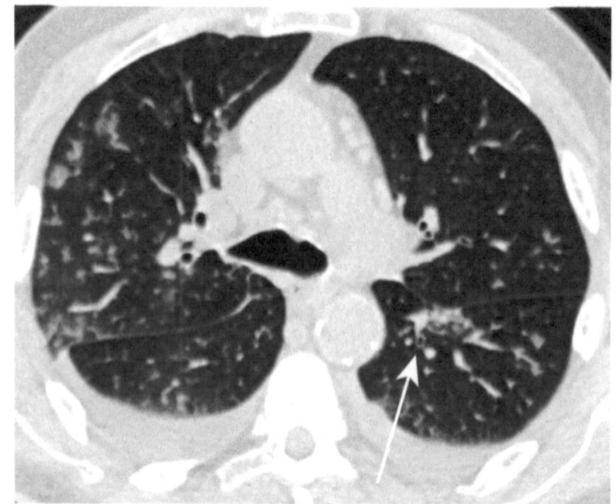

FIGURE 14.17 Human metapneumovirus pneumonia. Axial computed tomography image demonstrates tree-in-bud and centrilobular nodular opacities, bronchial wall thickening *(arrow),* and small bilateral pleural effusions typical of viral pneumonia.

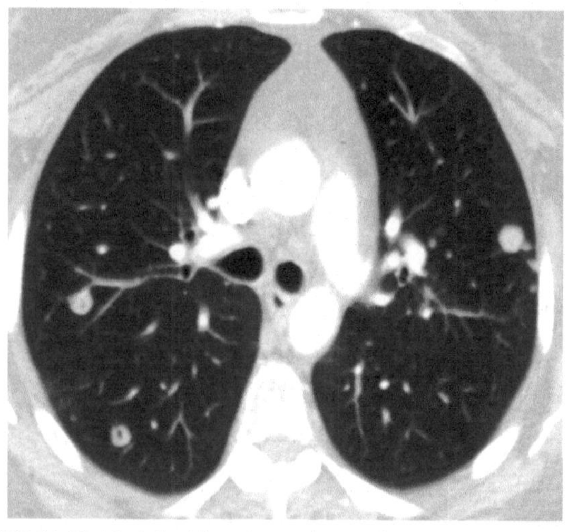

FIGURE 14.18 Nodular histoplasmosis. Axial computed tomography image in a patient with histoplasmosis demonstrates bilateral pulmonary nodules, some of which demonstrate central cavitation.

organisms from the *Actinomyces* and *Nocardia* genera, respectively; however, they share clinical and pathologic features with the fungi (and were previously characterized as such) and are considered in this section.

The most important endemic fungi in the United States are histoplasmosis, coccidioidomycosis, North American blastomycosis, and cryptococcus. These are dimorphic organisms that exist in mycelial form in nature and a pathologic yeast form in host tissue. As detailed in Table 14.4, most patients are asymptomatic, but there is wide heterogeneity in the clinical course, and both fulminant and chronic infections can occur. Likewise, imaging appearances are variable. There are several different forms that each infection can take, ranging from consolidation to masslike (see Fig. 14.14) to multiple nodules (Fig. 14.18). Persistence of any of these findings or progression to chronic cavitary disease (Fig. 14.19) should raise the suspicion of fungal infection, and "do-not-miss" mimics such as lung cancer and tuberculosis should also be considered. Any granulomatous disease, including fungal infection, can heal with residual scarring, calcified lymph nodes (see Fig. 14.11), and calcified or noncalcified parenchymal granulomas; histoplasmosis is the most common cause.

Aspergillus spp. are an important group of organisms in both immunocompromised and immunocompetent patients. The three forms that can be seen in immunocompetent patients are described in Table 14.4.

Actinomycosis and nocardiosis are relatively rare causes of pneumonia in the community setting. Actinomycosis should be considered along with mycobacterial and fungal organisms when soft tissue invasion is associated with parenchymal infection (Fig. 14.20). Similar to the endemic fungi, nocardiosis should be considered when infection is suspected in the setting of multiple nodules and masses,

TABLE 14.3 Common Viral Infections

Organism	Epidemiology and Risk Factors	Clinical Characteristics	Imaging Characteristics
Influenza	• Can affect patients of any age • Sporadic, epidemic, and pandemic infections are seen • During outbreaks, it is the most common cause of community-acquired pneumonia warranting hospitalization	• Variable severity • Dry cough, fever, myalgia, and headache are common • Pulmonary infection is progressive, usually beginning with bronchitis with rapid progression to severe illness, including shortness of breath and hypoxemia • ARDS and bacterial superinfection are important complications	• Variable, ranging from bronchial wall thickening to scattered ground-glass opacities to multifocal centrilobular nodules and consolidations • Superimposed diffuse alveolar damage and bacterial infection can be seen
Adenovirus	• Sporadic infection is most often seen in children • Epidemic outbreaks can be seen in close living quarters (e.g., military recruits)	• Presents with pharyngitis and flulike symptoms • Usually self-limited but can progress to hypoxemic respiratory failure • Can lead to chronic bronchitis, bronchiectasis, or bronchiolitis obliterans, particularly in children	• Variable; multifocal bronchopneumonia or consolidations can be seen • Bronchial wall thickening is common with resultant air-trapping or atelectasis • Can result in scarring, particularly in children
Respiratory syncytial virus	• Most common respiratory viral pathogen in the first 6 months of life • Rare in adults	• Can cause upper or lower respiratory tract disease • Pneumonia results in coughing, dyspnea, wheezing, and intercostal retractions	• Imaging can be unimpressive relative to clinical signs and symptoms • Radiographs show air trapping, perihilar linear opacities, and bronchial wall thickening • CT demonstrates interstitial thickening and ground-glass opacities
Human metapneumovirus	• Can be seen at any age but more commonly in children and older adult patients • Second most common cause of lower respiratory tract infection in children	• Ranges from asymptomatic to severe pneumonia • Usually simulates RSV infection	• Bronchiolitis, ground-glass opacities, or multifocal nodular opacities can be seen • Airspace consolidation in fewer than half of patients
Varicella-herpes zoster	• Causes varicella (chickenpox) more commonly in children and zoster (shingles) more commonly in adults • Pneumonia is more commonly seen in the adult varicella form (approximately one in six patients)	• High fever, chest pain, and dry cough • Can cause severe respiratory disease, particularly when seen in adults	• Diffuse ill-defined nodules measuring 4–6 mm • Can rapidly progress to airspace consolidation • Hilar lymphadenopathy is common • Relatively slow radiographic resolution can be seen • Diffuse discrete pulmonary calcifications measuring 2-3 mm can remain after the infection
Epstein-Barr virus	• Common infection but rarely causes pneumonia	• Upper respiratory symptoms predominate; dry cough can be seen	• Usually normal • Mediastinal and hilar lymphadenopathy are the most common intrathoracic manifestations • Occasionally, diffuse reticular opacities are seen
Coronavirus	• Before 2002, was considered an unimportant pathogen • Coronavirus-associated SARS emerged in 2002 and infected more than 8000 patients on multiple continents; no documented cases since 2004 • In 2012, MERS coronavirus emerged in Saudi Arabia; all cases have been linked to residence or travel within the Arabian peninsula	• Severe respiratory illness occurs in SARS and MERS, with mortality rates approximating 10% and 30%, respectively	• Early radiographs can be normal followed by rapid appearance of multifocal ground-glass opacities or consolidations • Sometimes lower and peripherally predominant • Degree of and response to diffuse alveolar damage determines ultimate imaging manifestations
Hantavirus	• Most commonly seen in rural areas in the southwestern United States • Infection results from inhalation of aerosolized rodent feces or urine	• Hantavirus pulmonary syndrome initially presents with fever, headache, and myalgia progressing to shortness of breath and hypoxia • Endothelial lung damage can result in ARDS • Mortality rate is nearly 50%	• Early disease demonstrates reticular opacities or interstitial thickening • Imaging manifestations of noncardiogenic alveolar pulmonary edema appear (perihilar- and basilar-predominant airspace opacities) as endothelial damage progresses

ARDS, Acute respiratory distress syndrome; *CT*, computed tomography; *MERS*, Middle Eastern respiratory syndrome; *RSV*, respiratory syncytial virus; *SARS*, severe acute respiratory syndrome.

TABLE 14.4 **Common Fungal Infections**

Organism	Epidemiology and Risk Factors	Clinical Characteristics	Imaging Characteristics
Histoplasma capsulatum (histoplasmosis)	• Similar to all of the endemic fungi, the most important risk factor is living or traveling in endemic areas, where lifetime incidence is up to 80% • Distribution is worldwide; in the United States, it occurs along river valleys, particularly the Ohio, Mississippi, and St. Lawrence • The organism exists in the soil, particularly that contaminated by bird or bat excrement • Massive exposure can occur with cleaning or destruction of areas containing droppings, such as chicken houses or attics of old buildings	• Most individuals are asymptomatic; constitutional symptoms and nonproductive cough can occur • Spore inhalation causes a localized infection with subsequent migration to locoregional lymph nodes and then to the spleen and liver • Most infections are cleared without treatment, but a chronic cavitary infection can occur	• Acute phase can consist of (1) single or multifocal consolidation, (2) multiple 1- to 5-mm poorly marginated nodules, or (3) solitary granuloma (histoplasmoma) • Ipsilateral mediastinal or hilar lymphadenopathy can occur with parenchymal disease or independently • Healing of nodules or lymphadenopathy often leaves persistent granulomas, which can be calcified; calcified granulomas can also be seen in the liver or spleen • Broncholiths and fibrosing mediastinitis are complications of calcified lymph nodes (see Chapter 6) • A chronic cavitary form of histoplasmosis can simulate TB
Coccidioides immitis (coccidioidomycosis)	• Endemic to the desert areas of the southwestern United States and Central and South America	• Most individuals are asymptomatic; a mild flulike illness is possible, and acute, severe disease can cause fever, cough, and pleuritic chest pain • Inhalation causes local pneumonitis; usually the spores are destroyed without sequelae • ≈5% of patients can have a chronic, often asymptomatic nodule or cavity • Reactivation of the initial focus can occur (similar to TB) • Dissemination to hilar or mediastinal lymph nodes is common; diffuse dissemination is rare but nearly universally fatal	• Pneumonic form: most common form; results in patchy consolidation, usually lower lobe, possibly bilateral; lymphadenopathy in 20% • Chronic form: "classic" form but only seen in 10%–15% of cases; results in solitary or multiple nodules that usually cavitate with resultant very thin walls • Disseminated form: rare; multiple nodules 5–10 mm in diameter or miliary pattern
Blastomycosis dermatitidis (North American blastomycosis)	• Endemic in North America, predominantly the southeastern United States and the regions where histoplasmosis occurs • Associated with hunters and those living or working in wooded areas • Infection can result from inhalation or skin inoculation of mycelia from the soil	• Asymptomatic infection is possible but less common than other endemic fungi • Symptomatic infection can result in a flulike illness or a more acute typical pneumonia syndrome • Musculoskeletal and skin signs and symptoms can be present	• Most often results in a bronchopneumonia pattern • Rapidly progressive disease, including progression to ARDS, is possible • Solitary or multifocal nodules and disseminated disease with a miliary pattern are less common manifestations
Cryptococcus neoformans (cryptococcosis)	• Typically found in pigeon droppings • 70% of patients with clinical disease are immunocompromised (see Chapter 15)	• Often asymptomatic in otherwise healthy patients; a mild flulike illness can occur • CNS is the most frequently affected site	• Most common manifestations in healthy adults are single or multiple nodules; a bronchopneumonia pattern can occur, and miliary nodules are rare in healthy individuals • Lymphadenopathy and pleural effusion are rare
		Aspergillosis	
Aspergilloma or mycetoma	• Requires a preexisting cyst, cavity, bulla, or area of bronchiectasis • High prevalence in patients with cavitary TB, end-stage sarcoidosis, or CF • Patients usually have normal immunity but underlying chronic conditions	• Often patients are asymptomatic • Cough, weight loss, and hemoptysis can occur; the latter can be life threatening • Parenchymal invasion is rare • Pathologically consists of aspergillus hyphae, mucus, and cellular debris	• Opacity, usually round, within a cavity or cyst • Air may dissect inside, producing the *air crescent sign* • Prone and supine CT acquisitions can increase diagnostic confidence if mobility of the fungus ball is demonstrated • Often accompanied by extensive pleural thickening at the apices (adjacent to the mycetoma)

TABLE 14.4 **Common Fungal Infections—cont'd**

Organism	Epidemiology and Risk Factors	Clinical Characteristics	Imaging Characteristics
Semi-invasive aspergillosis, or chronic necrotizing aspergillosis	• Patients are usually mildly immunosuppressed from chronic disease (e.g., alcoholism, chronic diabetes mellitus, malignancy, COPD, or corticosteroid use) • Preexisting structural lung disease is an additional risk factor	• Infection occurs after inhalation of spores • A chronic pneumonia results, which progresses to a cavitary lesion over months • Usually patients demonstrate low-grade fever and progressive cough; hemoptysis is possible	• Initial infection results in a consolidation, usually at the apices • The consolidation becomes cavitary, may contain an air crescent, and eventually becomes thick walled with an internal fungus ball • The evolving cavitary consolidation simulates TB initially and later mycetoma
Allergic bronchopulmonary aspergillosis (see Chapter 6)	• Occurs almost exclusively in people with asthma	• *Aspergillus* spores contained within mucous plugs in the tracheobronchial tree incite an allergic reaction • Peripheral eosinophilia and elevated IgE antibodies are seen • Treatment is with corticosteroids	• Mucoid impaction of the bronchus, with central branching opacities ("finger-in-glove" pattern) • Residual bronchiectasis is present when mucous plugs are expectorated
Actinomyces israelii (actinomycosis)	• Normal colonizer of the oropharynx • Disease may occur in any patients, but people with alcoholism and those with poor dentition or oral hygiene may have increased risk	• Thoracic disease results from aspiration of organisms with resultant focal abscess • Nonproductive cough often progresses to productive cough and fever • Hemoptysis, pleuritic pain, and musculoskeletal and skin signs and symptoms can develop • Destructive extension into local soft tissues, including the pleura, chest wall, and mediastinum, can occur with resultant complications (e.g., bronchopleural fistula, osteomyelitis, or pericarditis, respectively) • Anaerobic cultures are required to confirm the diagnosis	• Focal consolidation, usually lower lobe and often with central necrosis • Careful evaluation for local soft tissue and osseous invasion is required; fairly extensive periostitis of adjacent ribs in combination with parenchymal findings is highly suggestive • Pleural effusions are moderately common • Chronic disease can result in extensive architectural distortion
Nocardia asteroides (nocardiosis)	• Can occur in otherwise healthy patients but most common in patients with underlying immunodeficiency • Pulmonary alveolar proteinosis is a risk factor	• Acquired via inhalation of infected soil • Presents with cough, chest pain, and fever • Often takes a chronic course in normal or mildly immunosuppressed patients	• Bronchopneumonia pattern or solitary or multiple nodules or masses can be seen • Nodules and masses can be cavitary • Chest wall involvement is possible but rare • Pleural effusion in ≈50%

ARDS, Acute respiratory distress syndrome; *CF,* cystic fibrosis; *CNS,* central nervous system; *COPD,* chronic obstructive pulmonary disease; *CT,* computed tomography; *TB,* tuberculosis.

which is a rare appearance for bacterial pneumonia. Chronic disease and cavitation can be seen in actinomycosis or nocardiosis (Fig. 14.21).

PARASITIC INFECTION

Parasitic infection of the lung is rare in the United States, particularly in immunocompetent patients. Pulmonary pathology results from one of two mechanisms: direct lung invasion or a hypersensitivity reaction to the organisms resulting in pulmonary eosinophilia. Loeffler syndrome, or simple pulmonary eosinophilia, was first described by Wilhelm Loeffler in patients with roundworm and hookworm infections. Clinically, parasitic infection is suspected when patients demonstrate peripheral eosinophilia in combination with a compatible travel history.

The radiographic manifestations of parasitic lung disease are variable (Table 14.5). Nearly any parasitic organisms can result in the transient, peripheral opacities of simple pulmonary eosinophilia. Toxoplasmosis can cause a pattern simulating interstitial pneumonia, and schistosomiasis can result in signs of pulmonary hypertension. Amebiasis is suggested when right basilar disease is associated with hepatic involvement. Only echinococcus can produce more specific findings, including the *meniscus or air crescent sign*, seen when air dissects between endocysts and exocysts, or the *water lily sign*, seen when ruptured endocysts float on a fluid level within the exocyst (Fig. 14.22).

CONCLUSION

In most cases of community-acquired pneumonia, a specific pathogen will not be isolated, and our reports must balance a quest for specificity with the need for practicality. It is more important to identify a focus of cavitation than to posit a particular organism, especially on initial imaging.

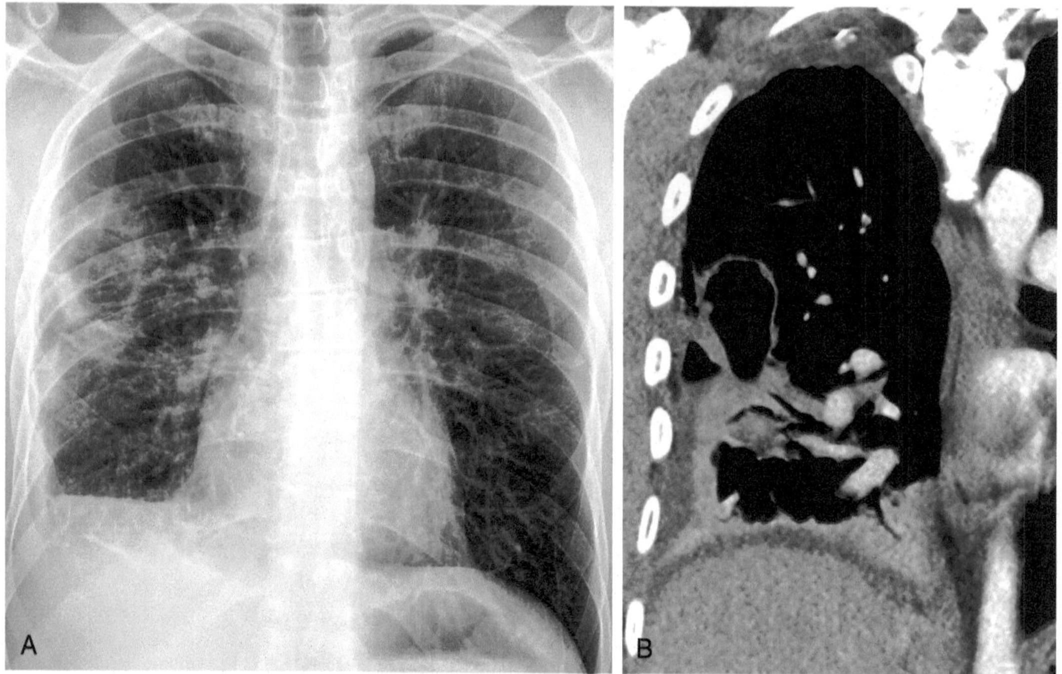

FIGURE 14.19 Cavitary coccidioidomycosis. **A,** Posteroanterior chest radiograph demonstrates a thick-walled cavity in the right mid lung with surrounding consolidation and adjacent pleural thickening. **B,** Coronal computed tomography reconstruction shows the asymmetrically thick-walled cavity with surrounding consolidation and a parapneumonic effusion secondary to subacute coccidioidomycosis.

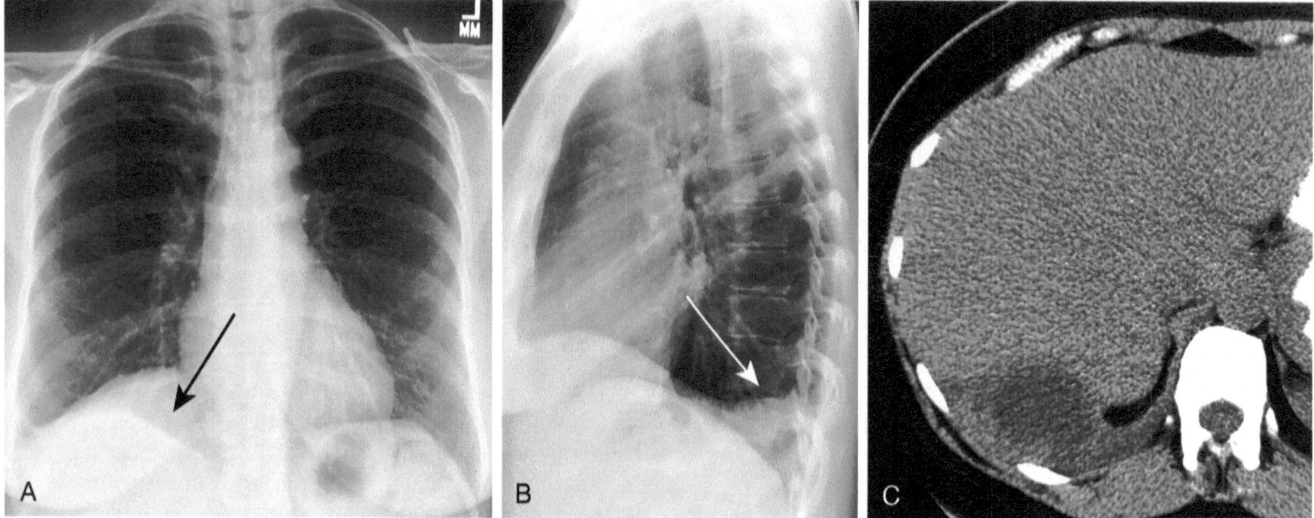

FIGURE 14.20 Actinomycosis invading the liver. **A,** Posteroanterior chest radiograph demonstrates a double density overlying the right hemidiaphragm *(arrow)*. **B,** Lateral radiograph shows convex blunting of the posterior right costophrenic angle *(arrow)*. **C,** Axial chest computed tomography reveals a low-density abscess within the left lower lobe, pleural thickening, and liver invasion. Surgical resection revealed pulmonary actinomycosis, likely related to aspiration, with transdiaphragmatic invasion into hepatic segment 7.

TABLE 14.5 Common Parasitic Infections

Organism	Epidemiology and Risk Factors	Clinical Characteristics	Imaging Characteristics
Toxoplasma gondii (toxoplasmosis)	• Infection is extremely common but usually asymptomatic • Congenital variety is most common, presenting with clinical disease • Cat is the definitive host; rats and mice can serve as intermediate hosts	• Infection is congenital or, in adults, via ingestion of the oocyte form of the parasite • Pulmonary infection in normal patients is very uncommon, as are symptoms • Low-grade fever can occur	• Radiographs demonstrate fairly diffuse reticulonodular opacities • CT shows patchy ground-glass opacities with possible foci of consolidation
Echinococcus granulosus (echinococcal or hydatid disease)	• Pastoral and sylvatic varieties with different geographic ranges and intermediate and definitive hosts • Pastoral variant (more common) is endemic in southeastern Europe, North Africa, the Middle East, and Russia and has domestic livestock and dogs as the intermediate and definitive hosts, respectively • Sylvatic variant is found in Alaska and Canada and has deer species and canines as the intermediate and definitive hosts, respectively	• Acquired via ingestion of eggs with subsequent dissemination: 65%–70% of cysts occur in the liver and 15%–30% in the lungs • Hydatid cyst is composed of two layers, the exocyst and endocyst, the latter of which may contain daughter cysts • Most patients are asymptomatic, but symptoms can arise from mass effect or cyst rupture into the lung parenchyma or bronchus with resultant intense inflammation or anaphylactic shock	• Single or multiple well-circumscribed spherical or oval masses • Usually located in the lower lobes • Air can enter between the endocyst and exocyst with resultant ***meniscus or air crescent sign*** • Occasionally, air crescent and air-fluid level can be seen, and the ruptured cyst membrane can float on the fluid, giving rise to the ***water lily sign***
Entamoeba histolytica (amebiasis)	• Pulmonary disease is rare and is usually a sequela of hepatic or GI (amebic dysentery) involvement • Amebic dysentery is found worldwide but usually in poorly developed regions or recent disaster areas, where fecal-oral transmission occurs	• Pulmonary involvement usually occurs via transdiaphragmatic spread from a liver abscess; therefore, patients usually present with right upper quadrant and right pleuritic pain, fever, and cough • Cough productive of "anchovy paste" or "chocolate sauce" material is a classic clinical sign, and biliptysis can rarely occur	• Usually there is a right pleural effusion with a right basal consolidation • Pulmonary abscess formation can rarely occur
Schistosomiasis	• Common and important disease worldwide, with varying species and associated clinical syndromes	• Infection results from drinking infected water or direct burrowing • Parasites reach the circulation and grow within the mesenteric or pelvic venous plexus • Worms mature and lay eggs, resulting in a host inflammatory response that causes clinical disease • Pulmonary symptoms can occur from a hypersensitivity reaction during the larval migration phase, or pulmonary hypertension can develop from impaction of and inflammation surrounding ova within and surrounding the pulmonary capillaries	• Transient eosinophilic pneumonia (Loeffler syndrome) manifesting as multifocal peripheral consolidation can occur • Signs of pulmonary hypertension: dilated central pulmonary arteries with peripheral tortuosity or dilated bronchial arteries; can be seen in chronic disease
Paragonimiasis	• Endemic in Southeast Asia, West Africa, and South America	• Acquired by eating infected crustaceans and water snails • The immature flukes penetrate the GI tract and migrate to the lung • Can result in a hypersensitivity reaction or direct inflammation from the migratory process, resulting in hemoptysis, chest pain, or chronic cough	• Imaging manifestations can result from eosinophilic reaction or direct inflammation from the migrating fluke, including chronic masslike consolidation or cavitation or pleural effusion or empyema • There are reports of direct visualization of the fluke tract
Other metazoan infections: ascariasis, strongyloidiasis, trichinosis, ancylostomiasis, and filariasis	• A number of additional worms cause clinical disease but are rare in the United States • A high level of suspicion and good medical history are keys to making the diagnosis	• Most pulmonary disease results from an HSR	• Usually transient eosinophilic pneumonia (Loeffler syndrome) manifesting as multifocal peripheral consolidation

CT, Computed tomography; *GI,* gastrointestinal; *HSR,* hypersensitivity reaction;

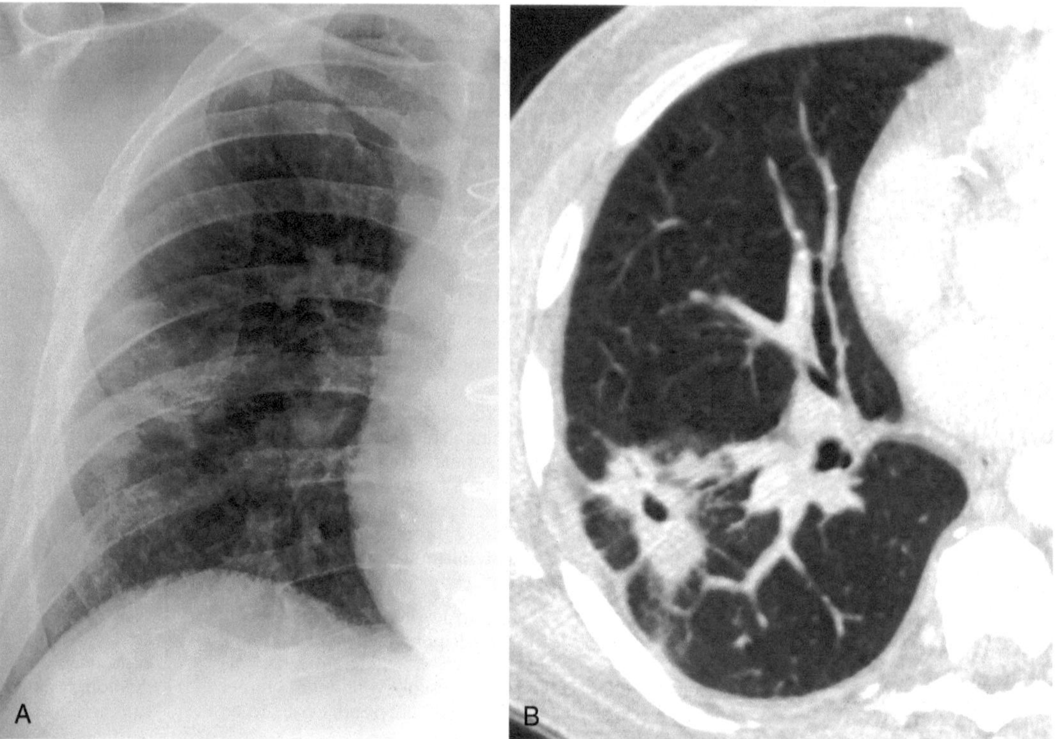

FIGURE 14.21 Actinomycosis. **A,** Posteroanterior chest radiograph demonstrates an irregular rounded opacity in the right mid lung. **B,** Axial chest computed tomography better demonstrates the irregular nodular consolidation and central cavitation.

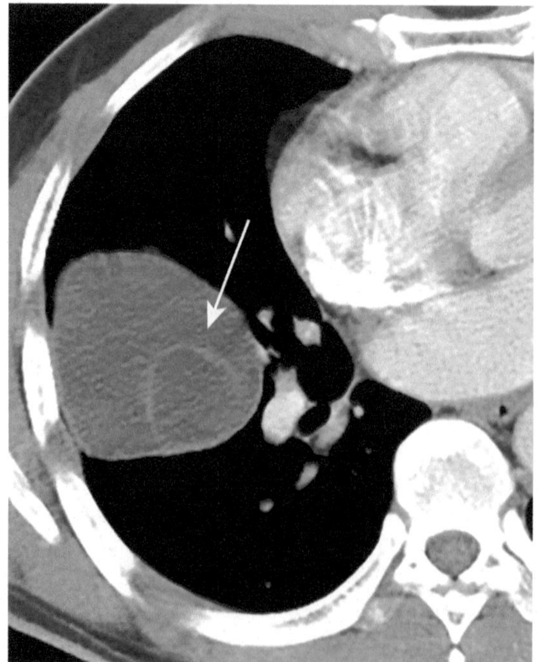

FIGURE 14.22 Echinococcus. Axial computed tomography image reveals an endocyst *(arrow)* within an exocyst.

TABLE 14.6 Radiographic Clues to Pulmonary Infections

Radiographic Finding	Suggested Infection
Consolidation (i.e., lobar pneumonia pattern)	Typical bacterial pneumonia, some fungi
Bronchopneumonia pattern	*Staphylococcus aureus,* gram-negative and anaerobic organisms
Interstitial pattern	*Mycoplasma pneumoniae, Chlamydia,* viruses
Chronic consolidation, nodule or mass, or cavitation	Actinomycosis, nocardiosis, granulomatous organisms (mycobacteria and fungi)
Patchy posterior or lower lung (i.e., dependent) consolidation	Aspiration pneumonia
Lymphadenopathy (i.e., detectable radiographically; any infection can cause mild reactive lymphadenopathy detectable on CT)	Granulomatous organisms, viruses, *Mycoplasma pneumoniae,* bacterial infection with subsequent abscess, *Yersinia pestis, Francisella tularensis, Bacillus anthracis*
Cavitation	*S. aureus, Streptococcus pneumoniae,* gram-negative and anaerobic organisms, granulomatous organisms
Pneumatoceles	Anything that causes cavitation, most commonly *S. aureus*
Lobar expansion/bulging fissure	*Klebsiella pneumoniae, Streptococcus pneumoniae, S. aureus, Haemophilus influenzae*
Pulmonary gangrene	*K. pneumoniae, Escherichia coli, H. influenzae,* granulomatous organisms, *S. pneumoniae,* anaerobes
Rounded pneumonia	*S. pneumoniae, Legionella pneumophila, Coxiella burnetii,* fungi, early septic emboli
Septic emboli	*S. aureus,* occasionally gram-negative bacilli or anaerobes from extrathoracic nidus
Empyema	*S. aureus,* mixed infections, gram-negative and anaerobic organisms, occasionally *S. pneumoniae*
Chest wall involvement	*Actinomycosis* spp., *Nocardia* spp., granulomatous organisms

CT, Computed tomography.

When asked directly about potential etiologies, all available clinical and radiographic information should be used. Clues that can suggest specific organisms can be found in Table 14.6. Do not neglect to use available serial imaging. Consider a new basilar consolidation without associated volume loss: Complete resolution in 48 hours is highly suggestive of bland aspiration, but cavitation appearing over 48 hours suggests aspiration pneumonia with virulent organisms. Progressive resolution over 3 weeks is typical of uncomplicated lobar pneumonia. Persistence through antibiotics with progressive volume loss warrants careful scrutiny for an obstructing mass, but persistence with progressive cavitation should prompt consideration of atypical organisms, including fungal.

The most important questions to consider when approaching a patient with suspected or known pneumonia are presented in Box 14.2.

BOX 14.2 Approach to Suspected or Known Pneumonia

CLINICAL QUESTIONS TO ASK

Where was the infection acquired?
Is the patient immunocompromised?
What are the age and sex of the patient?
What comorbid disease processes are present?
What is the dominant clinical pneumonia syndrome (see Table 14.1)?
What relevant travel or exposure history is available?
Could this infection be part of a known clustered or epidemic outbreak?
How long has the patient been ill?
What antimicrobial therapy has the patient received?

IMAGING FINDINGS AND CONSIDERATIONS

Are there findings compatible with pneumonia?
Do the findings suggest an alternative diagnosis?
What is the extent of disease?
What is the dominant radiographic pattern?
Are any specific imaging findings present to narrow the list of potential pathogens (see Table 14.6)?
Are underlying structural abnormalities present?
Are complications present?
Is the process evolving as expected?
Is the infection chronic?

SUGGESTED READINGS

Dunn JJ, Miller MB. Emerging respiratory viruses other than influenza. *Clin Lab Med.* 2014;34:409–430.

Herold CJ, Sailer JG. Community-acquired and nosocomial pneumonia. *Eur Radiol.* 2004;14(suppl 3):E2–E20.

Mandell LA, Wunderink RG, Anzueto A, et al. Infectious Diseases Society of America/American Thoracic Society consensus guidelines on the management of community-acquired pneumonia in adults. *Clin Infect Dis.* 2007;44(suppl 2):S27–S72.

Miller WT Jr, Mickus TJ, Barbosa E Jr, et al. CT of viral lower respiratory tract infections in adults: comparison among viral organisms and between viral and bacterial infections. *AJR Am J Roentgenol.* 2011;197:1088–1095.

Muller NL, Franquet T, Kyung SL. *Imaging of Pulmonary Infections.* Philadelphia: Lippincott Williams and Wilkins; 2006.

Musher DM, Thorner AR. Community-acquired pneumonia. *N Engl J Med.* 2014;371:1619–1628.

Prather AD, Smith TR, Poletto DM, et al. Aspiration-related lung diseases. *J Thoracic Imaging.* 2014;29:304–309.

Reimer LG. Community-acquired bacterial pneumonias. *Semin Respir Infect.* 2000;15:95–100.

Vilar J, Domingo ML, Soto C, et al. Radiology of bacterial pneumonia. *Eur J Radiol.* 2004;51:102–113.

Walker CM, Abbott GF, Greene RE, et al. Imaging pulmonary infection: classic signs and patterns. *AJR Am J Roentgenol.* 2014;202:479–492.

Chapter 15

Pulmonary Disease in the Immunocompromised Patient

Hristina Natcheva

INTRODUCTION

Infection with the human immunodeficiency virus (HIV) that causes the acquired immunodeficiency syndrome (AIDS) has been and continues to be a serious health threat around the globe. Despite great advances in the treatment of HIV/AIDS, such as the aggressive use of prophylactic antimicrobial therapies and the introduction of highly effective antiretroviral therapies, it remains a major cause of morbidity and mortality in populations with limited access to care, such as in sub-Saharan Africa, Eastern Europe, and Central Asia.

Highly active antiretroviral therapy (HAART) has been associated with a dramatic reduction in HIV-associated morbidity and mortality among patients with access to this treatment. By suppressing viral replication, it decreases the viral load and increases the CD4 cell count. Patients receiving HAART have a reduced prevalence of opportunistic infections and certain neoplasms. However, restoration of the immune system in patients treated with antiretroviral therapy may sometimes result in the immune reconstitution inflammatory syndrome (IRIS), which can cause considerable morbidity. Moreover, ART itself is increasingly implicated as a cause of respiratory symptoms and disease, including nucleoside-induced lactic acidosis, an increased incidence of bacterial pneumonia, and hypersensitivity reactions.

In April 2014, the Centers for Disease Control and Prevention (CDC) revised the definition of HIV infection to address multiple issues, the most important of which was the need to adapt to recent changes in diagnostic criteria. Laboratory criteria for defining a confirmed case now accommodate new multitest algorithms, including criteria for differentiating between HIV-1 and HIV-2 infection and for recognizing early HIV infection. A confirmed case can be classified in one of five HIV infection stages (0, 1, 2, 3, or unknown); early infection, recognized by a negative HIV test within 6 months of HIV diagnosis, is classified as stage 0, and acquired immunodeficiency syndrome (AIDS) is classified as stage 3, when the immune system of a person infected with HIV becomes severely compromised (CD4 cell count <200 cells/μL) or the person becomes ill with an opportunistic infection. Criteria for stage 3 (AIDS) have been simplified by eliminating the need to differentiate between definitive and presumptive diagnoses of opportunistic illnesses. Stage 1 is defined as acute infection, a time during which large amounts of the virus are being produced, and is characterized by flulike symptoms. Stage 2 is defined as clinical latency during which the virus replicates at very low levels but is still active. During this stage, the patient may be asymptomatic and with proper treatment can live for decades. Without treatment, this period lasts on average 10 years, but some patients may progress faster.

There is considerable overlap in the imaging manifestations of the various pulmonary complications of HIV/AIDS. Furthermore, the chest radiograph may be normal even when pulmonary disease is present. However, by carefully correlating clinical, laboratory, and imaging data with results of sputum analysis, bronchoalveolar lavage, and transbronchial biopsy, a confident diagnosis can usually be made. Computed tomography (CT) is useful in diagnosis or exclusion of pulmonary complications when radiographs are normal. It is also helpful in limiting the differential diagnosis when radiography is abnormal.

Box 15.1 summarizes the respiratory disorders associated with HIV/AIDS.

PULMONARY DISEASES

Major categories of disease involving the lungs in HIV-infected patients include infections, neoplastic entities, such as Kaposi sarcoma, lymphoma, and lung cancer, and lymphoproliferative disorders.

Pulmonary Infections

Bacterial Infection

The rate of bacterial pneumonia in HIV-infected patients has dropped considerably since the introduction of ART. However, this decline was not as dramatic as the overall decline in opportunistic pneumonia in the ART era. ART has thus transformed the epidemiology of pulmonary infections, particularly in developed countries, and bacterial pneumonia has become the most common cause of respiratory infection in HIV-infected individuals. Bacterial pneumonia is 10 to 25 times more common in HIV-infected patients than in the general population. Recurrent bacterial pneumonia is an AIDS-defining disease. A variety of HIV-induced immune abnormalities increase the risk of infection, particularly by encapsulated bacteria. Cigarette smoking and intravenous

BOX 15.1 HIV-Associated Respiratory Disorders

INFECTION

Bacterial Pneumonia

Streptococcus pneumoniae
Haemophilus influenzae
Pseudomonas aeruginosa
Staphylococcus aureus
Moraxella catarrhalis

Mycobacteria

Mycobacterium tuberculosis
Mycobacterium kansasii
Mycobacterium avium complex
Other non-tuberculous mycobacteria

Fungal Infections

Pneumocystis jirovecii
Cryptococcus neoformans
Histoplasma capsulatum
Aspergillus fumigatus
Coccidioides immitis
Blastomyces dermatitides

Protozoal Infections

Strongyloides stercoralis
Toxoplasma gondii

Viral Infections

Cytomegalovirus
Adenovirus
Herpes simplex virus

MALIGNANCY

Kaposi sarcoma
Non-Hodgkin lymphoma
Lung cancer

OTHER CONDITIONS

Sinusitis
Bronchitis
Bronchiectasis
Emphysema
LIP, NSIP, COP
Pulmonary hypertension
IRIS

COP, cryptogenic organizing pneumonia; *IRIS*, immune reconstitution inflammatory syndrome; *LIP*, lymphocytic interstitial pneumonitis; *NSIP*, nonspecific interstitial pneumonia.

drug use also increase the risk. Bacterial pneumonia can occur at any CD4 count, but the risk increases as the count drops. The median CD4 count in patients with bacterial pneumonia is 200 cells/μL.

Clinical features of bacterial pneumonia in HIV-infected patients are similar to those in non–HIV-infected patients, but the infection may progress more rapidly, and bacteremia can occur more frequently. *Streptococcus pneumoniae* is the most common cause of community-acquired pneumonia in both HIV-infected patients and the general population, but pneumococcal septicemia is 100 times more common in HIV-infected patients. *Haemophilus influenzae* is the second most common cause, followed by *Staphylococcus aureus*. *S. aureus* and *Pseudomonas aeruginosa* are the main pathogens causing nosocomial bacterial pneumonia in HIV-infected patients, although infection by *P. aeruginosa*

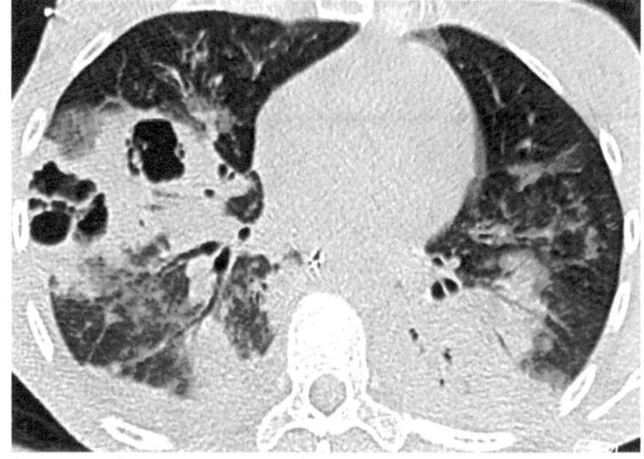

FIGURE 15.1 Fulminant pneumonia caused by multidrug-resistant *Staphylococcus aureus* in a patient with HIV, a history of intravenous drug abuse, and infectious endocarditis. Axial computed tomography image demonstrates multifocal consolidation with cavitation and a right pleural effusion.

has declined in the ART era. *Legionella* infection, although uncommon, has been reported to have a 40-fold higher incidence in AIDS patients.

Similar to its presentation in the general population, bacterial pneumonia typically is seen radiographically as focal consolidation in a segmental or lobar distribution. However, in HIV-positive patients, there is a higher propensity for multilobar and bilateral disease. Bacterial infection may also manifest as cavitary nodules or consolidation that resembles mycobacterial or fungal infection. This pattern usually results from infection with *P. aeruginosa* or *Staphylococcus aureus* (Fig. 15.1). The latter organism is usually responsible for septic emboli, which typically occur in patients with a history of intravenous drug use and tricuspid endocarditis. *S. aureus* infection may also predispose to empyema. More than half of *H. influenzae* infections manifest with bilateral interstitial opacities, mimicking *Pneumocystis* pneumonia.

HIV-infected patients are also at increased risk for developing infectious airways disease, such as bacterial tracheobronchitis and bronchiolitis. Chest radiographs are usually normal, but they may demonstrate bronchial wall thickening or a subtle reticulonodular pattern. Chest CT, particularly high-resolution CT (HRCT), is more sensitive than radiographs for detecting inflammation of the bronchi and bronchioles, and it may demonstrate bronchial wall thickening and tree-in-bud opacities even when the chest radiograph appears normal.

Despite the availability of ART and the plateauing of mortality rates for HIV infection, *M. tuberculosis* remains a major threat to HIV-infected patients. Tuberculosis (TB)-related deaths in people living with HIV have fallen by 32% since 2004, but it remains the leading cause of death among people living with HIV, accounting for around one in three AIDS-related deaths. The risk of developing TB is 50 times higher for an HIV-infected patient than for the average person. Moreover, drug-resistant TB is more common among HIV-infected patients than non–HIV-infected patients.

The imaging patterns of TB in HIV-infected patients vary depending on CD4 count. Above 200 cells/μL, a reactivation TB pattern predominates, with classic findings of upper lung consolidation and nodules, which may cavitate (Fig. 15.2). Endobronchial spread of TB manifests as centrilobular nodules in a tree-in-bud configuration. At a CD4 count of

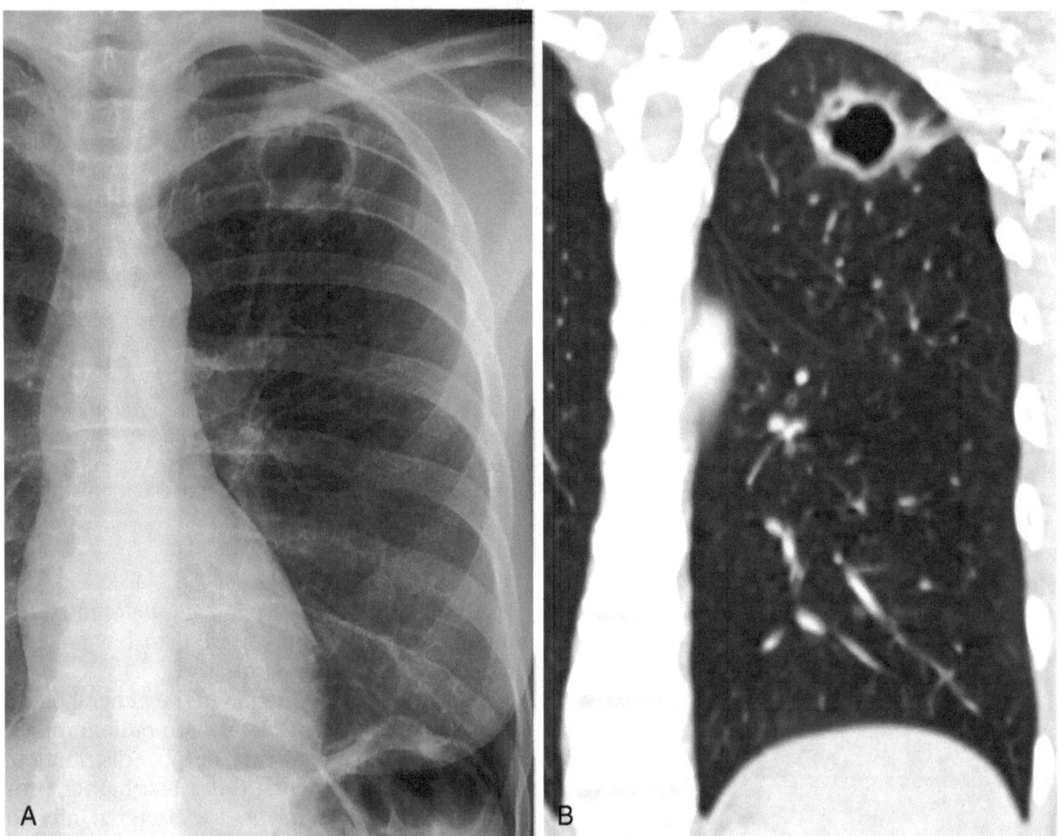

FIGURE 15.2 Tuberculosis in an HIV-infected patient. Frontal radiograph **(A)** demonstrates a cavitary nodule in the left upper lobe. Coronal computed tomography reformatted image **(B)** shows a thick-walled irregular cavity in the left upper lobe that on bronchoscopy revealed abundant acid-fast bacilli consistent with tuberculosis.

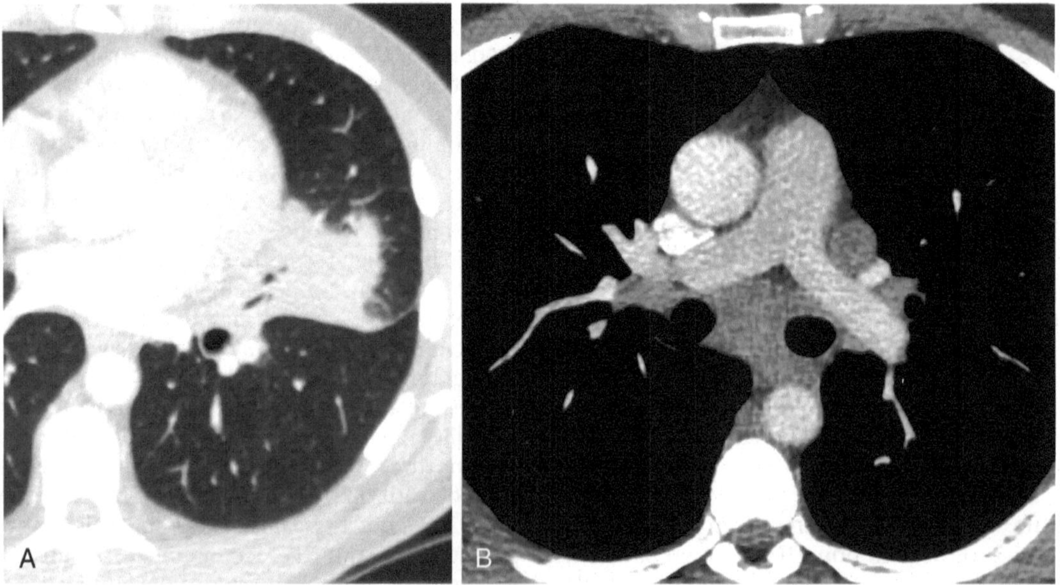

FIGURE 15.3 Tuberculosis in an HIV-infected patient. **A,** Axial computed tomography (CT) image demonstrates perihilar consolidation in the lingula. **B,** Axial CT image demonstrates bilateral hilar and subcarinal lymphadenopathy.

50 to 200 cells/μL, reactivation TB resembles primary TB at imaging and can manifest as mediastinal lymphadenopathy occasionally with rim enhancement and low-attenuation central necrosis (Fig. 15.3). A miliary pattern of TB can also be seen at this stage of HIV infection. Below 50 cells/μL, findings are not specific and include diffuse consolidation, ground-glass opacities, and pleural effusion. Compared with normal hosts, AIDS patients with TB are more likely to present with diffuse lung disease, bronchogenic spread, miliary disease, and extrapulmonary disease. The chest

radiograph may be normal for up to 20% of patients with TB who are in the advanced stages of AIDS.

Infection by atypical mycobacteria such as *Mycobacterium avium-intracellulare* (MAC) and *Mycobacterium kansasii* organisms is also an important cause of morbidity and mortality in people with AIDS. In this setting, MAC is a disseminated disease, with the gastrointestinal tract serving as the main entry site in most cases. Only 5% of patients have pulmonary involvement. Radiologic manifestations include adenopathy, nodules, and focal consolidation with cavitation.

Mycobacteria are the most commonly implicated infectious organisms in the paradoxical symptomatic deterioration of patients recently started on ART. IRIS should be considered when a patient recently started on ART develops fever accompanied by new thoracic abnormalities, such as lymphadenopathy, parenchymal consolidation, or pleural effusion. Treatment is aimed at the underlying infection, but severely symptomatic patients may also benefit from steroid therapy.

Fungal Infection

Fungi are ubiquitous and a common cause of recurrent symptoms during the course of AIDS-related illnesses because efficient eradication is difficult without a competent cell-mediated immune response. Despite a substantial decline in prevalence because of widespread prophylaxis, *Pneumocystis jirovecii* pneumonia (PJP) is still the most common life-threatening opportunistic respiratory infection in patients with HIV or AIDS, even in developed countries, where it may be the first presenting illness in patients with previously unrecognized HIV infection. It occurs predominantly in patients with a CD4 count less than 200 cells/mm^2. The diagnosis can often be made on induced sputum samples or bronchoalveolar lavage. Several polymerase chain reaction (PCR)-based molecular assays have been developed to aid the diagnosis of this organism, which cannot be grown in culture.

On chest radiographs, PJP typically manifests with diffuse or perihilar fine reticular or ground-glass opacities (Fig. 15.4, *A*). Untreated, these opacities may progress to diffuse homogeneous opacification in 3 to 4 days. Chest radiography may appear normal at presentation in up to 6% of symptomatic patients. Hilar and mediastinal lymphadenopathy is rare, as is pleural fluid in the absence of extrapulmonary pneumocystosis.

The CT appearance of PJP usually consists of scattered or diffuse ground-glass opacities, which may be identified even when the radiograph is normal (Fig. 15.4, *B* and *C*). Other CT findings may include consolidation and thickening of the interlobular septa. Atypical manifestations of PJP include nodules, focal lesions, adenopathy, and miliary disease. Up to one third of patients develop thin-walled air cysts (i.e., pneumatoceles), which may lead to pneumothorax (Fig. 15.5). These pneumothoraces are often refractory to chest tube drainage and are associated with an increased mortality rate.

Other fungal infections are rare and account for fewer than 5% of pneumonias in HIV-positive patients, although a higher prevalence may be observed in endemic areas. They include infections with *Cryptococcus*, *Candida*, and *Aspergillus* spp. and endemic fungi such as *Coccidioides*, *Histoplasma*, and *Blastomyces* spp., and they often take

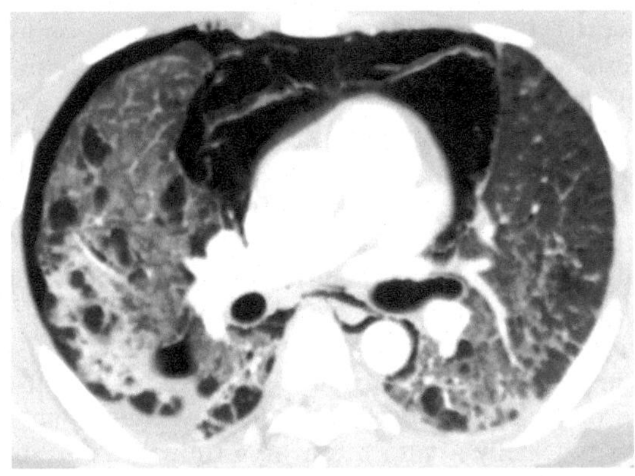

FIGURE 15.5 An axial computed tomography image of the chest in a patient with HIV and *Pneumocystis jirovecii* pneumonia demonstrates diffuse ground-glass opacity, interlobular septal thickening, patchy consolidation, and scattered cysts. Also noted are a small right pneumothorax and moderate pneumomediastinum.

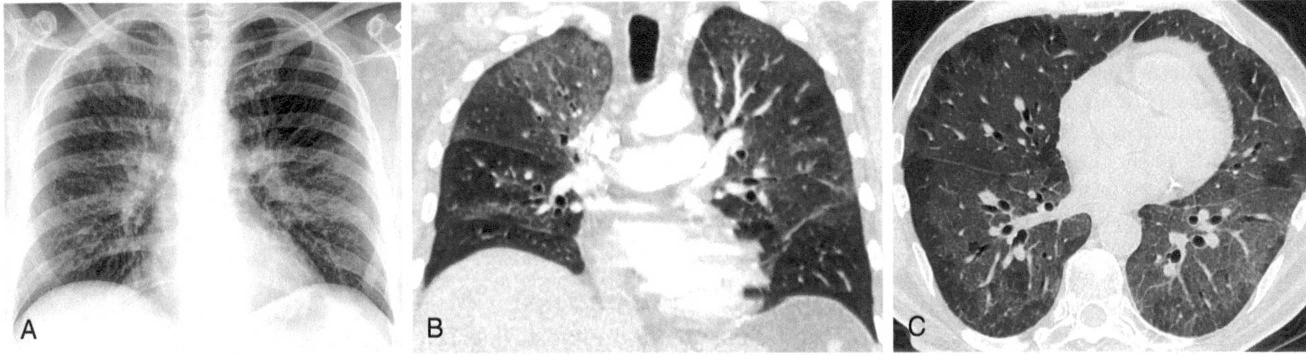

FIGURE 15.4 *Pneumocystis jirovecii* pneumonia (PJP) in an HIV-infected patient with a markedly low CD4 count. **A,** Frontal radiograph of the chest demonstrates diffuse hazy and reticular opacities throughout both lungs, more pronounced in the mid and upper lung zones. **B,** Coronal computed tomography (CT) from the same patient shows a corresponding diffuse ground-glass opacity in the mid and upper lung zones with relative sparing of the lung bases. **C,** Axial high-resolution CT image from a different patient with PJP shows bilateral diffuse ground-glass opacity.

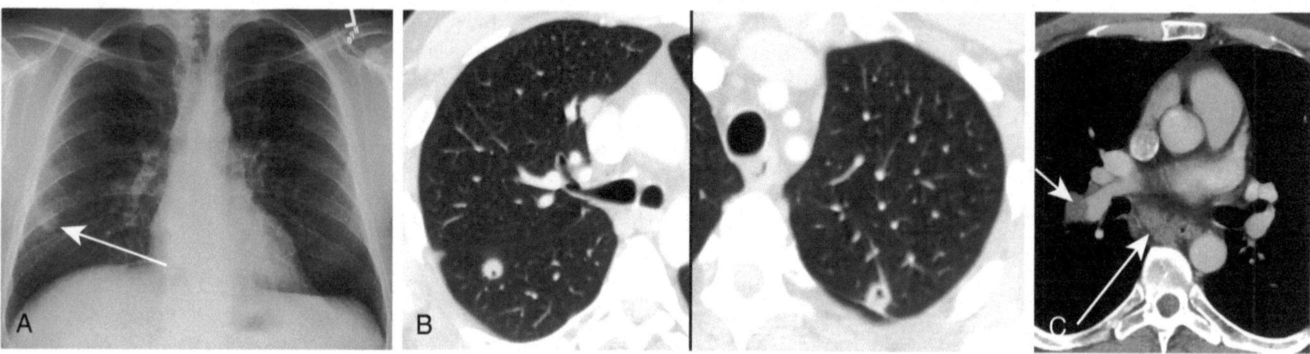

FIGURE 15.6 *Cryptococcus neoformans* pulmonary infection in an HIV-positive patient. **A,** Frontal chest radiograph demonstrates a peripheral nodule in the right lower lung zone *(arrow)*. **B,** Axial computed tomography (CT) images of the right and left lungs from the same patient demonstrate multiple pulmonary nodules, some of which are cavitary. **C,** Axial CT image shows right hilar and subcarinal lymphadenopathy *(arrows)*.

the form of disseminated disease. Radiologic findings are nonspecific, and pleural effusions are common, as is adenopathy, which is rare with *Pneumocystis* pneumonia and bacterial pneumonias.

Cryptococcus neoformans is a ubiquitous fungus that infects up to 2% of HIV-infected patients with markedly reduced CD4 count (<100 cells/μL) and most commonly manifests with meningitis. The lungs are the most common site of involvement outside the central nervous system (CNS), affected in 2% to 15% of AIDS patients with respiratory tract infection. Radiologic features include diffuse heterogeneous or reticulonodular opacities, as well as discrete nodules with or without cavitation (Fig. 15.6). Pleural effusions and adenopathy may occur. Miliary disease, indistinguishable from TB, has also been reported.

Candida albicans is a normal commensal organism of the skin and mouth. In advanced cases of AIDS, it usually causes oral and esophageal candidiasis. Pulmonary candidiasis is usually a late, often preterminal manifestation of HIV infection in the setting of disseminated disease. The imaging manifestations are nonspecific, with diffuse heterogeneous or homogeneous opacities or nodules with or without cavitation.

Histoplasmosis is important in the HIV-positive patient in endemic areas. *Histoplasma* lung disease usually represents a disseminated infection, and the typical radiographic pattern is micronodular (miliary) (Fig. 15.7).

Viral Infection

Viral infections are a rare cause of significant clinical disease in HIV-positive patients. Most cases of viral disease are caused by cytomegalovirus (CMV) and are usually reactivations of latent infection. Although frequently recovered from the lungs, CMV is not considered a significant pathogen in most cases. Clinically significant cases of CMV pneumonitis may rarely occur, typically in the setting of advanced immune suppression and extrathoracic CMV infection. CT findings include ground-glass opacities, dense consolidation, nodules, bronchial wall thickening or bronchiectasis, and diffuse reticular opacities.

Malignant Neoplasms

Kaposi sarcoma and non-Hodgkin lymphoma are the major neoplasms encountered in patients with AIDS and are probably mediated by viral infection. Therefore, they may be considered as a complication of opportunistic infection. Decreased cytotoxic T cells and natural killer cells may also predispose HIV-infected patients to development of neoplasms.

Kaposi Sarcoma

Kaposi sarcoma remains the most common malignancy in AIDS patients worldwide, but its prevalence has markedly declined in the Western world with the advent of ART. It is mostly seen in homosexual and bisexual men and is associated with the human herpesvirus 8 (HHV8), also referred to as Kaposi sarcoma herpesvirus. It manifests as proliferations of vascular or lymphatic endothelial cells with associated spindle cells, which form multiple slitlike spaces trapping erythrocytes and giving the lesions their purple color. One third of AIDS patients with Kaposi sarcoma have pulmonary involvement, and in 10% to 15% of cases, it is clinically apparent. Pulmonary involvement is associated with mucocutaneous involvement in 85% of cases. Most patients with pulmonary involvement have CD4 counts less than 100 cells/mm^2.

Radiographic features of Kaposi sarcoma include segmental, lobar, or masslike pulmonary opacities caused by tumor infiltration, usually in a perihilar and peribronchovascular distribution. Endobronchial disease may cause atelectasis or postobstructive pneumonia. Disseminated pulmonary disease is frequent and is usually bronchocentric in distribution (Fig. 15.8). Pleural effusions and lymphadenopathy are common. On HRCT, the pattern consists of an axial distribution of nodular or more confluent opacities, with thickening of the bronchovascular bundles. These opacities are sometimes described as "flame shaped" and may have a surrounding rim of ground-glass opacity, which is thought to represent hemorrhage (Fig. 15.9). Thickened interlobular septa are frequently observed.

Lymphoma

Lymphoma typically is seen in the late stages of AIDS and is usually disseminated at the time of diagnosis, involving the CNS, liver, or gastrointestinal tract. It is usually extranodal in distribution, and 25% of patients have thoracic involvement. The prognosis is extremely poor. Non-Hodgkin rather than Hodgkin lymphoma predominates in patients with AIDS and is typically of high-grade B-cell origin, associated with

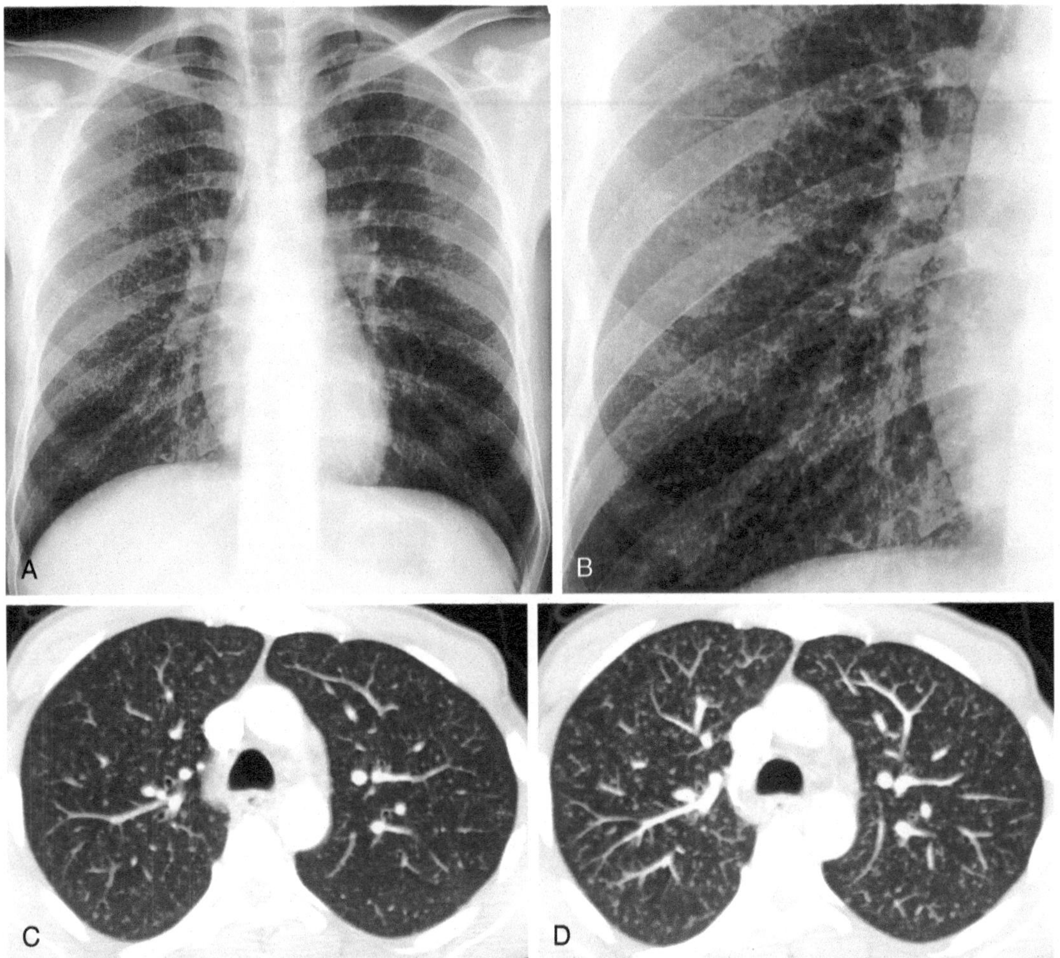

FIGURE 15.7 Disseminated *Histoplasma capsulatum* infection in an HIV-positive patient. Frontal radiograph **(A)** of the chest demonstrates diffuse miliary nodular opacities throughout both lungs, with a magnified view of the right lower lung shown in **(B)**. Axial computed tomography image **(C)** and axial maximum intensity projection reconstructed image **(D)** from the same patient reveal innumerable small randomly distributed nodules throughout both lungs in a miliary pattern.

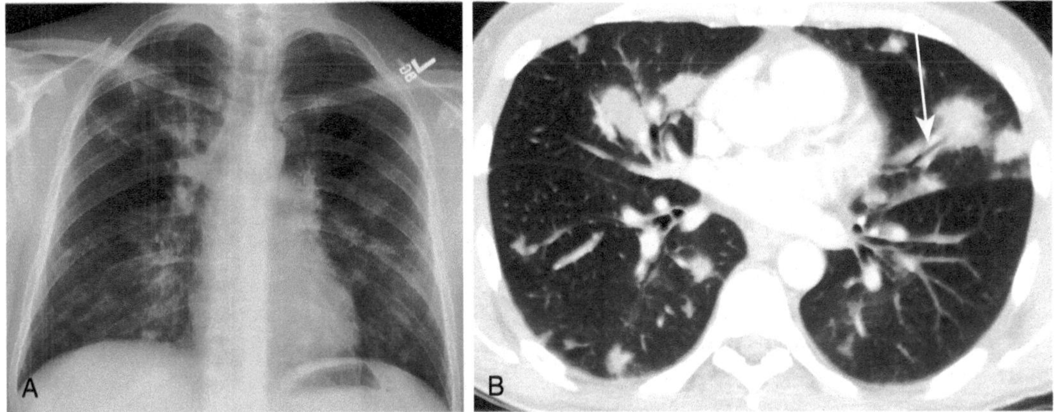

FIGURE 15.8 Kaposi sarcoma in an HIV-infected patient. **A,** Frontal radiograph of the chest demonstrates bilateral predominantly perihilar patchy opacities with poorly defined margins. **B,** Axial computed tomography image from the same patient reveals multiple bilateral nodules in a peribronchovascular distribution, some of which demonstrate air bronchograms *(arrow)*.

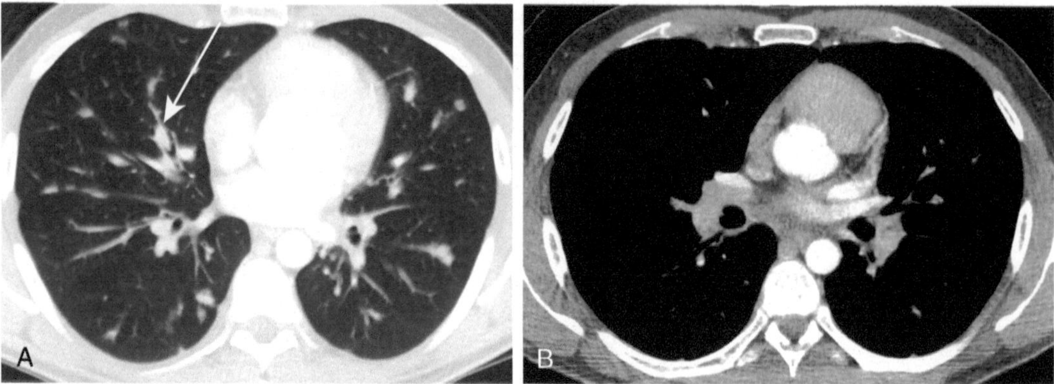

FIGURE 15.9 Kaposi sarcoma with lymphadenopathy. **A,** Axial computed tomography image demonstrates multiple bilateral peribronchovascular nodules, some of which are elongated and "flame shaped" *(arrow)*. **B,** Bilateral hilar lymphadenopathy is present.

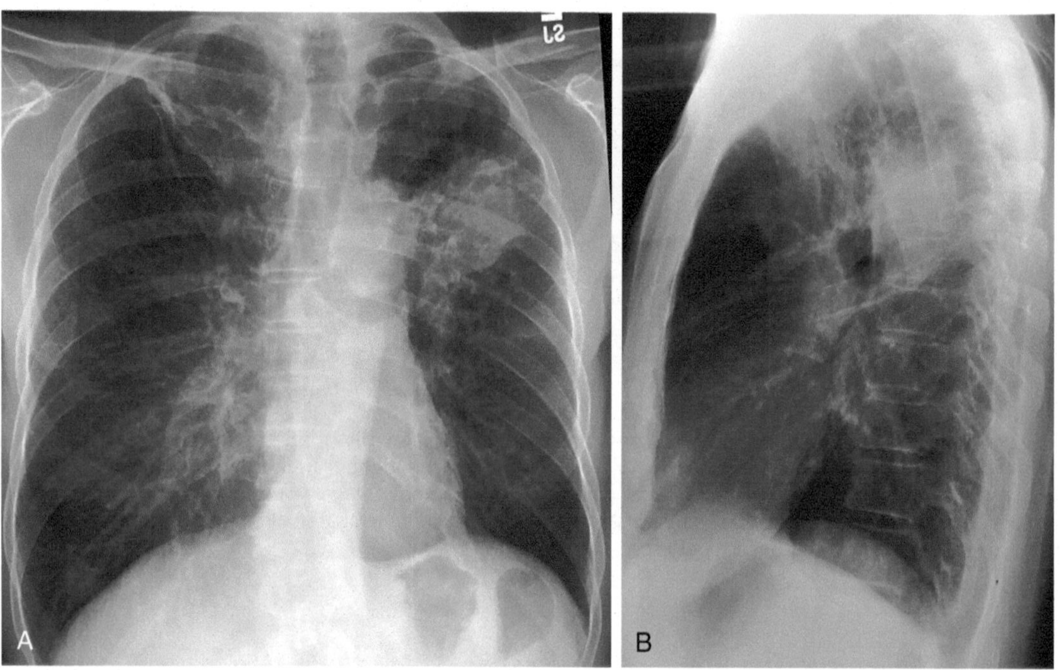

FIGURE 15.10 Frontal **(A)** and lateral **(B)** radiographs of the chest in a patient with AIDS demonstrating a posterior left upper lobe mass, which was found to be a primary lung cancer.

Epstein-Barr virus. Radiologically, lymphoma may manifest as nonspecific, bilateral, diffuse opacities, discrete nodules or masses or pleural effusions. Mediastinal adenopathy may occur, but it is less common than in non-AIDS patients.

Lung Cancer

Although not considered an AIDS-related neoplasm, the overall rate of lung cancer is increased among patients infected with HIV with a history of cigarette smoking compared with the general population of smokers. Unlike Kaposi sarcoma and lymphoma, there is no association with progressive immunosuppression. Lung cancer may occur at any stage of HIV infection. Patients with lung cancer and HIV infection are often younger and present at a more advanced stage of disease compared with the general population. However, the thoracic radiologic manifestations of lung cancer in HIV are similar to those in the general population and include a lung nodule or mass, often accompanied by intrathoracic lymphadenopathy (Fig. 15.10).

Lymphoproliferative Disorders

Lymphoproliferative disorders include lymphocytic interstitial pneumonitis (LIP), atypical lymphoproliferative disorder, and mucosa-associated lymphoid tissue (MALT). These are pulmonary complications of HIV that may occur in the absence of a detectable opportunistic infection or neoplasm.

Lymphocytic interstitial pneumonitis is a diffuse pulmonary disorder characterized by infiltration of the interstitium by lymphocytes, plasma cells, and histiocytes. It is thought to represent a lymphoid hyperplasia in response to chronic antigenic stimulus by HIV. It is much more common in children. Radiologic features are similar to, and often indistinguishable from, those of other infectious and noninfectious entities. LIP may present as a diffuse pattern with nodules 1 to 5 mm in diameter or a reticulonodular pattern. CT can reveal a variety of findings, including micronodules, thickening of the bronchovascular bundles and interlobular septa, and small cysts. Less common is patchy airspace disease. LIP is steroid responsive and not premalignant.

Atypical lymphoproliferative disorder is characterized by infiltration of the interstitium by a polymorphous population of atypical cells. MALT is characterized by infiltration of the bronchial epithelium by atypical lymphoid tissue (see Chapter 21).

Other Pulmonary Disorders

Other pulmonary disorders that may be observed in patients with HIV infection or AIDS include nonspecific interstitial pneumonitis, bronchiolitis obliterans, cryptogenic organizing pneumonia, emphysema, and bronchiectasis. These entities have similar manifestations in HIV-infected patients and the general population, and they are discussed separately in other chapters.

OTHER FORMS OF IMMUNOCOMPROMISE

Non–HIV-positive immunocompromised hosts include patients with hematologic malignancies such as lymphoma and leukemia, recipients of organ transplants, patients treated aggressively with cytotoxic drugs for solid tumors, and those receiving high-dose corticosteroid therapy for collagen vascular and other disorders.

Seventy-five percent of pulmonary complications in the immunocompromised patient are caused by infection. When the patient has severe neutropenia, the proportion increases to 90%. In the remaining few, pulmonary complications are caused by other conditions such as extension of malignancy (e.g., lymphoma or metastases), drug toxicity, or other noninfectious processes such as pulmonary edema or emboli. The mortality rate associated with pulmonary disease in the immunocompromised patient is often as high as 50%. Imaging yields a specific diagnosis in a minority of cases. In most instances, all that can be expected is a reasonable differential diagnosis that must be correlated with clinical and laboratory findings. The role of imaging includes detection of an abnormality, analysis of its imaging features with regard to differential diagnosis or possible diagnostic intervention (e.g., percutaneous needle biopsy), and monitoring response to therapy or development of complications.

Although the imaging features in most opportunistic infections are relatively nonspecific, there are three major patterns that should be considered because they generally correlate with the microorganism producing the pneumonia. These include (1) lobar or segmental consolidation, (2) nodules with rapid growth and/or cavitation, and (3) diffuse lung disease.

Radiologic Patterns of Pulmonary Infections

Lobar or Segmental Consolidation

Bacteria are the most common cause of pneumonia in immunocompromised hosts. In general, the clinical and imaging characteristics of bacterial pneumonia do not differ from those seen in the general population. Patients with neutropenia may show a slight lag in the appearance of pulmonary consolidation. On occasion, bacterial pneumonias may become widely disseminated in the lungs of immunocompromised patients. Radiographic features include localized dense consolidation, which may be lobar or segmental. Cavitation is frequently seen. Cavities may be solitary or multiple. Patchy multilobar pneumonia may also occur. Pleural effusions if present are typically small, and empyemas are unusual. Occasionally, the chest radiograph may be normal, especially in the setting of neutropenia. Colonization of the oral pharynx by altered flora in the presence of reduced lung defense mechanisms leads to a preponderance of gram-negative bacillary pneumonias. They include *Escherichia coli* and *Klebsiella*, *Enterobacter*, *Pseudomonas*, *Proteus*, and *Serratia* spp. Among gram-positive organisms, staphylococci are the most common. Fungal infection and TB may also manifest as consolidation in this patient population.

Legionnaires disease bacterium (*Legionella pneumophila*) and Pittsburgh pneumonia agent (*Legionella micdadei*) are causes of acute bronchopneumonia in the immunocompromised host, particularly in patients receiving corticosteroid therapy and renal transplant recipients. *L. pneumophila* pneumonia is a rapidly progressive disease that begins with focal consolidation but may spread to involve both lungs diffusely. CT shows multifocal peribronchovascular consolidation and scattered ground-glass opacities. Cavitation and pleural effusion are uncommon in the immunocompetent population but may occur in the compromised host. The Pittsburgh agent is particularly associated with dialysis patients and has a tendency to produce fairly well-circumscribed nodular opacities, which commonly cavitate.

Nocardia asteroides infection is fairly common in immunocompromised patients, particularly those receiving corticosteroids. It generally does not cause a fulminant, rapidly progressive pulmonary infection. It is a filamentous, gram-positive bacillus that grows very slowly on aerobic culture and causes single or multiple chronic cavitating lung lesions similar to those caused by pyogenic bacteria or TB. Mediastinal adenopathy and pleural involvement, either fibrous thickening or empyema, are frequent. Radiographic findings are variable, with consolidation being the most common feature, although nodular manifestations may occur. Consolidation can be unifocal, multifocal, lobar, segmental, or nodular. Cavitation, when present, may result in the formation of a thick-walled abscess, which may be hard to distinguish from malignancy. Chest wall invasion occasionally occurs (Fig. 15.11). The diagnosis can occasionally be made on sputum smears or cultures, but invasive procedures are usually required.

Tuberculosis and non-tuberculous mycobacterial infections, although important in the AIDS population, are uncommon in other immunosuppressed patients. TB, when it occurs in this setting, has a high fatality rate. The radiologic features of pulmonary TB are usual and consist of apical and posterior segmental disease in the upper lobes with or without the development of cavitation. These features are more thoroughly discussed in Chapter 16 on mycobacterial infections.

There is a limited differential diagnosis of lobar or segmental consolidation in the immunosuppressed patient.

Pulmonary lymphoma may appear as a chronic focal consolidation with air bronchograms.

Nodules and Masses With Rapid Growth or Cavitation

Multiple nodules with rapid growth or cavitation are most frequently caused by fungal infection in the immunocompromised host, but *Staphylococcus* and *Pseudomonas* can also manifest as growing nodules. The fungi typically isolated include the commensals such as *Aspergillus*, *Candida*, and *Mucor* spp. and true pathogenic fungi such as *Cryptococcus* spp. Fungal pneumonia characteristically develops in patients with hematologic malignancies who are neutropenic from cytotoxic drugs or who are receiving or have just completed a course of broad-spectrum antibiotics for fever of unknown origin.

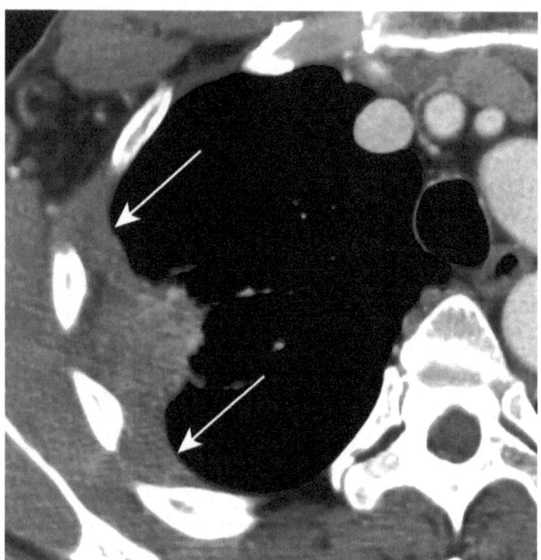

FIGURE 15.11 *Nocardia asteroides* pulmonary infection in a severely neutropenic patient. An axial computed tomography image demonstrates a large subpleural masslike consolidation that mimics a primary lung cancer. There is pleural thickening *(arrows)* and effacement of the extrapleural fat suggestive of chest wall invasion.

Aspergillus fumigatus is the most common fungal pulmonary infection in immunosuppressed patients, particularly those with hematologic malignancies. It causes an invasive necrotizing pneumonia secondary to invasion of small and medium-sized blood vessels with accompanying in situ pulmonary infarction, hemorrhage, and ultimately systemic dissemination. It may also infect the airways, causing a necrotizing tracheobronchitis.

Airway-invasive aspergillosis varies in its radiographic appearance based on the stage, severity, and extent of disease. In its early stages, imaging may be normal. As the disease progresses, either focal or diffuse nodular opacities are seen on radiography, with CT showing bronchocentric abnormalities such as bronchial wall thickening, peribronchial consolidation or ground-glass opacity, centrilobular nodules, and rarely bronchiectasis.

Angioinvasive aspergillosis is the most feared form of pulmonary aspergillosis and occurs in only the most severely immunocompromised patients. The radiographic features consist of multiple nodular areas of consolidation often abutting the pleural surfaces, which may demonstrate air bronchograms and may invade adjacent soft tissue structures. These frequently cavitate and may show crescentic radiolucencies around the parenchymal opacities, the *air crescent* sign that may mimic a mycetoma. This sign can also be identified on CT studies (Fig. 15.12). Another characteristic finding is nodular or masslike consolidation surrounded by ground-glass opacity, the *halo sign,* related to adjacent hemorrhage (Fig. 15.13). Although the halo sign is a very consistent and early finding of angioinvasive aspergillosis,

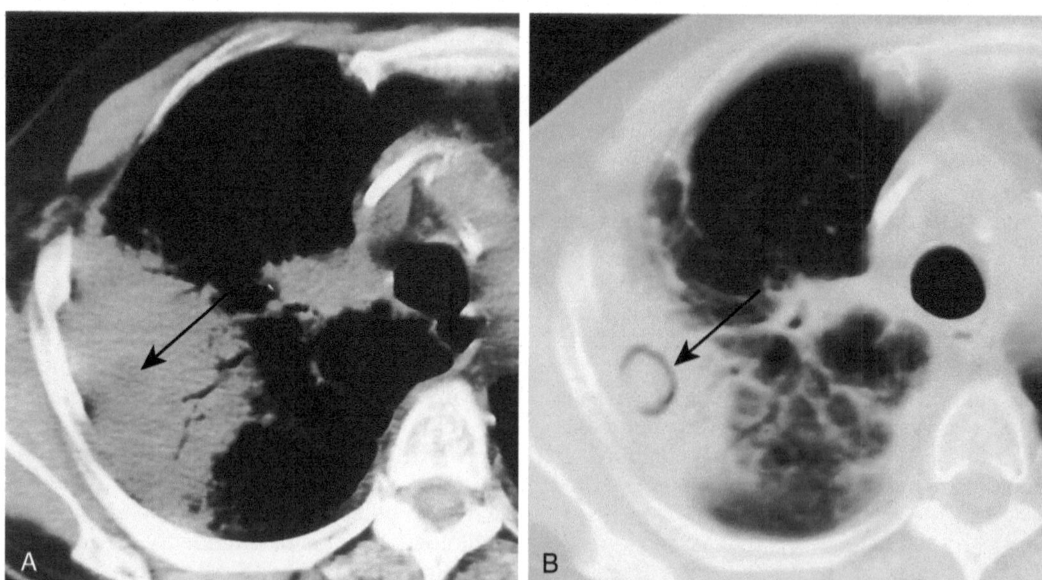

FIGURE 15.12 *Aspergillus fumigatus* infection in a severely immunocompromised patient on chemotherapy. **A,** Axial computed tomography image demonstrates a large area of consolidation in the right lung with a central hypodensity *(arrow)* and air bronchograms. **B,** A subsequent computed tomography shows a nondependent crescentic lucency, the *air crescent sign (arrow),* which indicates parenchymal infarction in the setting of invasive aspergillosis.

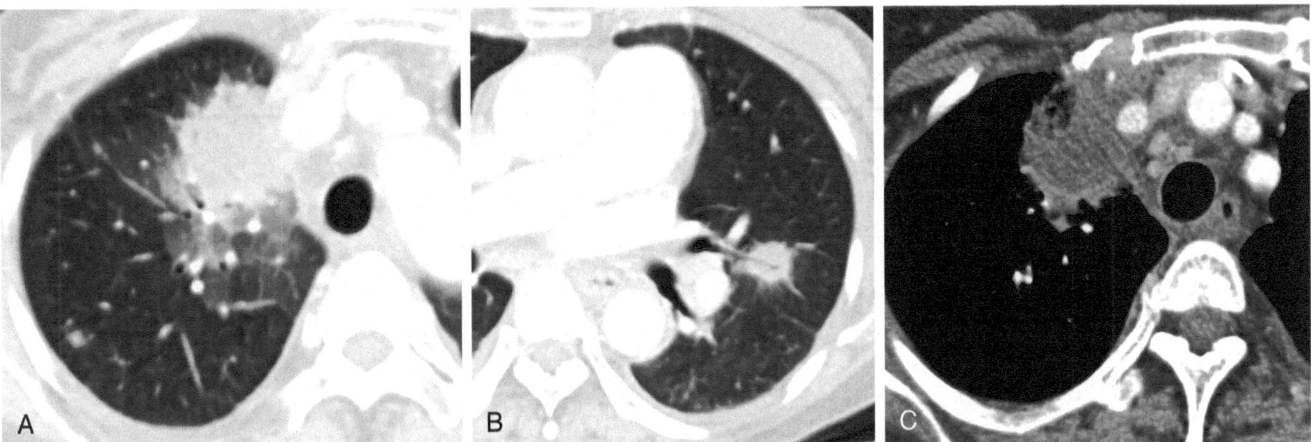

FIGURE 15.13 Invasive aspergillosis in a severely neutropenic patient. **A,** Axial computed tomography (CT) image demonstrates a rounded paramediastinal consolidation in the right upper lobe with surrounding ground-glass opacity known as the *halo sign,* indicative of surrounding hemorrhage. **B,** A left perihilar nodule with an air bronchogram is seen in the contralateral lung. **C,** Axial CT image in soft tissue window shows effacement of the mediastinal fat indicating mediastinal invasion by *Aspergillus.*

it has been described in a variety of other infectious and noninfectious entities. However, in the specific clinical setting of severe neutropenia and fever, it is very suggestive of early invasive fungal infection. Because prognosis is closely linked to early recognition and treatment, the halo sign plays a critical role for early intervention. The diagnosis of *Aspergillus* pneumonia usually requires invasive procedures such as needle aspiration or open-lung biopsy. Fungal hyphae are thin and septate and branch at acute angles of approximately 45 degrees.

Pulmonary disease caused by *Mucor* spp. is clinically and radiographically indistinguishable from that caused by *Aspergillus* spp. because the organism has a predilection for blood vessel invasion with resultant pulmonary infarction. Infection with *Mucor* spp. may demonstrate a rapidly progressive clinical course. It is frequently seen in patients with lymphoproliferative disease, leukopenia, and diabetes, as well as in patients after organ transplantation (Fig. 15.14). The diagnosis depends on identifying the organism by culture or by showing histopathologic evidence of fungal invasion on biopsy. Fungal hyphae are broad and nonseptate and branch at right angles.

Candida spp. may cause pneumonia alone but more commonly do so in association with other fungal pathogens, particularly *Aspergillus* spp. Primary candidal pneumonias are rare in immunosuppressed patients; the lung is more likely to be involved by a disseminated fungemia. The radiologic appearance is nonspecific, and there may be areas of airspace consolidation or nodular opacities (Fig. 15.15). Invasive biopsy is usually required for diagnosis.

Cryptococcal pneumonia, much less common than *Aspergillus* pneumonia, generally occurs in patients with defective cellular immunity rather than in neutropenic hosts. Pulmonary involvement occurs in disseminated disease and is usually overshadowed by cryptococcal meningitis. The radiographic manifestations of pulmonary cryptococcosis consist of single or multiple nodules with or without cavitation. Well-defined lobar or segmental consolidation is uncommon (Fig. 15.16). *Cryptococcus* spp. may be isolated from the sputum or more frequently from the cerebrospinal fluid on lumbar puncture. In some cases, a lung biopsy is required.

The differential diagnosis of the radiographic appearance of multiple nodules in the immunocompromised host is limited and includes metastatic disease or occasionally lymphoma involving the lung parenchyma. In both instances, rapid growth is usually not a feature.

Diffuse Lung Disease

A radiologic pattern of diffuse infiltration of the lungs in the immunocompromised host can be produced by a number of microorganisms, the most common of which are the fungus *P. jiroveci* (formerly *P. carinii*) and a variety of viral agents, including herpes zoster and CMV. A diffuse interstitial pattern can also be seen in nonspecific interstitial pneumonitis, drug reactions, radiation pneumonitis, pulmonary edema or hemorrhage, or lymphangitic carcinomatosis.

Pneumonia caused by *P. jiroveci* has decreased in prevalence after widespread prophylaxis in both HIV and non-HIV immunocompromised patients but remains a major cause of morbidity and mortality. Diagnosis in non-HIV patients can be difficult because the entity may not be initially considered. Also, many affected patients have underlying conditions such as sarcoidosis, Wegener granulomatosis, or drug toxicity, conditions whose imaging characteristics could mask the appearance of PJP. The pneumonia it produces in the non-AIDS population is acute and fulminating, with a mortality rate up to 50%. Therefore, the diagnosis should be strongly suspected in patients with risk factors such as high-dose corticosteroid or cytotoxic therapy who develop characteristic imaging findings. The classic radiographic appearance of PJP includes bilateral perihilar or diffuse symmetric interstitial opacities, which may be finely granular, reticular, or ground glass in appearance. If left untreated, these findings may progress over 3 to 5 days to homogeneous diffuse alveolar consolidation. Hilar adenopathy and pleural effusion are very unusual. CT may reveal areas of *Pneumocystis* pneumonia when the standard chest radiograph is normal. The affected lung parenchyma demonstrates ground-glass opacity without

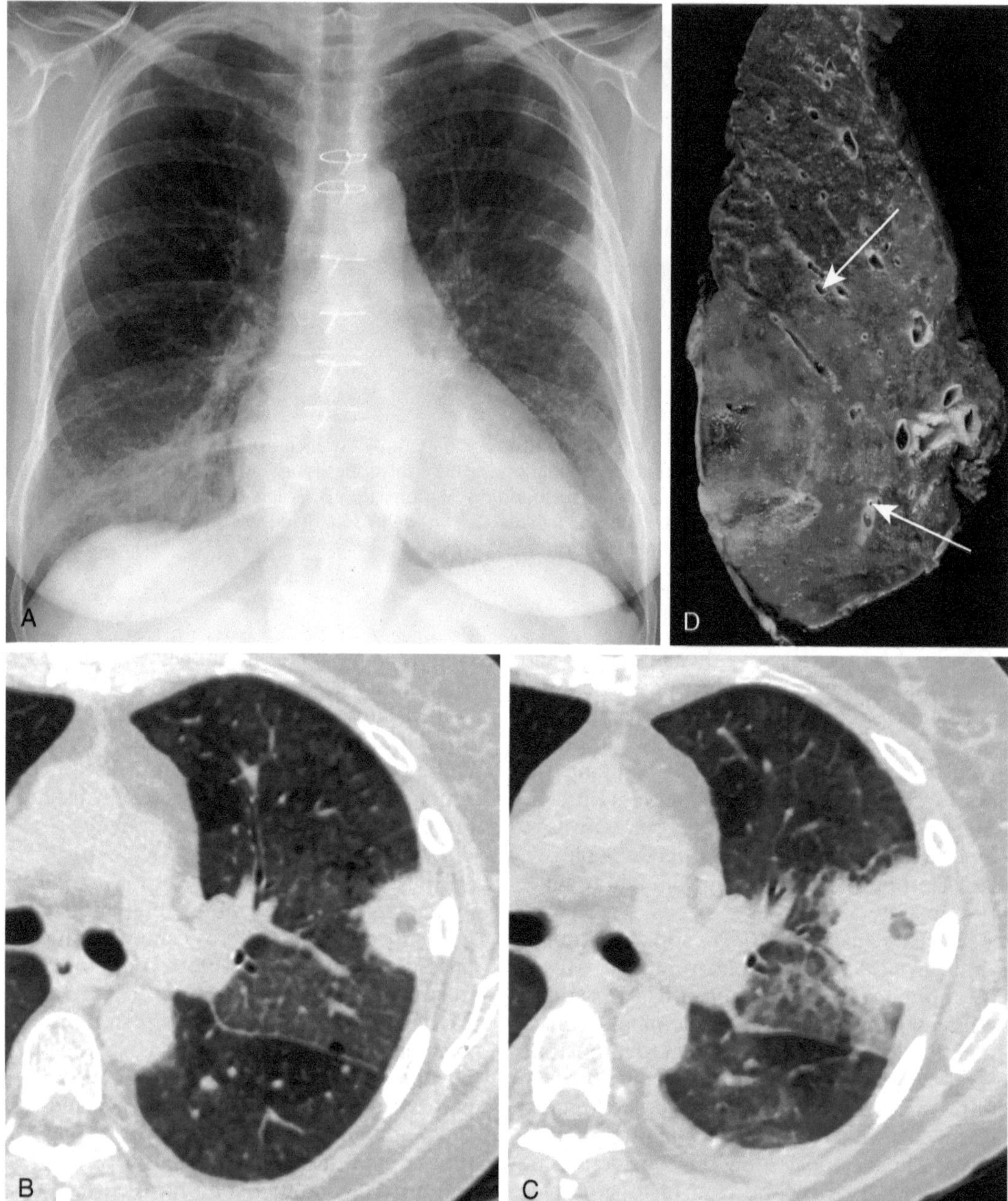

FIGURE 15.14 Pulmonary mucormycosis in an immunocompromised heart transplant recipient. **A,** Frontal radiograph of the chest demonstrates a peripheral nodule in the left upper lobe. **B,** Computed tomography (CT) confirms the presence of a subpleural nodule with adjacent ground-glass opacity and early central cavitation, the differential diagnosis for which includes malignancy or fungal infection. **C,** CT obtained several days later shows rapid growth of the nodule and progressive central necrosis, confirming its infectious etiology. Needle biopsy revealed mucormycosis, and the patient was successfully treated with surgical resection and antibiotics. **D,** Gross specimen reveals central necrosis with surrounding hemorrhage *(arrows)*. Chest wall invasion was identified at surgery.

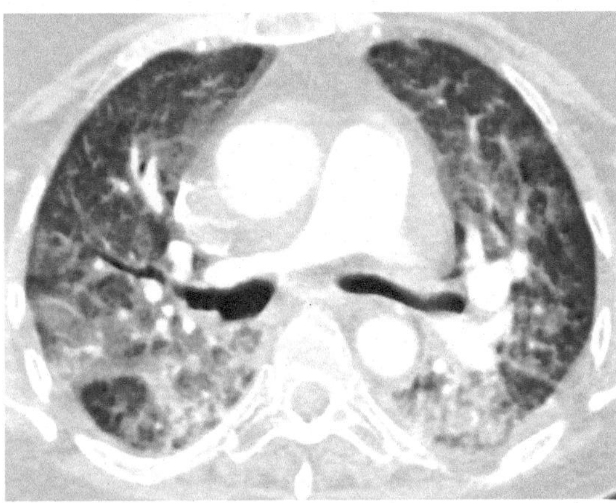

FIGURE 15.15 *Candida albicans* pneumonia in a severely immunocompromised patient on long-term steroid therapy. An axial computed tomography image demonstrates diffuse ground-glass opacities throughout both lungs, with consolidative opacities in the dependent lungs.

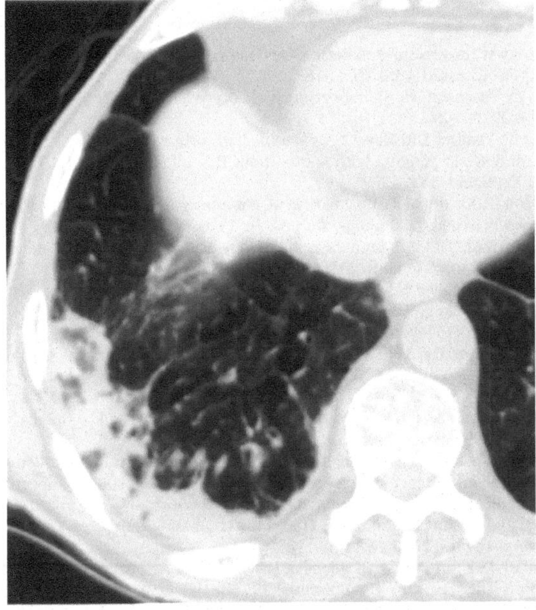

FIGURE 15.16 Cryptococcal pneumonia in an immunocompromised patient on long-term steroids. Axial computed tomography image shows patchy peripheral consolidation in the right lower lobe.

obliteration of normal pulmonary vessels. Because it is not possible to culture these organisms, the diagnosis depends on morphologic identification of *Pneumocystis* in respiratory secretions obtained by bronchoalveolar lavage or from lung tissue.

Organ transplant recipients and patients with hematologic malignancies are at high risk for viral pneumonia. By far, the most common agent of viral pneumonia in these patients is CMV. Infection results from defects in cell-mediated immunity. The diagnosis is complicated by the fact that CMV infection is very common in the general population, and many immunosuppressed patients are latent carriers of the virus. Clinical symptoms and imaging features of CMV pneumonia are nonspecific, and it may often coexist with or even predispose to other pneumonias, particularly PJP. The radiographic appearance of CMV pneumonia is varied. It most commonly manifests as bibasilar patchy opacities, although focal confluent opacities mimicking bacterial pneumonia are occasionally seen, as are pleural effusions. Less common appearances include diffuse reticular or reticulonodular opacities. The chest radiograph can also be normal even in biopsy-proven cases. CT manifestations can be equally varied, ranging from normal to focal or diffuse ground-glass opacities, nodules, masses, consolidations, or reticular opacities (Fig. 15.17). Confirmation of the diagnosis usually requires lung biopsy with identification of characteristic intranuclear inclusion bodies or isolation of virus directly from lung tissue.

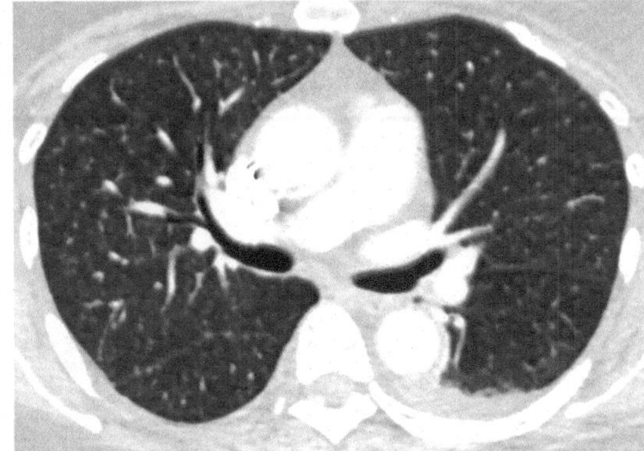

FIGURE 15.17 Pulmonary cytomegalovirus in a severely immunocompromised patient. Axial computed tomography image demonstrates innumerable miliary nodules throughout both lungs and a small left pleural effusion.

Other viral pathogens capable of causing severe pneumonia, especially in patients with lymphoma, are the varicella zoster and herpes simplex viruses. Radiographic findings reflect the fulminant clinical course of disease and include multiple nodular opacities and airspace consolidation (Fig. 15.18). Diagnosis is facilitated if the patient has coincident disseminated herpes zoster or varicella.

The noninfectious causes that produce fever and interstitial opacities in immunocompromised hosts include lymphangitic carcinomatosis, radiation pneumonitis, drug toxicity, and nonspecific interstitial pneumonitis.

Diagnostic and Therapeutic Approach

With regard to host factors, it is important to be aware of the time course for heightened susceptibility to specific infections among certain immunocompromised hosts, especially patients who have received solid organ or hematopoietic stem cell transplants.

Chest radiography is usually the first-line imaging technique used to detect and evaluate respiratory disease in the immunocompromised patient but is limited in its ability to elucidate a specific etiology. In many instances, CT may provide additional information and is particularly useful in identifying complications in immunocompromised patients with symptoms of pneumonia but a normal chest radiograph. Focal abnormalities may be identified on CT in areas that are difficult to evaluate with chest radiography; these areas include the apical, retrocardiac, and subdiaphragmatic lung. CT is also useful in characterizing the nature of radiographically evident abnormalities and in planning diagnostic procedures such as bronchoscopy or percutaneous biopsy.

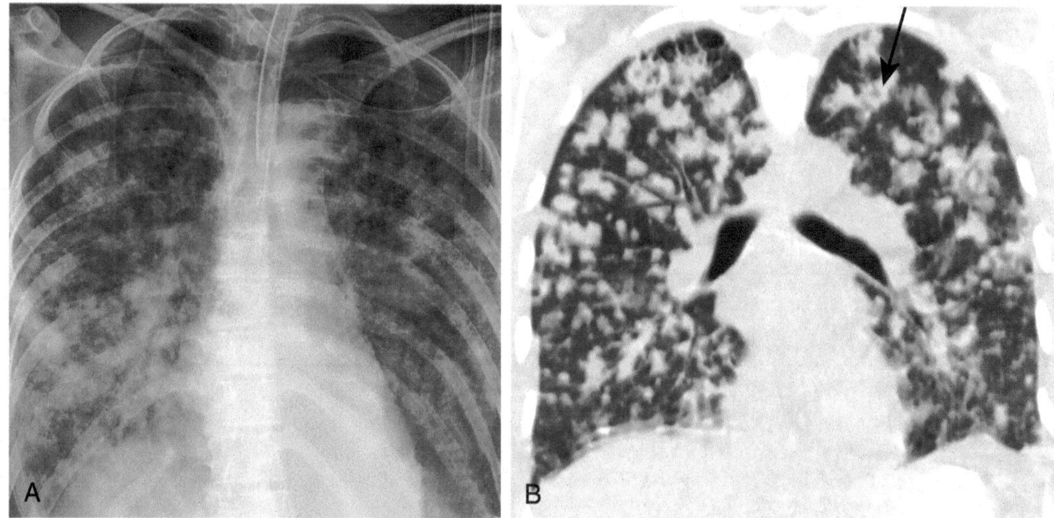

FIGURE 15.18 Fulminant varicella pneumonia in a severely immunocompromised patient. **A,** Frontal chest radiograph demonstrates multiple bilateral nodular and confluent opacities. **B,** Coronal computed tomography image confirms bilateral pulmonary nodules, some of which contain air bronchograms *(arrow)*.

SUGGESTED READINGS

Allen CM, et al. Imaging lung manifestations of HIV/AIDS. *Ann Thorac Med.* 2010;5(4):201-216.

Benito N, Moreno A, Miro JM, et al. Pulmonary infections in HIV-infected patients: an update in the 21st century. *Eur Respir J.* 2012;39(3):730-745.

Boiselle PM, Tocino I, Hooley RJ, et al. Chest radiograph interpretation of *Pneumocystis carinii* pneumonia, bacterial pneumonia, and pulmonary tuberculosis in HIV-positive patients: accuracy, distinguishing features and mimics. *J Thorac Imaging.* 1997;12:47-53.

Brecher CW, Aviram G, Boiselle PM. CT and radiography of bacterial respiratory infections in AIDS patients. *AJR Am J Roentgenol.* 2003;180(5):1203-1209.

CDC. Revised Surveillance Case Definition for HIV infection - United States, 2014. Recommendations and Reports, April 11, 2014 / 63(RR03); 1-10.

Chou SHS, Prabhu SJ, Crothers K, et al. Thoracic diseases associated with HIV infection in the era of antiretroviral therapy: clinical and imaging findings. *Radiographics.* 2014;34:895-911.

Conces DJ. Bacterial pneumonia in immunocompromised patients. *J Thorac Imaging.* 1998;13:216-270.

D'Avignon LC, Schofield CM, Hospenthal DR. Pneumocystis pneumonia. *Semin Respir Crit Care Med.* 2008;29:132-140.

Eisner MD, Kaplan LD, Herndier B, et al. The pulmonary manifestations of AIDS-related non-Hodgkin's lymphoma. *Chest.* 1996;110(3):729-736.

Franquet T, Lee KS, Muller NL. Thin section CT findings in 32 immunocompromised patients with cytomegalovirus pneumonia who do not have AIDS. *AJR Am J Roentgenol.* 2003;181:1059-1063.

Grubb JR, Moorman AC, Baker RK, et al. The changing spectrum of pulmonary disease in patient with HIV on antiretroviral therapy. *AIDS.* 2006;20:1095-1107.

http://www.unaids.org/en/resources/campaigns/HowAIDSchangedeverything/factsheet. Accessed April 26, 2016.

http://www.unaids.org/sites/default/files/media_asset/AIDS_by_the_numbers_2015_en.pdf. Accessed April 26, 2016.

Jarvis JN, Harrison TS. Pulmonary cryptococcosis. *Semin Respir Crit Care Med.* 2008;29:242-274.

Kanne JP, Yandow DR, Meyer CA. *Pneumocystis jirovecii* pneumonia: high-resolution CT findings in patients with and without HIV infection. *AJR Am J Roentgenol.* 2012;198:555-561.

Kuhlman JE, Kavuru M, Fishman EK, et al. *Pneumocystis carinii* pneumonia: spectrum of parenchymal CT findings. *Radiology.* 1990;175:711-714.

Lederman MM, Valdez H. Immune restoration with antiretroviral therapies: implications for clinical management. *JAMA.* 2000;284:223-228.

Marchiori E, Müller NL, Soares Souza A Jr, et al. Pulmonary disease in patients with AIDS: high-resolution CT and pathologic findings. *AJR Am J Roentgenol.* 2005;184(3):757-764.

Moon JH, Kim EA, Lee KS, et al. Cytomegalovirus pneumonia: high-resolution CT findings in ten non-AIDS immunocompromised patients. *Korean J Radiol.* 2000;1:73-78.

Naidich DP, Tarras M, Garay SM, et al. Kaposi's sarcoma. CT-radiographic correlation. *Chest.* 1989;96:723-728.

Oh YW, Effmann EL, Godwin JD. Pulmonary infections in immunocompromised hosts: the importance of correlating the conventional radiologic appearance with the clinical setting. *Radiology.* 2000;217:647-656.

Restepo C, Martinez S, Lemos J, et al. Imaging manifestations of Kaposi sarcoma. *Radiographics.* 2006;26:1169-1185.

Rosen MJ. Pulmonary complications of HIV infection. *Respirology.* 2008;13:181-190.

Saurborn DP, Fishman JE, Boiselle PM. The imaging spectrum of pulmonary tuberculosis in AIDS. *J Thorac Imaging.* 2002;17(1):28-33.

Segal LN, Methé BA, Nolan A, et al. HIV-1 and bacterial pneumonia in the era of antiretroviral therapy. *Proc Am Thorac Soc.* 2011;8(3):282-287.

Walker CM, Abbott GF, Greene RE, et al. Imaging pulmonary infections: classic signs and patterns. *AJR Am J Roentgenol.* 2014;202:479-492.

Chapter 16

Mycobacterial Infection

Thomas Keimig, Jo-Anne O. Shepard, and Gerald F. Abbott

INTRODUCTION

The genus *Mycobacterium* contains numerous acid-fast staining aerobic bacilli that result in a variety of infections in human hosts. Pulmonary infections by *Mycobacterium* spp. are characterized as *tuberculous (TB) mycobacterial infection* and *nontuberculous mycobacterial (NTM) infection*.

TUBERCULOUS MYCOBACTERIAL INFECTION

Tuberculosis is an infection caused by the inhalation of the aerosolized aerobic bacillus *Mycobacterium tuberculosis*. According to the World Health Organization (WHO) 2015 annual report on TB, there were an estimated 9.6 million new cases of TB worldwide in 2014, with an estimated 1.5 million deaths from TB. However, through strong public health measures, the TB mortality and prevalence rates have dropped nearly 50% and 42%, respectively, since 1990, with an estimated 43 million lives saved through diagnosis and treatment between 2000 and 2014.

The Centers for Disease Control list a number of risk factors for developing tuberculous infection, which are broadly divided into high exposure risks and states of a weakened immune system (Box 16.1). The relationship of TB and HIV/AIDS is of particular importance. According to the 2015 WHO Global Report on Tuberculosis, it is estimated that HIV-positive individuals are 26 times more likely to develop TB than HIV-negative individuals, that of the 9.6 million new cases of TB in 2014, 1.2 million (12%) were in HIV-positive individuals, that 25% of deaths attributed to TB were in HIV-positive individuals, and that TB accounted for one third of the estimated 1.2 million deaths from HIV/AIDS.

Although several laboratory tests are available for the diagnosis of TB, imaging remains an effective tool for the early diagnosis and treatment of TB as well as early isolation in patients suspected of TB, helping prevent further dissemination among the public. TB has traditionally been characterized as *primary TB*, *postprimary TB*, and *miliary TB*, but in recent years, this approach has been challenged on the basis of DNA fingerprinting. This research suggests that time from acquisition of infection to the development of clinical disease does not reliably predict the imaging features of TB. It further suggests that severely immunocompromised patients tend to have the *primary* form of TB, but immunocompetent individuals tend to have the *reactivation* form.

BOX 16.1 Risk Factors for Developing Tuberculosis

CONTACT WITH RECENTLY INFECTED PATIENTS

- Close contact of a person with infectious TB disease
- Emigration from area with high TB rate
- Children younger than 5 years old with a positive TB test result
- Groups with high rates of TB transmission (homeless persons, injection drug users, HIV positive)
- Persons who reside or work with people at high risk for TB (hospitals, homeless shelters, correctional facilities, nursing homes, residential homes for those with HIV)

WEAKENED IMMUNE SYSTEM

- Substance abuse
- HIV
- Silicosis
- Diabetes
- Severe kidney disease
- Low body weight
- Organ transplants
- Head and neck cancer
- Corticosteroid treatment
- Specialized treatments for rheumatoid arthritis or Crohn disease

TB, Tuberculosis.
From the Centers for Disease Control and Prevention. https://www.cdc.gov/tb/topic/basics/risk.htm

Primary Tuberculosis

Inhalation of aerosolized *M. tuberculosis* bacilli and subsequent pulmonary infection is referred to as *primary TB* (Box 16.2). Symptoms of primary TB include cough, fever, and chills, similar to typical bacterial pneumonias. Patients with mild symptoms may not seek health care treatment. Gram stains of sputum specimens are negative because of the high lipid content of tuberculous bacilli; therefore, an acid-fast stain is performed to evaluate specimens suspected of mycobacteria. Hence, mycobacteria are often referred to as *acid-fast bacteria*.

The host immune system response to TB infection is complex and involves caseous granuloma formation surrounding areas of infection in an attempt to contain the bacilli and prevent infection spread. Bacilli frequently spread via lymphatic drainage, leading to lymphadenopathy in a

BOX 16.2 Imaging Findings in Primary Tuberculosis

Airspace opacity
Hilar or mediastinal lymphadenopathy
Endobronchial nodules
Pleural effusion

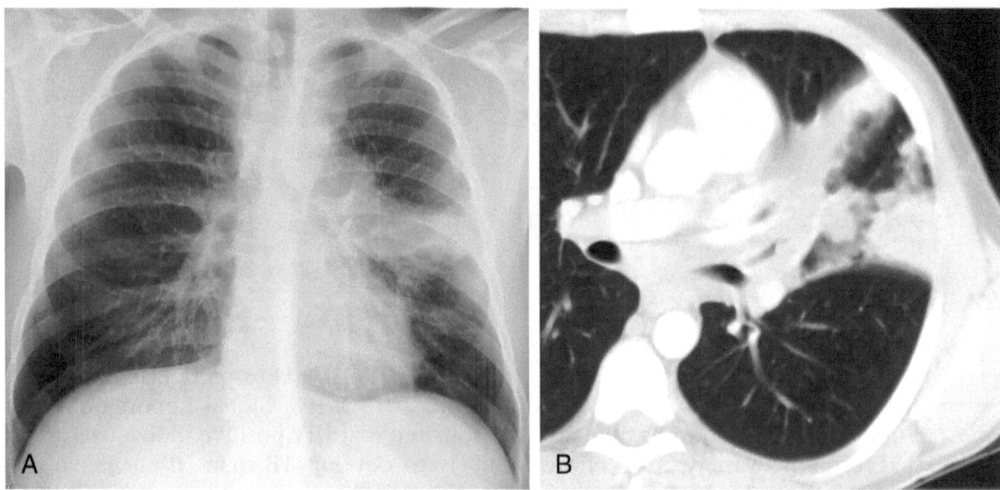

FIGURE 16.1 Consolidation. **A,** Posteroanterior chest radiograph shows patchy consolidation in the lingular portion of the left upper lobe. **B,** Computed tomography image shows dense consolidation in the lingula without evidence of cavitation. Primary tuberculosis may manifest as consolidation with or without cavitation.

predictable drainage pattern. Hematogenous dissemination may remain in the lungs (miliary TB) or disseminate to any site in the body.

Consolidation

Imaging of primary TB demonstrates airspace opacity, typically in a segmental or lobar distribution similar to typical bacterial pneumonia (Fig. 16.1). Tuberculous airspace opacities frequently involve the mid to lower lungs; however, any lobe may be involved, and multifocal disease may be found at time of presentation.

Lymphadenopathy

The presence of significant hilar and mediastinal lymphadenopathy in the setting of pulmonary consolidation raises the possibility of tuberculous infection rather than typical bacterial pneumonia. Lymph nodes are frequently identified by hilar enlargement or abnormal hilar contours, widening of the mediastinal silhouette and nodular contours of the mediastinum, and widened paratracheal stripe. On computed tomography (CT), the enlarged nodes may present with a round configuration, losing normal reniform shape and fatty hila. These enlarged lymph nodes may exhibit low attenuation centrally with peripheral enhancement, a finding suggesting central necrosis (Fig. 16.2). Tuberculous mediastinal and hilar lymphadenopathy may invade the central airways (Fig. 16.3). Cervical tuberculous lymphadenitis, also referred to as scrofula, may be visible on the superior images of a standard thoracic CT examination (Fig. 16.4).

Pleural Infection

Extension of primary lung TB into the pleural space may result in a tuberculous parapneumonic effusion (Fig. 16.5). Laboratory analysis of a tuberculous effusion typically demonstrates increased leukocyte counts with negative Gram stain. Negative acid-fast staining of pleural fluid is not uncommon and does not exclude a tuberculous effusion. In cases of inconclusive pleural fluid laboratory testing, pleural biopsy with culture and acid-fast staining may be necessary to confirm pleural TB. If primary TB progresses, a tuberculous empyema may develop (Fig. 16.6). Rarely, the empyema violates the parietal pleura and extends into adjacent spaces such as the mediastinum or chest wall, a finding referred to as *empyema necessitans*.

Pericardial Effusion

Pericardial effusion may develop at the time of primary TB infection. On radiographs, a pericardial effusion is characterized by increased size of the cardiac silhouette frequently resembling a "water bottle" on frontal radiographs. Lateral radiographs may depict a radiopaque stripe (pericardial fluid) separating a radiolucent retrosternal line (epicardial fat) and a second, more posterior radiolucent line (pericardial fat).

Healed Tuberculosis

Imaging of patients with resolved primary TB demonstrates a variety of findings. A calcified parenchymal scar or nodule may be present at the site of primary parenchymal involvement, sometimes referred to as a Ghon focus. The presence of a Ghon focus with a calcified ipsilateral lymph node is referred to as a Ranke complex (Fig. 16.7). Airway involvement may lead to bronchial stenosis (Fig. 16.8). Foci of pleural thickening or pleural calcification are consistent with fibrous tissue, termed *fibrothorax* (Fig. 16.9). Rarely, TB-related fibrothorax may progress to malignancy such as pyothorax-related lymphoma. Other types of malignant transformations, including squamous cell carcinoma and mesothelioma, have been reported. Pericardial calcifications and pericardial thickening are sequelae of prior tuberculous pericarditis and may result in imaging and clinical findings of constrictive pericarditis (Fig. 16.10).

Extrapulmonic Thoracic Tuberculosis

Hematogenous and lymphatic spread of TB can seed and infect any part of the body. A detailed discussion of extrathoracic TB is beyond the scope of this text; however, routine thoracic imaging may demonstrate foci of extrapulmonic infection.

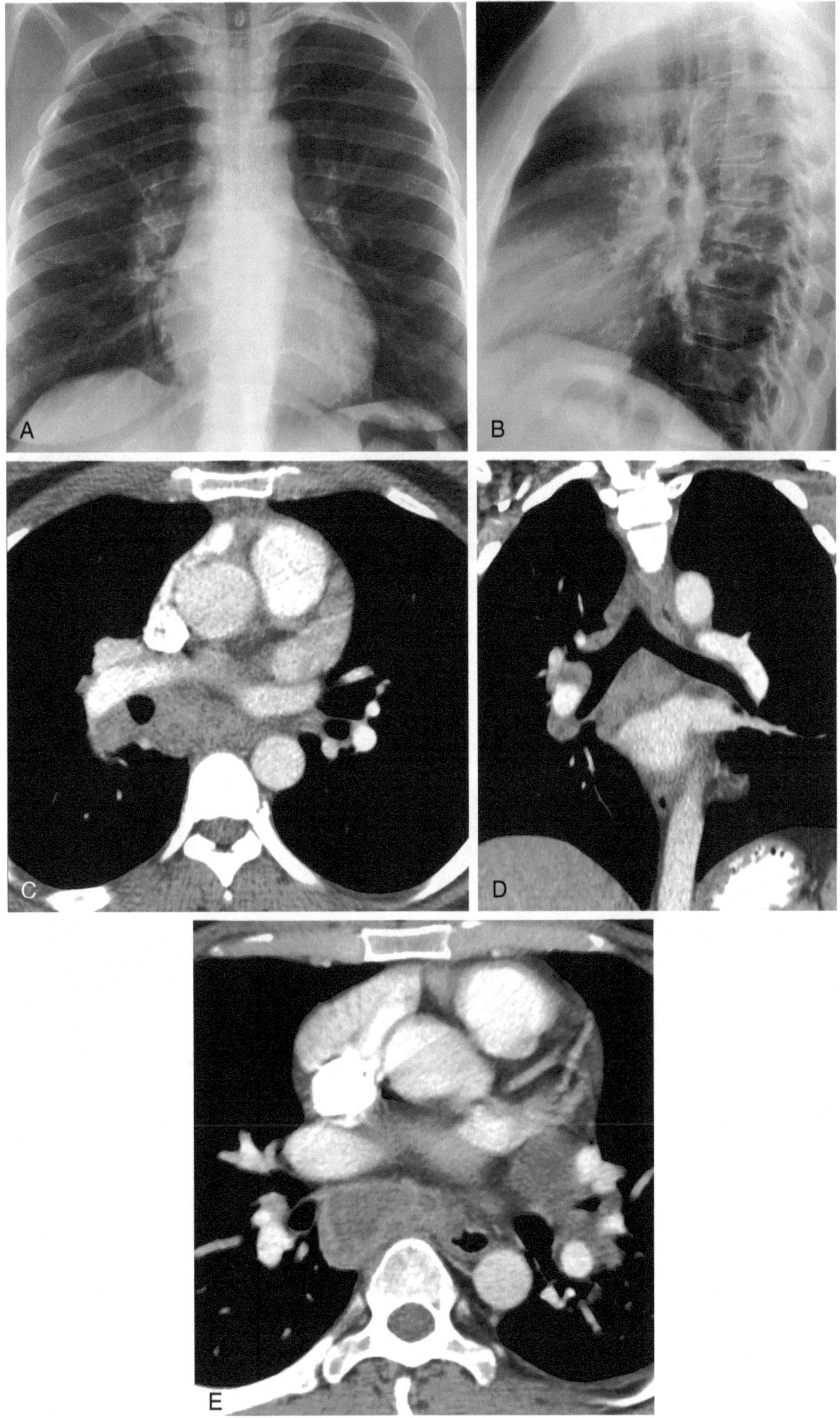

FIGURE 16.2 Lymphadenopathy. Posteroanterior **(A)** and lateral **(B)** chest radiographs show right hilar lymphadenopathy, with thickening of the intermediate stem line on the lateral radiograph. Axial **(C)** and coronal **(D)** reformatted chest computed tomography (CT) images of the same patient show right hilar and subcarinal lymphadenopathy with heterogeneous attenuation. **E,** Chest CT of a different patient with active tuberculosis shows subcarinal lymphadenopathy with peripheral enhancement and central low attenuation, a characteristic feature of tuberculous lymphadenopathy, and left hilar lymphadenopathy that does not demonstrate peripheral enhancement. Tuberculous lymphadenitis may manifest with homogeneous attenuation or exhibit necrosis with peripheral enhancement.

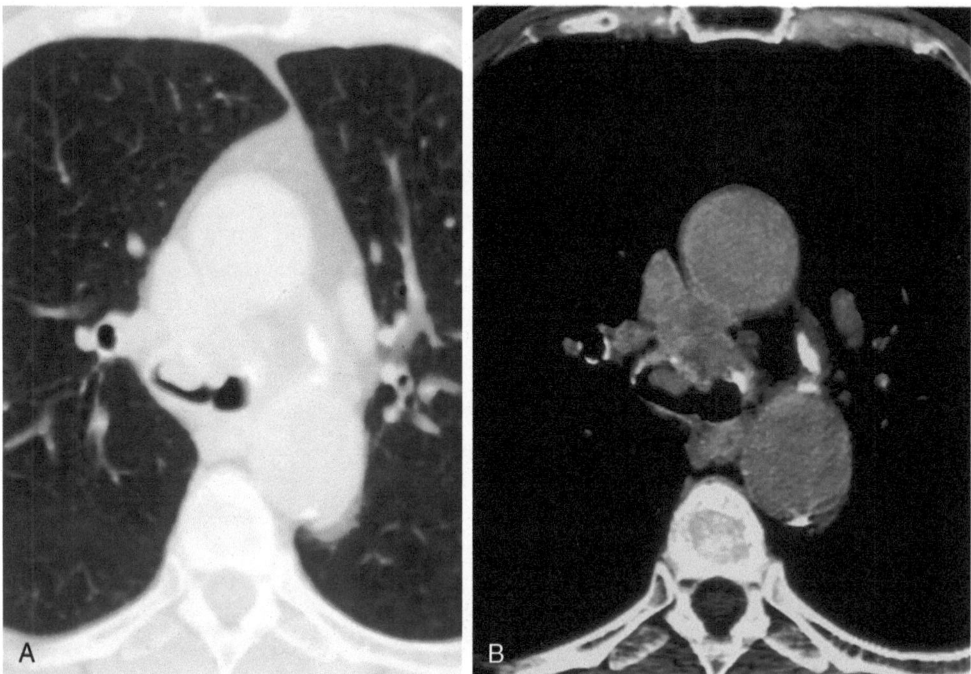

FIGURE 16.3 Airway invasion in a patient with drug-resistant tuberculosis. Composite image of chest computed tomography lung window **(A)** and mediastinal window **(B)** images show tuberculous lymphadenopathy in the lower paratracheal region that invades the right main bronchus at the level of the carina.

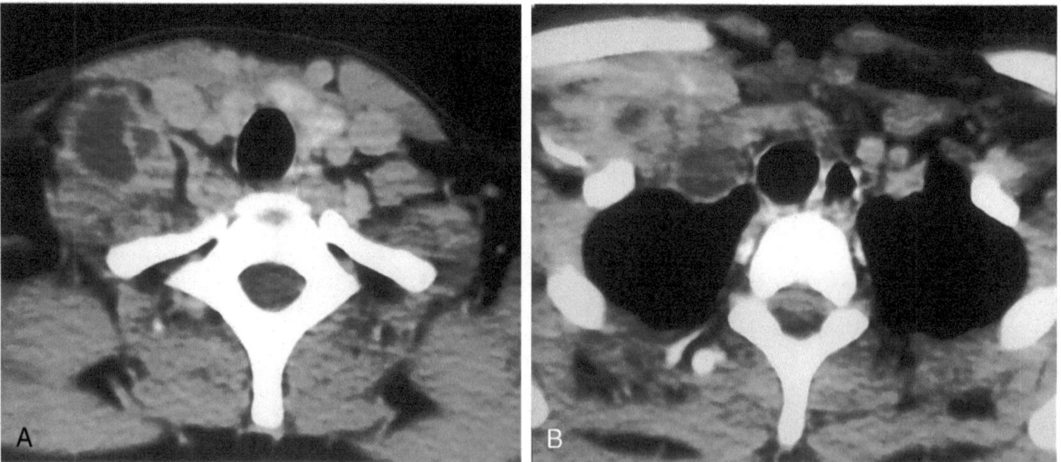

FIGURE 16.4 Scrofula. Composite image of axial contrast-enhanced chest computed tomography image shows low-attenuation lymphadenopathy with peripheral enhancement in the right lower neck **(A)** that is contiguous with lymphadenopathy in the right supraclavicular region and right anterior chest wall **(B)** that exhibits heterogeneous enhancement.

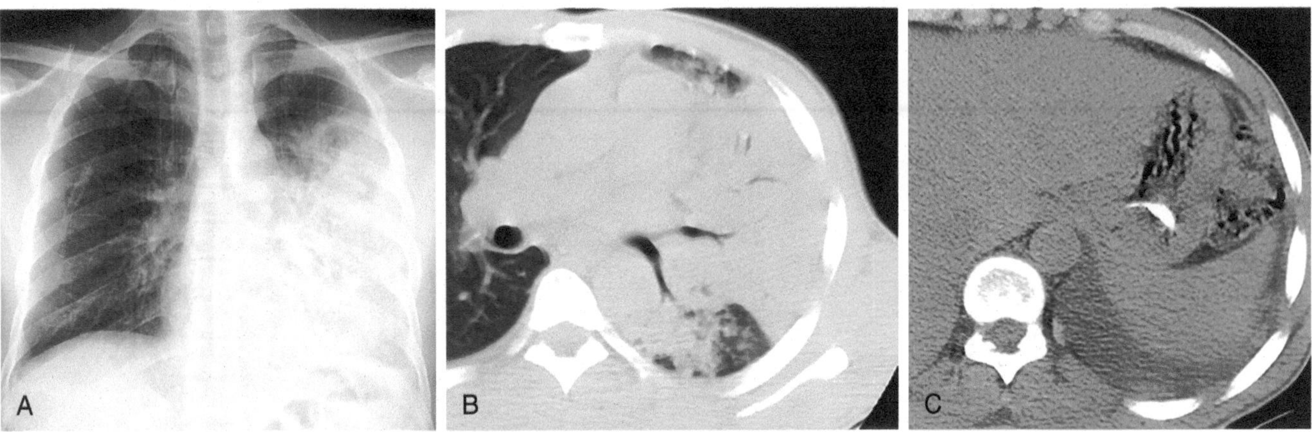

FIGURE 16.5 Pleural effusion. Composite image of posteroanterior chest radiograph **(A)** and chest computed tomography lung window **(B)** and mediastinal window **(C)** images show tuberculosis manifesting as consolidation in the left upper and lower lobes with a parapneumonic left pleural effusion **(C)**.

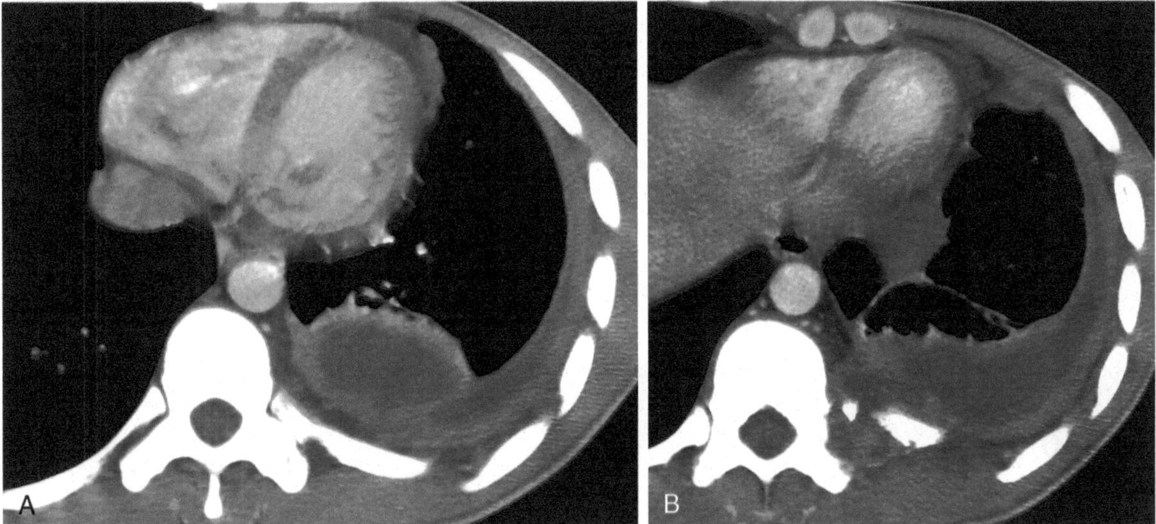

FIGURE 16.6 Empyema. **A,** Contrast-enhanced chest computed tomography (CT) image shows a loculated pleural effusion in the left lower hemithorax surrounded by pleural thickening. The thickened visceral and parietal pleura diverge around the fluid collection, forming the "split pleura" sign that is characteristic of an empyema. **B,** Axial CT image at a more caudal level shows the effusion extending into the adjacent left paraspinal soft tissues consistent with *empyema necessitans.*

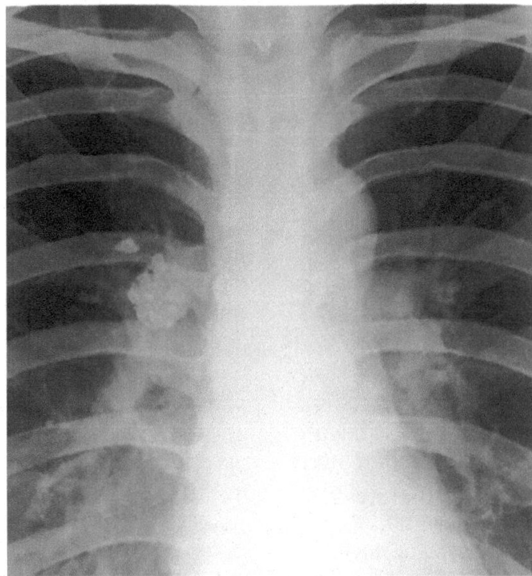

FIGURE 16.7 Ranke complex. Posteroanterior chest radiograph (detail) shows a calcified right hilar lymph node and an adjacent small calcified pulmonary nodule in the right upper lobe. This constellation of imaging findings forms the Ranke complex, a sign of healed primary tuberculosis.

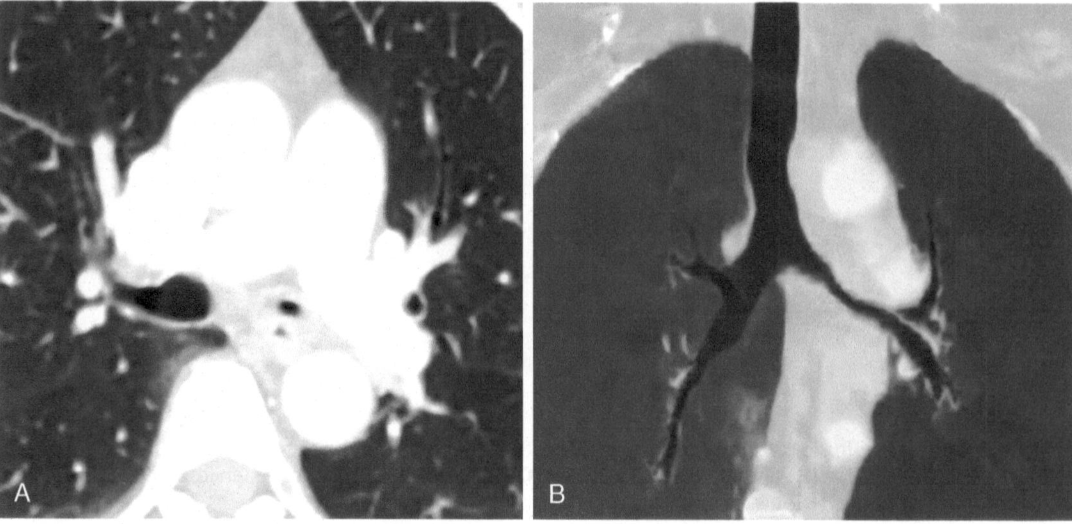

FIGURE 16.8 Bronchial stenosis, chronic. Composite image of axial contrast-enhanced chest computed tomography (CT) image **(A)** and reformatted coronal CT minimum-intensity projection image **(B)** shows diffuse smooth stenosis of the left main bronchus.

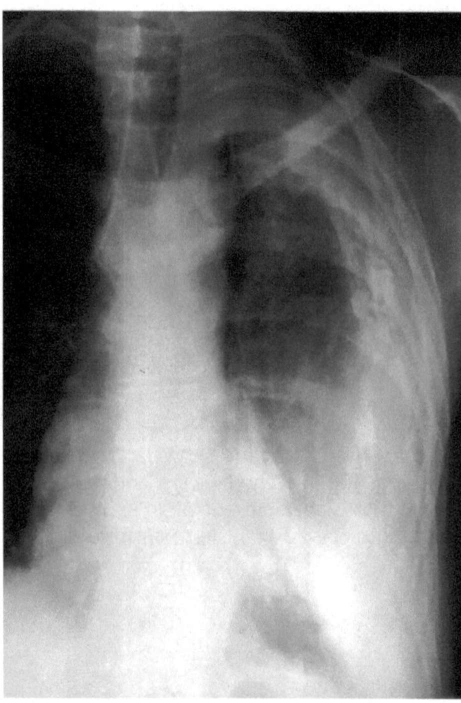

FIGURE 16.9 Fibrothorax. Posteroanterior chest radiograph (detail) shows extensive circumferential pleural thickening with calcification (fibrothorax), a sequela of a healed tuberculous empyema.

Tuberculous spondylitis, or Pott disease, results from hematogenous spread to the vertebral body (Fig. 16.11). Classically, tuberculous spondylitis results in vertebral destruction with relative sparing of the intervertebral disk, an unusual finding in typical bacterial diskitis with osteomyelitis. The resulting vertebral collapse with anterior wedging has been termed the *gibbus deformity*. The infection often spreads along the longitudinal ligaments involving multiple contiguous vertebral levels, another unusual finding for typical bacterial diskitis or osteomyelitis. Spread of infection into the paraspinal tissues may result in abscess formation.

BOX 16.3 Imaging Findings in Postprimary Tuberculosis

Airspace opacity +/− cavitary lesion
- Upper lobes (apical and posterior segments) and/or
- Lower lobes (superior segments)

Nodular, tree-in-bud opacities
- Endobronchial spread of disease
- May involve multiple segments or lobes

Pleural thickening

Postprimary Tuberculosis

Postprimary TB occurs when previously contained tuberculous infection spreads or when a host is unable to contain a primary TB infection, often during states of immune compromise, at times of extreme physical stress, or in advanced age. Postprimary TB may spread throughout the lungs or to other sites of the body through lymphatic and hematogenous dissemination.

Postprimary TB frequently presents as cough, fatigue, anorexia, and weight loss. Hemoptysis may or may not be present.

On chest radiographs, the classic finding of postprimary TB is one or more cavitary lesions in the mid to upper lungs, most commonly the apical and posterior segments of the upper lobes and the superior segments of the lower lobes (Box 16.3). Interspersed patchy airspace opacities may or may not be apparent. Disease involvement can be unilateral or bilateral (Fig. 16.12, *A*). Subtle findings on radiographs are often striking on CT (Fig. 16.12, *B*). Small cavitary lesions not appreciated on radiographs are well demonstrated by CT. Areas of consolidative opacity may be interspersed between cavitary lesions. Tree-in-bud and centrilobular nodules indicate endobronchial spread of mycobacteria into the small airways and may be found in multiple lobes or even the contralateral lung (Fig. 16.13).

A cavitary focus of infection may invade into an adjacent pulmonary artery, resulting in vessel wall weakening and eventual pseudoaneurysm formation (Rasmussen aneurysm)

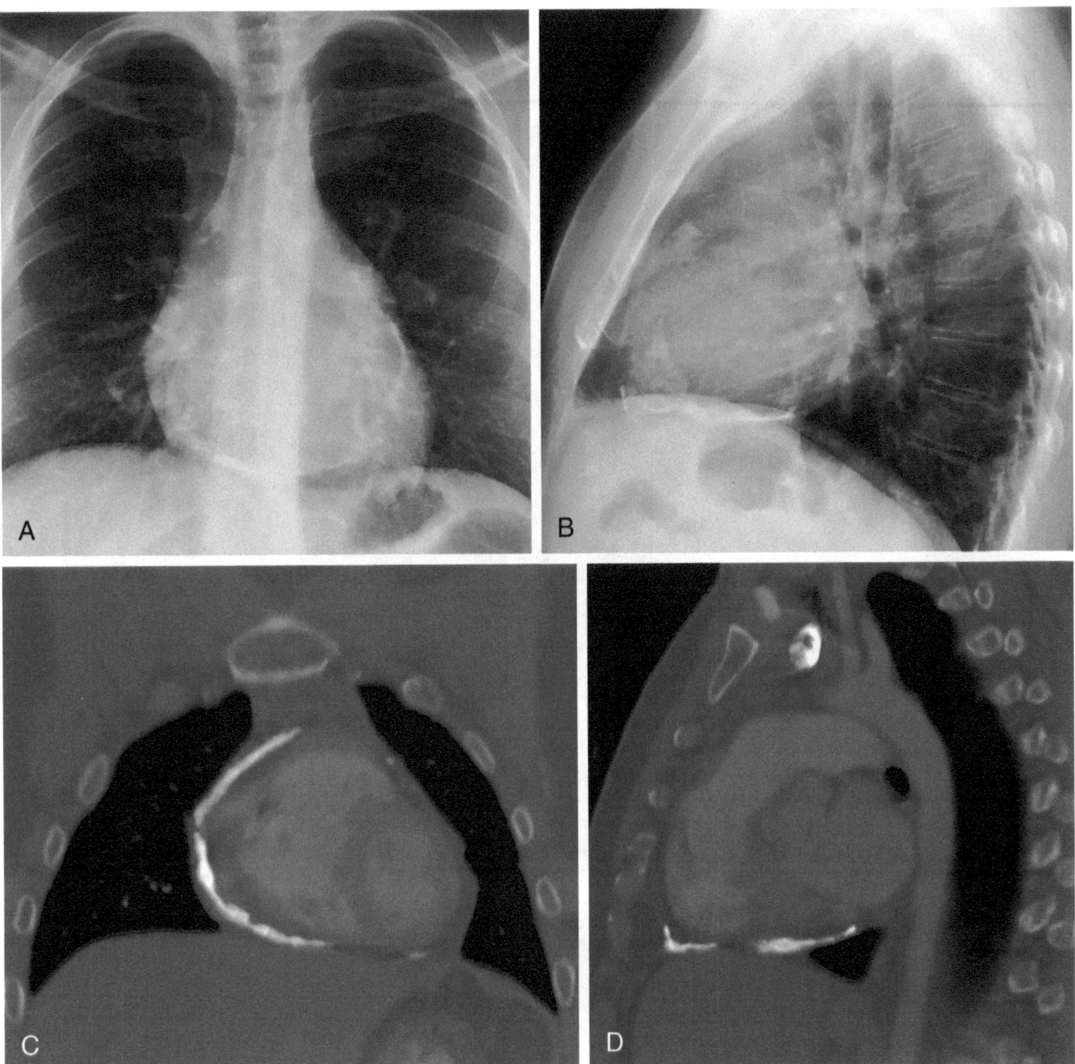

FIGURE 16.10 Pericardial calcification. Posteroanterior **(A)** and lateral **(B)** chest radiographs show pericardial calcification coursing along the right inferolateral aspect of the pericardium. Reformatted coronal **(C)** and sagittal **(D)** computed tomography images of the same patient shows the pericardial calcification extending along the right superolateral, lateral, and inferior pericardial surfaces.

(Fig. 16.14). These pseudoaneurysms may rupture, resulting in hemoptysis, which can be massive and life threatening. On contrast-enhanced CT, Rasmussen aneurysms are characterized by focal dilation of segmental or subsegmental pulmonary arteries adjacent to a tuberculous cavity.

Imaging sequelae of inactive postprimary TB include those of healed primary TB previously described. Other findings are upper lung fibrosis with associated volume loss and traction bronchiectasis (Fig. 16.15) as well as broncholith formation. Bronchiectasis may be associated with bronchial artery dilatation and resultant hemoptysis. Cavities can resolve after successful treatment but may persist as thin-walled cystlike structures. The stability of such thin-walled cysts over time reflects their etiology of treated infection rather than persistent areas of active infection. Detection of a new nodular opacity within such a cyst suggests the presence of a mycetoma (Fig. 16.16).

Collapse therapy was a form of treatment used before the discovery and implementation of antituberculous medication in which an infected cavity containing the upper lobe was surgically collapsed. One hypothesis for this treatment was that collapsing the cavities would limit oxygen to the infected lobe and therefore inhibit the growth and spread of the obligate aerobic tuberculous bacilli. The first collapse therapy treatments were achieved through iatrogenic pneumothorax. Later methods of collapse therapy included phrenic nerve paralysis, thoracoplasty, and plombage (Fig. 16.17) and the placement of material such as Lucite balls, paraffin, or sponges into the extrapleural space to collapse the lung.

Miliary Tuberculosis

Miliary TB is the result of hematogenous spread of *M. tuberculosis* throughout the host's lungs and may be present at the time of primary infection or manifest as a form of postprimary TB (Box 16.4). Named for the resemblance to millet seeds, miliary TB manifests as innumerable 1- to 3-mm nodules scattered in a random distribution throughout the lung parenchyma, consistent with foci of hematogenous

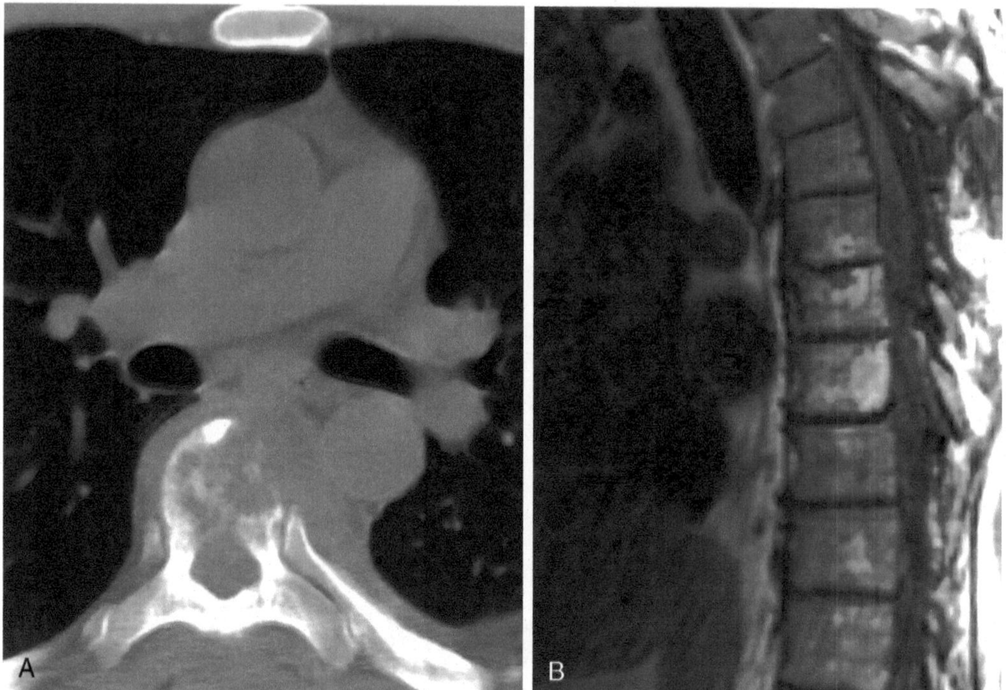

FIGURE 16.11 Potts disease. **A,** Unenhanced chest computed tomography image shows destruction of a thoracic vertebral body with adjacent bilateral paraspinal soft tissue, representing tuberculous osteomyelitis of the spine (Potts disease). **B,** Sagittal magnetic resonance T1-weighted contrast-enhanced image shows abnormal increased signal intensity in the same vertebral body without evidence of collapse deformity.

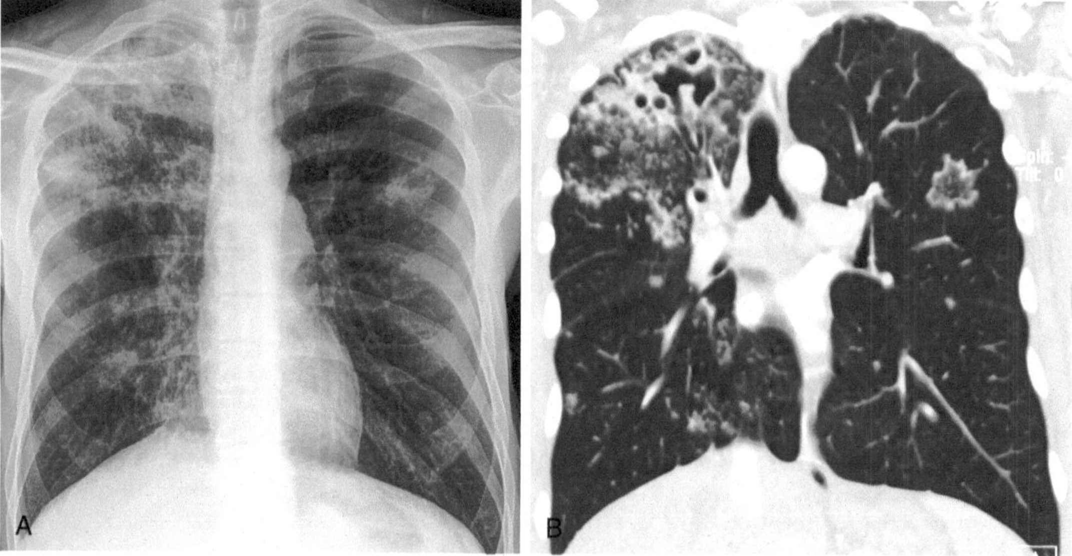

FIGURE 16.12 Postprimary tuberculosis (TB). **A,** Posteroanterior chest radiograph shows patchy consolidation in the right lung apex with an area of cavitation and a focal indistinct nodular opacity in the left upper lobe. **B,** Reformatted coronal computed tomography image shows the cavitation with surrounding consolidation, patchy ground-glass opacity, and nodular opacities. A focal area of ground-glass opacity in the left upper lobe is surrounded by a rim of consolidation (reverse-halo sign), representing spread of TB to the contralateral lung. Centrilobular tree-in-bud opacities are demonstrated in the right lower lobe.

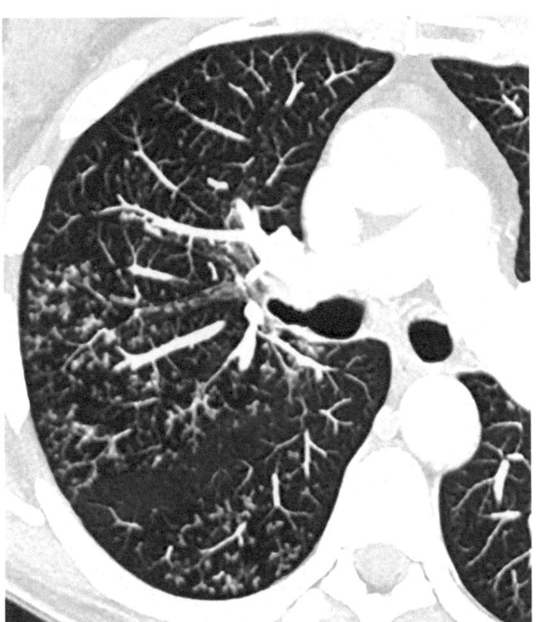

FIGURE 16.13 Centrilobular tree-in-bud nodules. Chest computed tomography (minimum-intensity projection image, lung window) image shows multiple centrilobular nodules and tree-in-bud opacities in the right upper and lower lobes in a patient with active tuberculosis.

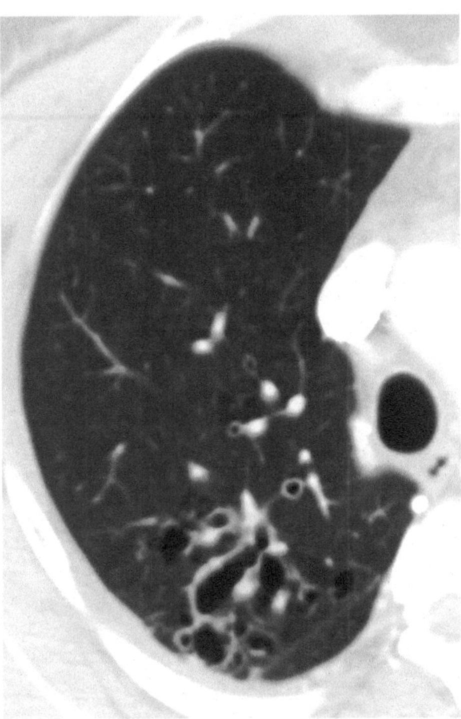

FIGURE 16.15 Bronchiectasis. Chest computed tomography image shows a patchy area of bronchiectatic airways in the posterior segment of the right upper lobe of a patient with healed tuberculosis.

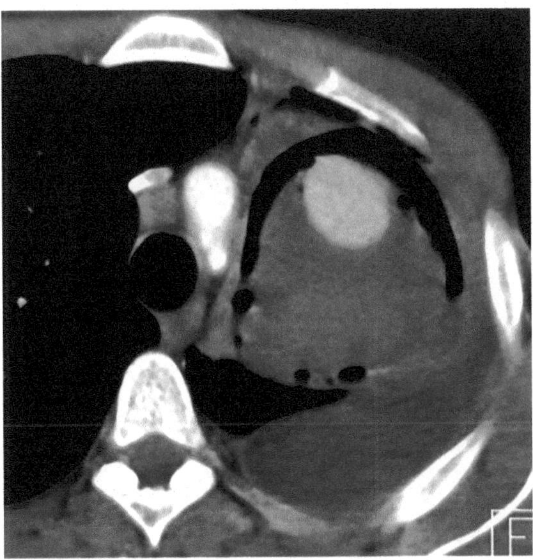

FIGURE 16.14 Rasmussen aneurysm. Contrast-enhanced chest computed tomography image shows a focal area of dense enhancement in a mass within a cavity in the left upper lobe, characteristic findings of an aneurysm resulting from tuberculous infection. (Courtesy of Rosane Martins, MD. Brasília, Brazil.)

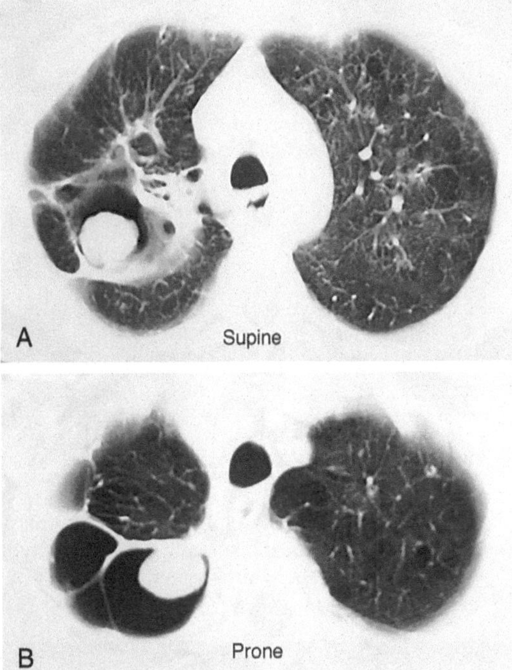

FIGURE 16.16 Mycetoma. **A,** Supine chest computed tomography (CT) image shows a spherical mass within a right upper lobe cavity. The mass is in contact with the posterior wall of the cavity. **B,** Prone chest CT image shows the mass in contact with the anterior wall of the cavity, indicating its free mobility within the cavity. The imaging findings are characteristic of a fungus ball (mycetoma) that moves freely within a cavity when imaged during prone and supine imaging.

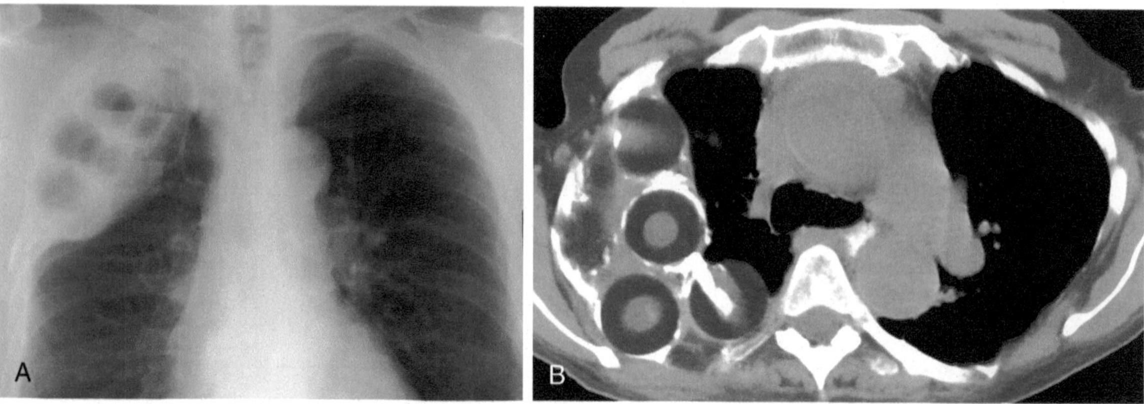

FIGURE 16.17 Plombage. **A,** Posteroanterior chest radiograph (detail) image shows Lucite balls manifesting as spherical filling defects within an extrapleural opacity in the right apical region. **B,** Chest computed tomography image of a different patient shows Lucite balls (plombage) forming an extrapleural mass in the right apical region that compresses the adjacent lung, a form of collapse therapy.

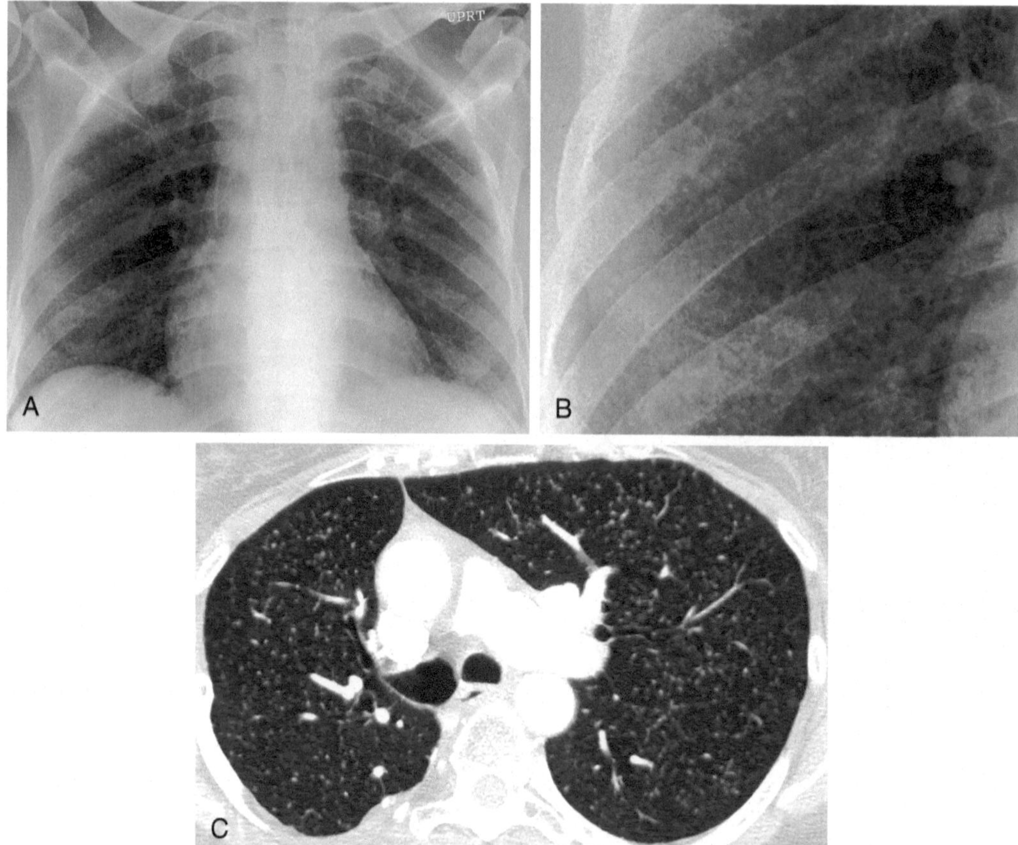

FIGURE 16.18 Miliary tuberculosis. Posteroanterior chest radiograph **(A)** and detailed view of the same image **(B)** show a diffuse, bilateral micronodular pattern. **C,** Contrast-enhanced chest computed tomography image of the same patient shows numerous small pulmonary nodules involving both lungs in a random distribution.

BOX 16.4 Differential Diagnosis for Miliary Nodules

Miliary tuberculosis
Disseminated fungal infection (histoplasmosis)
Metastatic disease (renal, thyroid, breast, lung)
Viral infection
Sarcoidosis
Silicosis

dissemination. Chest radiographs demonstrate a diffuse nodular pattern that may be subtle or striking in appearance (Fig. 16.18, *A* and *B*). On CT, numerous 1- to 3-mm nodules are diffusely scattered throughout the lung parenchyma and within the secondary pulmonary lobule in a random distribution (Fig. 16.18, *C*). In the setting of primary TB with hematogenous spread, there may be superimposed airspace opacity or lymphadenopathy. In the setting of postprimary TB with miliary disease, sequelae of past primary TB and of active postprimary TB, such as cavitation, may be present.

The primary differential diagnosis for miliary TB is diffuse, nodular metastatic disease, diffuse fungal or viral infection, and an atypical manifestation of sarcoidosis. Renal and thyroid carcinomas are typical malignancies, producing diffuse small nodular opacities; however, the nodules tend to be slightly larger, measuring 3 to 5 mm, than miliary nodules. Rarely, diffuse metastatic lung adenocarcinoma may present with hematogenously spread nodules. Nodular metastatic lung adenocarcinoma may also present with lymphadenopathy and a dominant mass that may bear resemblance to a tuberculoma. An upper lung cavitary lung cancer could be mistaken for a cavitary postprimary tuberculous focus.

Hematogenous spread of the fungal infection histoplasmosis can also present with numerous small parenchymal nodules, indistinguishable from miliary TB nodules. Sarcoidosis may present with numerous bilateral nodules with hilar and mediastinal lymphadenopathy. However, the parenchymal nodules in sarcoidosis are perilymphatic in distribution and not randomly distributed as in miliary TB.

NONTUBERCULOUS MYCOBACTERIAL INFECTION

The nontuberculous mycobacteria (NTM) are a collection of more than 100 organisms present in soil and water that are capable of causing an indolent pulmonary infection. The most common human NTM pathogens are *Mycobacterium avium-intracellulare* complex (MAC, so called because it is frequently difficult to isolate one species from the other) and *Mycobacterium kansasii*. NTMs are classified by the Runyon classification, which separates the many NTMs into groups based on growth rate (fast or slow), yellow pigment production, and whether this pigment is produced in the dark or after exposure to light.

The clinical diagnosis of NTM can be challenging because of the ubiquity of NTMs in the environment. NTMs are frequent airway colonizers and contaminants of sputum and lavage samples limiting diagnostic specificity of these specimens. Therefore, the presence of NTM in specimens alone is not sufficient for diagnosis. The clinical diagnosis of NTM infection requires a combination of clinical, radiographic, and microbiologic findings as described by the American Thoracic Society. Furthermore, NTM infections frequently require prolonged treatment (>12 months) with antibiotics that have potentially serious toxic side effects, emphasizing the importance of accurate diagnosis and appropriate selection of patients to undergo treatment. NTM infection is commonly classified as cavitary (*classic*) and bronchiectatic (*nonclassic*) (Table 16.1).

TABLE 16.1 Imaging Findings in Nontuberculous Mycobacterial Infection (NTBMI)

Cavitary (Classic) NTM	Bronchiectatic (Nonclassic) NTM
Airspace opacity +/− cavitary lesion	Bronchiectatic airways
Nodular, tree-in-bud opacities	Bronchial wall thickening Middle lobe and lingula predominance
Pleural thickening	Tree-in-bud opacities
	Centrilobular nodules

Cavitary Form (Classic)

The cavitary form of nontuberculous mycobacterial infection often affects patients, usually older men, with prior lung disease such as chronic obstructive pulmonary disease, prior TB or fungal infection, cystic fibrosis, or aspiration or gastroesophageal reflux disease. The imaging of cavitary NTM infection demonstrates many of the same features as postprimary TB, and the two may be indistinguishable (Fig. 16.19). Chest radiographs may reveal one or more upper lung cavitary lesions with surrounding nodular opacities suggestive of endobronchial spread. As in TB, signs of volume loss may be present secondary to scarring. Pleural thickening secondary to fibrothorax may also be apparent.

Cavitary lesions suspected on radiographs are well demonstrated with CT. Frequently, smaller cavitary lesions not visible on radiographs are well demonstrated with CT. Centrilobular and tree-in-bud opacities are consistent with endobronchial spread. Bronchiectasis may or may not be present.

Bronchiectatic Form (Nonclassic)

The bronchiectatic form of NTM infection is a disease process characterized by bronchiectatic airways and centrilobular and tree-in-bud nodules. The classic patient is a thin older woman without prior lung disease who suppresses her cough, sometimes termed *Lady Windermere syndrome*. Controversy exists regarding whether the infection causes bronchiectasis or develops in preexisting bronchiectatic airways.

Chest radiographs may be normal in patients with subtle disease. Typical findings on chest radiographs include cylindrical or cystic bronchiectasis with a superimposed nodular pattern. The lingula and middle lobe are most commonly the sites of disease, but any lobe may be involved. Larger nodules may measure up to 1.5 cm.

Computed tomography more accurately depicts the distribution and degree of bronchiectasis and pulmonary nodules. Subtle or inconspicuous nodular opacities on radiographs are clearly demonstrated by CT as centrilobular nodules and tree-in-bud opacities (Fig. 16.20). Occasionally, patchy airspace opacities may be present.

Serial imaging plays a key role in the management of patients with NTM. Clinicians may decide to follow asymptomatic patients without progressive disease and spare them potentially toxic antituberculous medication, but patients with increasing symptoms or disease burden may begin medical therapy. Serial imaging in patients undergoing therapy assesses response to treatment and possible need for changes in the medication regimen.

CONCLUSION

Mycobacterial infections remain an important group of infectious diseases despite great strides in diagnosis, treatment, and public health initiatives. Radiology continues to have a key role in the diagnosis and treatment of these patients and, in the case of TB, a vital function in the early detection of infection and protection of public exposure.

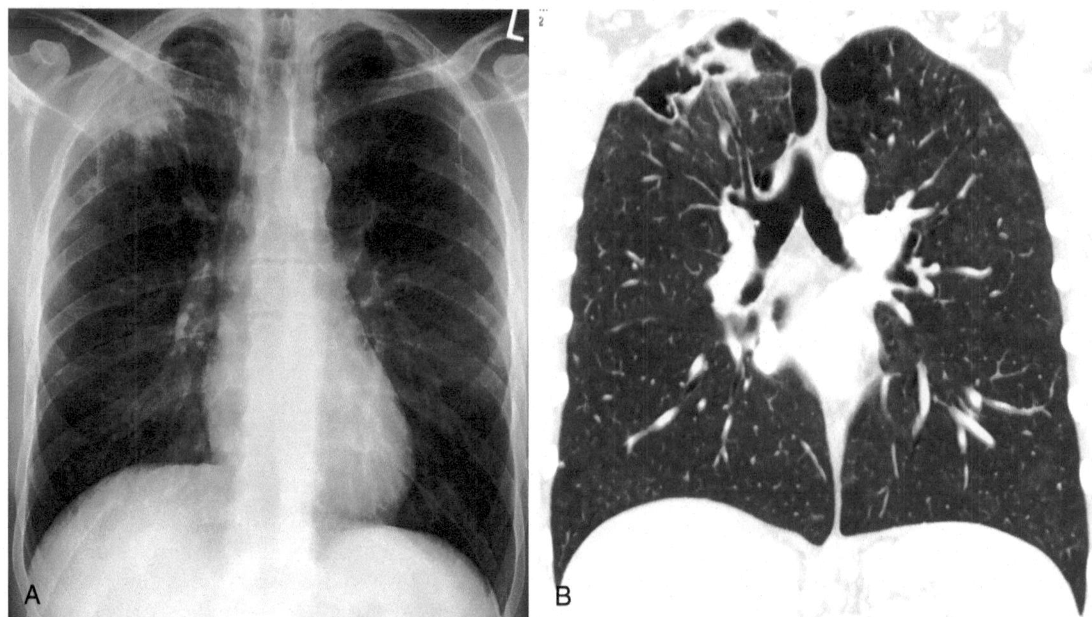

FIGURE 16.19 Cavitary ("classic") nontuberculous mycobacterial infection. **A,** Posteroanterior chest radiograph shows focal consolidation with evidence of cavitation in the right lung apex. **B,** Reformatted coronal computed tomography image shows a cavitary lesion in the right lung apex with an adjacent cavitary nodule.

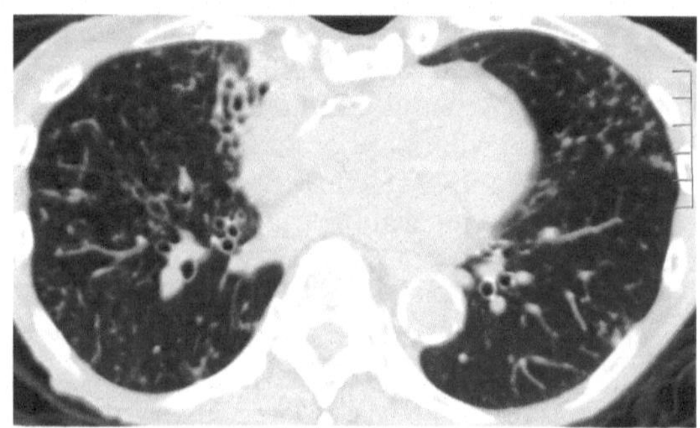

FIGURE 16.20 Bronchiectatic ("nonclassic") nontuberculous mycobacterial infection. Chest computed tomography image shows bronchiectasis in the middle and right lower lobes with numerous centrilobular nodules and tree-in-bud opacities in the right lower lobe and lingula.

SUGGESTED READINGS

Burrill J, Williams CJ, Bain G, et al. Tuberculosis: a radiologic review. *Radiographics*. 2007;27(5):1255-1273.

Erasmus JJ, McAdams HP, Farrell MA, et al. Pulmonary nontuberculous mycobacterial infection: radiologic manifestations. *Radiographics*. 1999;19(6):1487-1505.

Griffith DE, Aksamit T, Brown-Elliott BA, et al. An official ATS/IDSA statement: diagnosis, treatment, and prevention of nontuberculous mycobacterial diseases. *Am J Respir Crit Care Med*. 2007;175(4):367-416.

Hansell DM. *Imaging of Diseases of the Chest*. Edinburgh: Mosby; 2010.

Harisinghani MG, McLoud TC, Shepard JA, et al. Tuberculosis from head to toe. *Radiographics*. 2000;20(2):449-470.

Kim HY, Song KS, Goo JM, et al. Thoracic sequelae and complications of tuberculosis. *Radiographics*. 2001;21(4):839-858, discussion 859-860.

Lee Y, Song JW, Chae EJ, et al. CT findings of pulmonary non-tuberculous mycobacterial infection in non-AIDS immunocompromised patients: a case-controlled comparison with immunocompetent patients. *Br J Radiol*. 2013;86(1024).

Leung AN. Pulmonary tuberculosis: the essentials. *Radiology*. 1999;210(2):307-322.

Martinez S, McAdams HP, Batchu CS. The many faces of pulmonary nontuberculous mycobacterial infection. *AJR Am J Roentgenol*. 2007;189(1):177-186.

WHO Global tuberculosis report 2017.

Yeon JJ, Lee KS. Pulmonary tuberculosis: up-to-date imaging and management. *AJR Am J Roentgenol*. 2008;191(3):834-844.

Chapter 17

Approach to Diffuse Lung Disease: Anatomic Basis and High-Resolution Computed Tomography

Amita Sharma and Gerald F. Abbott

INTRODUCTION

Diffuse lung diseases are often detected and initially evaluated on chest radiographs (CXR). A CXR can provide valuable clues regarding pulmonary pathology such as the lung volume, distribution, and characterization of abnormalities. Radiographs assess lung volumes and distribution of disease. Whereas low volumes suggest the presence of a restrictive defect such as pulmonary fibrosis, large lung volumes suggest hyperinflation or obstructive lung disease. Ancillary findings such as lymphadenopathy, pleural effusions, and pleural plaques can assist in determining the cause of the pulmonary abnormality. Serial radiographs allow assessment of the acuity of abnormalities; those that persist for more than 4 weeks often indicate a chronic etiology. Findings on a CXR are often nonspecific, and necessitate further evaluation with thin-section chest computed tomography (CT) or high-resolution CT (HRCT).

High-resolution CT is a noninvasive cross-sectional examination of the whole lung. The distribution and characteristics of HRCT findings can indicate which group of differential diagnoses to consider or point to a specific disease without the need for biopsy. HRCT can suggest further tests for a definitive diagnosis or, if tissue sampling is required, can direct the site of biopsy. After diagnosis, follow-up HRCT scans monitor disease activity, the response to treatment, or the development of complications. Evolution of abnormalities over time may have prognostic implications.

HIGH-RESOLUTION COMPUTED TOMOGRAPHY PROTOCOL

The protocol for an HRCT scan is described in detail in Chapter 1. The principle of HRCT is acquisition of thin transverse sections (1–1.5-mm thickness) with a high spatial resolution technique and lung kernel algorithms to visualize the lung parenchyma (Fig. 17.1). Multiplanar reformatting in the coronal and sagittal planes facilitates evaluation of the distribution of parenchymal abnormalities. Maximum-intensity projection (MIP) and minimum-intensity projection (MinIP) images aid detection of multiple nodules and decreased attenuation, respectively. Prone images are routinely included in the HRCT protocol to differentiate early reticular abnormalities in the dependent peripheral portions of the lower lobes that persist from gravity-dependent density that resolves on prone imaging (Figs. 17.2 and 17.3).

Expiratory HRCT images are performed either dynamically (during expiration) or on static images (after end-expiration) (Fig. 17.4). The attenuation of the lung parenchyma on expiratory images is compared with inspiratory images at equivalent levels in the thorax. During normal expiration, the lung parenchyma decreases in volume and increases in attenuation. Areas of air trapping can be easily visualized on expiratory HRCT images as regions that remain similar in volume and attenuation when compared with the inspiratory images. Adequate expiration is confirmed if the posterior membrane of the trachea and main bronchi becomes flat or concave. It is important to consider normal expiration as the cause for increased parenchymal attenuation before suggesting a diagnosis of lung pathology. Respiratory motion can result in artifacts that mimic bronchiectasis, pulmonary embolism, and pulmonary nodules (Fig. 17.5).

HIGH-RESOLUTION COMPUTED TOMOGRAPHY EVALUATION

Many lung diseases involve the lung parenchyma, interstitium, or both. The key to diagnosis is recognition of the distribution of disease in relation to various anatomic regions (Table 17.1). Craniocaudal distribution refers to the preference of a disease process for the upper, mid, or lower zones (Fig. 17.6). Inhalational diseases, including smoking-related lung disease, have a predilection for the upper zones. This is because of the relative paucity of lymphatic drainage in the upper zones clearing inhaled pathogens. Hematogenous diseases, such as miliary metastases, have a predilection for the lower zones, where blood flow is greatest. *Axial distribution* refers to distribution on a single transverse image; certain diseases are central in distribution, and others predominantly involve the peripheral third of the lung

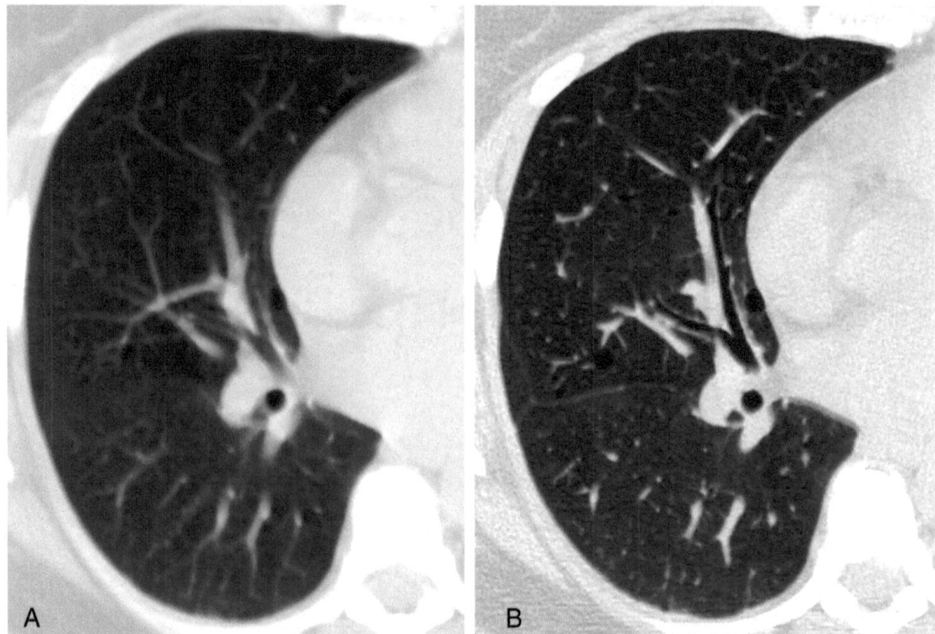

FIGURE 17.1 Effects of slice thickness. **A,** A 5-mm axial section through the middle lobe. **B,** A 1.5-mm axial section through the same region. The thinner slice results in less partial volume averaging and creates a sharper image. There is improved definition of the walls of the vessels and airways and the fissures. Subcentimeter cystic lucencies in the middle lobe are also more clearly visualized in this patient with lymphangioleiomyomatosis.

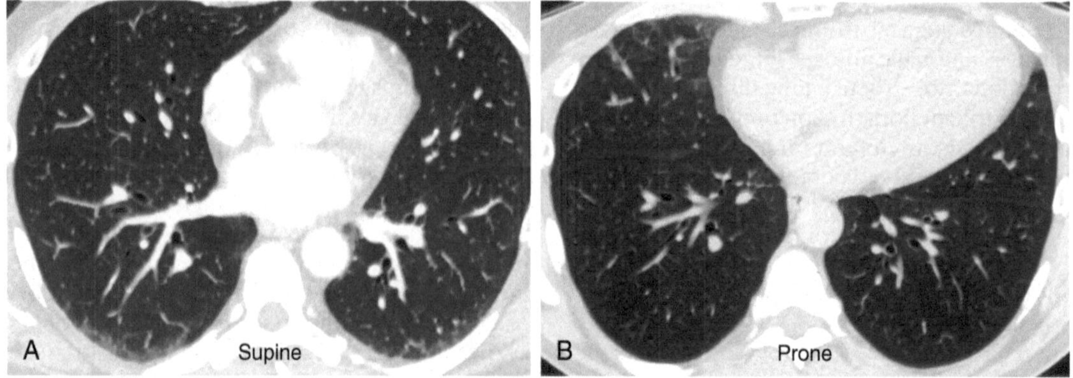

FIGURE 17.2 Effects of technique: supine versus prone. **A,** A 1.25-mm axial section in the supine position demonstrates lower lobe posterior ground-glass opacities representing dependent atelectasis. **B,** Axial image that is flipped but was obtained in the prone position at the same level shows clearing of the posterior ground-glass opacities that now lie anteriorly as this is now the dependent position. Gravity-dependent changes can increase attenuation of the posterior lung parenchyma by up to 100 Hounsfield units.

(Fig. 17.7). A dependent distribution of disease involves the posterior portion of the lung in supine patients and anterior portion in the prone position. Most importantly, thin-section CT permits evaluation of the distribution of disease at the level of the secondary pulmonary lobule (SPL), a key step in the accurate assessment and diagnosis of diffuse lung disease.

Anatomy of the Secondary Pulmonary Lobule

The SPL is the functional unit of lung where gaseous exchange occurs. The SPL contains bronchioles, branches of the pulmonary artery and veins, lymphatics, and interstitial tissue. The SPL measures approximately 1 to 2.5 cm in diameter, is roughly polyhedral in shape, and is outlined by an interlobular septum (Fig. 17.8). The structures in the center of the SPL, the centrilobular structures, consist of a lobular bronchiole and pulmonary artery that course and divide together. The pulmonary artery forms a dot approximately 0.5 to 1 mm in diameter, visible on HRCT in the center of the SPL. The wall of the bronchiole is 0.05 to 0.15 mm and beyond the resolution of HRCT to be normally visible unless thickened or fluid filled. Lobular bronchioles divide into terminal bronchioles, the most

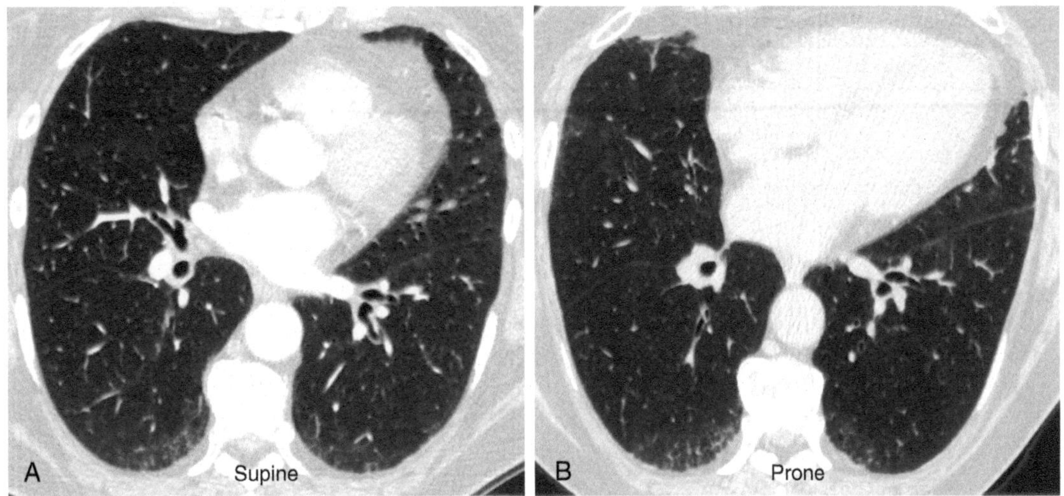

FIGURE 17.3 Effects of technique: supine versus prone. **A,** Supine 1.25-mm axial section demonstrates posterior lower lobe–dependent ground-glass opacities. **B,** Axial image that is flipped but was obtained in the prone position at the same level does not show resolution of the ground-glass opacities that represent changes of interstitial lung disease.

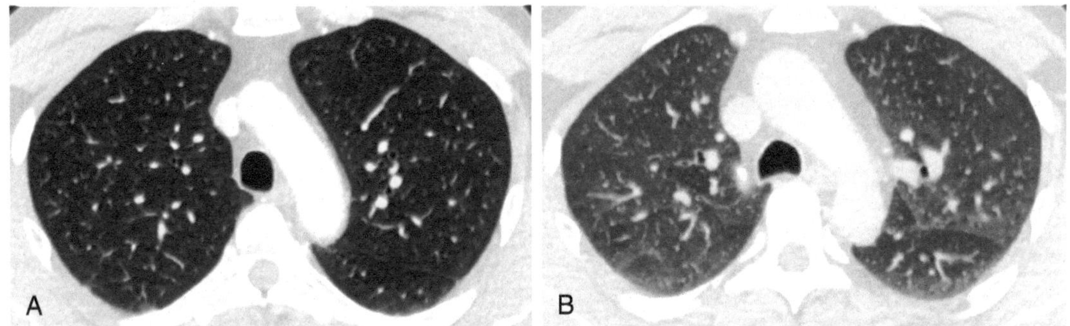

FIGURE 17.4 Effects of technique: inspiration versus expiration. **A,** Axial 1.5-mm computed tomography scan through the upper zones in inspiration demonstrates posterior gravity-dependent changes that can increase the attenuation of the lung by up to 100 Hounsfield units. **B,** Expiration images at the same level show decrease in volume of the lung parenchyma, crowding of the vasculature, and a diffuse increase in attenuation throughout the lung parenchyma. There is concavity of the posterior membranous wall of the trachea.

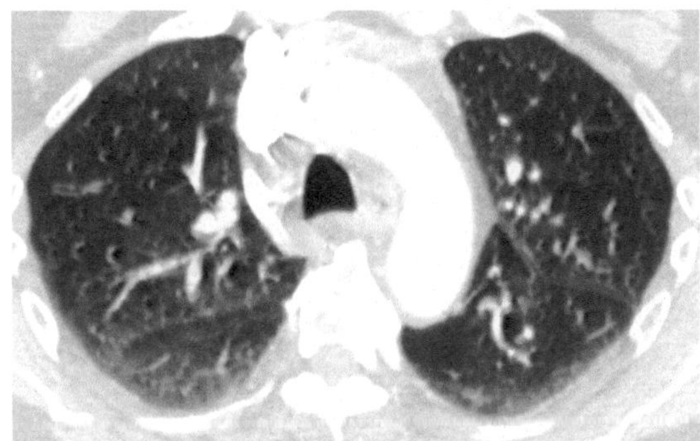

FIGURE 17.5 Respiratory motion artifact. The patient is breathing during acquisition of the scan, which caused a diffuse increase in attenuation and created a double exposure of the fissures and vessels. Artifacts seen adjacent to the vessels and airways mimic lung nodules and bronchiectasis as seen in the right upper lobe.

distal conducting airways that then divide into several respiratory bronchioles in the center of the SPL. Respiratory bronchioles open into several alveolar ducts to form an acinus. The 10 to 15 acini in each SPL participate in gas exchange and surround the centrilobular bronchovascular structures. Deoxygenated blood in the pulmonary artery passes through the rich capillary network surrounding the acini, where gas exchange occurs. The SPL is outlined by a connective tissue septum, the interlobular septum, within which course pulmonary veins and pulmonary lymphatics. Interlobular septa measure 0.1 cm and are often identified on HRCT by the pulmonary veins that course through the septa and measure 0.5 cm in diameter. The capillary network connects the centrilobular structures to the septal pulmonary veins that carry oxygenated blood back to the heart.

TABLE 17.1 Differentiation of Diseases by Distribution

Distribution	Disease
Upper zone	Pulmonary Langerhans cell histiocytosis
	Emphysema
	Respiratory bronchiolitis
	Cystic fibrosis
	Hypersensitivity pneumonitis
	Sarcoidosis
	Reactivation tuberculosis
	Pneumoconioses (silicosis, coal worker's pneumoconiosis, berylliosis)
	Ankylosing spondylitis, neurofibromatosis 1
Lower zone	Hematogenous metastases
	Aspiration
	Usual interstitial pneumonitis
	Nonspecific interstitial pneumonitis
	Asbestosis
Central	Pulmonary edema
	Pulmonary hemorrhage
	Pneumocystis pneumonia
	Lymphoma
	Kaposi sarcoma
Peripheral	Organizing pneumonia
	Chronic eosinophilic pneumonia
	Aspiration pneumonia
	Pulmonary infarction
	Septic emboli
	Sarcoidosis
	Adenocarcinoma
	Lymphoma
	IgG4-related lung disease
Dependent	Aspiration
	Diffuse alveolar damage (noncardiogenic pulmonary edema or acute lung injury)

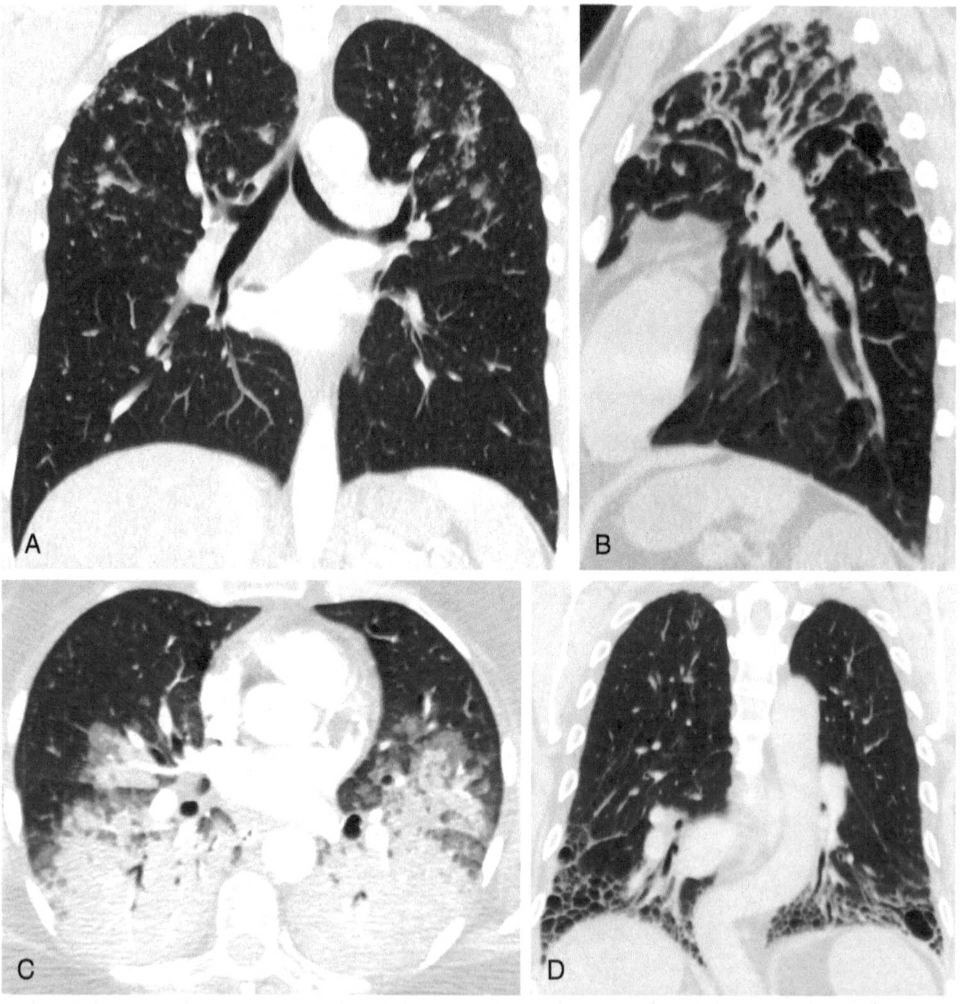

FIGURE 17.6 Distribution of disease in separate patients. **A,** Coronal image shows upper and mid-zone–predominant nodules in this patient with sarcoidosis. **B,** Sagittal image shows volume loss in the upper lobes associated with bronchiectasis and mosaic attenuation secondary to cystic fibrosis. **C,** Axial image shows dependent consolidation in this patient with aspiration pneumonia. Aspiration may cause peripheral and dependent distribution of changes. **D,** Coronal image shows lower zone honeycomb cysts and traction bronchiolectasis in this patient with a usual interstitial pneumonitis pattern of pulmonary fibrosis and a clinical syndrome of idiopathic pulmonary fibrosis.

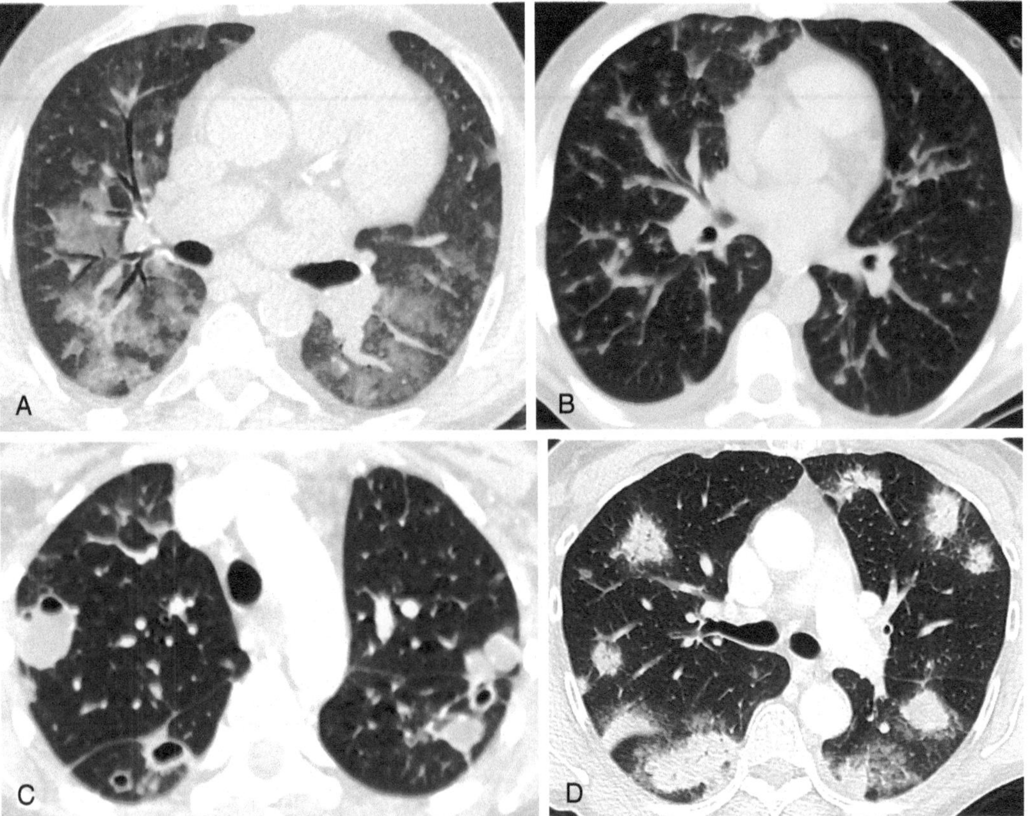

FIGURE 17.7 Distribution of disease in four separate patients: central versus peripheral. **A,** A 1.25-mm axial section in the upper lobes demonstrates central ground-glass opacities representing pulmonary edema in this patient with cardiac failure awaiting heart transplant. **B,** Axial sections in a patient with Kaposi sarcoma show central peribronchovascular nodules and flame-shaped opacities. **C,** Axial section in a patient with septic emboli secondary to endocarditis of the tricuspid valve shows multiple solid and cavitary peripheral nodules of variable size. **D,** Axial image through the mid zone in this patient with organizing pneumonia demonstrates multiple peripheral and peribronchiolar consolidative opacities with air bronchograms. This appearance is typical of organizing pneumonia.

Lung Interstitium

The lung interstitium forms a support system of connective tissue surrounding the lung parenchyma. The interstitium is divided into a central, peripheral, and intralobular interstitium. The central (axial) interstitium extends from the hila into the lung parenchyma, enveloping the bronchovascular bundles like a sheath and dividing as the bronchovascular bundles branch and arborize. The axial interstitium eventually reaches and terminates in the center of the SPL, surrounding the centrilobular pulmonary artery and bronchiole. The peripheral interstitium forms a subpleural cloak around the lung and extends along the fissures and forms the interlobular septa that outline the SPL. Between the central, centrilobular interstitium and the peripheral interlobular interstitium runs a fine meshwork of interstitial lines, the intralobular interstitium, that supports the structures within the SPL. The septa are most easily identified on CT in the subpleural region, along the fissures, and at the lung apices and bases.

Lymphatics are present in the interstitium. They course along the bronchovascular bundles surrounding the bronchiole and pulmonary artery that supply each lobule and within the interlobular septa. Lymphatic obstruction from tumor or edema can result in thickening of the bronchovascular interstitium and interlobular septa. Because the interlobular septa are best developed in the subpleural region and along the fissures, these areas are often involved with perilymphatic diseases, but centrilobular diseases involve structures in the center of the SPL; do not extend to the pleura, fissures, or interlobular septa; and are located approximately 5 to 10 mm from those surfaces. This distinction is helpful in localizing the site of abnormality on HRCT and directing the differential diagnosis.

HIGH-RESOLUTION COMPUTED TOMOGRAPHY PATTERNS

Most abnormalities identified on thin-section CT can be categorized into one of four main patterns: nodular, reticular, increased, or decreased attenuation. The predominant pattern as well as its anatomic location are extremely helpful in determining the imaging differential diagnosis. Diseases may show a craniocaudal and axial distribution as well as a predisposition to particular areas at the level of the SPL.

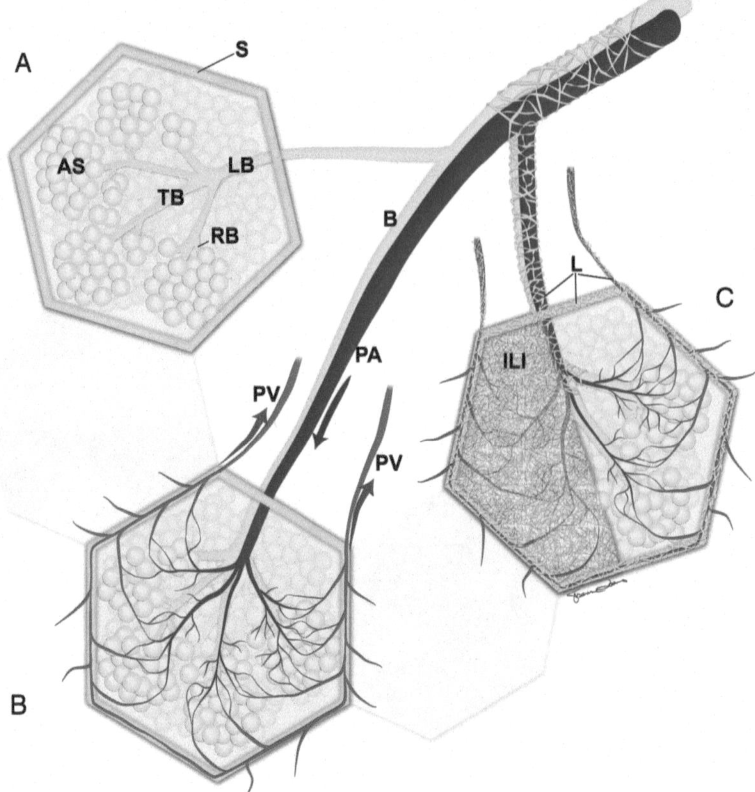

FIGURE 17.8 Diagram depicting the anatomy of the secondary pulmonary lobule (SPL). **A,** Airways. An SPL is surrounded by interlobular septa (S). Within the SPL, a lobular bronchiole (LB) divides into several terminal bronchioles (TBs) that in turn divide into multiple respiratory bronchioles (RBs). Several alveolar sacs (ASs) communicate with the RBs. This is the site of gaseous exchange within the lungs. **B,** Lobular pulmonary vessels. The pulmonary artery (PA in *blue*) branches course into the SPL alongside the bronchioles. The PA carries deoxygenated blood into the SPL and divides into a rich capillary network that surrounds the alveolar sacs. The capillary network transfers oxygenated blood to the periphery of the SPL. Pulmonary veins (PV in *red*) lie within the interlobular septa and transmit blood back to the heart. **C,** Interstitium. The lymphatics (L in *green*) course within a sheath that surrounds the bronchovascular bundle and course within the interlobular septa together with the pulmonary veins. There is an internal framework of connective tissue within the SPL that surrounds the alveolar sacs, known as the intralobular interstitium (ILI in *gray*).

Nodular Pattern (Table 17.2)

A nodular pattern consists of multiple well-defined rounded soft tissue or ground-glass nodules. The nodules usually measure between 2 and 10 mm in diameter, and their distribution can be related to the structures of the SPL (Fig. 17.9).

Perilymphatic Nodules

Perilymphatic nodules are located in the lymphatics that course along the peribronchovascular interstitium, interlobular septa, fissures, and subpleural interstitium. These nodules are often clustered, well defined, and of soft tissue attenuation. On HRCT, the subpleural space should be devoid of any structures and the walls of the bronchovascular structures as well as the fissures should be thin and sharp. Therefore, nodules in those regions are readily identified. At times, a collection of nodules in the subpleural space can mimic a pleural plaque, forming a "pseudo-plaque." The most common cause of perilymphatic nodules is sarcoidosis (Fig. 17.10). Other causes include lymphangitic carcinomatosis, berylliosis, silicosis, and coal worker's pneumoconiosis.

Random Nodules

Random nodules may be ground glass, solid, or cavitary in appearance. Random nodules may involve all areas of the lungs but predominate in the lower zones because of their hematogenous route of spread. The subpleural or perifissural space may also be minimally involved with a random pattern of nodules, and such findings should prompt a differential diagnosis that includes metastatic disease and miliary infection (Fig. 17.11). Multiple diffuse miliary nodules may be difficult to appreciate on thin-section CT, but their detection may be optimized by the use of MIP images.

Centrilobular Nodules

Centrilobular nodules occur in the center of the SPL and therefore do not contact the pleural space and spare the most peripheral 5 mm of the subpleural region, including the interlobar fissures. In some cases, larger centrilobular

TABLE 17.2 Causes of Multiple Nodular Opacities

Type	Causes
Perilymphatic	Sarcoidosis
	Lymphangitic carcinomatosis, lymphoma
	Silicosis, coal worker's pneumoconiosis
Rare	Berylliosis
	Amyloidosis
	Lymphocytic interstitial pneumonia
Random	Metastases
	Miliary infection: tuberculosis, fungal
Centrilobular: nonbranching	Respiratory bronchiolitis
	Hypersensitivity pneumonitis
	Pulmonary hemorrhage
	Infection
	Pulmonary edema
	PLCH
Rare	Follicular bronchiolitis
	Pulmonary arterial hypertension
	Invasive mucinous adenocarcinoma
	Organizing pneumonia
	Capillary hemangioendotheliosis
	Metastatic calcification, talcosis
	Pneumoconiosis (coal worker's pneumoconiosis, silicosis)
Centrilobular: branching (tree-in-bud)	Infection: bacterial, mycobacterial, viral, fungal, ABPA, panbronchiolitis
	Aspiration
	Bronchiectasis, cystic fibrosis
Rare	Invasive adenocarcinoma
	Follicular bronchiolitis
	Organizing pneumonia

ABPA, Allergic Bronchopulmonary Aspergillasis; *PLCH,* pulmonary Langerhans cell histiocytosis.

TABLE 17.3 Causes of Multiple Reticular Opacities

Type	Causes
Septal thickening	
Smooth	Pulmonary edema
	Pulmonary hemorrhage
	Lymphangitis carcinomatosis or lymphomatosis
	PAP
	AEP
Rare	Lymphangioleiomyomatosis
	Pulmonary venoocclusive disease
	Erdheim Chester disease
Nodular	Lymphangitis carcinomatosis or lymphomatosis
	Sarcoidosis, silicosis, coal worker's pneumoconiosis
Rare	Lymphoproliferative disease
	Amyloidosis
Irregular	Fibrosis secondary to UIP, HP, sarcoidosis, asbestosis
Intralobular interstitial thickening	UIP
	NSIP
	Transplant rejection
	PAP, DAH, AIP, DAD
Honeycombing	UIP (primary, secondary to drug reaction, connective tissue disease)
	HP
	Asbestosis
	Sarcoidosis
Traction bronchiectasis	UIP
	NSIP
	HP
	Sarcoidosis
	DAD

AEP, Acute eosinophilic pneumonia; *AIP,* Acute Interstitial Pneumonia; *DAD,* Diffuse Alveolar Damage; *DAH,* Diffuse Alveolar Hemorrhage; *HP,* hypersensitivity pneumonitis; *NSIP,* nonspecific interstitial pneumonia; *PAP,* pulmonary alveolar proteinosis; *UIP,* usual interstitial pneumonitis.

nodules may contact these areas, but their epicenter is centrilobular in location. Centrilobular nodules typically appear evenly spaced from each other because of their distribution in the center of adjacent SPLs. Centrilobular nodules may be branching and form tree-in-bud opacities or manifest as discrete nonbranching nodules. Centrilobular nonbranching nodules are often of ground-glass attenuation but may be of soft tissue or solid attenuation (Fig. 17.12).

Centrilobular nonbranching ground-glass nodules are typically a manifestation of respiratory bronchiolitis in a smoker and often indicate hypersensitivity pneumonitis in a nonsmoker. Any cause of bronchiolitis or vasculitis can cause centrilobular nonbranching nodules, and the differential diagnosis may be extensive.

Centrilobular branching, or tree-in-bud opacities, almost always represent inflammation and fluid filling of the small airways, and the most common causes are infection or aspiration. Viral, bacterial, fungal, and mycobacterial infections may all cause tree-in-bud opacities (Fig. 17.13). Panbronchiolitis results in diffuse tree-in-bud opacities throughout the lung parenchyma. Rare causes of tree-in-bud opacities include organizing pneumonia and invasive adenocarcinoma. Tree-in-bud opacities can be mimicked by other conditions (Fig. 17.14). Tumor emboli can grow within distal pulmonary arteries and veins and cause a branching, beaded appearance of the vessel, termed *vascular tree-in-bud.* The adjacent airway appears normal. Also, perilymphatic conditions, such as sarcoidosis, can mimic tree-in-bud opacities because there is nodularity along the walls of airways. However, the lumen of the airways is patent, and nodules also occur along the subpleural space and fissures, which indicate that the distribution is perilymphatic rather than centrilobular.

Reticular Opacities (Table 17.3)

Reticular or linear opacities can be secondary to interlobular septal thickening, intralobular lines, and honeycombing (Fig. 17.15). Bronchiectasis can also result in linear opacities.

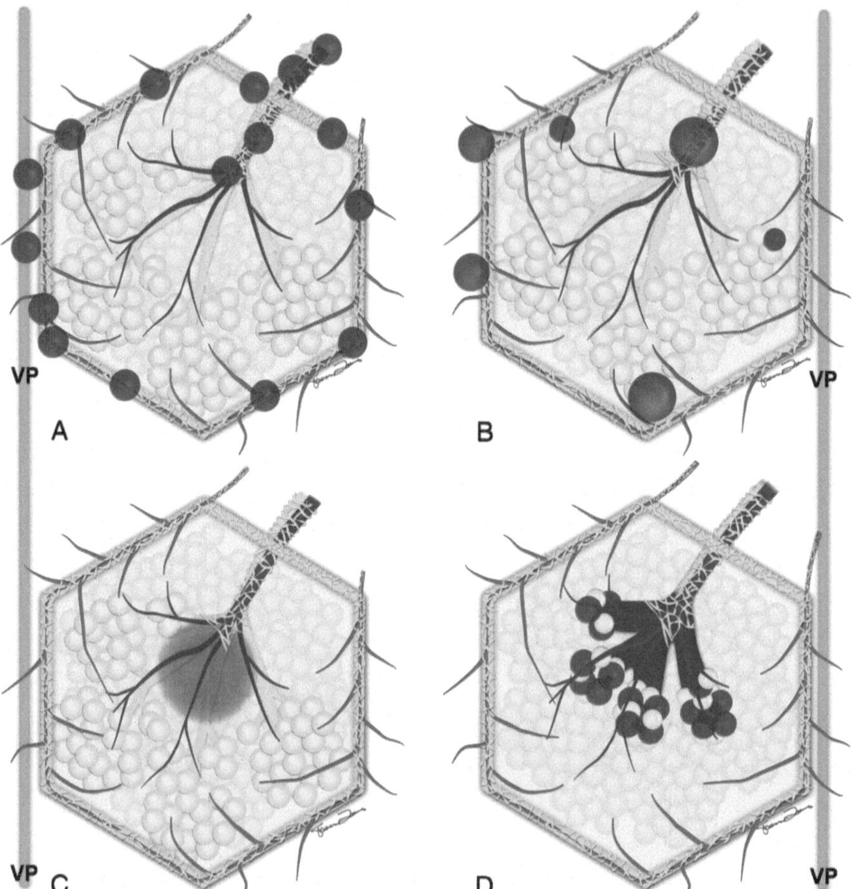

FIGURE 17.9 Diagram depicting the different nodular patterns at the level of the secondary pulmonary lobule (SPL). **A,** Perilymphatic pattern. Multiple nodules course along the bronchovascular bundle, interlobular septa, adjacent subpleural or fissural visceral pleura (VP in *pink*). **B,** Random pattern. Nodules do not correspond to any anatomic structure and vary in size. Some may abut the fissure and subpleural region **C,** Centrilobular nonbranching pattern. These nodules lie in the center of the SPL. They are most frequently of ground-glass attenuation but occasionally are solid or cavitary. They do not extend into the interlobular septa, the subpleural, or fissural regions. **D,** Centrilobular branching nodules. These are also known as tree-in-bud opacities. The opacity is the result of inflammation and fluid filling of the small airways.

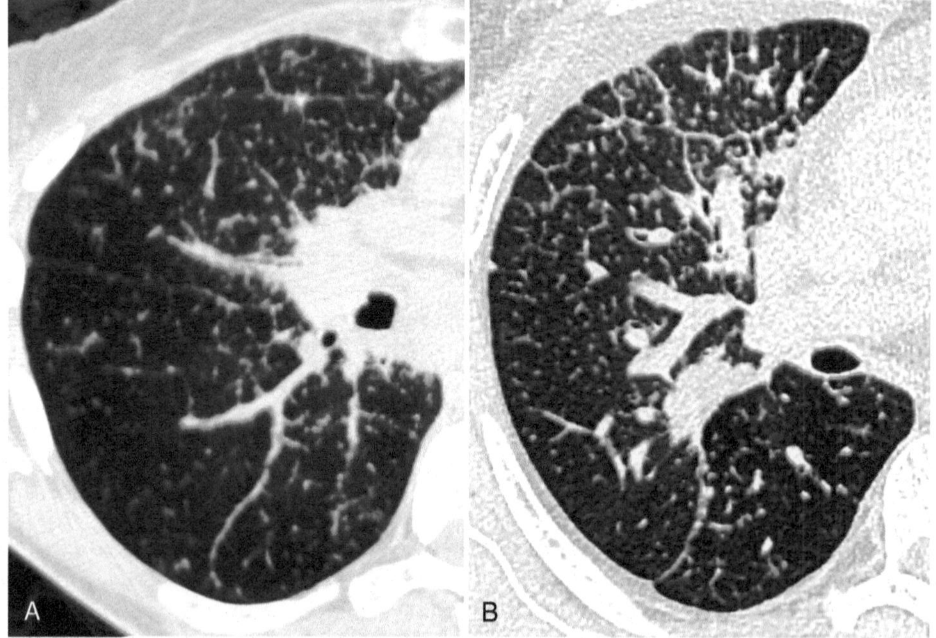

FIGURE 17.10 Perilymphatic nodules in two separate patients. **A,** Coned axial image of the right lung shows nodules along the bronchovascular bundle, fissures, and subpleural space and in the interlobular septa in a patient with sarcoidosis. **B,** Coned axial image of the right lung shows thickening and nodularity of the interlobular septa and visceral pleura in a patient with pulmonary lymphangitic carcinomatosis.

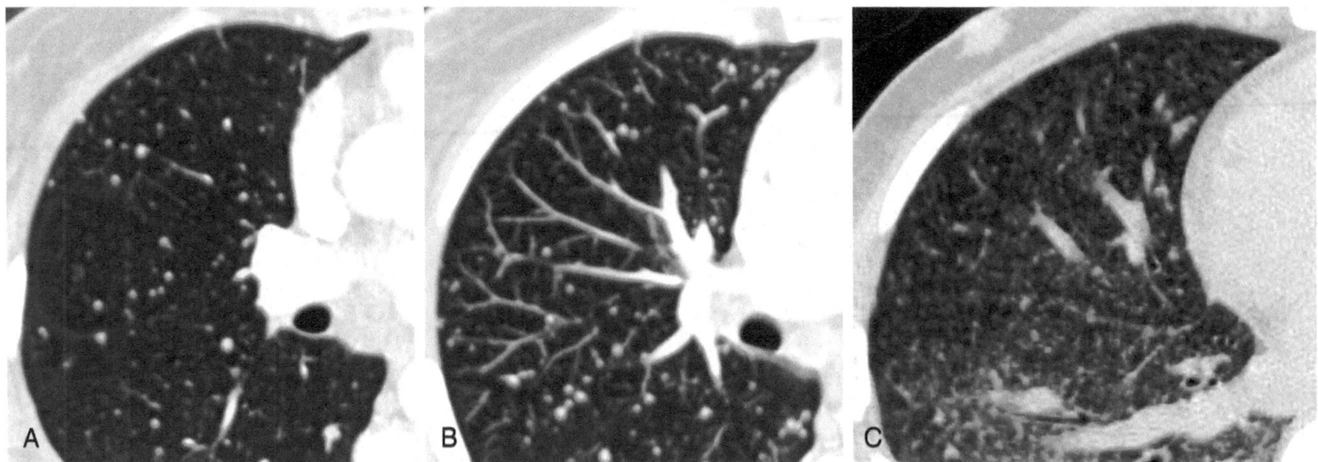

FIGURE 17.11 Random nodules in two separate patients. **A,** Axial image shows randomly distributed and variable sized nodules in a patient with metastatic melanoma. **B,** Maximum-intensity potential images in the same patient show improved visualization and characterization of multiple solid nodules that can be easily distinguished from adjacent vessels. **C,** Axial image shows random nodules in a patient with miliary tuberculosis.

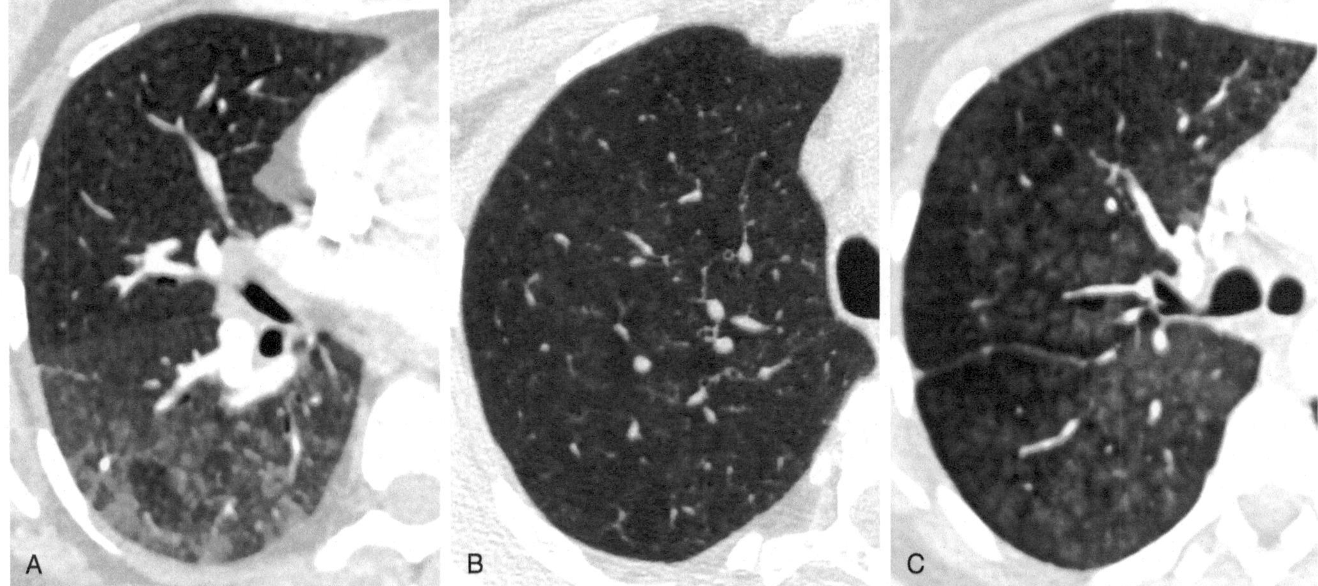

FIGURE 17.12 Centrilobular nonbranching nodules in three separate patients. **A,** Axial image shows multiple centrilobular ground-glass nodules in a patient with hypersensitivity pneumonitis secondary to mold in his home. There are lucent lobular areas in the lower lobes that demonstrated air trapping on expiration studies. **B,** Axial image shows multiple centrilobular ground-glass nodules in an asymptomatic heavy smoker with respiratory bronchiolitis. There is associated centrilobular emphysema. **C,** Axial image shows multiple centrilobular ground-glass nodules in a patient with pulmonary hemosiderosis. Note the sparing of the subpleural space and fissures in all the cases.

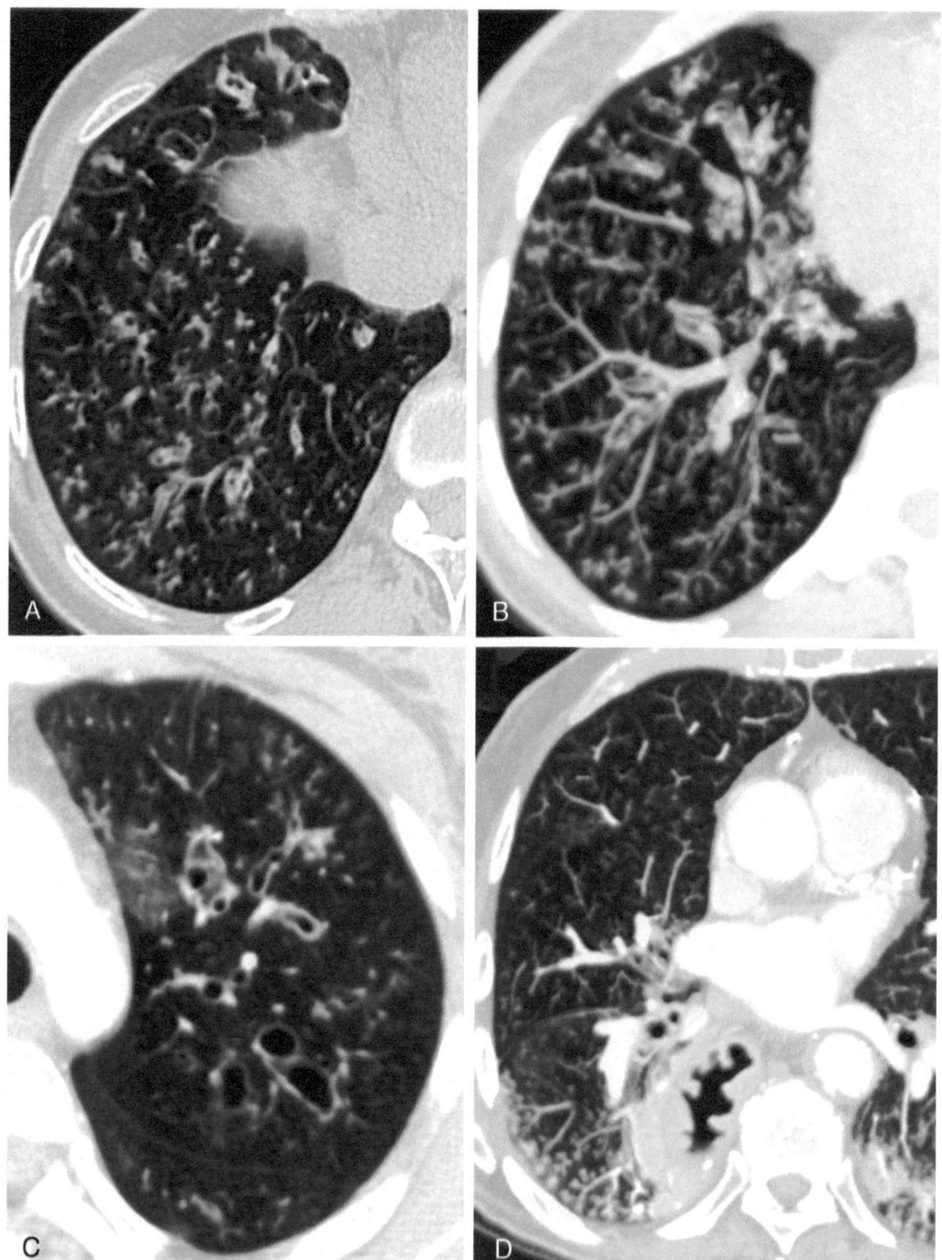

FIGURE 17.13 Centrilobular branching nodules or tree-in-bud opacities in three separate patients. **A,** Axial image shows tree-in-bud opacities and bronchial wall thickening in the right lung secondary to *Haemophilus influenzae* infection. **B,** Maximum-intensity projection (MIP) images in the same patient improve characterization of the branching opacities. **C,** Axial image of the left upper lobe shows bronchiectasis and tree-in-buad opacities in a patient with cystic fibrosis. **D,** Axial MIP image shows aspiration pneumonia in a patient with a gastric pull-up.

Interlobular Septal Thickening

Interlobular septal thickening creates multiple well-defined polygonal-shaped thickened outlines of SPLs and is most easily identified where the septa are best developed—at the lung apices, bases, subpleural space, and adjacent to the fissures. Coronal reformatted images are often helpful in confirming the presence of interlobular septal thickening. Thickening of the interlobular septa is associated with lymphatic and pulmonary venous diseases. Associated thickening of the bronchovascular bundles secondary to thickening of the axial interstitium results in prominence of the centrilobular arterioles and bronchioles. Septal thickening may be smooth, nodular, or irregular. Smooth thickening is most commonly seen with pulmonary edema and nodular thickening with lymphangitic carcinomatosis or sarcoidosis (Fig. 17.16). There may be associated ground-glass opacity, particularly with certain conditions, such as pulmonary edema, pulmonary hemorrhage, or pulmonary alveolar proteinosis (PAP).

Intralobular Lines

Reticular opacities may occur as a result of thickening of the interstitium within the SPL. Reticular opacities are often irregular and best seen along the fissures, subpleural space, and surrounding the bronchovascular bundles.

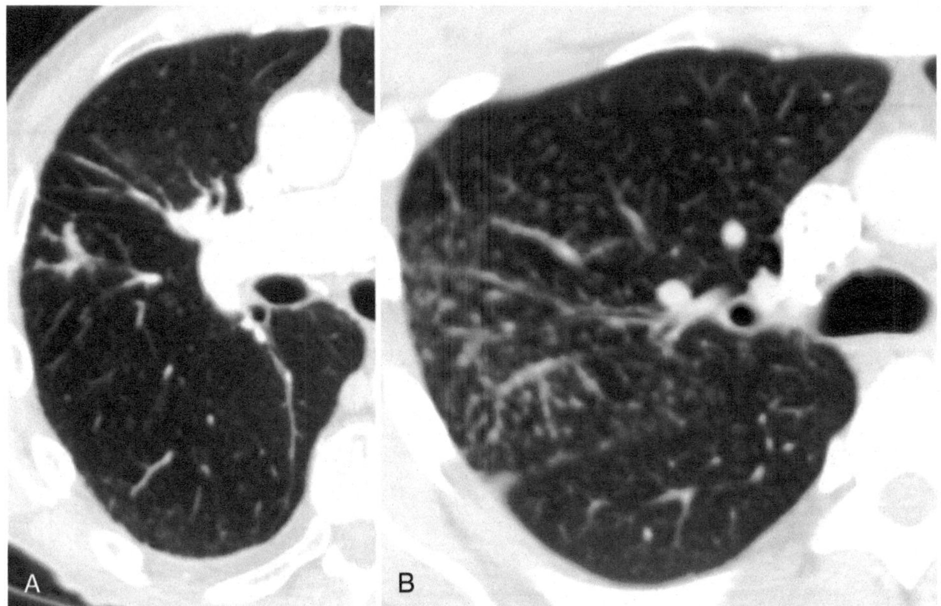

FIGURE 17.14 Mimics of tree-in-bud opacities in two separate patients. **A,** Axial image in a patient with tumor emboli from renal cell carcinoma. Tumor emboli manifest as dilated, beaded peripheral pulmonary arteries that can mimic airway disease. **B,** Axial image of the right upper lobe in a patient with sarcoidosis. The perilymphatic nodules course along the bronchovascular interstitium and can mimic tree-in-bud opacities. Note that the vessels and airways both appear nodular. Nodules are also present along the fissures and subpleural space, which is not a feature of centrilobular abnormalities.

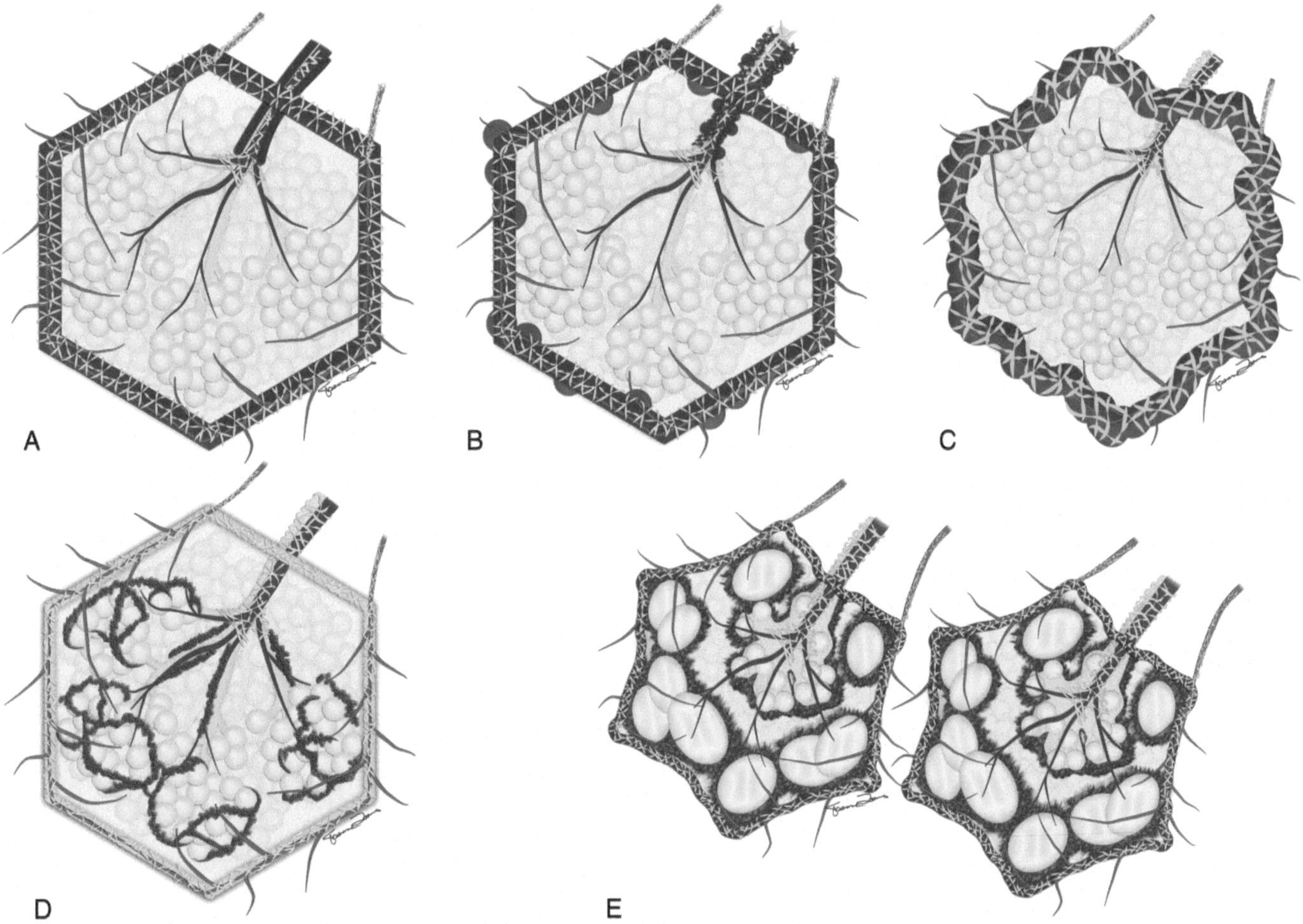

A B C

D E

FIGURE 17.15 Diagram depicting the different reticular patterns that can occur at the level of the secondary pulmonary lobule (SPL). **A,** Smooth septal thickening results in a meshwork pattern of polyhedral shapes outlining the SPL. **B,** Nodular septal thickening. **C,** Irregular septal thickening results in distortion and loss of volume of the SPL. **D,** Fine intralobular lines within the SPL. **E,** Honeycomb cystic change. There is volume loss of the SPL associated with irregular septal thickening and cysts. Traction bronchiectasis is also present.

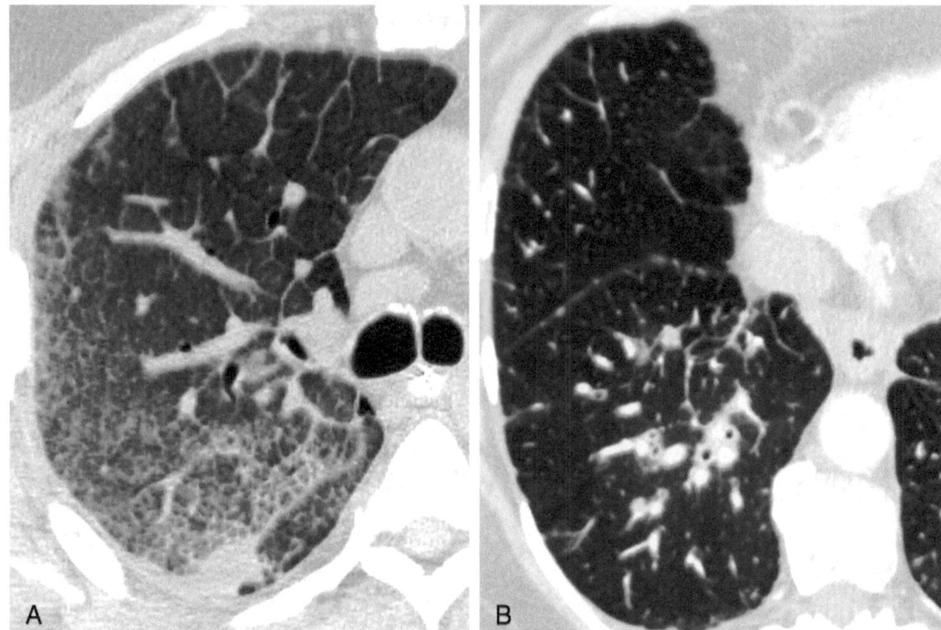

FIGURE 17.16 Septal thickening resulting in reticular opacities in two separate patients. **A,** Axial computed tomography scan shows smooth interlobular septal thickening and intralobular lines, resulting in reticular opacities secondary to pulmonary edema. Note the small bilateral pleural effusions and diffuse ground-glass opacity. **B,** Nodular septal thickening in the right lung is associated with thickening of the bronchovascular interstitium and fissural and subpleural nodules secondary to lymphangitic carcinomatosis in this patient with metastatic lung cancer.

Isolated lower lobe peripheral reticular opacities may be a sign of aging in asymptomatic older individuals. However, when associated with architectural distortion and traction bronchiectasis, intralobular interstitial thickening reflects fibrosis (Fig. 17.17). It is commonly seen with a usual interstitial pneumonitis (UIP) pattern of pulmonary fibrosis, a nonspecific interstitial pneumonia (NSIP) pattern, hypersensitivity pneumonitis, and sarcoidosis. In the absence of findings of fibrosis, intralobular interstitial thickening may be secondary to pulmonary edema, pulmonary hemorrhage, alveolar proteinosis, or atypical infection.

Honeycombing

Honeycombing represents end-stage pulmonary fibrosis. On HRCT, honeycombing is typically located in the subpleural space and often in the lower lobes. The cystic spaces of honeycombing range from 3 mm to 3 cm in diameter, have thick clearly defined walls, and share their walls with contiguous cysts in the subpleural region of the lung. They may occur as a single tier of honeycomb cysts but more often form multiple layers, often with associated areas of traction bronchiectasis. Detection of honeycombing as a predominant pattern in the lower lobes strongly suggests a UIP pattern of pulmonary fibrosis.

Increased Attenuation (Table 17.4)

Increased lung attenuation on CT may manifest as ground-glass opacity or consolidation. These terms refer to CT findings rather than a diagnosis and have many causes (Fig. 17.18).

Ground-glass opacity is defined as increased opacification of the lung parenchyma that does not obscure the underlying pulmonary vessels. *Consolidation* is defined as complete opacification of the lung that does obscure underlying vessels. Both ground-glass opacity and consolidation may be associated with air bronchograms. Increased lung opacity may appear anatomic in location by involving one or several SPLs, pulmonary segments, lobes, or the whole lung.

Ground-Glass Opacity

Ground-glass opacity may be a normal physiologic finding. When a patient is supine, there is a normal anteroposterior gradient within the lung parenchyma of up to 100 Hounsfield units (HU). In the supine position, there is also dependent density secondary to subpleural partial atelectasis of lung parenchyma that can mimic interstitial lung disease, changes that resolve on prone images. In addition, normal parenchymal changes during expiration can be misinterpreted as ground-glass opacity. In expiration, the lung has proportionately less air, and lung attenuation on HRCT may increase by 150 to 300 HU.

Pathologic causes for ground-glass opacity may be related to partial filling of the airspaces, thickening of the intralobular interstitium, increased blood flow, or partial alveolar collapse (Fig. 17.19). Partial filling of the airspaces can occur because of fluid such as edema, blood, infection, tumor, macrophages, or protein. Fine fibrosis beyond the resolution of HRCT can also result in ground-glass opacity caused by mild interstitial thickening of the alveolar walls. Clues to the diagnosis of fibrosis include the presence of adjacent traction bronchiectasis and evidence of architectural distortion. Alveolar collapse is associated with increased ground-glass in its early phase. Increased capillary blood volume may also increase the attenuation of lung parenchyma.

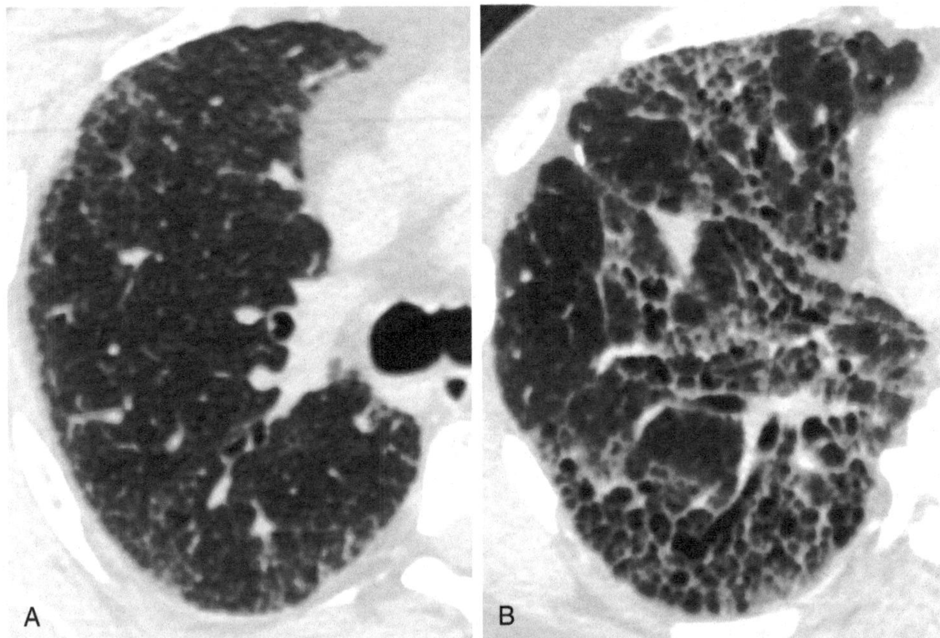

FIGURE 17.17 Reticular opacities in two separate patients. **A,** Axial computed tomography (CT) scan shows peripheral distribution of irregular intralobular interstitial thickening in this patient with an early usual interstitial pneumonitis pattern of pulmonary fibrosis. **B,** Axial CT scan demonstrates peripheral, multilayered honeycombing cystic changes associated with traction bronchiectasis. There is irregular septal thickening outlining several secondary pulmonary lobules.

TABLE 17.4 Causes of Diffuse Increased Attenuation

Type	Cause
Ground-glass opacity: acute	Infection: atypical: viral, mycobacterial, PCP
	Pulmonary edema
	Pulmonary hemorrhage
	Aspiration pneumonitis
	AIP or DAD
	Acute exacerbation of ILD
	AEP
Ground-glass opacity: chronic	RB, DIP
	HP, NSIP, LIP
	OP, CEP
	PAP
	Tumor: invasive adenocarcinoma
Consolidation: acute	Infection
	Aspiration
	DAD, AIP
	Severe edema, hemorrhage
	HP
	AEP
Consolidation: chronic	Malignancy: adenocarcinoma
	Lymphoma
	OP, CEP
	Granulomatosis with polyangiitis
	Sarcoidosis

AEP, acute eosinophilic pneumonia; *AIP*, acute interstitial pneumonia; *CEP*, chronic eosinophilic pneumonia; *DAD*, diffuse alveolar damage; *DIP*, desquamative interstitial pneumonia; *HP*, hypersensitivity pneumonitis; *LIP*, lymphocytic interstitial pneumonitis; *NSIP*, nonspecific interstitial pneumonia; *OP*, organizing pneumonia; *PAP*, pulmonary alveolar proteinosis; *PCP*, *Pneumocystis* pneumonia; RB, respiratory bronchiole.

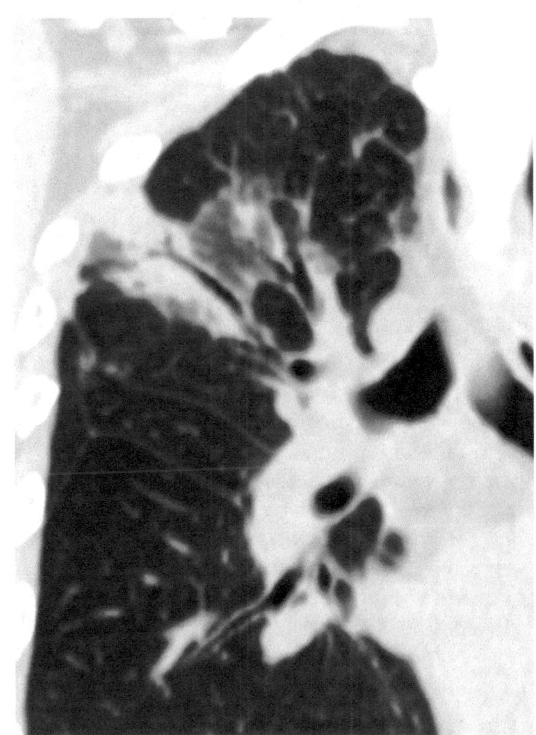

FIGURE 17.18 Coronal image of a patient with multifocal pneumonia demonstrates both consolidation and ground-glass opacity in the right upper lobe. Vessels remain visible through the ground-glass opacity and are obscured by the consolidation. Both conditions are associated with air bronchograms.

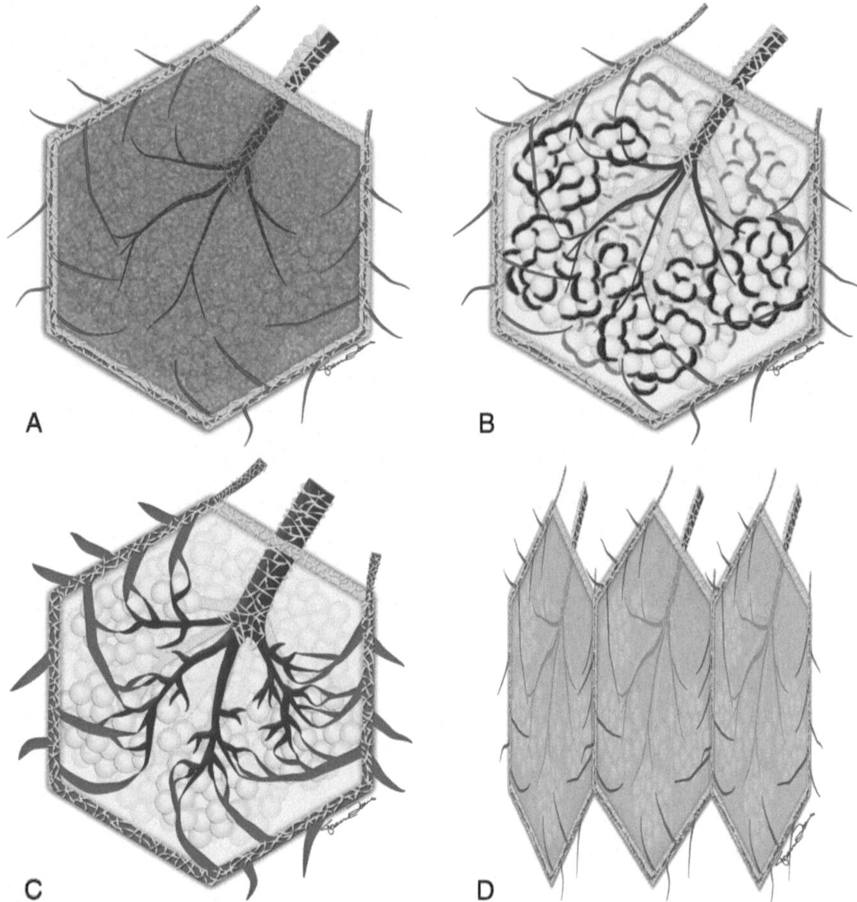

FIGURE 17.19 Diagram depicting causes of increased attenuation or ground-glass opacity. **A,** Partial filling of the secondary pulmonary lobule (SPL) with fluid that displaces air results in ground-glass opacity. **B,** Thickening of the intralobular interstitium around the alveolar walls can result in ground-glass opacity. **C,** Increased blood flow or venous engorgement results in relatively greater vascularity within the SPL, resulting in ground-glass opacity. **D,** Partial volume loss results in relatively less air within the SPL, causing ground-glass opacity.

The differential diagnosis for ground-glass opacity depends on the acuity or chronicity of findings and their distribution in the lungs (Fig. 17.20). Acute, central, perihilar ground-glass opacity is most commonly caused by pulmonary edema or pulmonary hemorrhage. Aspiration pneumonitis, acute eosinophilic pneumonia, diffuse alveolar damage, and diffuse pneumonia (e.g., viral pneumonia, *Pneumocystis jirovecii* pneumonia) can have a similar appearance. A multifocal, patchy distribution of ground-glass opacity is usually secondary to infection.

When ground-glass opacity is chronic, likely causes include interstitial lung disease (e.g., hypersensitivity pneumonitis, organizing pneumonia, NSIP, desquamative interstitial pneumonia, lymphocytic interstitial pneumonitis [LIP]), PAP, and malignancy (i.e., adenocarcinoma).

Consolidation

Consolidation is caused by complete replacement of air within the SPL by fluid or tumor, resulting in obscuration of the underlying pulmonary vessels. In the acute phase, pneumonia, aspiration, and diffuse alveolar damage are the most common causes; chronic causes include organizing pneumonia, eosinophilic pneumonia, malignancy (e.g., adenocarcinoma, lymphoma), vasculitis (e.g., granulomatosis with polyangiitis), and radiation pneumonitis (Fig. 17.21).

Decreased Attenuation (Table 17.5)

Decreased lung opacities or low-attenuation lesions include cystic lung disease, emphysema, and a mosaic pattern of pulmonary attenuation secondary to pulmonary vascular disease or small airway disease (Fig. 17.22).

Emphysema

Emphysema is a smoking-related disease, the result of irreversible destruction of the lung parenchyma beyond the terminal bronchiole (Fig. 17.23). The earliest findings of emphysema are poorly defined centrilobular lucencies within an SPL. Remnants of the pulmonary parenchyma are often seen coursing within the lucencies, including the centrilobular pulmonary artery or remnants of interlobular septa. As the emphysema progresses, further breakdown of lung parenchyma results in large bullous spaces, which may have a mass effect on adjacent structures and result in architectural distortion and compressive atelectasis. Paraseptal emphysema is also smoking related and refers to subpleural, paramediastinal, or parafissural lucencies. These lucencies typically occur in the upper lobes as a single row of multiple well-defined lucencies separated by thin walls that represent interlobular septa. There is often associated centrilobular emphysema. Differentiation

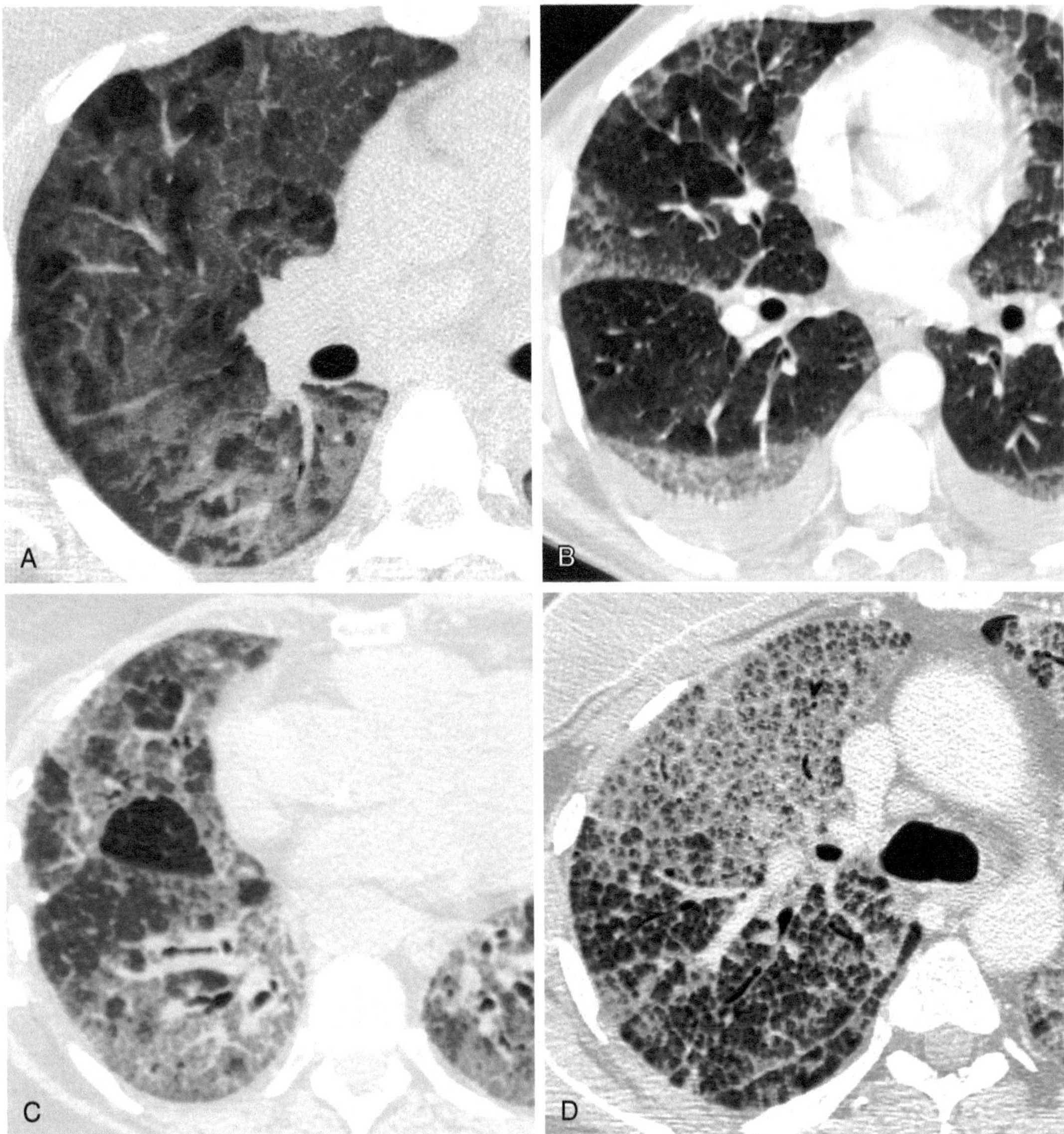

FIGURE 17.20 Causes of ground-glass opacity in four separate patients. **A,** Diffuse ground-glass opacity secondary to *Pneumocystis jirovecii* pneumonia in a patient with AIDS. **B,** Patchy multifocal and dependent ground-glass opacities, septal thickening, and small bilateral pleural effusions in a new heavy smoker presenting with respiratory failure secondary to acute eosinophilic pneumonia. **C,** Chronic ground-glass opacity, lobular lucencies, and fibrosis in a patient with hypersensitivity pneumonitis. Expiration studies showed air trapping. **D,** Chronic ground-glass opacity, septal thickening, and intralobular lines in a patient with pulmonary alveolar proteinosis.

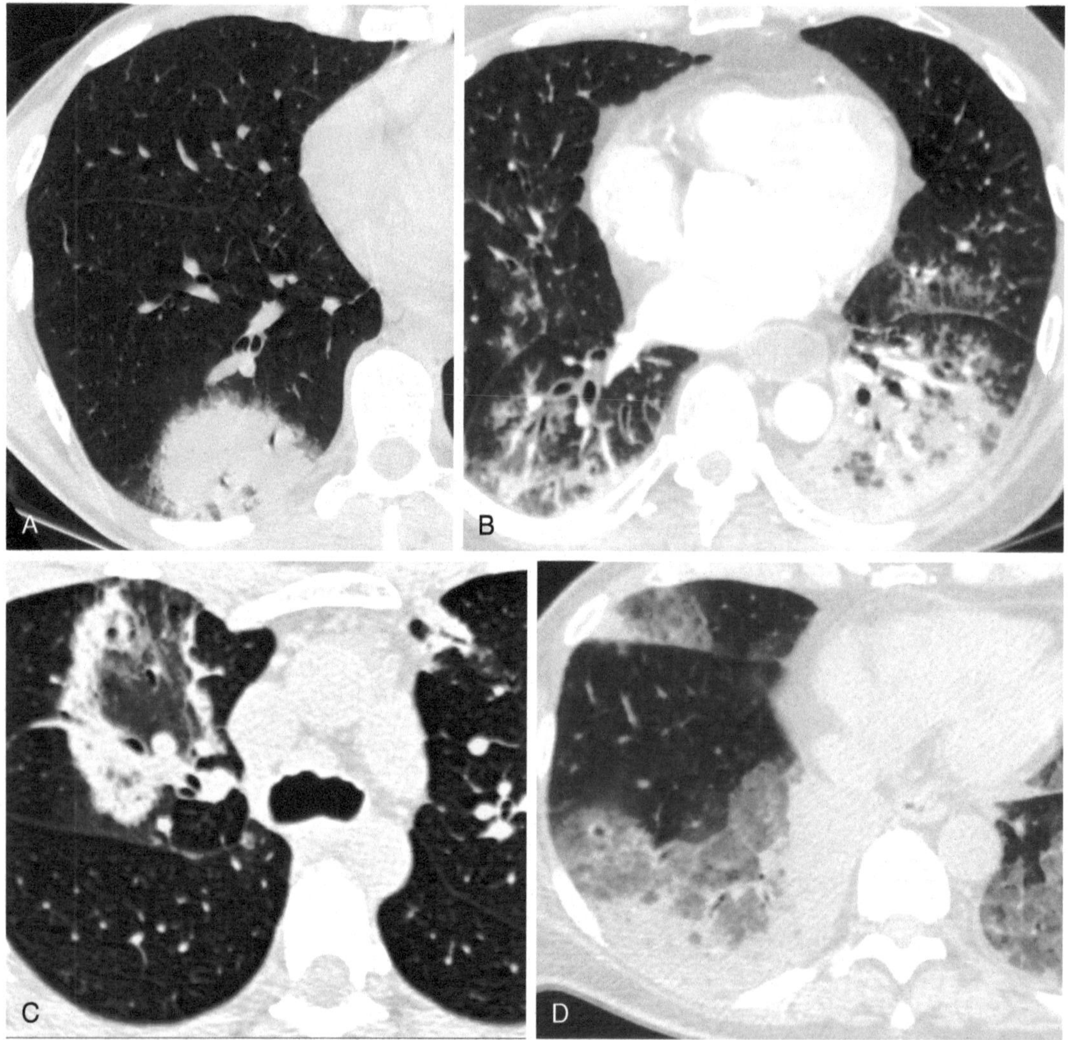

FIGURE 17.21 Causes of consolidation in four separate patients. **A,** Right lower lobe rounded consolidation secondary to community-acquired pneumonia. **B,** Bilateral lower lobe–dependent consolidation secondary to aspiration pneumonia. **C,** Right upper lobe peripheral consolidation surrounding central ground-glass opacity resulting in a reverse halo sign. There is also consolidation in the anteromedial aspect of the left upper lobe in this patient with organizing pneumonia. **D,** Multifocal peripheral consolidation and ground-glass opacity secondary to multifocal adenocarcinoma of the lung.

TABLE 17.5 Causes of Decreased Attenuation

Type	Cause
Emphysema	Centrilobular
	Paraseptal
	Pan lobular
Cysts	PLCH
	LAM
	LAM and tuberous sclerosis complex
	LIP
	Pneumatoceles: treated infection, trauma
	Birt-Hogg-Dube syndrome
Rare	Light-chain deposition disease
	Amyloidosis
	Neurofibromatosis
	Treated metastatic disease
Mosaic attenuation: vascular	Chronic pulmonary thromboembolic disease
	Vasculitis
Mosaic attenuation: airways	HP
	Obliterative bronchiolitis
	Asthma

HP, Hypersensitivity pneumonitis; *LAM,* lymphangioleiomyomatosis; *LIP,* lymphocytic interstitial pneumonitis; *PLCH,* pulmonary Langerhans cell histiocytosis.

from honeycombing can be challenging, but the cysts in paraseptal emphysema are larger in size, with thinner walls than honeycomb cysts (Fig. 17.24). The cysts in paraseptal emphysema are not in multiple stacks or arcades and are not associated with architectural distortion, traction bronchiectasis, or volume loss.

Cystic Disease

Cystic lung diseases cause regions of decreased lung attenuation. The cyst has a thin well-defined wall (<4 mm), and there is complete absence of normal anatomic structures within the cyst. These features differentiate cysts from centrilobular emphysema in which the low-attenuation areas have imperceptible walls, and centrilobular remnants of lung parenchyma are commonly seen (Fig. 17.25). Cystic lung disease may result in thin-walled cysts such as with lymphangioleiomyomatosis (LAM), LIP, Birt-Hogg-Dube syndrome, or pneumatoceles. Thick-walled bizarre-shaped cysts are a feature of pulmonary Langerhans cell histiocytosis (PLCH) (Fig. 17.26). Occasional scattered thin-walled cysts have also been described in older patients and may be a normal finding older than the age of 75 years.

A multitiered peripheral honeycomb cystic pattern is seen secondary to fibrosing chronic interstitial lung disease, most notably with the UIP pattern of pulmonary fibrosis.

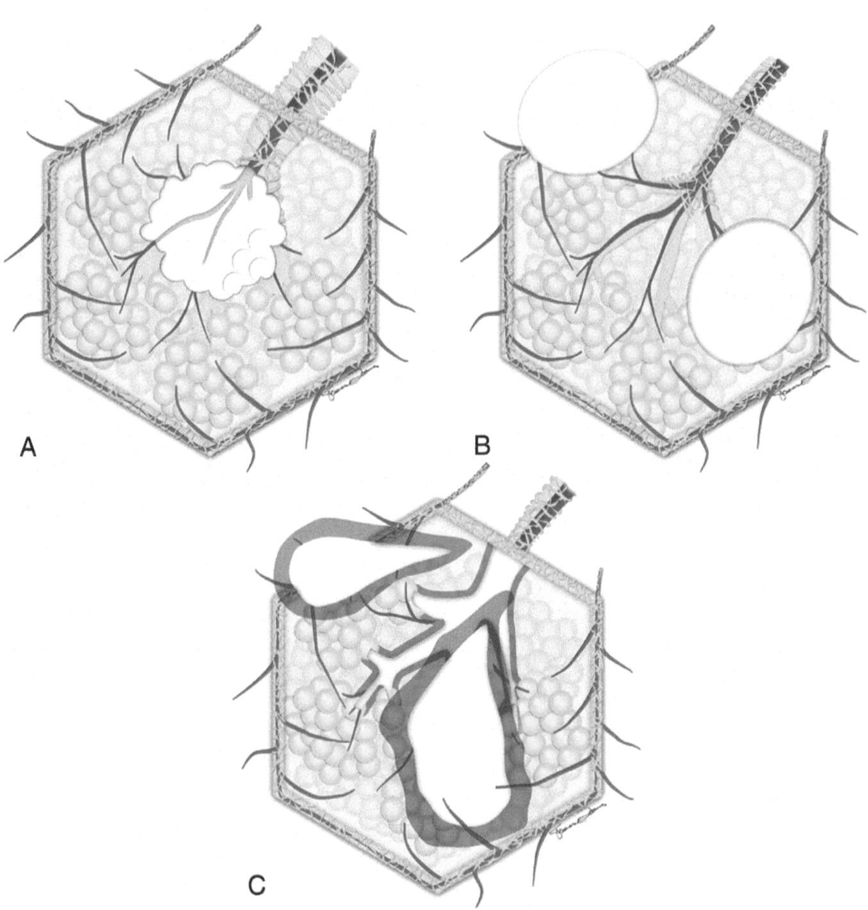

FIGURE 17.22 Diagram depicting causes of focal decreased attenuation or lucency. **A,** Centrilobular emphysema. **B,** Multiple thin-walled cysts differ from centrilobular emphysema because they have a definable wall and are randomly located relative to the secondary pulmonary lobule. **C,** Bronchiolar dilation associated with thick-walled irregular bizarre-shaped cysts as seen in pulmonary Langerhans cell histiocytosis.

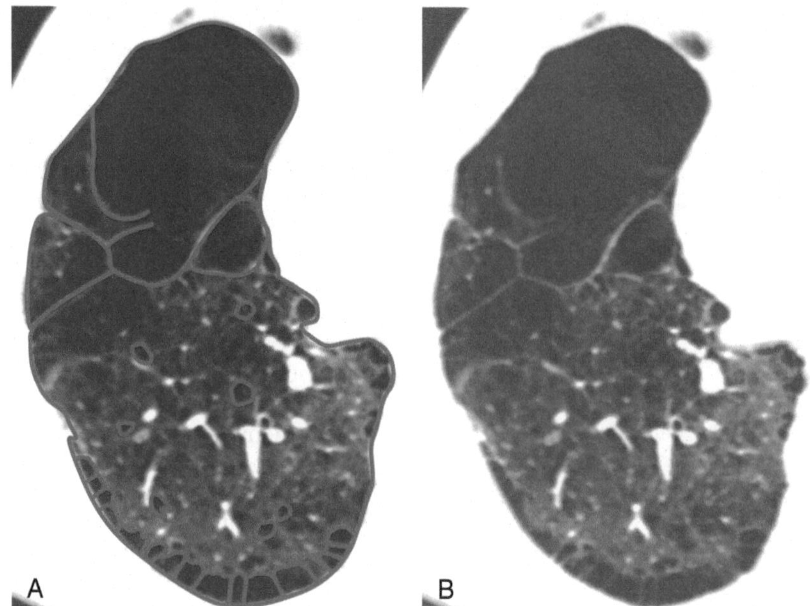

FIGURE 17.23 **A,** Diagrammatic overlay outlining the different forms of emphysema. **B,** Corresponding axial computed tomography scan of a patient with emphysema depicting paraseptal emphysema in the periphery, centrilobular emphysema in the lower lobes posteriorly, and bullous emphysema in the anterior aspects of both lungs.

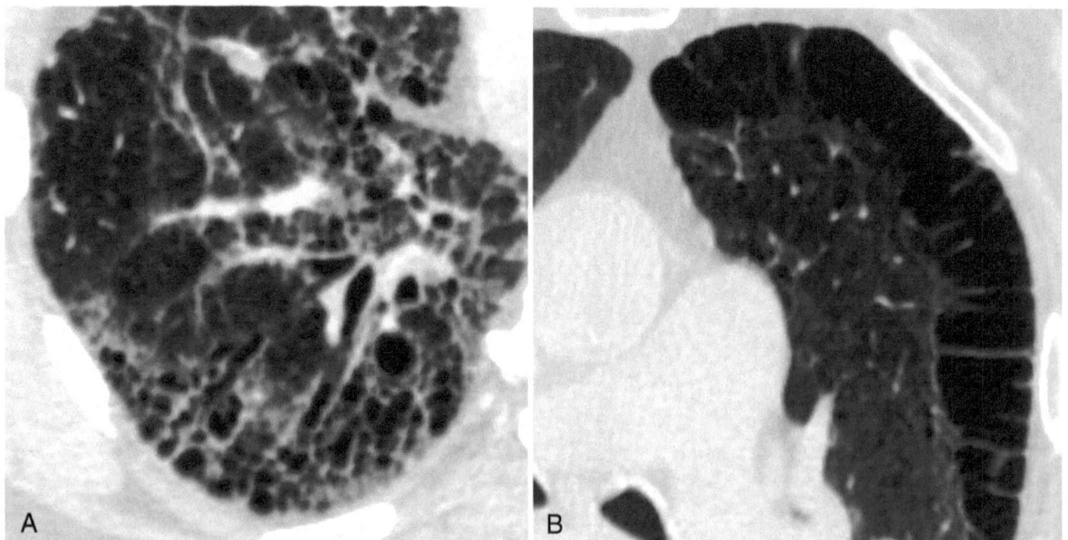

FIGURE 17.24 Causes of peripheral cystic lucencies in two separate patients. **A,** Axial scans through the right lower lobe shows honeycomb cysts. The cysts are usually in the lower lobes and posterior. They are associated with pulmonary fibrosis and appear as multiple, smaller cysts with irregular thick walls. The cysts share walls and often occur in multiple layers. Associated architectural distortion, traction bronchiectasis, and bronchiolectasis are present. **B,** Axial computed tomography scan in the left upper lobe shows extensive paraseptal emphysema that results from dilatation of the air sacs in the secondary pulmonary lobule surrounded by intact interlobular septa.

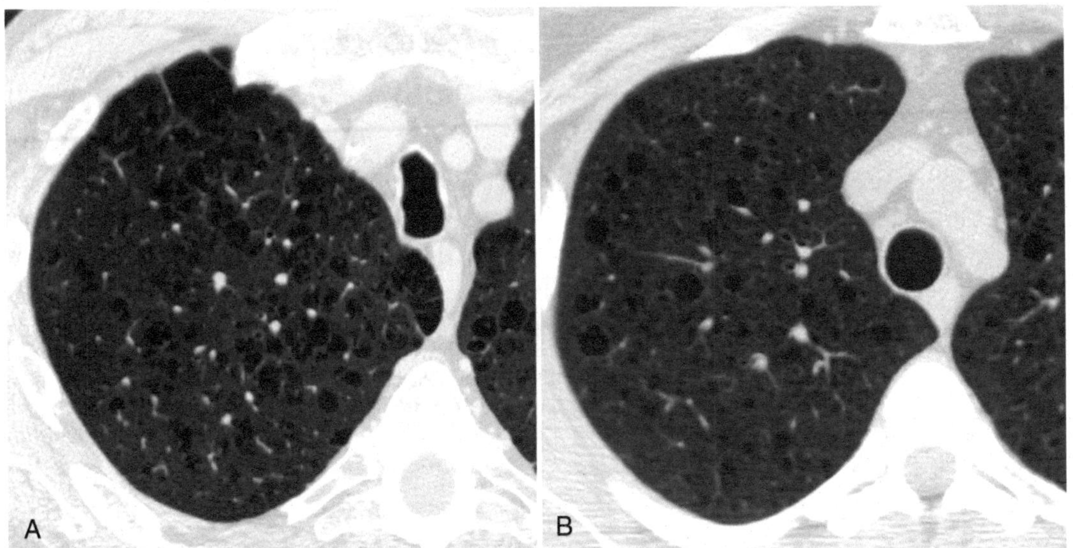

FIGURE 17.25 Comparison of emphysema and cysts in two separate patients. **A,** Axial image through the right upper lobe in a patient with centrilobular emphysema demonstrates upper lobe–predominant poorly defined lucencies lacking discrete walls. Remnants of the secondary pulmonary lobular structures are visible within the lucencies. Note that the trachea has a saber-sheath configuration. **B,** Axial computed tomography scan through the right upper lobe demonstrates well-defined spherical cysts with thin walls in a patient with lymphangioleiomyomatosis.

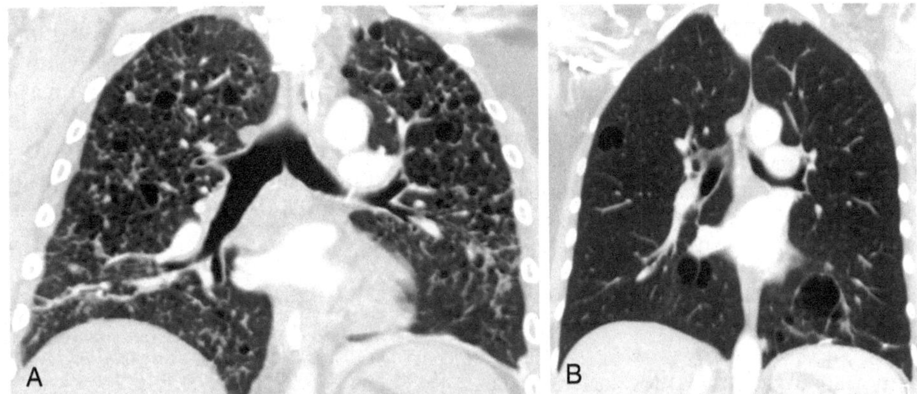

FIGURE 17.26 Distribution of cysts in two separate patients. **A,** Coronal image in a patient with pulmonary Langerhans cell histiocytosis (PLCH). There are upper lobe–predominant, variable-sized, bizarre-shaped, thick-walled cysts that spare the lung bases and costophrenic angles. This distribution is an extremely helpful finding in suggesting PLCH. **B,** Coronal image in a patient with Sjögren syndrome and lymphoid interstitial pneumonitis. Cysts in this condition show lower lobe predominance and often have an elliptical shape. There are associated ground-glass opacities and pulmonary nodules. The wedge resection site is present at the left base.

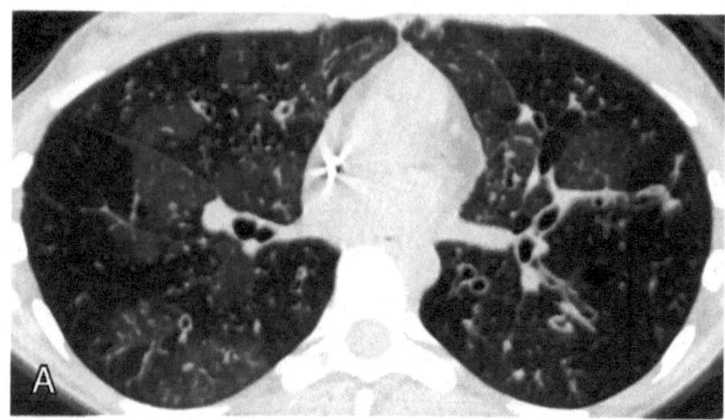

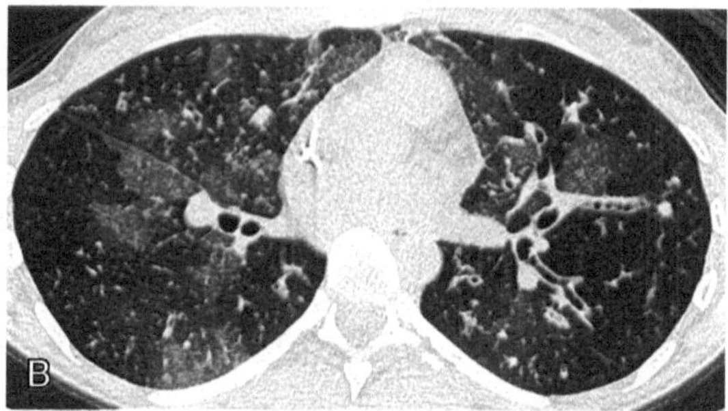

FIGURE 17.27 Mosaic attenuation secondary to air trapping in a patient with cystic fibrosis. **A,** Axial inspiratory images through the middle lobe and lower lobes demonstrate mosaic attenuation of the lung parenchyma. There are constricted vessels caused by decreased perfusion that manifests as abnormally lucent lung. There are also bronchiectasis and airway wall thickening. **B,** Axial expiratory image through the middle lobe and lower lobes shows decreases in volume and an increase in attenuation of the normal lung while the relatively lucent lung remains of large volume and lucent.

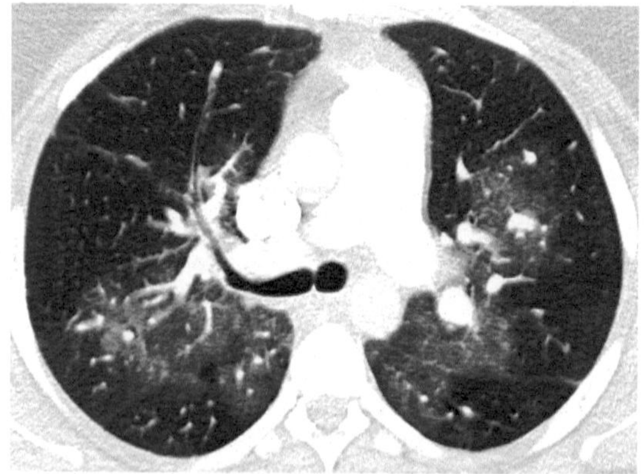

FIGURE 17.28 Axial computed tomography scan in a patient with chronic pulmonary embolic disease. There is mosaic attenuation of the lung parenchyma. Areas of relatively lucent lung are secondary to decreased perfusion following vascular occlusion. The relatively opaque lung is normally perfused. The pulmonary arterial vessels in normal lung are enlarged, as is the main pulmonary artery.

Mosaic Attenuation

The CT finding of mosaic lung attenuation refers to a patchwork of increased and decreased attenuation of the lung parenchyma. Mosaic lung attenuation often has a well-defined geographic distribution that follows the boundaries of SPLs. The abnormal lung may be due to areas of increased attenuation, as is seen with conditions that cause ground-glass opacity. When the abnormal lung is due to areas of decreased attenuation or lucent lung, it is secondary to vasoconstriction and reduced blood flow. This finding may be as a result of small airways disease, in which secondary vasoconstriction is a response to a primary ventilatory abnormality or caused by occlusive pulmonary vascular disease. The two causes of lucent lung can be differentiated with expiration images.

In cases of small airways disease, the areas of lucent lung remain of decreased attenuation and have relatively increased volume on expiration compared with the normal lung that collapses its volume and increases in its attenuation on expiration (Fig. 17.27). In patients with pulmonary thromboembolic disease, areas of lucent lung occur as a result of decreased vascular perfusion. On expiration, these regions decrease in size and do increase somewhat in attenuation (Fig. 17.28).

CONCLUSION

Thin-section CT and HRCT can provide specific radiographic clues to the diagnosis of diffuse lung diseases. Correct interpretation of the abnormality involves simultaneous pattern identification and distribution assessment within the whole lung and at the level of the SPL. Comparison with prior studies to evaluate the chronicity of the findings and evaluation of ancillary features are also helpful in refining the differential diagnosis.

SUGGESTED READINGS

Aquino SL, Gamsu G, Webb WR, et al. Tree-in-bud pattern: frequency and significance on thin section CT. *J Comput Assist Tomogr*. 1996;20:594-599.

Copley SJ, Wells AU, Hawtin KE, et al. Lung morphology in the elderly: comparative CT study of subjects over 75 years old versus those under 55 years old. *Radiology*. 2009;251:566-573.

Hansell DM, Bankier AA, MacMahon H, et al. Fleischner Society: glossary of terms for thoracic imaging. *Radiology*. 2008;246:697-722.

Kang EY, Grenier P, Laurent F, et al. Interlobular septal thickening: patterns at high-resolution tomography. *J Thorac Imaging*. 1996;11:260-264.

Kligerman SJ, Henry T, Lin CT, et al. Mosaic attenuation: etiology, methods of differentiation, and pitfalls. *Radiographics*. 2015;35:1360-1380.

Levesque MH, Montesi SB, Sharma A. Diffuse parenchymal abnormalities in acutely dyspneic patients: a pattern-based approach. *J Thorac Imaging*. 2015;30:220-232.

Miller WT Jr, Shah RM. Isolated diffuse ground-glass opacity in thoracic CT: causes and clinical presentations. *AJR Am J Roentgenol*. 2005;184:613-622.

Murata K, Itoh H, Todo G, et al. Centrilobular lesions of the lung: demonstration by high-resolution CT and pathologic correlation. *Radiology*. 1986;161:641-645.

Raoof S, Bondalapati P, Vydyula R, et al. Cystic lung diseases: algorithmic approach. *Chest*. 2016;150:945-965.

Webb WR. Thin-section CT of the secondary pulmonary lobule: anatomy and the image–the 2004 Fleischner lecture. *Radiology*. 2006;239:322-338.

Worthy SA, Muller NL, Hartman TE, et al. Mosaic attenuation pattern on thin-section CT scans of the lung: differentiation among infiltrative lung, airway, and vascular diseases as a cause. *Radiology*. 1997;205:465-470.

Chapter 18

Diffuse Lung Diseases

Jonathan H. Chung

INTRODUCTION

There are innumerable causes of chronic diffuse lung disease. This chapter reviews the common causes of diffuse lung disease, including the idiopathic interstitial pneumonias (IIPs), connective tissue disease (CTD), hypersensitivity pneumonitis (HP), sarcoidosis, cystic lung disease, eosinophilic lung disease, collagen vascular diseases, and drug reaction.

IDIOPATHIC INTERSTITIAL PNEUMONIAS

The IIPs are a group of diffuse lung diseases that present similarly. The classification system of IIPs is grounded on underlying histology-specific idiopathic conditions. However, many known nonidiopathic conditions may lead to histologic patterns identical to those in the IIPs. Other common conditions to consider include collagen vascular diseases, HP, and drug-related lung disease. The IIPs are subcategorized into the chronic fibrotic conditions, the subacute and acute conditions, the smoking-related conditions, and the rare conditions.

Chronic Fibrosing Interstitial Pneumonias

Idiopathic Pulmonary Fibrosis

Idiopathic pulmonary fibrosis (IPF) is the most common type of pulmonary fibrosis and is also the most common of the IIPs. As implied by its name, the cause of IPF is unknown. The imaging and histopathologic pattern of IPF is usual interstitial pneumonia (UIP). All cases of IPF are UIP, and most cases of UIP are IPF; a minority of UIP cases are caused by collagen vascular disease (usually rheumatoid arthritis [RA]), chronic HP, drug-related pulmonary fibrosis, or occupational lung disease. IPF usually affects older male patients in the sixth and seventh decades of life; two thirds are current or former smokers.

Timely diagnosis requires a high level of clinical suspicion in all adult patients presenting with chronic exertional dyspnea or dry cough with inspiratory crackles. Inspiratory crackles and digital clubbing are often present on physical examination. Hiatal hernias are common; gastroesophageal reflux disease (GERD) may worsen pulmonary fibrosis and is associated with worse patient survival. Restrictive physiology and reduced diffusion capacity are typical on pulmonary function testing. IPF has a poor prognosis with a median survival time of approximately 3 years.

The histopathologic findings of UIP are characterized by spatially and temporally heterogeneous fibrosis with adjacent spared areas of normal lung. The subpleural lung is most severely affected. Fibroblast foci are a key finding in UIP and are associated with worse survival.

The low-contrast resolution of chest radiography limits its utility in the assessment of pulmonary fibrosis. UIP most commonly presents with reduced lung volumes and reticular and linear opacities in the basilar portions of the lungs (Fig. 18.1, *A*). In severe cases, traction bronchiectasis and honeycombing may be evident even on radiography.

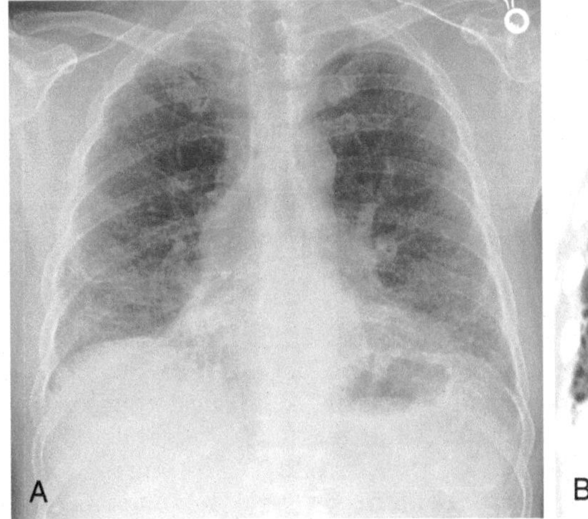

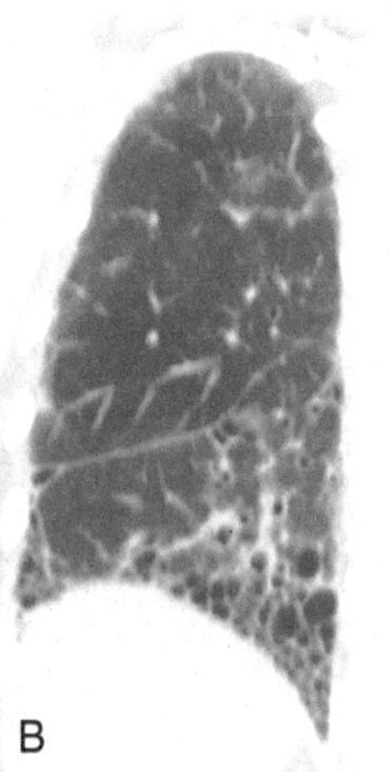

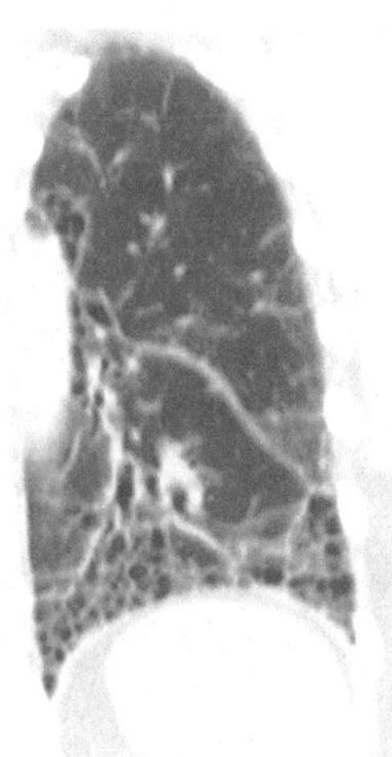

FIGURE 18.1 Usual interstitial pneumonitis on radiography **(A)** and computed tomography **(B)**. Posteroanterior chest radiograph **(A)** demonstrates low lung volumes and basilar-preponderant lung reticulation in this patient with idiopathic pulmonary fibrosis. Coronal image from noncontrast chest CT **(B)** from another patient demonstrates basilar and peripheral preponderant pulmonary fibrosis characterized by reticulation, traction bronchiectasis and bronchiolectasis, and exuberant honeycombing consistent with usual interstitial pneumonitis.

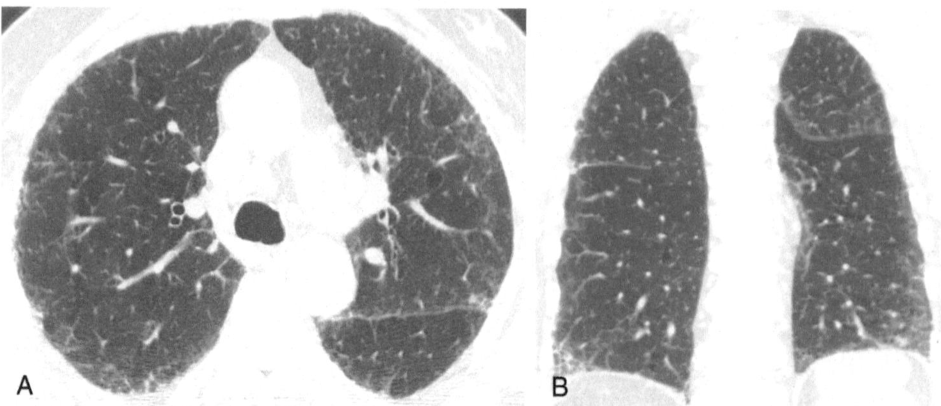

FIGURE 18.2 Possible usual interstitial pneumonitis pattern on chest computed tomography (CT). Axial **(A)** and coronal **(B)** images from noncontrast chest CT demonstrate basilar- and peripheral-preponderant pulmonary fibrosis characterized by reticulation and traction bronchiectasis as well as traction bronchiolectasis without honeycombing consistent with a possible usual interstitial pneumonitis pattern.

Full characterization of lung disease is best performed on thin-section chest computed tomography (CT).

Chest CT plays a central role in the clinical workup of patients with suspected pulmonary fibrosis. A UIP pattern on chest CT is highly accurate for UIP on pathology, obviating lung biopsy. However, only half of cases of IPF have a UIP pattern on chest CT. A UIP pattern on chest CT is defined as reticulation in the peripheral and basilar aspects of the lungs with associated subpleural honeycombing without other features that are "inconsistent with UIP" (Fig. 18.1, *B*). Traction bronchiectasis or bronchiolectasis often coexists with other findings of pulmonary fibrosis. Fibrosis in UIP may be asymmetric as opposed to the distribution in nonspecific interstitial pneumonia (NSIP), which is almost always symmetric. A "possible UIP" pattern on chest CT has all the characteristics of a UIP pattern except there is no honeycombing (Fig. 18.2). An inconsistent-with-UIP pattern on chest CT should be considered if there are any of the specific CT findings listed in Box 18.1 suggestive of an alternative diagnosis. In cases of possible UIP and inconsistent with UIP, biopsy should be considered for diagnosis (Fig. 18.3).

Honeycombing is a finding of localized end-stage pulmonary fibrosis. Honeycombing on CT is an important finding because it is the single most specific finding of UIP and has poor prognostic ramifications. In certain cases, differentiating paraseptal emphysema from honeycombing on CT can be challenging because smoking is associated with both entities. Honeycombing usually manifests as rows or stacks of thin-walled subcentimeter lung cysts and adjacent reticulation, often in the mid and lower lung zones; paraseptal emphysema presents as longer and often larger cystic regions often in the upper lung zone and often contain subtle internal septations, which would be highly unusual for honeycombing (Fig. 18.4). Unfortunately, differentiation of these two entities may be impossible in a minority of cases.

Combined pulmonary fibrosis and emphysema (CPFE) is a distinct clinical entity and is separate from the IIP classification system. Approximately one third of IPF patients have concomitant emphysema. On pulmonary function tests, lung volumes are typically normal or near-normal because of the offsetting effects of fibrosis (restriction) and emphysema (obstruction). However, diffusion capacity is typically markedly reduced. Emphysema is usually upper lung preponderant, and fibrosis is usually basilar in distribution and often has a UIP-like configuration, although other fibrotic patterns may also predominate (see Fig. 18.4). The majority of patients have some degree of diffuse ground-glass opacity likely reflecting superimposed smoking-related respiratory bronchiolitis (RB) or desquamative interstitial pneumonitis (DIP). Patients with CPFE are at increased risk of pulmonary hypertension and lung cancer.

BOX 18.1 Idiopathic Pulmonary Fibrosis

CHARACTERISTICS

Clinical features
40–60 years old
Dyspnea, dry cough
Histologic feature: temporal heterogeneity

RADIOGRAPHIC FINDINGS

Reticulation
Lower zones
Honeycombing
Small lungs

CHEST COMPUTED TOMOGRAPHY FINDINGS

Reticulation
Honeycombing
Traction bronchiolectasis
Traction bronchiectasis
Peripheral and subpleural distribution

CHEST COMPUTED TOMOGRAPHY FINDINGS INCONSISTENT WITH USUAL INTERSTITIAL PNEUMONITIS

Upper, mid, or peribronchovascular distribution
Extensive ground-glass opacity
Consolidation
Discrete cysts
Diffuse mosaic attenuation or air trapping
Profuse micronodules

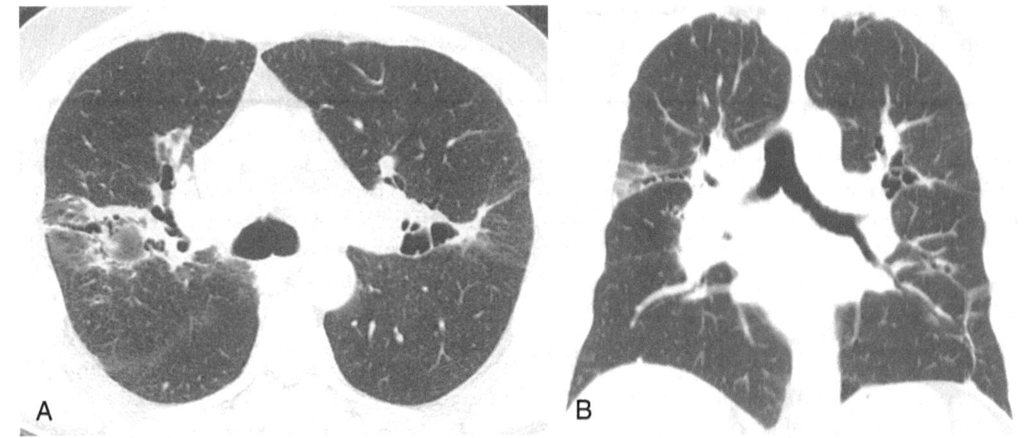

FIGURE 18.3 Inconsistent with usual interstitial pneumonitis pattern on chest computed tomography (CT). Axial **(A)** and coronal **(B)** images from noncontrast chest CT demonstrate mid and central-lung–predominant pulmonary fibrosis characterized by reticulation, ground-glass opacity, and traction bronchiectasis inconsistent with usual interstitial pneumonitis. The patient was shown to have sarcoidosis.

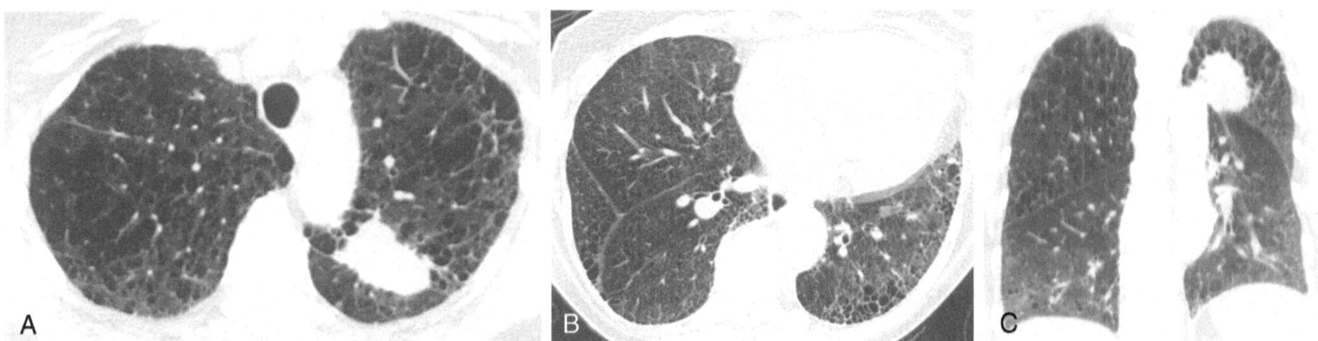

FIGURE 18.4 Combined pulmonary fibrosis and emphysema on chest computed tomography (CT). Axial (**A** and **B**) and coronal **(C)** images from noncontrast chest CT demonstrate upper lung centrilobular, paraseptal, and confluent emphysema with associated basilar-preponderant pulmonary fibrosis consistent with usual interstitial pneumonitis. There is also a mass within the left upper lobe, highly suggestive of primary lung cancer. Patients with combined pulmonary fibrosis and emphysema are at increased risk for development of lung malignancy.

Nonspecific Interstitial Pneumonia

Nonspecific interstitial pneumonia is most often secondary to an underlying condition, most often collagen vascular diseases (particularly scleroderma, myositis, and mixed connective tissue disease [MCTD]), drug-induced pneumonitis, and HP. Idiopathic NSIP is a distinct clinical entity with a good prognosis and typically responds well to steroid treatment.

The histologic features consist of various amounts of interstitial inflammation and fibrosis with a uniform appearance. There are two distinct types: cellular NSIP, with mild to moderate inflammation and little fibrosis, and fibrosing NSIP, with interstitial thickening by uniform fibrosis and preservation of alveolar architecture. The fibrosis is of the same age, unlike the temporal heterogeneity seen in UIP.

Nonspecific interstitial pneumonia is more common in women and is diagnosed at a younger age (average age of 50 years at diagnosis) than UIP and IPF. There is no strong association with smoking. The clinical presentation is nonspecific and includes dyspnea, cough, and weight loss.

The plain radiographic features consist of reticular opacities in the lower lungs without honeycombing (Box 18.2). Chest CT findings are more specific. Typical findings include basilar-predominant ground-glass opacity, reticulation, and traction bronchiectasis—at times quite exuberant and above expected for the severity of adjacent lung disease (Fig. 18.5). The distribution of disease is invariably symmetric in contrast to the often asymmetric distribution of UIP. The axial distribution may be central or peripheral but with subpleural sparing (see Fig. 18.5). Subpleural sparing is highly suggestive of NSIP and essentially excludes UIP as the predominant pattern of lung injury. Honeycombing is uncommon in NSIP and, if present, should be mild.

Acute and Subacute Fibrosing Interstitial Pneumonia

Organizing Pneumonia

Cryptogenic organizing pneumonia (COP), formerly known as bronchiolitis obliterans with organizing pneumonia (OP), is the idiopathic form of OP. Slightly more than half of cases of OP are idiopathic. The more common secondary causes of OP include collagen vascular disease, radiation therapy, medication, aspiration, pneumonia, and solid organ as well as stem cell transplantation. OP typically has a good prognosis and usually responds very well to corticosteroid therapy, although relapses are common. Histologically, OP is characterized by organizing cellular infiltrate and collections of young myxoid colagen with fibroblasts in the distal alveoli, which extend into the distal airways.

The imaging findings of OP are somewhat heterogeneous and diverse. Consolidation with a variable degree of ground-glass opacity is the most common finding. The changes are usually in a peripheral or peribronchovascular distribution and may be migratory. Airways within areas of lung opacity may transiently dilate. The borders of lung opacity are often "wispy" on CT, which is suggestive of the diagnosis (Fig. 18.6). A reasonably specific finding for OP on imaging is a "perilobular pattern" consisting of irregular opacity with or without septal thickening that surrounds the secondary pulmonary lobule, often in the lower lung zones (Fig. 18.7). Another frequent finding of OP is the atoll or reversed halo sign: a central region of ground-glass opacity with a circumferential border of consolidation (Fig. 18.8). The presence of a substantial degree of reticulation in OP suggests a worse prognosis.

BOX 18.2 Nonspecific Interstitial Pneumonitis

CHARACTERISTICS

Clinical features
Average age, 50 years
More women than men affected
Dyspnea, dry cough
Histologic feature: temporal homogeneity

RADIOGRAPHIC FINDINGS

Reticulation
Lower zones
Absent or rare honeycombing
Small lungs

CHEST COMPUTED TOMOGRAPHY FINDINGS

Reticulation
Traction bronchiectasis
Ground-glass opacity
Almost always basilar
Axial central or subpleural sparing highly suggestive; often peripheral

Acute Interstitial Pneumonia

Acute interstitial pneumonia (AIP) is essentially idiopathic acute respiratory distress syndrome (ARDS) and is most often characterized by a diffuse alveolar damage pattern. Affected patients often present with a viral-like prodrome followed by rapid respiratory decompensation. The diagnosis of AIP is that of exclusion, and secondary causes of ARDS such as pneumonia, trauma, transplant rejection, and blood transfusion must be excluded.

As in ARDS, there are typical stages of AIP. First, during the exudative phase, histology will demonstrate edema, hyaline membranes, acute lung inflammation, and alveolar hemorrhage. The organizing phase can develop within a few days with type II pneumocyte hyperplasia and organizing fibrosis. If patients survive their acute illness, some patients may progress to a chronic phase of pulmonary fibrosis.

Imaging findings mirror the histologic stages. On radiography, patchy bilateral consolidation is present during the early exudative phase. On CT, there are diffuse or dependent ground-glass opacities and consolidation (Fig. 18.9). Usually the zonal distribution of disease is diffuse, although there may be a slight basilar preponderance. In the organizing stage, consolidation usually improves both

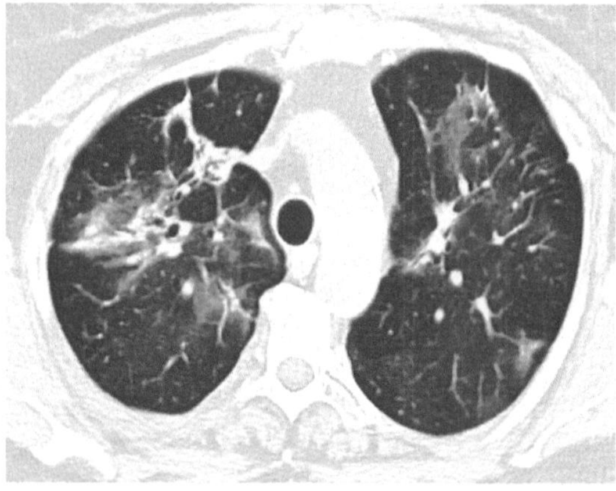

FIGURE 18.6 Organizing pneumonia on chest computed tomography (CT). Axial image from noncontrast chest CT demonstrates peribronchovascular consolidation and ground-glass opacity with "wispy" margins, consistent with organizing pneumonia as a manifestation of drug reaction from chemotherapy.

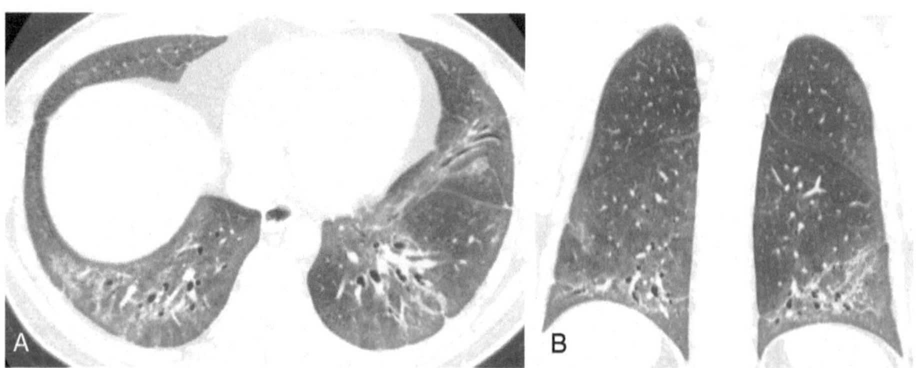

FIGURE 18.5 Nonspecific interstitial pneumonitis pattern on chest computed tomography (CT). Axial **(A)** and coronal **(B)** images from noncontrast chest CT demonstrate basilar- and central-preponderant pulmonary fibrosis characterized by ground-glass opacity, reticulation, and traction bronchiectasis without honeycombing highly suggestive of nonspecific interstitial pneumonitis in this patient with underlying connective tissue disease.

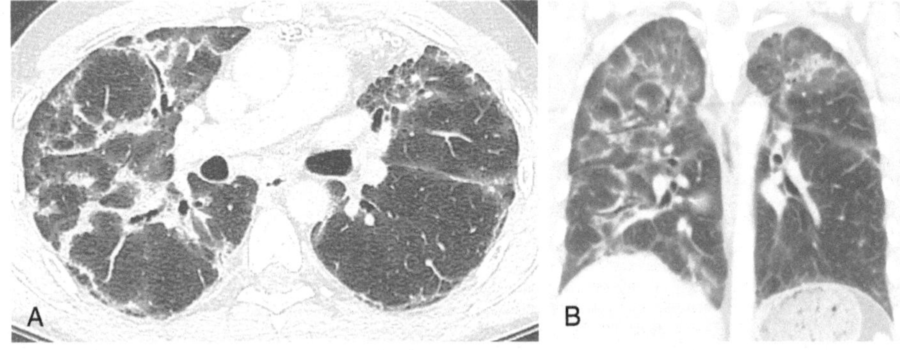

FIGURE 18.7 Organizing pneumonia on chest computed tomography (CT). Axial **(A)** and coronal **(B)** images from noncontrast chest CT demonstrate right lung–predominant, perilobular consolidation and mild ground-glass opacity highly suggestive of organizing pneumonia related to stem cell transplantation and chronic graft-versus-host disease.

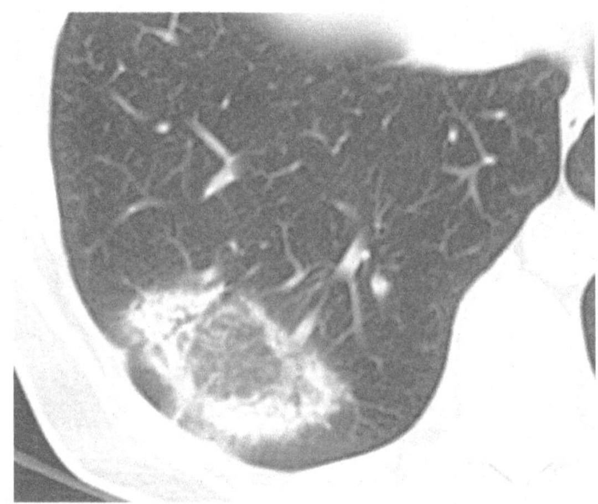

FIGURE 18.8 Organizing pneumonia on chest computed tomography (CT). Axial image from noncontrast chest CT demonstrates right lower lobe focus of ground-glass opacity and reticulation with a near complete circumferential ring of consolidation (reverse halo sign). This sign is not pathognomonic for organizing pneumonia but is highly suggestive of the diagnosis.

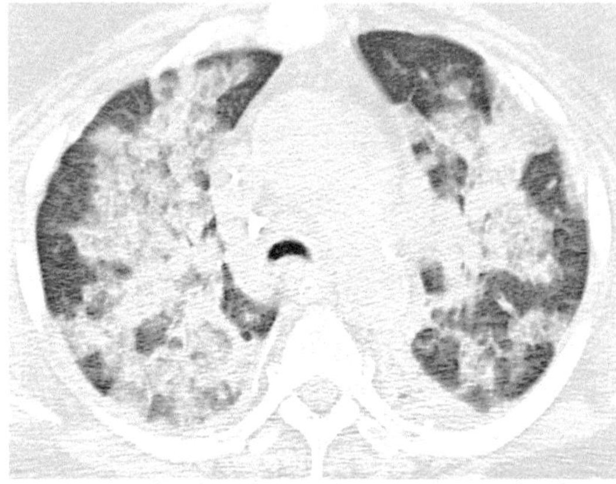

FIGURE 18.9 On computed tomography, there are diffuse or dependent ground-glass opacities and consolidation.

on radiography and CT. A peribronchovascular distribution and bronchial dilation may be evident on CT. In patients who survive and develop fibrosis, the anterior and upper aspects of the lungs are usually more severely affected.

Smoking-Related Interstitial Pneumonias

Respiratory Bronchiolitis–Interstitial Lung Disease

Interstitial pneumonias associated with smoking represent a spectrum of lung disease ranging from the asymptomatic RB to symptomatic respiratory bronchiolitis–interstitial lung disease (RB-ILD) to DIP. RB is very common in smokers and is found on pathology in the vast majority of patients with significant smoking history. Histologically, RB is characterized by collections of pigmented macrophages primarily within a bronchiolar distribution. In patients with RB, RB-ILD is diagnosed if patients have associated symptoms or functional impairment. Radiologic and histologic findings in RB and RB-ILD are essentially identical.

Respiratory bronchiolitis is usually not apparent on radiography, although more severe cases of may manifest as diffuse increased interstitial opacities sometimes referred to as "dirty lungs" or "dirty chest." CT findings of RB typically include upper lung or diffuse centrilobular ground-glass nodules (Fig. 18.10), similar to findings in subacute HP. A history of smoking is highly suggestive of RB as opposed to HP. The mild immunosuppressant effects of cigarette smoke protect from HP, but smoking is the causative agent in RB. Although most patients improve clinically and on imaging with smoking cessation, a substantial minority of patients will not respond or even worsen over time.

Desquamative Interstitial Pneumonia

Desquamative interstitial pneumonitis is much less common than RB, and up to 40% of patients with DIP have no history of smoking. Other less common causes of DIP include autoimmune disease, hepatitis C infection, and drug toxicity. The histologic finding in DIP is characterized by a diffuse alveolar infiltration of pigmented macrophages.

A chest radiograph may appear normal or demonstrate a subtle diffuse or basilar-predominant increased opacity in the lungs. On CT, DIP usually manifests as confluent areas of ground-glass opacity primarily in the lung periphery and at the lung bases (Fig. 18.11, *A*). In most cases, small clustered cystic lesions are superimposed on ground-glass opacity; these cysts may represent mild emphysema or very early traction bronchiolectasis caused by pulmonary fibrosis (Fig. 18.11, *B*). Indeed, a minority of cases of DIP progress to frank pulmonary fibrosis, although progression to a classic UIP pattern is not common. Given the relatively nonspecific imaging appearance of DIP, surgical lung biopsy may be necessary to achieve an accurate diagnosis.

Rare Entities

Lymphocytic Interstitial Pneumonitis

Lymphocytic interstitial pneumonitis (LIP) is one of the rare interstitial pneumonias and is almost always secondary to an underlying condition. Most cases of LIP in adults occur in association with Sjögren syndrome. Other causes include human immunodeficiency virus (usually in children) and hematopoietic stem cell transplantation. The histologic pattern is marked by polymorphic lymphocyte infiltration in the pulmonary interstitium and lymphatics. Imaging findings on radiography are nonspecific, with most cases being normal. On chest CT, a variable degree of patchy ground-glass opacity and nodules may be present, often in the lung periphery and along the bronchovascular tree. In chronic cases, LIP manifests most commonly as a diffuse cystic lung disease, which is basilar and peribronchovascular predominant (Fig. 18.12).

Idiopathic Pleuroparenchymal Fibroelastosis

Idiopathic pleuroparenchymal fibroelastosis (IPPFE) is a recent addition to the IIP classification but is poorly

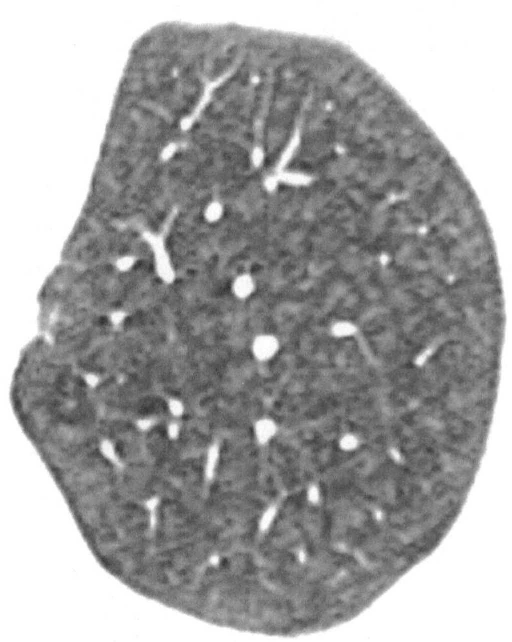

FIGURE 18.10 Respiratory bronchiolitis on chest computed tomography (CT). Axial image from noncontrast chest CT demonstrates diffuse centrilobular ground-glass nodules consistent with respiratory bronchiolitis in this long-time smoker. The imaging appearance is identical to subacute hypersensitivity pneumonitis (HP). History of smoking is protective for HP and is causative for respiratory bronchiolitis. Additionally, supportive respiratory exposure history (usually to birds or molds) is also suggestive of HP.

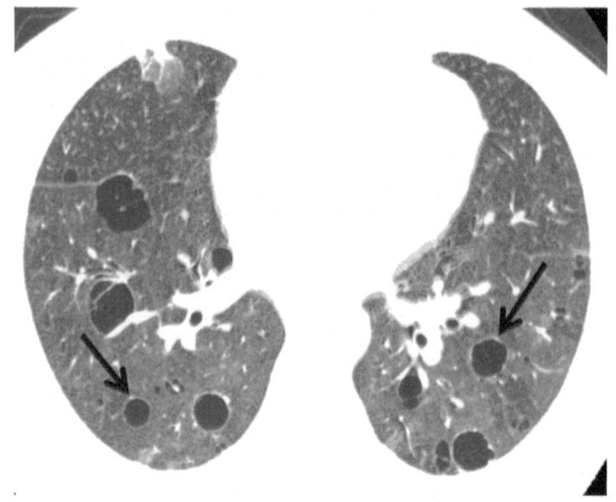

FIGURE 18.12 Lymphocytic interstitial pneumonitis on chest computed tomography (CT). Axial image from noncontrast chest CT demonstrates multiple cysts within the lower lobes in a peribronchovascular distribution as indicated by the eccentric pulmonary artery branches *(arrows)*. This patient had an underlying diagnosis of Sjögren syndrome, which is a common cause of lymphocytic interstitial pneumonitis in adults.

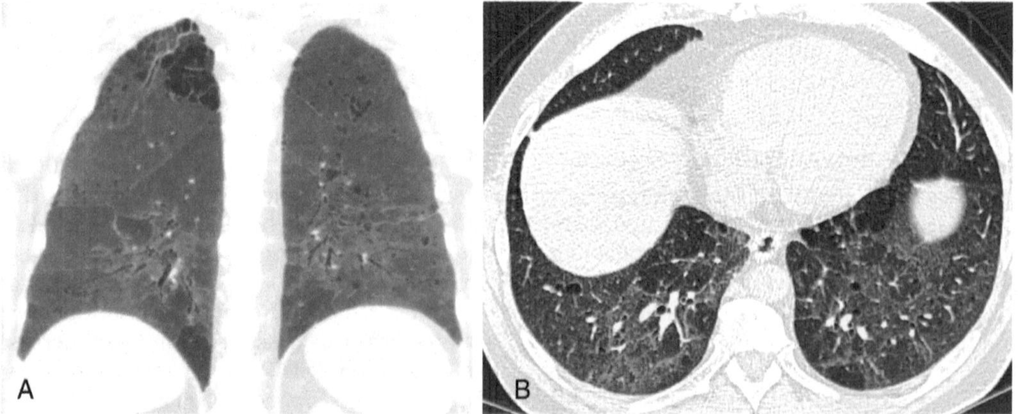

FIGURE 18.11 Desquamative interstitial pneumonitis on chest computed tomography (CT). Coronal minimum intensity projection image **(A)** demonstrates basilar-preponderant ground-glass opacity consistent with desquamative interstitial pneumonitis. Emphysema is noted primarily within the upper lobes in centrilobular, confluent, and paraseptal distributions, indicating a smoking history. Axial image from noncontrast chest CT image **(B)** from another patient demonstrates diffuse ground-glass opacity with superimposed microcystic abnormality highly suggestive of desquamative of interstitial pneumonitis in this long-time smoker.

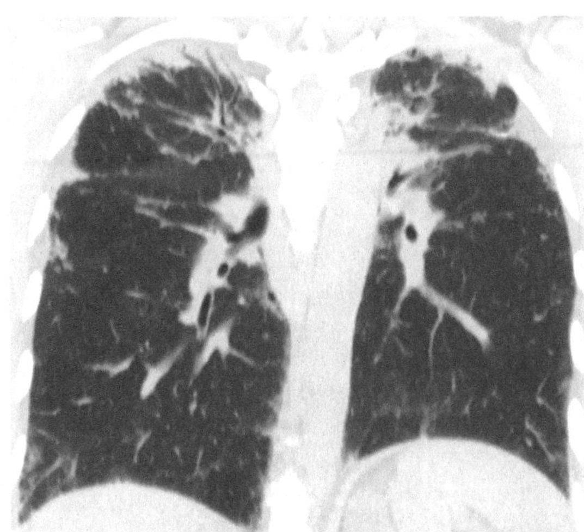

FIGURE 18.13 Idiopathic pleuroparenchymal fibroelastosis on chest computed tomography (CT). Coronal image from noncontrast chest CT demonstrates exuberant by apical pleural parenchymal scarring in this patient with idiopathic pleuroparenchymal fibroelastosis. (From Hobbs S, Lynch D. The idiopathic interstitial pneumonias: an update and review. Radiol Clin North Am 2014;52:105-120.)

understood. Although it is an idiopathic condition, an association with chronic infection and stem cell transplantation has been described. On histology, there is exuberant biapical subpleural fibrosis. CT mirrors the histology; dense pleural and subpleural lung fibrosis affects the lung apices symmetrically and often extends along the superior margins of the upper lobes (Fig. 18.13). A similar imaging appearance occurs in the setting of chronic lung transplant rejection, known as restrictive allograft syndrome (RAS).

CONNECTIVE TISSUE DISEASES

Thoracic involvement in CTD is quite common. Each CTD is associated with a particular autoantibody or collection of antibodies; indeed, often serology is the main means by which diagnosis is achieved (Table 18.1). Thoracic involvement from CTD may be pulmonary, airway, pleural, gastrointestinal, or vascular. The pulmonary manifestations of CTD usually mirror the patterns described in the IIPs (Fig. 18.14 and Table 18.2). In approximately 15% of cases, lung disease may be the initial manifestation of CTD and can precede overt clinical presentation by 5 years. Other common manifestations of CTD in the thorax that aid in achieving accurate diagnosis are the presence of pleural or pericardial effusion, esophageal dilation, pulmonary arterial enlargement (from pulmonary hypertension), soft tissue calcification (more common in scleroderma or dermatomyositis), and shoulder or acromioclavicular joint erosive arthritis in RA.

TABLE 18.1 Common Autoantibodies in Connective Tissue Diseases

Disease	Autoantibodies
RA	RF, anti-CCP
Scleroderma	Anti-centromere antibody, anti-SCL-70
MCTD	Anti-RBNP
DM, PM, AS	Anti-Jo-1, anti-aminoacyl-tRNA synthetases
SLE	Anti-ds DNA, anti-Smith, antiphospholipid

AS, Antisynthetase syndrome; *DM*, dermatomyositis; *MCTD*, mixed connective tissue disease; *PM*, polymyositis; *RA*, rheumatoid arthritis; *SLE*, systemic lupus erythematosus.
Adapted from Lynch DA. Lung disease related to collagen vascular disease. J Thorac Imaging. 2009;24(4):299-309.

Rheumatoid Arthritis

The most common ILD pattern to affect patients with RA is a UIP pattern. Often, the imaging manifestation of UIP in RA is indistinguishable from that in IPF. However, there are some CT findings that are more suggestive of RA than IPF: substantial fibrosis in the anterior upper lobes (in addition to basilar fibrosis), exuberant honeycombing that affects the vast majority of fibrotic lung, and isolation of fibrosis to the lung bases without substantial extension along the lateral margins of the lungs on coronal images. NSIP and OP may also occur in RA but are less common patterns.

Patients with RA may also be affected by obliterative bronchiolitis (OB). Although it may be difficult to differentiate OB from severe asthma on CT because both conditions present with severe air trapping, a history of RA and nonreversibility are suggestive of OB rather than asthma. Follicular bronchiolitis is a rare condition that manifests as centrilobular or tree-in-bud nodularity on imaging and can affect patients with RA but should only be considered after more common causes of tree-in-bud opacity (aspiration or pneumonia) have been thoroughly excluded.

Systemic Lupus Erythematosus

Interstitial lung disease is rare in systemic lupus erythematosus (SLE), although patients with SLE are predisposed to development of pulmonary hemorrhage and pulmonary infections. SLE more often presents with pleural or pericardial effusions or thickening. Pleural thickening may result in restrictive thoracic physiology that mimics pulmonary fibrosis on pulmonary function testing and can lead to substantial patient morbidity. Some patients develop diaphragmatic weakness, which leads to chronically low lung volumes—the so-called shrinking lung syndrome that may mimic mild ILD on radiography caused by vascular crowding and atelectasis.

Mixed Connective Tissue Disease

Mixed connective tissue disease is a distinct clinical entity defined by the presence of the antiribonucleoprotein (RNP) antibody. ILD in MCTD is common and occurs in up to 60% of patients with MCTD; NSIP is the most common ILD pattern in MCTD. It differs from interstitial pneumonia with autoimmune features (IPAF), which is a heterogeneous group of conditions that present with ILD and suspected autoimmune disease not meeting criteria for a well-defined CTD.

Scleroderma

Patients with scleroderma are especially susceptible to the development of ILD, with some series showing that the majority of patients develop ILD. The most common CT

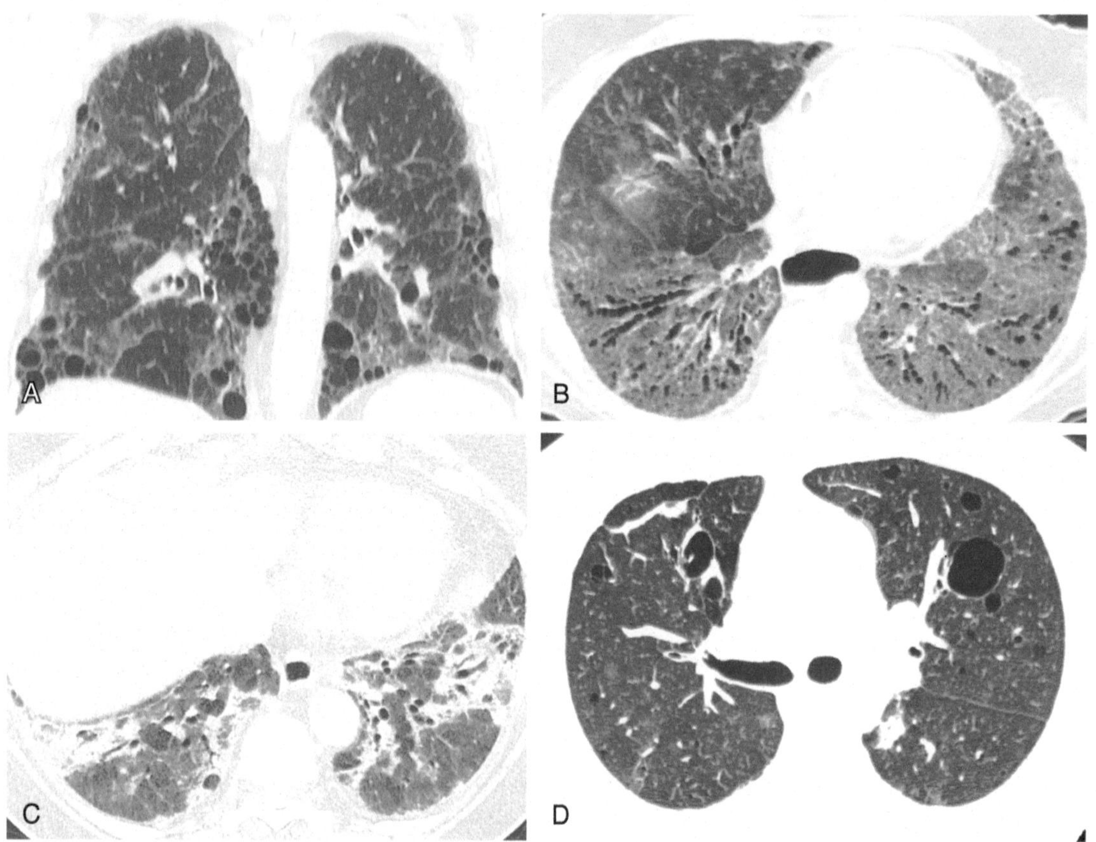

FIGURE 18.14 Connective tissue diseases (CTDs) on chest CT. **A,** Usual interstitial pneumonitis (UIP) pattern in rheumatoid arthritis presenting with a typical peripheral and basilar distribution of fibrosis. Note the large degree of macrocystic honeycombing, which is more common in UIP seen in CTD than in idiopathic pulmonary fibrosis. **B,** Nonspecific interstitial pneumonitis (NSIP) pattern in scleroderma characterized by ground-glass opacity, reticulation, and traction bronchiectasis. The esophagus is severely dilated with an internal gas–fluid level consistent with esophageal dysmotility, a common finding in scleroderma. **C,** Combined organizing pneumonia and NSIP in antisynthetase syndrome presenting with basilar-predominant consolidation and ground-glass opacity. **D,** Lymphocytic interstitial pneumonitis pattern in Sjögren syndrome presenting as a diffuse cystic lung disease.

TABLE 18.2 Common Thoracic Manifestations of Connective Tissue Diseases

Imaging Pattern	RA	SLE	MCTD	Scleroderma	PM, DM, AS	Sjögren
UIP	++	+	+	++	+	+
NSIP	+	+	++	++++	++	+
OP	++	+	+	+	++	–
LIP	–	–	–	–	–	++
PH	+	+	+	++	–	+
Bronchiectasis	++	–	–	–	–	++
OB	++	+	–	–	–	–

AS, Antisynthetase syndrome; *DM,* dermatomyositis; *LIP,* lymphocytic interstitial pneumonitis; *MCTD,* mixed connective tissue disease; *NSIP,* nonspecific interstitial pneumonitis; *OB,* obliterative bronchiolitis; *OP,* organizing pneumonia; *PH,* pulmonary hypertension; *PM,* polymyositis; *RA,* rheumatoid arthritis; *SLE,* systemic lupus erythematosus; *UIP,* usual interstitial pneumonitis.
Adapted from Lynch DA. Lung disease related to collagen vascular disease. J Thorac Imaging 2009;24(4):299-309.

pattern is NSIP followed by UIP. Given the high prevalence of esophageal dysmotility and pulmonary hypertension in scleroderma, findings of dysmotility (esophageal dilation, gas–fluid level, open esophageal sphincter) and pulmonary hypertension (pulmonary artery size and cardiac chamber enlargement) should be specifically addressed.

Myositis

Inflammatory myositis (dermatomyositis, polymyositis, and antisynthetase syndrome) commonly cause ILD, occurring in 50% to 75% of cases. The Jo-1 antibody is associated with ILD in the setting of myositis and can predict the development of ILD in the future as well as response to therapy. Most patients with ILD present initially with NSIP and OP—CT shows basilar ground-glass opacity, mild reticulation, mild traction bronchiectasis, and superimposed bronchovascular or peripheral lung consolidation. With corticosteroid therapy, consolidation (OP) often resolves, leaving residual ground-glass opacity and reticulation (NSIP). This disease course is typical and highly suggestive of myositis-related ILD.

Sjögren Syndrome

Sjögren syndrome is a relatively rare disease; the most common ILD to develop in this setting is LIP as described previously. Mild bronchiectasis is also common in this condition.

HYPERSENSITIVITY PNEUMONITIS

Hypersensitivity pneumonitis (Box 18.3), also known as extrinsic allergic alveolitis, describes a spectrum of granulomatous and interstitial pulmonary disorders associated with intense and often prolonged exposure to a wide range of inhaled organic or inorganic dusts, gases, or organisms. The site of inflammatory host response in these disorders is located primarily in the alveolar air exchange portion of the lung and not in the large conducting airways that are involved in asthmatic diseases.

An innumerable number of antigens may cause HP. However, the most common antigens to cause HP are avian and mold related. These antigens, usually disseminated as aerosol dust, can be derived from animal dander and proteins; saprophytic fungi (i.e., spores) in contaminated vegetables, wood, bark, or water reservoir vaporizers; and dairy and grain products. The exposure is often occupational. The organic antigen may be a microbial organism, and the most commonly incriminated microbe is thermophilic *Actinomyces,* a ubiquitous bacterium that has the morphologic features of a fungus. This is the offending antigen in one of the most common types of HP, farmer's lung.

Hypersensitivity pneumonitis is often categorized into acute, subacute, and chronic stages. However, there is often substantial overlap in the presentation of patients. Acute HP is caused by intermittent high-intensity antigenic exposure, with symptoms occurring hours after antigen exposure and with resolution within 1 day to 2 weeks of antigen withdrawal. Subacute HP is caused by continuous low-intensity antigen exposure; repeated exposure; or, rarely, the manifestation of long-standing undiagnosed acute HP. Chronic HP may occur as progression of known acute or subacute HP but may also arise from chronic low-level exposures to an antigen without any acute or subacute events.

The first clue to the diagnosis of HP is a good clinical history that suggests the temporal relationship between the patient's symptoms and certain activities, including hobbies and occupation. The acute form of the disease is characterized by cough, dyspnea, and fever, which usually begin 4 to 6 hours after exposure to large quantities of the causative agent. There is often a leukocytosis, and pulmonary function studies reveal restrictive dysfunction. Usually characterized by dyspnea and chronic cough, subacute and chronic disease associated with low-grade exposure to the offending antigen may be confused with other forms of ILD. Laboratory studies consistent with the diagnosis include precipitating antibodies reactive to the offending dust antigen and a positive inhalational challenge that can reproduce the symptoms.

The imaging features of HP vary with the stage of the disease. A minority of patients with acute or subacute HP have a normal or near-normal CT scan.

In the *acute stage*, consolidation may be observed, especially in the lower lung zones. This reflects pathologic findings of alveolar filling by polymorphonuclear leukocytes, eosinophils, lymphocytes, and large mononuclear cells. Consolidation may be quite extensive, simulating pulmonary edema, but it is transitory and usually clears within hours or days. It is uncommon to image patients during the acute stage of disease.

The *subacute stage* is characterized by a fine nodular or reticulonodular pattern, although the radiographic appearance is largely nonspecific and usually not helpful in achieving a specific diagnosis. This nodular appearance corresponds pathologically with alveolitis, interstitial infiltration, small granulomas, and some degree of bronchiolitis. Histologic abnormalities are usually most severe in a peribronchiolar distribution. CT is very helpful in the diagnosis of the subacute HP. Characteristic findings include ground-glass opacity, often in a centrilobular distribution (see Fig. 18.10), with superimposed mosaic attenuation and air trapping. The "head cheese" sign manifests as three distinct densities demarcated by the margins of secondary

BOX 18.3 Hypersensitivity Pneumonitis

CHARACTERISTICS

Causes
Inhaled organic dust
Occupational antigens
Animal proteins
Saprophytic fungi
Dairy and grain products
Water vaporizers

Stages
Acute (4–6 hours)
Subacute: after resolution of acute stage, between episodes
Chronic: fibrosis, occurring months or years after exposure

Diagnosis
History related to exposure
Precipitating antibodies
Positive inhalational challenge

RADIOGRAPHIC FEATURES

Acute
Airspace consolidation (diffuse)
Rapid clearing

Subacute
Nodular or reticular nodular opacities
Upper zones
Centrilobular nodules on computed tomography
Ground-glass opacity on computed tomography

Chronic
Medium to coarse linear opacities
Honeycombing
Upper zones

pulmonary lobules on expiratory chest CT and is nearly pathognomonic for HP in the subacute to chronic setting (Fig. 18.15).

In the *chronic stage* of HP, continued exposure to the antigen results in changes characteristic of pulmonary fibrosis: reticulation, traction bronchiectasis, traction bronchiolectasis, volume loss, and honeycombing. Although upper lung preponderance is a helpful finding in differentiating HP from UIP and NSIP, HP is only upper lung preponderant in a minority of cases (Fig. 18.16). In many cases, the distribution of chronic HP is basilar preponderant,

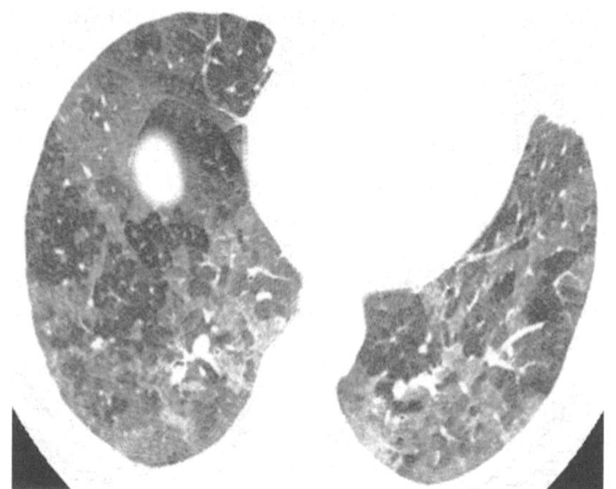

FIGURE 18.15 Hypersensitivity pneumonitis (HP) on expiratory chest computed tomography (CT). Axial image from expiratory phase chest CT demonstrates three distinct different densities demarcated by the margins of secondary pulmonary lobule, consistent with the head cheese sign, which is highly suggestive of HP. The most hypodense areas represent areas of air trapping, the intermediate-density regions represent normal lung, and the most hyperdense areas represent localized areas of lymphocytic inflammation.

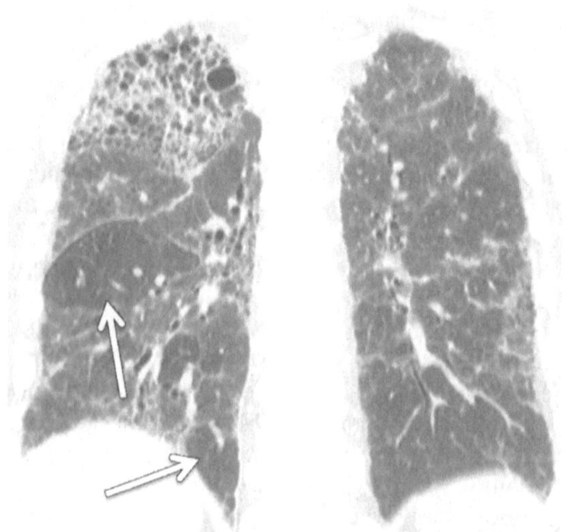

FIGURE 18.16 Fibrotic hypersensitivity pneumonitis (HP) on chest computed tomography (CT). Coronal image from noncontrast chest CT demonstrates asymmetric right greater than left, upper lung–predominant pulmonary fibrosis characterized by reticulation, traction bronchiectasis and bronchiolectasis, and early subpleural honeycombing. Mosaic attenuation within the lower lobes is consistent with air trapping in this patient with HP. *Arrows* indicate areas of air trapping.

mimicking UIP or NSIP. However, residual imaging findings of subacute HP (centrilobular ground-glass opacity or air trapping) may be present and suggest the correct diagnosis in these cases. In a minority of chronic HP cases, emphysema may develop even in the absence of smoking history, particularly in farmer's lung.

If the environmental source of the inhaled antigen is identified, simple avoidance is usually sufficient treatment; however, in up to 50% of cases, the antigen is never definitively identified. The acute form of the disease abates without specific therapy. With chronic forms of disease, a trial of corticosteroids can be given. A small proportion of cases may progress despite antigen avoidance and corticosteroids.

Hypersensitivity Pneumonitis–Specific Diseases

Farmer's Lung

Farmer's lung was the first occupationally related form of HP to be clearly described and understood. *Thermoactinomyces vulgaris* is the most important antigen in farmer's lung. It is found in moldy hay that has been improperly dried for storage. Farmer's lung typically affects men between 40 and 50 years old. The disease occurs in late winter or early spring, when the lower levels of hay, which have had the longest time to compost, are reached. A classic acute onset occurs in one third of cases, but a more common clinical presentation is insidious and is characterized by gradual progression of cough and dyspnea, weight loss, and fever. Prevalence of the syndrome among farmers is estimated to be between 1% and 10%.

Humidifier Lung

Equipment used to heat, humidify, or cool air may harbor microorganisms responsible for HP. Humidifier lung can develop in unsuspecting people who do not have obvious known exposure, and it may affect large numbers of people in an epidemic form. The diagnosis may be obvious when exposure occurs at home. However, contamination of heating and air conditioning or humidifying equipment with microorganisms in an office or commercial establishment is difficult to prove. The causative agents are usually thermophilic *Actinomyces* species. An accurate diagnosis requires a thorough history and detailed environmental probing, including a visit to suspicious areas and cultures from contaminated appliances.

Pigeon Breeder's Lung

Pigeon breeder's lung (i.e., bird fancier's disease) differs from farmer's lung or humidifier lung in that it is caused by inhaled proteins rather than microbial antigens and spores. Exposure to excreta and proteinaceous material from pigeons and other fowl and birds provokes the disease. It may produce an acute or chronic reaction.

Hot Tub Lung

Water within hot tubs may be contaminated by nontuberculous mycobacterial organisms that may become aerosolized and inhaled, resulting in HP. *Mycobacterium avium* complex is by far the most common type of nontuberculous mycobacteria found on culture in affected patients, with other species only rarely detected. This condition is reportedly more common after exposure to enclosed indoor hot tubs, which are at greater risk for causing HP than those located outdoors.

SARCOIDOSIS

Sarcoidosis (Box 18.4) is a systemic disorder of unknown cause that is characterized pathologically by widespread noncaseating granulomas. These granulomas are not unique to sarcoidosis and may appear in many other conditions. The diagnosis therefore must be based on consistent clinical and laboratory findings, tissue biopsy, and exclusion of other diseases, particularly granulomatous infections. Sarcoidosis is associated with hypercalcemia caused by high serum vitamin D levels as well as elevated angiotensin-converting enzyme (ACE) levels. The noncaseating granulomas may resolve spontaneously or may progress to fibrosis.

Most patients are young (20–40 years old), and at least one half of them are asymptomatic. The disease is more common among blacks. When symptoms occur, they are usually systemic rather than respiratory.

The chest radiograph is abnormal in more than 90% of patients. Lymph node enlargement, parenchymal abnormalities, or a combination of the two constitute the major radiographic changes. Approximately 20% of patients with radiographic evidence of ILD eventually develop fibrosis. Sarcoidosis is often categorized based on chest radiographic appearance using the Scadding stage schema: stage 0, no disease; stage 1, isolated lymphadenopathy; stage 2, lymphadenopathy and lung disease; stage 3, isolated lung disease; and stage 4, pulmonary fibrosis. Although disease progression does not reliably follow sequentially from stage 1 to stage 4, increasing Scadding stage has been associated with worsening prognosis.

The majority of patients with sarcoidosis have intrathoracic lymphadenopathy at some time during the course of their disease. On the initial chest radiograph, approximately half of the patients have this finding exclusively (stage 1); the others have lymphadenopathy plus parenchymal disease (stage 2). Bilateral hilar adenopathy occurs in almost all patients with nodal enlargement (Fig. 18.17, *A*). Bilateral, symmetric mediastinal adenopathy is also common. The parenchymal lung disease in sarcoidosis typically consists of a nodular or a reticulonodular pattern, which predominates in the upper lung zones (Fig. 18.17, *B*). It is common for

BOX 18.4 Sarcoidosis

CHARACTERISTICS

Cause unknown
Clinical features
20–40 years old
50% asymptomatic
Elevated angiotensin-converting enzyme levels
Pathologic features: Noncaseating granulomas

RADIOGRAPHIC FEATURES

Symmetric adenopathy
Nodular or reticular nodular opacities
Upper lung zones
Fibrosis in upper lobes with hilar retraction
Bullae

HIGH-RESOLUTION COMPUTED TOMOGRAPHY

Axial interstitial thickening
Nodular thickening along lymphatics
Interlobular septa, fissures, subpleural zones
Reticular opacities
Fibrosis: upper lobes, architectural distortion, fibrotic masses, traction bronchiectasis

DIFFERENTIAL DIAGNOSIS

Granulomatous infections
Silicosis: progressive massive fibrosis

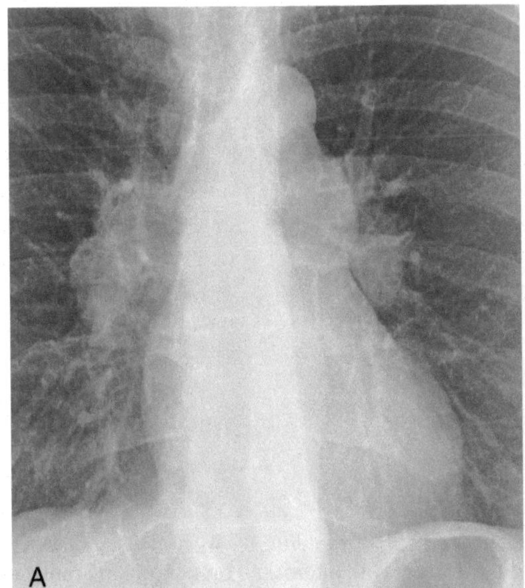

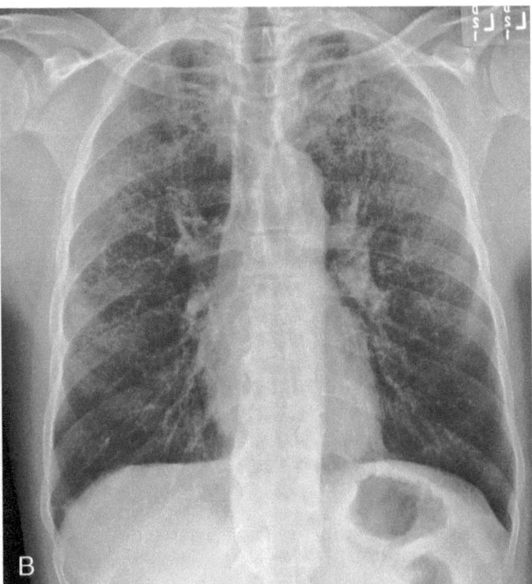

FIGURE 18.17 Sarcoidosis on posteroanterior (PA) radiograph. **A,** PA radiograph demonstrates symmetric hilar and anteroposterior window lymphadenopathy consistent with sarcoidosis. **B,** PA radiograph in another patient demonstrates upper lung–predominant reticulonodular opacities in this patient with known sarcoidosis.

adenopathy to decrease as the parenchymal disease becomes worse. Radiographic findings may be atypical in up to a quarter of cases and include diffuse airspace disease or large parenchymal nodules simulating metastases.

Sarcoid granulomas are distributed primarily along the lymphatics, and this distribution is more easily recognized on CT than on radiographs (Fig. 18.18). On CT, the classic pattern consists of small nodules identified along the axial interstitium, emanating from the hila along the bronchovascular bundles, within the interlobular septa, adjacent to the major fissures, and in the subpleural regions. The nodules vary from 2 mm to 1 cm in diameter. There is often a characteristic clustering of nodules such that a portion of lung will be severely affected while an adjacent region of lung will be completely free of disease. "Pseudoplaques" refer to a confluence of subpleural granulomas that mimic pleural plaques. Confluence of sarcoid granulomas may result in large opacities with ill-defined contours, some of which may appear nodular (nummular sarcoidosis) and others of which may contain air bronchograms (Fig. 18.19, *A*). A characteristic imaging finding in cases of confluent granulomas is the "CT galaxy sign," which manifests as a focal nodular opacity, usually in a peribronchovascular distribution with surrounding very small reticulonodular opacities, reminiscent of a cluster of stars as viewed through a high-powered telescope (Fig. 18.19, *B*). The differential diagnosis includes lymphangitis carcinomatosis that can cause a nodular perilymphatic pattern; septal thickening is usually the major pattern in lymphangitic carcinomatosis in contrast to the predominantly nodular pattern in sarcoidosis.

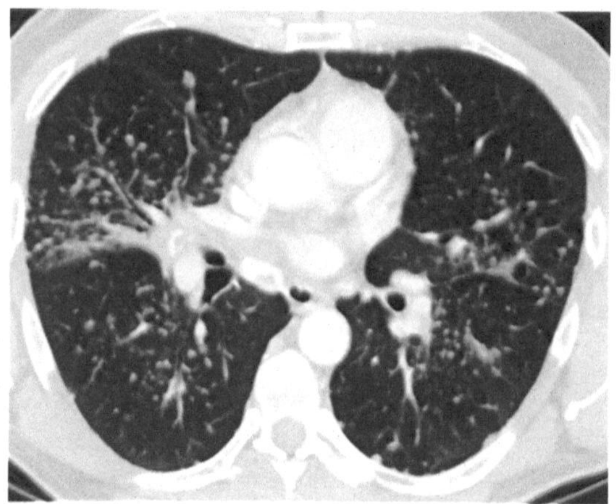

FIGURE 18.18 Sarcoidosis on chest computed tomography (CT). Axial image from contrast-enhanced chest CT demonstrates clustered nodularity along the interlobular septa, pulmonary fissures, and bronchovascular tree consistent with a perilymphatic distribution. This pattern of nodularity is essentially diagnostic of sarcoidosis or chronic beryllium disease. Although lymphangitic carcinomatosis can also manifest with perilymphatic nodularity, septal thickening (rather than nodularity) predominates.

The fibrosis in sarcoidosis is quite characteristic (stage 4). It is typically identified in the upper lobes, which show evidence of hilar retraction and bullae. The bullous component may be quite pronounced and predispose patients to develop mycetomas; sarcoidosis is the most common condition associated with mycetoma formation in the United States. The fibrosis is more pronounced in the apical and posterior portions of the upper lobes and the superior segments of the lower lobes. Chest CT (Fig. 18.20) shows the fibrosis as irregular reticular opacities, which usually predominate along the bronchovascular bundles. Loss of volume in the upper lobes occurs with distortion of lung architecture. Large masses of fibrous tissue may develop centrally along the perihilar bronchi and vessels, particularly in the upper lobes; this is often associated with traction bronchiectasis (Fig. 18.21). Because of this appearance, silicosis, HP, and tuberculosis must be considered in the differential diagnosis in upper lung fibrosis.

CYSTIC LUNG DISEASES

Lymphangioleiomyomatosis

Lymphangioleiomyomatosis (LAM) (Box 18.5) is a rare cystic disease of the lungs that occurs in women of childbearing age. It can occur as a rare sporadic disease, with a prevalence

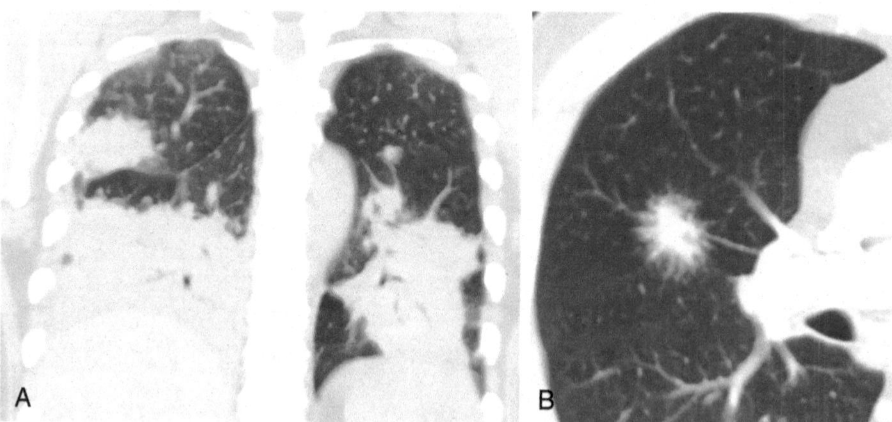

FIGURE 18.19 Nummular (alveolar) sarcoidosis on chest computed tomography (CT). **A,** Coronal image from noncontrast chest CT demonstrates multiple masses throughout the lungs with internal air bronchograms consistent with nummular sarcoidosis. **B,** Axial image from contrast-enhanced chest CT in another patient demonstrates a focal nodule within the right upper lobe with surrounding fine linear and nodular opacities consistent with the CT galaxy sign in this patient with known sarcoidosis. This sign is highly suggestive of a granulomatous process such as sarcoidosis or granulomatous infection and argues against malignancy.

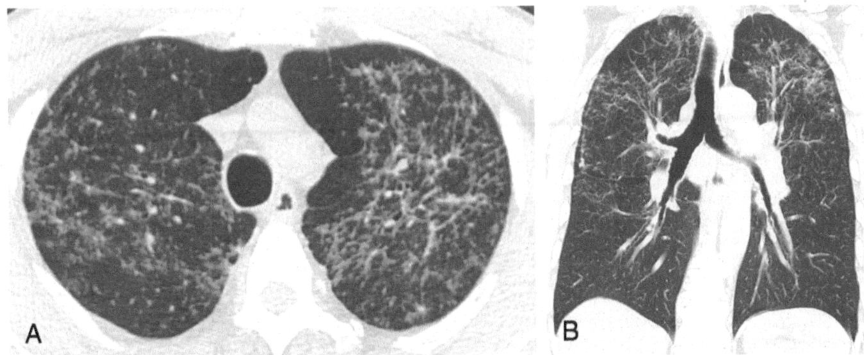

FIGURE 18.20 Fibrotic sarcoidosis on chest computed tomography (CT). Axial **(A)** and coronal **(B)** images from noncontrast chest CT demonstrate upper lung–predominant nodularity and reticulation with mild traction bronchiectasis and architectural distortion consistent with fibrotic sarcoidosis.

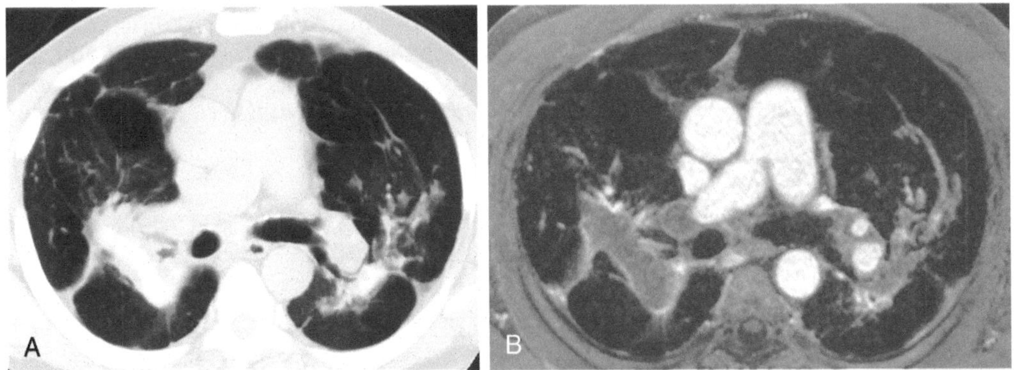

FIGURE 18.21 Masslike fibrosis in the setting of sarcoidosis on noncontrast chest computed tomography (CT) and contrast-enhanced magnetic resonance imaging (MRI). Axial chest CT image **(A)** and axial postgadolinium contrast-enhanced MRI image **(B)** demonstrate masslike areas of fibrosis within the upper lungs with adjacent paracicatricial emphysema. Low density within fibrotic masses on MRI is typical of focal areas of fibrosis on this modality and may even be seen within the lymph nodes.

BOX 18.5 Lymphangioleiomyomatosis

CHARACTERISTICS

Clinical features
Young women, reproductive age, tuberous sclerosis
Chylothorax
Pneumothorax
Hemoptysis
Pathologic features
Proliferation of immature smooth muscle

RADIOGRAPHIC FINDINGS

Linear pattern
Thin-walled cysts
Normal or increased lung volumes

HIGH-RESOLUTION COMPUTED TOMOGRAPHY FINDINGS

Thin-walled cysts
Diffuse
Otherwise normal parenchyma

of 1 in 1,000,000, or as a manifestation of tuberous sclerosis (TSC), with a prevalence of 30% to 40% in women with this genetic disease. TSC-related LAM is up to five times more common than sporadic LAM, although those with TSC-related disease often have a milder subclinical disease. Sporadic disease is seen exclusively in women, but the genetic form may also affect men, albeit rarely.

The pathologic feature is accumulation and proliferation of abnormal smooth muscle cells. These LAM cells contain receptors for estrogen and progesterone. The cells form nodules and progressively accumulate in the airways and lymphatics. Cystic change likely results from tissue destruction from LAM cell–derived matrix metalloproteinases. In the lymphatics, LAM cells form haphazard clumps of cells, leading to thickening of lymphatic walls, obliteration of the vessel lumen, and cystic dilation. Nodules may compress venules and capillaries. The LAM lesions are lined with type II pneumocytes, and in patients with TSC, focal proliferations of type II pneumocytes (i.e., multifocal micronodular pneumocyte hyperplasia [MMPH]) may occur.

Most patients present with progressive dyspnea or pneumothorax. Less common presentations are cough, hemoptysis, or chylous pleural effusions caused by compression of airways, lymphatics, and venules. The clinical course of LAM is highly variable; the 10-year survival rate is between 55% and 71%. The pulmonary complications increase during pregnancy.

Standard radiographic features include a diffuse linear pattern that may be associated with thin-walled cysts. The lung volumes are normal or increased. The increase in lung volumes correlates with evidence of airway obstruction on pulmonary function testing. Pneumothorax and chylous pleural effusions develop in the majority of patients during the course of disease. The high-resolution CT findings consist of thin-walled spherical cysts that are difficult to recognize on standard radiography. The cysts are distributed diffusely throughout the lungs (Fig. 18.22), in contrast to honeycombing, in which the cysts are thicker walled and are predominantly subpleural. The intervening lung parenchyma is usually normal, without evidence of lung distortion, although there may be occasional septal thickening and linear or ground-glass opacities. Nodules are extremely unusual, but adenopathy occurs occasionally. Nodules caused by MMPH may be seen in patients with TSC (Fig. 18.23). Fatty lesions within the heart are not uncommon in TSC. In the upper abdomen, renal angiomyolipomas are the most common extrathoracic manifestation of LAM and are much more common in TSC-LAM, although they may also occur in sporadic cases. Soft tissue lymphangiomas may also occur in association with the axial lymphatics.

The prognosis for LAM has improved; sirolimus has been shown to have efficacy in patients with LAM. Severe disease is treated with lung transplantation.

Pulmonary Langerhans Cell Histiocytosis

Langerhans cell histiocytosis (LCH) represents a diverse group of diseases of unknown origin that affect several organs with different clinical outcomes. These diseases can affect single or multiple organs. Multiorgan involvement is seen in children and adolescents. Single-system LCH can affect the bone, lung, or skin; has a more benign course; and can regress spontaneously. Isolated pulmonary involvement is the most common form in adults and is characterized by distinct clinical, epidemiologic, and radiologic features (Box 18.6). Langerhans cells are found in the tracheobronchial epithelium. In patients with pulmonary Langerhans cell histiocytosis (PCLH), these cells infiltrate the interstitium around the terminal and respiratory bronchioles to form granulomas, eventually destroying the bronchioles. The granulomas are focal and patchy, with normal intervening lung parenchyma. The alveoli contain macrophages that resemble RB and desquamative interstitial pneumonia changes. The adjacent arterioles may be involved. Later in the disease, cavitary nodules develop, representing

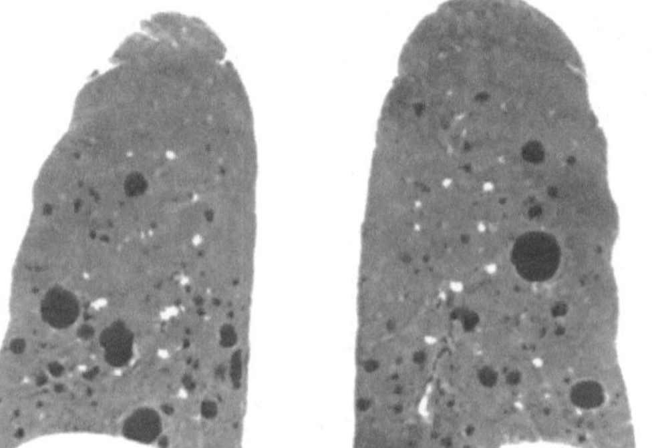

FIGURE 18.22 Lymphangioleiomyomatosis on chest computed tomography (CT). Coronal minimum-intensity projection image from noncontrast chest CT demonstrates diffuse, thin-walled cysts scattered throughout the lungs in this patient with lymphangioleiomyomatosis.

BOX 18.6 Langerhans Cell Histiocytosis

CHARACTERISTICS

Clinical features
Young adults
Smokers

PATHOLOGIC FEATURES

Benign proliferation of histiocytes
Granulomas

RADIOGRAPHIC FEATURES

Reticulonodular pattern
Predominance in upper zone
Pneumothorax
Cysts

HIGH-RESOLUTION COMPUTED TOMOGRAPHY FINDINGS

Thin-walled cysts
Nodules with or without cavitation
Predominance in upper zone

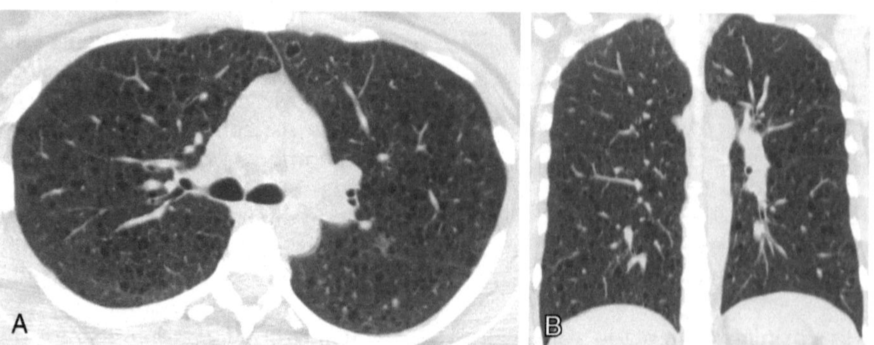

FIGURE 18.23 Multifocal micronodular pneumocyte hyperplasia in a patient with diffuse cystic lung disease from tuberous sclerosis (TSC) on chest computed tomography (CT). Axial **(A)** and coronal **(B)** images from noncontrast CT demonstrate multiple subsolid nodules and innumerable cysts within the lungs of this patient with known multifocal micronodular pneumocyte hyperplasia and TSC.

the destroyed bronchiolar lumens. In the advanced stage, there is confluence of adjacent cavities forming irregular cysts. The nodules are replaced by fibrotic scars, enlarged abnormal airways, and adjacent cicatricial emphysema causes bizarre-shaped cysts.

There is a strong epidemiologic association with smoking, but the exact mechanism is unknown. LCH is an uncommon disease that occurs in young and middle-aged adults, and more than 90% of the patients are smokers. The presenting symptoms usually consist of dyspnea and a nonproductive cough. The natural history of disease is variable and unpredictable. 50% of patients have a favorable outcome, with regression of symptoms spontaneously or with cessation of smoking. Between 30% and 40% have persistence or progression of symptoms and progression of radiologic findings. In 10% to 20%, respiratory failure and recurrent pneumothoraces may occur.

Features seen on standard radiographs include a reticulonodular pattern. These findings are bilateral and symmetric. The apical areas are affected, with relative sparing of the bases and particular sparing of the costophrenic sulci. The lung volumes are normal or increased. Occasionally, thin-walled cysts can be recognized. Pneumothorax is a common complication, occurring in 20% to 30% of cases, and it may be recurrent.

Chest CT findings (Fig. 18.24) include centrilobular or peribronchial nodules that measure 1 to 10 mm in diameter early in the disease. The disease is focal, with normal intervening lung parenchyma. With disease progression, thin-walled lung cysts are seen, usually measuring less than 1 cm in diameter. Longitudinal studies have shown evolution of nodules to cavitary nodules, the so-called Cheerio sign (Fig. 18.25), and then to thick- and thin-walled cysts. The cysts may coalesce and lead to bizarre shapes. The nodules and cavitated nodules can resolve, but the cysts persist or progress. There is upper lobe predominance of the disease and sparing of costophrenic angles. Given the strong association between PLCH and pulmonary hypertension, the pulmonary artery should be carefully assessed in all cases of suspected PLCH. The differential diagnosis includes LAM, but there are several distinguishing features. The distribution of disease is diffuse in LAM but upper zone predominant with PLCH, with sparing of the costophrenic angles. The cysts in LAM are thin walled and spherical; cysts in PLCH are bizarre shaped and thick walled, and the presence of nodules in PLCH is a highly useful distinguishing feature. As in LAM, the cysts of PLCH must be differentiated from the emphysema and honeycombing seen in pulmonary fibrosis. The differential diagnosis of PLCH includes other diseases characterized by nodules, and if cysts are not present, differentiation may be difficult. The treatment consists primarily of smoking cessation. In some cases, glucocorticoid therapy is successful.

Other Diffuse Cystic Lung Diseases

Lymphocytic interstitial pneumonia (LIP) is another cause of diffuse cystic lung disease and is discussed in the IIP section of this chapter. Cysts in this condition tend to be basilar and peribronchovascular in distribution (see Fig. 18.12). Birt-Hogg-Dube (BHD) syndrome is an autosomal dominant disorder caused by mutations in the FLCN gene on chromosome 17p11.2, encoding the tumor-suppressor protein folliculin, and classically presents with the triad of fibrofolliculomas, trichodiscomas, and skin tags. BHD syndrome is also associated with renal tumors, specifically renal cell carcinoma and oncocytomas, diffuse cystic lung disease, and pneumothoraces. Cysts in BHD syndrome are usually basilar predominant and range in size from 0.2 to 8 cm with variable shapes. The axial distribution of cysts is typically subpleural, perivascular, and paramediastinal; paramediastinal involvement is relatively specific for BHD syndrome cysts. In contrast to other cystic lung diseases, cysts may be multiseptated (Fig. 18.26, *A*). The cysts may be round, oval, or lentiform; lentiform shape is a helpful differentiator from LIP-related cysts (Fig. 18.26, *B*).

Light chain deposition disorder (LCDD) is a multisystem process associated with plasma cell dyscrasia, particularly multiple myeloma and Waldenström macroglobulinemia. The kidneys are invariably affected, with heart and liver involvement common. The lungs are uncommonly affected and usually asymptomatic. Imaging manifestations include

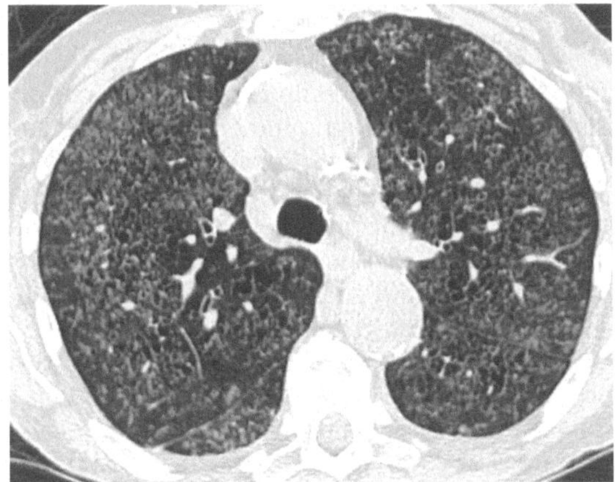

FIGURE 18.24 Langerhans cell histiocytosis (LCH) on chest computed tomography (CT). Axial image from noncontrast chest CT demonstrates innumerable small nodular opacities throughout the lungs with superimposed emphysema or early cystic changes in this patient with LCH.

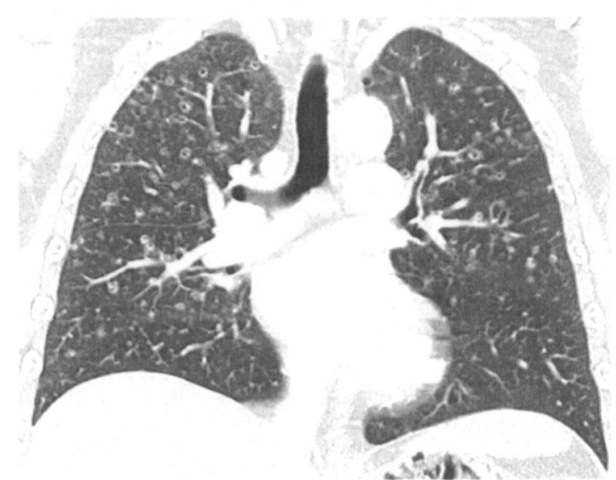

FIGURE 18.25 Langerhans cell histiocytosis on chest computed tomography (CT). Baseline coronal chest CT from contrast-enhanced chest CT demonstrates mid and upper lung–preponderance of small cavitary nodules throughout the lungs in this patient with a long smoking history.

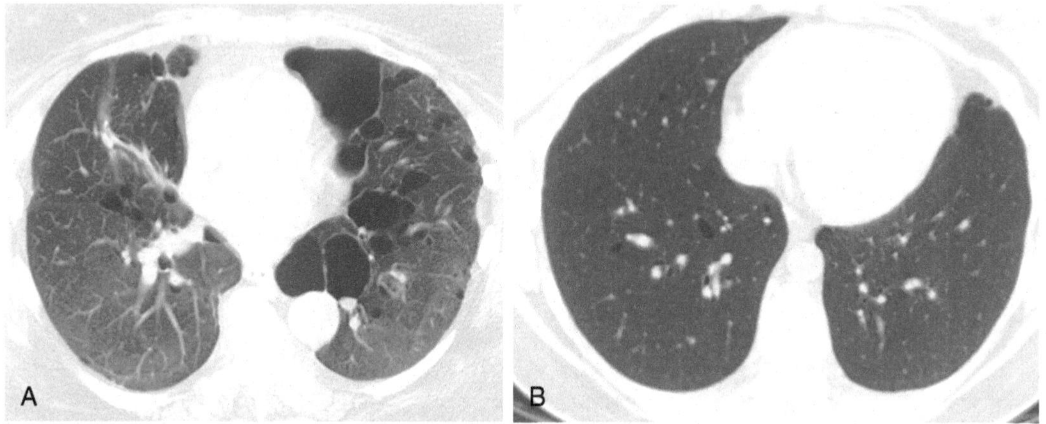

FIGURE 18.26 Birt-Hogg-Dube (BHD) syndrome on chest computed tomography (CT). Axial image from noncontrast chest CT **(A)** demonstrates multiseptated cysts along the mediastinum highly suggestive of BHD syndrome. Noncontrast chest CT image **(B)** from another patient demonstrates the lentiform shape of cysts in the peribronchovascular aspects of the lower lobes, which is suggestive of BHD syndrome as opposed to lymphocytic interstitial pneumonitis.

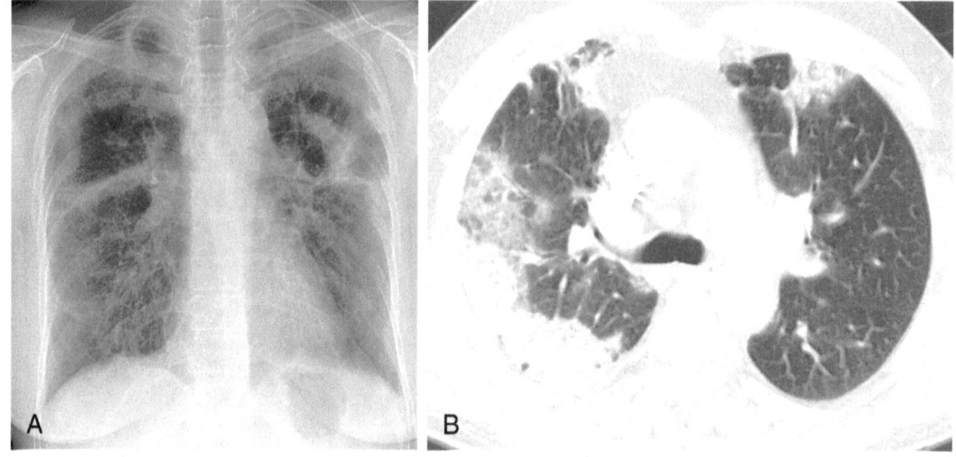

FIGURE 18.27 Loeffler syndrome on chest radiography. Frontal chest radiograph **(A)** demonstrates multiple areas of ground-glass opacity and consolidation within the peripheral aspects of the lungs. Axial image from noncontrast chest computed tomography **(B)** from another patient demonstrates multiple areas of ground-glass opacity and consolidation within the peripheral aspects of the lungs.

variable-sized nodules and basilar-predominant cysts. Rarely, amyloidosis may present with a similar pattern of cystic lung disease, often with concomitant calcified nodules. Spherical, thin-walled cysts, or pneumatoceles, may occur as a sequela of previous infection (staphylococcal infection, *Pneumocystis pneumoniae*), inflammation (HP), or trauma.

EOSINOPHILIC LUNG DISEASE

Characteristics

The term *pulmonary eosinophilia* was originally used to describe a group of diseases in which radiographic abnormalities were seen in association with blood eosinophilia. The descriptive term of *pulmonary infiltration with eosinophilia,* or *PIE syndrome,* is sometimes used to identify these disorders. However, eosinophilic infiltration of the lung can exist in the absence of blood eosinophilia and includes a series of disorders.

Loeffler Syndrome

Loeffler syndrome (i.e., simple pulmonary eosinophilia) consists of fleeting radiographic opacities associated with blood eosinophilia (Box 18.7). Most patients have a background of atopy. Loeffler syndrome may be idiopathic or secondary to drug therapy or parasites, such as *Ascaris lumbricoides*. Patients may be asymptomatic or present with cough, fever, and chest pain. A low-level eosinophilia can be identified in the peripheral blood.

Radiographic features of Loeffler syndrome consist of single or multiple ill-defined air space opacities in the peripheral or axillary portions of the lungs (Fig. 18.27, *A*). The areas of consolidation are transient and frequently shift from one area to another, although stability may occur over several days. Cavitation, pleural effusion, and lymphadenopathy do not occur. CT typically shows ground-glass attenuation and consolidation in the upper and middle lung regions, with a subpleural distribution (Fig. 18.27,

B). Single or multiple small nodules with a ground-glass halo (similar in appearance to nodules associated with angioinvasive *Aspergillus* infection) may be seen in some cases. The prognosis is excellent, and the opacities and blood eosinophilia usually resolve spontaneously. Careful search for a parasite or drug reaction should be undertaken and the underlying disease treated.

Chronic Eosinophilic Pneumonia

Chronic eosinophilic pneumonia (Box 18.8) is a serious disease that requires treatment. Most patients are middle-aged women. Prominent symptoms include dyspnea, fever, chills, night sweats, and weight loss. Asthma is present in only 50% of cases. The disease is often insidious. Peripheral blood eosinophilia (>6% of total white cell count) occurs in most patients, but it is often mild or moderate.

The typical radiographic pattern consists of subpleural, poorly defined opacities without lobar or segmental distribution. The opacities are usually in an apical or axillary location, but they occasionally may be basal. When the opacities surround the lung, the appearance is that of a photographic negative or reversal of opacities usually seen in pulmonary edema. The opacities sometimes disappear and recur in exactly the same location. Oblique or vertical lines with no anatomic reference occasionally appear during resolution. CT shows peripheral consolidation even when the chest radiograph fails to show the peripheral location of the opacities (Fig. 18.28). Less common CT findings, which are typically seen in the later stages of this condition, include ground-glass opacities, nodules, and reticular opacities. Half of the patients have mediastinal adenopathy on CT that is also not apparent on standard radiographs. Histologic examination demonstrates eosinophil and leukocyte accumulation in the alveoli and in the interstitium with thickened alveolar walls.

The prognosis for patients with this disease is excellent, although if untreated, it is likely to be protracted and may be fatal. One of the characteristic features of chronic eosinophilic pneumonia is a dramatic response to corticosteroid treatment, with clinical improvement occurring in hours and radiographic resolution occurring within a few days. A trial of corticosteroids may be used as a diagnostic tool when infection has been excluded.

Acute Eosinophilic Pneumonia

Idiopathic acute eosinophilic pneumonia (Box 18.9) was first described in 1989 and represents a clinical entity distinct from other idiopathic eosinophilic lung disease,

BOX 18.7 Loeffler Syndrome*

CHARACTERISTICS

Atopy
Causes
Idiopathic
Parasites
Drug induced
Mild symptoms and eosinophilia

RADIOGRAPHIC FEATURES

Peripheral consolidation
Fleeting opacities

*Also called simple pulmonary eosinophilia.

BOX 18.8 Chronic Eosinophilic Pneumonia

CHARACTERISTICS

Middle-aged women
Mild or moderate eosinophilia
More severe disease than Loeffler syndrome; insidious onset
Rapid response to steroids

RADIOGRAPHIC FEATURES

Peripheral consolidation
Upper zones
Photographic negative of pulmonary edema
Differential diagnosis: organizing pneumonia

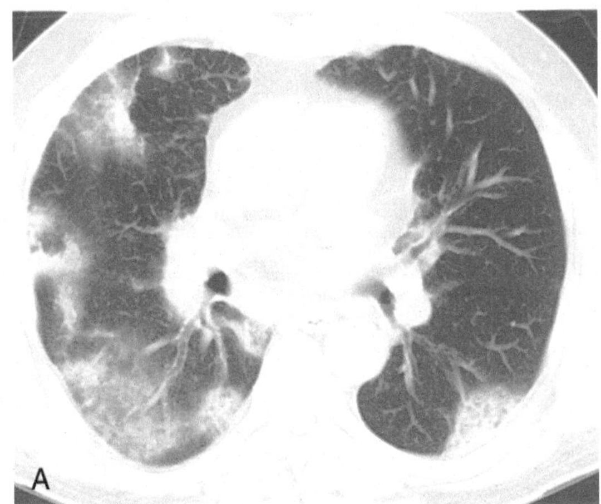

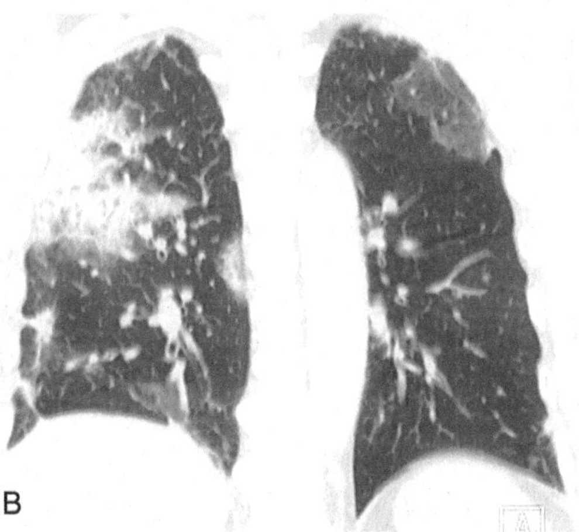

FIGURE 18.28 Chronic eosinophilic pneumonia on chest computed tomography (CT). Axial **(A)** and coronal **(B)** images from noncontrast chest CT demonstrates peripheral regions of ground-glass opacity and consolidation in this patient with known chronic eosinophilic pneumonia.

BOX 18.9 Acute Eosinophilic Pneumonia

CHARACTERISTICS

Acute febrile illness
Respiratory failure
Complete response to steroids
Absence of atopic history

RADIOGRAPHIC FEATURES

Diffuse consolidation
Not peripheral

COMPUTED TOMOGRAPHY FEATURES

Diffuse parenchymal consolidation
Septal thickening
Effusion
No lymphadenopathy

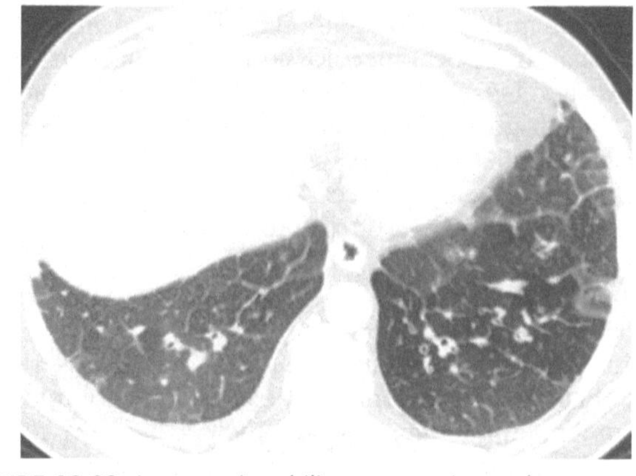

FIGURE 18.29 Acute eosinophilic pneumonia on chest computed tomography (CT). Axial image from noncontrast CT demonstrates interlobular septal thickening and a small right-sided pleural effusion in this patient with acute eosinophilic pneumonia.

such as chronic eosinophilic pneumonia. Diagnostic criteria include an acute febrile illness of less than 5 days' duration; respiratory failure; eosinophils greater than 25% on bronchoalveolar lavage; absence of parasitic, fungal, or other infection; prompt and complete response to corticosteroids; and failure to relapse after discontinuation of corticosteroids. Patients do not usually have a history of atopy or asthma, but a recent history of smoking or a change in smoking habit is often seen.

Radiographic findings usually include subtle linear opacities, which progress to a consolidative pattern that is usually bilateral and extensive and involves all lobes. Unlike chronic eosinophilic pneumonia and many of the other eosinophilic syndromes, the opacities are usually not located peripherally. CT shows diffuse parenchymal consolidation, ground-glass attenuation, pleural effusions, pronounced thickening of the interlobular septa, and normal-size lymph nodes (Fig. 18.29). Less commonly, focal areas of consolidation or poorly defined nodules may be seen.

The cause of this disease is unknown, but it may represent an acute hypersensitivity phenomenon to an unidentified inhaled antigen; many patients have recently started smoking or increased their rate of smoking. In the differential diagnosis, infectious disease must be excluded. Patients respond rapidly to high doses of corticosteroids, usually within 24 to 48 hours. If untreated, they may progress rapidly to acute respiratory failure.

Idiopathic Hypereosinophilic Syndrome

Idiopathic hypereosinophilic syndrome is a rare and fatal disorder characterized by blood eosinophilia of greater than 1500 cells/mL for more than 6 months and an absence of parasitic or other causes of secondary eosinophilia. Initially, this disease was called *eosinophilic leukemia*. The disease usually occurs in the third or fourth decades of life, and there is marked 7 : 1 male-to-female predominance. Symptoms include night sweats, anorexia, weight loss, cough, and fever. There is a profound peripheral eosinophilia of 30% to 70%, with a total white blood cell count greater than 10,000 cells/mL. Cardiac involvement may occur, and it is a major cause of morbidity and mortality. Pulmonary involvement occurs in up to 40% of patients and typically manifests with cough. It is usually caused by pulmonary edema related to cardiac failure.

The chest radiograph shows interstitial linear or nodular opacities that are nonlobar in distribution, and approximately half of patients have pleural effusions. CT findings include septal thickening, ground-glass attenuation, and alveolar opacities related to pulmonary edema. CT may show poorly defined nodules, with or without surrounding ground-glass attenuation. Thromboembolic disease occurs in two thirds of patients. About half of the patients have a good clinical response to steroids alone, but others may require cytotoxic therapy.

Parasitic Infections

Many parasites can cause pulmonary consolidation with blood or alveolar eosinophilia or both. Those causing infection in the United States include *Strongyloides, Ascaris, Toxocara,* and *Ancylostoma* spp. Radiographic features for most of parasitic infections are typically those of fleeting and migratory peripheral areas of consolidation. Tropical pulmonary eosinophilia is caused by filarial worms.

DRUG-INDUCED LUNG DISEASE

Drug-induced lung toxicity is common and may result from complex chemotherapeutic regimens or the abuse of illicit drugs. Many drugs may produce a similar clinical syndrome, and individual drugs may cause a variety of reactions. Many drug reactions are immunologically mediated, although some may occur as a result of direct toxicity. Direct toxicity is usually dose related. The pathologic reaction consists of permeability pulmonary edema, which may progress to diffuse alveolar damage and pulmonary fibrosis. The injury may be mediated by the generation of reactive oxygen species. Hypersensitivity reactions are not dose related and require prior sensitization to the drug. This reaction is the result of the interaction between the drug and humeral antibodies or sensitized lymphocytes. Idiosyncratic toxicity is not dose related and does not require prior sensitization. These reactions are

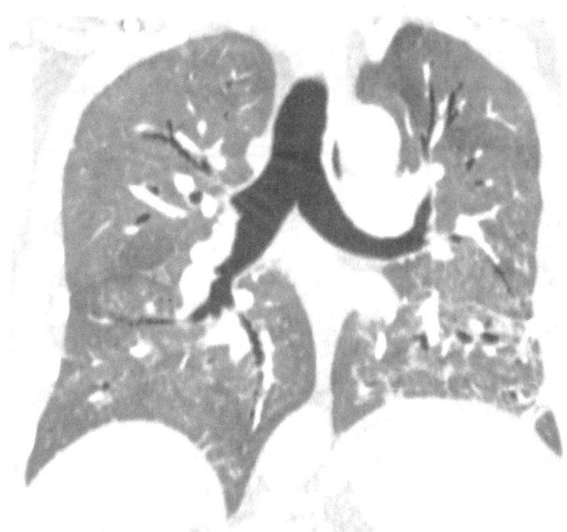

FIGURE 18.30 Noncardiogenic pulmonary edema on chest computed tomography (CT). Coronal image from noncontrast chest CT demonstrates diffuse ground-glass abnormality within the lungs in this patient who had overdosed on heroin.

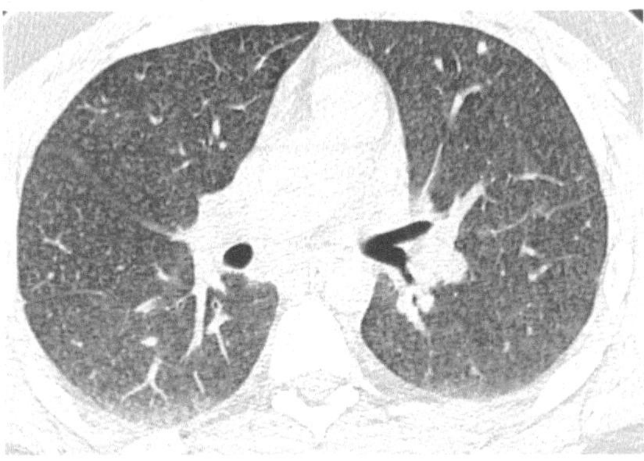

FIGURE 18.31 Excipient lung on chest computed tomography (CT). Axial image from noncontrast chest CT demonstrates diffuse centrilobular ground-glass nodularity in this patient who had been injecting medications illicitly through his central venous line.

usually acute, manifesting with noncardiogenic pulmonary edema.

Patterns of Injury

Noncardiogenic Pulmonary Edema

Noncardiogenic pulmonary edema is a common complication of a variety of drugs, particularly hydrochlorothiazide and cytotoxic agents, such as interleukin, methotrexate, cytosine, and arabinoside. The pulmonary edema typically occurs within hours of administration. It is also a well-recognized complication of opiate (heroin) and salicylate overdose (Fig. 18.30).

Pulmonary Hemorrhage

Pulmonary hemorrhage is most commonly a complication of anticoagulant therapy or drug-induced thrombocytopenia. Penicillamine may rarely cause a pulmonary renal syndrome similar to Goodpasture syndrome. Acute and even fatal pulmonary hemorrhage has been reported with nitrofurantoin therapy, but more commonly, this drug is associated with HP or pulmonary fibrosis. Cocaine abuse is increasingly recognized as a cause of intra-alveolar hemorrhage.

Pulmonary Fibrosis

Pulmonary fibrosis usually develops as a chronic insidious process and is typically seen with a wide variety of cytotoxic and noncytotoxic drugs, such as busulfan and bleomycin. Several new chemotherapy agents, including gemcitabine, have been associated with pulmonary fibrosis.

Eosinophilic Pneumonia

Drug reactions are one of the most commonly reported causes of pulmonary opacities associated with blood or alveolar eosinophilia. One of the most common is sulfasalazine, which is used for inflammatory bowel disease. Eosinophilia-myalgia syndrome is an interesting multiorgan disorder caused by contaminants found in batches of L-tryptophan that were manufactured in the late 1980s. The disease involved approximately half of the persons ingesting the contaminated drug, who developed acute peripheral blood eosinophilia accompanied by severe myalgias. Approximately half of the patients had respiratory symptoms. Typical peripheral pulmonary consolidation was identified on chest radiographs. Drug-induced eosinophilia may be mild or manifest as a fulminant, acute eosinophilic pneumonia-like syndrome. Most patients respond to withdrawal of the drug, although steroid therapy may be necessary.

Exogenous Lipoid Pneumonia

Exogenous lipoid pneumonia has been described as a complication of accidental aspiration of mineral oil. Endogenous phospholipidosis induced by amiodarone is an important cause of pulmonary toxicity.

Drug-Induced Lupus Syndrome

Drug-induced lupus syndrome is more common than the idiopathic form of SLE. It has, however, a more benign course and is usually reversible. Common manifestations include pleural and pericardial effusions. Subsegmental atelectasis and basilar consolidation are typical radiographic findings. Drugs implicated include hydralazine, procainamide, and phenytoin. Most patients have a positive antinuclear antibody (ANA) result.

Obliterative Bronchiolitis

Obliterative bronchiolitis is characterized pathologically by the proliferation of granulation tissue in the small airways and obliteration of their lumens. It is an uncommon drug-induced complication, most frequently associated with penicillamine therapy prescribed for RA.

Illicit Drug Use

The pulmonary manifestations of drug abuse include a wide variety of infectious and inflammatory complications. The adverse effects are related to the route of administration and to the type of drug. Excipient lung may result from intravenous injection of aqueous solutions of oral preparations containing talc, methylcellulose, or other inert fillers. Talc is a filler used in the manufacturing of tablets to prevent them from sticking to the mouth. When injected, these particles become lodged in peripheral pulmonary arterioles and capillaries, producing pulmonary hypertension and vasculitis. Imaging shows centrilobular and tree-in-bud nodularity throughout the lungs (Fig. 18.31).

Specific Drugs

Clinical and radiologic features of drug-induced lung disease are summarized in Box 18.10.

Amiodarone

Amiodarone is a tri-iodinated compound used in the treatment of cardiac arrhythmias. Pulmonary toxicity is a common complication, occurring in up to 18% of patients. Toxicity appears to be dose related. The onset is usually subacute. Several forms of pulmonary toxicity have been reported among patients treated with amiodarone. The most common presentation is a chronic interstitial pneumonitis with imaging features of reticular opacities that may be difficult to distinguish from congestive heart failure. If the diagnosis is delayed, the interstitial process may progress to end-stage pulmonary fibrosis. In some cases, patchy alveolar and interstitial opacities may be present diffusely. Upper lobe predominance has been described in some cases, which can be helpful for differentiating this condition from congestive heart failure. A less common presentation is solitary or multiple peripheral areas of consolidation, nodules, or both that may mimic COP, chronic eosinophilic pneumonia, and pulmonary infarction. A rare but potentially fatal form of pulmonary toxicity is ARDS. A pleural reaction may occur, but effusions are uncommon. CT may demonstrate the characteristic high density of the pleuropulmonary lesions as a result of the iodine content of amiodarone (Fig. 18.32). When areas of consolidation, nodules, or both with high attenuation are seen on unenhanced CT scans, amiodarone pulmonary toxicity should be considered. Because amiodarone therapy is frequently associated with high attenuation of the liver, evaluation of the hepatic parenchyma may provide an important clue to the diagnosis.

Nitrofurantoin

Nitrofurantoin is a drug that is widely used in the treatment of urinary tract infections. It is an important cause of pulmonary eosinophilia, which occurs in the majority of patients. It may cause acute onset of pneumonitis and chronic interstitial pneumonia, often with an OP component. Imaging demonstrates bilateral, patchy, and occasionally peripheral or perilobular consolidation (Fig. 18.33). Pleural effusions may occur. Pulmonary fibrosis develops with prolonged use of nitrofurantoin, and the fibrosis probably results from chronic drug toxicity rather than a hypersensitivity reaction.

Methotrexate

This drug is used to treat a variety of inflammatory diseases, such as RA and psoriasis, and malignant disorders. Methotrexate toxicity is unique is several respects. Discontinuation of the drug is not always required for recovery, and reintroduction of the drug is not necessarily associated with recurrent symptoms. Toxicity may occur with low-dose therapy, and it appears to be related to the frequency of administration. The features are usually that of an allergic response with a subacute illness associated with pulmonary

BOX 18.10 Clinical and Radiologic Features of Drug- and Chemical-Induced Lung Disease

HYDROCHLOROTHIAZIDE

Noncardiogenic pulmonary edema

INTERLEUKIN-2

Noncardiogenic edema
Pleural effusions and ascites

AMIODARONE

Treatment of cardiac arrhythmias
Patchy alveolar and diffuse linear opacities
Upper lobe and peripheral distribution
Solitary or multiple nodules and consolidation
High attenuation (iodine) on computed tomography

NITROFURANTOIN

Treatment of urinary tract infections
Eosinophilia
Patchy and peripheral airspace consolidation
Fibrosis (with chronic use)

METHOTREXATE

Treatment of inflammatory diseases and malignancy
Allergic response
Diffuse, reticulonodular opacities or widespread consolidation
Adenopathy
Distribution in lung bases and middle zones

BUSULFAN

Treatment of chronic granulocytic leukemia
Diffuse, reticulonodular opacities

BLEOMYCIN

Treatment of lymphoma, solid tumors
Dose-related effects
Pulmonary fibrosis
Linear subpleural basilar opacities

CYCLOSPORINE

Prevention of transplant rejection
Lymphoproliferative disorder (3%–5%)
Lungs, nodes, gastrointestinal tract distribution
Solitary mass, multiple nodules, with or without adenopathy

INTERFERON

Treatment for hepatitis B and C; hematologic malignancy; melanoma
Secondary sarcoidosis

CHECKPOINT INHIBITOR IMMUNOTHERAPY

Treatment for various malignancies
Nonspecific pneumonitis

ASPIRATED OILY SUBSTANCES

Lipoid pneumonia
Chronic multifocal basal areas of consolidation
Air bronchograms
Attenuation of fat on computed tomography

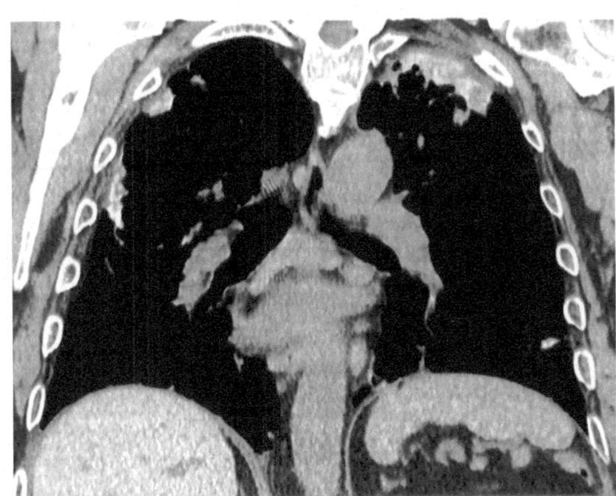

FIGURE 18.32 Amiodarone lung on chest computed tomography (CT). Coronal image from noncontrast chest CT demonstrates subpleural consolidation in the upper lung zones, which are hyperdense. The liver is also hyperdense relative to the spleen. The patient had been treated chronically with amiodarone for cardiac arrhythmia.

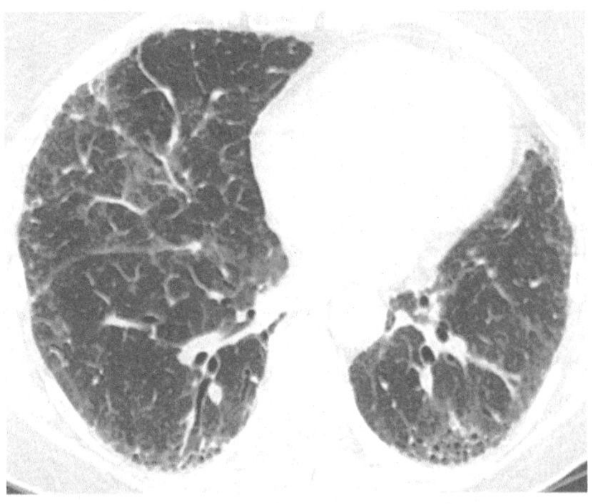

FIGURE 18.34 Bleomycin pulmonary toxicity on chest computed tomography (CT). Axial image from noncontrast chest CT demonstrates a mild usual interstitial pneumonitis pattern of pulmonary fibrosis in this patient who has been treated with bleomycin.

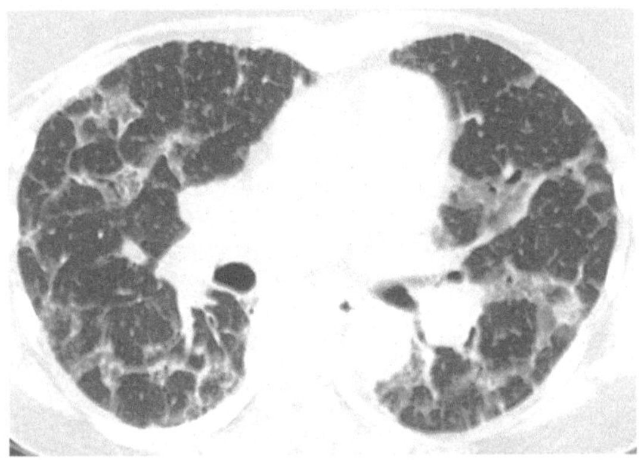

FIGURE 18.33 Nitrofurantoin lung on chest computed tomography (CT). Axial image from noncontrast chest CT demonstrates perilobular ground-glass opacity and mild reticulation in this patient with known nitrofurantoin lung toxicity.

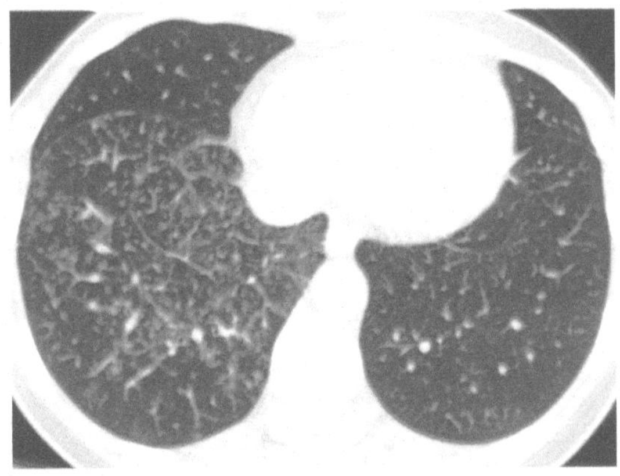

FIGURE 18.35 Secondary sarcoidosis caused by interferon therapy on chest computed tomography (CT). Axial image from noncontrast chest CT demonstrates diffuse perilymphatic nodularity within the right lower lobe in this woman treated with interferon for melanoma.

eosinophilia. The imaging manifestations are diverse but typically follow a diffuse alveolar damage, NSIP, or OP pattern. A predilection for the lung bases and middle zones has been described. Most patients recover completely, even if the drug is continued, and residual pulmonary fibrosis is uncommon.

Bleomycin

Bleomycin is used in the treatment of lymphomas, squamous cell cancer, and testicular tumors. Pulmonary toxicity occurs in about 4% of patients and is an important factor limiting dosage. The incidence of toxicity is related to the cumulative dose. Pulmonary fibrosis is the most serious complication, although acute hypersensitivity reaction has been described. Bleomycin is so effective at causing pulmonary fibrosis that it is ubiquitously used as the fibrosis model in mouse studies. The chest radiograph may be normal or may show typical basal subpleural reticular opacities similar to those seen in IPF (Fig. 18.34). CT may demonstrate abnormalities even when the chest radiograph is normal. In the early stages of the disease, regression may occur after stopping therapy, but fibrosis may progress, resulting in death.

Interferon

Interferon therapy aims to alter the immune response and is used in the treatment of some malignancies (hematologic malignancy and melanoma) and hepatitis B and C. Approximately one third of patients treated with interferon develop cough, fever, and malaise, although macroscopic evidence of lung disease on imaging is rare. However, imaging manifestations of lung disease are quite rare and may present as mild pneumonitis to severe diffuse alveolar damage. A characteristic complication of interferon therapy, however, is secondary sarcoidosis, which shares similar imaging manifestations as idiopathic sarcoidosis (Fig. 18.35).

Checkpoint Inhibitor Immunotherapy

Checkpoint inhibitor immunotherapy is a new and promising therapy for malignancy that aims to boost the immune response to tumor cells. A small proportion of patients (5%–10%) treated with immunotherapy develop pneumonitis. The imaging and histologic pattern of lung injury has not been clearly defined and may very well be inconsistent (Fig. 18.36).

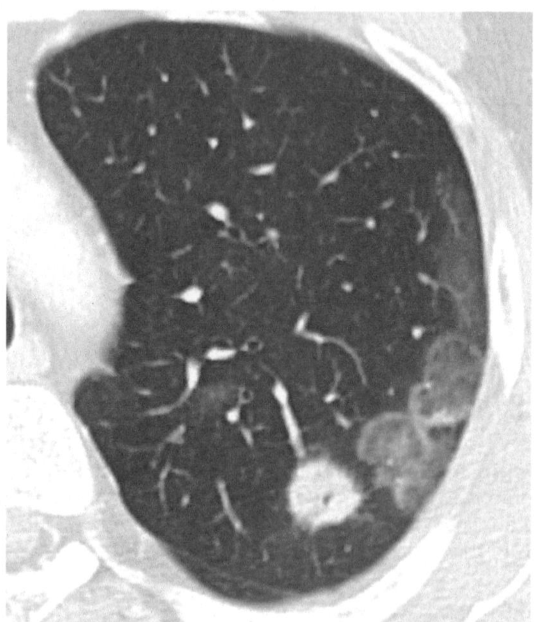

FIGURE 18.36 Checkpoint inhibitor immunotherapy toxicity on chest computed tomography (CT). Axial image from noncontrast chest CT demonstrates a poorly defined solid nodule in the left upper lobe with adjacent subsolid nodules, some demonstrating the reverse halo sign (central ground-glass opacity with a peripheral rim of consolidation). The CT findings are strongly suggestive of organizing pneumonia in this patient with history of mesothelioma treated with checkpoint inhibitor immunotherapy.

SUGGESTED READINGS

Hobbs S, Lynch D. The idiopathic interstitial pneumonias: an update and review. *Radiol Clin North Am.* 2014;52(1):105-120.

Lynch DA. Lung disease related to collagen vascular disease. *J Thorac Imaging.* 2009;24(4):299-309.

Martin MD, Chung JH, Kanne JP. Idiopathic pulmonary fibrosis. *J Thorac Imaging.* 2016;31(3):127-139.

Raghu G, Collard HR, Egan JJ, et al. An official ATS/ERS/JRS/ALAT statement: idiopathic pulmonary fibrosis: evidence-based guidelines for diagnosis and management. *Am J Respir Crit Care Med.* 2011;183(6):788-824.

Raoof S, Bondalapati P, Vydyula R, et al. Cystic lung diseases: algorithmic approach. *Chest.* 2016;150(4):945-965.

Webb WR. Thin-section CT of the secondary pulmonary lobule: anatomy and the image—the 2004 Fleischner lecture. *Radiology.* 2006;239:322-338.

Chapter 19
Pneumoconioses

Rydhwana Hossain, Subba R. Digumarthy, and Victorine V. Muse

INTRODUCTION

Industrial and technological advancements have made occupational lung diseases a major cause of work-related illness. The pneumoconioses are a set of lung diseases caused by the repeated inhalation and retention of small particles within the lung. The resultant lung injury depends on many factors, including particle size, cumulative dose, clearance rate, and inherent toxicity of the substance. The fact that only a proportion of similarly exposed workers develop the disease suggests a genetic component.

Broadly, pneumoconiosis can be divided into fibrotic and nonfibrotic lung diseases (Table 19.1). The classic fibrotic particles include silica, coal, beryllium, and asbestos. Some diseases such as silicosis, coal worker's pneumoconiosis (CWP), and asbestosis have reemerged not only in unregulated developing countries but also in the United States because of new industrial techniques such as fracking and denim sandblasting. Nonfibrotic pneumoconioses are caused by metal dusts such as iron, tin, and barium. Newly recognized pneumoconioses such as dental technician's pneumoconiosis and World Trade Center lung reflect both the novel exposures and the emerging importance of high-resolution computed tomography (HRCT) in the early diagnosis of pneumoconiosis.

PATHOPHYSIOLOGY

Inhaled dust has turbulent flow in the proximal large airways and gradually converts to laminar flow in the peripheral airways. The larger particles are cleared in the proximal airways by mucociliary transport. Smaller particles measuring 1 to 5 μm deposit at the level of the respiratory bronchioles. Some of these particles reach the alveoli, where they are phagocytized by macrophages, which then drain into the lymphatics and are cleared. If there are a large number of particles, this pathway fails, and dust-ingesting macrophages collect in the perivascular and peribronchiolar interstitium. These can remain in situ and eventually be covered by type 1 pneumocytes and remain entirely in the interstitium of the lung. In the case of fibrogenic dusts such as silica and asbestos, there is a proliferation of collagen fibers secondary to released inflammatory cytokines with development of a fibrotic nodule. Nonfibrotic inert dusts such as iron and tin induce a supporting network of fine reticulin fibers. When the macrophages die, the particles are released and the process repeats, with slow migration to the lymphatics or bronchioles. Therefore, the distribution of the pneumoconiotic nodule is a reflection of the lymphatic clearance of the lung. The lymphatic clearance in turn is affected by pulmonary arterial pressure, blood

TABLE 19.1 Fibrogenic and Nonfibrogenic Dust Diseases

Agent	Disease	Occupation
	Fibrogenic	
Asbestos	Asbestosis	Asbestos mining, ship building, textile, construction
Silica	Silicosis	Mining, drilling, ceramic, sandblasting, tunneling, glass manufacture, roadwork
Coal	Coal worker's pneumoconiosis	Coal mining
Talc	Talc pneumoconiosis	Ceramic, paint, paper, cosmetic
Beryllium	Berylliosis	Aerospace, ceramic, fluorescent light manufacturing
Aluminum	Aluminosis	Explosives manufacturing
Cobalt or tungsten	Hard metal pneumococcosis, giant cell interstitial pneumonitis	Diamond-cutting industry, jet engine exhaust, oil well drilling
Mix of chromium-cobalt-molybdenum	Dental technician's pneumoconiosis	Dental prosthesis manufacturing
Mix of cement dust, asbestos, microscopic shards of glass, silica, heavy metals, and numerous organic compounds	World Trade Center lung	9/11 workers, volunteers, and first responders
	Nonfibrogenic	
Tin	Stannosis	Mining, welding, pesticides
Iron	Siderosis	Polishing, welding, foundry work, mining
Barium	Baritosis	Glass and paper manufacturing

flow, and lung movement. The pulmonary flow is gravity dependent with relatively greater blood flow to the lower lungs. The thoracic cage has greater movement along the anterior and lateral walls compared with the posterior wall. These dynamics of lymphatic clearance result in weakest clearance in the upper posterior lungs, more so on the right side.

Whereas immune-mediated fibrosis is the predominant pattern in dusts from cobalt and beryllium, mixed dusts cause immune-mediated chronic interstitial pneumonitis.

INTERNATIONAL LABOUR ORGANIZATION CLASSIFICATION OF PNEUMOCONIOSIS

Screening of dust-exposed workers with chest radiographs has been and remains the standard of care throughout the world for the past 50 years because of its widespread availability, low cost, and low radiation dose despite its known low sensitivity and specificity in detection of early disease. The International Labour Organization (ILO) developed a systematic classification system that has been in use for more than 50 years to classify pneumoconiosis (Fig. 19.1). In 2011, the ILO system was revised with help from the American College of Radiology (ACR) and the National Institute for Occupational Safety and Health (NIOSH). The opacities seen on the standard chest radiograph are divided into two basic types, small and large opacities. The small opacities are further categorized based on shape into small round or irregular opacities (Fig. 19.2). Each of these categories are subdivided into three types based on size (Table 19.2) and further subdivided based on frequency or profusion. The profusion is defined as opacities per unit area. The large opacities measure more than 1 cm and are also divided in to three categories: A (1-5 cm), B (>5 cm to the lower limit of the right upper long zone), and C (equal to or greater than the right upper lung zone) (Fig. 19.3). Pleural abnormalities are described separately and divided into pleural plaques, calcification, costophrenic angle obliteration, and diffuse pleural thickening.

Any physician may become certified by NIOSH to become a "B-reader," which permits him or her to classify, but not interpret, screening standard chest radiographs for pneumoconioses using a set of 22 standard comparison films. New guidelines now allow use of digital radiography with correlative software to directly compare digital chest radiographs with the set of standard radiographs, providing better uniformity and reproducibility in classification. Reader variability, however, continues to be an important issue, and computer-assisted classification is being pursued.

High-resolution CT is more sensitive for detecting the early changes of pneumoconioses and has improved our understanding of airway, pleural, and parenchymal changes

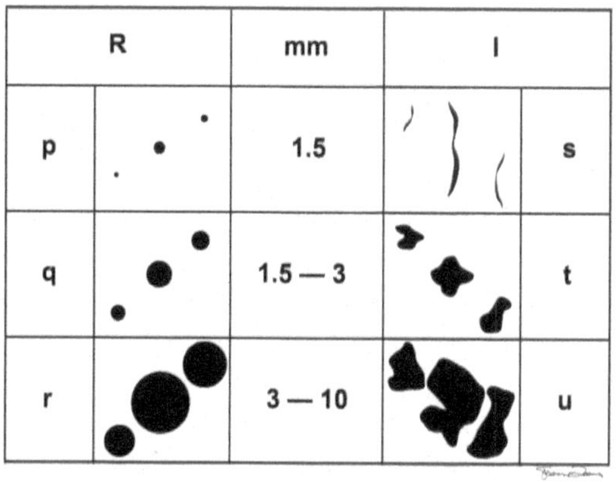

R		mm	I	
p		1.5		s
q		1.5—3		t
r		3—10		u

FIGURE 19.1 Diagrammatic representation of small opacities in the International Labour Organization classification. The small, rounded nodules (R) are divided into p, q, and r subsets based on size. The small, irregular (linear and reticular) lesions (I) are divided in to s, t, and u subsets based on thickness in millimeters.

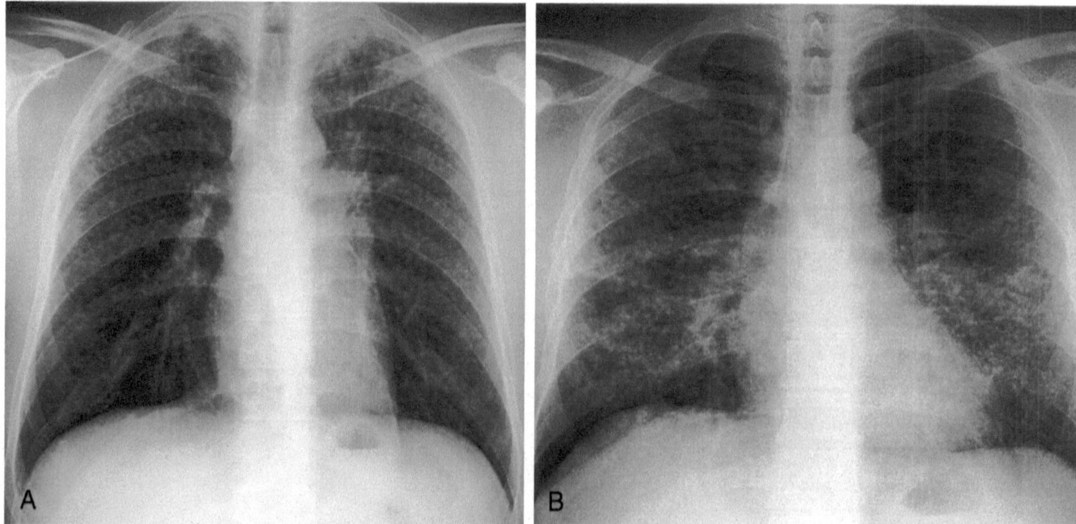

FIGURE 19.2 International Labour Organization (ILO) classification of small rounded opacities in silicosis. **A,** Posteroanterior radiograph demonstrates innumerable small rounded bilateral upper lobe–predominant nodules (ILO classification p, q). **B,** Mid to lower lung zone–predominant nodules (ILO classification q, r). (Courtesy of Fatih Alper, MD, PhD, professor, Department of Radiology, Ataturk University, School of Medicine, Erzurum, Turkey, and Metin Akgun, MD, professor, Department of Pulmonary Medicine, Ataturk University, School of Medicine, Erzurum, Turkey.)

and progression of established pneumoconiosis. HRCT is also aiding in identifying new causes of occupational lung diseases. There are no data to support the use of low-dose chest CT for screening in pneumoconiosis as there is for lung cancer screening among heavy smokers. There is potential application of lung cancer screening using CT in patients who are exposed to dusts, such as asbestos, that increase the risk of cancer

TABLE 19.2 International Labour Organization Classification of Pneumoconioses

Opacities	Profusion (Severity)
Small	0 (normal: 0/–, 0/0, 0/1)
Rounded (p, q, r)*	1 (slight: 1/0, 1/1, 1/2) 2 (moderate: 2/1, 2/2, 2/3)
Irregular (s, t, u)	3 (severe: 3/2, 3/3, 3/+)
Large	
A (1-5 cm)	
B (cm^2 = RU)	
C (cm^2 >RU)	
Zones	
RU	LU
RM	LM
RL	LL

*The size of small, round opacities is characterized by a diameter of p (≤1.5 mm), q (1.5-3 mm), or r (3-10 mm). Irregular, small opacities are classified by width and appearance as s (≤1.5 mm, fine), t (1.5-3 mm, medium), or u (3-10 mm, coarse or blotchy).

LL, Left lower; *LM*, left middle; *LU*, left upper; *RL*, right lower; *RM*, right middle; *RU*, right upper.

MINERAL DUST PNEUMOCONIOSIS

Silicosis

Silicosis is the most common and oldest recognized occupational lung disease, also known as widow maker's disease. Silica crystals are an abundant component on Earth's crust. Silicon dioxide has been found in many rocks such as marble, sandstone, flint, and slate. Occupations such as mining, quarrying, drilling, foundry working, ceramics manufacturing, sandblasting, construction, roadwork, glass manufacture, and tunneling are all associated with silicosis. A new application with a high incidence of silicosis was recently described in Turkish men employed in sandblasting denim.

Silicone particles of diameters greater than 5 μm can be easily expelled with the help of ciliary movement, preventing accumulation within the lung alveoli. Silicone particles smaller than 5 μm are not as effectively expelled and consequently have a higher probability of leading to silicosis. There are three subtypes of silicosis: acute, classic, and accelerated.

Acute Silicosis

Primarily described among sandblasters, acute silicosis or silicoproteinosis is the result of a very large exposure to silicone over a short period of time. Patients may be asymptomatic or present with severe dyspnea, cough, fever, and weight loss. This disease usually manifests within a short period of time after exposure and may rapidly progress, resulting in respiratory failure. Bronchoalveolar lavage shows a considerable amount of proteinaceous material with a positive reaction to periodic acid–Schiff stain. Unlike

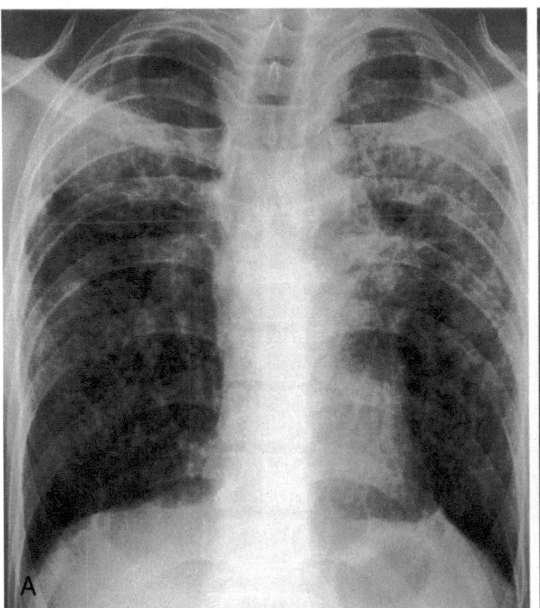

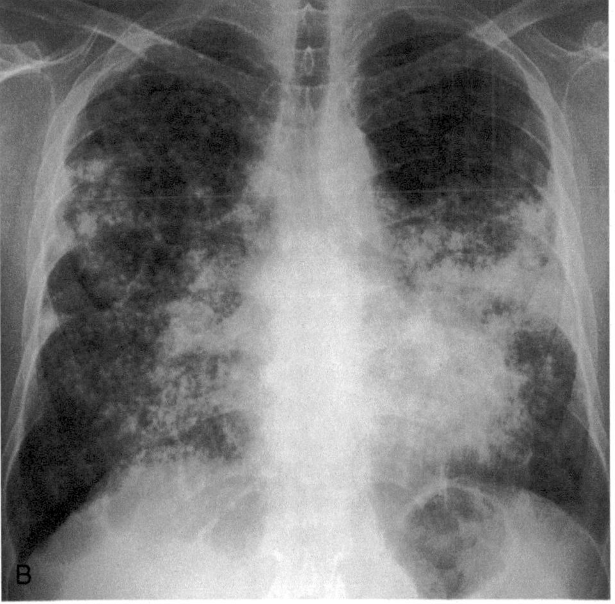

FIGURE 19.3 International Labour Organization (ILO) classification of large opacities in silicosis. **A,** Posteroanterior radiograph demonstrates bilateral upper lobe large opacities (ILO classification b). **B,** Mid to lower lung zone–predominant large opacities (ILO classification b, c). (Courtesy of Fatih Alper, MD, PhD, professor, Department of Radiology, Ataturk University, School of Medicine, Erzurum, Turkey, and Metin Akgun, MD, professor, Department of Pulmonary Medicine, Ataturk University, School of Medicine, Erzurum, Turkey.)

classic silicosis, silicoproteinosis is associated with minimal collagen deposition and fibrosis.

Imaging Findings

The findings include ground-glass opacification with prominent reticulation and septal thickening ("crazy paving") similar to alveolar proteinosis, perihilar or diffuse consolidations with air bronchograms, and multiple bilateral centrilobular opacities.

Classic or Chronic Silicosis

The classic or chronic form of silicosis usually manifests 10 to 20 years after exposure to low concentrations of silica. Classic silicosis is subdivided into two radiologic forms, simple silicosis and complicated (progressive massive fibrosis [PMF]).

Simple Silicosis

Simple silicosis usually has no symptoms and is not associated with significant changes in pulmonary function tests.

Imaging Findings

Multiple bilateral small nodular opacities are seen measuring approximately 2 to 5 mm in diameter (Fig. 19.4). These nodules may be more defined than those in coal worker's pneumoconiosis, with an upper perihilar distribution. Silicotic nodules may contain weakly birefringent silicate crystals. Occasionally, these nodules may calcify. Lymphadenopathy is common and may precede pulmonary parenchymal findings. Eggshell calcification of lymph nodes is a characteristic appearance and highly suggestive of silicosis (Fig. 19.5).

Complicated Form or Progressive Massive Fibrosis

PMF occurs when there is confluence of individual nodules creating larger opacities greater than 1 cm with irregular margins. These opacities tend to migrate toward the hilum. As this process continues, paracicatricial emphysema can be seen predominantly in the upper lungs.

Imaging Findings

Upper lobe-predominant volume loss with architectural distortion is seen. Additionally, large focal masses with irregular margins and calcifications are seen surrounded by emphysematous tissue (Fig. 19.6). As these large masses coalesce, it may result in cavitation due to ischemia, allowing for superimposed infections (Fig. 19.7). Mediastinal and hilar lymphadenopathy is again seen, but the eggshell calcification pattern is less common.

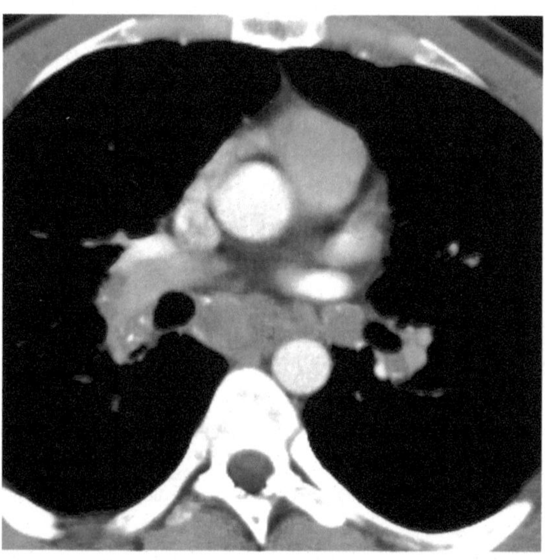

FIGURE 19.5 Simple silicosis. Computed tomography using mediastinal windows demonstrates calcified subcarinal and hilar lymphadenopathy. (Courtesy of Fatih Alper, MD, PhD, professor, Department of Radiology, Ataturk University, School of Medicine, Erzurum, Turkey, and Metin Akgun, MD, professor, Department of Pulmonary Medicine, Ataturk University, School of Medicine, Erzurum, Turkey.)

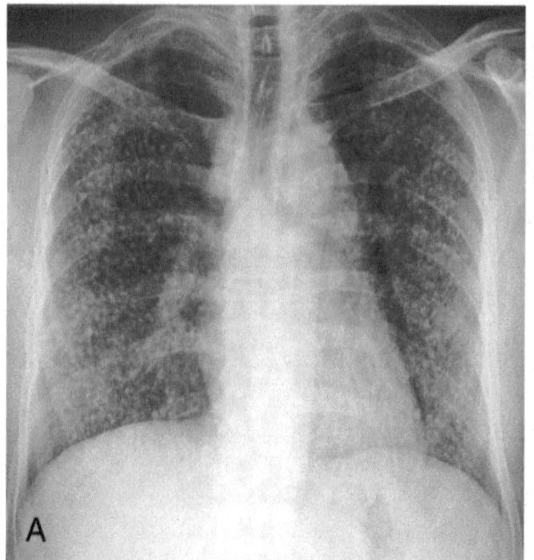

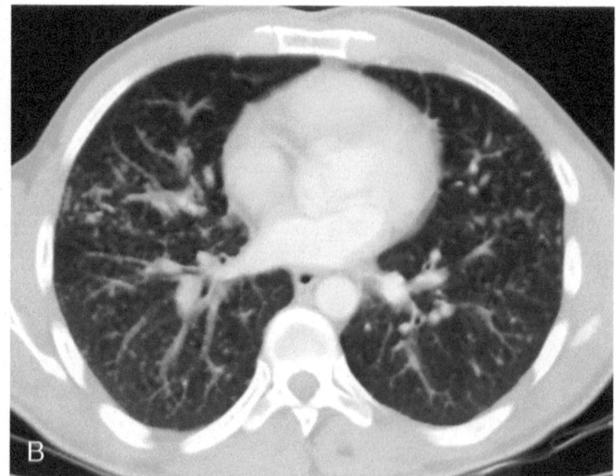

FIGURE 19.4 Simple silicosis. **A,** Posteroanterior radiograph demonstrates innumerable small diffuse rounded 1- to 5-mm nodules throughout the lungs. **B,** Axial chest computed tomography image demonstrates multiple randomly distributed nodules throughout all lobes. (Courtesy of Fatih Alper, MD, PhD, professor, Department of Radiology, Ataturk University, School of Medicine, Erzurum, Turkey, and Metin Akgun, MD, professor, Department of Pulmonary Medicine, Ataturk University, School of Medicine, Erzurum, Turkey.)

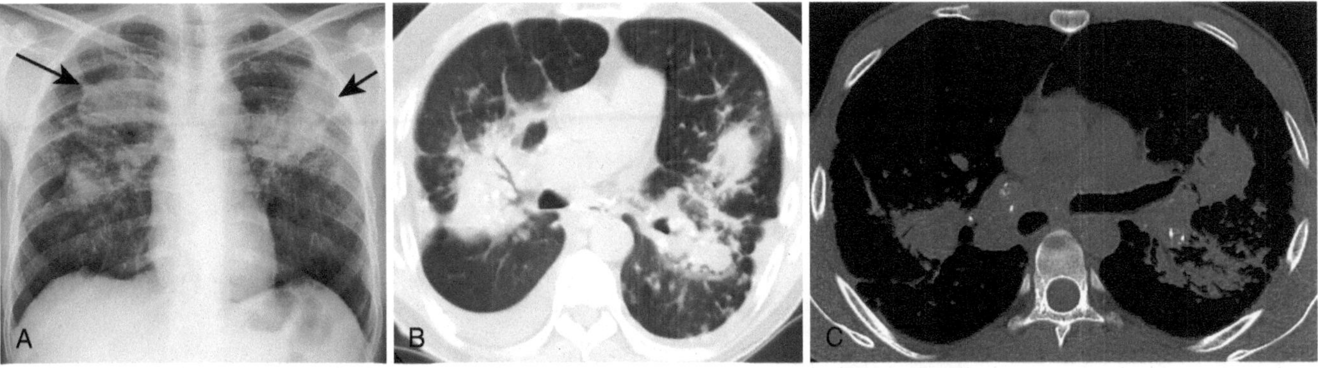

FIGURE 19.6 Complicated silicosis with progressive massive fibrosis. **A,** Large, vertically oriented mass like opacities paralleling the chest wall are seen in the upper lung zones midway between the hila and lateral pleura *(arrows)*. Notice the tenting of bilateral hemidiaphragms resulting from upper lobe volume loss. Computed tomography using lung **(B)** and mediastinal **(C)** windows shows calcified conglomerate masses consistent with fibrosis in the perihilar regions. Notice the calcified mediastinal and hilar nodes. (Courtesy of Fatih Alper, MD, PhD, professor, Department of Radiology, Ataturk University, School of Medicine, Erzurum, Turkey, and Metin Akgun, MD, professor, Department of Pulmonary Medicine, Ataturk University, School of Medicine, Erzurum, Turkey.)

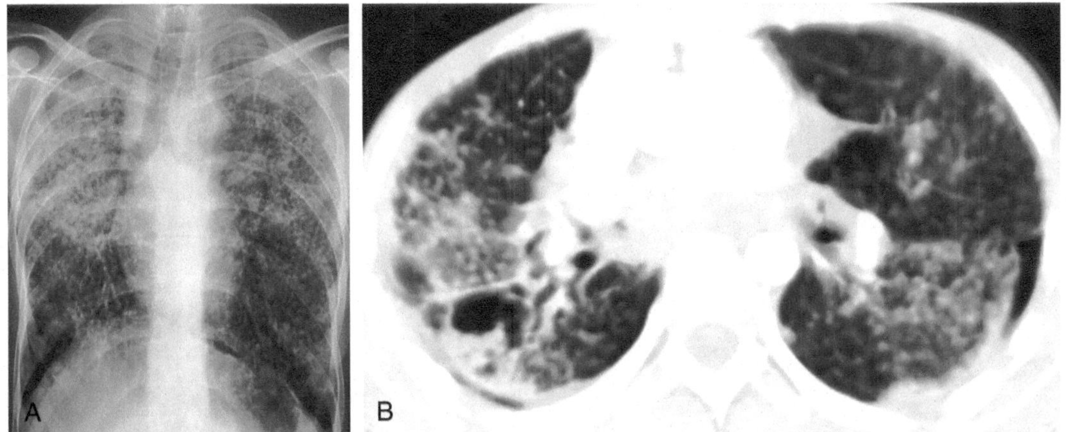

FIGURE 19.7 Complicated silicosis. **A,** Posteroanterior radiograph shows bilateral medium-sized pulmonary nodules primarily in the upper zone with associated upper lobe volume loss. There is hyperinflation of the lower lung zone caused by emphysema. **B,** Computed tomography image through the mid lung demonstrates innumerable small bilateral pulmonary nodules. There is a cavitary lesion in the right lower lobe from ischemic necrosis and a small left pneumothorax. (Courtesy of Fatih Alper, MD, PhD, professor, Department of Radiology, Ataturk University, School of Medicine, Erzurum, Turkey, and Metin Akgun, MD, professor, Department of Pulmonary Medicine, Ataturk University, School of Medicine, Erzurum, Turkey.)

Silicosis and Mycobacterial Disease

Tuberculous and nontuberculous mycobacterial infections develop in up to 25% of patients with acute or classic silicosis. Superimposed tuberculosis (TB) is difficult to detect radiographically; however, findings such as rapid radiographic changes with or without cavitation should raise suspicion. Risk of mycobacterial infection is higher in patients with acute silicosis rather than classic silicosis.

Accelerated Silicosis

Accelerated silicosis occurs over a short period of time, usually 4 to 8 years after exposure to large amounts of silica. Symptoms, as well as radiographic manifestations of accelerated silicosis, develop more rapidly than in chronic simple silicosis (Fig. 19.8). Pathologically, it is more cellular than fibrotic in nature.

Prognosis and Treatment of Silicosis

Complications of silicosis include pulmonary hypertension, spontaneous pneumothorax, broncholithiasis, tracheobronchial obstruction, lung cancer, TB, and respiratory failure. To date, there is no specific therapy for silicosis aside from prevention of further exposure to silica dust. Patients should be strongly advised to quit smoking.

COAL WORKER'S PNEUMOCONIOSIS

Coal remains an important source of energy in the United States as well as globally despite movement toward renewable energy. Although the presence of CWP has declined steadily, there has been a slight increase in the prevalence rate since 2000, reported between 9% and 27%. Radiographic manifestations of CWP does not appear until after at least 10 years of exposure. The federally mandated upper limit of

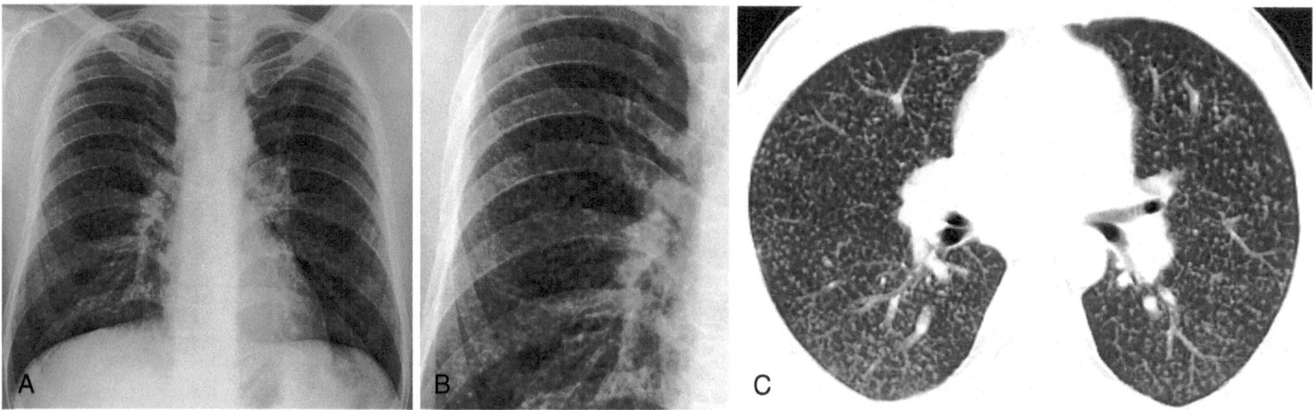

FIGURE 19.8 Accelerated silicosis in a denim sandblaster after 2 years of exposure. Posteroanterior chest radiograph **(A)** with detailed view **(B)** demonstrates diffuse small nodular opacities. **C,** High-resolution computed tomography image demonstrates innumerable nodules primarily in a centrilobular distribution. (Courtesy of Fatih Alper, MD, PhD, professor, Department of Radiology, Ataturk University, School of Medicine, Erzurum, Turkey, and Metin Akgun, MD, professor, Department of Pulmonary Medicine, Ataturk University, School of Medicine, Erzurum, Turkey.)

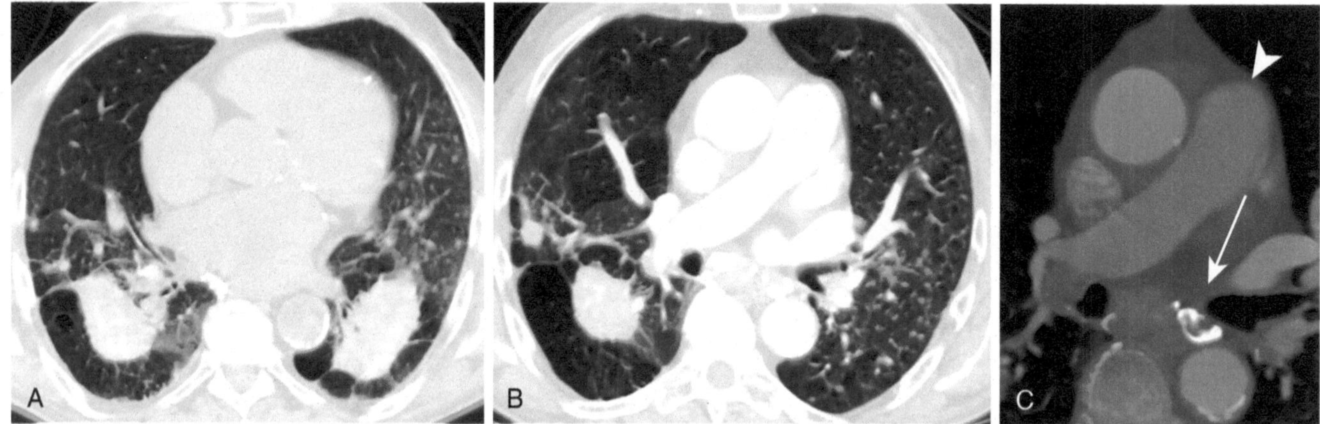

FIGURE 19.9 Complicated coal worker's pneumoconiosis. **A,** Axial high-resolution computed tomography image on lung windows demonstrates large opacities in the superior segment of bilateral lower lobes with associated surrounding paracicatricial emphysema. **B,** Nodules of varying size measuring up to 12 mm are seen in the right upper lobe. **C,** Eggshell calcification in noted within the lymph nodes *(arrow)*. There is also dilation of the pulmonary artery *(arrowhead)*.

occupational exposure to coal is 2 mg/m^3 and is maintained with adequate ventilation. These individuals are at a higher risk for developing cor pulmonale and gastric cancer. There are two forms of CWP, simple and complicated.

Simple Coal Worker's Pneumoconiosis

Simple CWP microscopically appears as a coal macule. These are carbon-containing macrophages surrounded by a network of collagen fibers and fibroblasts. These nodules accumulate in the upper lobes and calcify in 10% to 20% of patients. These patients usually do not demonstrate any functional or physiologic impairment.

Imaging Findings

Parenchymal and subpleural micronodules are seen with an upper right lung predominance. Subpleural focal linear areas of increased attenuation measuring less than 7 mm in width are also seen and represent pseudoplaques. Larger nodules measuring up to 20 mm can be seen on a background of smaller micronodules. Eggshell calcifications of both mediastinal and hilar lymph nodes are also seen in CWP.

Complicated Coal Worker's Pneumoconiosis

As the coal macules coalesce with dense collagen, central areas become necrotic because of ischemia. This relates to the development of PMF (which is also seen with silica exposure). Unlike simple CWP, these individuals are symptomatic, and the condition can lead to respiratory failure as well as premature death. If the patient is symptomatic with a cough, the sputum may appear black.

Imaging Findings

Imaging findings of complicated CWP are identical to those found with silicosis, with upper lobe-predominant opacities greater than 1 cm. There are two categories of lesions of PMF, depending on the borders of the mass (i.e., regular vs irregular borders). Irregular borders are usually associated with scar emphysema and occasional bulla formation (Fig. 19.9). Masses with regular borders are not associated with emphysema. Superimposed infections may occur with cavitary lesions such as TB and aspergilloma.

Differentiating Silicosis and Coal Worker's Pneumoconiosis

Although it is often difficult to make the distinction between these two pneumoconioses, clinical history is the key in differentiating the diagnoses. Silicotic nodules are better defined than those found in CWP. However, both are upper lobe predominant and may coalesce to form PMF.

CAPLAN SYNDROME

There is an increased prevalence of several connective tissue diseases in patients with silicosis and CWP. Caplan syndrome, also called rheumatoid pneumoconiosis, is the combination of seropositive rheumatoid arthritis and pneumoconiosis. Radiographically, multiple necrobiotic nodules are superimposed on typical changes of chronic silicosis or CWP. The nodules are well defined; measure between 0.5 and 5 cm; and can coalesce, cavitate, or calcify. Pathologically, the nodules are a granulomatous reaction composed of macrophages within a necrotic core, histiocytes, pigmented plaque, and fibroblasts.

ASBESTOS-RELATED DISEASE

Asbestos fibers are a group of naturally occurring fibrous silicate that have been widely used because of their heat resistance, durability, and strength. Although asbestos use is currently strictly regulated in the Western world, given the long latent (20 years) pathophysiologic response to the inhaled fibers, asbestos remains an important public health issue. Major sources of asbestos exposure are both occupational and industrial, including the shipbuilding, textile, construction, and mining industries.

There are two primary groups of asbestos, amphibole and serpentine fibers. Amphibole fibers can be subdivided into commercial (crocidolite, blue asbestos, brown asbestos) and noncommercial (anthophyllite, tremolite, actinolite). Chrysotile (or white asbestos) is the only form of serpentine asbestos and accounts for nearly 90% of the asbestos used in the United States.

The adverse effects of asbestos within the lung can be generally categorized into three categories: pleural, parenchymal, and malignant neoplasms.

Pleural Manifestations

Pleural changes are the most common finding and include pleural effusions, plaques, and diffuse pleural thickening.

Benign Asbestos Pleural Effusions

Benign pleural effusion is the earliest manifestation of pleural disease and usually occurs within 5 to 10 years of exposure. The effusion may be hemorrhagic or exudative and unilateral or bilateral and usually resolves within a few months but may recur. It is a diagnosis of exclusion, particularly in regard to mesothelioma.

Chest radiographs can detect most benign pleural effusions. Pleural thickening is commonly seen after resolution of pleural effusion with residual blunting of the costophrenic angle (Fig. 19.10).

Pleural Plaques

Pleural plaques are the most common manifestation of asbestos exposure and tend to occur 15 to 30 years after exposure. The size and number of plaques are variable and increase with both time and intensity of exposure. The plaques are composed of acellular collagen and are primarily localized to the parietal pleura but occasionally can involve the visceral pleura, including the fissures. Pleural plaques are not considered premalignant and are generally incidentally discovered and asymptomatic.

On chest radiographs, plaques are identifiable as localized, plateau-like, smooth, and nodular areas of pleural thickening. Characteristic radiographic distribution of pleural plaques includes the bilateral lower half of the thorax between the sixth and ninth ribs, dome of the

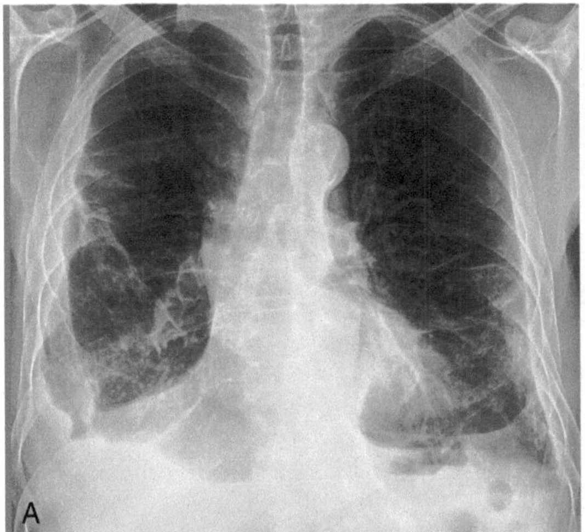

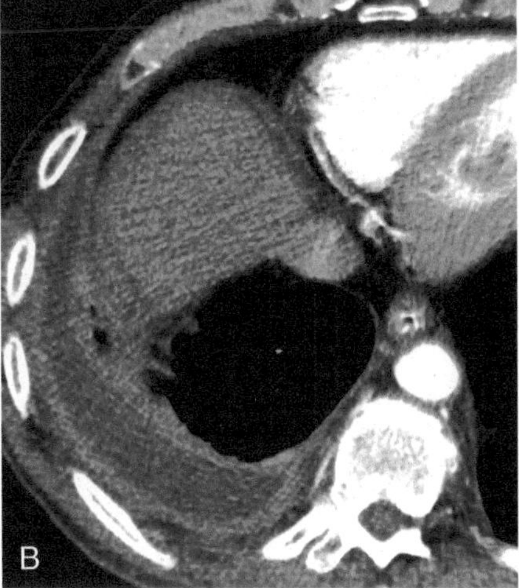

FIGURE 19.10 Asbestos-related benign pleural effusion. **A,** Posteroanterior chest radiograph demonstrates a right pleural effusion, left calcified pleural plaques, and bilateral parenchymal bands. **B,** Computed tomography defines the chronic pleural effusion with associated pleural thickening.

diaphragm, and mediastinal pleura. The costophrenic angles and lung apices are usually spared. If the plaque is seen in profile, it appears as a well-marginated soft tissue band along the parallel lateral thoracic wall. If seen en face, it appears ill defined with irregular edges and veil-like (Fig. 19.11). Plaques with a nodular configuration may mimic a pulmonary nodule on chest radiograph. Calcification of plaques, which occurs up to 15% of the time, can make the plaques easier to see on chest radiography.

Pleural plaque calcifications usually manifest 30 to 40 years after exposure and can increase over time. Calcifications can occur along the chest wall, cardiac border, or diaphragm (Fig. 19.11). Viewed en face, they have an irregular, uneven dense pattern likened to the fringe of a holly leaf. Although calcifications can be seen on chest radiographs, CT may be needed to differentiate from underlying lung nodules.

Diffuse Pleural Thickening

Diffuse pleural thickening is less specific for asbestos and is uncommon, with a latency of 10 to 40 years. It is secondary to thickening and fibrosis of the visceral pleura and may follow a pleural effusion. In contrast to pleural plaques, which are usually asymptomatic, diffuse pleural thickening may result in respiratory impairment caused by the fibrothorax and can calcify.

On chest radiographs, pleural thickening is described as a smooth, uninterrupted (nonnodular) opacity that extends to at least one quarter of the chest wall with or without obliteration of the costophrenic angle (Fig. 19.12).

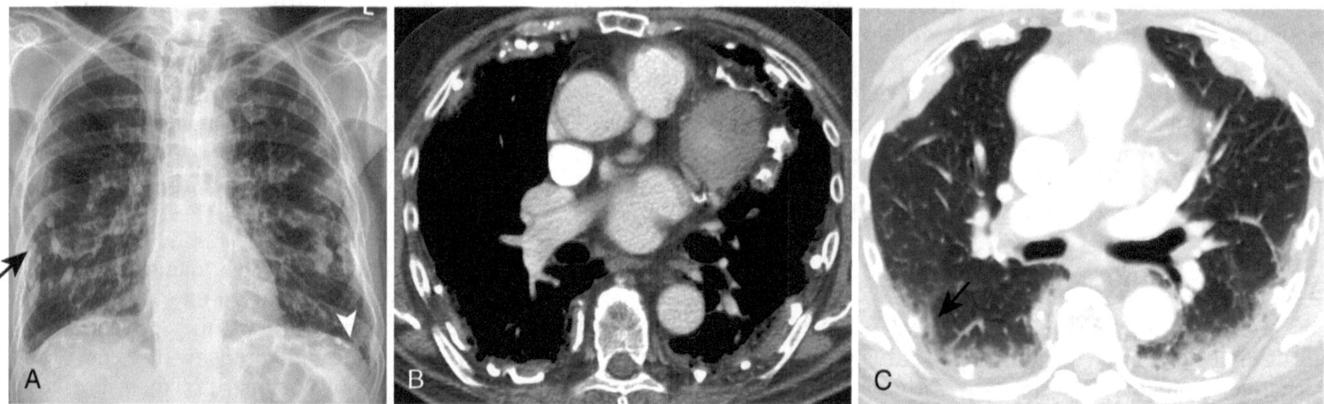

FIGURE 19.11 Calcified bilateral pleural plaques. **A,** Posteroanterior radiograph demonstrates extensive bilateral pleural plaques *(arrow)* sparing the apices and costophrenic angles. Plaques are also seen along the diaphragm *(arrowhead)*. **B,** Contrast-enhanced chest computed tomography (CT) using mediastinal window demonstrates classic distribution of calcified pleural plaques along the cardiac border and chest wall. **C,** Axial high-resolution CT using lung windows demonstrates the appearance of pseudofibrosis adjacent to the calcified pleural plaques *(arrow)*.

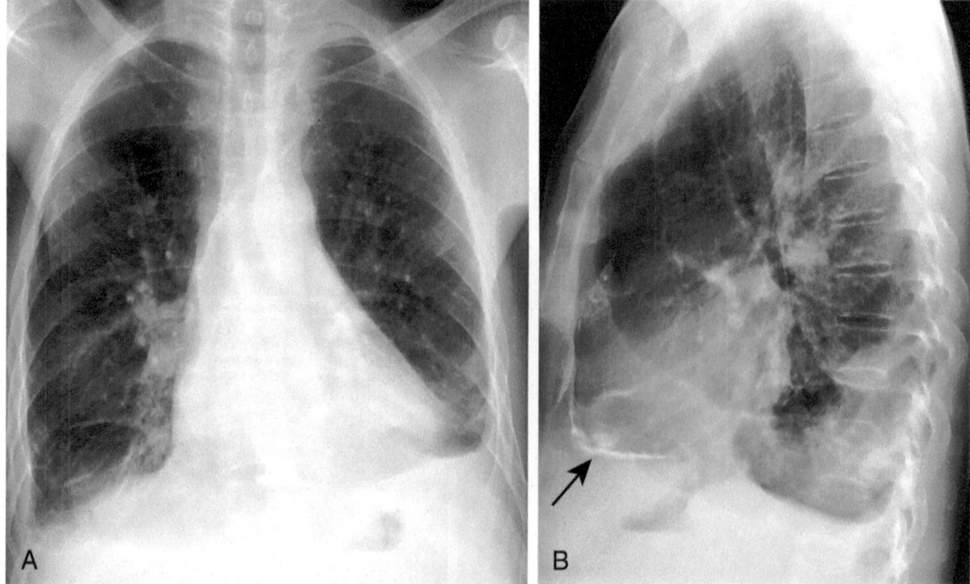

FIGURE 19.12 Diffuse pleural thickening. Posteroanterior **(A)** and lateral **(B)** chest radiographs demonstrate blunting of the costophrenic angles caused by bilateral pleural thickening. Pleural calcifications are also seen along the anterior pleural and along the diaphragm *(arrow)*, better appreciated on the lateral view.

Suggested CT criterion is that of a continuous sheet of pleural thickening more than 5 cm wide, more than 8 cm in craniocaudal extent, and more than 3 mm thick.

In contrast to pleural plaques, pleural thickening has ill-defined, irregular margins and usually involves less than four interspaces. Increased pleural fat in obese patients may mimic pleural thickening on chest radiographs. CT is more sensitive for the detection of pleural thickening than chest radiography.

Parenchymal Manifestations

Asbestosis

Asbestosis is the term used for the diffuse interstitial lung fibrosis and has a dose-response relationship between exposure and severity. Symptoms, functional abnormalities, and imaging findings usually lag more than 20 years after exposure but can be seen as early as three years after exposure to high doses.

The pathogenesis of asbestosis is hypothesized to be related to tissue damage caused by chemotactic factors and fibrogenic mediators. Fibrogenesis occurs in and around the respiratory bronchioles and alveolar ducts. Asbestos bodies and asbestos fibers may be seen adjacent to areas of fibrosis. Imaging changes of fibrosis usually are more pronounced in the lower lobes. In more advanced cases, it may progress to upper lobes and lead to honeycombing.

Imaging

Radiographic findings include primarily reticular opacities in bilateral lower lobes. Volume loss and honeycombing may be seen with more advanced disease. Partial obscuration of the heart border caused by parenchymal and pleural changes is called the "shaggy" heart sign. Up to 80% of patients with asbestosis have pleural changes. History of asbestos exposure combined with radiologic manifestations such as pleural abnormalities and other parenchymal abnormalities assist in the diagnosis of asbestosis.

High-resolution CT is superior for the diagnosis of asbestosis compared with conventional radiography. Five major parenchymal findings that may be seen with asbestos exposure on HRCT are curvilinear subpleural lines; thickened, interstitial short lines; subpleural-dependent density; parenchymal bands; and honeycombing. However, these findings are not specific for asbestosis and may also be seen with usual interstitial pneumonitis (UIP) (Fig. 19.13).

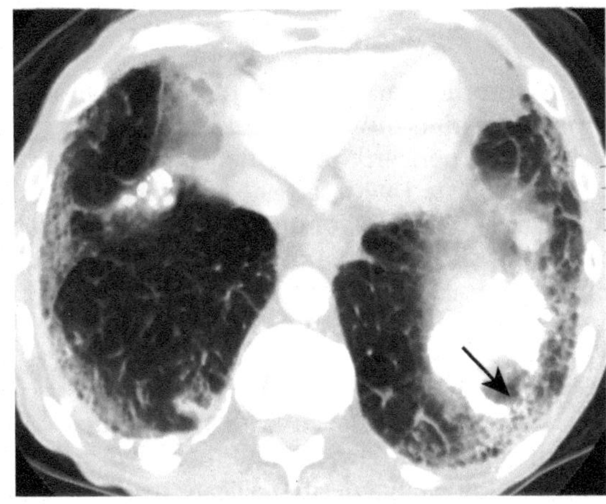

FIGURE 19.13 Asbestosis. Axial high-resolution computed tomography image through the lung bases demonstrates subpleural reticulation, traction bronchiolectasis, and honeycombing *(arrow)*. Calcified pleural plaques are also present.

A subpleural curvilinear line runs parallel to the pleura, separated by 1 cm (Fig. 19.14). Parenchymal bands course the lung and contact the pleura and can range between 2 and 5 cm. These bands are related to pleural thickening, fibrosis, and atelectasis (Fig. 19.15). These may lead to the development of rounded atelectasis. Progression of multiple bands radiating from a single point on the pleura has a similar appearance to crow's feet. Other imaging features include reticulation, interlobular septal thickening, and ground-glass opacities. Honeycombing is seen in advanced fibrosis.

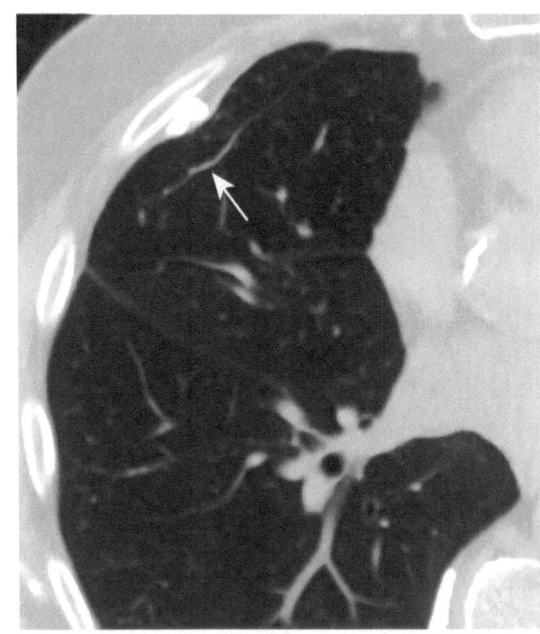

FIGURE 19.14 Subpleural, curvilinear opacity. High-resolution computed tomography image shows a linear opacity paralleling the chest wall *(arrow)*, a finding indicating fibrosis. When seen along with pleural plaques, this finding is suggestive of asbestosis.

Benign Parenchymal Lesions

Rounded Atelectasis

Asbestos-related rounded atelectasis is also known Blesovsky syndrome and is the most common benign parenchymal lesion and is a form of peripheral lobar collapse that develops in patients with pleural disease. This is fully discussed in the chapter on atelectasis (see Chapter 2).

Malignant Neoplasms

Bronchogenic Carcinoma

Correlation between asbestos exposure and lung cancer was first proven in the 1950s, with a variable latency period between 10 to 30 years. Smoking has an additive effect with as much as an 80- to 100-fold risk compared with nonsmokers. Amphiboles have a much greater potency than chrysotile in inducing lung cancer. Please refer to the neoplasm chapter (see Chapter 21).

Malignant Mesothelioma

Malignant mesothelioma is a rare tumor that most commonly occurs within the pleura but can also arise within the peritoneum, pericardium, or tunica vaginalis testis. It is strongly associated with asbestos exposure, especially amphibole fibers. The risk of developing mesothelioma is approximately 10% in an exposed individual. Please refer to the pleural disease chapter (see Chapter 7).

TALCOSIS

Exposure to talc can be seen with two groups of individuals, intravenous drug users and those working in the talc industry. Talc is magnesium silicate hydroxide and is usually contaminated with other substances such as silica and asbestos. Injection of medications prepared for the sole purpose of oral usage results in granulomatous reaction caused by the presence of insoluble fillers such as talc. Microscopically, birefringent particles within granulomas can be seen. Pathologically, injection talcosis results in endothelial injury secondary to occlusion of the arterioles and capillaries. In severe cases, it may result in pulmonary arterial hypertension.

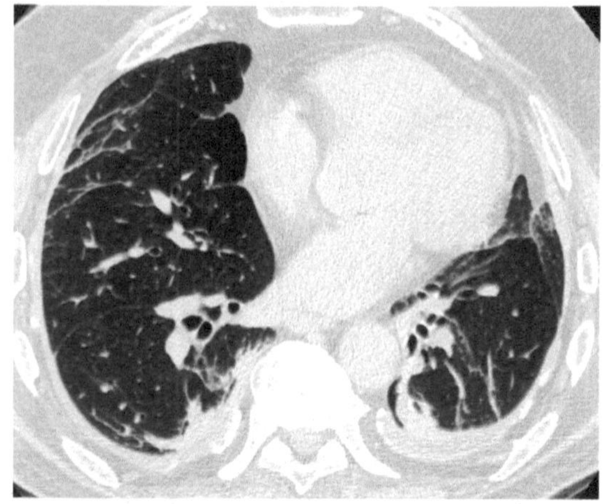

FIGURE 19.15 Parenchymal bands. Axial computed tomography image demonstrates long, linear bands that extend into lung parenchyma from areas of pleural thickening. Note the diffuse bilateral pleural thickening and calcified pleural plaques.

Imaging Findings

Inhalation talcosis has a similar appearance to silicosis or asbestosis, depending on the contaminant. Pleural thickening, calcifications, parenchymal bands, and interstitial fibrosis may be seen with talcoasbestosis. In talcosilicosis, calcified lymph nodes, diffuse small nodules, and perihilar conglomerate masses may be seen (Fig. 19.16). In intravenous drug users who inject crushed tablets, the imaging appearance includes diffuse, randomly distributed micronodules and consolidation (Fig. 19.17). As the disease progresses, the nodules may coalesce to form upper lobe–predominant perihilar masses, similar in appearance to PMF, that contain high-density foci. After repetitive intravenous exposure to talc, lower lobes may demonstrate emphysema caused by ischemia with alveolar wall necrosis.

BERYLLIUM

Although beryllium-related lung disease was first described in 1946 among fluorescent lamp workers, current occupational risk exposures include dental laboratory technicians and those working in aeronautic, telecommunication, computers, and electronics manufacturing. There are three classified forms of beryllium lung diseases: beryllium sensitization, chronic berylliosis, and acute toxic chemical pneumonitis.

Beryllium disease is unique in that there is both a bronchioalveolar lavage and blood test for T-lymphocyte response called the beryllium lymphocyte transformation test (BeLT). This test can be used to detect early disease in patients with no radiographic abnormality. The BeLT is used as a screening test to detect beryllium sensitization as well as subclinical disease. Beryllium sensitization can be seen in 2% to 10% of patients within a few weeks after beryllium exposure. These individuals are usually asymptomatic with no radiographic abnormality. If the BeLT result is positive among high-risk individuals, the only treatment is removal from further exposure. Acute beryllium disease may manifest as diffuse pulmonary edema and likely represents acute chemical pneumonitis. Chronic

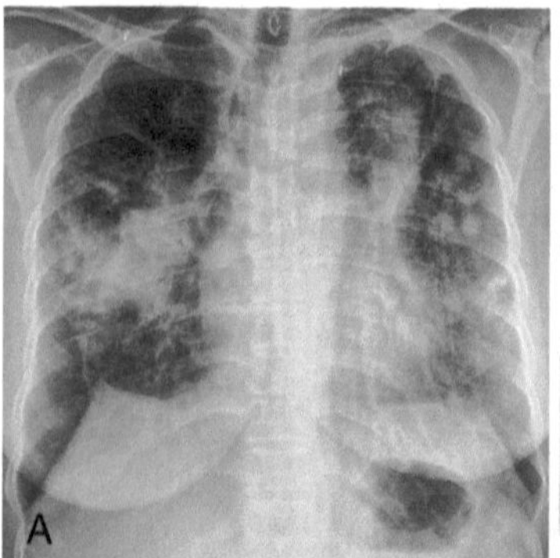

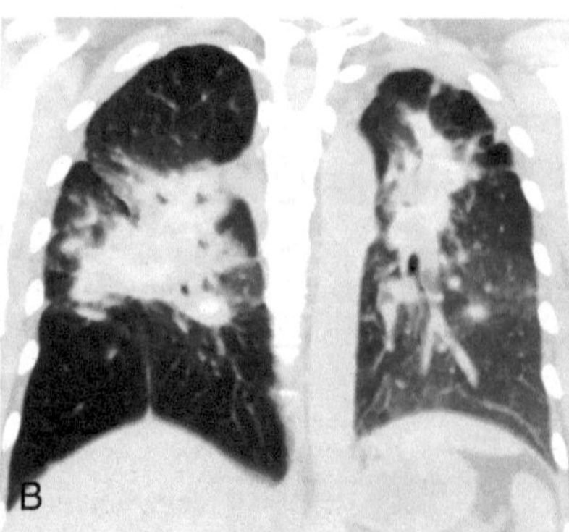

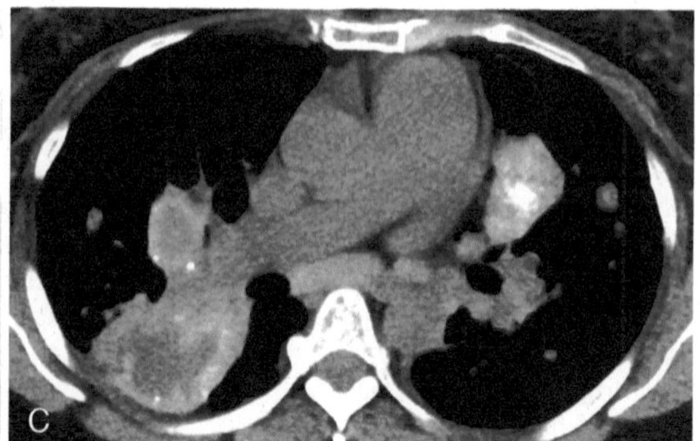

FIGURE 19.16 Inhalational talcosis. **A,** Portable chest radiograph shows masslike, confluent opacities in the perihilar regions with adjacent smaller nodules in the upper lung zones similar to progressive massive fibrosis seen with silicosis. **B,** Coronal high-resolution computed tomography image shows masslike consolidation in bilateral perihilar regions with architectural distortion and volume loss. Smaller nodules are seen in the left perihilar regions. **C,** Mediastinal window shows characteristic high attenuation peripherally within the masses secondary to talc deposition. Note the central areas of hypoattenuation representing necrosis.

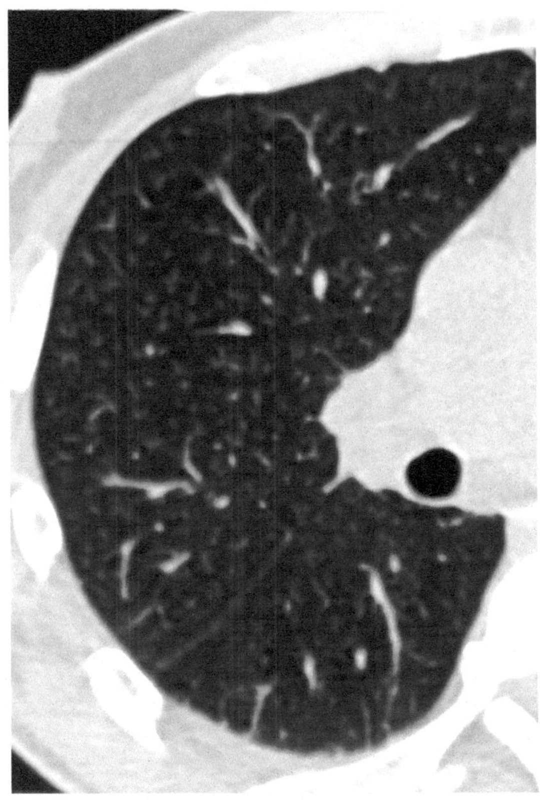

FIGURE 19.17 Talcosis in an intravenous drug abuser. Axial computed tomography image reveals diffuse centrilobular and tree-in-bud nodules consistent with embolized talc throughout the pulmonary arterial vasculature.

berylliosis can be seen in sensitized patients after months to years of exposure. It may manifest as a multisystem granulomatous disease predominantly involving the lung. Long-term corticosteroids are used for the treatment of chronic berylliosis.

Imaging

Beryllium is a granulomatous disease with a similar appearance to sarcoid. The two most common parenchymal abnormalities are septal lines and small nodules. Very small nodules up to 2 mm in diameter occur most commonly, and they can produce a granular or sandpaper appearance. After treatment with steroids, these small nodules may gradually decrease over time. Similar to sarcoid, noncaseating granulomas are found along the bronchovascular bundles and pleura in a perilymphatic distribution. Mediastinal and hilar lymphadenopathy is also a common feature, occurring in up to 25% of patients. The lymph nodes can calcify and have a similar pattern as sarcoidosis. Similar to sarcoidosis and silicosis, upper lobe-predominant confluent opacities may develop, with associated volume loss, traction bronchiectasis, and cicatricial emphysema (Fig. 19.18). As in most pneumoconioses, airway involvement of berylliosis results in bronchial wall thickening.

HARD METAL DISEASE

Hard metal lung disease (HMLD) is an uncommon disease seen in workers exposed to dust when creating hard metals. The hard metal, not to be confused for heavy metal, is produced by compacting tungsten carbide and cobalt. The typical pathologic pattern is that of giant cell interstitial pneumonitis. The symptoms include cough, asthma-like symptoms, and dyspnea on exertion. The radiologic findings include reticulation, ground-glass opacities, consolidation, traction bronchiectasis, and honeycombing (Fig. 19.19).

ALUMINUM

Aluminum exposure-induced lung pathology is rare but can be seen among aluminum production workers exposed to various particles, gases, fumes, and airborne materials. Aluminosis is a rare rapidly progressive lung fibrosi, characterized by upper lobe-predominant emphysema and blebs, which may rupture, causing a pneumothorax. The etiology is unclear, but it causes granulomatosis pneumonitis. Various parenchymal changes can be seen, including granulomas, pulmonary alveolar proteinosis, desquamative interstitial pneumonia, and UIP.

NONFIBROGENIC PNEUMOCONIOSIS

Iron

Siderosis is caused by iron oxide accumulation within macrophages. Workers who are exposed to metal fumes during welding and mining are at risk for the development of siderosis. It is important to note that siderosis is not associated with functional impairment or fibrosis. However, mixed iron may be contaminated with silica, resulting in silicosiderosis, which is associated with pulmonary fibrosis. Iron accumulation within macrophages on imaging appears as small nodules along the perivascular and perilymphatic vessels. Imaging findings are reversible after cessation of exposure.

Tin

Stannosis is the term given to pneumoconiosis caused by inhalation of tin oxide. Similar to iron, this condition does not result in functional impairment. Tin oxide is extremely dense on imaging and appears as evenly distributed small micronodules.

Barium

Baritosis is the term for pulmonary disease caused by exposure to barium and its salts, particularly barium sulfate. Similar to tin, barium is extremely dense on imaging because of the high radiopacity of barium. On imaging, these lesions are usually nodular, sparing the lung apices and bases. Imaging findings regress after the patient is removed from the environment.

COMPLEX DUST DISEASES

Dental Technician's Pneumoconiosis

Pneumoconiosis among dental technicians has been reported since 1939, with prevalence rates up to 15% after 20 years of exposure. Dental pneumoconiosis is caused by a complex mix of dust containing chromium-cobalt-molybdenum

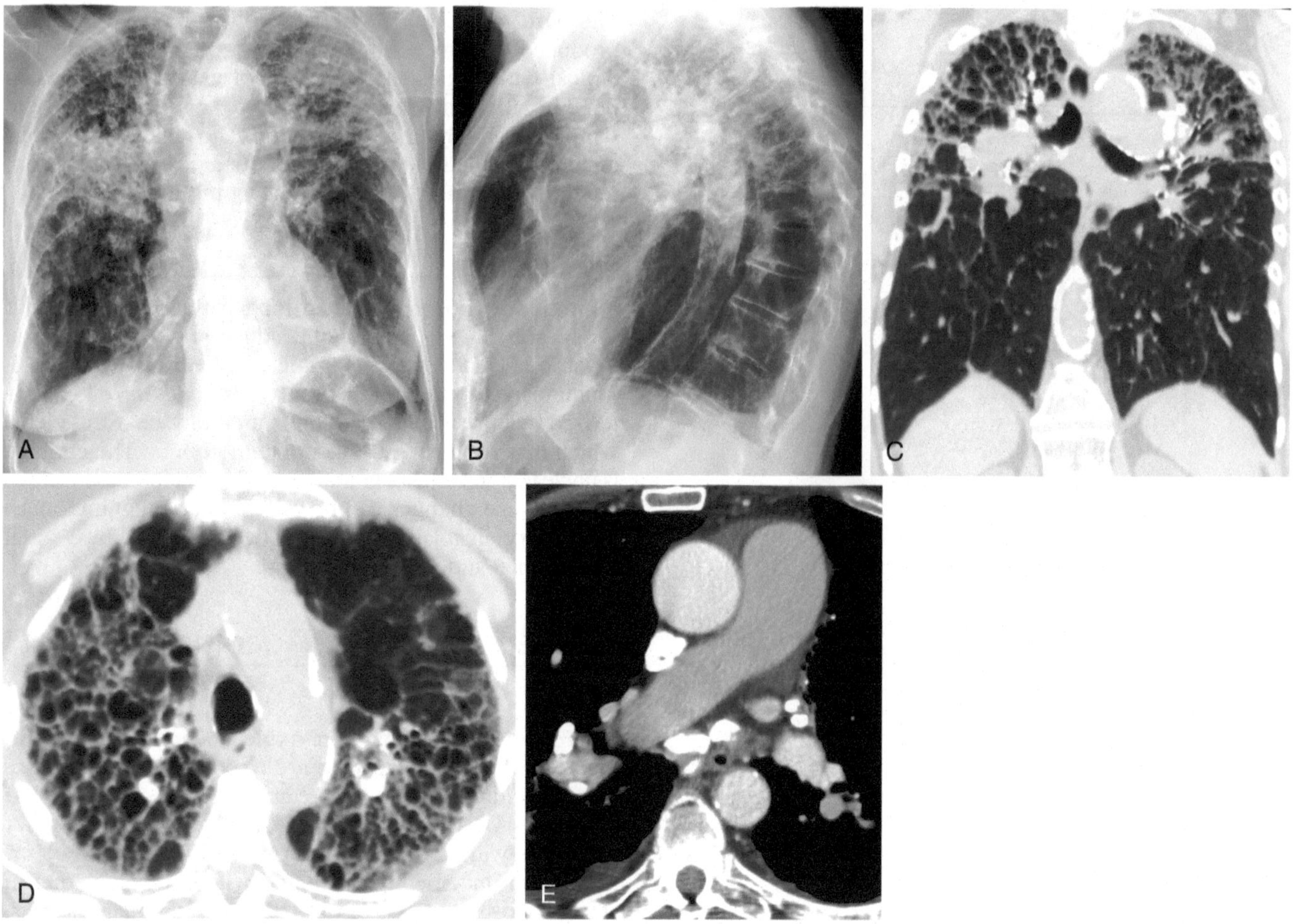

FIGURE 19.18 Posteroanterior **(A)** and lateral **(B)** chest radiographs show upper lobe–predominant coalescing reticular nodular opacities with volume loss, architectural distortion, traction bronchiectasis, and paracicatricial emphysema. Coronal **(C)** and axial **(D)** high-resolution computed tomography (CT) images show upper lobe coarse reticulation associated with architectural distortion and adjacent paracicatricial emphysema. Axial CT in mediastinal window **(E)** shows calcified lymph nodes *(arrows)* and an enlarged pulmonary artery.

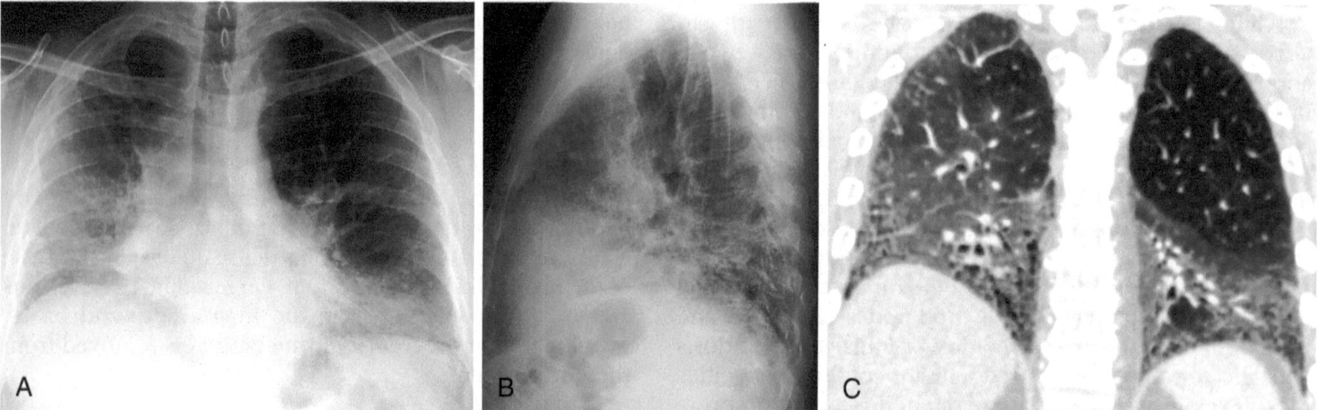

FIGURE 19.19 Heavy metal exposure. Posteroanterior **(A)** and lateral **(B)** chest radiographs show lower lobe–predominant hazy and reticular opacities with volume loss. Coronal high-resolution computed tomography image **(C)** shows lower lobe–predominant subpleural reticulation, ground-glass opacities, and traction bronchiolectasis.

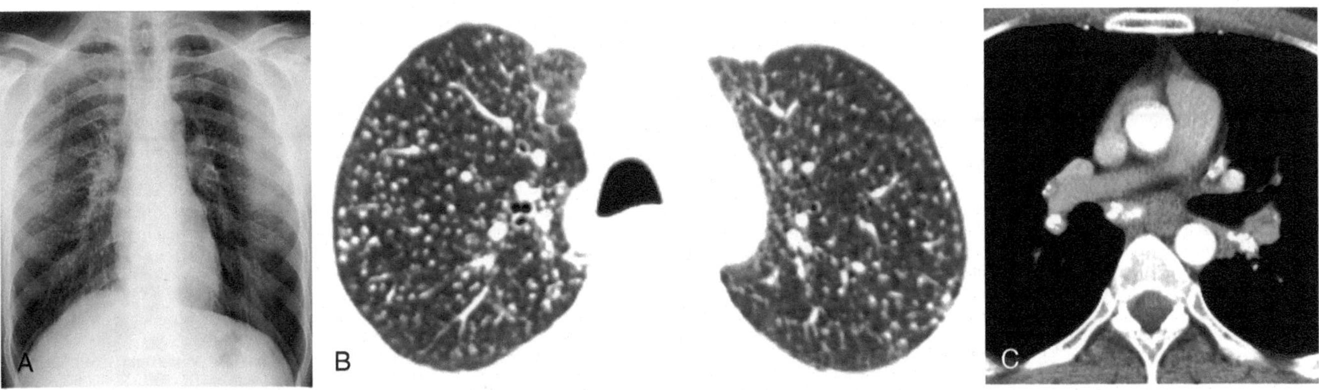

FIGURE 19.20 Dental technician's lung. **A,** Posteroanterior chest radiograph shows small, diffuse rounded nodules throughout both lungs. **B,** High-resolution computed tomography image on lung window demonstrates upper lobe–predominant small, dense centrilobular nodules. **C,** Axial soft tissue window shows calcified hilar and mediastinal lymph nodes.

particles, dental alloy, acrylic, resin, quartz, carbon, silica, and hard metal dust while working on dental frameworks. In addition, these individuals are exposed to various gases, vapors, and chemical hazards. Both the physiologic and radiographic manifestations are largely dependent on the amount and duration of exposure to causative agents. The most common presenting symptoms are dyspnea, cough, and sputum production.

Imaging

Chest radiography may reveal increased reticular or reticular nodular opacities. The early stage of the disease is characterized by small, irregular, rounded opacities with upper lobe predominance (Fig. 19.20). With time and increased exposure, these lesions can increase in number and size and result in massive fibrosis.

WORLD TRADE CENTER LUNG

On September 11, 2001, when the twin towers of the World Trade Center collapsed, a large, dense cloud of dust containing high levels of complex mixed airborne pollutants was released. Multiple studies since 9/11 have reported a wide variety of pollutants, including jet fuel, pulverized building materials, cement dust, asbestos, microscopic shards of glass, silica, heavy metals, and numerous organic compounds. This dust cloud covered Manhattan and extended to the other New York boroughs. The first responders to the scene were exposed to the dust cloud without appropriate respiratory protection. It is estimated that nearly 11,000 firefighters worked at the scene of Ground Zero. A large number developed clinical symptoms of aerodigestive tract mucosal damage and cough. This is largely due to decreased mucociliary clearance and alveolar macrophage defense mechanisms.

Pathology and Imaging

A database was created to provide standardized monitoring and treatment of first responders or volunteers called the Mount Sinai WTC Medical Monitoring and Treatment Program. A review of pathology from the database demonstrates a variety of pathology, including UIP, nonspecific interstitial pneumonia, hypersensitivity pneumonitis, and sarcoidlike findings. Small airways disease characterized by areas of mosaic attenuation was found to be present in all cases of World Trade Center lung disease. A few other case reports of acute eosinophilic pneumonia have also been reported after the immediate event. Among rescue workers, the incidence of sarcoidosis or sarcoidlike granulomatous disease is also increased (Fig. 19.21). A wide variety of radiologic manifestations of World Trade Center lung disease has been reported, including obstructive airway disease, miliary nodules, calcified lymph nodes, bronchiectasis, and interstitial opacities with and without honeycombing.

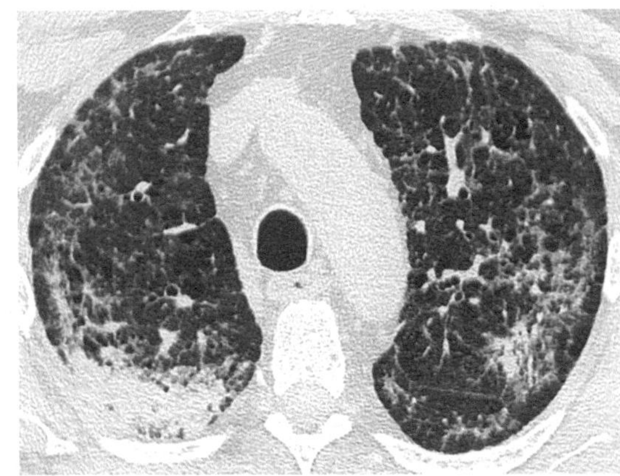

FIGURE 19.21 World Trade Center lung. Axial computed tomography image shows sarcoidlike reaction with upper lobe–predominant consolidations on the right greater than on the left, with associated volume loss, paracicatricial emphysema, ground-glass opacities, and reticulations.

SUGGESTED READINGS

Akira M, Kozuka T, Yamamoto S, et al. Inhalational talc pneumoconiosis: radiographic and CT findings in 14 patients. *AJR Am J Roentgenol*. 2007;188(2):326–333.

Alper F, Akgun M, Onbas O, et al. CT findings in silicosis due to denim sandblasting. *Eur Radiol*. 2008;18(12):2739.

Bacchus L, Shah RD, Chung JH, et al. ACR appropriateness Criteria® occupational lung diseases. *J Thorac Imaging*. 2016;31(1):W1–W3.

Balmes JR, Abraham JL, Dweik RA, et al. An official American Thoracic Society statement: diagnosis and management of beryllium sensitivity and chronic beryllium disease. *Am J Respir Crit Care Med*. 2014;190(10):e34–e59.

Bauer TT, Heyer CM, Duchna HW, et al. Radiological findings, pulmonary function and dyspnea in underground coal miners. *Respiration*. 2007;74(1):80-87.

Cox CW, Rose CS, Lynch DA. State of the art: imaging of occupational lung disease. *Radiology*. 2014;270(3):681-696.

dos Santos Antao VC, Pinheiro GA, Terra-Filho M, et al. High-resolution CT in silicosis: correlation with radiographic findings and functional impairment. *J Comput Assist Tomogr*. 2005;29(3):350-356.

Girvin F, Zeig-Owens R, Gupta D, et al. Radiologic features of World Trade Center-related sarcoidosis in exposed NYC Fire Department rescue workers. *J Thorac Imaging*. 2016;31(5):296-303.

Halldin CN, Blackley DJ, Petsonk EL, et al. Pneumoconioses radiographs in a large population of US coal workers: variability in A reader and B reader classifications by using the International Labour Office classification. *Radiology*. 2017;162437.

International Labour Office. Guidelines for the Use of the ILO International Classifications of Radiographs of Pneumoconioses Revised Edition; 2011. Geneva: International Labour Office.

Kahraman H, Koksal N, Cinkara M, et al. Pneumoconiosis in dental technicians: HRCT and pulmonary function findings. *Occup Med*. 2014;64(6):442-447.

Knoop H, Million P, Weber A, et al. Distribution of pleural plaques and pulmonary fibrosis due to asbestos exposure: radiological patterns in asbestos-related disorders (ARDs). *European Respiratory Journal*. 2015;46:PA816.

Laney AS, Attfield MD. Coal workers' pneumoconiosis and progressive massive fibrosis are increasingly more prevalent among workers in small underground coal mines in the United States. *Occup Environ Med*. 2010;67(6):428-431.

Laney AS, Blackley DJ, Halldin CN. Radiographic disease progression in contemporary US coal miners with progressive massive fibrosis. *Occup Environ Med*. 2017;74(7):517-520.

Mayer A, Hamzeh N. Beryllium and other metal-induced lung disease. *Curr Opin Pulm Med*. 2015;21(2):178-184.

Mayer AS, Hamzeh N, Maier LA. Sarcoidosis and chronic beryllium disease: similarities and differences. In: *Seminars in Respiratory and Critical care Medicine*. Vol 35. No. 03. Stuttgart, Germany: Thieme Medical Publishers; 2014:316-329.

Ollier M, Garcier JM, Naughton G, et al. CT Scan procedure for lung cancer screening in asbestos-exposed workers. *Chest*. 2014;146(2):e76-e77.

Ooi GC, Tsang KW, Cheung TF, et al. Silicosis in 76 men: qualitative and quantitative CT evaluation—clinical-radiologic correlation study 1. *Radiology*. 2003;228(3):816-825.

Prazakova S, Thomas PS, Sandrini A, et al. Asbestos and the lung in the 21st century: an update. *Clin Respir J*. 2014;8(1):1-10.

Reichert M, Bensadoun ES. PET imaging in patients with coal workers pneumoconiosis and suspected malignancy. *J Thorac Oncol*. 2009;4(5):649-651.

Seaman DM, Meyer CA, Kanne JP. Occupational and environmental lung disease. *Clin Chest Med*. 2015;36(2):249-268.

Sharma N, Patel J, Mohammed TLH. Chronic beryllium disease: computed tomographic findings. *J Comput Assist Tomogr*. 2010;34(6):945-948.

Silva CIS, Müller NL, Neder JA, et al. Asbestos-related disease: progression of parenchymal abnormalities on high-resolution CT. *J Thorac Imaging*. 2008;23(4):251-257.

Weissman DN. Role of chest computed tomography in prevention of occupational respiratory disease: review of recent literature. In: *Seminars in Respiratory and Critical Care Medicine*. Vol 36. No. 03. Stuttgart, Germany: Thieme Medical Publishers; 2015:433-448.

Chapter 20

Obstructive Lung Diseases

Carol C. Wu, Brett W. Carter, and Jo-Anne O. Shepard

INTRODUCTION

Obstructive lung diseases consist of a heterogeneous group of chronic respiratory illnesses characterized by airway obstruction and air trapping (Box 20.1). The most common causes include chronic obstructive pulmonary disease (COPD), which includes emphysema and chronic bronchitis, followed by asthma and bronchiectasis. Bronchiectasis is discussed in Chapter 6. Constrictive or obliterative bronchiolitis is a less common cause of obstructive lung disease. Patients with obstructive lung diseases often present with nonspecific symptoms such as dyspnea, particularly during exertion, and cough. Pulmonary function tests (PFTs) characteristically show disproportionate reduction in the forced expiratory volume in 1 second (FEV_1) compared with the forced vital capacity (FVC) as reflected in the decreased FEV_1/FVC ratio.

BOX 20.1 Obstructive Lung Diseases

Emphysema
Chronic bronchitis
Asthma
Bronchiectasis
Constrictive bronchiolitis

The presence of air trapping is common to all obstructive lung diseases, which in its mild form is difficult to detect on plain radiography. When severe, air trapping can be detected radiographically as hyperinflation with more than 6 anterior or 10 posterior ribs visualized above the diaphragm at the midclavicular line (Fig. 20.1). Hyperinflation is also characterized by a low, flat diaphragm, particularly on the lateral view. The diaphragm is considered to be flattened when the highest level of the dome is less than 1.5 cm above a straight line drawn between the costophrenic junction and the vertebral phrenic junction. The angle formed by the diaphragm and the anterior chest wall is often 90 degrees or greater compared with the acute angle seen with a normal upwardly curved diaphragm. Another criterion of overinflation is a widened retrosternal air space greater

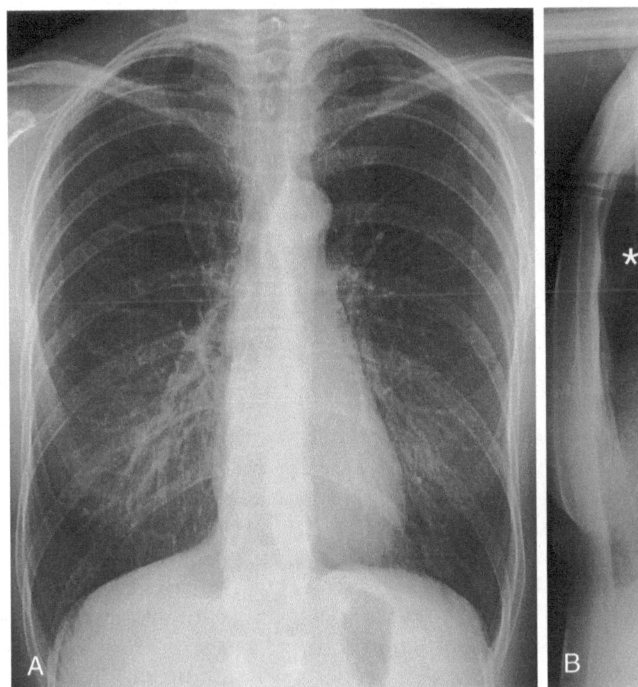

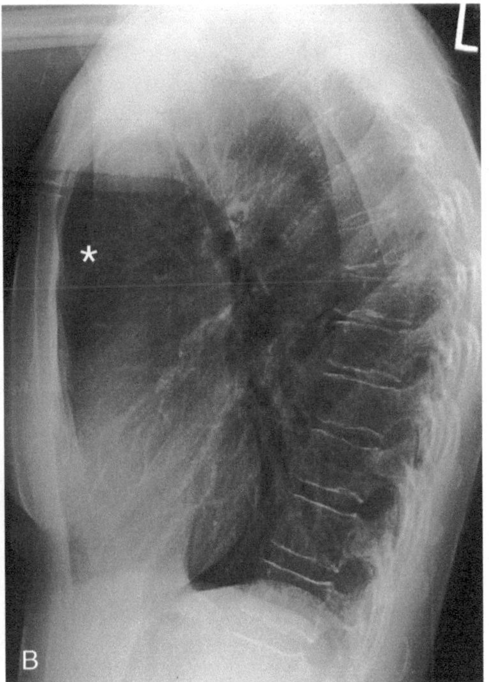

FIGURE 20.1 Hyperinflation of lungs in a smoker with chronic bronchitis. **A,** Posteroanterior radiograph demonstrates hyperlucent lungs and low diaphragm with more than 10 posterior ribs seen above the diaphragm at the midclavicular line. The cardiac silhouette appears long and narrow. **B,** Lateral radiograph shows increased anterior–posterior diameter of the thorax, widening of retrosternal clear space *(asterisk),* and flattening of the diaphragm.

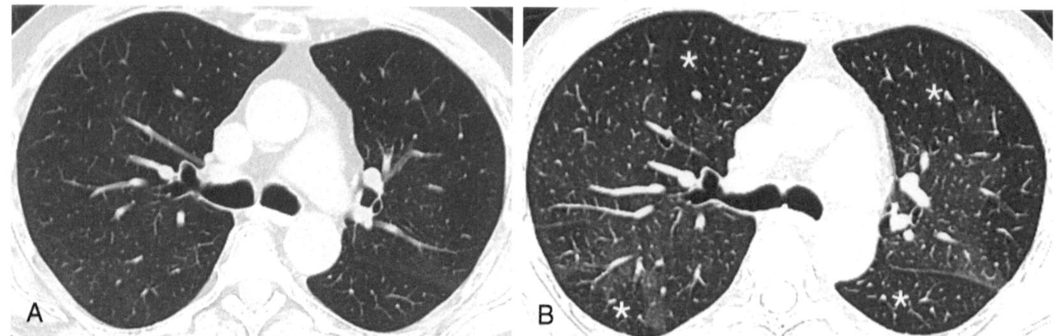

FIGURE 20.2 Air trapping on computed tomography (CT) image in a patient with post–stem cell transplant graft-versus-host disease and constrictive bronchiolitis. **A** The inspiratory CT image is nearly normal with very subtle mosaic attenuation of pulmonary parenchyma. **B,** Expiratory CT image shows anterior bowing of posterior wall of mainstem bronchi as expected during expiration. The normal areas of lung show increased attenuation because of decreased amount of air in the alveoli. Areas of lungs affected by air trapping remain lucent *(asterisks).*

than 2.5 cm in diameter. The cardiac silhouette tends to be long and narrow. High-resolution computed tomography (HRCT) has significantly improved our ability to image morphologic abnormalities associated with obstructive lung diseases, particularly in emphysema and bronchiectasis. On inspiratory CT, air trapping manifests as mosaic attenuation of the lungs, with areas involved by air trapping manifesting as hypoattenuation compared with the normal lung parenchyma. Air trapping can be distinguished from mosaic attenuation caused by vascular and interstitial lung disease on expiratory CT images where the hypoattenuating areas caused by air trapping are accentuated (Fig. 20.2) (see Chapter 17).

CHRONIC OBSTRUCTIVE PULMONARY DISEASE

Chronic obstructive pulmonary disease includes chronic bronchitis, which is defined in clinical terms, and emphysema, which is defined anatomically. Although asthma is also characterized by airflow obstruction, it differs from COPD in its pathogenic and therapeutic responses. Asthma is therefore considered a separate clinical entity from COPD, and it is discussed separately. However, there is some overlap between these conditions, and some patients have COPD and asthma. COPD is predominantly a disease of smokers, although only about 15% of smokers develop disabling airflow obstruction.

The chest radiograph is an important imaging modality in the assessment of patients with COPD. However, it has limitations in the detection and differential diagnosis of obstructive airway disease. It is relatively insensitive in the detection of early emphysema, and it is frequently normal for patients with pure chronic bronchitis and asthma. HRCT has improved our ability to differentiate between emphysema and bronchitis. CT also can delineate functional abnormalities such as air trapping and decreased perfusion.

EMPHYSEMA

Emphysema is a condition of the lung characterized by abnormal, permanent enlargement of the airspaces distal to the terminal bronchiole, accompanied by destruction of their walls without obvious fibrosis (Box 20.2).

BOX 20.2 Emphysema

CLINICAL FEATURES

Cigarette smoking
Dyspnea
Chronic airflow obstruction

PATHOLOGIC FEATURES

Permanent enlargement of the airspaces distal to the terminal bronchiole and destruction of their walls
- Centrilobular (central lobule)
- Panlobular (entire lobule)
- Paraseptal (distal lobule, subpleural)

IMAGING FEATURES

Radiography
- Overinflation
- Low, flat diaphragm
- Increased retrosternal clear space
- Vascular deficiency shown by areas of irregular lucency
- Bullae

Computed tomography
- Centrilobular
- Multiple, small areas of low attenuation without walls
- Upper lobes > lower lobes

Panlobular
- Fewer and smaller vessels
- Lower lobes

Paraseptal
- Subpleural and along fissures
- Thin walls
- Single row

Clinical Features

Emphysema is defined anatomically and pathologically. Emphysema may occur without detectable chronic airway obstruction. Mild degrees of emphysema are frequently found in smokers at autopsy. Widespread and severe emphysema is usually associated with a history of cigarette smoking, chronic airflow obstruction, and dyspnea. The airflow obstruction can be measured with PFT by a diminution of the FEV_1 or the ratio of the FEV_1 to the FVC. Lung volumes increase in emphysema as a result of hyperinflation with increases in the total lung capacity (TLC), functional residual capacity, and residual volume, with a concomitant decrease in vital capacity as the emphysema becomes more severe. The loss of the internal surface area of the lung and of the alveolar capillary bed, two components of emphysema, is reflected in a decrease in the diffusing capacity of the lung for carbon monoxide (D_{LCO}).

Pathologic Features

The four anatomically defined types of emphysema are centrilobular (centriacinar), panlobular (panacinar), paraseptal (distal acinar), and paracicatricial (irregular) emphysema. The acinus is the air-exchanging unit of the lung, and it is located distal to the terminal bronchiole. It includes the respiratory bronchioles, alveolar ducts, alveolar sacs, and alveoli (Fig. 20.3). Although this classification relies on the relationship of emphysema to the acinus, acini cannot be resolved on HRCT, and it may be more useful for the radiologist to consider the types of emphysema relative to their location at the lobular level. Centrilobular, panlobular, and paraseptal emphysema often can be distinguished morphologically, but as emphysema becomes severe, distinction among the three types becomes more difficult.

Centrilobular emphysema affects predominantly the respiratory bronchioles in the central portion of the secondary pulmonary lobule (Fig. 20.4). It is usually identified in the upper lung zones, and it is associated with cigarette smoking.

Panlobular emphysema involves all of the components of the acinus and therefore involves the entire lobule (Fig. 20.5). It is classically associated with α_1-antitrypsin deficiency (AATD), although panlobular emphysema may also be seen without AATD in smokers, in older adults, and distal to bronchial and bronchiolar obstruction. Thurlbeck described this entity as a "diffuse simplification of the lung structure with progressive loss of tissue until little remains but the supporting framework of vessels, septa, and bronchi." α_1-Antitrypsin (AAT) is a potent inhibitor of neutrophil elastase, which is released as part of an inflammatory pathway triggered by smoking. In smokers with genetic mutations resulting in deficiency of AAT, unchecked activities of neutrophil elastase cause alveolar destruction at an accelerated rate compared with those normal with a AAT level.

Paraseptal emphysema is characterized by involvement of the distal part of the secondary lobule (i.e., alveolar ducts and sacs), and it therefore occurs in a subpleural location (Fig. 20.6). It can be seen in the periphery of the lung adjacent to the chest wall and along the interlobular septa and the fissures. Paraseptal emphysema, which can be an isolated phenomenon in young adults, is associated with spontaneous pneumothorax without other evidence of restriction in lung function. However, it can also be seen in older patients with centrilobular emphysema.

Paracicatricial or irregular emphysema refers to abnormal airspace enlargement associated with pulmonary fibrosis. This is most frequently a localized phenomenon and not necessarily associated with smoking or airflow obstruction.

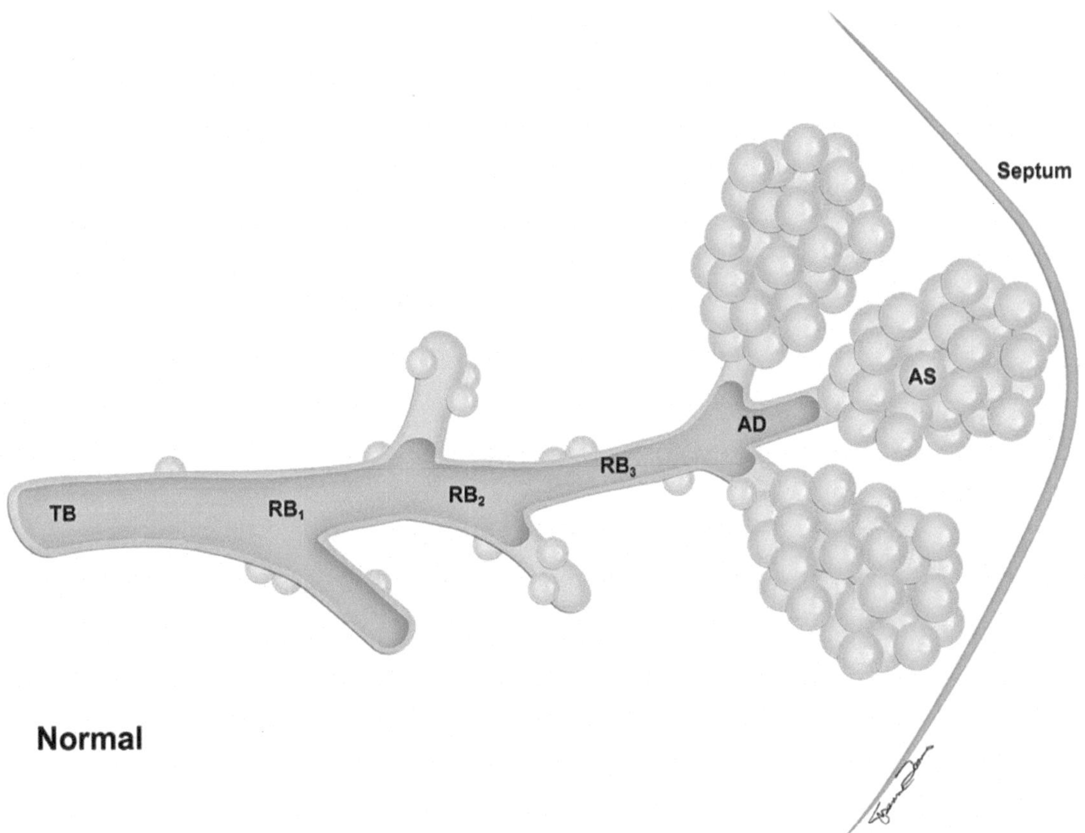

FIGURE 20.3 Normal lung. The acinus is the part of the lung distal to the terminal bronchiole (TB). *AD,* Alveolar duct; *AS,* alveolar sac; *RB,* respiratory bronchiole. (Adapted from Thurlbeck WM: Chronic Airflow Obstruction in Lung Disease. Philadelphia: WB Saunders, 1976.)

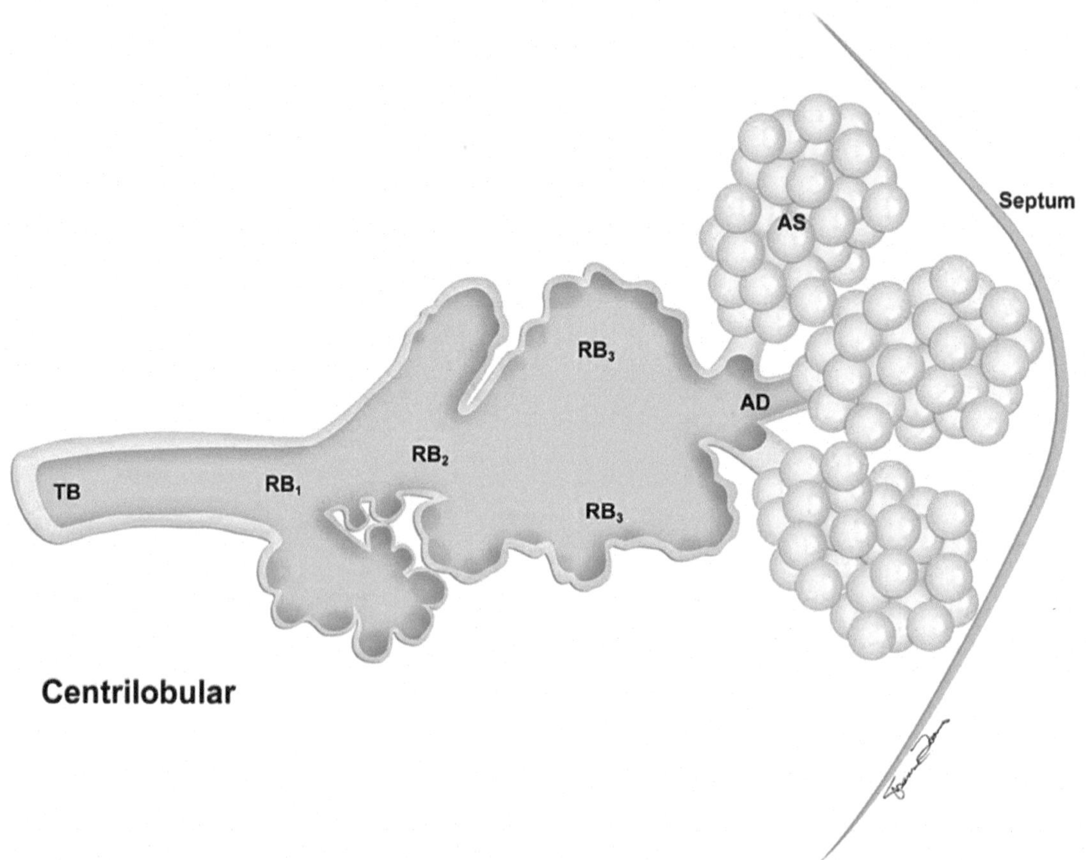

FIGURE 20.4 Centrilobular emphysema. The respiratory bronchioles are selectively and dominantly involved. *AD,* Alveolar duct; *AS,* alveolar sac; *RB,* respiratory bronchiole; *TB,* terminal bronchiole. (Adapted from Thurlbeck WM: Chronic Airflow Obstruction in Lung Disease. Philadelphia: WB Saunders, 1976.)

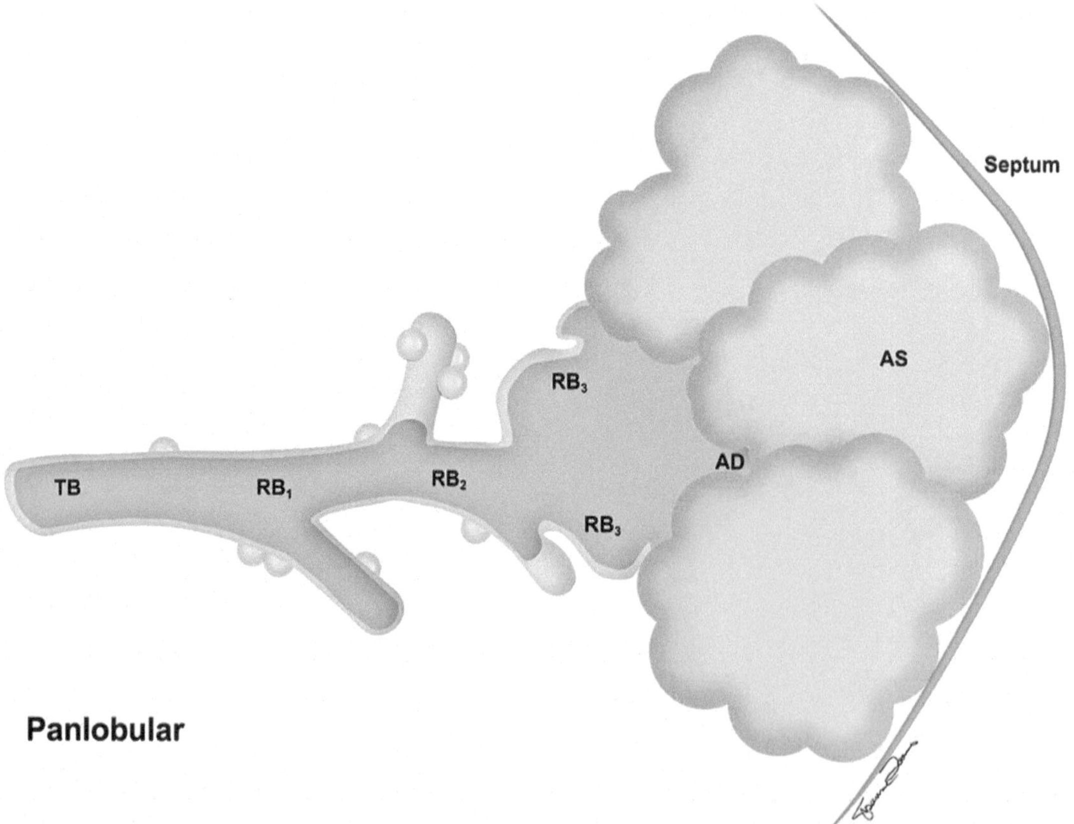

FIGURE 20.5 Panlobular emphysema. The enlargement and destruction of airspaces (A) involve the acinus more or less uniformly. *AD,* Alveolar duct; *AS,* alveolar sac; *RB,* respiratory bronchiole; *TB,* terminal bronchiole. (Adapted from Thurlbeck WM: Chronic Airflow Obstruction in Lung Disease. Philadelphia: WB Saunders, 1976.)

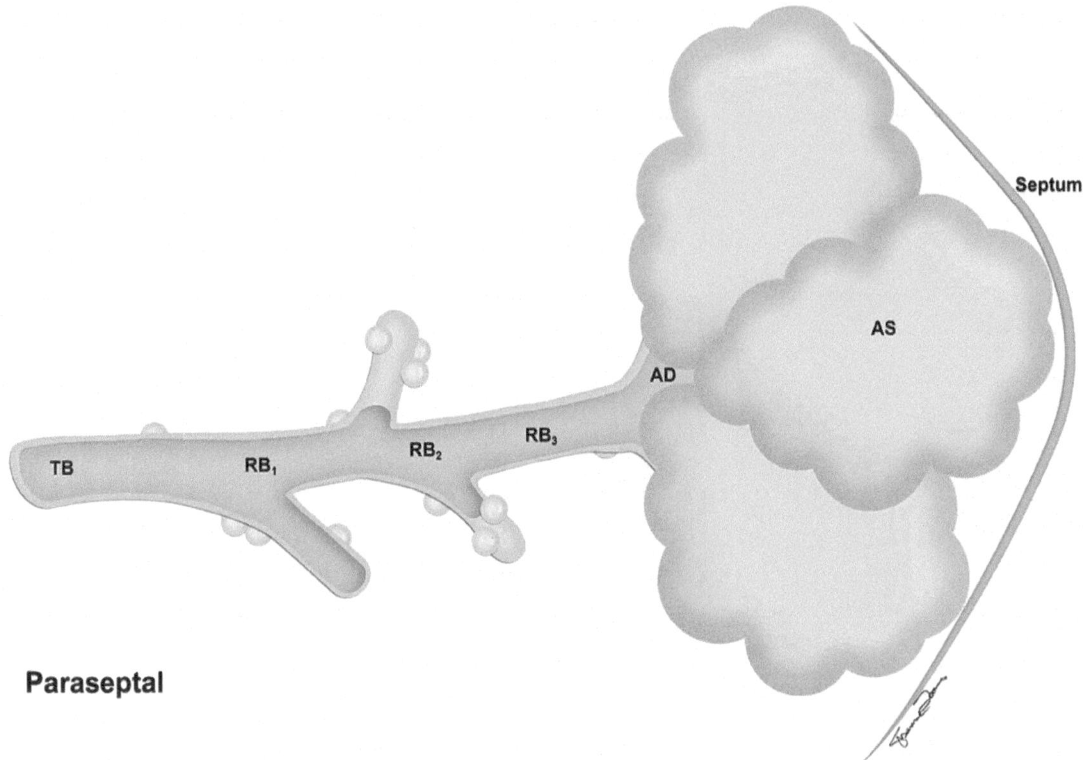

FIGURE 20.6 Paraseptal emphysema. The peripheral part of the acinus (alveolar ducts and sacs) is dominantly and selectively involved. (Adapted from Thurlbeck WM: Chronic Airflow Obstruction in Lung Disease. Philadelphia: WB Saunders, 1976.)

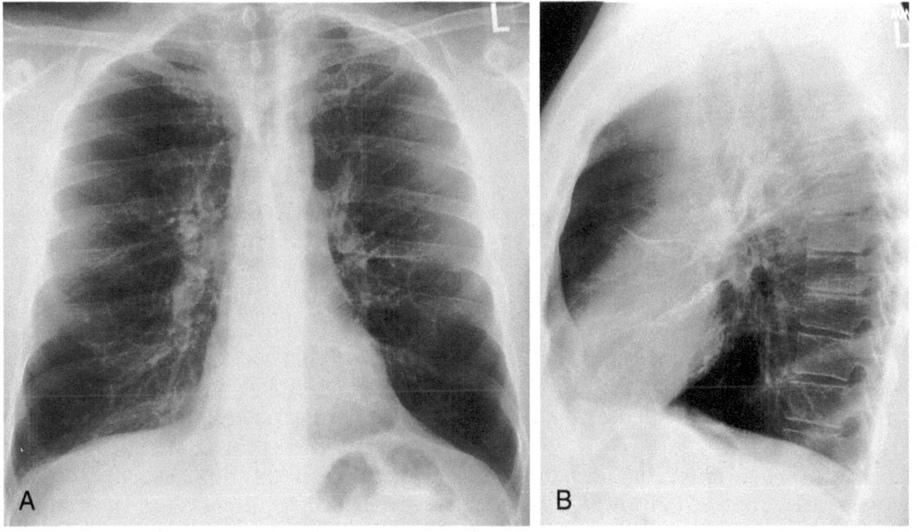

FIGURE 20.7 Emphysema in a patient with α_1-antitrypsin deficiency. Posteroanterior **(A)** and lateral **(B)** chest radiographs show attenuation of pulmonary vessels at the lung bases compared with the upper lungs characteristic of panlobular emphysema. Notice the flattening of the diaphragm and increased retrosternal air.

Imaging Features

Radiography

Emphysema can be diagnosed by standard radiography when the disease is severe. If the lungs are mildly affected by emphysema, the chest radiograph is usually normal. Only about half of cases of moderately severe emphysema are diagnosed radiologically. The standard radiograph is not considered a reliable tool for diagnosing and quantitating emphysema. However, certain radiographic signs are accurate in the diagnosis of emphysema. The first sign is overinflation of the lungs. Similar radiographic findings are seen in patients with severe asthma, but the signs of overexpansion abate with clinical improvement. In emphysema, they persist. The second major sign of emphysema is a rapid tapering and attenuation of pulmonary vessels accompanied by irregular radiolucency of affected areas (Fig. 20.7). Although this is an important radiographic

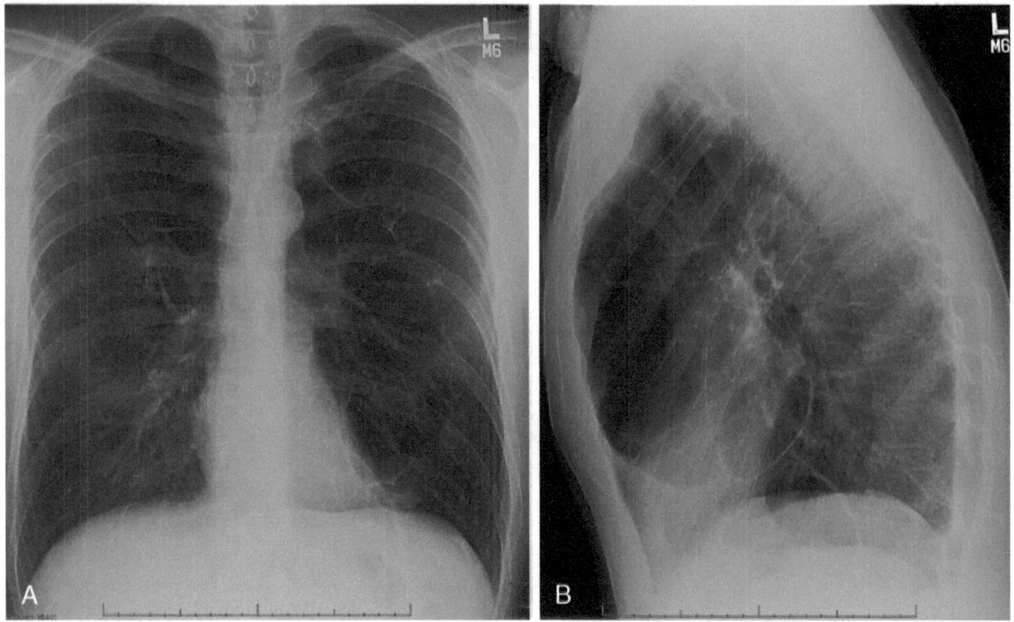

FIGURE 20.8 Bullae in a patient with vanishing lung syndrome. Posteroanterior **(A)** and lateral **(B)** chest radiographs show bilateral upper lobe bullae characterized by large lucent space with thin walls.

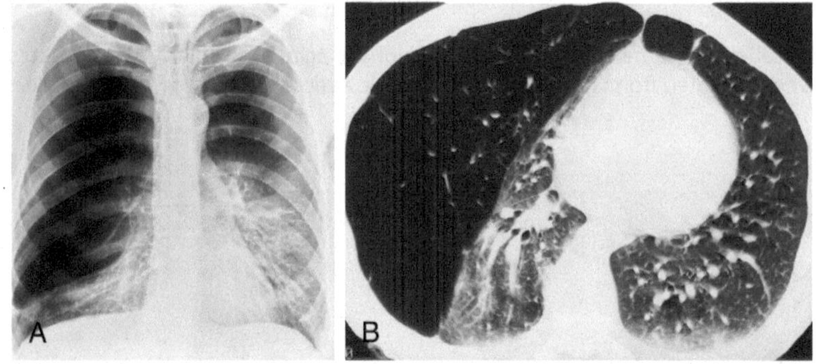

FIGURE 20.9 Vanishing lung syndrome in a 30-year-old man. **A,** The posteroanterior chest radiograph shows bilateral upper lobe bullae with compression of the basilar lung. The minor fissure is depressed. **B,** Computed tomography image at the level of lung bases demonstrates compression of the middle and lower lobes, which are relatively free of emphysema.

finding, it is subjective and difficult to detect before the disease is severe. Localized lucent areas, particularly if they are surrounded by consolidation, may be apparent in the periphery of the lungs.

Bullae may occur in emphysema (Figs. 20.8 and 20.9). A bulla is a sharply demarcated area of emphysema that is 1 cm or more in diameter and that has a wall less than 1 mm thick. Evidence of bullae should be sought on standard radiographs to support the diagnosis of emphysema. Bullae reflect only locally severe involvement and do not necessarily mean that the disease is widespread.

Computed Tomography

Computed tomography is superior to chest radiography in showing the presence, extent, and severity of emphysema. CT has high sensitivity and specificity for emphysema. It is also possible with CT to distinguish among the anatomic types of emphysema (see Box 20.2).

Centrilobular emphysema is characterized on CT by the presence of multiple small round areas of abnormally low attenuation that are several millimeters to 1 cm in diameter and distributed throughout the lung, usually with an upper lobe predominance (Fig. 20.10). The centrilobular location of these lucencies can sometimes be recognized. The lucencies tend to be multiple, small, and "spotty." Classically, the areas of low attenuation of centrilobular emphysema lack visible walls. A central dot, representing the central bronchovascular bundle, is sometimes visible. As the disease becomes more severe, the areas of lung destruction become more confluent, and the centrilobular distribution may no longer be recognizable. The HRCT appearance can then closely simulate panlobular emphysema.

Panlobular emphysema is characterized on CT by the presence of fewer and smaller-than-normal pulmonary vessels (Fig. 20.11). It is almost always more severe in the lower lobes but may appear diffuse. When it is advanced, extensive lung destruction can be identified, and the associated paucity of vessels is readily detectable. However, in moderate disease, increased lucency of the lung parenchyma and a limited, slight decrease in the caliber of the pulmonary

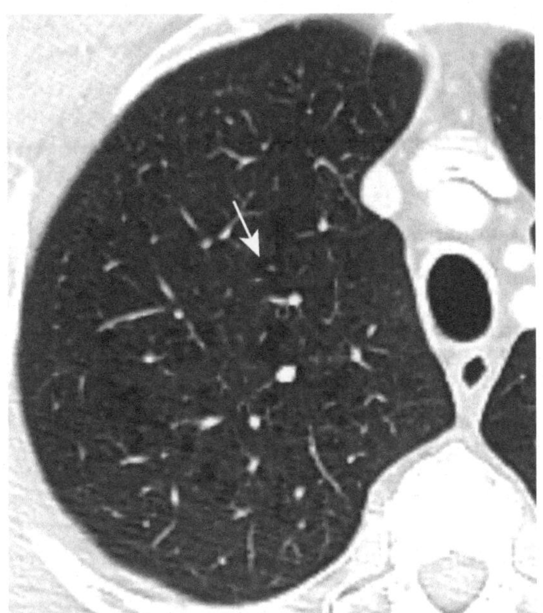

FIGURE 20.10 Centrilobular emphysema. Axial computed tomography image shows multiple, round lucent areas without visible walls in the upper lobes. A "central dot" *(arrow)* can be identified in the lucent area, signifying a centrilobular bronchovascular bundle.

vessels may be more difficult to recognize. When lower lobe-predominant panlobular emphysema is identified, the possibility of AATD should be raised. The disease can be confirmed by genetic and blood tests, and treatments with smoking cessation and possible AAT augmentation therapy can be initiated.

Paraseptal emphysema (Fig. 20.12) is easily detected by CT. The appearance is that of multiple areas of subpleural emphysema, often with visible thin walls that correspond to interlobular septa. The emphysema is localized in the subpleural zones and along the interlobar fissures. When larger than 1 cm, areas of paraseptal emphysema are most appropriately called *bullae*. Subpleural bullae are manifestations of paraseptal emphysema, although they may be seen in all types of emphysema. They are often associated with spontaneous pneumothorax.

Paracicatricial or irregular emphysema (Fig. 20.13) is focal emphysema that is usually found adjacent to parenchymal scars in diffuse pulmonary fibrosis, sarcoidosis, and pneumoconioses, particularly when progressive, massive fibrosis is present. It is usually recognized on CT when the associated fibrosis is identified.

Bullous emphysema does not represent a specific pathologic entity but refers to the presence of emphysema

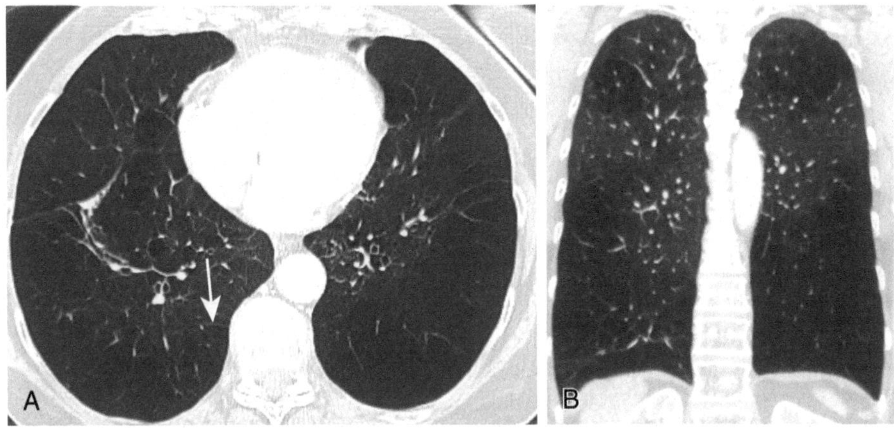

FIGURE 20.11 Panlobular emphysema in a patient with α_1-antitrypsin deficiency and a history of cigarette smoking. **A,** Axial computed tomography image shows a pronounced paucity of vessels in both lower lobes, sometimes referred to as a simplification of lung architecture. "Empty" secondary pulmonary lobules nearly devoid of vessels can be identified *(arrow)*. **B,** Coronal reformation image shows the lower lobe predominance of panlobular emphysema and less severe centrilobular emphysema in the upper lobes.

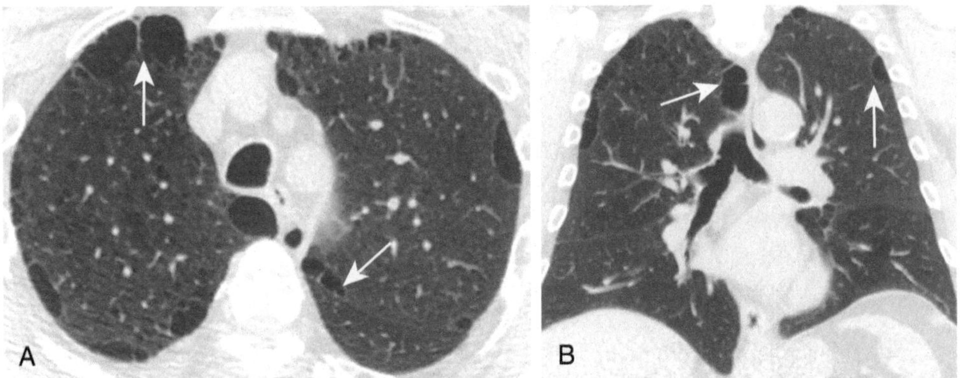

FIGURE 20.12 Paraseptal emphysema. Axial **(A)** and coronal **(B)** computed tomography images show lucent areas localized to the subpleural region *(arrows)*. The patient also has mild centrilobular emphysema.

associated with large bullae. Bullae can develop in association with any type of emphysema, but they are most common in paraseptal emphysema and centrilobular emphysema. A bulla is a sharply demarcated area of emphysema that is more than 1 cm in diameter and that possesses a well-defined wall less than 1 mm thick. Bullae occasionally can become quite large and may be rather focal and may result in atelectasis of normal adjacent lung; occasionally, they are not associated with diffuse emphysema. Large bullae may result in compromised respiratory function. This syndrome has been referred to as bullous emphysema, vanishing lung syndrome, and primary bullous disease of the lung (see Fig. 20.8 and Fig. 20.14). This entity may occur in young men and is characterized by large progressive upper lobe bullae. Most are smokers, but the entity may occur in nonsmokers.

Clinical Indications, Applications, and Implications. The diagnosis of emphysema is usually based on a combination of clinical features, a smoking history, and compatible pulmonary function abnormalities. However, HRCT may be useful in diagnosing patients whose clinical findings suggest another disease process, such as interstitial lung disease or pulmonary vascular disease. For these patients, HRCT can be valuable in detecting the presence of emphysema and in excluding other abnormalities in the chest. More recently, combined pulmonary fibrosis and emphysema is increasingly recognized in smokers. The presence of both obstructive and restrictive lung diseases can mask the degree of airway obstruction on PFT, which often shows disproportionately impaired D_{LCO}, and CT is helpful in uncovering the abnormalities. With increasing utilization of chest CT for various clinical indications, such as evaluating traumatic injuries and screening for lung cancer, emphysema is sometimes incidentally detected before clinical symptoms become apparent.

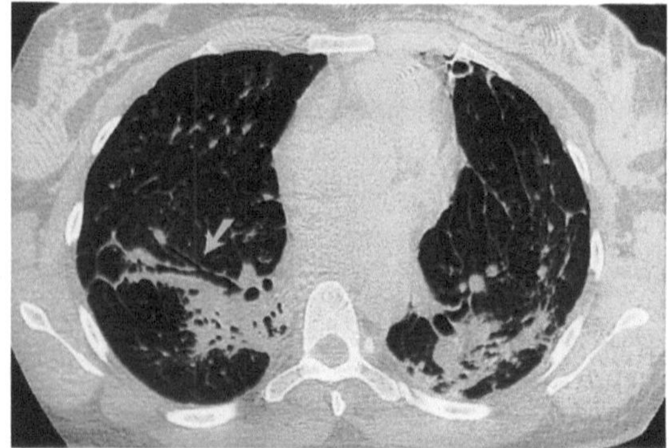

FIGURE 20.13 Paracicatricial emphysema in a patient with sarcoidosis and pulmonary fibrosis. Axial computed tomography image demonstrates bilateral parahilar fibrosis, architectural distortion, and traction bronchiectasis. Notice the dilated medial and lateral segmental bronchi in the right middle lobe *(arrow)*, which represent traction bronchiectasis, and areas of hyperlucency in the adjacent lung consistent with paracicatricial emphysema.

With its excellent capability in showing the distribution of emphysema, CT plays an important role in the preoperative evaluation of patients with severe emphysema who are selected for lung volume-reduction surgery (LVRS). This surgery typically involves the resection of target areas of emphysema to reduce lung volume, restore elastic recoil, and improve ventilation-perfusion matching. In selected patients, this procedure has improved respiratory mechanics, diminished oxygen requirement, reduced dyspnea, increased exercise capacity, improved the quality of life, and extended survival. Based on the results of the National Emphysema Treatment Trial, which randomized patients to LVRS or to maximal medical therapy, patients with upper lobe-predominant emphysema are candidates for this procedure.

Various bronchoscopic techniques have been introduced as an alternative to LVRS. Most of these methods attempt to occlude the conducting airways to regions of severe emphysema by using a variety of techniques, including endobronchial airway sealants, coils, and one-way valves. The goal of most of these approaches is to achieve atelectasis of the targeted lung segments, resulting in nonsurgical volume reduction. Similar to LVRS, these methods are designed to treat patients with heterogeneous distribution of emphysema rather than diffuse disease. In contrast, airway bypass is a new bronchoscopic technique under investigation for treating patients with homogeneous distribution of emphysema. This method aims to decrease hyperinflation by placing shunts between the lung parenchyma and central airways, creating new conducting expiratory airways to bypass high-resistance, collapsing airway segments. CT plays an important role in preprocedural delineation of distribution of emphysema and patient selection. The presence of incomplete fissures should be reported because

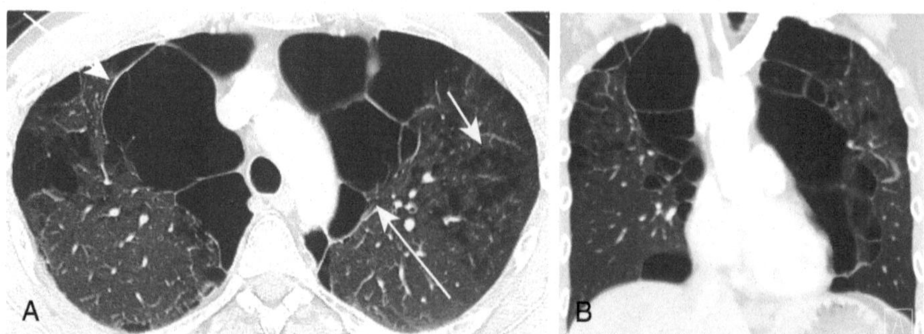

FIGURE 20.14 Vanishing lung syndrome in a 38-year-old man. **A,** Axial computed tomography (CT) image through the upper lobes shows bilateral bullae *(long arrow)* and centrilobular emphysema *(short arrow)*. **B,** Coronal reformation CT image demonstrates more severe destruction of the upper lobe parenchyma than the lower lobes.

collateral ventilation through bridging lung parenchyma can prevent successful collapse of the targeted lobe with endoscopic lung reduction. CT is also useful for evaluation of procedural effectiveness and complications.

Emphysema is an independent risk factor for lung cancer, and about 5% of patients evaluated by CT before LVRS had incidentally detected lung cancer. When evaluating patients with emphysema, it is important to report incidental lung nodules and recommend appropriate imaging follow-up.

Several HRCT methods are available to quantitate the degree and severity of emphysema. The most common quantitative method is lung densitometry analysis. This technique provides histograms of lung attenuation values and calculates the area of lung occupied by pixels within a predetermined range of attenuation values. A percentage of low-attenuation area under -950 Hounsfield units has been shown to have the strongest associations with microscopic and macroscopic emphysema. Previous studies have shown that visual and quantitative CT methods for estimating severity of emphysema correlate well with findings on pathologic specimens of emphysematous lungs. However, quantitative methods have been shown to provide more objective and reliable assessment than visual scoring.

Although not routinely employed, postprocessing of CT data using a minimum-intensity projection technique, which highlights the lowest attenuation voxels on CT, has been shown to enhance the detection of mild emphysema (Fig. 20.15). This method may help to improve the detection of mild emphysema when conventional CT images are equivocal.

Differential Diagnosis. Several entities should be considered in the differential diagnosis of emphysema on HRCT. The first is honeycombing, which occurs in pulmonary fibrosis and is characterized by areas of subpleural cystic lesions that somewhat mimic the appearance of paraseptal emphysema. However, honeycomb cysts are usually smaller; occur in several layers along the pleural surface, often localized in the lung bases; and are associated with other findings of fibrosis. Paraseptal emphysema is often associated with bullae, and the areas of emphysema are larger and occur in a single layer. They predominate in the upper lobes without evidence of fibrosis.

The second feature to be considered in the differential diagnosis of emphysema is pneumatoceles. A pneumatocele is a thin-walled, gas-filled space within the lung that usually is associated with a prior pneumonia or a pulmonary laceration. It can be identical to a bulla on CT. However, the association with previous infection or trauma should suggest the diagnosis.

The third entity is cystic lung disease. Multiple thin-walled lung cysts can be seen in a variety of disorders, such as lymphangioleiomyomatosis and Langerhans cell histiocytosis. These cysts usually can be differentiated from centrilobular emphysema because the walls of cysts are more distinct and appear larger. When the lucency can be clearly identified as within the center of the pulmonary lobule, it is diagnostic of centrilobular emphysema. Cystic bronchiectasis can be readily differentiated from lung cysts and emphysema based on connectivity with the proximal airways and a constant relationship with its accompanying pulmonary artery.

The fourth possibility is bronchiolitis obliterans. Constrictive bronchiolitis, a disease of the small airways described in more detail later in this chapter, can result in increased lung volume and oligemia that is similar to that of panlobular emphysema. However, it usually has a patchy distribution, which is an important distinguishing feature.

CHRONIC BRONCHITIS

Clinical Features

Chronic bronchitis, unlike emphysema, is defined in clinical rather than pathologic terms. It is defined as a productive cough occurring on most days for at least 3 consecutive months and for not less than 2 consecutive years. Other causes of chronic productive cough, including bronchiectasis, tuberculosis, and other chronic infections, must be

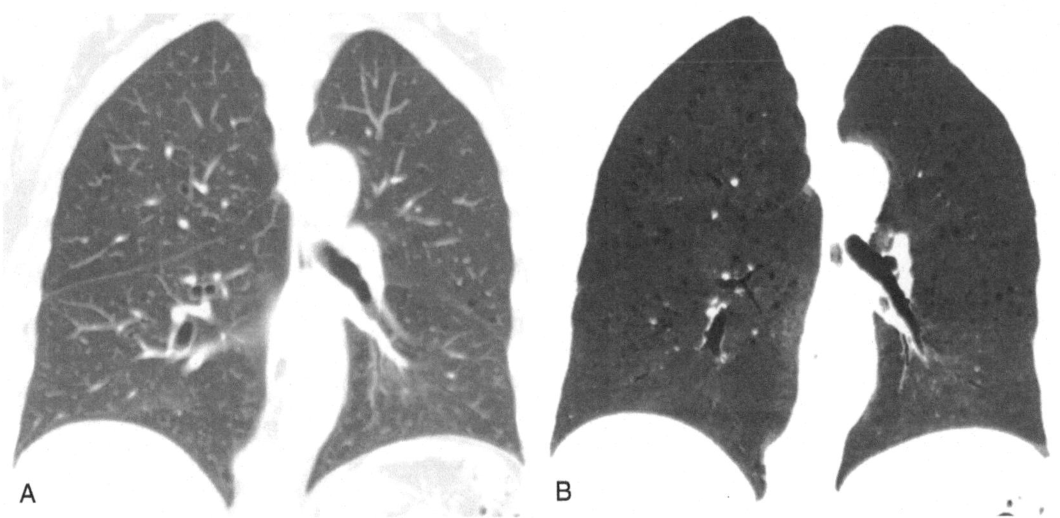

FIGURE 20.15 Mild emphysema better seen on minimum-intensity projection image (minIP). **A,** Coronal reformation computed tomography image demonstrates small lucent areas consistent with centrilobular emphysema. **B,** Coronal minIP shows the emphysema to better advantage.

excluded before the diagnosis of chronic bronchitis can be made. Most patients with chronic bronchitis are smokers, and they often have coexisting emphysema. Air pollution is also a culprit. Treatments include smoking cessation, bronchodilators, and steroids.

Pathologic Features

Pathologically, the hallmark of chronic bronchitis is hyperplasia of mucous glands. They have increased volumes, which can be assessed by the ratio of the bronchial gland to the bronchial wall, called the *Reid index*. Airflow obstruction in the small airways is related to reversible mucous plugging and smooth muscle hypertrophy and irreversible fibrosis and stenosis.

Imaging Features

The radiographic features of chronic bronchitis are nonspecific, and the chest radiograph is most frequently normal. Described features include thickened bronchial walls seen end-on in cross section (peribronchial cuffing) or in profile (i.e., tram lines) and hyperinflation of the lungs (see Fig. 20.1). Bronchial wall thickening is a nonspecific finding that may be seen in patients with infection, interstitial pulmonary edema or other interstitial diseases, asthma, and bronchiectasis, and it is occasionally seen in healthy subjects. On CT, bronchial wall thickening (Fig. 20.16), mosaic attenuation, and air trapping can be observed. Mucous plugging can be seen. Patients often have coexisting emphysema. The diagnosis of chronic bronchitis is based on clinical rather than imaging findings.

ASTHMA

Clinical Features

Asthma is a chronic illness that causes widespread narrowing of the tracheobronchial tree (Box 20.3). It is characterized by reversible bronchospasm that may be provoked by a variety of stimuli. Acute exacerbations often resolve spontaneously or with therapy. It is a common disease, estimated to affect 3% to 5% of the population of the United States. At least two thirds of patients are atopic, and the pathogenesis of asthma in these individuals is related to a reaction to different types of allergens. Although death is rare, the mortality rates have been increasing for several years. Treatments usually consist of bronchodilators and antiinflammatory agents.

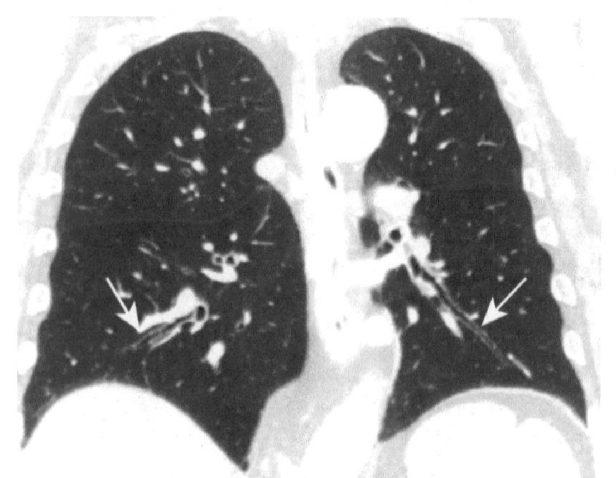

FIGURE 20.16 Chronic bronchitis. Coronal reformation computed tomography image demonstrates bronchial wall thickening *(arrows)*, which would correspond to tram tracking on radiography. Subtle mosaic attenuation of the lungs is also present.

Pathologic Features

Pathologically, asthma is characterized by an active inflammatory process in the airways, even when patients are asymptomatic. Other features include edema of the bronchial mucosa and excessive mucous production.

Imaging Features

Uncomplicated Asthma

There is some controversy regarding the indications for chest radiography in asthma. For adults, a chest radiograph should be obtained when asthma is first suspected and when conventional treatment is ineffective to exclude other causes of wheezing, such as neoplasm, congestive heart failure, bronchiectasis, and foreign bodies. In pediatric patients, chest radiographs are seldom abnormal and should be obtained only when there is no improvement or there is worsening of symptoms despite conventional therapy, when there is fever associated with auscultatory findings that persist after treatment, and when there is a clinical suspicion of a complication such as pneumothorax.

For most patients with asthma, the chest radiograph is normal. Radiographic changes, more common in children than in adults, usually consist of signs of hyperinflation, flattening of the hemidiaphragms (best identified on the lateral radiograph), and an increase in the retrosternal airspace. Another radiographic feature of asthma is that of bronchial

BOX 20.3 Asthma

CLINICAL FEATURES

Reversible bronchospasm
Two thirds of cases atopic

PATHOLOGIC FEATURES

Active inflammation and edema of the airways

IMAGING FEATURES

Uncomplicated
- Normal in most patients
- Signs of hyperinflation
- Bronchial wall thickening

Complicated
- Pneumonia
- Lobar or segmental atelectasis
- Mucoid impaction
- Allergic bronchopulmonary aspergillosis
- Bronchiectasis
- Mucous plug (can be hyperdense on computed tomography)
- Pneumomediastinum
- Pneumothorax

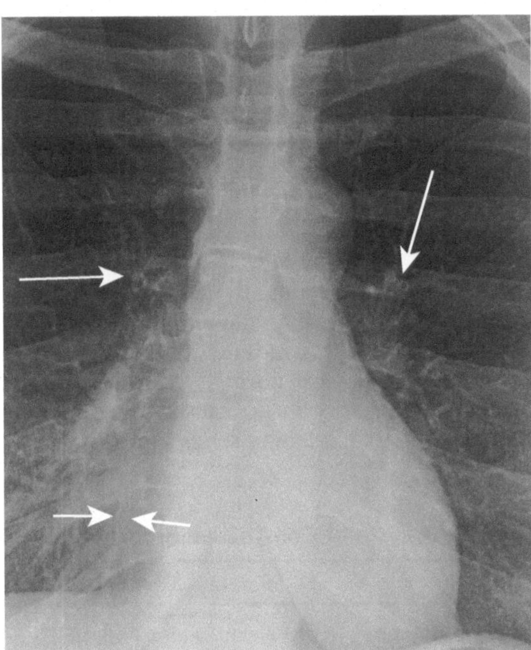

FIGURE 20.17 Asthma. Magnified view of posteroanterior chest radiograph shows ring shadows *(long arrows)* caused by bronchial wall thickening of airways seen on end and tram lines *(short arrows)* of airways seen in profile.

wall thickening. In children, the walls of secondary bronchi are normally not discernible beyond the mediastinum and hila; when visualized more peripherally in the lung, they are considered abnormal. In adults and children, the thickening of the bronchial walls can best be detected in bronchi seen in cross section, most commonly in the perihilar areas (Fig. 20.17). Bronchi seen in the longitudinal plane often appear as *tram lines*, which are paired parallel lines separated by lucency. Occasionally, the thickening of the bronchial walls may produce a perihilar haze or stringy linear opacities in the perihilar areas. Transient pulmonary hypertension during severe attacks of asthma increases the size of the central pulmonary arteries on standard radiographs. This effect is probably caused by alveolar hypoxia.

On CT, mild bronchial dilation has been reported in 15% to 77% of patients with asthma, and more than 90% may have bronchial wall thickening. Less common CT findings include branching or nodular centrilobular opacities and a mosaic perfusion pattern. Expiratory HRCT may detect areas of regional air trapping, even in the absence of inspiratory HRCT abnormalities. The severity of HRCT findings correlates with the severity of asthma as measured by PFTs. Hyperpolarized gas magnetic resonance imaging techniques have been used to assess regional ventilation in patients with asthma. Studies have shown that patients with asthma have more ventilation defects than the general population and that the number of defects increases proportionately with the severity of asthma.

Complicated Asthma

The most frequent complication in asthma is pneumonia. In the pediatric age group, most exacerbations are caused by viral infections, particularly respiratory syncytial virus in infants and parainfluenza and rhinoviruses in older children. The radiographic appearance is similar to viral pneumonias in the nonasthmatic population. Lobar or segmental atelectasis can occur in cases of asthma, but it is unusual. It is seen more commonly in children and most frequently involves the right middle lobe because of retention of mucus in the large airways.

Allergic bronchopulmonary aspergillosis is discussed in more detail in Chapter 6. The most characteristic finding is the presence of central bronchiectasis, which frequently involves or predominates in the upper lobes. The dilated bronchi are often filled with mucoid material that contains *Aspergillus* organisms. Radiographic findings of mucoid impaction include a bandlike opacity that appears like a gloved finger; it can also be V shaped, Y shaped, or round. Mucous plugs are typically located centrally in the perihilar areas and upper lobes and can be hyperdense on CT.

Pneumomediastinum is a complication of asthma that occurs in approximately 1% to 5% of asthma cases. It has a bimodal distribution that peaks at ages 4 to 6 and 13 to 18 years. The postulated mechanism is a mucous plug or infection that causes a check-valve obstruction that increases intraalveolar pressure. With deep inspiration or cough, the alveolar wall may rupture, with tracking of interstitial air along the perivascular sheaths toward the hilum and eventual extension into the mediastinum (the Macklin effect). Patients usually have symptoms of chest or neck pain. Radiographic findings are described in Chapter 10. Air encircling major bronchi and hilar vessels and outlining the trachea and the esophagus, the aorta, and the heart is characteristic. It may be observed more easily on the lateral view. Air eventually dissects into the neck, and examination should include a careful search of the soft tissues of the neck for evidence of air, which can often be more easily detected than air in the mediastinum. Occasionally, inferior dissection of air may result in a pneumoperitoneum or an extraperitoneal air collection.

Pneumothorax may occur in conjunction with pneumomediastinum, and although rare, it may be fatal. It can be caused by barotrauma in intubated asthmatic patients (Fig. 20.18). It usually occurs with long-standing disease. A small pneumothorax may become significant in patients who are intubated and maintained on intermittent positive-pressure breathing. The chest radiograph is diagnostic.

Although the presence of patchy consolidative or ground-glass opacities on imaging most likely represents infection in patients with asthma, eosinophilic granulomatosis with polyangiitis, formerly known as Churg-Strauss syndrome, can be considered. It is a rare vasculitis associated with severe asthma, sinusitis, and blood or tissue eosinophilia. The pulmonary opacities are often bilateral, transient, patchy, or nodular with peripheral and upper lung predominance, similar to those seen in chronic eosinophilic pneumonia (see Chapter 11).

CONSTRICTIVE AND OBLITERATIVE BRONCHIOLITIS

Clinical Features

Constrictive bronchiolitis, also known as obliterative bronchiolitis or bronchiolitis obliterans, is characterized by submucosal fibrosis, resulting in narrowing or occlusion of the bronchioles and obstruction. Patients usually present with progressive dyspnea and cough, similar to other obstructive lung diseases. The obstructive ventilator defect is not reversed by inhaled bronchodilator. Causes include childhood infection, lung transplant rejection, graft-versus-host disease in stem cell transplant recipients, inhalational lung disease, and connective tissue disease (Table 20.1). It is estimated that bronchiolitis obliterans syndrome occurs in up to 50% of lung transplant patients 5 years after transplant and 5% of hematopoietic stem cell transplant recipients. Some cases are idiopathic. The diagnosis is often made based on clinical history, PFTs, and imaging findings. Immunosuppressants such as steroids are often used for treatment. Many patients eventually require lung transplantation.

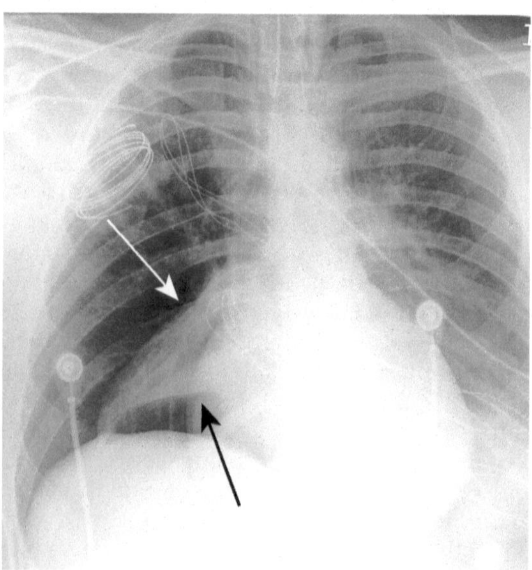

FIGURE 20.18 Asthma exacerbation with complications. Portable radiograph in supine position shows lucency at the right basilar thorax outlining the collapsed right middle lobe *(arrows)* and right hemidiaphragm consistent with an anterior pneumothorax. Note also left lower lobe pneumonia.

Pathologic Features

Pathologically, injury to the respiratory epithelium leads to excessive accumulation of fibroblasts and fibroproliferation. Fibrosis between the epithelium and muscular mucosa of the bronchioles results in concentric luminal narrowing.

Imaging Features

Chest radiographs are frequently normal in patients with constrictive bronchiolitis showing only mild hyperinflation. The key finding on CT is mosaic attenuation where the high-attenuation areas are normal. The lucent areas are accentuated on expiratory images caused by air trapping (see Figs. 20.2 and 20.19). Expiratory series should be performed

TABLE 20.1 Causes of Constrictive Bronchiolitis

Cause	Clinical Features
Chronic lung transplant rejection	>3 months after transplant ≤50% of patients affected at 5 years posttransplant Leading cause of death beyond the first year
Chronic graft-versus-host disease	~5% of hematopoietic stem cell transplant recipients Most occur within 18 months of transplant ≤97% have extrapulmonary (i.e., skin and gastrointestinal tract) involvement
Inhalational lung disease	Exposure to popcorn or other flavoring agent, smoke, nitrous oxide, sulfur gas, and so on
Autoimmune	Rheumatoid arthritis most common, systemic lupus erythematosus, IgA nephropathy, inflammatory bowel disease
Postinfectious	Viral, *Mycoplasma* spp., *Nocardia* spp., *Legionella* spp.
Drug induced	Penicillamine, gold, cocaine, talc, busulfan, sulfasalazine, and so on

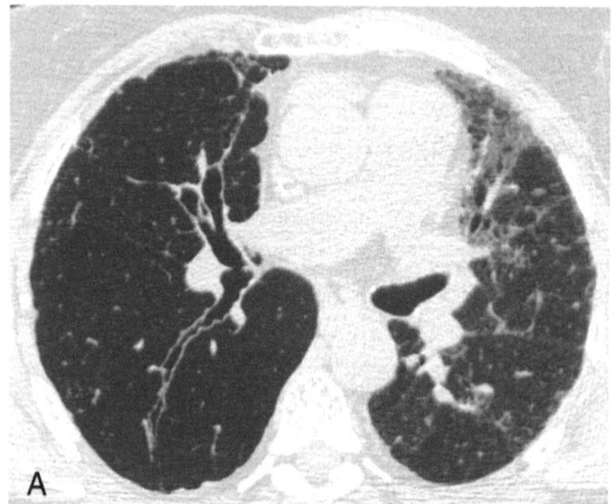

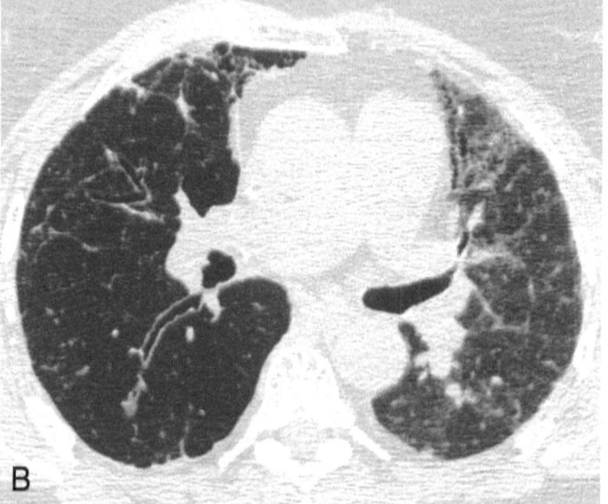

FIGURE 20.19 Obliterative bronchiolitis in a transplanted right lung. Inspiratory **(A)** and expiratory **(B)** computed tomography images show uniform lucency in the transplanted right lung, indicating air trapping. Notice the bronchiectasis in the right lung. The native left lung has pulmonary fibrosis.

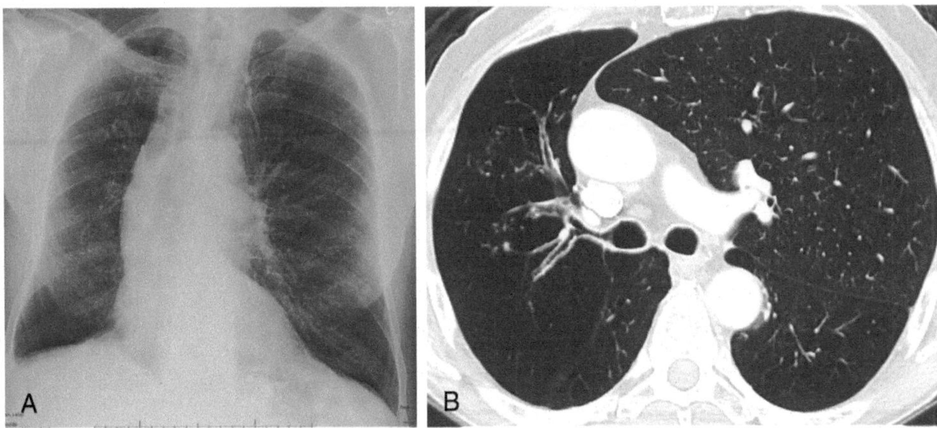

FIGURE 20.20 Swyer-James-MacLeod syndrome. **A,** Posteroanterior chest radiograph shows hyperlucent right lung with small volume. Note the small caliber of the right lung pulmonary vessels compared with the left lung. **B,** Axial computed tomography confirms radiographic findings and demonstrates bronchiectasis and bronchial wall thickening caused by airway injury from prior infection as well as vascular attenuation throughout the right lung.

in all clinically suspected cases of constrictive bronchiolitis and in routine follow-up of lung transplant recipients. Mild bronchial wall thickening or bronchiectasis is occasionally present. Unlike in other small airway diseases, tree-in-bud opacities or centrilobular nodules are usually absent.

SWYER-JAMES-MACLEOD SYNDROME

Clinical Features

Swyer-James-MacLeod syndrome is an advanced form of constrictive bronchiolitis, usually involving an entire lobe or lung and sometimes both lungs, caused by childhood infection, usually viral etiologies.

Pathologic Features

Infection before alveolar maturation, around 8 years of age, results in disruption of alveoli and impaired development of pulmonary vessels.

Imaging Features

The classic radiographic finding is a hyperlucent lung or lobe with associated volume loss and decreased vascularity (Fig. 20.20). On CT, findings characteristics of constrictive bronchiolitis, including mosaic attenuation and air trapping, can be seen. Bronchiectasis and hypoplasia of the pulmonary artery branches of affected lobe or lung, not typically seen in other causes of constrictive bronchiolitis, are often present.

DIFFUSE IDIOPATHIC PULMONARY NEUROENDOCRINE CELL HYPERPLASIA

Clinical Features

Diffuse idiopathic pulmonary neuroendocrine cell hyperplasia (DIPNECH) often affects middle-aged or older women and is not associated with smoking. Patients may be asymptomatic or present with insidious onset of nonproductive cough, dyspnea, and wheezing. The symptoms are often erroneously attributed to asthma or COPD. PFTs often reveal an obstructive or mixed obstructive and restrictive ventilator defect. The disease is usually slowly progressive or stable and rarely life threatening.

Pathologic Features

Constrictive bronchiolitis with narrowing and obstruction of small airway lumens caused by progressive fibrosis is the result of neuroendocrine cell proliferation in DIPNECH. It is also considered a preneoplastic condition in the spectrum of pulmonary neuroendocrine tumors commonly found in patients with carcinoid tumors (see Chapter 21).

Imaging Features

Plain radiographs are often normal or may demonstrate hyperinflation or small pulmonary nodules. Multiple small solid or ground-glass pulmonary nodules are the predominant abnormalities on CT (Fig. 20.21). The nodules often remain stable or enlarge very slowly. Mosaic attenuation is also a common finding, with air trapping confirmed by expiratory images.

CONCLUSION

Obstructive lung diseases present with nonspecific clinical findings. Imaging is helpful in identifying the underlying anatomic abnormalities and causes of obstructive defects detected on PFTs. In the setting of COPD and asthma, imaging is helpful in the evaluation of disease severity and detection of complications. In cases of AATD, Swyer-James-MacLeod syndrome, and DIPNECH, characteristic imaging findings should prompt radiologists to suggest the diagnoses and guide further workup and management.

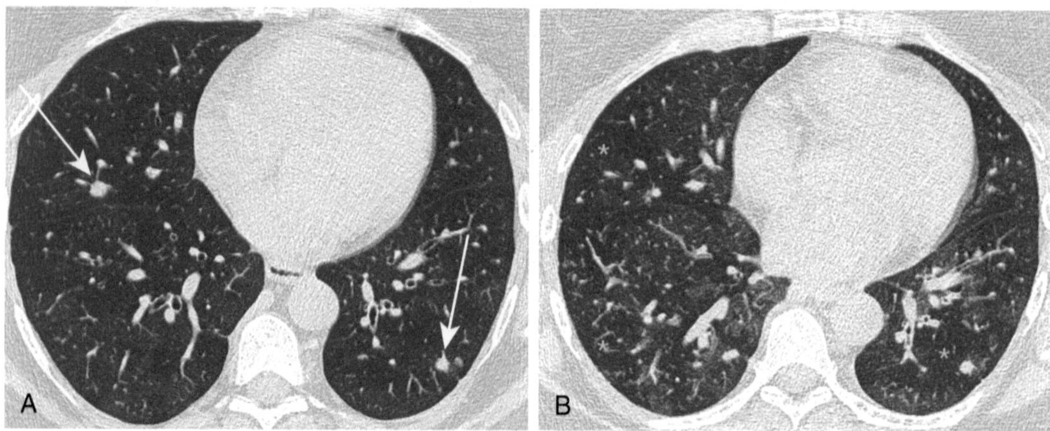

FIGURE 20.21 Diffuse idiopathic pulmonary neuroendocrine cell hyperplasia in 55-year-old woman. **A,** Inspiratory computed tomography (CT) image shows bilateral small pulmonary nodules *(arrows)* and subtle mosaic attenuation of lungs. **B,** Expiratory CT image shows hyperlucent areas *(asterisks)* consistent with air trapping.

SUGGESTED READINGS

Aguilar PR, Michelson AP, Isakow W. Obliterative bronchiolitis. *Transplantation*. 2016;100:272-283.

Edwards RM, Kicska G, Schmidt R, et al. Imaging of small airways and emphysema. *Clin Chest Med*. 2015;36:335-347.

Grabenhorst M, Schmidt B, Liebers U, et al. Radiologic manifestations of bronchoscopic lung volume reduction in severe chronic obstructive pulmonary disease. *AJR Am J Roentgenol*. 2015;204:475-486.

Kligerman SJ, Henry T, Lin CT, et al. Mosaic attenuation: etiology, methods of differentiation, and pitfalls. *Radiographics*. 2015;35:1360-1380.

Richards JC, Lynch D, Koelsch T, et al. Imaging of asthma. *Immunol Allergy Clin North Am*. 2016;36:529-545.

Rossi G, Cavazza A, Spagnolo P, et al. Diffuse idiopathic pulmonary neuroendocrine cell hyperplasia syndrome. *Eur Respir J*. 2016;47:1829-1841.

Stern EJ, WebbW R, Weinacker A, et al. Idiopathic giant bullous emphysema (vanishing lung syndrome): imaging findings in nine patients. *AJR Am J Roentgenol*. 1994;162:279-282.

Storbeck B, Schröder TH, Oldigs M, et al. Emphysema: imaging for endoscopic lung volume reduction. *Rofo*. 2015;187:543-554.

Strange C, Beiko T. Treatment of alpha-1 antitrypsin deficiency. *Semin Respir Crit Care Med*. 2015;36:470-477.

Thurlbeck WM, Simon G. Radiographic appearance of the chest in emphysema. *AJR Am J Roentgenol*. 1978;130:429-440.

Zompatori M, Sverzellati N, Gentile T, et al. Imaging of the patient with chronic bronchitis: an overview of old and new signs. *Radiol Med*. 2006;111:634-639.

Chapter 21

Pulmonary Tumors and Lymphoproliferative Disorders

Mylene T. Truong, Carol C. Wu, Brett W. Carter, and Bradley S. Sabloff

Lung cancer is the leading cause of cancer mortality in the United States, accounting for more than 150,000 deaths each year. In addition to lung cancer, the chapter reviews primary malignant and benign pulmonary tumors more commonly encountered in clinical practice based on the latest 2015 World Health Organization (WHO) Classification of Lung Tumors (Box 21.1). Pulmonary lymphoproliferative disorders and benign entities that mimic tumors in the lungs are also discussed. Posttreatment changes related to chemotherapy, radiation therapy, and immunotherapy are briefly described.

LUNG CANCER

More than 200,000 patients are diagnosed with lung cancer in the United States each year. Lung cancer is the leading cause of cancer death in men and has surpassed breast cancer as the leading cause of cancer death in women. Lung cancer is one of the most common diseases of the lungs that radiologists encounter in practice. Plain radiography, computed tomography (CT), positron emission tomography (PET), and magnetic resonance imaging (MRI) all play important roles in the imaging evaluation of patients with lung cancer. Please refer to Chapters 3 and 4 for more detailed discussion of PET and MRI findings.

BOX 21.1 Classification of Lung Tumors

EPITHELIAL TUMORS

Adenocarcinoma
Squamous cell carcinoma
Neuroendocrine tumors
- Carcinoid tumors
- Small cell carcinoma
- Large cell neuroendocrine carcinoma

Sarcomatoid carcinomas
- Carcinosarcoma
- Adenosquamous carcinoma
- Pulmonary blastoma

MESENCHYMAL TUMORS

Pulmonary hamartoma
Chondroma
Synovial sarcoma
Epithelioid hemangioendothelioma

LYMPHOHISTIOCYTIC TUMORS

Mucosa-associated lymphoid tissue lymphoma
Diffuse large cell lymphoma
Lymphomatoid granulomatosis

METASTATIC TUMORS

Adapted from 2015 World Health Organization Classification.

Risk Factors

The strongest risk factor for the development of lung cancer is cigarette smoking. An estimated 85% to 90% of lung cancers are directly attributable to smoking. The risk is related to the number of pack-years of smoking, the age at which smoking began, and the depth of inhalation. The risk decreases with cessation of smoking but never completely disappears.

In recent years, genome-wide association studies have helped identify lung cancer susceptibility risk foci mapped to various chromosomal regions, such as 15q and 5p, in different ethnic populations.

Various occupational and environmental exposures are known to increase the risk of lung cancer, including exposure to asbestos, radon, and silica as well as prior radiation. The combination of asbestos exposure (Fig. 21.1) and cigarette smoking is synergistic and results in a markedly

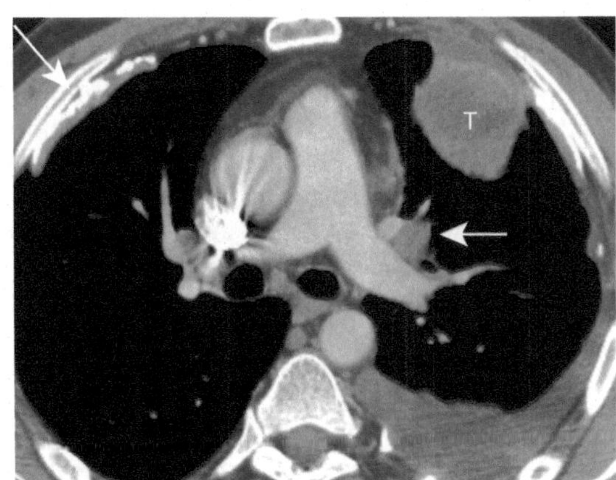

FIGURE 21.1 Lung cancer and asbestos exposure. Computed tomography image shows left upper lung cancer (T) with right anterior calcified pleural plaques *(long arrow)*. Note left hilar adenopathy *(short arrow)* and small left pleural effusion.

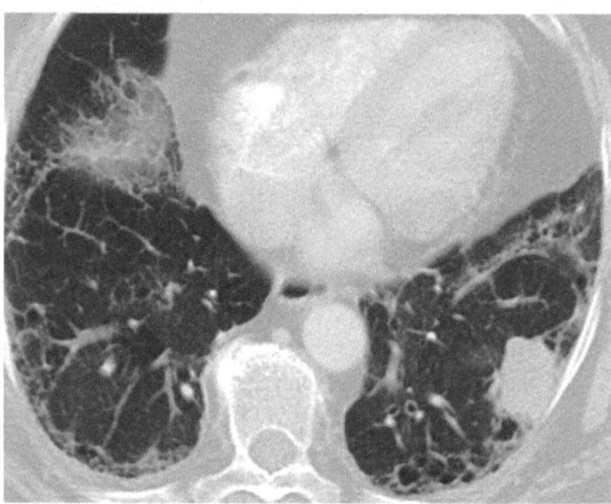

FIGURE 21.2 Lung cancer and pulmonary fibrosis. Computed tomography image shows left lower lobe lung cancer with honeycombing and reticular opacities in the lung bases consistent with fibrosis.

increased risk of lung cancer, particularly if asbestosis is present in the lung parenchyma.

Most of the concomitant lung diseases associated with lung cancer reflect the presence of pulmonary fibrosis, which can be diffuse, as in idiopathic pulmonary fibrosis (Fig. 21.2), or localized, as in tuberculosis. The presence of emphysema on CT has also been linked to increased lung cancer risks among smokers and never-smokers.

Clinical Presentation

Only 10% of patients with lung cancer are asymptomatic. Typically, symptoms are caused by central tumors that result in obstruction of a major bronchus (Box 21.2). This leads to cough, wheezing, hemoptysis, and postobstructive pneumonia. Invasion or compression of adjacent thoracic structures by the tumor may result in pleuritic or chest wall pain, Pancoast syndrome, and symptoms related to obstruction of the superior vena cava. Occasionally, patients may have symptoms that result from distant metastases (e.g., a seizure caused by brain metastases).

Several paraneoplastic syndromes are associated with lung carcinoma, including clubbing; migratory thrombophlebitis; and ectopic hormone production, including Cushing syndrome from adrenocorticotropic hormone (ACTH) production, hyponatremia associated with syndrome of inappropriate antidiuretic hormone secretion (SIADH), and hypercalcemia caused by excessive parathyroid hormone-related protein (PTHrP) production by the tumor. Hypertrophic pulmonary osteoarthropathy consists of periosteal new bone formation that typically involves the bones of the lower arms and legs and can be painful (Fig. 21.3). There are also a variety of neurologic paraneoplastic syndromes.

Classifications

Lung cancer is traditionally divided into non-small cell lung cancer (NSCLC) and small cell lung cancer (SCLC) based on histologic features and differences in treatment strategy. NSCLC in the early stages can be treated with surgery alone. The most common NSCLC include adenocarcinoma and squamous cell carcinoma (SCC). SCLC usually presents in the late stage and requires treatment with a combination of chemotherapy and radiation therapy. Based on the latest 2015 WHO classification (see Box 21.1), SCLC, large cell neuroendocrine carcinoma (LCNEC), and carcinoid tumors all belong to the category of neuroendocrine tumors.

BOX 21.2 Signs and Symptoms of Lung Carcinoma

NO SYMPTOMS

10% of patients

CENTRAL TUMORS

Hemoptysis
Cough
Fever caused by postobstructive pneumonia

INVASION OR COMPRESSION OF THORACIC STRUCTURES

Pleuritic and chest wall pain
Pancoast syndrome (see Box 21.8)
Superior vena cava syndrome
- Dyspnea
- Facial swelling
- Arm swelling
- Chest pain

PARANEOPLASTIC SYNDROMES

Clubbing
Hypertrophic pulmonary osteoarthropathy
Migratory thrombophlebitis
Ectopic hormone production
- Adrenocorticotropic hormone: Cushing syndrome
- Antidiuretic hormone: hyponatremia
- Parathyroid hormone–related protein: hypercalcemia

Neurologic symptoms

BOX 21.3 Adenocarcinoma

CLINICAL FEATURES

Most common cell type
- Predominant cell type in women and nonsmokers

Occasionally asymptomatic
Bronchorrhea in a small subset of patients
Pulmonary fibrosis is a risk factor

PATHOLOGIC FEATURES

Can be slow growing
Peripheral, subpleural location
±Mucin

IMAGING FEATURES

Peripheral location
Solitary nodule or mass
- Spiculated, lobulated, or ill-defined border
- ±Air bronchogram
- Solid, ground-glass, or mixed attenuation

Consolidation
Multiple nodules

Adenocarcinoma

Clinical Features. Adenocarcinoma (Box 21.3) is the most frequent histologic type and accounts for approximately 50% of all lung cancers. It is the most common histologic type in women and in nonsmokers. Typically

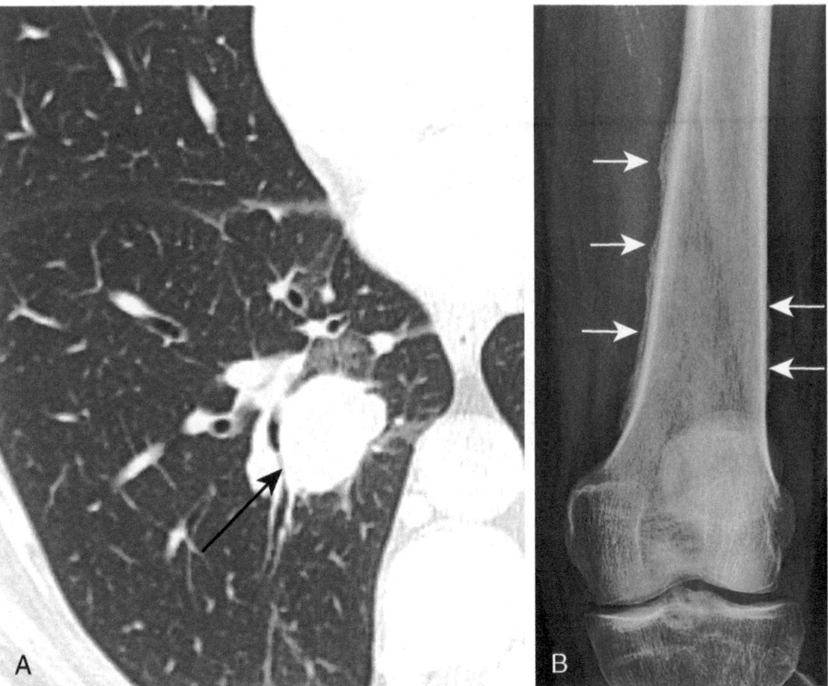

FIGURE 21.3 Hypertrophic pulmonary osteoarthropathy. Computed tomography image **(A)** shows right lower lobe non–small cell lung cancer with an air bronchogram *(arrow)*. Frontal view of the distal femur **(B)** shows smooth periosteal reaction medially and laterally *(arrows)*.

located in the periphery of the lung, these lesions may not produce symptoms and are found incidentally on routine chest radiography. One of the more unusual symptoms of adenocarcinoma is bronchorrhea, which is the production of more than 100 mL/day of watery sputum.

Pathologic Features. Adenocarcinomas typically show slow growth and tend to metastasize early. They can occur in areas of preexisting pulmonary fibrosis. They are most frequently peripheral and subpleural in location and may arise endobronchially.

The classification of lung adenocarcinoma by the 2011 International Association for the Study of Lung Cancer (IASLC), American Thoracic Society (ATS), and European Respiratory Society (ERS) includes a multidisciplinary diagnostic approach using data from pathology, imaging, and molecular biology. The IASLC/ATS/ERS system introduces the use of clearer terminology with respect to the degree of growth along the alveolar surface (lepidic growth) and invasive components to define pre-invasive and invasive lesions. Preinvasive lesions include atypical adenomatous hyperplasia (AAH) and adenocarcinoma in situ (AIS), both defined as lesions with lepidic growth. AAH is a localized, small (≤5 mm) proliferation of mildly to moderately atypical type II pneumocytes or Clara cells lining alveolar walls. AIS is a localized small (≤3 cm) adenocarcinoma with lepidic growth without evidence of stromal, vascular, or pleural invasion. AAH and AIS are pathologic entities considered to be part of a spectrum and cannot be reliably differentiated on cytology. The term *bronchioloalveolar carcinoma* (BAC) is no longer used.

Invasive lesions include minimally invasive adenocarcinoma (MIA) and invasive adenocarcinoma. MIA is defined as a predominantly lepidic lesion lacking necrosis and invasion of lymphatics, blood vessels, or pleura and measuring less than 3 cm with an invasive component measuring no more than 5 mm in any one location. Invasive adenocarcinomas are further classified into histologic subtypes according to the predominant histology present: lepidic, acinar, papillary, micropapillary, or solid-predominant patterns. For example, lepidic-predominant adenocarcinoma (LPA) is defined as a lepidic lesion that may have necrosis, invade lymphatics or blood vessels, and the focus of invasion is greater than 5 mm. The nonmucinous adenocarcinomas are more common than mucinous forms. The term *invasive mucinous adenocarcinoma* has replaced *mucinous bronchoalveolar carcinoma*.

Various gene mutations have been identified in lung adenocarcinoma. There is a strong association between *KRAS* mutations in white smokers. Mutations in the epidermal growth factor receptor (EGFR) are more often seen in adenocarcinomas of nonsmokers and Asian women. Rearrangements of the gene encoding anaplastic lymphoma kinase (ALK) are uncommon, mostly seen in young never- or light smokers with adenocarcinoma. Testing of adenocarcinoma for various mutations has become increasingly important because of availability of targeted drug therapies and prognostic significance.

Imaging Features. Adenocarcinoma may manifest distinct radiologic patterns. The most common is a solitary peripheral nodule or mass often with lobulated, spiculated, and ill-defined borders. On CT, they may present with pure ground-glass, solid, or mixed (both ground-glass and solid) attenuation. AAH and AIS present as pure ground-glass nodules (Figs. 21.4 and 21.5). MIA is usually of ground-glass or mixed attenuation. Correlation of CT features with histopathologic diagnosis using the IASLC/ ERS/ATS system is still evolving, and studies describing CT manifestations of mixed attenuation nodules relating to the more common nonmucinous forms of adenocarcinoma are summarized in Table 21.1. In contradistinction, the less common

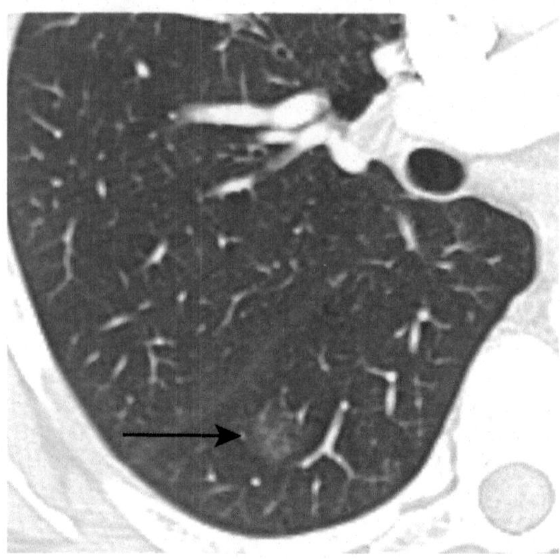

FIGURE 21.4 Adenocarcinoma in situ (AIS). Computed tomography (CT) image shows a 2-cm pure ground-glass nodule in the right lower lobe *(arrow)*, and surgical pathology showed AIS. Note that atypical adenomatous hyperplasia (AAH) and AIS are pathologic entities considered to be part of a spectrum and cannot be differentiated on cytology. The differentiation of AAH and AIS is not possible on CT when the lesion is a small pure ground-glass nodule.

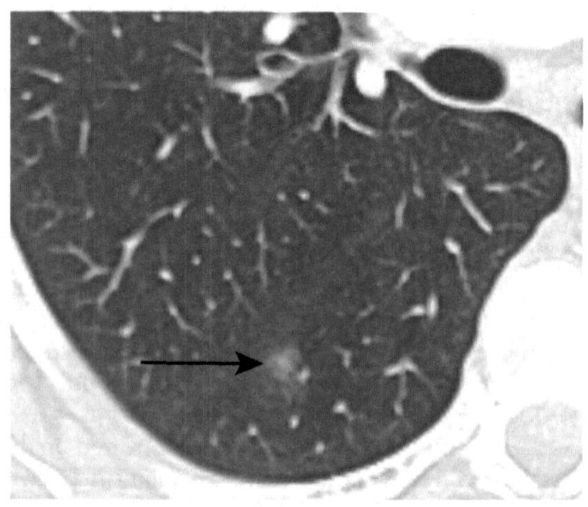

FIGURE 21.5 Minimally invasive adenocarcinoma (MIA). Computed tomography image shows 1-cm ground-glass nodule *(arrow)* in the right lower lobe with a soft tissue component measuring less than 3 mm consistent with MIA.

mucinous form of AIS, MIA, and LPA and other forms of invasive adenocarcinomas can manifest as solid nodules. The soft tissue component of mixed attenuation lesions can represent the invasive component or fibrosis and alveolar collapse (Fig. 21.6). The degree of invasion is reported to correlate directly with the size of the soft tissue component on CT. The solitary nodule is associated with an excellent prognosis when it is resected in early-stage disease. Bubbly internal lucencies termed *pseudocavitation* is caused by alveoli or bronchi spared by tumor infiltration (Fig. 21.7). An air bronchogram may be identified on standard radiography and CT.

The second appearance is an area of consolidation, which occurs in approximately 20% of cases (Fig. 21.8). This appearance can mimic pneumonia, which is more common than lung cancer. Differential considerations for chronic consolidation also include lymphoma, organizing pneumonia, and chronic infection. The consolidation may be associated with nodules in the same lobe or in other lobes of either lung, reflecting tumor dissemination via the tracheobronchial tree.

TABLE 21.1 Classification of Nonmucinous Adenocarcinoma and Corresponding Computed Tomography Features

IASLC/ATS/ERS 2011	Computed Tomography Features
Atypical adenomatous hyperplasia	Ground-glass nodule
Adenocarcinoma in situ	Ground-glass nodule (possible solid component)
Minimally invasive adenocarcinoma	Ground-glass nodule Part solid nodule
Lepidic-predominant adenocarcinoma	Part solid nodule Solid nodule
Invasive adenocarcinoma classified by predominant subtype	Part solid nodule with ↑↑ solid component Solid nodule

ATS, American Thoracic Society; *ERS*, European Respiratory Society; *IASLC*, International Association for the Study of Lung Cancer.

The third appearance is that of multiple nodules and masses scattered throughout the lungs (Fig. 21.9).

There is also increased awareness in recent years that adenocarcinoma and SCC can initially present as cystic lesions with progressive increase in wall nodularity, thickness, or size (Fig. 21.10).

Adenocarcinoma can have variable degree of fludeoxyglucose (FDG) avidity. Pre- or minimally invasive, ground-glass attenuation, and small-sized lesions are known to have minimal or absent FDG uptake on PET. The degree of FDG avidity pretreatment has been found to have prognostic value for recurrence and survival in those with stage I NSCLC treated with stereotactic body radiotherapy (SBRT). Please see additional detail regarding PET in Chapter 4.

Squamous Cell Carcinoma

Clinical Features. Squamous cell carcinoma represents approximately 30% of all lung cancers (Box 21.4). There is a strong association with cigarette smoking. SCC is the histologic type most commonly associated with hypercalcemia caused by PTHrP production by the tumor.

Pathologic Features. Squamous cell carcinoma often arises in areas of squamous metaplasia, and there appears to be an orderly progression of alterations in bronchial mucosa in cigarette smokers from squamous metaplasia to invasive carcinoma. Typically, these tumors occur in main, segmental, or subsegmental bronchi, and they grow endobronchially. Bronchial wall invasion occurs with growth proximally along the bronchial mucosa. Spread to regional lymph nodes is common and may occur by direct extension. Central necrosis is a common feature. Histologic features typical for SCCs include the formation of keratin pearls and intercellular bridges.

Imaging Features. The radiologic presentation depends on the location of the tumor. The most common presentation is a central mass in the hilar or perihilar region obstructing the bronchus (Fig. 21.11). Involvement of the

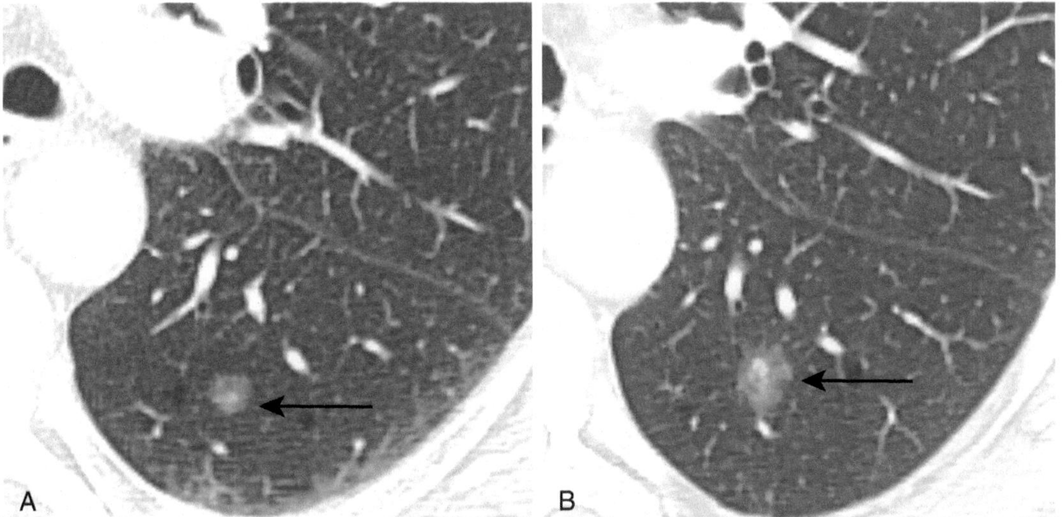

FIGURE 21.6 Lepidic predominant adenocarcinoma (LPA). Computed tomography (CT) image **(A)** shows left lower lobe mixed attenuation lesion *(arrow)* with a soft tissue component measuring less than 3 mm. CT image **(B)** 4 years later shows an increase in the overall size of the lesion *(arrow)* as well as an increase in the size of the soft tissue component now measuring greater than 3 mm. At resection, pathology revealed LPA, with the soft tissue area representing the invasive component.

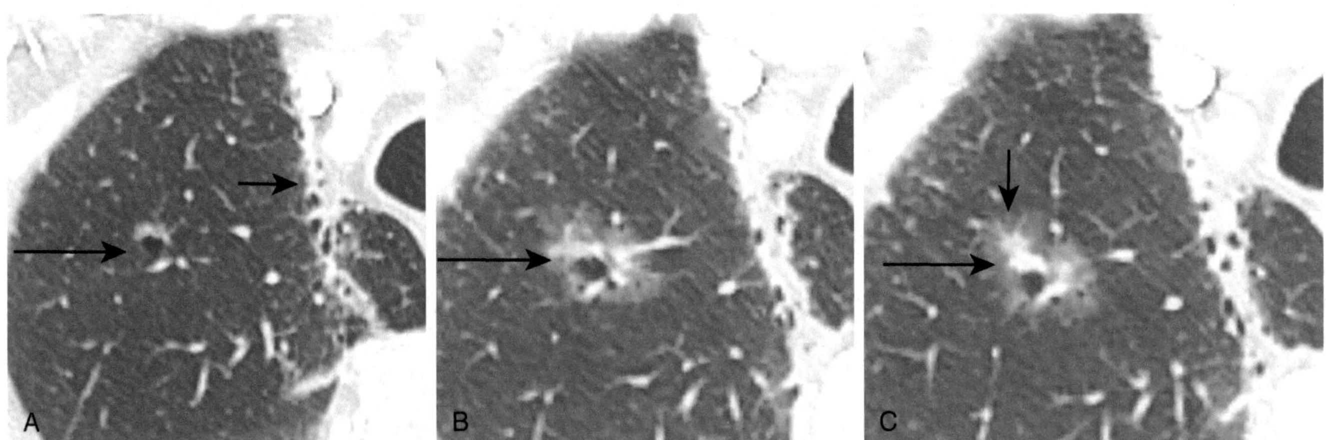

FIGURE 21.7 Lepidic predominant adenocarcinoma (LPA). **A,** Computed tomography (CT) image shows a small lucency *(long arrow)* bordered posteriorly by a vessel and anteriorly by ground-glass opacity. Note radiation fibrosis in the right apex *(short arrow)* with straight margin and traction bronchiectasis. The patient had undergone selective right neck dissection followed by radiation therapy for melanoma 11 years earlier. **B,** CT image 4 years later shows increased ground-glass opacity surrounding the lucency *(arrow)*. **C,** CT image at a level superior to **B** shows a solid component measuring more than 3 mm *(vertical arrow)*. At resection, pathology revealed the mixed attenuation lesion represents LPA, with the soft tissue area representing the invasive component. Adenocarcinomas can show indolent growth and internal bubbly lucencies.

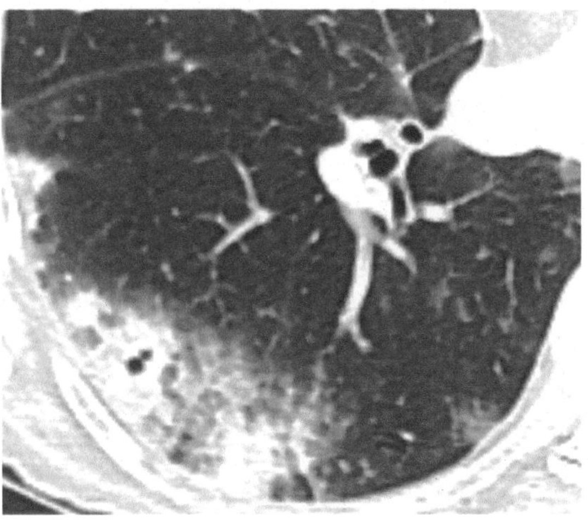

FIGURE 21.8 Adenocarcinoma as consolidative opacity. Computed tomography image shows area of consolidation in the periphery of the right lower lobe consistent with adenocarcinoma.

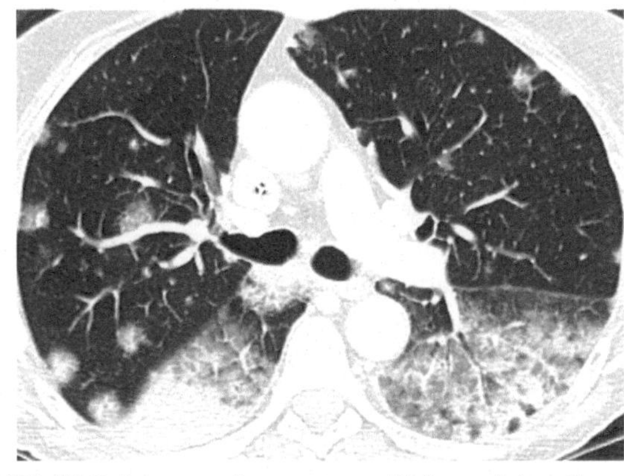

FIGURE 21.9 Adenocarcinoma as multiple nodules. Computed tomography image shows multifocal adenocarcinoma with consolidative and ground-glass opacities in the lower lobes and mixed attenuation nodules in the upper lobes.

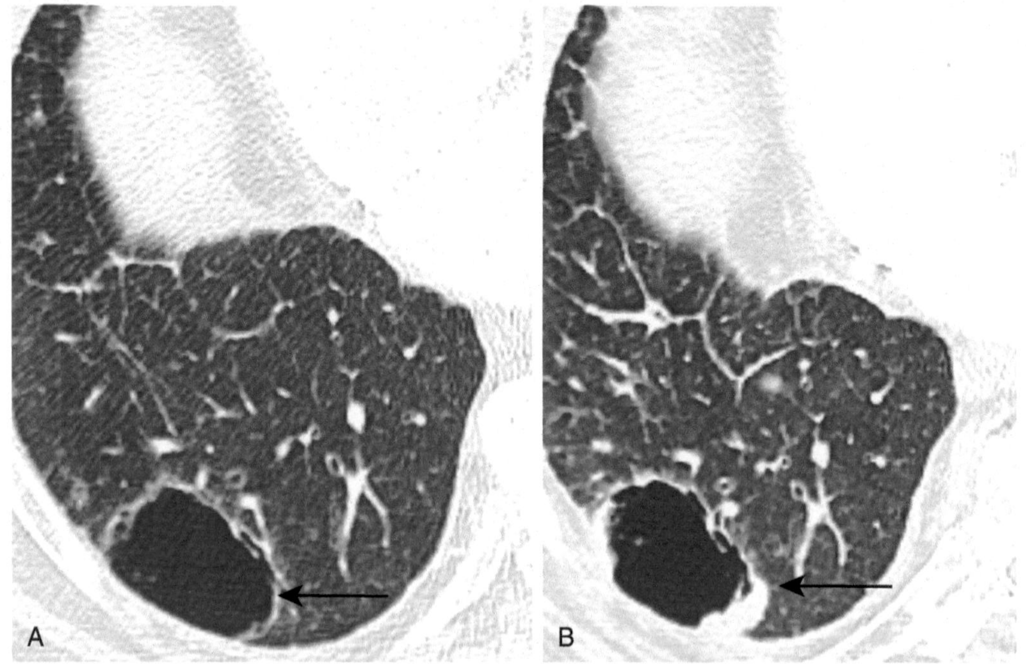

FIGURE 21.10 Adenocarcinoma as nodular thickening of wall of cystic airspace. **A,** Computed tomography (CT) image shows air-filled thin wall cyst in the right lower lobe *(arrow)*. **B,** Follow-up CT 1 year later shows nodular thickening of the wall of the air-filled cyst *(arrow)*. Biopsy confirmed adenocarcinoma.

BOX 21.4 Squamous Cell Carcinoma

CLINICAL FEATURES

One third of all lung cancers
Hypercalcemia related to parathyroid hormone–related protein production

PATHOLOGIC FEATURES

Central, endobronchial location
Local metastases to lymph nodes
Central necrosis

IMAGING FEATURES

Two thirds in central location
Endobronchial lesion best seen on computed tomography
Postobstructive atelectasis or pneumonia of the lung or lobe
One third in peripheral location
Thick-walled, cavitary mass
Solitary nodule

BOX 21.5 Superior Sulcus Tumor

CLINICAL FEATURES

Pain in shoulder and ulnar nerve distribution
Horner syndrome: stellate ganglion involvement
Bone destruction (upper thoracic vertebral bodies, ribs)
Atrophy of hand muscles

PATHOLOGIC FEATURES

Most common: adenocarcinoma

IMAGING FEATURES

Apical mass or asymmetric thickening
Bone destruction
Magnetic resonance imaging best for brachial plexus involvement

central bronchus may range from focal thickening to complete occlusion. When the lesion is small, the tumor may not be evident on chest radiography, but the bronchial wall abnormalities are more readily detected on CT. Atelectasis or postobstructive pneumonia is usually identified distal to the obstructed bronchus. Any patient presenting with lobar collapse and signs of infection should be followed radiographically to complete resolution with reexpansion of the involved lobe. Persistent atelectasis strongly suggests a central lung carcinoma.

Approximately one third of SCC occurs in the lung periphery. The most characteristic appearance is a thick-walled cavitary nodule or mass that usually does not contain an air–fluid level. The diameter ranges from 2 to 10 cm (Fig. 21.12). The cavitary malignancy may be indistinguishable from a lung abscess based on imaging. A solitary nodule or mass without cavitation can occur in the periphery of the lung parenchyma.

Squamous cell carcinoma is usually FDG avid, although the central necrotic region can be photopenic. PET, MRI, or dual-energy CT is often helpful in distinguishing central tumor from adjacent postobstructive atelectasis.

Superior Sulcus Tumor

Clinical Features. Superior sulcus tumor (Box 21.5) is not a distinct pathologic entity. It refers to NSCLC arising in the lung apex and is also known as Pancoast tumor. In recent series, adenocarcinomas have accounted for the majority of superior sulcus tumors, although in earlier series, SCC were predominant. Superior sulcus tumors

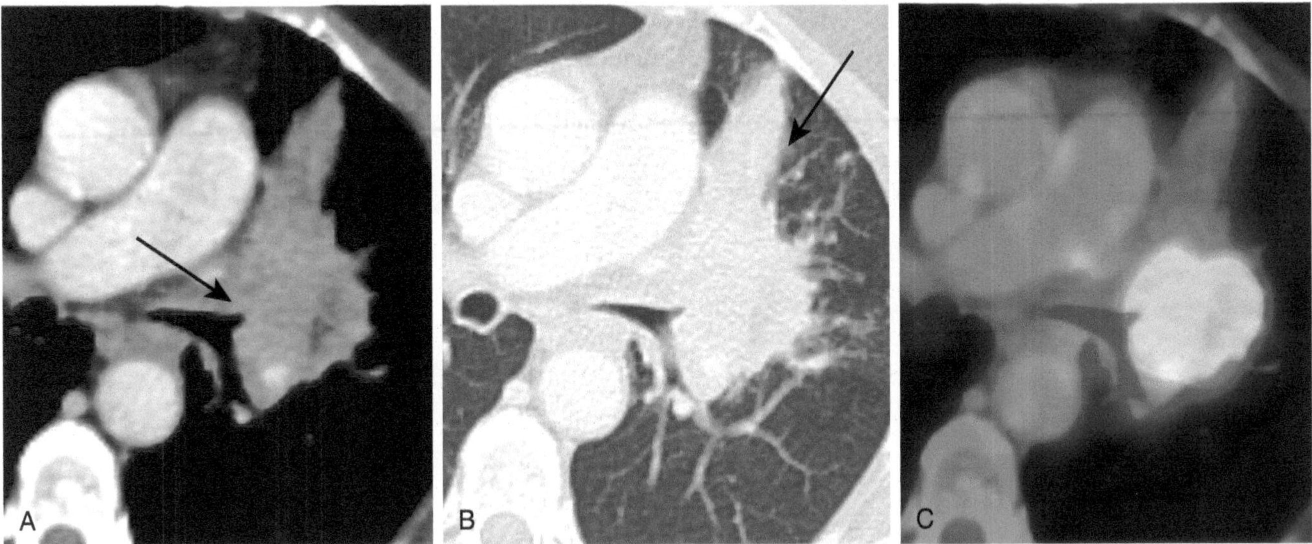

FIGURE 21.11 Squamous cell lung cancer. Computed tomography (CT) **(A)** shows a partially necrotic central left upper lobe mass with cut-off of the left upper lobe bronchus *(arrow)* and **(B)** associated wedge-shaped postobstructive atelectasis *(arrow)*. Positron emission tomography/CT **(C)** is useful in delineating the primary tumor from the adjacent atelectasis.

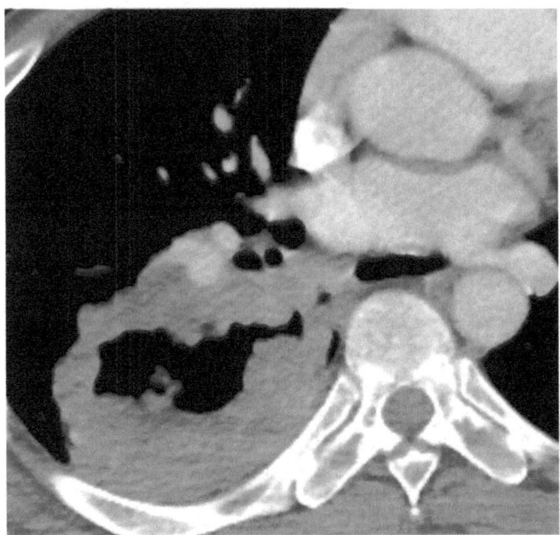

FIGURE 21.12 Squamous cell lung cancer. Computed tomography image shows a large cavitary mass in the right lower lobe consistent with squamous cell lung cancer.

BOX 21.6 Small Cell Lung Carcinoma

CLINICAL FEATURES

Most aggressive subtype
Strongest association with smoking
Poorest survival
Accounts for 15% to 20% of cancers
Treated with chemotherapy
Inappropriate ADH production, ectopic ACTH

PATHOLOGIC FEATURES

Central tumor
Tumor necrosis

IMAGING FEATURES

Hilar or perihilar mass
Massive adenopathy, often bilateral
Lobar collapse
Peripheral nodule

ACTH, Adrenocorticotropic hormone; *ADH,* antidiuretic hormone.

often cause Pancoast syndrome, which is pain in the shoulder girdle and ulnar nerve distribution of the arm and hand. Horner syndrome, characterized by ipsilateral anhidrosis of the face, miosis, and ptosis with narrowing of the palpebral fissure caused by paralysis of the Muller muscle, is seen when the stellate ganglion is involved. These tumors typically invade the chest wall and extend into the neck. Local extension may result in involvement of the brachial plexus, spread to the vertebral bodies and spinal canal, involvement of the sympathetic ganglion, and anterior extension with invasion of the subclavian artery. In patients with potentially resectable tumor, multimodality treatment in which surgery (en bloc resection of the tumor and chest wall) is combined with pre- or postoperative radiation therapy, with or without chemotherapy now forms the standard of care for patients with superior sulcus tumors.

Imaging Features. Brachial plexus involvement is suspected when tumor infiltration of the interscalene triangle and around the subclavian artery is observed on CT. MRI is the preferred modality for evaluating superior sulcus tumors because it allows visualization of structures at the apex of the thorax in multiple planes (Fig. 21.13).

Neuroendocrine Tumors

Small Cell Lung Carcinoma

Clinical Features. Small cell lung carcinoma, the most aggressive form of lung cancer, is characterized by rapid growth and early metastases, which are seen in two thirds of patients at the time of presentation (Box 21.6). It is associated with the poorest prognosis and has the strongest association with cigarette smoking. It accounts for approximately 15% to 20% of all lung cancers.

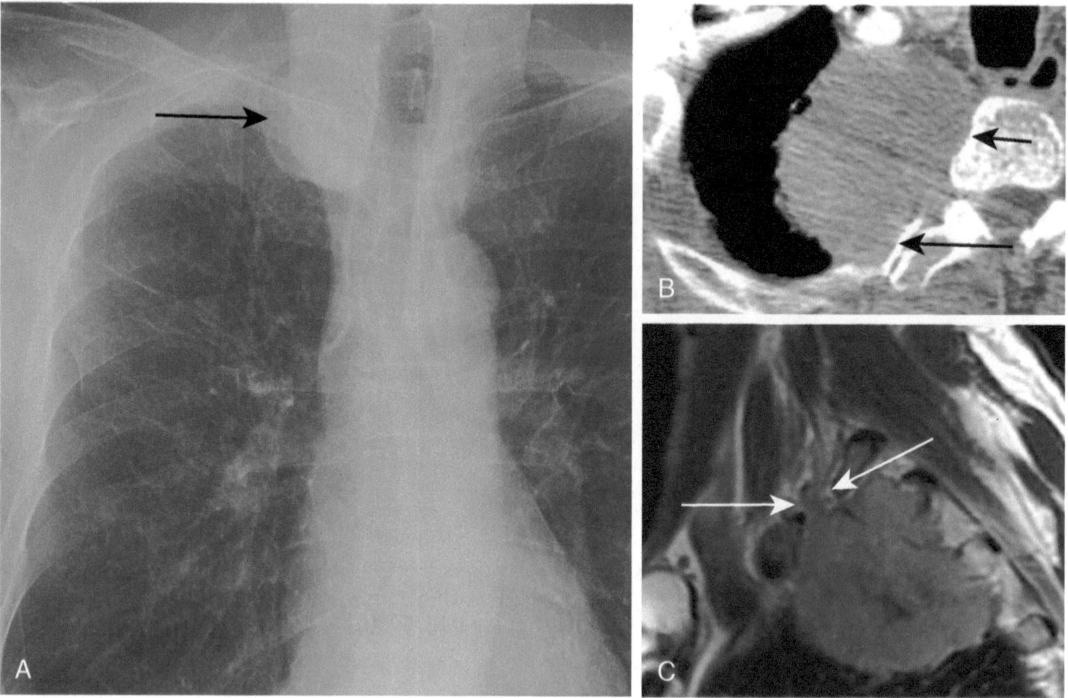

FIGURE 21.13 Pancoast tumor. **A,** Frontal chest radiograph shows right apical mass *(arrow)*. **B,** Computed tomography image shows the right superior sulcus tumor invading the right posterior third rib (long arrow) and right lateral aspect of the T3 vertebra *(short arrow)*. **C,** Sagittal T1-weighted non–contrast-enhanced magnetic resonance image of the brachial plexus shows invasion of the chest wall fat and brachial plexus *(arrows)*.

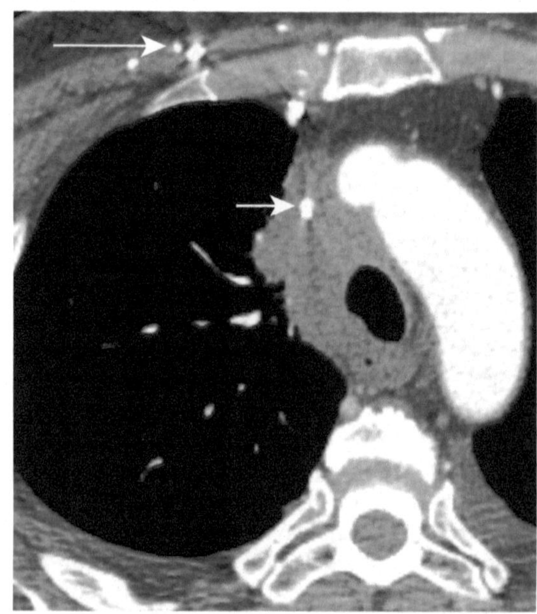

FIGURE 21.14 Small cell lung cancer with superior vena cava (SVC) syndrome. Computed tomography image shows bulky right paratracheal adenopathy encasing and narrowing the SVC *(short arrow)* and multiple collaterals in the right anterior chest wall *(long arrow)*.

Bulky lymphadenopathy associated with SCLC can cause compression of the superior vena cava (SVC) and lead to SVC syndrome (facial swelling, dyspnea, and headache) (Fig. 21.14). SCLC is also associated with Cushing syndrome (central obesity, hypertension, glucose intolerance, plethora, and hirsutism) and SIADH, resulting in hyponatremia and serum hyposmolarity.

When found in the early stage as an isolated pulmonary nodule, SCLC can be resected and is associated with a better prognosis. However, most patients present in the late stage and are often managed with chemotherapy with or without radiation. The long-term survival is extremely poor because of a high rate of recurrence. Even when treated, the median survival time is 9 to 18 months.

Pathologic Features. Small cell lung carcinoma is a high-grade neuroendocrine tumor with more than 10 mitoses per 2 mm^2 that manifests histologically as sheets of small oval to slightly spindle-shaped cells with scant cytoplasm and hyperchromatic nuclei with small to absent nucleoli. SCLC is characterized by extensive tumor necrosis and hemorrhage.

Imaging Features. The primary tumor is typically small and often central in location with extensive and bulky hilar and mediastinal adenopathy (Fig. 21.15). Rarely, SCLC manifests as a small, peripheral, solitary nodule. SCLC tends to exhibit avid FDG uptake.

Large Cell Neuroendocrine Carcinoma

Clinical Features. Large cell neuroendocrine carcinomas (LCNEC) account for 3% of lung cancers in surgical series and have a strong association with cigarette smoking. They are characterized by rapid growth, early metastases, and a poor prognosis.

Pathologic Features. Similar to SCLC, LCNEC is a high-grade neuroendocrine tumor with more than 10 mitoses per 2 mm^2. It is characterized by large cells with low nuclear to cytoplasmic ratio. Typically, these tumors are peripheral

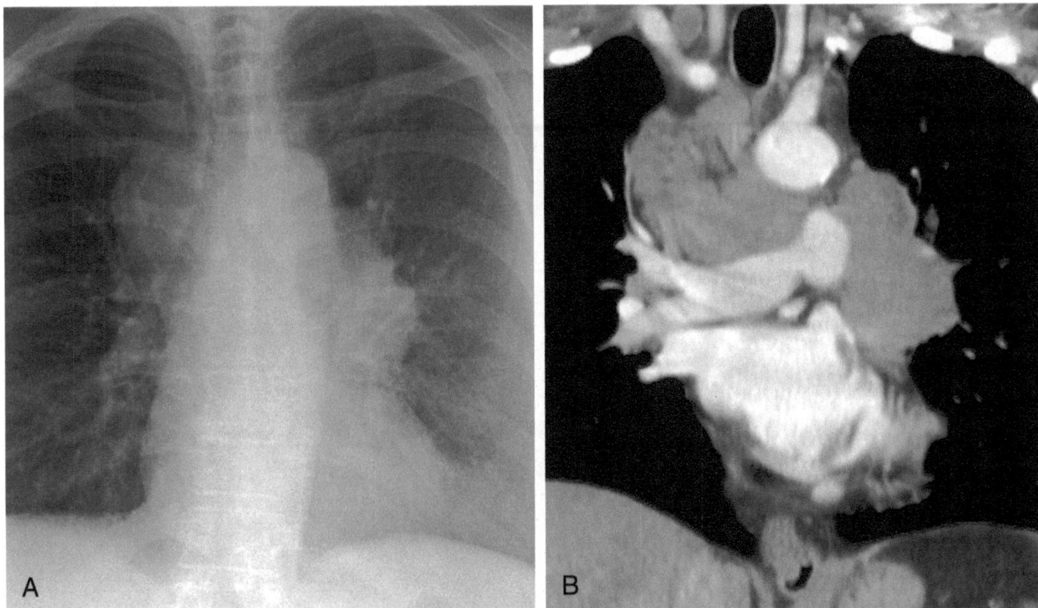

FIGURE 21.15 Small cell lung cancer. Frontal radiograph **(A)** and coronal contrast-enhanced computed tomography **(B)** images show left upper lobe central mass with bulky mediastinal adenopathy. Biopsy showed small cell lung cancer.

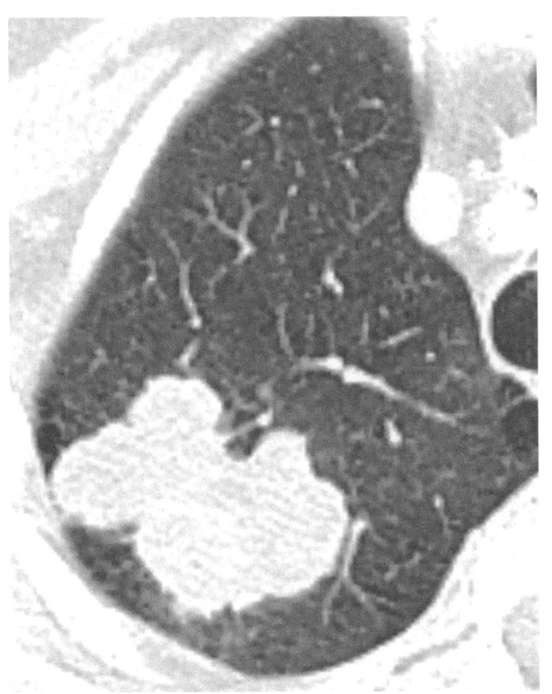

FIGURE 21.16 Large cell lung cancer. Computed tomography image shows a lobular mass in the right upper lobe consistent with large cell lung cancer.

in location. On gross inspection, they are large, with mean diameter of 3 to 4 cm with areas of necrosis.

Imaging Features. The lesions are usually peripheral and quite large (Fig. 21.16).

Carcinoid Tumors

Clinical Features. Carcinoid tumors are low-grade malignant neoplasms that represent between 1% and 2% of all primary pulmonary malignancies (Box 21.7). Males and females are equally affected over a wide age range. The median age is 50 years. There is no association with cigarette smoking. Patients may present with cough and hemoptysis. Carcinoid tumors may be associated with ectopic hormone production, specifically ACTH. However, these tumors do not produce the clinical carcinoid syndrome unless liver metastases are present. Typical carcinoid (TC) tumors rarely metastasize, but atypical carcinoid (AC) tumors metastasize in 40% to 50% of patients. AC tumors are usually peripheral in location and account for 10% of carcinoid

BOX 21.7 Carcinoid Tumors

CLINICAL FEATURES

Median age at diagnosis: 50 years
Men and women equally affected
Cough, hemoptysis
Good prognosis

PATHOLOGIC FEATURES

Typical carcinoid: <2 mitoses per 2 mm^2
Atypical carcinoid: 2–10 mitoses per 2 mm^2
- Rare; 10% of carcinoid tumors
- Lymph node involvement and distant metastases more likely

Neurosecretory granules

IMAGING FEATURES

Central location in 80% of cases
- Lobar, segmental, subsegmental bronchi
- Hilar mass
- Postobstructive atelectasis or pneumonia

Peripheral location in 20% of cases
- Slow growth if typical
- Faster growth if atypical

Avid contrast enhancement
Calcification on computed tomography

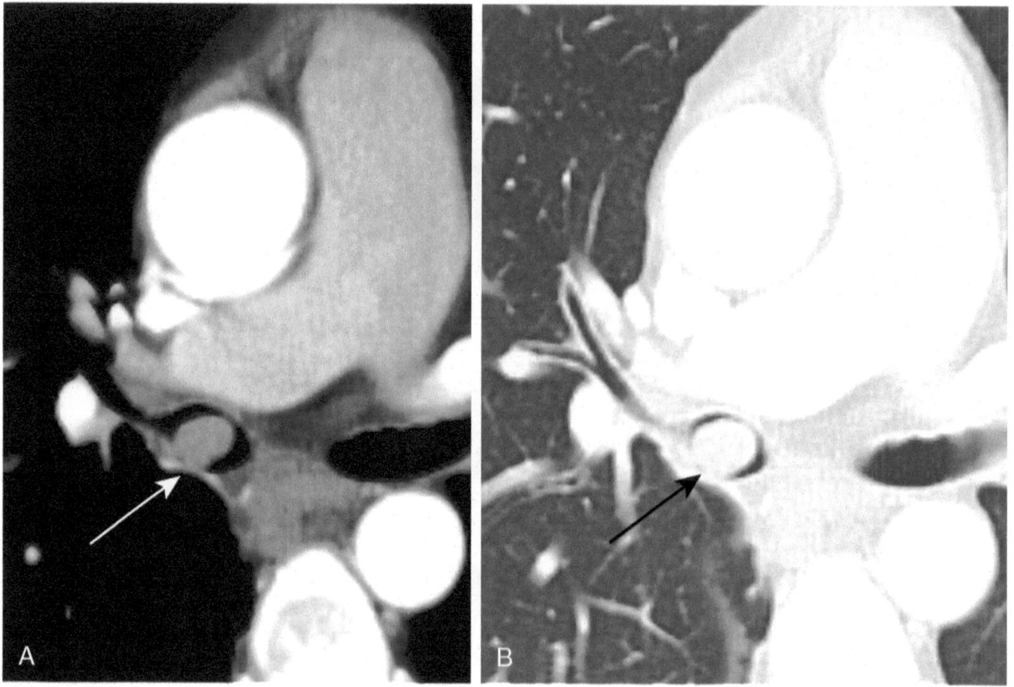

FIGURE 21.17 Carcinoid. Computed tomography images (**A** and **B**) show a mildly enhancing soft tissue nodule in the right mainstem bronchus consistent with carcinoid *(arrow).*

tumors. They may be associated with involvement of hilar and mediastinal lymph nodes and distant metastases, such as the liver or bone.

The prognosis is good, with a 5-year survival rate of approximately 90% for TC and up to 80% for AC tumors.

Pathologic Features. Typical carcinoid tumors are low-grade neuroendocrine tumors with less than 2 mitoses per 2 mm^2. AC tumors are intermediate-grade neuroendocrine tumors with 2 to 10 mitoses per 2 mm^2. Carcinoid tumors are composed of small cells that are arranged in nests or trabeculae separated by thin fibrovascular stroma. Electron microscopy studies show an ultrastructure consisting of neurosecretory granules.

Imaging Features. Carcinoid tumors may be centrally (80%) or peripherally (20%) located and can arise in the lobar, segmental, or subsegmental bronchi. They may appear as a small endobronchial nodule or a hilar or perihilar mass with associated postobstructive pneumonia and atelectasis (Fig. 21.17). Because of their indolent growth, carcinoid tumors may produce low-grade infection with bronchiectasis in the involved lobe. TC tumors in the lung periphery show a slow rate of growth, and carcinoid tumors should be considered in the differential diagnosis of slow-growing solitary pulmonary nodules. AC tumors also occur in the lung periphery and are usually large. Only a small percentage of carcinoid tumors contain visible calcification on CT. Carcinoid tumors may demonstrate intense enhancement after intravenous contrast administration because of their increased vascularity (Fig. 21.18). When present, osseous metastases are usually sclerotic.

Carcinoid tumors usually demonstrate no or low-level FDG uptake, with higher uptake in AC than TC tumors. PET with Ga-68–labeled somatostatin analogues is more sensitive for detecting TC than AC tumors. Octreotide scan can also be used to diagnose and locate occult carcinoid tumors.

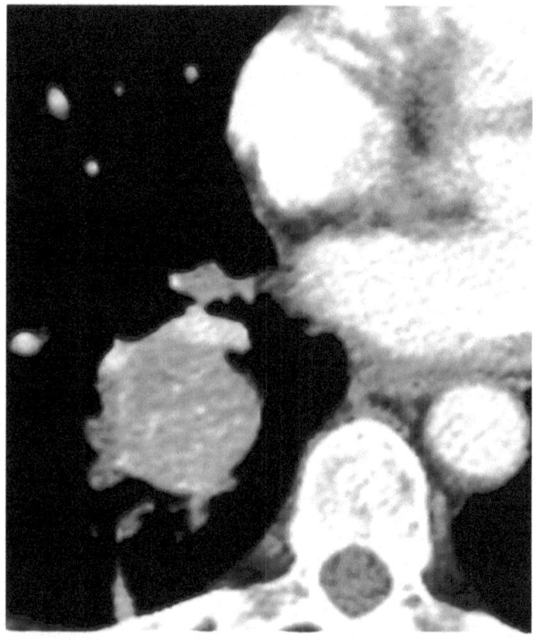

FIGURE 21.18 Carcinoid. Axial computed tomography image shows a lobular right lower lobe mass with enhancement. Biopsy showed atypical carcinoid.

Sarcomatoid Carcinoma

These are rare tumors accounting for fewer than 1% of all lung cancers.

Carcinosarcoma

Clinical Features

Carcinosarcomas are rare tumors that occur mainly in middle-aged and elderly men. They are aggressive tumors with a poor prognosis and are characterized by locoregional invasion and widespread metastases.

Pathologic Features

These tumors consist of an epithelial component of SCC or adenocarcinoma and a mesenchymal component, most commonly of the spindle cell type. TP53 mutations are often present.

Imaging Features

The radiologic features vary according to tumor location and may consist of a large, peripheral, well-circumscribed mass or a central lesion with atelectasis and postobstructive pneumonia. There is an upper lobe predominance. Disease may extend to the pleura, chest wall, and mediastinum.

Pulmonary Blastoma

Clinical Features

The tumor shows a biphasic age distribution occurring predominantly in males in the first and seventh decades of life. It is associated with a poor prognosis.

Pathologic Features

Pulmonary blastoma consists of fetal adenocarcinoma and primitive mesenchymal stroma.

Imaging Features

The radiologic findings consist of a well-circumscribed, large, peripheral mass with occasional pleural invasion and metastases (Fig. 21.19).

MESENCHYMAL TUMORS

Pulmonary hamartoma is the most common benign mesenchymal tumor in the lungs. Chondroma is also a benign mesenchymal tumor. Malignant mesenchymal tumors are rare, including synovial sarcoma and pulmonary artery intimal sarcoma (see Chapter 11).

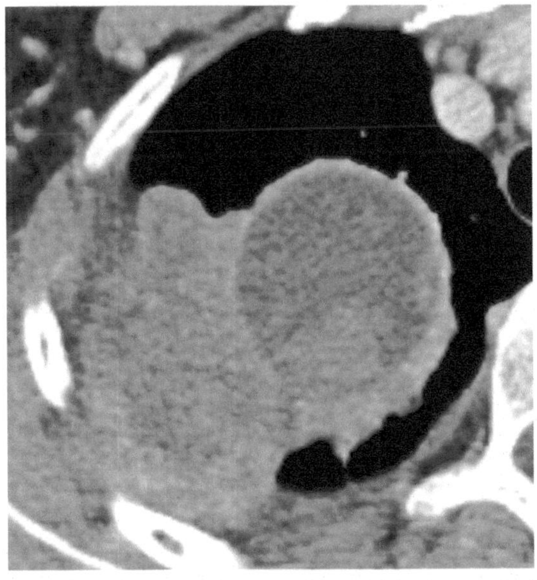

FIGURE 21.19 Pulmonary blastoma. Computed tomography image shows a large necrotic mass in the right upper lobe with pleural invasion.

Pulmonary Hamartoma

Clinical Features

Hamartoma accounts for 5% to 8% of solitary pulmonary nodules (Box 21.8). The peak incidence occurs in the sixth decade of life, with an age range of 30 to 70 years. The lesions show slight predominance in women. Most patients are asymptomatic, and the hamartoma is discovered on routine chest radiography as a solitary pulmonary nodule. Occasionally, hamartomas can arise in a bronchus and may produce obstructive symptoms.

Pathologic Features

Based on genetic studies, pulmonary hamartomas are now considered neoplasms. They are composed of varying amounts of at least two mesenchymal elements (cartilage, fat, myxoid fibrous connective tissue, bone, or smooth muscle), combined with entrapped respiratory epithelium.

Imaging Features

Pulmonary hamartomas typically appear as well-defined, solitary, round nodules or masses, usually less than 4 cm in diameter. Calcification is seen in 10% to 15% of cases on standard radiographs and 25% of the cases on CT. The calcification has a characteristic "popcorn" appearance. Hamartomas typically show slow growth and in rare cases can be multiple.

Thin-collimation CT can be valuable in diagnosing pulmonary hamartomas. The presence of focal deposits of fat on CT (−50 to −150 HU) in a well-circumscribed lesion with slow growth is diagnostic of hamartoma (Fig. 21.20). Internal fat can also be demonstrated on MRI.

METASTATIC TUMORS

Pulmonary metastases represent the most common lung neoplasms. The most common sites of primary malignancies include the lung, breast, colon, pancreas, stomach, skin (i.e., melanoma), head and neck, and kidney. The probability of lung metastasis increases with advanced tumor stage.

Metastatic disease to the lungs may occur via three routes of spread: hematogenous, lymphatic, and endobronchial.

Hematogenous Metastases

Clinical Features

Hematogenous spread via the pulmonary arterial system is the most common cause of pulmonary involvement.

BOX 21.8 Pulmonary Hamartomas

CLINICAL FEATURES

Patients 30 to 70 years old
Usually asymptomatic

PATHOLOGIC FEATURES

Nests of cartilage surrounded by fibrous tissue and mature fat cells
May contain bone, vessels, and smooth muscle

IMAGING FEATURES

Solitary, well-defined pulmonary nodule
Popcorn calcification
Internal fat density on computed tomography diagnostic

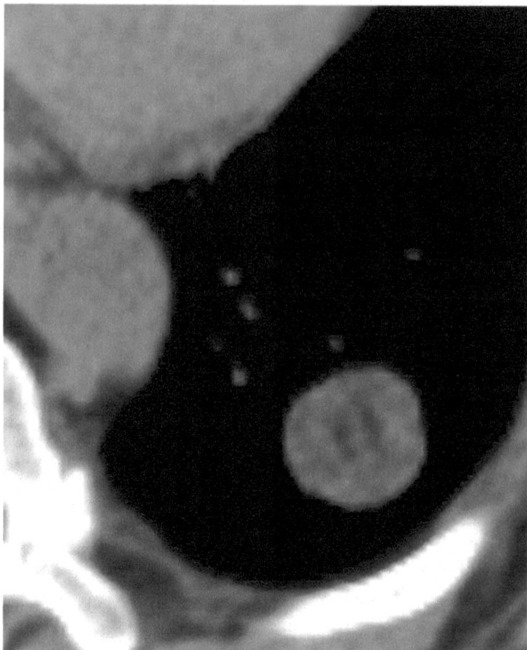

FIGURE 21.20 Hamartoma. Computed tomography image shows well-circumscribed nodule in the left lower lobe with internal fat attenuation of -50 Hounsfield units consistent with a hamartoma.

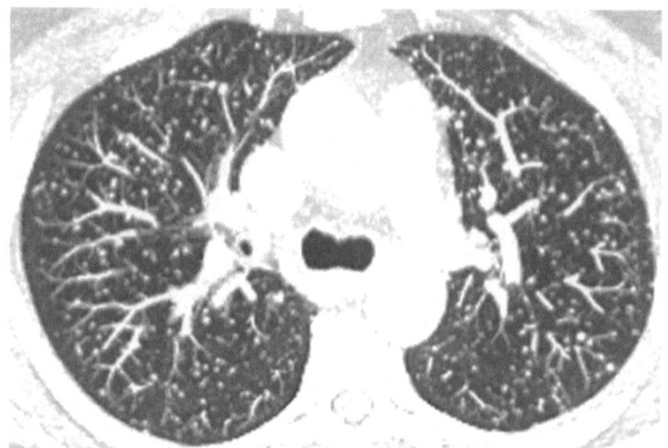

FIGURE 21.21 Hematogenous metastases with miliary pattern. Computed tomography maximal intensity projection image shows small lung nodules in a random distribution caused by metastatic disease from thyroid cancer.

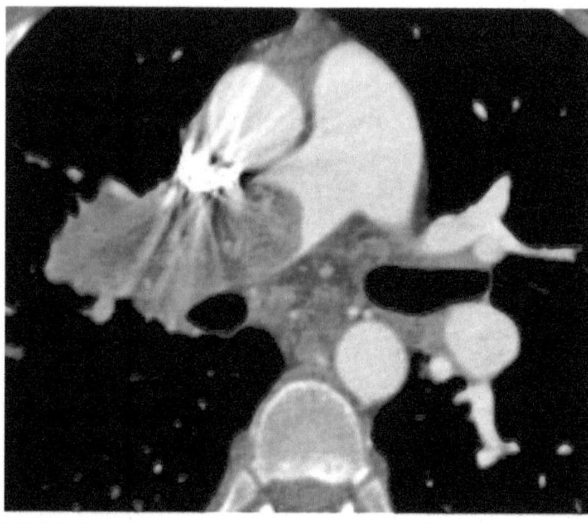

FIGURE 21.22 Hematogenous metastasis with tumor emboli in a patient with sarcoma of the forearm. Computed tomography image shows enhancing soft tissue mass within and expanding the right main pulmonary artery and right upper lobe pulmonary artery.

Incidence of malignant lung metastasis presenting as a solitary nodule is less than 10% and can occur in patients with sarcoma and carcinomas of the colon, breast, bladder, kidney, and testicle. In an adult with a head and neck primary SCC, a solitary nodule is more likely to represent a primary lung cancer than a metastasis. If the primary tumor is an adenocarcinoma, the likelihood of the lung nodule representing a solitary metastasis is equal to the incidence of a second primary tumor. In contradistinction, in a patient with melanoma or sarcoma, a solitary metastasis is more likely.

Pathologic Features

In addition to the malignancies mentioned earlier, benign tumors including leiomyoma of the uterus, hydatidiform mole (a gestational trophoblastic neoplasm), giant cell tumor of bone, chondroblastoma, pleomorphic adenoma of the salivary glands, and meningioma can also produce hematogenous metastases.

Imaging Features

Metastases typically present with multiple bilateral round and well-circumscribed solid lung nodules and masses with predominance in the lower lobes caused by the increased blood flow to the lung bases. Between 80% and 90% of metastases occur in the lung periphery near the pleura. Lung metastases can vary in size from 1 mm to 5 cm or larger. Small miliary nodules are seen in metastases from hypervascular primary tumors such thyroid cancer, renal cell cancer, and melanoma (Fig. 21.21).

On CT, pulmonary metastases usually appear as solid lesions. Vascular tumors such as choriocarcinoma, angiosarcoma, melanoma, and renal cell carcinoma can have metastases with perilesional hemorrhage, resulting in ground-glass halos. Irregular margins can be seen in treated or hemorrhagic metastases. Calcification may occur in metastatic lesions from osteosarcoma, chondrosarcoma, and papillary and mucinous adenocarcinomas of the gastrointestinal tract or breast. Sometimes a pulmonary artery can be seen leading to a metastasis. In cases of tumor embolization to the pulmonary arterial vessels, the arterial vascular branches may be thickened and beaded and demonstrate incremental growth over time (Figs. 21.22 and 21.23). Cavitation is uncommon but can be seen in metastases from SCC (arising from the head and neck in men and the cervix in women) and transitional cell carcinoma, which may be thin walled. Occasionally, a metastasis, particularly in osteosarcoma, located in the subpleural location may rupture into the pleural space, resulting in a pneumothorax.

The growth rates of hematogenous metastases show considerable variation, with volume doubling time ranging from 1 to 2 weeks for some sarcomas (Fig. 21.24) and melanomas to years for some thyroid carcinomas.

Lymphangitic Metastases

Clinical Features

Common primary sites of origin include carcinomas of the lung, breast, stomach, and pancreas. The process can be

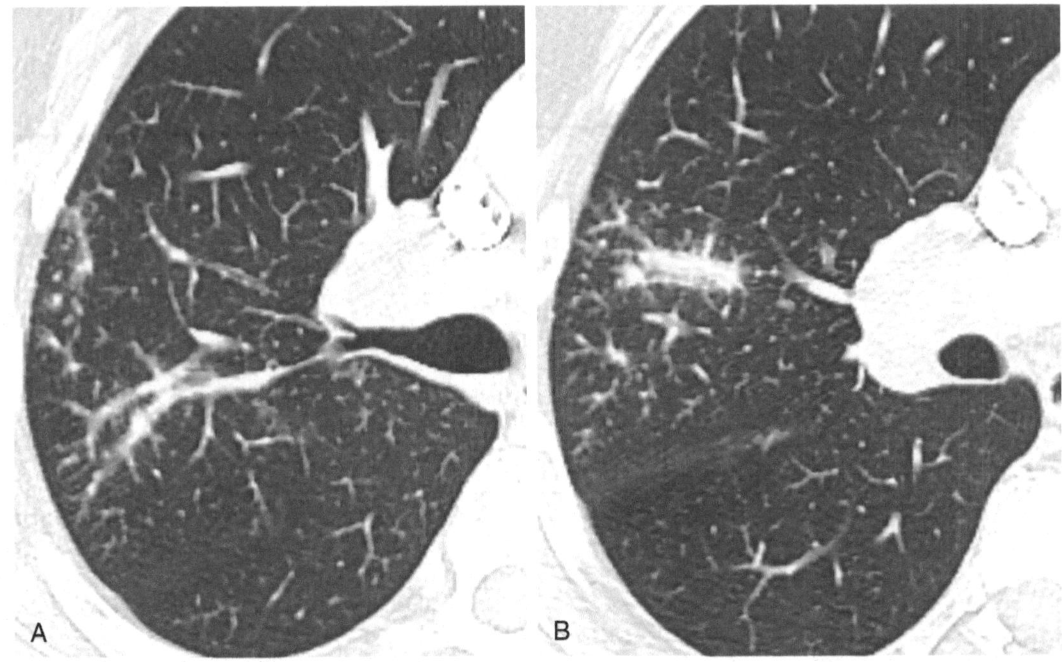

FIGURE 21.23 Tumor emboli in metastatic renal cell cancer. Computed tomography images (**A** and **B**) show dilation and beading of the branches of the right upper lobe posterior segmental pulmonary artery consistent with tumor emboli.

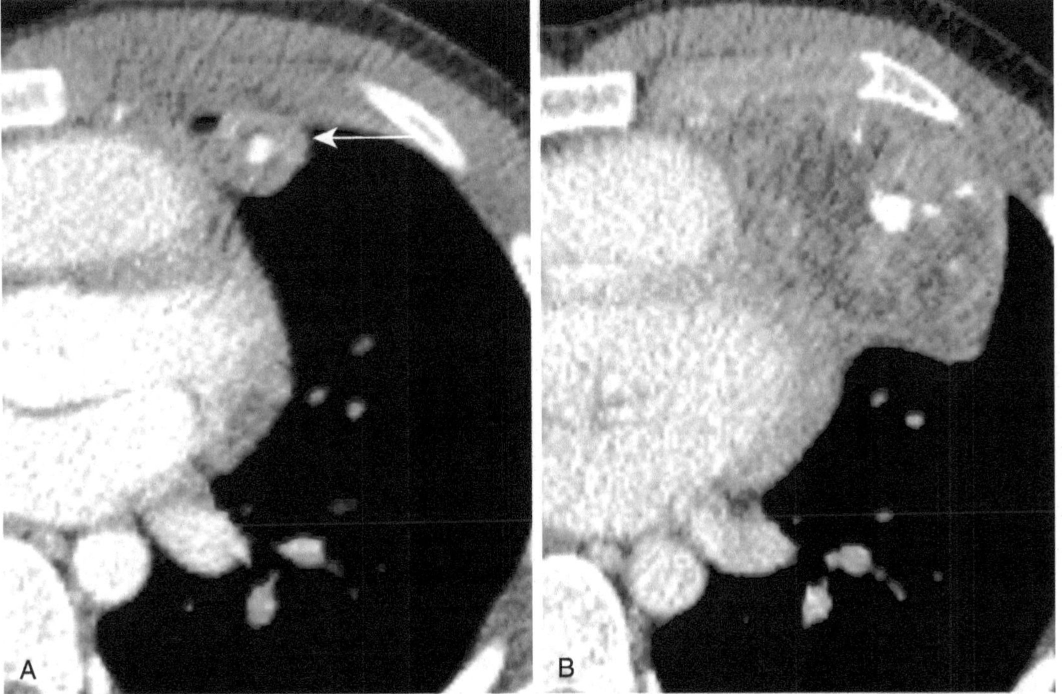

FIGURE 21.24 Hematogenous metastasis with calcification and rapid growth. Computed tomography (CT) image **(A)** shows an osteosarcoma metastasis in the lingula *(arrow)*. Central calcification mimics the calcification pattern of granulomatous disease. Follow-up CT image **(B)** demonstrates rapid growth of the nodule consistent with a metastasis.

unilateral or bilateral. In lung cancer, lymphangitic spread may occur in the ipsilateral or contralateral lung.

Pathologic Features

Usually the result of hematogenous dissemination with secondary invasion of the lymphatic system, lymphangitic spread of tumor involves the pulmonary capillaries, lymphatics, and surrounding interstitium. Less frequently, lymphangitic carcinomatosis can result from retrograde spread from the mediastinal and hilar lymph nodes.

Imaging Features

The mixed reticulonodular pattern on radiography represents thickening of the interlobular septae (Kerley B lines).

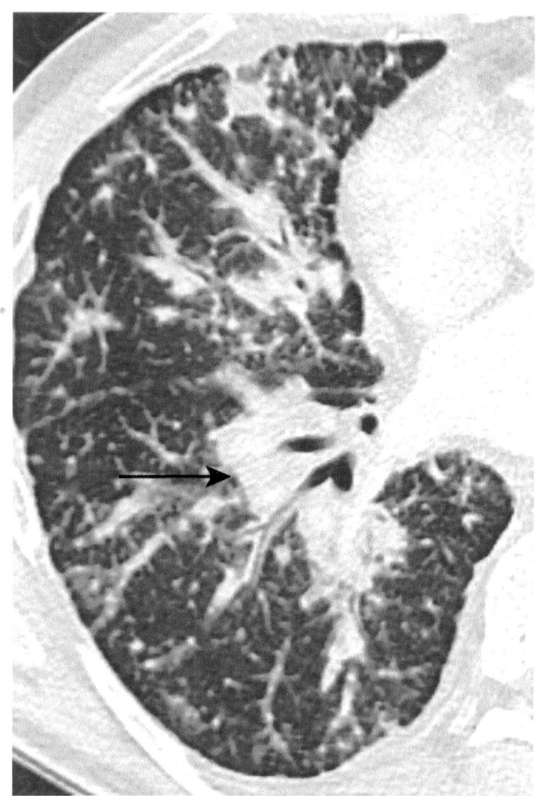

FIGURE 21.25 Lymphangitic carcinomatosis diffusely in the right lung caused by non–small cell lung cancer. Computed tomography shows the primary tumor in the right infrahilar region *(arrow)* with diffuse lymphangitic spread in the right middle and lower lobes with nodular thickening of the bronchovascular bundles, bronchial wall thickening, and septal thickening.

Lymphangitic spread of tumor is associated with pleural effusion in 60% of cases and hilar adenopathy in fewer than 25% of cases.

Computed tomography is more sensitive than chest radiography in the diagnosis of lymphangitic carcinomatosis (see Chapter 17). On CT, the typical findings include nodular, irregular, or smooth thickening of the bronchovascular bundles and the interlobular septae (Fig. 21.25). The pattern can be diffuse or focal. Small, isolated nodules and pleural effusions may be identified. Lymphadenopathy is more commonly detected on CT than on standard radiographs. The differential diagnosis includes sarcoidosis and lymphoma.

Endobronchial Metastases

Metastases to major bronchi are uncommon and are discussed in Chapter 6.

Diagnostic Workup

The diagnosis of pulmonary metastases can often be made on standard chest radiographs, and comparison with previous examinations is important. Compared with radiography, CT has markedly higher sensitivity but lower specificity because of its inability to differentiate granulomas and intrapulmonary lymph nodes from small pulmonary metastases. PET imaging when combined with CT is even more sensitive for detecting metastases in the chest.

BOX 21.9 Mucosa-Associated Lymphoid Tissue Lymphoma

CLINICAL FEATURES

Extranodal, marginal zone B-cell lymphoma
Involves bronchus-associated lymphoid tissue
Associated with autoimmune disorders (e.g., Sjögren syndrome)

PATHOLOGIC FEATURES

Low-grade extranodal B-cell lymphoma
Proliferation of small lymphocytes in the bronchiolar mucosa

IMAGING FEATURES

Solitary or multiple, poorly defined nodules or consolidation
±Air bronchograms
±Ground-glass halos

Lung metastases from unknown primary tumors do occur. Unknown primary tumors, typically adenocarcinomas, account for 3% to 4% of all cancers. The average survival time from diagnosis is 3 to 7 months. An extensive imaging search for a primary tumor in these situations is controversial. Needle aspiration biopsy of a lung metastasis may establish the diagnosis and identify the types of adenocarcinomas that may be likely to respond to specific targeted therapies (i.e., hormonal therapy in prostate and breast carcinoma). See Chapter 25 for more details.

PULMONARY LYMPHOPROLIFERATIVE DISORDERS

Primary Pulmonary Lymphoma

Primary pulmonary lymphoma (PPL) is defined as clonal lymphoid proliferation affecting one or both lungs without evidence of extrapulmonary disease at diagnosis or during the 3 subsequent months. PPL is rare and accounts for 0.4% of all lymphomas. The more common subtypes are described here.

Mucosa-Associated Lymphoid Tissue Lymphoma

Clinical Features. Mucosa-associated lymphoid tissue (MALT) found along mucosal surfaces serves as a mucosal defense. MALT lymphoma (Box 21.9), the most common type of PPL, accounts for 70% to 90% of cases. The median age of diagnosis is 60 years. Approximately 40% of patients are asymptomatic and diagnosed incidentally by imaging. Cough, weight loss, and fatigue are also common. It is associated with autoimmune disorders such as Sjögren syndrome and systemic lupus erythematosus. Surgical resection or radiation therapy can be performed for localized disease. The 5-year survival rate is greater than 80%.

Pathologic Features. Mucosa-associated lymphoid tissue lymphoma is a non-Hodgkin, low-grade, extranodal B-cell lymphoma characterized by proliferation of small lymphocytes forming a masslike lesion in the bronchiolar mucosa.

Imaging Features. Computed tomography features of thoracic MALT lymphoma include solitary or multiple, poorly defined nodules and foci of consolidation (Fig. 21.26). Air bronchograms are frequently observed in this entity, and the lesions may demonstrate peripheral ground-glass halos. Pleural effusions are uncommon. FDG uptake on PET is usually absent or minimal.

High-Grade B-Cell Lymphoma

Clinical Features. High-grade B-cell lymphoma is the second most common type of PPL and accounts for 5% to 20% of cases. Patients usually present with dyspnea, fever, or weight loss. It is associated with solid organ transplantation, human immunodeficiency virus (HIV) infection, Sjögren syndrome, and Epstein-Barr virus (EBV) infection. Surgical resection can be performed for localized disease, and combination chemotherapy is used for more diffuse pulmonary involvement. The mean survival time is estimated to be 8 to 10 years.

Pathologic Features. High-grade B-cell lymphoma is characterized by blastlike lymphoid cells with high mitotic activity.

Radiographic Features. Computed tomography features of pulmonary high-grade B-cell lymphoma include peribronchial or subpleural consolidations or ground-glass opacities (Fig. 21.27). Pulmonary nodules and masses are reported in 50% of cases.

Lymphomatoid Granulomatosis

Clinical Features. Lymphomatoid granulomatosis (LG) is rare (Box 21.10), usually occurring in patients aged 30 to 50 years with a male-to-female ratio of 2:1. Patients may present with symptoms such as fever, cough, dyspnea, and hemoptysis. LG primarily involves the lungs but may also involve the kidneys, skin, and central nervous system. Surgical biopsy is usually required for diagnosis. It is treated with chemotherapy. Prognosis is highly variable depending on the histologic grade.

Pathologic Features. Lymphomatoid granulomatosis demonstrates angioinvasive lymphoid infiltration composed of lymphocytes, plasma cells, and histiocytes. The malignant B-cells frequently contain EBV. Testing for presence of EBV with in situ hybridization is therefore helpful in establishing the diagnosis. Reactive T cells are often identified. Grading is based on the number of neoplastic large B-cells and degree of cytologic atypia. Grade 3 lesions are treated as large B-cell lymphoma.

Imaging Features. The most common radiographic presentation consists of multiple pulmonary nodules and masses varying in size from 1 to 10 cm. On CT, these lesions have a perilymphatic distribution, occurring along bronchovascular bundles, interlobular septa, and subpleural region. There is a basal lung predominance. Central low attenuation or cavitation, peripheral enhancement, and ground-glass halos have been described for these nodules and masses (Fig. 21.28). These lesions may coalesce, producing a consolidative appearance. Hilar adenopathy is rare. Lesions can demonstrate avid FDG uptake on PET.

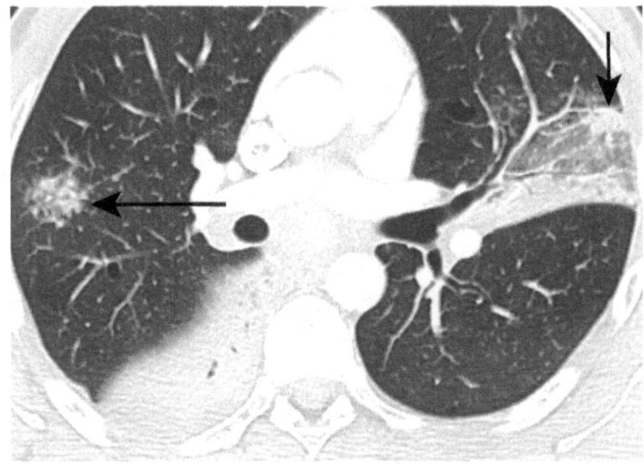

FIGURE 21.26 Mucosa-associated lymphoid tissue lymphoma. Computed tomography image shows consolidative opacities in the right lower lobe and left upper lobe, a mixed attenuation nodule in the right upper lobe *(long arrow)*, and a solid nodule in the left upper lobe *(short arrow)* adjacent to ground-glass opacities. Air bronchograms traverse all lesions.

BOX 21.10 Lymphomatoid Granulomatosis

CLINICAL FEATURES

Occurs in middle age
Men affected more than women

PATHOLOGIC FEATURES

Angioinvasive lymphoid infiltration of lymphocytes, plasma cells, and histiocytes
Frequently contain Epstein-Barr virus

IMAGING FEATURES

Nodules and masses
- Peripheral enhancement
- Central low attenuation
- Ground-glass halo

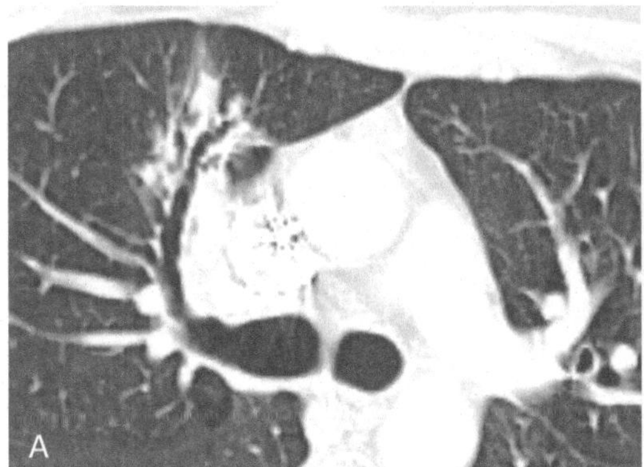

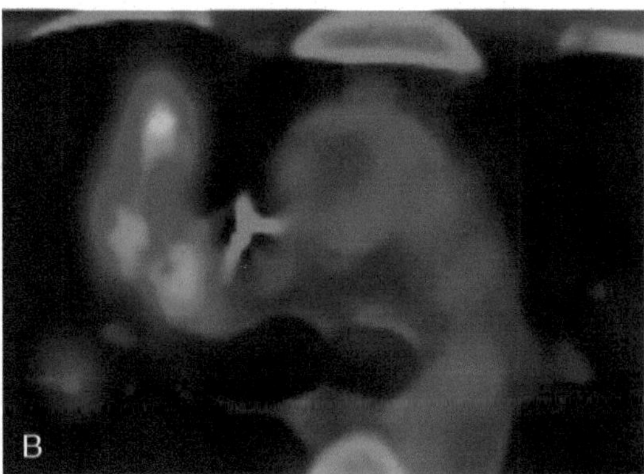

FIGURE 21.27 High-grade B-cell lymphoma. Computed tomography (CT) **(A)** and positron emission tomography/CT **(B)** images show fludeoxyglucose-avid lymphomatous involvement of the right upper lobe spreading out from the hilum in an axial distribution along the bronchovascular bundles.

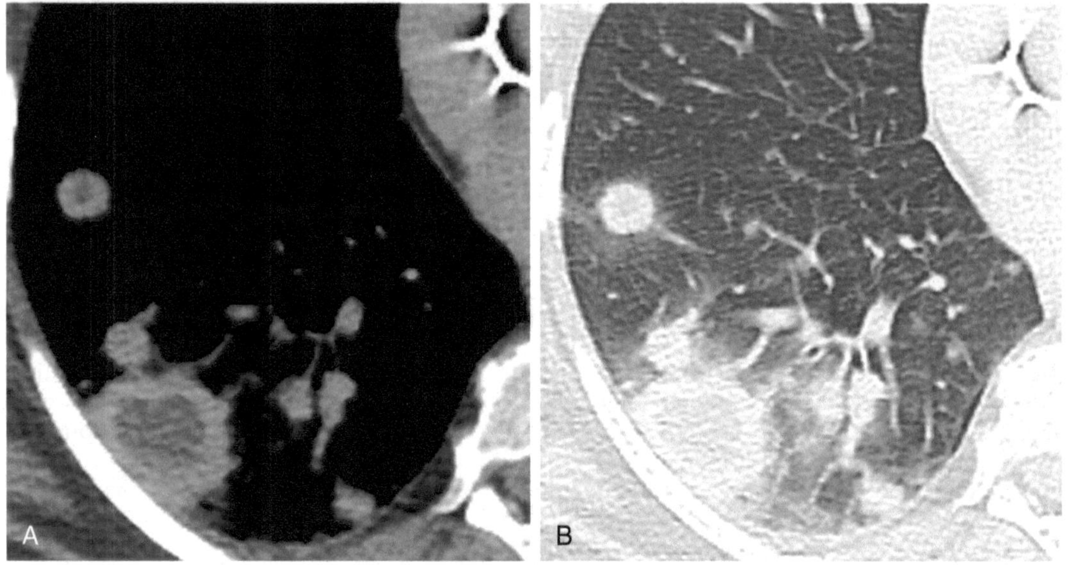

FIGURE 21.28 Lymphomatoid granulomatosis. Computed tomography (**A** and **B**) images show multiple lung nodules of various sizes. In the right lower lobe, some lesions have central low attenuation, subtle peripheral enhancement, and halos of ground-glass attenuation.

Pulmonary Involvement as Part of Systemic Lymphoma

Pulmonary involvement as part of systemic disease is more common than PPL, occurring in approximately 40% of patients with Hodgkin lymphoma (HL) and 25% of patients with non-Hodgkin lymphoma (NHL). The mechanisms include hematogenous dissemination and contiguous invasion from hilar and mediastinal lymph nodes. Imaging findings include single or multiple lung nodules and masses. Consolidative and ground-glass opacities are also common.

Nonneoplastic Pulmonary Lymphoproliferative Disorders

Various nonneoplastic lymphoproliferative disorders may occur in the lung. The lung contains abundant lymphoid tissue along the tracheobronchial tree, subpleural region, and interlobular septae. Bronchial MALT lymphomas are submucosal lymphoid aggregates along the bifurcation of bronchioles and along lymphatic chains. The nonneoplastic pulmonary lymphoproliferative disorders include a wide range of focal and diffuse abnormalities distinguished from neoplastic disorders on the basis of cellular morphology and clonality. Reactive lymphoproliferative diseases are thought to represent hyperplasia of the lymphoid system in response to chronic antigenic stimulation associated with abnormal immune response and includes nodular lymphoid hyperplasia, follicular bronchiolitis, lymphocytic interstitial pneumonia, and inflammatory pseudotumor. IgG4-related disease (IgG4-RD) is increasingly recognized as a systemic disorder that can involve various organ systems, including the lungs.

Nodular Lymphoid Hyperplasia

Clinical Features. Although most patients are asymptomatic, nodular lymphoid hyperplasia may be associated with a variety of autoimmune diseases (e.g., Sjögren syndrome) or dysgammaglobulinemias. It is usually found incidentally on imaging studies. It affects middle-aged patients with an equal sex distribution. It was previously described as pseudolymphoma because of its similarity to low-grade lymphoma. Surgical resection is sometimes necessary to establish the diagnosis. The prognosis is excellent.

Pathologic Features. Dense nodular infiltration of polyclonal T- and B-cell lymphocytes and plasma cells with multiple reactive germinal centers are observed in nodular lymphoid hyperplasia, usually along bronchovascular bundles and interlobular septa. In contrast, MALT lymphoma consists of a monoclonal population of lymphocytes.

Imaging Features. Nodular lymphoid hyperplasia usually manifests as a focal nodular consolidative opacity with or without air bronchograms (Fig. 21.29). The focal consolidation is typically 2 to 4 cm in diameter and may be subpleural in location. Rarely, multiple lesions can be seen. Lymphadenopathy and pleural effusions are usually absent.

Follicular Bronchiolitis

Follicular bronchiolitis is an uncommon lymphoproliferative disorder and is discussed in Chapter 6.

Lymphocytic Interstitial Pneumonia

Clinical Features. Lymphocytic interstitial pneumonia (LIP) is usually associated with underlying diseases with alterations of immune function, such as HIV infection, common variable immunodeficiency, and Sjögren syndrome. In the setting of HIV infection, LIP is predominantly seen in pediatric patients. LIP in the non-HIV population tends to occur between the ages of 40 and 70 years and is more common in women. Respiratory symptoms such as cough and progressive dyspnea are common. Corticosteroids and other immunosuppressants can be used for treatment. The disease course is variable, and subsequent development or transformation to lymphoma has been reported.

Pathologic Features. On microscopy, dense polymorphous interstitial inflammatory T lymphocytes, plasma cells,

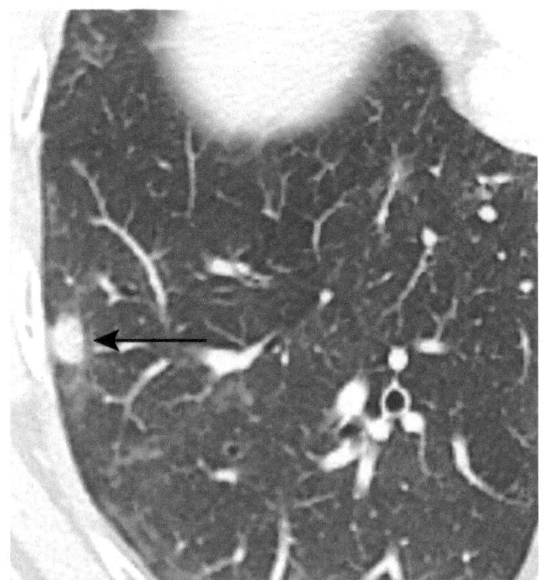

FIGURE 21.29 Nodular lymphoid hyperplasia. Computed tomography image shows a right lower lobe nodule *(arrow)*. Biopsy confirmed nodular lymphoid hyperplasia.

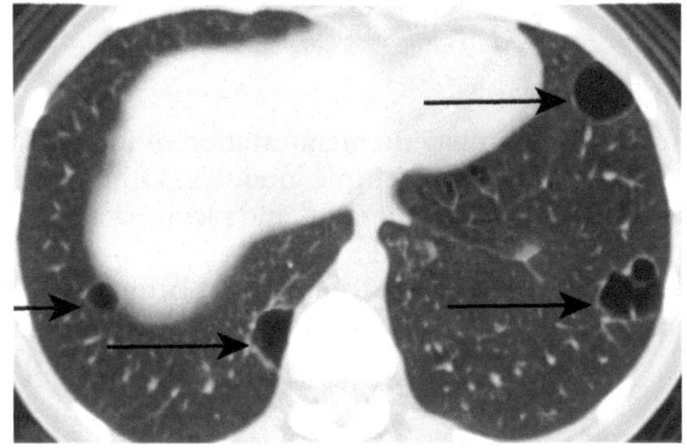

FIGURE 21.30 Lymphocytic interstitial pneumonia. Computed tomography image shows bilateral lung cysts *(arrows)* caused by lymphocytic interstitial pneumonia in a patient with Sjögren syndrome.

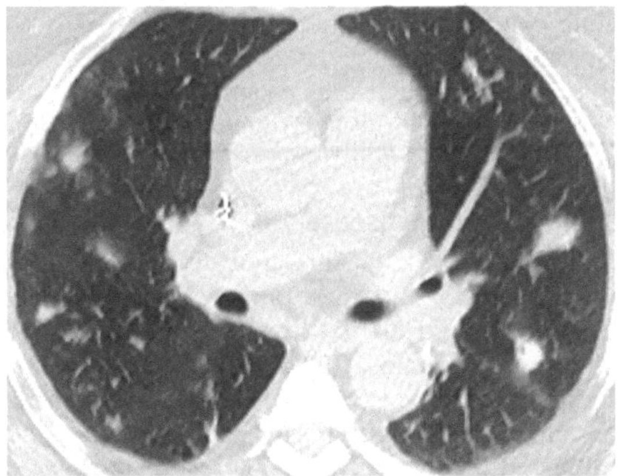

FIGURE 21.31 Inflammatory pseudotumor as multiple lung nodules. Computed tomography image shows bilateral small lung nodules and left hilar adenopathy.

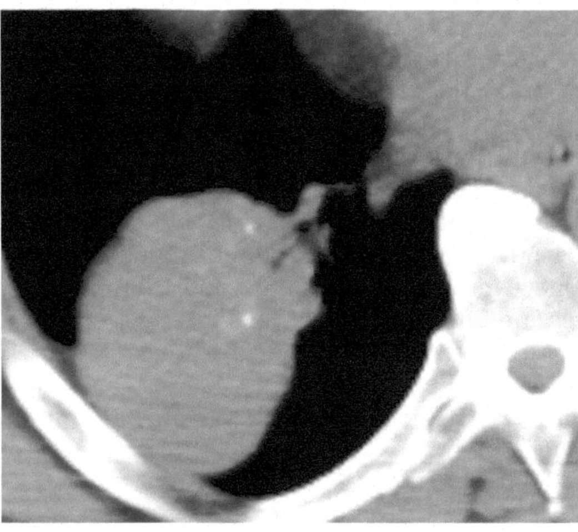

FIGURE 21.32 Inflammatory pseudotumor with calcification. Computed tomography image shows right lower mass with amorphous calcification. Surgical pathology from en bloc resection of the right lower lobe and right hemidiaphragm showed inflammatory pseudotumor with plasma cell variant.

and macrophages are found along alveolar septa and small airways. The cells are polyclonal. The findings are similar to those in follicular bronchiolitis but with extension along the alveolar septa within the pulmonary parenchyma.

Imaging Features. Bilateral reticular or reticulonodular opacities are observed on radiography. CT often demonstrates patchy or diffuse consolidative or ground-glass opacities and nodules in perilymphatic distribution. Cysts are often found in peribronchiolar regions, thought to result from compression of bronchiolar lumen by peribronchiolar lymphocytic infiltrate (Fig. 21.30). Unlike other interstitial pneumonias, bronchiectasis, honeycombing, and architectural distortion are uncommon in LIP.

Inflammatory Pseudotumor

Clinical Features. The cause of pulmonary inflammatory pseudotumors (IPT) is unknown, although they are thought to represent a localized form of organizing pneumonia in patients with subclinical infection. Patients are often asymptomatic, and antecedent infection can be documented in fewer than 20% of cases. It is often discovered incidentally on imaging. In plasma cell granuloma, a subtype of IPT, there is a slight female predominance, and most patients are younger than 30 years of age. IPT in the pediatric population is more likely to be a true neoplasm termed *inflammatory myofibroblastic tumor (IMT)*.

The treatment of choice is complete surgical resection.

Pathologic Features. Inflammatory pseudotumors include a wide spectrum of histopathologic features with spindle cell proliferations with inflammatory cells such as plasma cells, lymphocytes, and histiocytes. Plasma cells predominate in the plasma cell granuloma form. When the lesion is composed primarily of myelofibroblasts, it is considered an IMT, which is a true neoplasm.

Imaging Features. Inflammatory pseudotumor manifests as well-circumscribed peripheral pulmonary nodule(s) or mass(es) (Fig. 21.31). Calcification occurs in about 20% of cases (Fig. 21.32), and airway involvement is uncommon. Invasion of adjacent structures is rare but can be seen in children.

Plasma cell granuloma may range from 1 to 12 cm in diameter and occasionally may cavitate or calcify. Nodule growth is usually indolent and can span months to years. On CT, the nodule may show heterogeneous attenuation and enhancement after administration of intravenous contrast.

IgG4-Related Lung Disease

Clinical Features. IgG4-related disease is a systemic disease that can involve multiple sites such as the liver, pancreas, lungs, and mediastinum. It has been linked to autoimmune pancreatitis, Riedel thyroiditis, inflammatory pseudotumor, and retroperitoneal fibrosis. It affects middle-aged or elderly patients, and a male predominance has been reported. Pulmonary IgG4-RD results in nonspecific symptoms including cough, dyspnea, chest pain, and fever.

Elevated serum IgG4 concentration and IgG4-to-IgG ratio are usually observed.

The disease is usually treated with steroids. Cyclosporine or rituximab can be used in patients who are not responsive to steroid treatments.

Pathologic Features. Characteristic findings include lymphoplasmacytic infiltration with abundant IgG4-positive plasma cells and storiform fibrosis. Obliterative arteritis can be seen with or without luminal obliteration.

Imaging Features. Four different pulmonary manifestations have been described for IgG4-RD in the lungs, including (1) solid nodule or mass, (2) ground-glass nodule, (3) interstitial pneumonia with diffuse ground-glass opacities and honeycombing, and (4) thickening of bronchovascular bundles and interlobular septa (Fig. 21.33).

Mediastinal or hilar lymphadenopathy and pleural effusions have also been reported.

Intense FDG uptake can be seen on PET, mimicking malignancy.

Posttransplantation Lymphoproliferative Disorders

Clinical Features

Posttransplantation lymphoproliferative disorder (PTLD) occurs in up to 2% of all transplant patients. The incidence of PTLD involving the thorax is highest after lung, combined heart and lung, heart, and liver followed by kidney transplants. Closely associated with EBV, PTLD typically occurs within the first few years of transplantation. The risk is highest in EBV-positive donors and EBV-negative recipients and related to the overall degree of immunosuppression. The clinical findings are variable and include fever, adenopathy, and lethargy. In the early stage, the patients are often asymptomatic.

The disorder usually regresses with a decrease in immunosuppression. Concomitant treatment with chemotherapy, radiation therapy (for localized disease), or anti–B-cell monoclonal antibody therapy may be administered for cases that do not respond to reduction in immunosuppression.

Pathologic Features

This entity represents a heterogeneous group of lymphoproliferative disorders ranging from polyclonal benign B-cell proliferation to a monoclonal aggressive lymphoma. The majority of PTLD is of B-cell origin.

Imaging Features

The most common imaging manifestation of intrathoracic PTLD is lung mass or multiple nodules. Other findings include consolidation, adenopathy, and pleural or pericardial effusion (Fig. 21.34). FDG-PET is helpful to evaluate the extent of disease once the diagnosis has been confirmed. It is not particularly helpful for initial evaluation as FDG

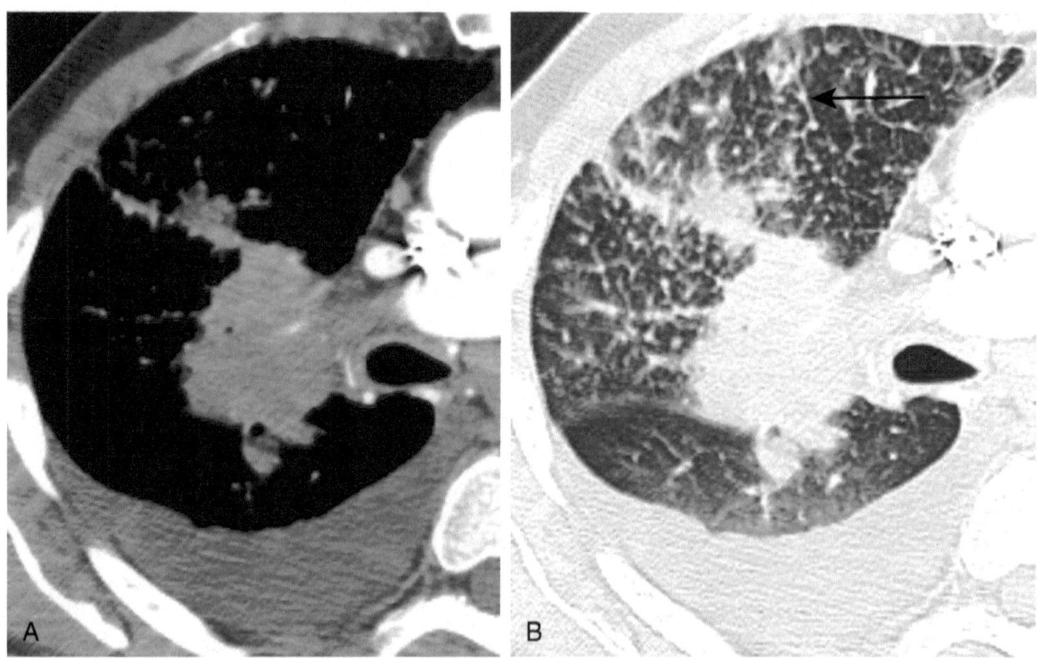

FIGURE 21.33 IgG4-related lung disease. **A,** Computed tomography (CT) image shows right central mass with small right pleural effusion. **B,** CT image shows thickening of the interlobular septae *(arrow)*. Surgical biopsy showed lymphoplasmacytic infiltration and granulomas in patient with elevated serum IgG4.

uptake can be seen in infectious lesions, which is common in transplant recipients.

Tumor Mimics

There is considerable overlap in the imaging features of benign and malignant pulmonary lesions. Many infectious and inflammatory conditions mimic tumors (Fig. 21.35). Specific morphologic characteristics useful in differentiating benign from malignant lesions include size, margins, contour, internal characteristics (including attenuation, wall thickness in cavitary nodules, and air bronchograms), presence of satellite nodules, halo sign, reverse halo sign, and growth rate. Awareness of the spectrum of potential mimics of lung tumors is important in preventing misinterpretation. The more tumor-like conditions are discussed here. Please also refer to Chapter 22.

Amyloid

Clinical Features. Amyloid (Box 21.11) occurs in two major forms, primary and secondary. Lung involvement in primary amyloidosis is estimated to occur in 30% to 90% of cases. Secondary amyloidosis is usually associated with rheumatoid arthritis, suppurative disease such as osteomyelitis, and malignant neoplasms. Amyloidosis may also be associated with multiple myeloma. In the thorax, amyloid occurs in two locations. The first is the tracheobronchial tree (discussed Chapter 6). Amyloidosis may also involve the lung parenchyma in a nodular form or as a diffuse, infiltrative process.

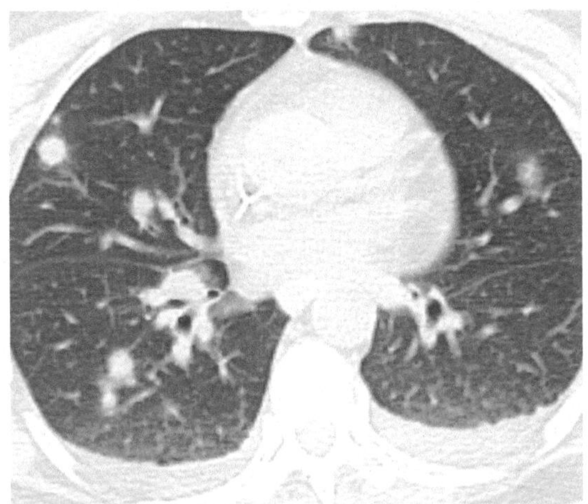

FIGURE 21.34 Posttransplantation lymphoproliferative disorder (PTLD). Computed tomography image shows multiple bilateral pulmonary nodules and pleural effusions in a patient with PTLD 2 years after stem cell transplantation for chronic myelogenous leukemia.

BOX 21.11 Amyloid

CLINICAL FEATURES

Nodular type
- Seventh decade of life
- Asymptomatic

Infiltrative type
- Sixth decade of life
- Symptomatic

PATHOLOGIC FEATURES

Waxy, pink material that stains with Congo red

IMAGING FEATURES

Nodular type
- Solitary or multiple nodules/masses
- Calcification in 30% to 50%
- Slow growth

Infiltrative type
- Diffuse reticular or nodular pattern

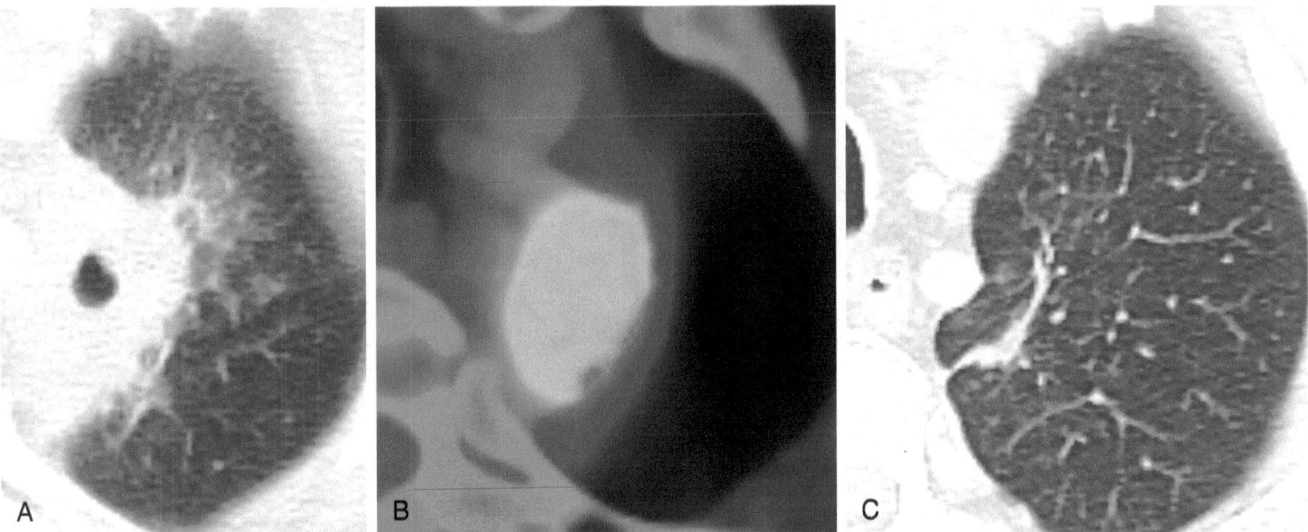

FIGURE 21.35 Cavitary pneumonia mimicking squamous cell lung cancer. **A,** Computed tomography (CT) image shows cavitary left apical mass. **B,** Positron emission tomography/CT image shows intense fludeoxyglucose uptake in the left apical mass suspicious for malignancy. **C,** CT image 3 months later shows linear scar and resolution of the mass.

Nodular disease usually occurs late in life (i.e., seventh decade), and it has an equal sex prevalence. Patients are usually asymptomatic, and the prognosis is excellent. The diffuse, infiltrative form is less common and usually occurs in the sixth decade. Patients with the diffuse form are symptomatic, with progressive dyspnea, respiratory insufficiency, and possibly death.

Pathologic Features. Amyloid, a waxy pink material that stains with Congo red, has a typical birefringence with polarization microscopy. Diffuse infiltration of amyloid associated with giant cells and plasma cells involves the vascular walls and interstitium of the lung.

Imaging Features. The radiologic appearance of the nodular form consists of solitary or multiple nodules and masses (Fig. 21.36), which can mimic primary or metastatic lung neoplasms. Calcification is common, occurring in 30% to 50% of patients, but cavitation is rare. The lower lobes are more frequently involved, often in a subpleural location. These lesions may demonstrate slow growth.

In the diffuse, infiltrative form, bilateral and fine linear, nodular, or reticulonodular patterns may occur. There is no specific distribution in the lung parenchyma. In the mediastinum, nodal calcification may be present.

Pulmonary amyloidosis can be hypermetabolic on FDG-PET.

Lipoid Pneumonia

Lipoid pneumonia, caused by accumulation of exogenous or endogenous lipid in the alveoli, can produce nodular or masslike opacities on chest radiograph or CT and mimic pulmonary neoplasm. The presence of fat attenuation on CT is suggestive of the diagnosis. Please refer to Chapter 14 for details.

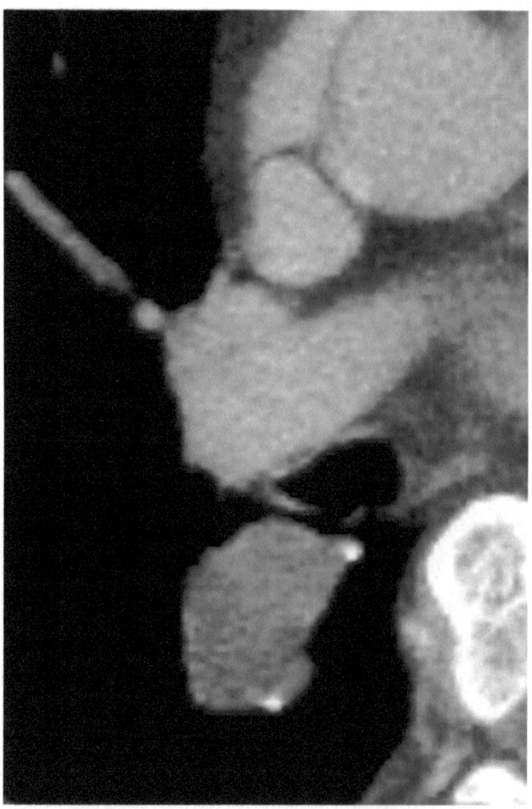

FIGURE 21.36 Amyloid. Computed tomography image shows right lower lobe mass with eccentric calcifications.

Rounded Atelectasis

Rounded atelectasis appears as a subpleural mass adjacent to thickened pleura or chronic pleural effusion and can also be mistaken for pulmonary neoplasm. Rounded atelectasis, in distinction from neoplasms, is associated with signs of volume loss. Please refer to Chapter 2.

POSTTREATMENT CHANGES

Many of the entities discussed in this chapter can be treated with surgical resection if found in the early stage or when localized. Details of normal and abnormal postoperative findings can be found in Chapter 12. Changes related to chemotherapy, radiation therapy, and immunotherapy are discussed here.

Chemotherapy-Induced Changes

After chemotherapy, primary or metastatic pulmonary lesions may decrease in size or completely resolve. Cavitation can also occur after treatment (Fig. 21.37). Dystrophic calcification can occur in areas of necrosis after therapy. Some lesions may initially respond to therapy and then remain stable in size. The residual nodules may contain only necrotic or fibrous tissue without viable tumor and represent sterilized metastases. Occasionally, biologic markers or FDG-PET may help distinguish viable tumor from residual fibrotic disease. Certain chemotherapy can result in drug-induced interstitial pneumonias, described in Chapter 18.

Radiation-Induced Changes

Clinical Features

Radiotherapy (RT) plays an important role in curative and palliative treatment of locoregional disease in various pulmonary neoplasms. SBRT, used frequently in early-stage lung cancer, isolated pulmonary lymphoma or metastases, is a hypofractionated high-dose technique in which the radiation conforms tightly to the target lesion to decrease injury to adjacent lung.

Acute radiation pneumonitis occurs in 5% to 40% of patients who receive RT. Risk factors include concurrent chemotherapy, high radiation dose, large target volume, poor pretreatment functional status, and preexisting pulmonary disease. Patients may be asymptomatic or present with dyspnea, low-grade fever, or cough. Patients with severe symptoms may require steroid therapy and supportive ventilation.

Over time, pulmonary fibrosis may develop, which may be asymptomatic or result in chronic dyspnea and reduced pulmonary function.

Pathologic Features

In radiation pneumonitis, injuries to the small vessels result in increased vascular permeability and infiltration of inflammatory cells and filling of alveolar space. Fibroblastic proliferation, septal thickening, and vascular sclerosis are seen in radiation fibrosis.

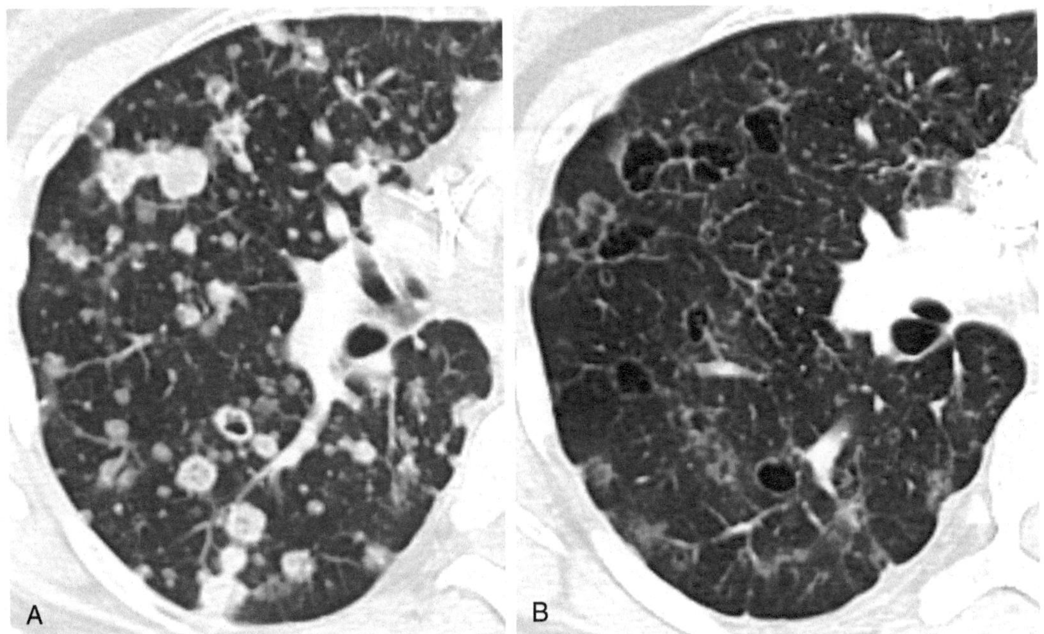

FIGURE 21.37 Hematogenous metastases cavitate after chemotherapy. **A,** Computed tomography (CT) image shows multiple right lung metastatic nodules from pancreatic adenocarcinoma. **B,** CT image 2 months later shows response to chemotherapy. The lung metastases have cavitated now and appear as thin-walled air-filled cysts.

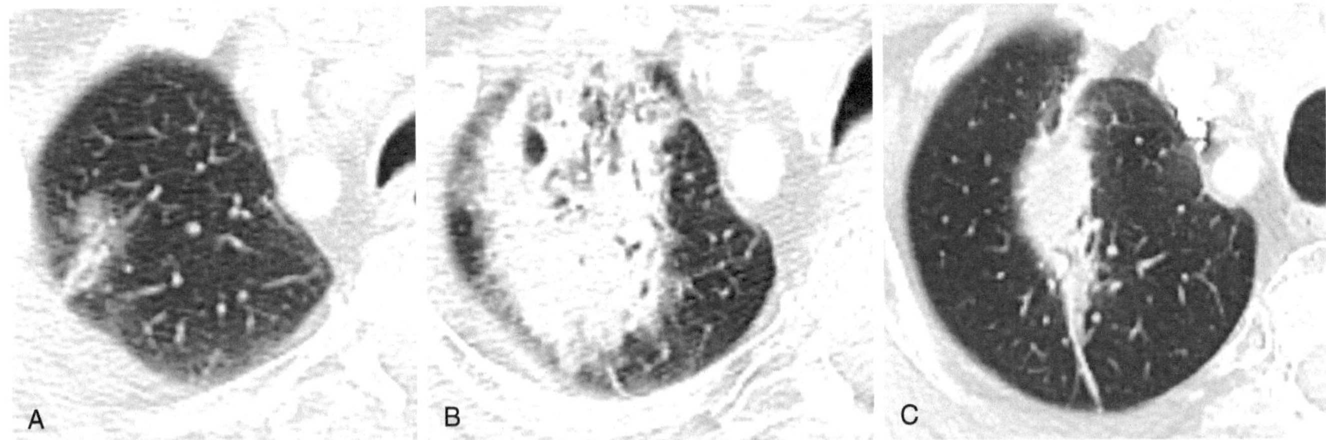

FIGURE 21.38 Evolution of radiation therapy changes. **A,** Computed tomography (CT) image shows the mixed attenuation nodule in the right upper lobe biopsy proven to be adenocarcinoma. **B,** Three months after radiation therapy, CT image shows masslike consolidation in the right upper lobe consistent with radiation pneumonitis. **C,** One year after radiation therapy, CT image shows evolution of radiation change to an area of residual soft tissue opacity and traction bronchiectasis.

Imaging Features

Classically, radiation pneumonitis can be identified within 6 to 8 weeks after the completion of treatment on standard radiographs and at an earlier time on CT. The consolidative and ground-glass opacities can demonstrate a sharp demarcation denoting the limits of the radiation portal (see Fig. 21.7). However, with SBRT, the margin is often not as well defined. Air bronchograms are common within areas of pneumonitis. Fibrosis usually develops within 6 to 12 months after radiation therapy, resulting in consolidation with characteristic volume loss, architectural distortion, and traction bronchiectasis (Fig. 21.38). The opacity may be linear or masslike, but the imaging appearance should stabilize 1 to 2 years after the completion of RT. Pleural effusion can be seen in both the acute and chronic phases.

The target lesion can be obscured by radiation-induced changes in the lung. Tumor lesion shrinkage may or may not occur. However, recurrence should be suspected if a previously stabilized area of radiation fibrosis increases in density or size and develops a convex margin (Fig. 21.39). Filling of previously aerated bronchi within an area of radiation fibrosis is another sign of recurrence.

Radiation pneumonitis can exhibit avid FDG uptake on PET caused by inflammation. The uptake should decrease over time. Focal areas of increased FDG uptake within the radiated field would be suspicious for residual or recurrent tumor.

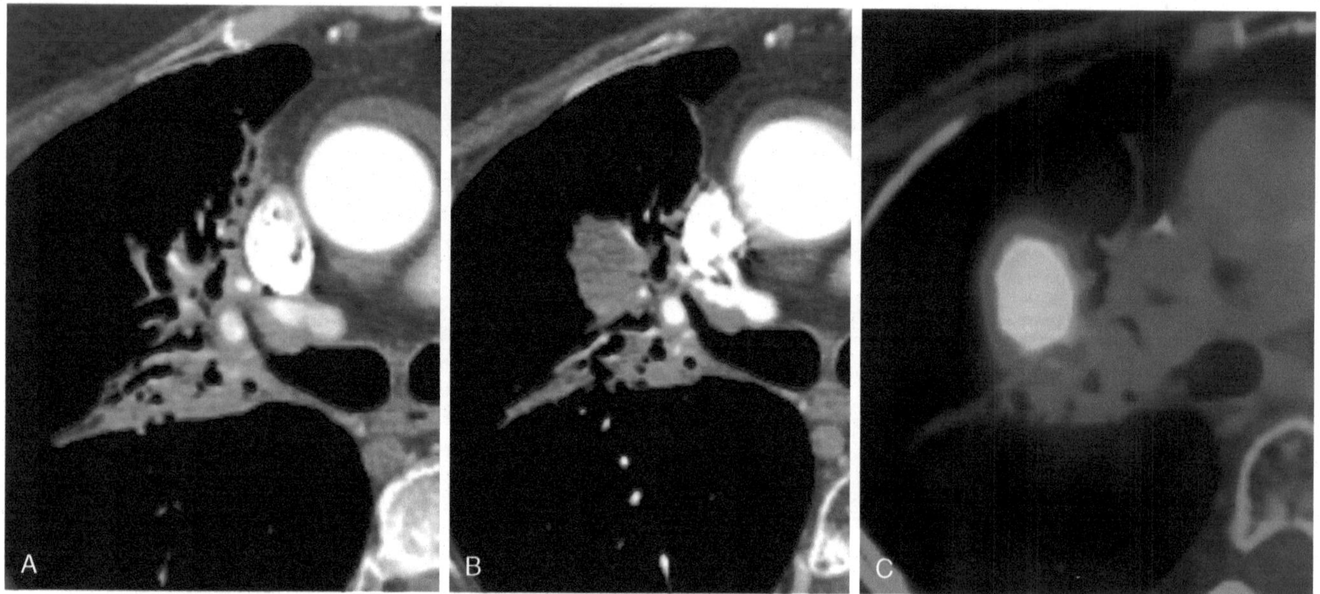

FIGURE 21.39 Small cell lung cancer recurs after radiation therapy. **A,** Computed tomography (CT) image shows the radiation fibrosis with a straight margin and traction bronchiectasis in the right perihilar region 18 months after radiation therapy. Six months later, CT image **(B)** and positron emission tomography/CT **(C)** show new fludeoxyglucose-avid soft tissue along the lateral aspect of the area of radiation change. Biopsy confirmed tumor recurrence.

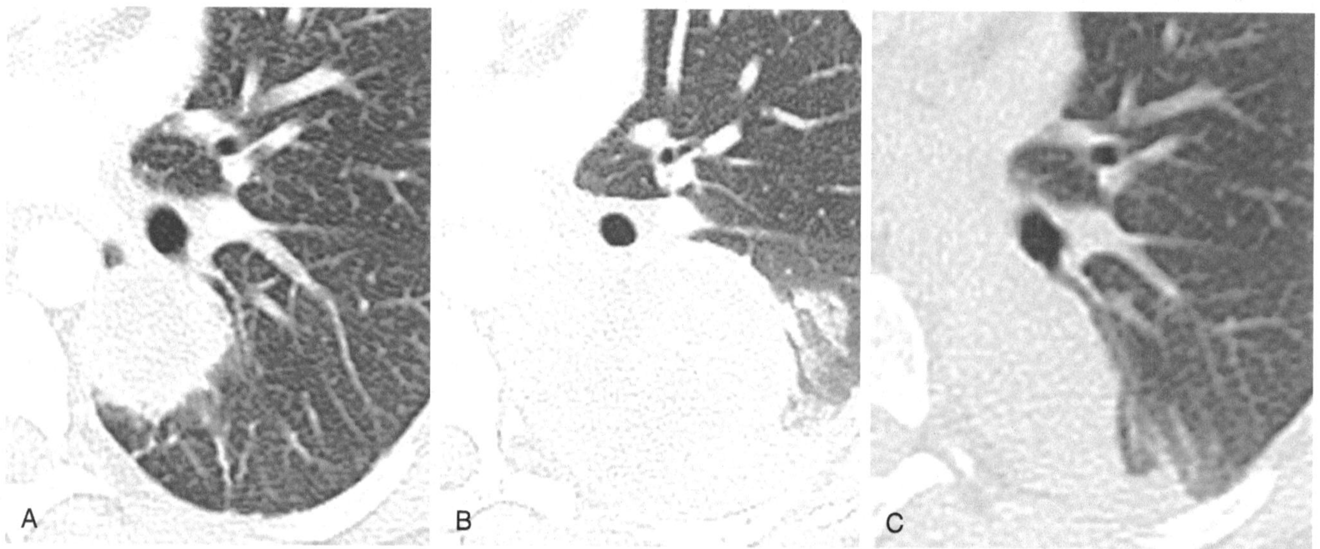

FIGURE 21.40 Immunotherapy changes as pseudoprogression. **A,** Computed tomography (CT) image shows the primary lung cancer in the left lower lobe. **B,** Six weeks after immunotherapy, CT image shows apparent increase in size of the treated primary tumor. **C,** Two months later, CT image shows response to therapy with decrease in size of the tumor, now more elliptical in shape.

Immunotherapy-Induced Changes

Clinical Features

Immunotherapy modulates the patient's immune system to fight cancer. Ipilimumab, a monoclonal antibody that works by targeting cytotoxic T-lymphocyte-associated protein 4 (CTLA-4), is used to treat metastatic and unresectable melanoma. It is also used to treat other cancers in clinical trials. Many other similar medications are now being used and developed.

Pathologic Features

In tumor biopsies, it has been observed that the immune response can lead to immune cell infiltration of the tumor with or without edema.

Imaging Features

In patients treated with immunotherapy agents, the response to treatment may be delayed. Transient enlargement of the tumor or pseudoprogression (Fig. 21.40) can occur, which is postulated to be caused by infiltration of the tumor by immune cells. Similarly, new lesions may become apparent on imaging as previously occult micrometastases become larger. These changes can also result in increased FDG avidity. Therefore, imaging assessment of treatment response or disease progression after completion of treatment requires two consecutive follow-up imaging studies performed at least 4 weeks apart.

CONCLUSION

Familiarity with the various imaging characteristics and posttreatment changes of lung cancer, the leading cause of cancer mortality in the United States, is vital in clinical practice. Awareness of other common pulmonary tumors and tumor mimics is also important in guiding diagnostic work-up. Pulmonary lymphoproliferative disorders, with a wide range of clinical presentations and imaging manifestations, should also be included in the differential considerations in the appropriate clinical settings.

SUGGESTED READINGS

Abbott GF, Fintelmann FJ. Lung cancer mimics. In: Rosado-de-Christenson ML, Carter BW, eds. *Specialty Imaging Thoracic Neoplasms*. Philadelphia: Elsevier; 2016:182-185.

Aquino SL. Imaging of metastatic disease to the thorax. *Radiol Clin North Am*. 2005;43:481-495.

Bruzzi JF, Komaki R, Walsh GL, et al. Imaging of non-small cell lung cancer of the superior sulcus. *Radiographics*. 2008;28:551-560.

Bueno J. Pulmonary Hodgkin lymphoma. In: Rosado-de-Christenson ML, Carter BW, eds. *Specialty Imaging Thoracic Neoplasms*. Philadelphia: Elsevier; 2016:288-289.

Carter BW, Glisson BS, Truong MT, et al. Small cell lung cancer: staging, imaging, and treatment considerations. *Radiographics*. 2014;34:1707-1721.

Hare SS, Souza CA, Bain G, et al. The radiological spectrum of pulmonary lymphoproliferative disease. *Br J Radiol*. 2012;85:848-864.

Kwak JJ, Tirumani SH, Van den Abbeele AD, et al. Cancer immunotherapy: imaging assessment of novel treatment response patterns and immune-related adverse events. *Radiographics*. 2015;35:424-437.

Suut S, Al-Ani Z, Allen C, et al. Pictorial essay of radiological features of benign intrathoracic masses. *Ann Thorac Med*. 2015;10:231-242.

Travis WD, Brambilla E, Nicholson AG, et al. The 2015 World Health Organization Classification of Lung Tumors: impact of genetic, clinical and radiologic advances since the 2004 classification. *J Thorac Oncol*. 2015;9:1243-1260.

Travis WD, Brambilla E, Noguchi M, et al. International Association for the Study of Lung Cancer/American Thoracic Society/European Respiratory Society International Multidisciplinary Classification of Lung Adenocarcinoma. *J Thorac Oncol*. 2011;6:244-285.

Viswanathan C, Carter BW, Shroff GS, et al. Pitfalls in oncologic imaging: complications of chemotherapy and radiotherapy in the chest. *Semin Roentgenol*. 2015;50:183-191.

Wu CC. Pulmonary non-Hodgkin lymphoma. In: Rosado-de-Christenson ML, Carter BW, eds. *Specialty Imaging Thoracic Neoplasms*. Philadelphia: Elsevier; 2016:290-293.

Chapter 22

Incidental Pulmonary Nodule

Milena Petranovic and Subba R. Digumarthy

INTRODUCTION

A pulmonary nodule is defined as a rounded or irregular opacity measuring up to 3 cm in diameter. There are many etiologies, both benign and malignant, of lung nodules (Table 22.1). Some opacities can resemble a nodule but are truly nodule mimics and can be identified as such in cross-sectional imaging. Lung nodules are extremely common, with some studies indicating that more than 50% of smokers older than 50 years of age demonstrate nodules on computed tomography (CT). There is also variation in incidence according to geography. People living in regions with endemic fungal infections such as histoplasmosis and coccidioidomycosis have a higher incidence of nodules. The prevalence of malignancy in incidentally detected nodules ranges widely but is estimated to be anywhere from 1% to 5%.

TABLE 22.1 Benign and Malignant Causes of Incidental Pulmonary Nodules

Benign Causes (Nodule Mimics)	Malignant Causes
Neoplastic	Primary lung cancer
Hamartoma	Pulmonary lymphoproliferative disorders
Fibroma	Carcinoid
Sclerosing hemangioma	Sarcoma
Neural tumor	Metastasis
Leiomyoma	
Endometriosis	
Infectious	
Granuloma (tuberculosis, histoplasmosis)	
Fungal infections	
Bacterial infections	
Parasites	
Round pneumonia	
Abscess	
Septic embolus	
Noninfectious inflammatory	
Intraparenchymal or subpleural lymph node	
Rounded atelectasis	
Rheumatoid nodule	
Amyloid	
Lipoid pneumonia	
Focal fibrosis	
Sarcoidosis	
Endometriosis	
Vascular	
Vasculitis	
Infarct	
Hematoma	
Arteriovenous malformation	
Vascular calcifications	
Congenital	
Bronchogenic cyst	
Bronchial atresia with mucoid impaction	
Sequestration	
Other	
Rib fracture	
Costochondral calcification	
Bone island	
Pleural thickening, fluid, or pleural plaques	
Soft tissue lesions	

APPROACH TO ASSESSMENT OF LUNG NODULES

Assessment of various features of nodules is helpful in determining the significance and may help in identifying potential malignant nodules. The major features include attenuation, shape and contour, size and evolution, location, and enhancement.

Attenuation

Pulmonary nodules are primarily classified by their attenuation into solid and subsolid nodules. Subsolid pulmonary nodules are further divided into pure ground-glass and part solid nodules. Pure ground-glass nodules demonstrate hazy increased attenuation without obscuring the bronchi and vessels within the nodule. Part-solid nodules contain components of both ground-glass and soft tissue (solid) attenuation (Fig. 22.1).

The presence of fat within a nodule can indicate a benign etiology such as a hamartoma or lipoid pneumonia. Fat appears as an area of low attenuation measuring between −50 to −150 HU (Fig. 22.2). If fat is suspected but the Hounsfield units are not at least −30 HU, a reliable diagnosis of hamartoma cannot be made on CT. Magnetic resonance imaging evaluation, however, may be considered for assessment of microscopic fat in large nodules.

Hounsfield values greater than +200 HU indicate the presence of calcification on CT. The pattern of calcification plays an important role in evaluating whether a nodule is benign or malignant (Fig. 22.3). Benign patterns include diffuse, central, laminar, and popcorn. Diffuse central and laminated calcifications are typical with granulomatous infection. Popcorn calcifications are seen in cartilaginous tumors and hamartomas. All other patterns of calcification, including punctate, eccentric, and amorphous, are considered nonspecific and are seen in up to 10% to 15%

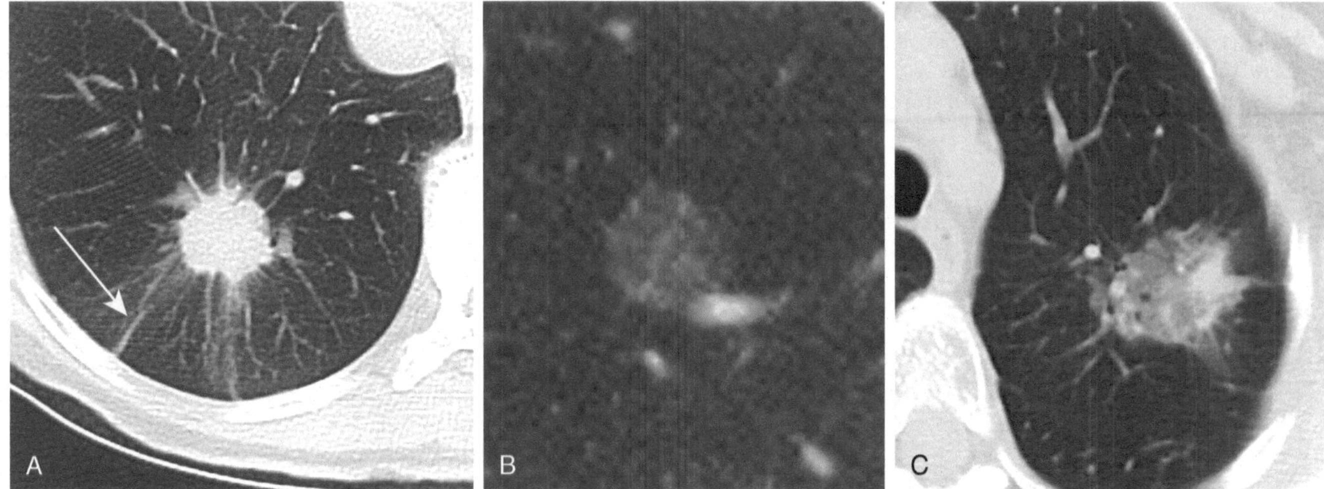

FIGURE 22.1 Solid and subsolid nodules. **A,** Computed tomography image of solid pulmonary nodules demonstrates soft tissue attenuation that obscures adjacent vessels and bronchi. This solid nodule also exhibits linear opacities extending to the pleural surface (pleural tags, *arrow*), a finding associated with malignancy. **B,** Pure ground-glass nodules demonstrate hazy increased attenuation without obscuring the bronchi and vessels within the nodule **(B)**. **C,** Part-solid nodules contain components of both ground-glass and solid attenuation.

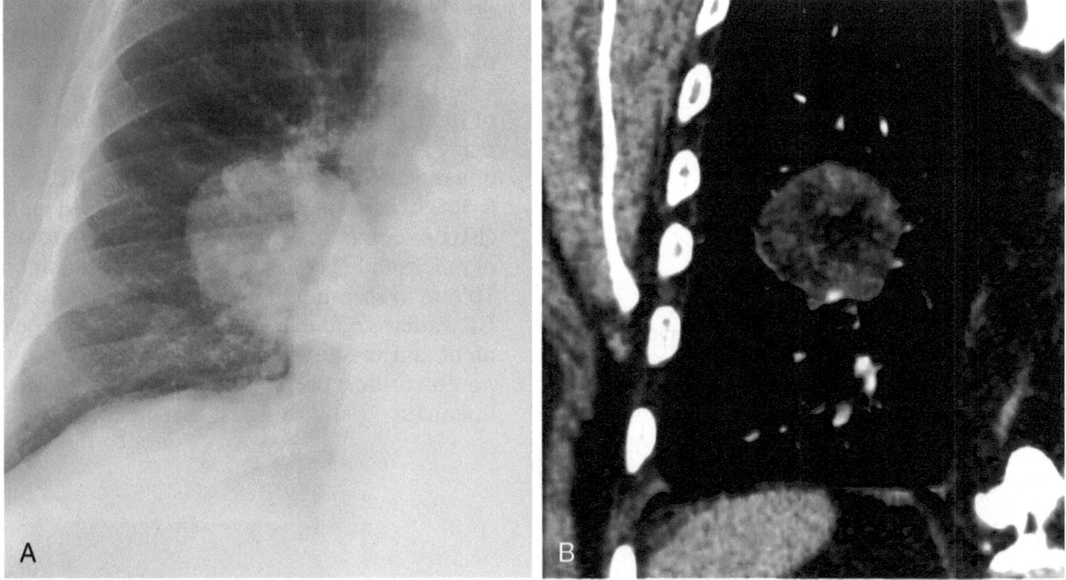

FIGURE 22.2 Fat-containing hamartoma. Chest radiograph **(A)** demonstrates a well-defined nodule that corresponds to a nodule with internal areas of low-attenuation measuring –40 HU on the coronal reformat chest computed tomography **(B)** consistent with a fat-containing hamartoma. Although not all hamartomas are fat containing, nodules with definite internal fat are considered benign with rare exceptions such as liposarcoma metastases.

of primary lung cancers (Fig. 22.4). Lung metastases from chondrosarcoma or osteosarcoma may also manifest with calcifications but should demonstrate interval growth unlike granulomas.

Cavitation is frequently found in infectious and inflammatory conditions (e.g., vasculitis). However, it can also be seen in malignancy, often of squamous cell histology. Cavitation is the result of necrosis, which may be related to ischemia or tissue destruction from coagulation or caseous necrosis. Cavitary nodules with smooth walls are more typical in benign lesions (Fig. 22.5). Thick, nodular, and irregular walls are more common with primary and metastatic tumors, but these are not specific for benign or malignant lesions.

Cysts should be distinguished from cavities. In contrast to cavities, the presence of a cyst does not imply necrosis. Cysts are smooth, thin-walled structures that are likely related to dilated airspaces from obstruction of distal bronchioles. Irregular nodular thickening of a cyst wall or interval development of a solid component is worrisome for malignancy (Fig. 22.6).

Some nodules demonstrate air bronchograms within them. This can be seen in association with certain infections and pulmonary lymphoma, as well as in lung adenocarcinoma (Fig. 22.7). Other nodules demonstrate what is known as a "reverse halo sign," which can be seen in organizing pneumonia as well as in certain infections, after radiation treatment, or in pulmonary neoplasms (Fig. 22.8).

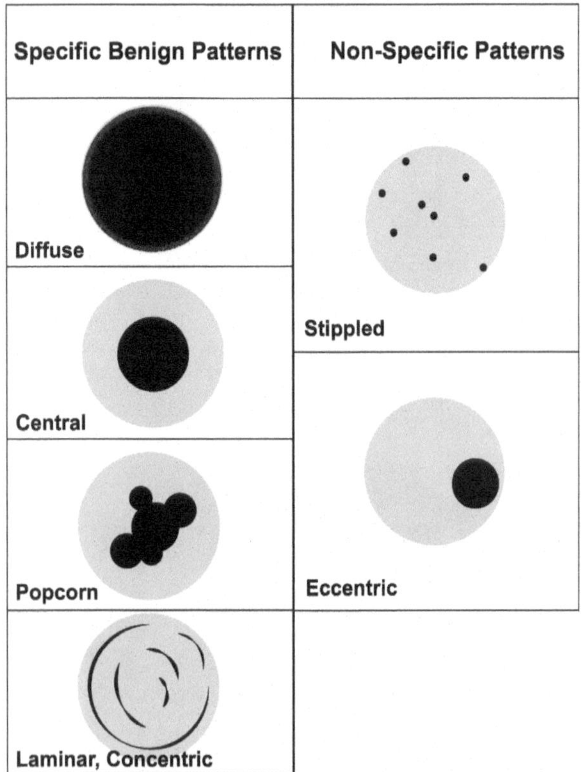

FIGURE 22.3 Patterns of calcification. Specific benign patterns of calcification include diffuse, central, popcorn, and laminar or concentric. Other patterns such as stippled and eccentric are considered nonspecific patterns.

Shape and Contour

Nodules can be categorized broadly into various shapes, including triangular, linear, oval, and spherical. Triangular and linear or oval shapes are more commonly associated with benign nodules. A triangular nodule along the pleural surface is virtually pathognomonic for an intrapulmonary lymph node (Fig. 22.9). Intraparenchymal nodes also have ovoid and reniform or kidney-bean shapes. A spherical shape, however, is less reassuring and needs careful analysis.

Nodule contour or margin may be described as smooth, lobulated, irregular, or spiculated (Fig. 22.10). Although both benign and malignant etiologies can take any of those forms, a spiculated contour or margin has a positive predictive value for malignancy of 90% and is thought to be related to growth of malignant cells along the pulmonary interstitium. Lobulated margins may appear to be caused by differential growth rates within nodules and are seen in both malignant and benign etiologies. Although in general benign nodules tend to have a smooth contour, up to 20% of primary lung malignancies also have smooth margins.

Enhancement

Enhancement after administration of intravenous contrast in a nodule can be helpful in differentiating benign and malignant nodules. An enhancement value of less than 15 HU is associated with 99% positive predictive value of benign lesion. Because increased blood flow is seen in many inflammatory conditions as well as in malignancy, an enhancement value greater than 15 HU is indeterminate (≈58% of cases are malignant). Decreased enhancement can also be seen in malignant nodules because of the presence of mucin and necrosis. Cavitary lesions and nodules less than 10 mm in size should not be evaluated for enhancement by CT. Patterns of enhancement such as rapid peak to enhancement and washout may also be used to predict malignant potential. Because it is not a standard practice to obtain unenhanced and contrast-enhanced chest CT, it is often

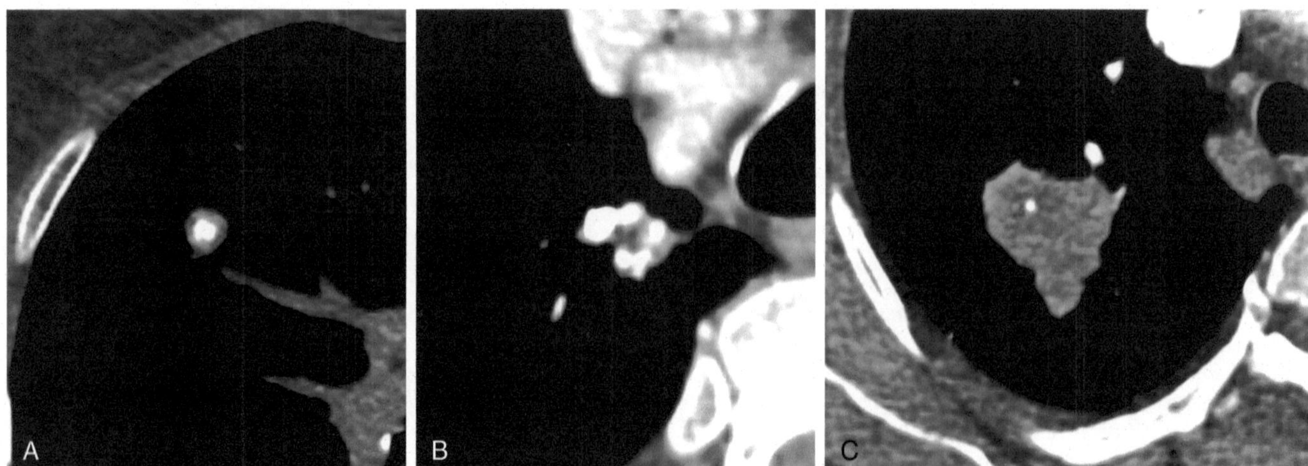

FIGURE 22.4 Patterns of calcification. **A,** Computed tomography (CT) image demonstrates a central or "bull's eye" pattern of calcification, which is considered a specific benign pattern and typical of a healed granuloma. **B,** CT image demonstrates a popcorn pattern of calcification found in hamartomas. **C,** Punctate calcifications on chest CT are an example of nonspecific calcifications, in this case seen within a large cell neuroendocrine carcinoma.

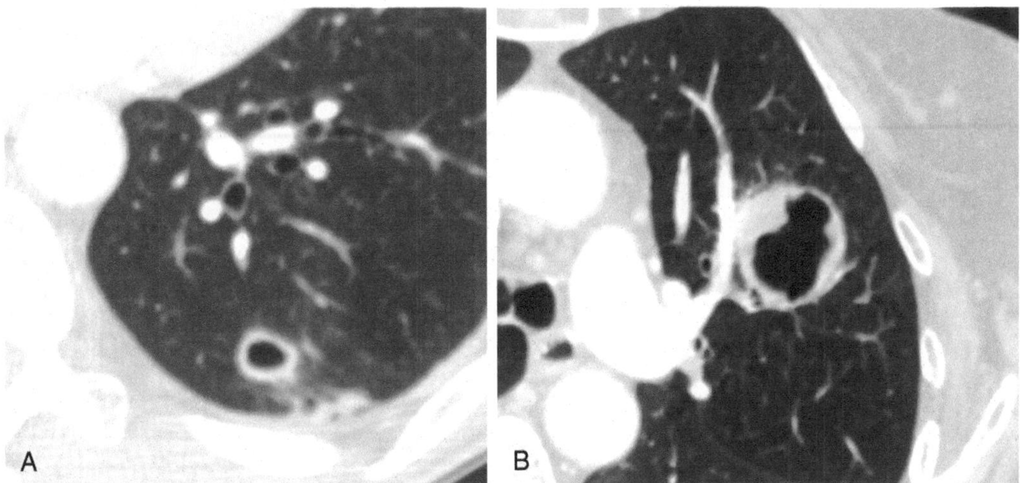

FIGURE 22.5 Cavitary nodules. Computed tomography images demonstrating cavitary nodule with smooth wall, which tends to be more typical in benign lesions such as this case of biopsy-proven Mycobacterium avium-intracellulare infection (MAI) **(A)** and cavitary lesion with thick and irregular walls, which are more common with primary and metastatic tumors such as this squamous cell carcinoma **(B)**.

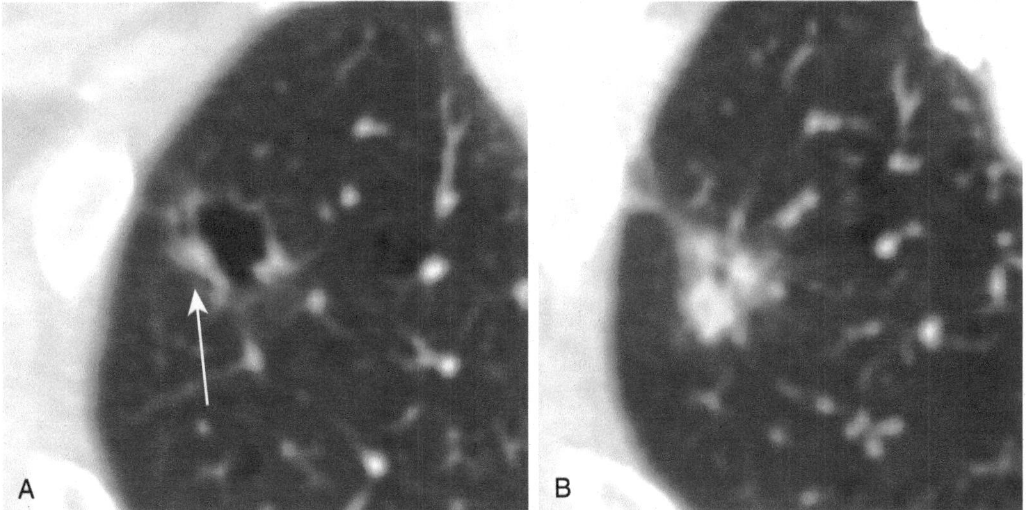

FIGURE 22.6 Cystic nodule. **A,** A cystic nodule containing mural nodularity *(arrow)* is noted in the periphery of the lung. **B,** Two years later, a follow-up computed tomography image demonstrates interval growth of a now solid nodule with spiculated borders replacing the previously demonstrated cyst. The nodule was subsequently resected and found to be an adenocarcinoma. This is a typical appearance for a rare cyst-associated lung cancer.

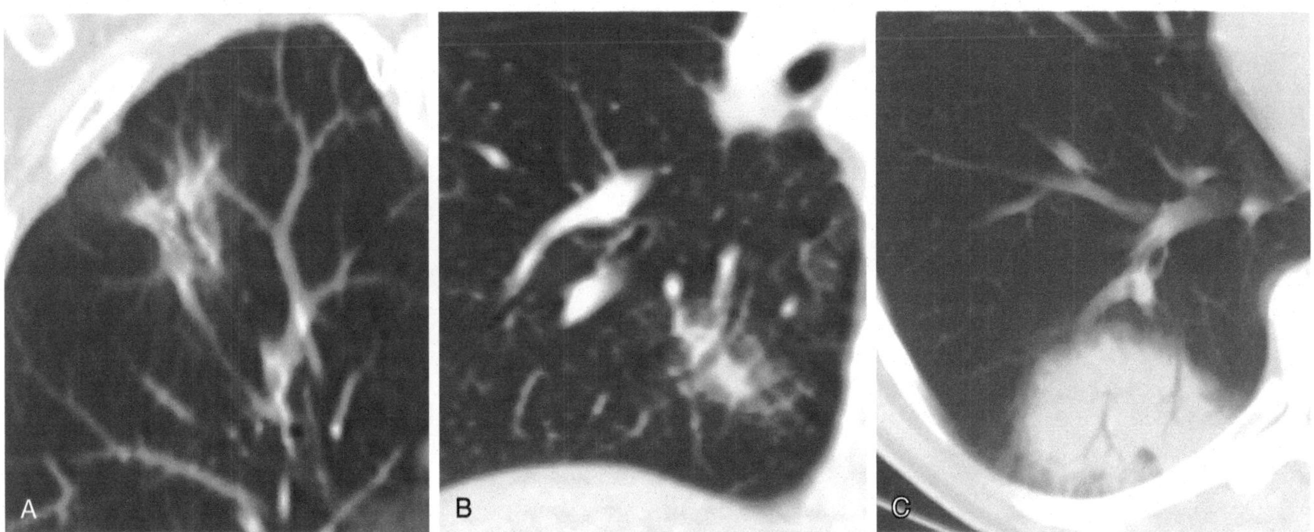

FIGURE 22.7 Air bronchogram. Coronal chest computed tomography reformats demonstrate two examples of subsolid nodules demonstrating prominent air bronchograms, also known as the "bronchus sign." One was an invasive adenocarcinoma in the right upper lobe **(A)**, and the other was a lymphoma in the right lower lobe **(B)**. A focal infection can also have this appearance, in this case, rounded pneumonia **(C)**.

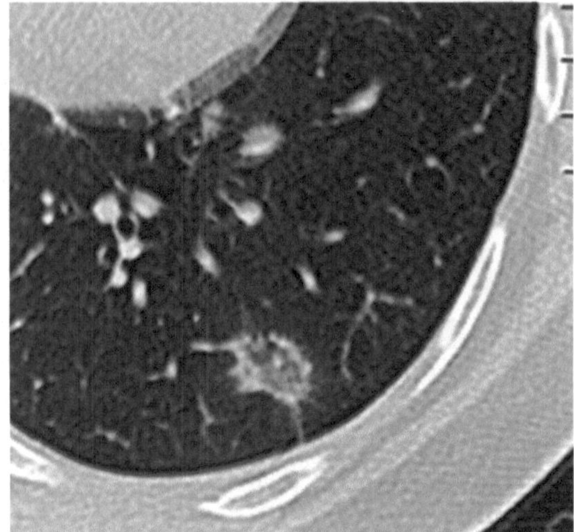

FIGURE 22.8 Reverse halo sign. Axial chest computed tomography image demonstrates a nodular area of ground glass in the left lower lobe with surrounding rim of soft tissue density consistent with a "reverse halo sign" in this patient with organizing pneumonia.

not possible to determinate the degree of enhancement. Dual-energy CT can generate virtual noncontrast images and can potentially help to better characterize pulmonary nodules (see Chapter 1).

Location

The location of a pulmonary nodule may also help in stratification of risk. Lung cancers tend to occur most frequently in the right upper lobe, but metastases tend to be lower lobe predominant and multiple and show greater variability in size. Perifissural and subpleural solid nodules often represent intrapulmonary lymph nodes. A central versus peripheral location may serve as a hint to type of pathology because certain cancers such as adenocarcinomas and metastases tend to be peripheral, but squamous cancers are more often found near the hila.

Size and Evolution

The size of a nodule and the change within a nodule over time is perhaps the most important diagnostic feature in

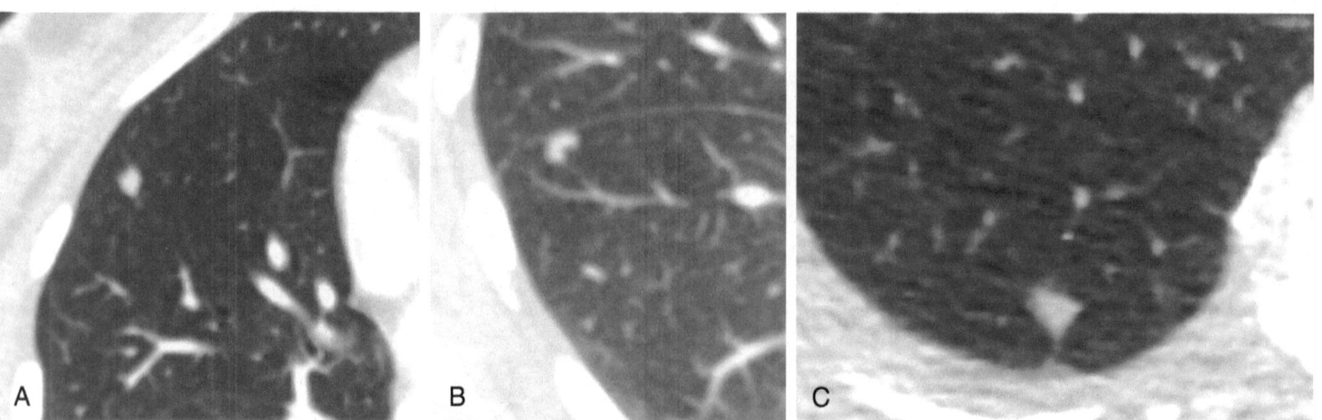

FIGURE 22.9 Intraparenchymal lymph nodes. Computed tomography images demonstrate an oval-shaped nodule adjacent to the right minor fissure **(A)**, a kidney-bean–shaped nodule adjacent to the major fissure **(B)**, and a triangular nodule associated with an interlobular septum extending to the pleural surface **(C)**. Perifissural location and association with an interlobular septum are characteristic features of benign intraparenchymal lymph nodes.

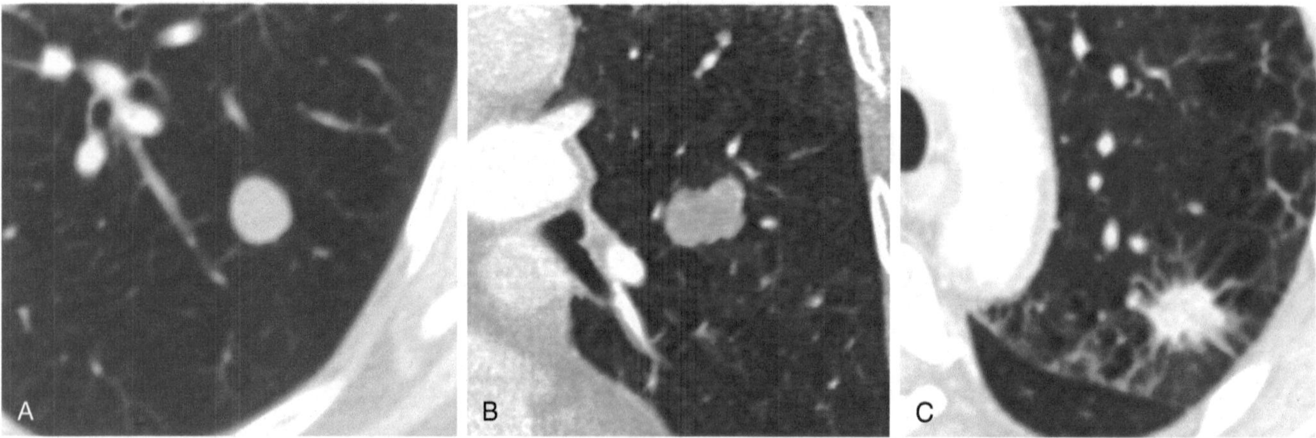

FIGURE 22.10 Nodule margins. Computed tomography images demonstrating examples of smooth margins of a nodule, in this case a benign metastasizing leiomyoma **(A)**, lobulated margins in a melanoma metastasis **(B)**, and spiculated margins in a lung adenocarcinoma **(C)**.

characterizing a nodule. Therefore, every attempt should be made to obtain and compare to oldest available study, and sometimes this may include comparing to imaging performed on other body parts such as the abdomen and neck. Additionally, comparison to prior imaging allows detection of preexisting abnormalities such as bronchiectasis and bullae. Awareness of these abnormalities helps in differentiating nodule mimics from true nodules.

To appreciate change in a nodule, proper and consistent measurements are crucial. Nodule evaluation is ideally performed on thin section CT (0.5–1.5 mm). This reduces the partial volume averaging, increases the sensitivity for the detection of calcification, and aids in correctly characterizing the nodules based on their attenuation. The sagittal and coronal reformats are helpful for discerning true nodule size and for differentiating nodule mimics such as scar and focal atelectasis.

The incidentally detected nodule size is expressed as the mean measurement of long- and short-axis measurements, obtained on the same axial, coronal, or sagittal image (Fig. 22.11). The decision to use axial, coronal, or sagittal images is made based on the greatest dimension of the nodule. Measurements should be performed on lung windows and recorded to the nearest whole millimeter. For subsolid nodules, both the mean diameter of the entire nodule as well as the mean diameter of the solid component should be recorded (Fig. 22.12). Volumetric assessment is more sensitive in capturing early changes in nodule size and should be used when following a nodule in time. Please also refer to the CT protocol for lung nodule follow-up in Chapter 1.

Nodule size is linked to risk of malignancy and is a dominant factor in management. Based on size alone, nodules smaller than 6 mm have a less than 1% risk of representing a primary lung malignancy, but nodules measuring 6 to 10 mm in size have a 6% to 28% risk for malignancy. Nodules larger than 20 mm have a prevalence of malignancy greater than 64%.

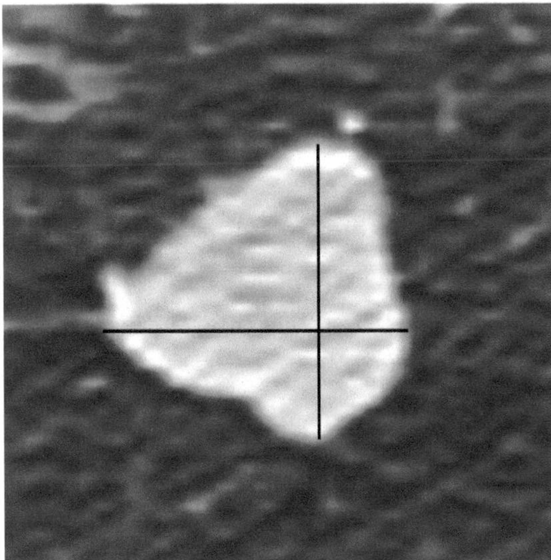

FIGURE 22.11 Solid nodule measurement. Solid pulmonary nodule size should be measured and recorded as the average of the long and short diameters, both of which should be obtained on the same axial, coronal, or sagittal reconstructed images, whichever yields the greatest dimension.

In terms of growth, doubling time plays an important role in determining whether a lesion is benign or malignant. Malignant pulmonary nodules usually have doubling time of less than 100 days with range of 20 to 400 days. Whereas infectious or inflammatory causes have a doubling time of less than 20 days, other benign conditions have a doubling time of longer than 400 days (Fig. 22.13). A growth rate with doubling time of less than 7 days is virtually diagnostic of a benign lesion. In a spherical nodule, an increase by 25% in diameter corresponds to doubling of volume.

In general, a solid nodule that decreases in size usually implies benign etiology, as does stability for longer than 2 years. A malignant subsolid nodule, however, may show a much more indolent growth pattern; for example, subsolid adenocarcinoma may take as many as 1346 days to double in volume. Furthermore, their growth is defined not only by a change in size and contour but also by an increase in attenuation (Fig. 22.14). Some lung cancers can also show a temporary regression in growth, possibly due to development of a fibrous component or resolution of superimposed infection or postobstructive component (Fig. 22.15).

MANAGEMENT OF SOLID NODULES

Radiograph

Nodules smaller than 9 mm are seldom evident on standard radiographs unless they are diffusely calcified. Diffuse calcification or stability for longer than 2 years is strongly indicative of benign etiology, and no further assessment is required. The probability of malignancy directly correlates with increasing size of the nodule. The identification of calcification in a nodule can be inaccurate on radiograph. Even in nodules larger than 1 cm, calcification can be missed in up to half of nodules; inversely, in a minority of nodules, false determination of calcification can be made.

Careful review and comparison with old studies and cross-sectional imaging are useful in separating true lung nodules from opacities in the ribs and soft tissues, such as bone island and skin nodules.

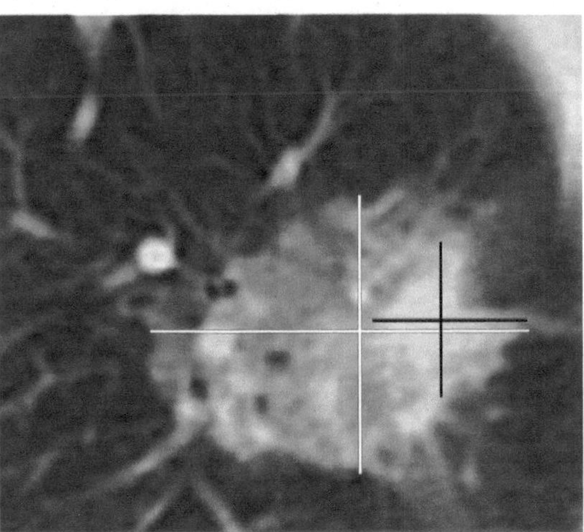

FIGURE 22.12 Subsolid nodule measurement. Subsolid pulmonary nodule size should specify both the average of the long and short diameters of the entire nodule (depicted in *white*) as well as the average of the long and short diameters of the largest solid component (depicted in *black*).

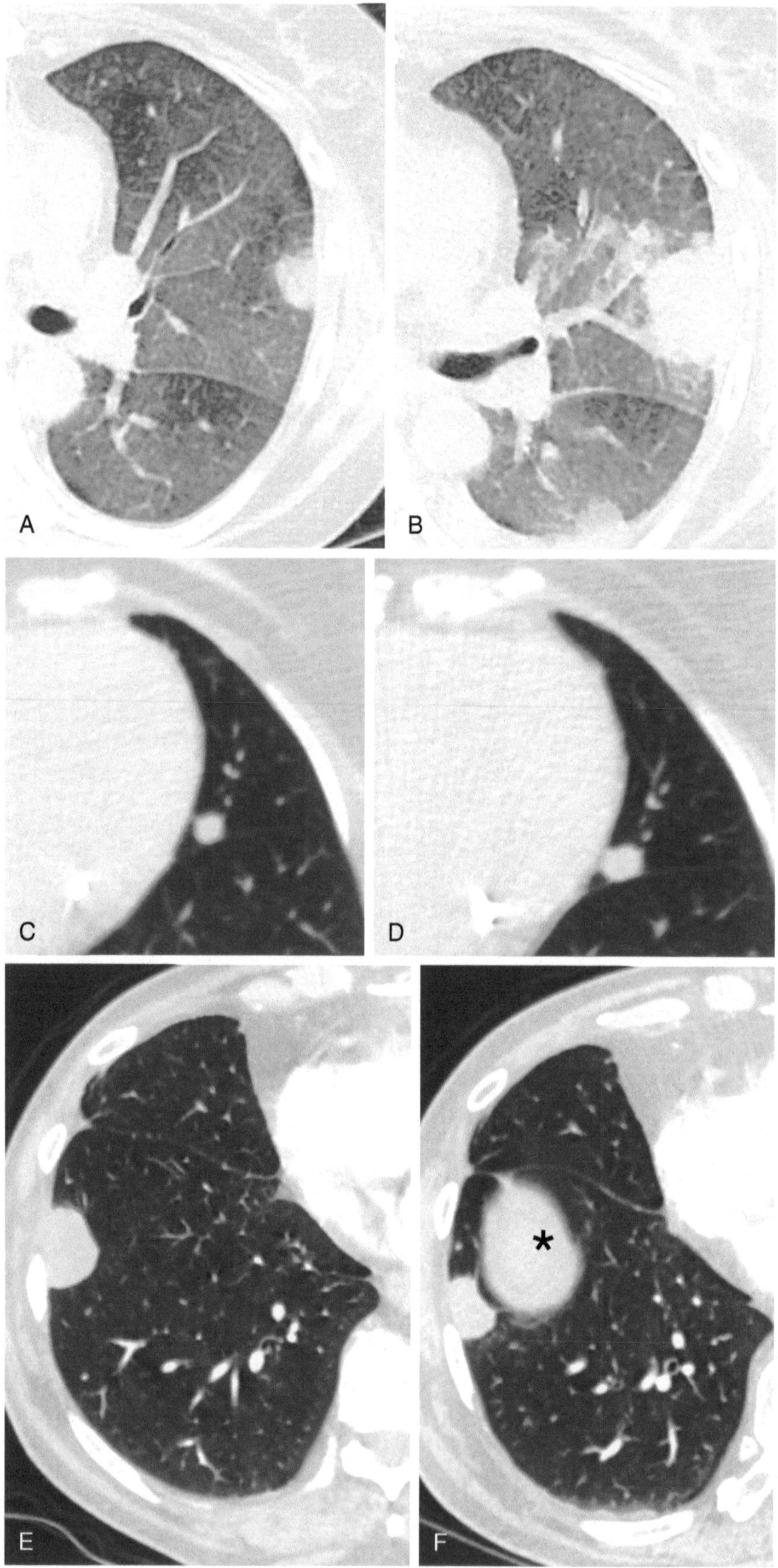

FIGURE 22.13 Nodule growth. Chest computed tomography (CT) images obtained 5 days apart show rapid growth of a peripheral nodule in the left upper lobe representing mucormycosis in a transplant patient (**A** and **B**). Chest CT images obtained 5 years apart show slow growth of a nodule in the lingula, which proved to be a carcinoid (**C** and **D**). Chest CT images obtained 4 months apart demonstrate decrease in size of a peripheral subpleural nodule suggestive of benign etiology, in this case a resolving pulmonary infarct (**E** and **F**) adjacent to the dome of the liver *(asterisk)*.

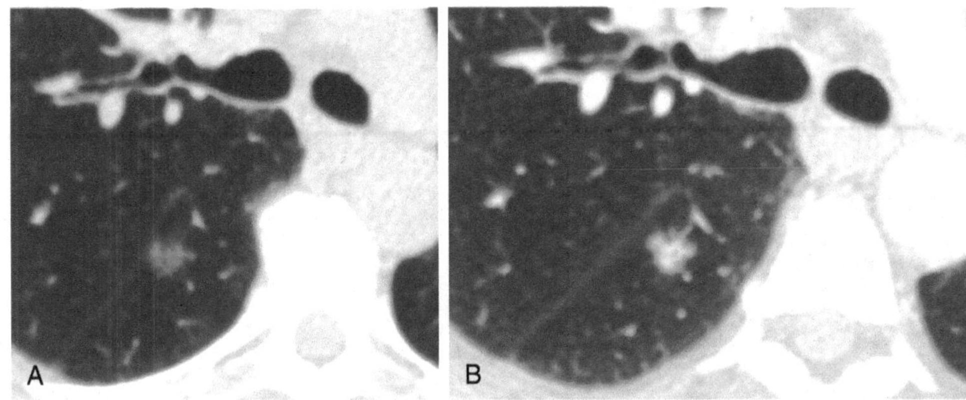

FIGURE 22.14 Increase in nodule attenuation. Axial chest computed tomography images (**A** and **B**) obtained 14 months apart demonstrate a ground-glass nodule in the superior segment of the right lower lobe that did not grow in overall size but increased in attenuation. The patient underwent a wedge resection, which demonstrated adenocarcinoma in situ.

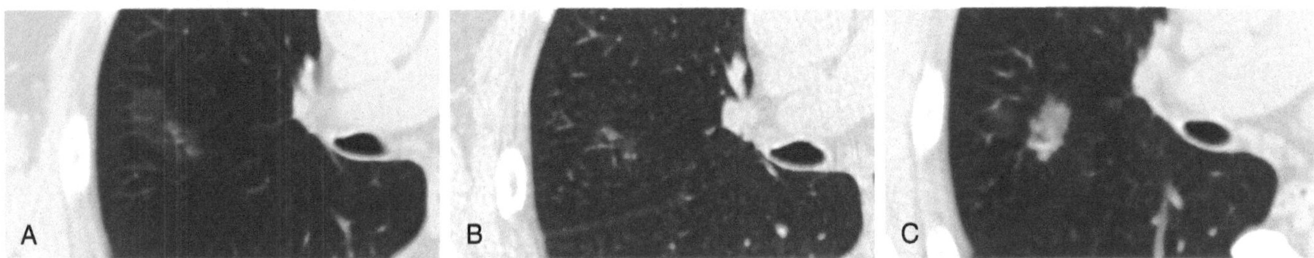

FIGURE 22.15 Temporary growth regression. Serial chest computed tomography images obtained over a course of 6 years demonstrate an initial decrease in the size of a mixed attenuation nodule over a 2-year period (**A** and **B**) and a subsequent increase in both size and density over the subsequent 4-year period (**B** and **C**). This nodule was found to be an invasive adenocarcinoma at resection. The temporary growth regression between *A* and *B* is thought to occur because of fibrosis.

The location of the nodule also affects its conspicuity on radiographs. Nodules that are located in upper lobes around the clavicles and first two ribs and costochondral cartilages are among the commonly missed cancers on standard radiographs. Subtraction of bones can enhance visibility and detection of lung nodules.

Computed Tomography

In contrast to a standard radiograph, CT is able to discern many more features of a nodule such as the various attenuations and shapes described earlier. It is also more sensitive in detecting incremental changes over time. Furthermore, CT may help identify specific diagnostic features of nodule mimics described later.

Guidelines

Incidentally detected solid nodules in low-risk patients that demonstrate benign features on chest CT such as benign patterns of calcification, regions of definite fat attenuation, or prolonged stability (>2 years), require no further follow-up (Fig. 22.16). If none of the definitively benign features is present, management of solid pulmonary nodules is guided by both the pretest probability in a specific patient as well as certain CT features. Factors that increase the chances of a malignancy in a nodule include age, presence of symptoms, history of smoking and other exposures (including asbestos, uranium, radon), having a first-degree relative with lung cancer, personal history of malignancy, and pulmonary fibrosis. Both the Fleischner Society and the American College of Chest Physicians have issued guidelines in the past, and a recent update to the Fleischner Society guidelines for solid nodule management was made (Table 22.2). It is important to note that these guidelines do not apply to patients younger than 35 years of age, immunosuppressed patients, patients with known primary malignancy, or patients undergoing CT as part of lung cancer screening. The current Fleischner Society guidelines also allow for greater latitude in follow-up based on clinical concerns or patient preference.

In cases with multiple solid nodules, management is guided by the mot suspicious nodule. With multiple nodules, patient history plays a particularly important role. History of malignancy, for instance, raises suspicion for metastases, immunocompromised state raises concern for atypical and fungal infections, and smoking history raises the possibility of smoking-related lung disease.

Although there are no convincing data yet to show that incidental solid or subsolid pulmonary nodules are higher risk than nodules found in lung cancer screening, the guidelines remain different. Please refer to Chapter 23.

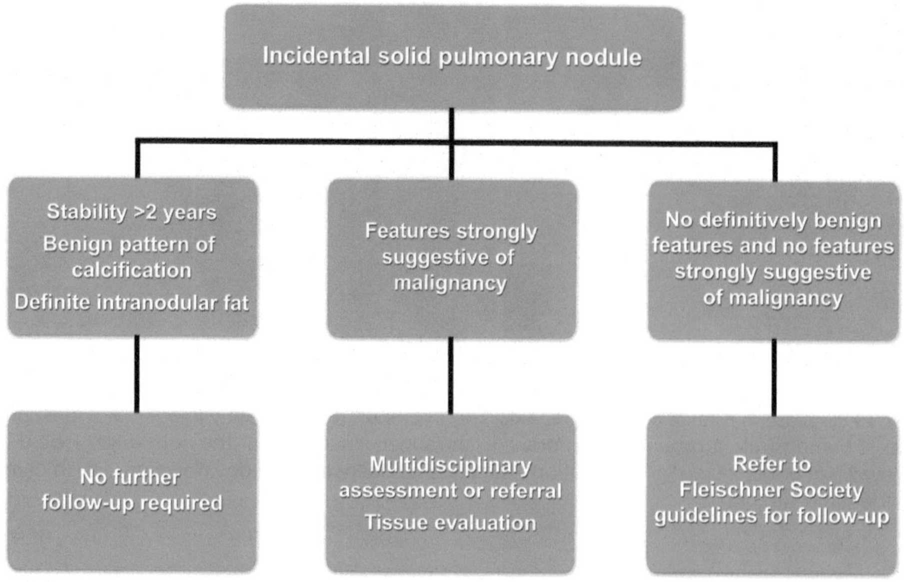

FIGURE 22.16 Approach to evaluating an incidental solid pulmonary nodule.

TABLE 22.2 Fleischner Society 2017 Guidelines for Management of Solid Pulmonary Nodules*

Nodule Type	<6 mm (<100 mm³)	6–8 mm (100–250 mm³)	>8 mm (>250 mm³)
Single			
Low risk†	No routine follow-up	CT at 6–12 mo; then consider CT at 18–24 mo	Consider CT, PET/CT, or tissue sampling at 3 mo
High risk†	Optional CT at 12 mo‡	CT at 6–12 mo; then CT at 18–24 mo	Consider CT, PET/CT, or tissue sampling at 3 mo
Multiple§			
Low risk†	No routine follow-up	CT at 3–6 mo; then consider CT at 18–24 mo	CT at 3–6 mo; then consider CT at 18–24 mo
High risk†	Optional CT at 12 mo	CT at 3–6 mo; then at 18–24 mo	CT at 3–6 mo; then at 18–24 mo

*These recommendations do not apply to lung cancer screening, patients with immunosuppression, or patients with known primary cancer.
†Consider all relevant risk factors.
‡Nodules <6 mm do not require routine follow-up, but certain patients at high risk with suspicious nodule morphology, upper lobe location, or both may warrant 12-month follow-up.
§Use most suspicious nodule as the guide to management. Follow-up intervals may vary according to size and risk.
CT, Computed tomography; *PET,* positron emission tomography.
From MacMahon H, Naidich DP, Goo JM, et al. Guidelines for management of incidental pulmonary nodules detected on CT images: from the Fleischner Society 2017. *Radiology*. 2017 Feb 23:161659. doi: 10.1148/radiol.2017161659. [Epub ahead of print]

Nodule Mimics

Because the goal of pulmonary nodule management is not only to identify small malignant nodules that can be resected with high survival rates but also to spare patients with benign disease from undergoing invasive procedures, one should first always consider the benign causes and mimics.

Certain lesions (Box 22.1) in the lung may produce the appearance of a nonspecific pulmonary nodule or lesion on chest radiography, but CT may help identify specific diagnostic features for these nodule mimics.

Symmetric nodular opacities projecting over the lower lung zones on a chest radiograph are often caused by nipple shadows and, when in doubt, can be confirmed with repeat radiographs obtained with nipple markers (see Chapter 1). Prominent calcifications within the first costochondral junction or vascular calcifications are also frequently mistaken for a nodule on radiograph but are clearly identified as such on CT. Bone islands may be identified on chest radiographs by

BOX 22.1 Mimics of Solid Pulmonary Nodule

Bone island
Nipple shadow
Pleural thickening, fluid, or pleural plaques
Soft tissue, costochondral, and vascular calcifications
Rib fractures
Hematoma
Arteriovenous fistula
Pseudoaneurysm
Mucous impaction
Pulmonary infarcts
Nodular atelectasis
Congenital lesions (sequestration, bronchogenic cyst, bronchial atresia)
Fluid-filled bullae
Fungus ball

their relationship with the osseous structures and consistent location relative to bone on old radiographs and on CT by their high CT attenuation, which is typically greater than 1100 HU. Pleural plaques often create a holly-leaf appearance on radiographs but can also be nodular. They are clearly identified by CT (Fig. 22.17).

Arteriovenous fistulas can be diagnosed by the presence of a feeding artery and draining vein as well as by intense enhancement after the administration of contrast material. Features of rounded atelectasis include a peripheral rounded lesion in the lung abutting pleural thickening associated with the classic comet tail sign, consisting of crowding of pulmonary vessels and bronchi leading to the mass (see Chapter 2). A fungus ball within a preexisting cavity may appear as a solitary pulmonary nodule on standard films, but CT can clearly identify the presence of a nodule within a cavity. Mucoid impaction on CT can be diagnosed by classic features of branching opacities located endobronchially and is often associated with bronchiectasis. Pulmonary infarcts classically abut the pleura and are round or wedge shaped. Furthermore, they demonstrate a characteristic evolution over time.

MANAGEMENT OF SUBSOLID NODULES

Radiography

Radiographs are usually not sensitive in the evaluation of subsolid nodules, particularly those that are of pure ground-glass attenuation.

Computed Tomography

Computed tomography plays a crucial role in determining subtle changes in a subsolid nodule, most importantly changes in attenuation and growth as discussed previously. The size of the solid component within a subsolid nodule has direct correlation with probability of adenocarcinoma and inverse correlation with prognosis.

In terms of growth, rapid growth of subsolid nodules may again be indicative of a benign lesion as it is for solid nodules. However, very long doubling times may be seen in subsolid malignant lesions. Also, an increase in density of a subsolid nodule should be considered growth even if the overall size does not change. An overall growth regression may also be observed and is thought to occur because of fibrosis.

Margin, shape, and internal features have not been confirmed as reliable differentiators of benign and malignant subsolid nodules. However, some features such as bubbly lucencies (pseudocavitation), presence of dilated bronchus, pleural tags, and convex margin are all thought to be more frequent in invasive adenocarcinoma compared with preinvasive or minimally invasive lesions (Fig. 22.18).

Transient Versus Persistent

Subsolid nodule frequency varies widely among reports, with frequency among all nodules ranging from 3% to 38% in screening CT study reports. Some of the benign etiologies of subsolid nodules, such as infectious or inflammatory and hemorrhage, are characterized by their transient nature, and one of the first questions when evaluating a subsolid nodule is whether it is transient or persistent. Transient nodules are defined as those that resolve spontaneously or following antibiotics. Between 38% and 70% of subsolid nodules are estimated to be transient. The precise etiology of these nodules is unknown as histology is frequently unavailable. However, some predictors of transient lesions include young age, blood eosinophilia, polygonal shape, lesion multiplicity, ill-defined borders, solid components, and location in lung bases.

When persistent, an estimated 19% of pure ground-glass and 63% of part-solid nodules are thought to be malignant. The malignant causes for persistent subsolid nodules include adenocarcinoma, metastases (including gastrointestinal, melanoma, and renal cell metastases), and pulmonary lymphoproliferative disorders.

Guidelines

Patients with subsolid nodules are not divided into high- and low-risk groups under current Fleischner guidelines as they are for solid nodules (Table 22.3). PET has a limited role in subsolid nodule management and is most useful in cases with a large solid component (>8 mm). The fludeoxyglucose uptake in malignant ground-glass and part-solid nodules varies and cannot be used to reliably distinguish between benign and malignant lesions. Apart from evaluating nodules by CT, radiologists also play a role in biopsy of suspicious nodules as well as percutaneous localization before surgery. These techniques are reviewed separately (see Chapter 25).

TABLE 22.3 Fleischner Society 2017 Guidelines for Management of Subsolid Pulmonary Nodules*

Nodule Type	<6 mm (<100 mm^3)	≥6 mm (>100 mm^3)
Single		
Ground glass	No routine follow-up[‡]	CT at 6–12 mo to confirm persistence; then CT every 2 yr until 5 yr
Part solid[†]	No routine follow-up[‡]	CT at 3–6 mo to confirm persistence; if unchanged and solid component remains <6 mm, annual CT should be performed for 5 yr
Multiple	CT at 6 mo; if stable, consider CT at 2 and 4 yr[§]	CT at 3–6 mo; subsequent management based on the most suspicious nodule(s)

*These recommendations do not apply to lung cancer screening, patients with immunosuppression, or patients with known primary cancer.

[†]In practice, part-solid nodules cannot be defined as such until ≥6 mm, and nodules <6 mm do not usually require follow-up. Persistent part-solid nodules with solid components ≥6 mm should be considered highly suspicious.

[‡]In certain suspicious nodules <6 mm, consider follow-up at 2 and 4 years. If solid component(s) or growth develops, consider resection.

[§]Multiple <6-mm pure ground-glass nodules are usually benign, but consider follow-up in selected patients at high risk at 2 and 4 years.

CT, Computed tomography.

From MacMahon H, Naidich DP, Goo JM, et al. Guidelines for management of incidental pulmonary nodules detected on CT images: from the Fleischner Society 2017. *Radiology.* 2017 Feb 23:161659. doi: 10.1148/radiol.2017161659. [Epub ahead of print]

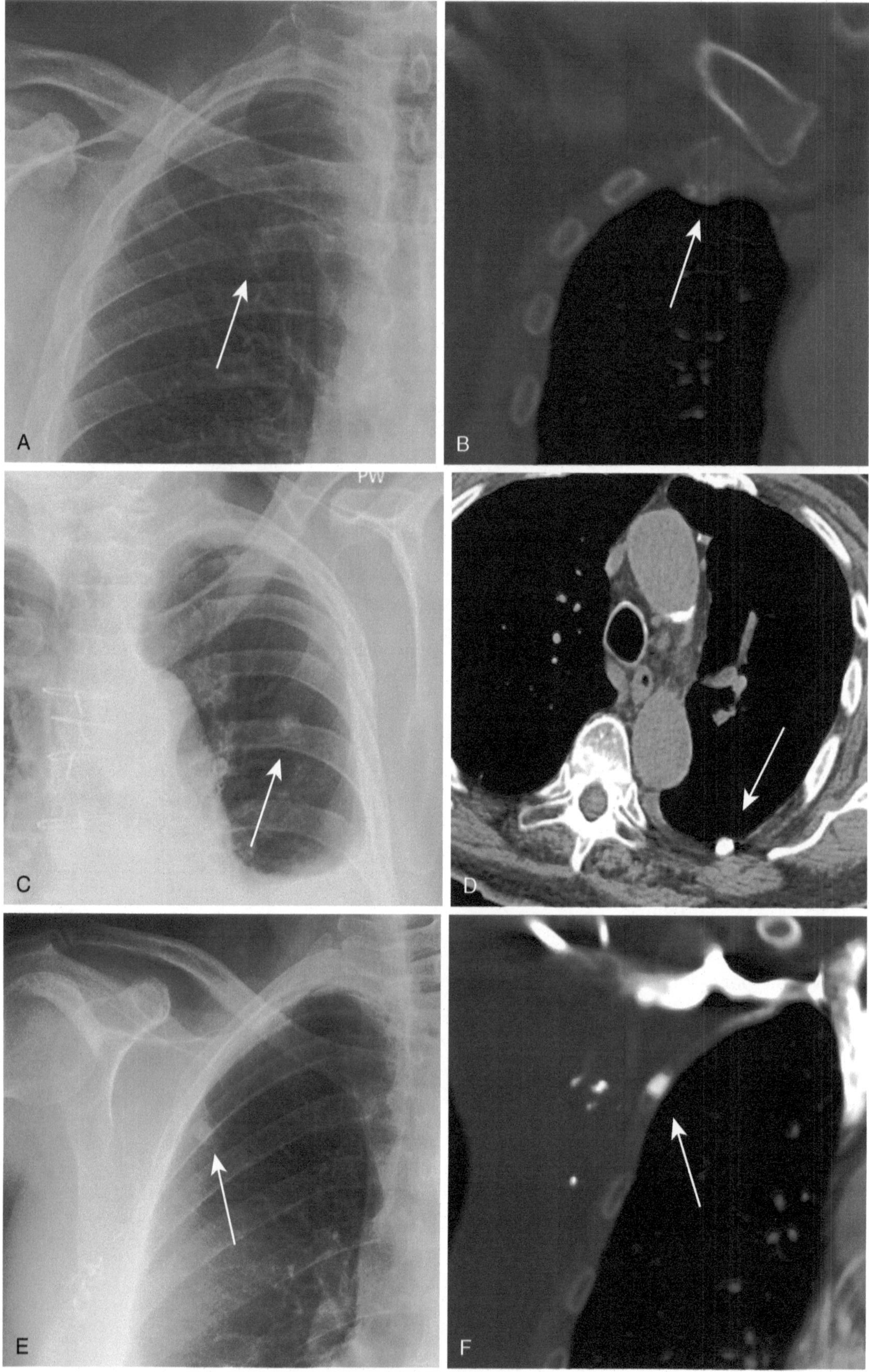

FIGURE 22.17 Solid nodule mimics. Chest radiographs demonstrating commonly seen solid nodule mimics with corresponding chest computed tomography images. Nodular appearance of prominent costochondral calcifications at the first costochondral junction (**A** and **B**), nodular pleural plaque creating the appearance of a nodule on chest radiograph (**C** and **D**), and a bone island within a rib presenting as a dense nodule on the radiograph (**E** and **F**). *Arrows* indicate nodule mimics and corresponding findings on CT.

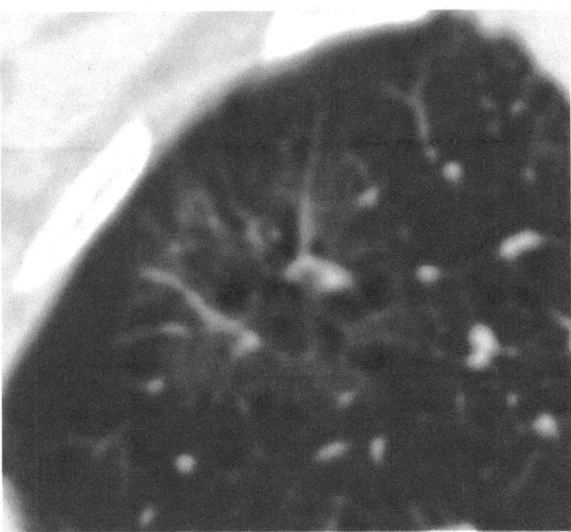

FIGURE 22.18 "Bubbly" lucencies. Chest computed tomography image demonstrates a subsolid nodule that had increased in both size and attenuation over several years and contained internal areas of "bubbly" lucencies, a characteristic pattern for adenocarcinoma.

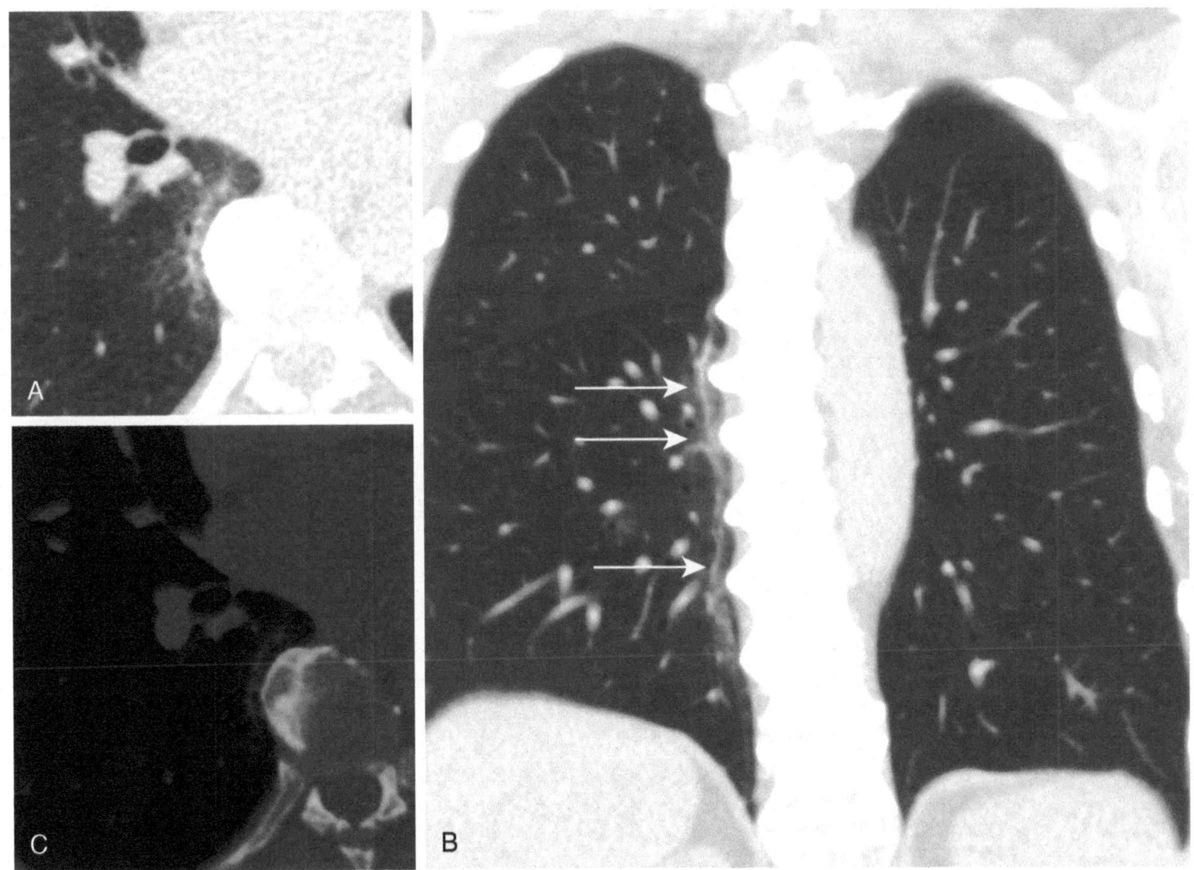

FIGURE 22.19 Subsolid nodule mimic. Axial chest computed tomography (CT) image demonstrates a focal mixed attenuation opacity in the right paraspinal region **(A)**. The coronal reformats demonstrate the linear extent of this opacity in the paraspinal region of the right lower lobe **(B)**, and bone windows on axial CT reveal a large osteophyte adjacent to the opacity **(C)** and at multiple levels in the thoracic spine (*arrows* in *B*). This lung opacity represents fibrosis related to irritation of the lung by the osteophytes during respiration.

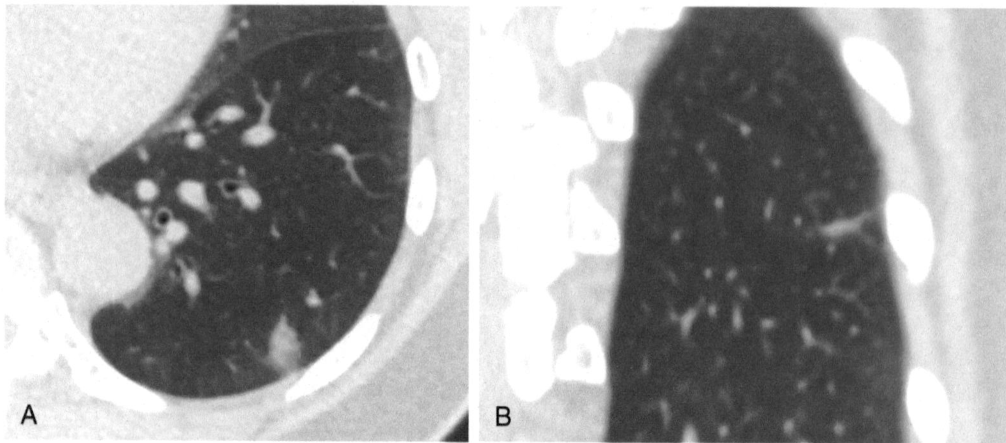

FIGURE 22.20 Subsolid nodule mimic. Axial chest computed tomography image demonstrates a mixed attenuation nodule in the periphery of the left lower lobe **(A)**. The coronal reformats reveal the linear configuration of the nodule **(B)**, which is suggestive of benign atelectasis or scarring and stable on subsequent studies.

Nodule Mimics

There are mimics to subsolid nodules as well. A mixed attenuation opacity in the paraspinal region, for example, is often attributable to focal lung fibrosis. Viewing the images on bone windows to confirm the presence of adjacent large osteophyte is helpful (Fig. 22.19). In the absence of focal nodular components, this finding does not warrant follow-up. Atelectasis may appear as a nodular subsolid opacity in axial cross section but in coronal or sagittal planes will appear as a linear opacity (Fig. 22.20).

SUGGESTED READINGS

Aoki T, Nakata H, Watanabe H, et al. Evolution of peripheral lung adenocarcinomas: CT findings correlated with histology and tumor doubling time. *AJR Am J Roengenol*. 2000;174(3):763–768.

Benjamin MS, Drucker EA, McLoud TC, et al. Small pulmonary nodules: detection at chest CT and outcome. *Radiology*. 2003;226(2):489–493.

Callister ME, Baldwin DR, Akram AR, et al. British Thoracic Society guidelines for the investigation and management of pulmonary nodules. *Thorax*. 2015;70(suppl 2):ii1–ii54. doi:10.1136/thoraxjnl-2015-207168. No abstract available. Erratum in: *Thorax*. 2015;70(12):1188.

Erasmus JJ, Connolly JE, McAdams HP, et al. Solitary pulmonary nodules: Part I. Morphologic evaluation for differentiation of benign and malignant lesions. *Radiographics*. 2000;20:43–58.

Godoy MCB, Naidich DP. Overview and strategic management of subsolid pulmonary nodules. *J Thorac Imaging*. 2012;27:240–248.

Godoy MC, Truong MT, Carter BW, et al. Pitfalls in pulmonary nodule characterization. *Semin Roentgenol*. 2015;50(3):164–174. doi:10.1053/j.ro.2015.01.011. [Epub 2015 Feb 4]

Gould MK, Donington J, Lynch WR, et al. Evaluation of individuals with pulmonary nodules: when is it lung cancer? Diagnosis and management of lung cancer, 3rd ed: American College of Chest Physicians evidence-based clinical practice guidelines. *Chest*. 2013;143(5 suppl):e93S–120S. doi:10.1378/chest.12-2351. Review.

Hodnett PA, Ko JP. Evaluation and management of indeterminate pulmonary nodules. *Radiol Clin North Am*. 2012;50:895–914.

MacMahon H, Naidich DP, Goo JM, et al. Guidelines for management of incidental pulmonary nodules detected on CT images: from the Fleischner Society 2017. *Radiology*. 2017;161659. doi:10.1148/radiol.2017161659. [Epub ahead of print]

Naidich DP, Bankier AA, MacMahon H, et al. Recommendations for the management of subsolid pulmonary nodules detected at CT: a statement from the Fleischner Society. *Radiology*. 2013;266:304–317.

Ost D, Fein AM, Feinsilver SH. Clinical practice. The solitary pulmonary nodule. *N Engl J Med*. 2003;348:2535–2542.

Raad RA, Suh J, Harari S, et al. Nodule characterization: subsolid nodules. *Radiol Clin North Am*. 2014;52(1):47–67.

Seidelman JS, Myers JL, Quinta LE. Incidental, subsolid pulmonary nodules at CT: etiology and management. *Cancer Imaging*. 2013;13(3):365–373.

Truong MT, Ko JP, Rossi SE, et al. Update in the evaluation of the solitary pulmonary nodule. *Radiographics*. 2014;34(6):1658–1679.

Wahidi MM, Govert JA, Gouldar RK, et al. American College of Chest Physicians. Evidence for the treatment of patients with pulmonary nodules: when is it lung cancer? ACCP evidence-based clinical practice guidelines. *Chest*. 2007;132(3 suppl):94S–107S.

Chapter 23

Lung Cancer Screening

Shaunagh McDermott, Jo-Anne O. Shepard, and Amita Sharma

Lung cancer is suitable for screening because of identifiable risk factors that allow targeted screening of high-risk individuals, its significant prevalence, the existence of a preclinical phase, its high morbidity and mortality, and evidence that treatment in early-stage disease is potentially curative.

WHY SCREEN?

Lung cancer is the third most common cancer in the United States but has the highest mortality rate among cancers. The 5-year survival rate from non-small cell lung cancer (NSCLC) is 16.8%, which is much lower compared with that of other common cancers such as breast cancer (89.2%) and colon cancer (64.7%). The high mortality rate is often due to the diagnosis of lung cancer at an advanced stage. The 5-year survival rate of NSCLC varies from 49% when detected at stage IA to 1% when detected at stage IV. Therefore, early diagnosis would be expected to reduce the mortality rate from this disease.

In 2011, the National Lung Screening Trial Research Group published results from the largest to date, randomized, multicenter study, which included more than 50,000 participants and tested the utility of low-dose computed tomography (LDCT) versus conventional chest radiography (CXR) for lung cancer screening in high-risk individuals. The primary outcome was lung cancer mortality, which was compared between the two arms of the trial. Secondary outcomes included the incidence of lung cancer and causes of death other than lung cancer. There was a relative reduction in the rate of death from lung cancer with LDCT of 20% (95% confidence interval, 6.8-26.7; $P = 0.004$). The number needed to screen with LDCT to prevent one death from lung cancer was 320. There was a reduction of 6.7% in the rate of death from any cause with LDCT screening ($P = 0.02$). The rate of lung cancer detection did not diminish between the screening years. However, fewer stage IV cancers were observed in the LDCT group than the CXR group during the second and third screening rounds, which suggests that the diagnosis of earlier-stage cancers reduces the occurrence of later-stage lung cancers.

Other randomized trials have not demonstrated a mortality benefit; however, these may be too small and therefore underpowered or still preliminary. Several observational studies of LDCT, such as the Early Lung Cancer Project (ELCAP), Mayo Clinic CT study, and Continuous Observation of Smoking (COSMOS) study, have demonstrated that screening with LDCT can identify early-stage asymptomatic lung cancer.

The potential of screening to detect early cancers and increase the overall cure rate can only be achieved in the context of a multidisciplinary program that ensures screening is properly performed, interpreted, and followed up and abnormal findings are appropriately managed.

WHO TO SCREEN?

Unfortunately, because of economic constraints, LDCT screening is directed to those considered to be at highest risk for lung cancer. Tobacco use remains the major modifiable risk factor for lung cancer, with an associated 20-fold relative increase in risk of lung cancer. Smoking cessation markedly reduces the risk of developing lung cancer over time; however, the level of risk never declines to that of a lifetime nonsmoker. Other risk factors for lung cancer include occupational exposures, residential radon exposures, personal cancer history (particularly smoking-related cancers such as head and neck cancers), family history of lung cancer (Fig. 23.1), and chronic lung disease (including chronic obstructive pulmonary disease and chronic interstitial lung disease).

Many professional societies have released screening guidelines based in part on NLST enrollment demographics (Box 23.1). For example, the Centers for Medicare & Medicaid Services covers screening with LDCT once per year in patients who are 55 to 77 years old, asymptomatic, current smokers or have quit smoking within the past 15 years, and have a tobacco smoking history of at least 30 pack-years. However, several other professional societies, including the National Comprehensive Cancer Network and the American Association of Thoracic Surgery, advocate for broader inclusion of at-risk individuals. A retrospective analysis of data from Surveillance, Epidemiology and End results (SEER), the U.S. Census, the 2010 National Health Interview Survey, and two statistical models of lung cancer risk found that only 26.7% of individuals with a diagnosis of lung cancer met NLST screening criteria.

BOX 23.1 Currently Approved Eligibility Criteria for Lung Cancer Screening

Age
- 55–77 years (CMS)
- 55–80 years (USPSTF)

Smoking pack-years
- 30 (CMS, USPSTF)

Current or former smoker

Years since quitting smoking
- 15 years (CMS, USPSTF)

Asymptomatic
- No signs or symptoms of lung cancer

CMS, Centers for Medicare & Medicaid Services; *USPSTF,* U.S. Preventive Services Task Force.

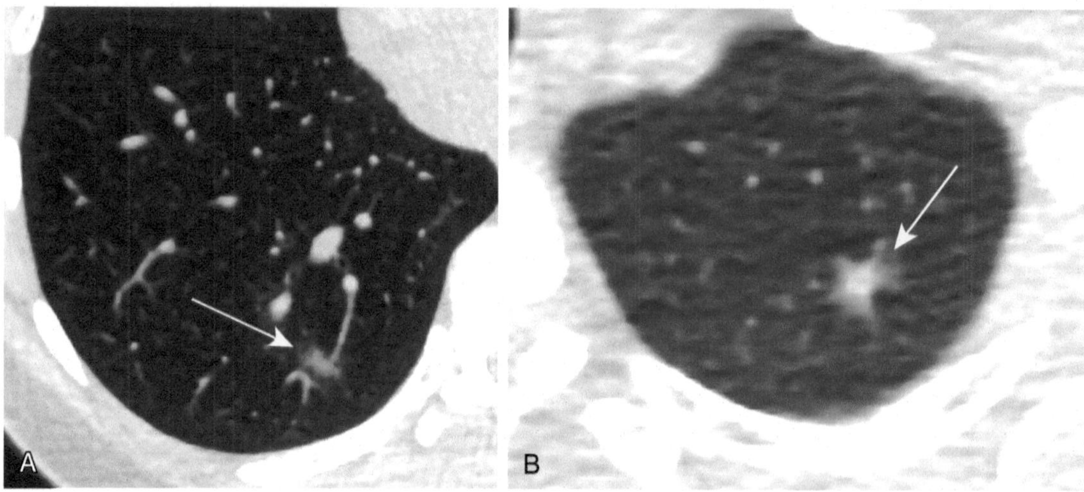

FIGURE 23.1 A 45-year-old woman who never smoked but with a strong family history of lung cancer (two generations of nonsmoking relatives). **A,** The dominant nodule in the right lower lobe *(arrow)* is a part solid nodule measuring 12 × 6 mm (mean diameter, 9 mm). **B,** There is a second smaller part solid nodule *(arrow)* in the left upper lobe. These persisted on a short-term follow-up computed tomography performed 3 months later. The patient underwent bilateral wedge resections, which found both lesions to be adenocarcinoma.

HOW TO SCREEN?

A shared decision-making visit between a patient and her or his provider should precede screening. The visit should incorporate discussion of eligibility criteria, the benefits and harms of screening, the likelihood of further diagnostic testing, the risk of overdiagnosis, and false-positive rates. A screening program must also be integrated with a smoking cessation program.

The American College of Radiology (ACR) and Society of Thoracic Radiology have published guidelines regarding how LDCT should be performed for lung cancer screening (see Chapter 1). A facility is eligible to receive the ACR Lung Cancer Screening Center designation if it meets a list of basic criteria (Box 23.2).

BOX 23.2 Criteria for Designation Through the American College of Radiology as a Lung Cancer Screening Center

Shared decision-making visit
Smoking cessation counseling
Screening protocol
- A CT dose index volume of <3 mGy for a standard patient
- Exposure values must be reduced for smaller sized patients and increased for larger sized patients, using manual or automated methods

Personnel
- Interpreting physicians must have read 200 chest CTs in the preceding 36 months
- Medical physicists and radiologic technologists continue to meet the requirements of the CT accreditation program

Equipment
- CT equipment specifications and performance must meet state and federal requirements and applicable ACR Practice Parameters and Technical Standards
- CT scanners used are multidetector helical CT scanners

Follow-up and reporting
- Must use structured reporting systems that includes management recommendations
- Facilities that accept self-referrals must have procedures for referring them to a qualified health care provider if abnormal findings are present
- Follow the ACR Practice Parameter for Communication of Diagnostic Imaging Findings

Data collection and research

ACR, American College of Radiology; *CT,* computed tomography.

LUNG NODULE ASSESSMENT

Computed tomography (CT) features that assess the malignant potential of a nodule include its morphology, size, presence of calcification or fat, border, and growth. The ACR has proposed a standardized, comprehensive, clinical decision-oriented system—namely, the Lung CT Screening Reporting and Data System (Lung-RADS) (Table 23.1), which combines a nodule's morphology (solid, part solid, nonsolid) with its average diameter and establishes categories that correlate with risk of malignancy and that determine recommended follow-up protocols. Whereas a screening examination may contain several nodules of varying categories, the overall Lung-RADS score is based on the most suspicious nodule.

Morphology

Nodule attenuation should be classified as solid or subsolid (part solid and nonsolid). A solid nodule consists of homogeneous soft tissue attenuation (Fig. 23.2). A nonsolid (ground-glass) nodule manifests as hazy increased attenuation in the lung that does not obliterate the bronchial and vascular margins (Fig. 23.3). A part solid nodule consists of both ground-glass and solid soft tissue attenuation components (Figs. 23.4 and 23.5). Although solid nodules are more common, part solid lesions have a higher likelihood of being malignant.

TABLE 23.1 Lung CT Screening Reporting and Data System (Lung-RADS) Version 1.0 Assessment Categories (2014)[a]

Category	Category Descriptor	Category	Findings	Management	Probability of Malignancy (%)	Estimated Population Prevalence (%)
Incomplete	—	0	Prior chest CT examination(s) being located for comparison Part or all of lungs cannot be evaluated	Additional lung cancer screening CT images and/or comparison to prior chest CT examinations is needed	N/A	1
Negative	No nodules and definitely benign nodules	1	No lung nodules	Continue annual screening with LDCT in 12 mo	<1	90
Benign appearance or behavior	Nodules with a very low likelihood of becoming a clinically active cancer because of size or lack of growth	2	Nodule(s) with specific calcifications: complete, central, popcorn, concentric rings, and fat-containing nodules Solid nodule(s): <6 mm new <4 mm Part solid nodule(s): <6-mm total diameter on baseline screening Nonsolid nodule(s) (GGN): <20 mm *or* ≥ 20 mm and unchanged or slowly growing Category 3 or 4 nodules unchanged for ≥ 3 mo			
Probably benign	Probably benign finding(s): short-term follow-up suggested; includes nodules with a low likelihood of becoming clinically active cancer	3	Solid nodule(s): ≥ 6 to <8 mm at baseline *or* new 4 mm to <6 mm Part solid nodule(s): ≥ 6-mm total diameter with solid component <6 mm *or* new <6-mm total diameter Nonsolid nodule(s) (GGN) ≥ 20 mm on baseline CT or new	6-mo LDCT	1–2	5

Continued

TABLE 23.1 Lung CT Screening Reporting and Data System (Lung-RADS) Version 1.0 Assessment Categories (2014)—cont'd

Category	Category Descriptor	Category	Findings	Management	Probability of Malignancy (%)	Estimated Population Prevalence (%)
Suspicious	Findings for which additional diagnostic testing or tissue sampling is recommended	4A	Solid nodule(s): ≥8 to <15 mm at baseline *or* growing <8 mm *or* Part solid nodule(s): ≥6 mm with solid component ≥6 mm to <8 mm *Or* with a new or growing <4-mm solid component Endobronchial nodule	3-mo LDCT; PET/CT may be used when there is a ≥8-mm solid component	5–15	2
		4B	Solid nodule(s) ≥15 mm *or* new or growing and ≥8 mm Part solid nodule(s) with: a solid component ≥8 mm *or* new or growing ≥4-mm solid component	Chest CT with or without contrast, PET/CT and/or tissue sampling depending on the probability[b] of malignancy and comorbidities; PET/CT may be used when there is a ≥8-mm solid component	>15	2
		4X	Category 3 or 4 nodules with additional features or imaging findings that increase the suspicion of malignancy			
Other	Clinically significant or potentially clinically significant findings (nonlung cancer)	5	Modifier: may add on to category 0–4 coding	As appropriate to the specific finding	N/A	10
Prior lung cancer	Modifier for patients with a prior diagnosis of lung cancer who return	C	Modifier: may add on to category 0–4 coding	—	—	—

[a]Important notes for use:
1. A negative screen does not mean that an individual does not have lung cancer.
2. Size: Nodules should be measured on lung windows and reported as the average diameter rounded to the nearest whole number; for round nodules, only a single diameter measurement is necessary.
3. Size thresholds apply to nodules at first detection and that grow and reach a higher size category.
4. Growth: an increase in size of >1.5 mm.
5. Exam category: Each exam should be coded 0–4 based on the nodule(s) with the highest degree of suspicion.
6. Exam modifiers: S and C modifiers may be added to the 0–4 category.
7. Lung cancer diagnosis: After a patient is diagnosed with lung cancer, further management (including additional imaging such as positron emission tomography [PET]/computed tomography [CT]) may be performed for the purposes of lung cancer staging; this is no longer screening.
8. Practice audit definitions: a negative screen is defined as categories 1 and 2; a positive screen is defined as categories 3 and 4.
9. Category 4B management: this is predicated on the probability of malignancy based on patient evaluation, patient preference, and risk of malignancy; radiologists are encouraged to use the McWilliams et al assessment tool[†] when making recommendations.
10. Category 4X: nodules with additional imaging findings that increase the suspicion of lung cancer, such as spiculation, GGN that doubles in size in 1 year, enlarged lymph nodes, and so on.
11. Nodules with features of an intrapulmonary lymph node should be managed by mean diameter and the 0–4 numerical category classification.
12. Category 3 and 4A nodules that are unchanged on interval CT should be coded as category 2 and individuals returned to screening in 12 months.

GGN, Ground glass nodule. *LDCT,* Low-dose chest computed tomography.

[b]Link to McWilliams Lung Cancer Risk Calculator: Upon request from the authors at: http://www.brocku.ca/lung-cancer-risk-calculator At UptoDate http://www.uptodate.com/contents/calculator-solitary-pulmonary-nodule-malignancy-risk-brock-university-cancer-prediction-equation.

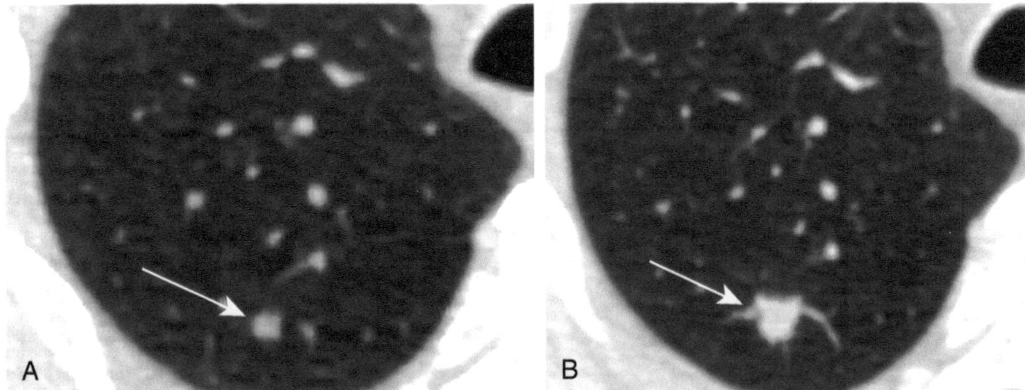

FIGURE 23.2 A 68-year-old man with a 40 pack-year history. **A,** The dominant nodule *(arrow)* on the initial screening low-dose computed tomography (LDCT) scan is a solid 5-mm nodule in the right upper lobe (category 2). **B,** On the next annual surveillance LDCT, the nodule *(arrow)* had increased in size to 11 × 9 mm (mean diameter, 10 mm) (category 4B). He underwent a right upper lobectomy, which revealed an adenocarcinoma.

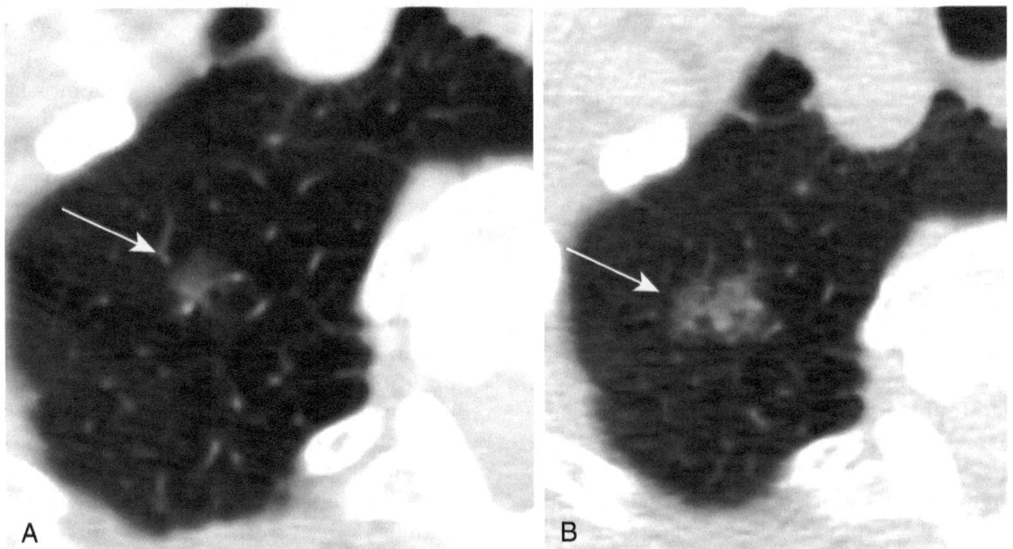

FIGURE 23.3 A 69-year-old man, a current smoker with a 35 pack-year history. **A,** The dominant nodule on the initial screening low-dose computed tomography image is a 22 × 15 mm (mean diameter, 19 mm) nonsolid nodule in the right upper lobe *(arrow)*. **B,** This had significantly increased in size since a prior study from 3 years previously *(arrow)* (category 4X). This was confirmed as an adenocarcinoma on resection.

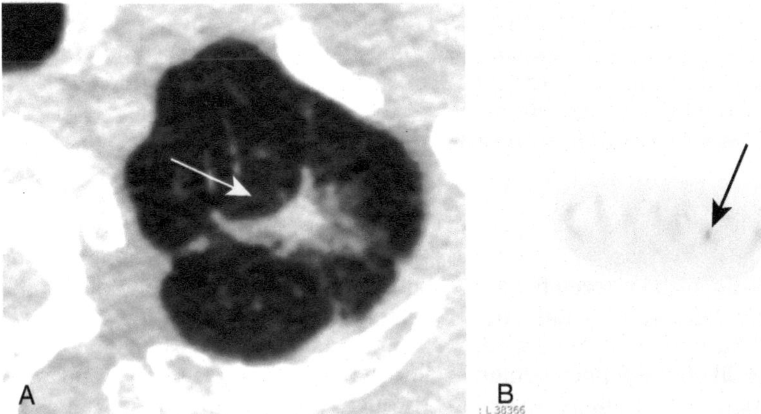

FIGURE 23.4 A 74-year-old man who quit smoking 3 years earlier with a 40 pack-year history. **A,** Initial screening computed tomography (CT) image demonstrates a part solid nodule in the left upper lobe measuring 38 × 18 mm (mean diameter, 28 mm) with a 10 × 8 mm (mean diameter, 9 mm) solid component *(arrow)* (category 4X). **B,** He underwent positron emission tomography/CT, which demonstrated intense fludeoxyglucose uptake associated with the solid component of the nodule *(arrow)*. The patient underwent a left upper lobe segmentectomy, which revealed an adenocarcinoma.

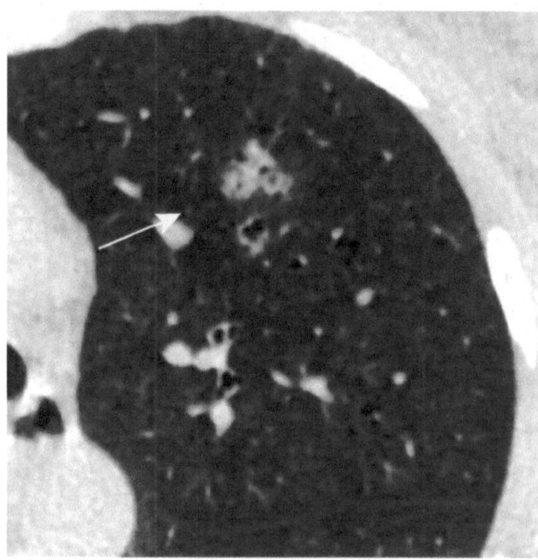

FIGURE 23.5 A 58-year-old woman, a current smoker with a 32 pack-year history. The dominant nodule *(arrow)* is a part solid nodule in the left upper lobe measuring 17 × 9 mm (mean diameter, 13 mm) with a solid component measuring 14 × 7 mm (mean diameter, 10 mm) (category 4B). She underwent short-interval contrast-enhanced computed tomography, and the nodule had resolved, consistent with an inflammatory nodule.

Size

Lung-RADS recommends that nodules and solid components of part solid nodules should be measured on thin sections in the axial plane on lung windows and reported as the average diameter rounded to the nearest whole number. Data from both retrospective series and prospective screening trials show that the risk of malignancy is related to nodule size. The risk of malignancy in a nonsolid nodule that persists beyond 3 months ranges from 10% to 60% and depends on its size and the presence of a solid component.

Growth

A nodule that has clearly increased in size on serial imaging is at high risk for malignancy. An increase in mean size of at least 1.5 mm is needed to identify nodule growth by Lung-RADS criteria. It is important to remember that lesions that partially decrease in size at short-term LDCT are not necessarily benign. It has been shown that adenocarcinomas can decrease temporarily in size owing to fibrosis or atelectasis.

Presence of Calcification or Fat

Calcification patterns can help distinguish between benign and malignant lesions. Eccentric calcifications raise the suspicion for malignancy, but diffuse, central, laminated, and popcorn patterns are more likely to reflect benign etiologies. Intranodular fat attenuation is typically associated with hamartomas (see Chapter 22).

PITFALLS IN LUNG CANCER SCREENING

Lung-RADS differentiates the categorization and management of screen-detected nodules based on their morphology. When a nodule is detected on the LDCT, the next step is to classify it as either solid or subsolid (which incorporates both part solid and nonsolid nodules). This classification leads to substantially different management, including selection of an appropriate imaging interval, modality for assessment, and need for intervention. However, studies have shown that both the inter- and intraobserver agreement among experienced thoracic radiologists in distinguishing solid from subsolid nodules is variable.

Although Lung-RADS incorporates different morphologic subtypes of nodules, including solid, part solid, and nonsolid nodules, it does not specifically mention how to categorize or manage cystic lung lesions (Fig. 23.6). There is increasing evidence that lung cancer could arise in association with pulmonary cystic airspaces, including cysts, bullae, and blebs. Progressive wall thickening or the development of or increase in size of a nodule inside or outside a cystic airspace should raise the suspicion of lung cancer. The cystic component could increase, decrease, or remain unchanged with tumor growth.

A subset of nodules not specifically mentioned in Lung-RADS are perifissural nodules. These are solid nodules that are adjacent to either the major or minor fissures and are often oval or triangular in shape with the broadest base along the fissure, and they are most often fissural lymph nodes. Currently, these nodules should be assessed the same way as any other nodule and categorized based on their mean diameter and attenuation.

Another entity that deserves specific consideration in lung cancer screening are the lung apices. Lung cancer has been found to be more prevalent in the upper lobes. The detection and interpretation of parenchymal abnormalities within the lung apices can be a challenge because apical regions are a frequent location of fibrotic scars that can be difficult to differentiate from early lung cancer. Lung cancer should be considered when a new lesion arises in a previously detected apical scar or when a focal apical abnormality shows progressive enlargement at annual screening LDCT.

The detection of a lung cancer can be difficult or even delayed when arising in abnormal lung such as interstitial lung disease. The tumor can be hidden or overlooked in the presence of underlying lung abnormalities. This is especially important because idiopathic pulmonary fibrosis is associated with an increased risk of lung cancer, and some studies have reported that the tumors preferentially occur in areas with lung fibrosis.

LUNG NODULE MANAGEMENT ALGORITHMS

A screening program should include a multidisciplinary team consisting of physicians with expertise in the management of lung nodules and the treatment of lung cancer, including thoracic surgeons, pulmonologists, medical and radiation oncologists, and diagnostic and interventional radiologists. The program must have lung nodule management pathways and have the expertise to evaluate concerning nodules through positron emission tomography (PET) imaging, nonsurgical and minimally invasive surgical approaches.

Because solid nodules smaller than 8 mm are unlikely to be malignant, are difficult to biopsy, and not reliably characterized by functional imaging with PET imaging, follow-up by CT is recommended. Subsolid nodules may also be falsely negative on PET because a critical mass of metabolically active malignant cells is required for detection.

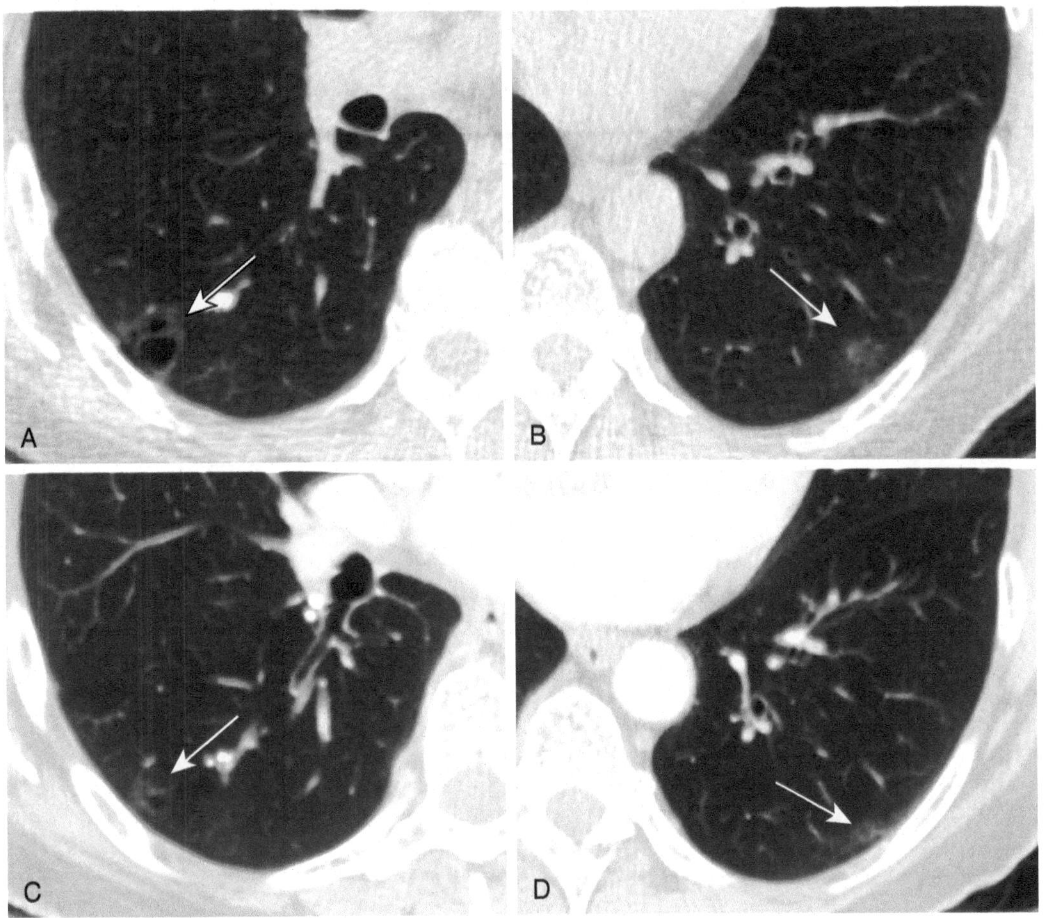

FIGURE 23.6 A 62-year-old woman, a current smoker with a 33 pack-year history. **A,** The dominant nodule is a multicystic nodule in the right lower lobe *(arrow)*. **B,** There is a part solid nodule in the left lower lobe measuring 18 × 15 mm (mean diameter, 17 mm) with a 3-mm solid component *(arrow)*. **C** and **D,** Both these nodules *(arrows)* had increased in size since a computed tomography scan from 5 years prior, making the dominant nodule a category 4X. Resection of the right lower lobe nodule confirmed adenocarcinoma. Currently, the left lower lobe nodule is being followed by LDCT.

A negative LDCT (category 1) and nodules with a benign appearance or behavior (category 2) should undergo annual screening in 12 months. Nodules that are probably benign (category 3) require LDCT within 6 months. A category 3 or 4 nodule that is unchanged for more than 3 months can be downgraded to a category 2 nodule and followed with annual screening, which should be performed 12 months after the initial screening LDCT.

The decision to perform a PET scan depends on the probability of malignancy and the size and attenuation of the nodule. In Lung-RADS, a PET scan is recommended for suspicious nodules, including solid nodules larger than 8 mm, or part solid nodules with a solid component greater than 8 mm (category 4A, 4B, and 4X nodules). False-negative results can also occur with less metabolically active tumors such as adenocarcinoma in situ, minimally invasive adenocarcinoma, mucinous adenocarcinoma, and carcinoid tumors. Unfortunately, false-positive findings can occur with infectious and inflammatory conditions, including pneumonia, mycobacterial disease, rheumatoid nodules, and sarcoidosis. Besides nodule characterization, PET can identify regional and distant disease, including normal sized fludeoxyglucose-avid lymph nodes.

Tissue sampling is recommended for solid nodules larger than 15 mm, new or growing nodules that are larger than 8 mm, part-solid nodules with a solid component larger than 8 mm, or a new or growing solid component larger than 4 mm (category 4B or 4X nodules). Tissue sampling can be performed using imaging or bronchoscopic guidance or surgical biopsy. Refer to Chapter 25.

A screening program must have a means to track nodule management and to collect and report data related to surveillance and diagnostic imaging and surgical and nonsurgical biopsies of screen-detected lung nodules.

INCIDENTAL FINDINGS

There is no universally accepted definition of a "significant incidental finding," but in general, these findings require some form of clinical or imaging evaluation before the next lung screening examination. Lung-RADS requires that the reading radiologist specifically code for significant incidental findings on each examination (category S) to highlight the finding for the referring physician and to facilitate auditing the resulting diagnostic workup. The radiologist should make a suitable recommendation based on the finding.

Among the lung cancer screening trials, lung findings excluding pulmonary nodules were common and included diagnoses such as bronchiectasis, pulmonary fibrosis, and infections. Other cancers have also been discovered,

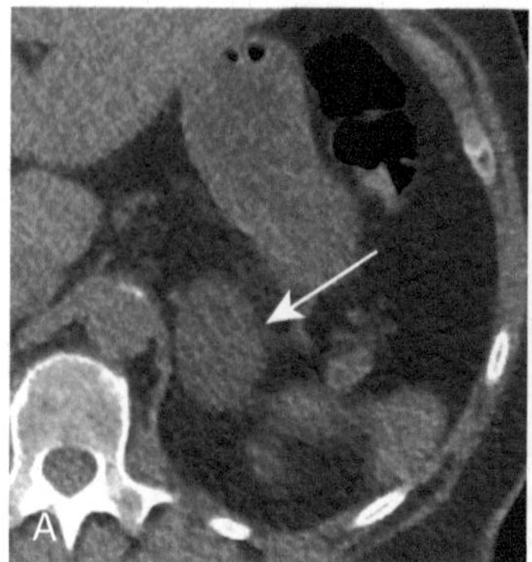

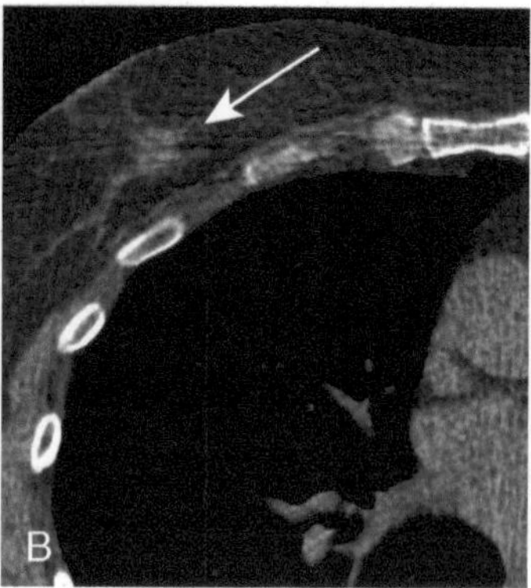

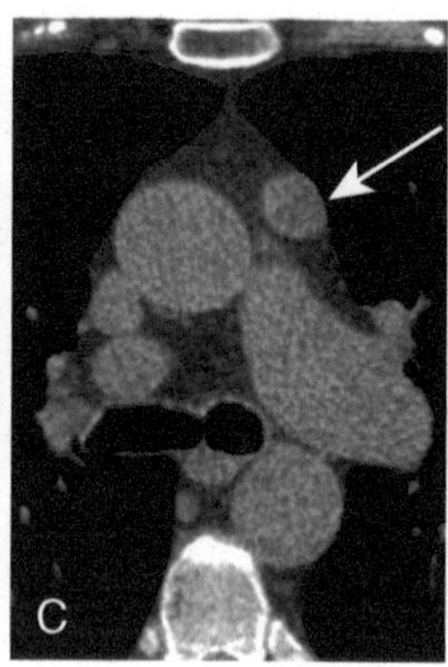

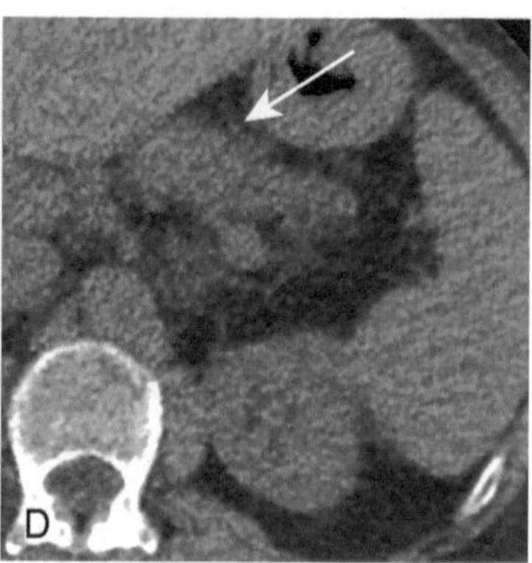

FIGURE 23.7 Incidental significant findings on screening computed tomography (CT). **A,** A 4 × 3-cm incompletely imaged left adrenal nodule *(arrow)*, which after dedicated adrenal computed tomography imaging was not diagnostic for an adenoma, was found to be an adrenocortical adenoma on resection. **B,** A 1-cm right breast nodule *(arrow)*, which was diagnosed as invasive ductal carcinoma after mammography and ultrasound-guided biopsy. **C,** A 2-cm soft tissue nodule in the left thymic bed *(arrow)*, which had increased in size from a prior study and was found to be a thymoma on resection. **D,** A 2.5-cm mass in the body of the pancreas *(arrow)* is difficult to appreciate on this unenhanced, low-dose CT image. Reports should have a caveat regarding how studies without contrast and with lower than standard dose have decreased sensitivity for the detection of small lesions in the upper abdomen.

including esophageal, breast, thyroid, and lymphomas (Fig. 23.7). Coronary artery calcifications or aortic aneurysms have also been identified. The ACR has white papers on managing incidental thyroid nodules detected on imaging and incidental findings on abdominal CT that could be translated to incidental findings in the thyroid gland and upper abdomen on LDCT.

STRUCTURED REPORTING

Variation in nodule characterization and subsequent management recommendations among radiologists is a well-known problem. The use of structured reports assists in more uniform documentation of pertinent findings and defines a positive finding. Structured reports with embedded nodule management, such as Lung-RADS, help provide a decision-orientated reporting system in which imaging findings are linked with standard guideline-based recommendations. They also result in improved communication among providers. Standardized reports can also be used to populate nodule registries and quality metrics.

POTENTIAL HARMS OF LOW-DOSE COMPUTED TOMOGRAPHY SCREENING FOR LUNG CANCER

The risks of low-dose CT screening for lung cancer include false-positive and false-negative results, potential unnecessary testing, overdiagnosis, radiation exposure, financial costs, and anxiety.

False-Positive Results in the NLST Trial

A false-positive result is the most common risk associated with CT screening for lung cancer. Notably, more than 96% of the positive test results, defined as detection of a nodule equal to or greater than 4 mm in diameter, in the CT group were false positives for lung cancer. Lung-RADS increased the solid diameter of a positive nodule to equal to or greater than 6 mm for solid and part solid nodules and to equal to or greater than 20 mm in nonsolid nodules to reduce the number of false positives but maintain sensitivity for malignancy. These changes have resulted in a considerable improvement in the performance of LDCT screening. By applying Lung-RADS to the NLST data, the false-positive rate for the baseline screen was 12.8% compared with 26.6% with the NLST criteria.

Overdiagnosis

Overdiagnosis refers to detection of indolent lung cancers that may never have become symptomatic and would not have been detected outside of a screening program. It is not possible to differentiate between cancers that a patient will die of from those that a patient will die with. Potentially curable lung cancers detected by screening are treated surgically, with the associated risks and mortality. Observational studies of screening for lung cancer with LDCT have estimated the extent of overdiagnosis to range between 13% and 27%. Other biases that can occur when clinicians fail to take into account the natural history of asymptomatic disease include lead-time bias and length-time bias.

Radiation

Radiation exposure is another risk from screening with CT. The effective dose of radiation of LDCT is estimated to be 1.5 mSv per examination. However, the use of diagnostic chest CT (~8 mSv) or PET/CT (~14 mSv) to further investigate detected lesions increases the exposure and accounts for most of the radiation exposure in screening studies. The risk for radiation-induced lung cancer depends on the age at which a person begins screening and the amount of cumulative radiation received. Using data from the NLST models predict approximately one cancer death caused by radiation from imaging per 2500 subjects screened. Therefore, the benefit in preventing lung cancer deaths in NLST considerably outweighs the radiation risk, which also only manifests 10 to 20 years later.

THE FUTURE OF LUNG CANCER SCREENING

The use of high-quality risk prediction models to select individuals for screening may save additional lives, reduce the number of false positives, and make screening more efficient and cost-effective. However, prospective studies are needed to determine whether risk models will identify a population in which screening would have greater benefit than the 20% lung cancer mortality benefit identified in the NLST.

Volumetric assessment may be used in the future to decide on the management of screen-detected nodules. Three-dimensional volumetric measurements are probably superior to two-dimensional diameter measurements in terms of accuracy and reproducibility because the whole nodule is analyzed. Growth rates can also be assessed using volume doubling time, which may be used to distinguish between positive screens that require additional diagnostic procedures and negative screens.

Computer-aided detection (CAD) systems may have a role to play in lung cancer screening. One study found that CAD systems detected 56% to 70% of lung cancers in the earlier round of screening when cancers were missed by radiologists. However, CAD systems missed about 21% of cancers in the round of screening when the cancers were first identified by radiologists. Therefore, the most appropriate role, at least for now, is for CAD to be used as a second reader.

The need to limit the number of false-positive results in LDCT screening has resulted in an effort to identify suitable diagnostic biomarkers. Potential biosamples for biomarker analysis include airway epithelium (including buccal mucosa), sputum, exhaled breath, and blood. The underlying rationale of a diagnostic biomarker based on biologic fluids is that molecular alterations within cancer cells lead to the synthesis of distinct molecular compounds, which, if detected, may signify the presence of cancerous transformation in an individual under investigation. Ideally, checking for a molecular biomarker in a lung cancer screening participant with a suspicious nodule should help in making diagnostic or therapeutic decisions.

CONCLUSION

There has been increasing implementation of lung cancer screening since the results of the NLST demonstrated improved lung cancer mortality and adoption of screening guidelines by both the U.S. Preventive Services Task Force and CMS. However, as screening becomes more disseminated, many challenges and areas of growth and improvement remain. These include identifying the most appropriate "at-risk" populations for screening, ensuring appropriate classification and management of screen-detected nodules, and defining the optimum duration of LDCT screening.

SUGGESTED READING

ACR. ACR designated lung cancer screening center. Available at: http://www.acr.org/Quality-Safety/Lung-Cancer-Screening-Center. Accessed May 12, 2016.

ACR. Lung cancer screening registry. Available at: http://www.acr.org/Quality-Safety/National-Radiology-Data-Registry/Lung-Cancer-Screening-Registry. Accessed May 12, 2016.

ACR-STR practice parameter for the performance and reporting of lung cancer screening thoracic computed tomography (CT). Available at: http://www.acr.org/~/media/ACR/Documents/PGTS/guidelines/LungScreening.pdf. Accessed May 13, 2016.

Bach PB, Mirkin JN, Oliver TK, et al. Benefits and harms of CT screening for lung cancer: a systematic review. *JAMA*. 2012;307(22):2418-2429.

Berland LL, Silverman SG, Gore RM, et al. Managing incidental findings on abdominal CT: white paper of the ACR incidental findings committee. *J Am Coll Radiol*. 2010;7(10):754-773.

Blanchon T, Brechot JM, Grenier PA, et al. Baseline results of the Depiscan study: a French randomized pilot trial of lung cancer screening comparing low dose CT scan (LDCT) and chest X-ray (CXR). *Lung Cancer*. 2007;58(1):50-58.

Centers for Medicare & Medicaid Services. Decision Memo for Screening for Lung Cancer with Low Dose Computed Tomography (LDCT)(CAG-00439N). Available at: https://www.cms.gov/medicare-coverage-database/details/nca-decision-memo.aspx?NCAId=274. Accessed May 12, 2016.

Field JK, Oudkerk M, Pedersen JH, et al. Prospects for population screening and diagnosis of lung cancer. *Lancet*. 2013;382(9893):732-741.

Gates TJ. Screening for cancer: concepts and controversies. *Am Fam Physician*. 2014;90(9):625-631.

Gohagan JK, Marcus PM, Fagerstrom RM, et al. Final results of the Lung Screening Study, a randomized feasibility study of spiral CT versus chest X-ray screening for lung cancer. *Lung Cancer*. 2005;47(1):9-15.

Hansell DM, Bankier AA, MacMahon H, et al. Fleischner Society: glossary of terms for thoracic imaging. *Radiology*. 2008;246(3):697-722.

Hoang JK, Langer JE, Middleton WD, et al. Managing incidental thyroid nodules detected on imaging: white paper of the ACR Incidental Thyroid Findings Committee. *J Am Coll Radiol*. 2015;12(2):143-150.

Infante M, Cavuto S, Lutman FR, et al. Long-term follow-up results of the DANTE Trial, a randomized study of lung cancer screening with spiral computed tomography. *Am J Respir Crit Care Med*. 2015;191(10):1166-1175.

Jaklitsch MT, Jacobson FL, Austin JH, et al. The American Association for Thoracic Surgery guidelines for lung cancer screening using low-dose computed tomography scans for lung cancer survivors and other high-risk groups. *J Thorac Cardiovasc Surg*. 2012;144(1):33-38.

Kazerooni EA, Armstrong MR, Amorosa JK, et al. ACR CT accreditation program and the lung cancer screening program designation. *J Am Coll Radiol*. 2015;12(1):38-42.

Lopes Pegna A, Picozzi G, Mascalchi M, et al. Design, recruitment and baseline results of the ITALUNG trial for lung cancer screening with low-dose CT. *Lung Cancer*. 2009;64(1):34-40.

Lung Cancer Alliance. National framework for excellence in lung cancer screening and continuum of care. Available at: http://www.lungcanceralliance.org/assets/docs/am-i-at-risk/NationalFramework2015.pdf. Accessed May 12, 2016.

Mascalchi M, Attina D, Bertelli E, et al. Lung cancer associated with cystic airspaces. *J Comput Assist Tomogr*. 2015;39(1):102-108.

McWilliams A, Tammemagi MC, Mayo JR, et al. Probability of cancer in pulmonary nodules detected on first screening CT. *N Engl J Med*. 2013;369(10):910-919.

Murugan VA, Kalra MK, Rehani M, et al. Lung Cancer screening: computed tomography radiation and protocols. *J Thorac Imaging*. 2015;30(5):283-289.

National Comprehensive Cancer Network. The NCCN Clinical Practice Guidelines in Oncology (NCCN Guidelines ®): Lung Cancer Screening (version 2.2016). Available at: https://www.nccn.org/professionals/physician_gls/pdf/lung_screening.pdf. Accessed May 12, 2016.

National Lung Screening Trial Research Group, Aberle DR, Adams AM, et al. Reduced lung-cancer mortality with low-dose computed tomographic screening. *N Engl J Med*. 2011;365(5):395-409.

Raji OY, Duffy SW, Agbaje OF, et al. Predictive accuracy of the Liverpool Lung Project risk model for stratifying patients for computed tomography screening for lung cancer: a case-control and cohort validation study. *Ann Intern Med*. 2012;157(4):242-250.

Rampinelli C, Calloni SF, Minotti M, et al. Spectrum of early lung cancer presentation in low-dose screening CT: a pictorial review. *Insights Imaging*. 2016;7(3):449-459.

Ridge CA, Yildirim A, Boiselle PM, et al. Differentiating between subsolid and solid pulmonary nodules at CT: inter- and intraobserver agreement between experienced thoracic radiologists. *Radiology*. 2016;278(3):888-896.

Saghir Z, Dirksen A, Ashraf H, et al. CT screening for lung cancer brings forward early disease. The randomised Danish Lung Cancer Screening Trial: status after five annual screening rounds with low-dose CT. *Thorax*. 2012;67(4):296-301.

Smith RA, Manassaram-Baptiste D, Brooks D, et al. Cancer screening in the United States, 2015: a review of current American Cancer Society guidelines and current issues in cancer screening. *CA Cancer J Clin*. 2015;65(1):30-54.

Tammemagi CM, Pinsky PF, Caporaso NE, et al. Lung cancer risk prediction: Prostate, Lung, Colorectal and Ovarian Cancer Screening Trial models and validation. *J Natl Cancer Inst*. 2011;103(13):1058-1068.

U.S. Preventive Services Task Force. Lung cancer: screening. Final recommendation Statement. Available at: http://www.uspreventiveservicestaskforce.org/Page/Document/RecommendationStatementFinal/lung-cancer-screening. Accessed May 12, 2016.

van Klaveren RJ, Oudkerk M, Prokop M, et al. Management of lung nodules detected by volume CT scanning. *N Engl J Med*. 2009;361(23):2221-2229.

Chapter 24

Lung Cancer Staging

Bojan Kovacina and Subba R. Digumarthy

INTRODUCTION

A standardized staging system is fundamental in delivering evidence-based treatment tailored to an individual patient. To determine the extent of a tumor and choose treatment strategies, an accurate staging system is essential. The stage of the tumor is the single most important factor in determining prognosis in patients with lung cancer. The American Joint Committee on Cancer (AJCC) and Union for International Cancer Control (UICC) are two international bodies that define and unify lung cancer staging classification. Periodic revisions of the staging system are required to include innovations in diagnostic methods and management strategies and are proposed by the Working Committee from the International Association for the Study of Lung Cancer (IASLC). The staging system most commonly used is the TNM classification, in which T refers to features of the primary tumor, N indicates metastasis to regional lymph nodes, and M describes the presence or absence of distal metastasis. The latest 8th edition of the TNM classification of malignant lung tumors took effect on January 2017 (Table 24.1).

TABLE 24.1 Tumor, Node, Metastasis Categories and Definitions

Descriptor	Category	Definition
Tumor (T)	Tx	Primary tumor cannot be assessed or cytologically proven primary tumor that is not visualized by imaging or bronchoscopy
	T0	No primary tumor
	Tis	Carcinoma in situ
	T1	Tumor <3 cm in greatest dimension
	T1a	Tumor <1 cm Minimally invasive adenocarcinoma Superficially spreading tumor of any size confined to bronchial or tracheal wall
	T1b	Tumor >1 cm but <2 cm
	T1c	Tumor >2 cm but <3 cm
	T2	Tumor >3 cm but <5 cm in greatest dimension or tumor <5 cm that is associated with: • Invasion of main bronchus • Invasion of visceral pleura • Atelectasis or obstructive pneumonitis extending to the hilum
	T2a	Tumor >3 cm but <4 cm
	T2b	Tumor >4 cm but <5 cm
	T3	Tumor >5 cm but <7 cm in greatest dimension or tumor <7 cm that is associated with: • Invasion of parietal pleura, pericardium, chest wall, or phrenic nerve • Separate nodules in the same lobe
	T4	Tumor >7 cm in greatest dimension or tumor of any size that is associated with: • Invasion of carina or trachea • Invasion of mediastinum, heart, esophagus, great vessels, or recurrent laryngeal nerve • Invasion of diaphragm or spine • Separate tumor nodules in different lobe in ipsilateral lung
Node (N)	Nx	Regional lymph nodes cannot be assessed
	N0	No regional lymph node involvement
	N1	Involvement of ipsilateral intrapulmonary and peribronchial or ipsilateral hilar lymph nodes
	N2	Involvement of ipsilateral mediastinal lymph nodes or subcarinal lymph nodes
	N3	Involvement of contralateral mediastinal or hilar lymph nodes or supraclavicular lymph nodes
Metastasis (M)	M0	No distant metastasis
	M1	Distant metastasis
	M1a	Malignant pleural effusion/nodules[a] or malignant pericardial effusion/nodules[a] or separate nodules in contralateral lung
	M1b	Single extrathoracic metastasis
	M1c	>1 extrathoracic metastases

[a]Most pleural and pericardial effusions in patients with lung cancer are caused by tumor. However, if multiple fluid analyses are negative for tumor cells, if fluid is not bloody, if fluid is not an exudate, and if clinical impression is concordant, then the effusion should not be considered in staging classification.

Modified from Goldstraw P, Chancky K, Crowley J, et al. The IASLC Lung Cancer Staging Project: Proposals for revision of the TNM stage groupings in the forthcoming (Eighth) edition of the TNM Classification for Lung Cancer. J Thoracic Oncol 2015;1:39-51.

IMAGING AND SURGICAL STAGING PROCEDURES (Table 24.2)

Imaging Modalities

The most common imaging modalities used for clinical staging of lung cancer are computed tomography (CT), magnetic resonance (MR), and positron emission tomography (PET). Given the fact that each of the modalities has pitfalls, these often need to be used in combination or be complemented by an additional surgical procedure to determine the correct tumor stage. The pitfalls apply particularly while assessing the N component of the TNM classification because the metastatic involvement of regional lymph nodes may be difficult to detect reliably by imaging alone. Combined CT/PET currently has the highest accuracy for nodal disease among imaging modalities and commonly is used not only to guide the management but also in the selection of the best approach for surgical staging if required. CT/PET has been shown to have high negative predictive value, particularly in the context of stage I or II lung cancers. Its specificity, however, is limited because many nonneoplastic processes may result in a false-positive scan. Therefore, mediastinal lymph nodes that are judged to be positive on PET/CT scan usually require histologic confirmation for accurate staging. The mediastinal and hilar lymph nodes are separated into 14 nodal levels (Fig. 24.1). Nodes numbered 1 to 9 are in the mediastinum, and nodes numbered 10 to 14 are in the hilum and lung. The left brachiocephalic vein and aortic arch divide the upper and lower paratracheal nodes (nodes 2R, L, and 4R, L)

TABLE 24.2 Noninvasive and Minimally Invasive Staging Procedures

Imaging	Bronchoscopic or Endoscopic	Surgical
CT	Rigid bronchoscope	Mediastinoscopy
MRI	Flexible (fiberoptic bronchoscope)	Anterior mediastinotomy
PET	Navigational bronchoscope	VATS
Combined PET/CT	EBUS	
Combined PET/MR	EUS	

CT, Computed tomography; *EBUS,* endobronchial ultrasound; *EUS,* endoscopic ultrasound; *MRI,* magnetic resonance imaging; *ET,* positron emission; *VATS,* video-assisted thoracoscopic surgery.

Surgical (Interventional) Procedures

Mediastinoscopy, anterior mediastinotomy (Chamberlain procedure), bronchoscopy (rigid, fiberoptic, and navigational), endobronchial ultrasound (EBUS), endoscopic ultrasound (EUS), and video-assisted thoracoscopy (VATS) are nonradiologic methods that allow additional assessment of the primary tumor and nodes (Table 24.3). Mediastinoscopy is considered the "gold standard" for the staging of mediastinal lymph nodes. It is performed under general anesthesia and requires a suprasternal incision with subsequent scope insertion into the pretracheal space, allowing sampling paratracheal and subcarinal nodes (Fig. 24.2). Routine mediastinoscopy has been shown to change the management in up to a quarter of patients with lung cancer and is indicated in all cases except for a peripheral tumor smaller than 2 cm in size that is surrounded with lung

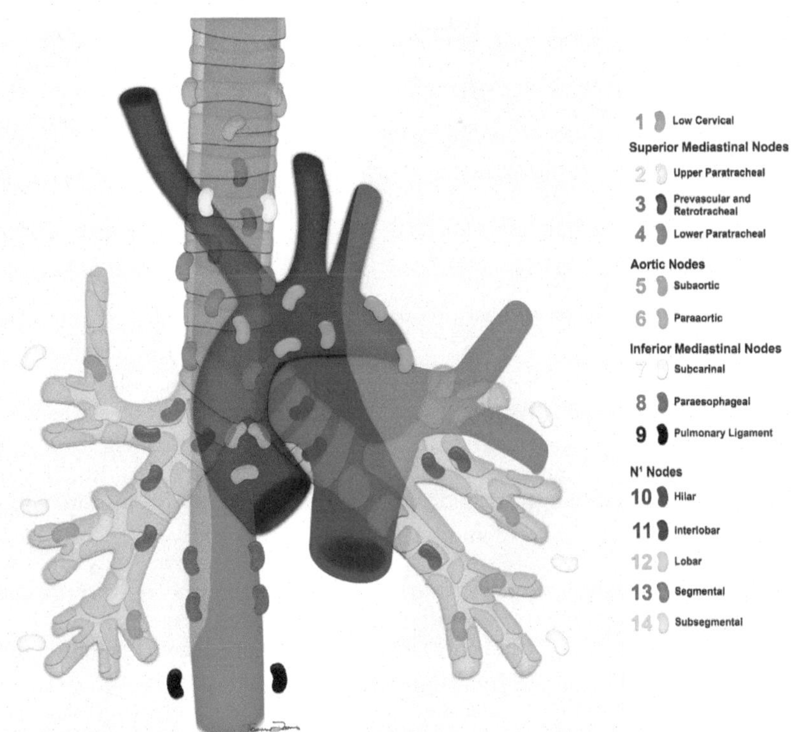

FIGURE 24.1 Mediastinal and hilar lymph nodes. The nodes are numbered to 14 levels in accordance with International Lung Cancer Staging.

TABLE 24.3 Interventional and Surgical Staging Procedures and Accessible Lymph Node Stations[a]

	Lymph Node Station									
Procedures	2	3	4	5	6	7	8	9	10	>10
ENDOBRONCHIAL OR ENDOSCOPIC										
Bronchoscopy	X		X			X			X	X
EBUS	X		X	X		X			X	X
EUS	X		X			X	X	X		
SURGICAL										
Mediastinoscopy	X		X			X				
Anterior mediastinotomy				X	X					
VATS				X	X					

[a]Lymph node stations: 2, high paratracheal; 3, prevascular; 4, low paratracheal; 5, aortopulmonary window; 6, paraaortic; 7, subcarinal; 8, paraesophageal; 9, inferior pulmonary ligament; 10, hilar; >10, intrapulmonary.
EBUS, Endobronchial ultrasound; *EUS*, endoscopic ultrasound; *VATS*, video-assisted thoracoscopic surgery.

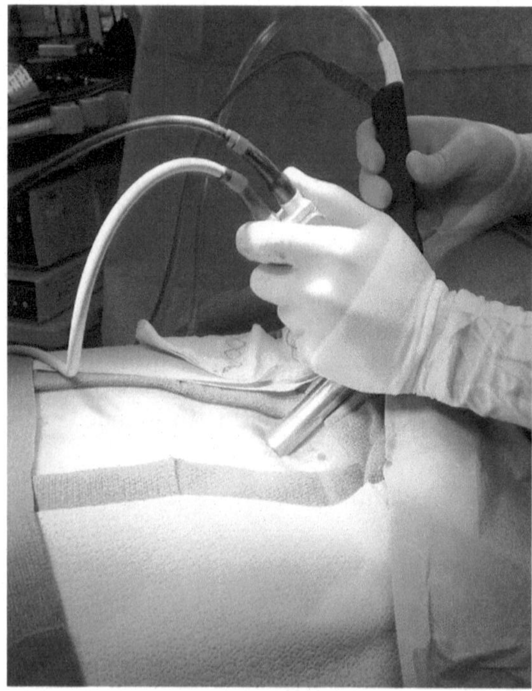

FIGURE 24.2 Mediastinoscopy. Intraoperative photograph shows a scope inserted through a suprasternal incision into the pretracheal space for sampling paratracheal and subcarinal nodes. The procedure is done under general anesthesia. (Courtesy of Michael Lanuti, MD, Boston, MA.)

parenchyma and has no pathologic regional lymph nodes on imaging modalities. Goiter is a relative contraindication, and hemorrhage and injury to the large mediastinal vessels, esophagus, and recurrent laryngeal nerve are the significant complications. It is not possible to access aortopulmonary and paraaortic nodes via mediastinoscopy.

Anterior mediastinotomy is performed via a short transverse incision in the left parasternal region of the second or third intercostal space and is done to access the left anterior mediastinal nodes and tumors. In addition to complications of mediastinoscopy, chylothorax, pneumothorax, and injury to the phrenic nerve may also complicate this procedure.

Different types of bronchoscopies are available for lung cancer diagnosis and staging; rigid, flexible (fiberoptic), and

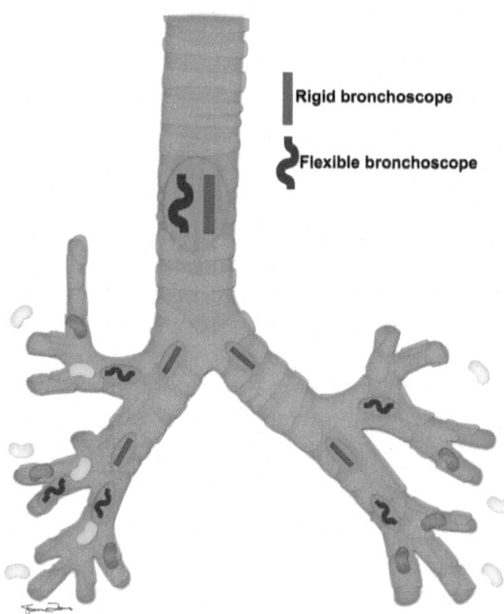

FIGURE 24.3 Rigid and flexible bronchoscopy. Schematic showing the reach of rigid and flexible bronchoscopy. Whereas rigid bronchoscopy is used for central airway tumors and nodes, a flexible scope is used for more distal lobar or segmental tumors and nodes.

navigational bronchoscopy. Rigid bronchoscopy is predominantly used for central airway tumors, and a flexible scope is used for more distal lobar or segmental tumors (Fig. 24.3). Both bronchoscopic methods are used for transbronchial biopsy targeting tumors or suspicious mediastinal, hilar, or peribronchial lymph nodes. The biopsies performed via these types of bronchoscopies are blind procedures; thus, their diagnostic yield is limited, particularly for smaller distal parenchymal lesions. Navigational bronchoscopy consists of manipulation of a steerable probe that can be tracked and directed by integrated virtual endobronchial images preobtained by multidetector CT scan. The virtual imaging and planning allow more optimal localization of the target lesion and considerable improvement in the diagnostic yield of biopsies (Fig. 24.4). This is especially useful for peripheral small lung lesions, which otherwise would not be accessible with more conventional bronchoscopic methods, and in patients with emphysema in whom percutaneous lung biopsy poses a high risk of pneumothorax. Hemorrhage and pneumothorax are the most common complications of these types of procedures. EBUS is a relatively new technique that has slowly become a preferred method for mediastinal lymph node staging in cases of lung cancer. It can be performed in an outpatient setting under conscious sedation and allows transbronchial fine-needle aspiration biopsy (FNAB) under sonographic guidance, thereby maximizing diagnostic yield and minimizing potential complications (Figs. 24.5 and 24.6). Its sensitivity and specificity range from 88% to 94% and 92% to 100%, respectively. In experienced hands, several studies have shown a similar accuracy of EBUS and mediastinoscopy. The latter remains justified in situations when EBUS-guided FNAB of suspicious mediastinal lymph nodes is negative. Esophageal endoscopic ultrasound and associated EUS-guided FNA can be combined with EBUS to cover almost entire mediastinal lymph node stations. It is the only noninvasive procedure that allows access to tissue

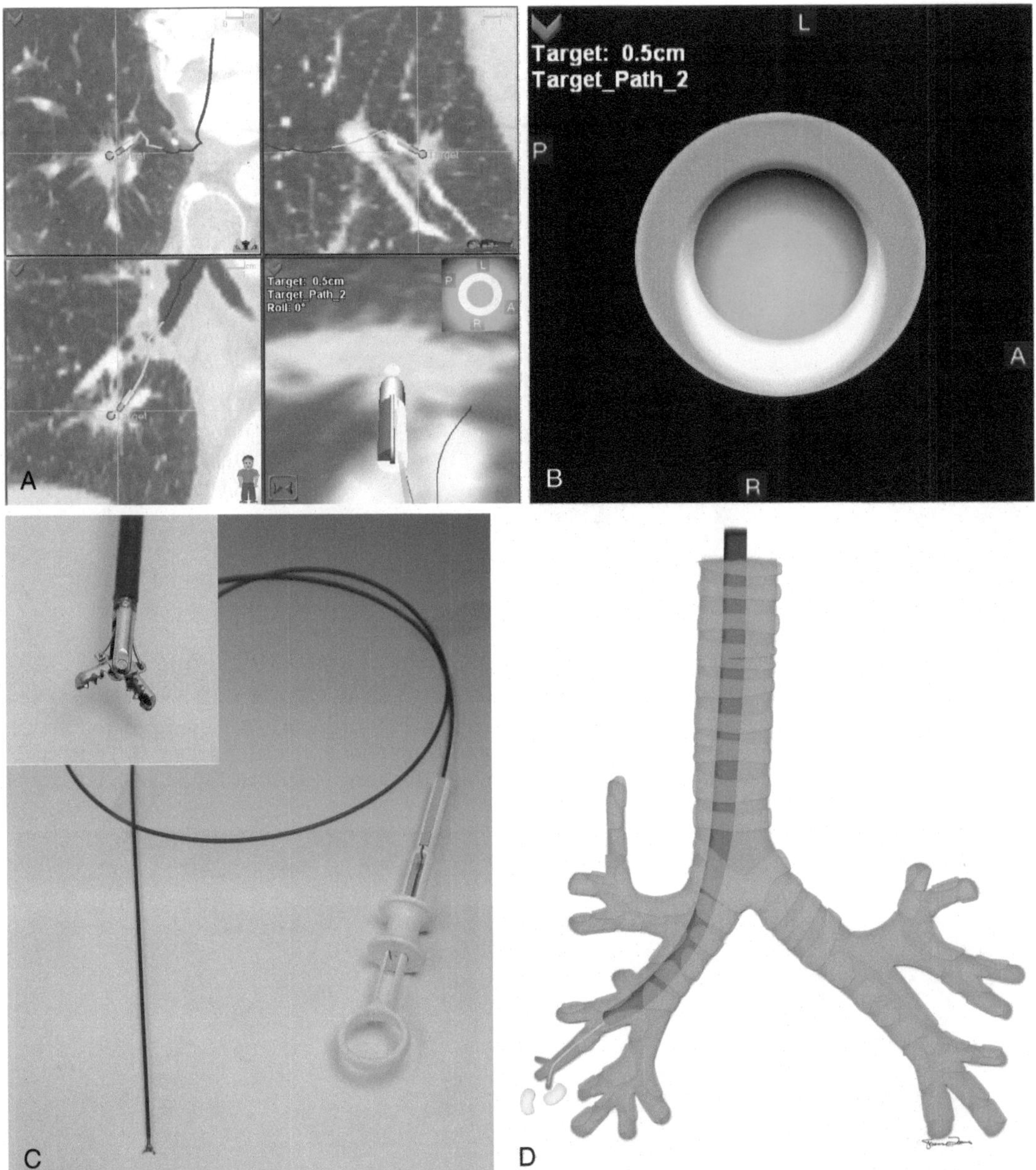

FIGURE 24.4 Navigational bronchoscopy. **A,** Image display. Image-guided navigational software aligns the computed tomography (CT) and bronchoscopy images. The *purple line* depicts the bronchoscope, the *blue line* depicts the steerable navigation probe, and the *green dot* highlights the sensor tip. The lesion is shown in coronal, sagittal, and axial CT images. **B,** CT-to-body divergence. The *green* and *yellow zones* represent the location of the target on mapped CT images and virtual position on real-time bronchoscopy, respectively. **C,** At the time of biopsy, the steerable navigational probe is exchanged for the biopsy forceps. **D,** Schematic diagram of navigational bronchoscopy showing the steerable wire inserted through the flexible bronchoscope.

sampling of low paraesophageal and pulmonary ligament lymph nodes. Sonographic guidance during FNA allows high diagnostic yield (90%) and specificity (approaching 100%). VATS is a minimally invasive surgical procedure used for sampling mediastinal lymph nodes that are suspicious on imaging but otherwise inaccessible by other noninvasive methods for histologic correlation. It usually is performed at the time of surgical resection of cancer. In addition to nodal staging, it also allows for further assessment of the primary tumor; in particular, it may determine tumor invasion into mediastinal structures, chest wall, and pleural metastasis.

TUMOR, NODE, METASTASIS CLASSIFICATION

Primary Tumor

A tumor can be classified into one of seven T categories. The size of the tumor, the presence of lung atelectasis, extension into the main bronchus, invasion of adjacent structures, and presence and location of satellite nodules determine the classification. Tis and T1 categories include carcinoma in situ and tumors smaller than 3 cm in size without additional findings, respectively. The T1 tumors are further subdivided based on the long axis diameter, in

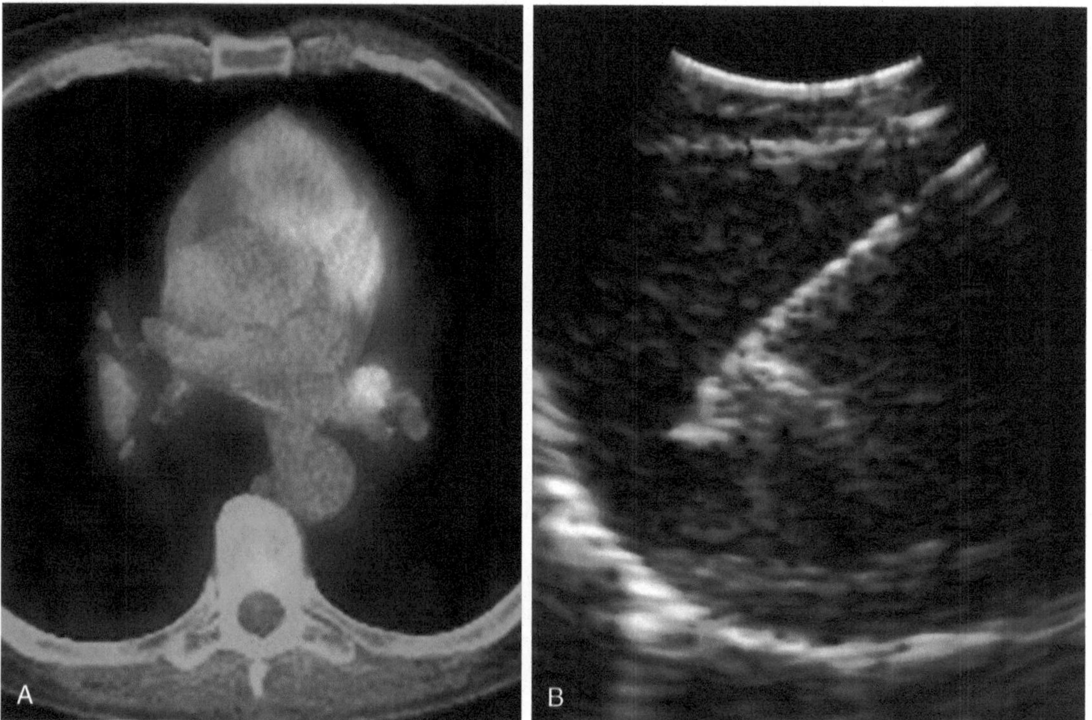

FIGURE 24.5 Metastatic left hilar (10 L) node from squamous cell carcinoma. **A,** Fused positron emission/computed tomography image shows a fludeoxyglucose-avid lymph node in the left hilum. **B,** Endobronchial ultrasound biopsy of the node with needle in the lymph node. (Courtesy of Michael Lanuti, MD, Boston, MA.)

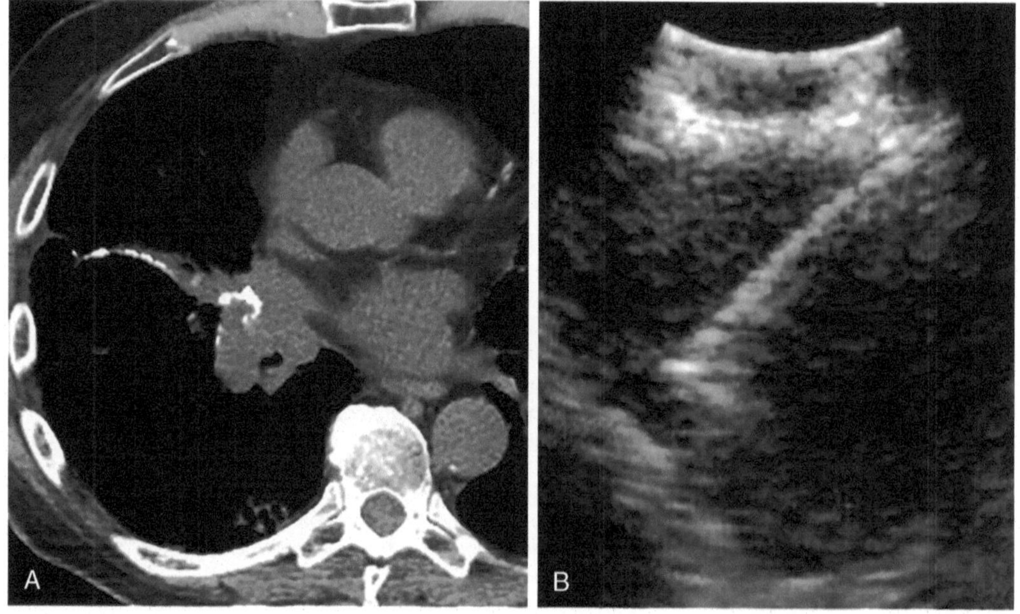

FIGURE 24.6 Recurrent non–small cell lung cancer after surgery. **A,** Axial computed tomography image shows recurrent mass in the right hilum at the suture line. **B,** Endobronchial ultrasound biopsy with a needle in the mass. (Courtesy of Michael Lanuti, MD, Boston, MA.)

1-cm increments. The T2 category includes cancers that are larger than 3 cm and smaller than 5 cm or any tumors smaller than 5 cm causing atelectasis to the hilum, invasion of the visceral pleura, or invasion of the main bronchus (Fig. 24.7). Cancers that are larger than 5 cm and smaller than 7 cm make part of the T3 classification. Similarly, any tumor smaller than 7 cm in size that invades the chest wall, parietal pericardium, or phrenic nerve or is associated with satellite nodule(s) in the same lobe is T3. Determining chest wall invasion in tumors of smaller than 5 cm is essential because of its importance in T classification; however, the presence of invasion may be challenging to detect by imaging tools. Unless there is a mass in the chest wall or rib destruction, several other CT findings are suggestive but not specific for chest wall invasion (Fig. 24.8). These additional CT findings include thickening of the parietal pleura adjacent to the tumor, large contact surface between the tumor and pleura (>3 cm), obliteration of extrapleural

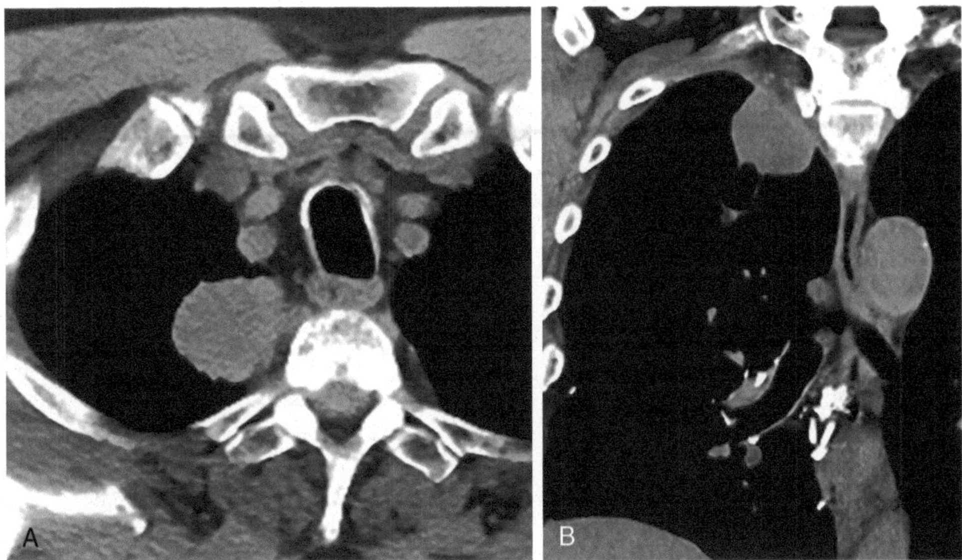

FIGURE 24.7 Non–small cell lung cancer with visceral pleural invasion. Axial **(A)** and coronal **(B)** chest computed tomography images demonstrate peripheral right apical mass with broad-based contact with pleura but without extrapleural extension or pleural effusion.

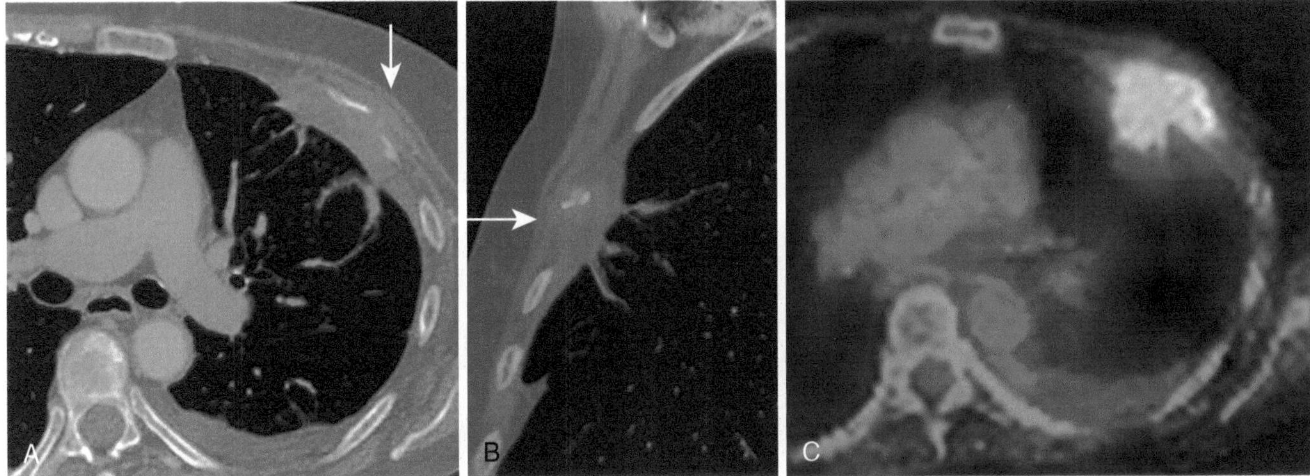

FIGURE 24.8 Non–small cell lung cancer with chest wall invasion. Axial **(A)** and sagittal **(B)** chest computed tomography (CT) images in the bone window demonstrate a mass in the anterior left upper lobe with definite signs of chest wall invasion, rib destruction, and soft tissue swelling bulging the chest wall musculature *(arrow)*. **C,** Fused positron emission tomography/CT image demonstrates contiguous increased fludeoxyglucose uptake in the mass in left upper lobe and chest wall.

fat, and the presence of an obtuse angle between the pleura and the cancer. Magnetic resonance imaging (MRI) with or without gadolinium administration is considered to have slightly higher accuracy than CT and may be beneficial in cases when subtle chest invasion is suspected. T4 tumors are tumors measuring larger than 7 cm in size or tumors of any size with invasion of vital structures such as carina, trachea, esophagus, aorta, heart, visceral pericardium, spine, diaphragm, or recurrent laryngeal nerve (Figs. 24.9 and 24.10). Additionally, tumors invading mediastinal fat and those associated with satellite nodules in the same lung but not the same lobe are also considered T4. One challenging area for exact determination of T factor is the fat overlying the parietal pericardium. Although invasion of mediastinal fat is considered T4, invasion of this fat is considered T3 because invasion of the underlying parietal pericardium itself falls under the T3 category. As with chest wall invasion, MRI may troubleshoot difficult cases in which mediastinal invasion cannot be reliably confirmed or excluded by CT or PET/CT. Given its higher contrast resolution, MR may more optimally demonstrate encasement or distortion of mediastinal structures by the tumor, which usually indicates their invasion. The superior sulcus (Pancoast) tumor is another particular situation in which MRI plays a significant role in reliably determining T classification. In fact, local extension of cancer, which commonly extends into extrapleural space at the time of diagnosis, is more reliably determined by MRI. This modality allows classifying tumors into a T3 category if they only invade adjacent muscles or thoracic nerve roots or into a T4 category if they invade cervical nerve roots, cords of brachial plexus, spine, and subclavian vessels. Sagittal and coronal MR

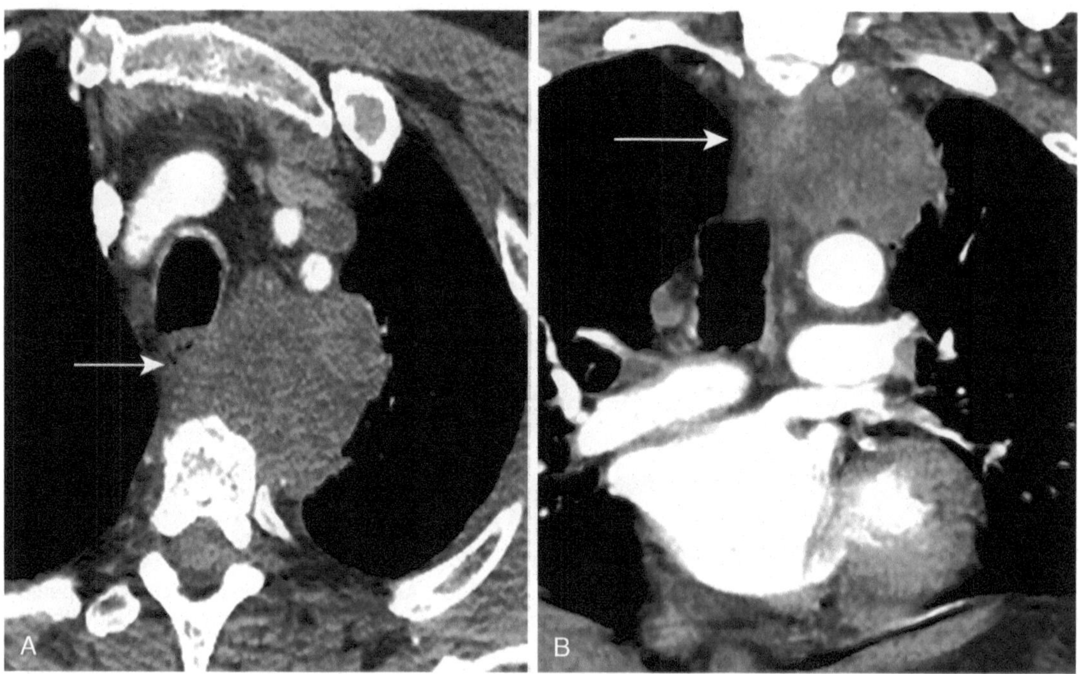

FIGURE 24.9 Non–small cell lung cancer with mediastinal invasion. Axial **(A)** and coronal **(B)** chest computed tomography images demonstrate a left apical mass with invasion of superior mediastinal fat. Note the loss of fat plane between the mass, T3 vertebral body, and esophagus *(arrow)*.

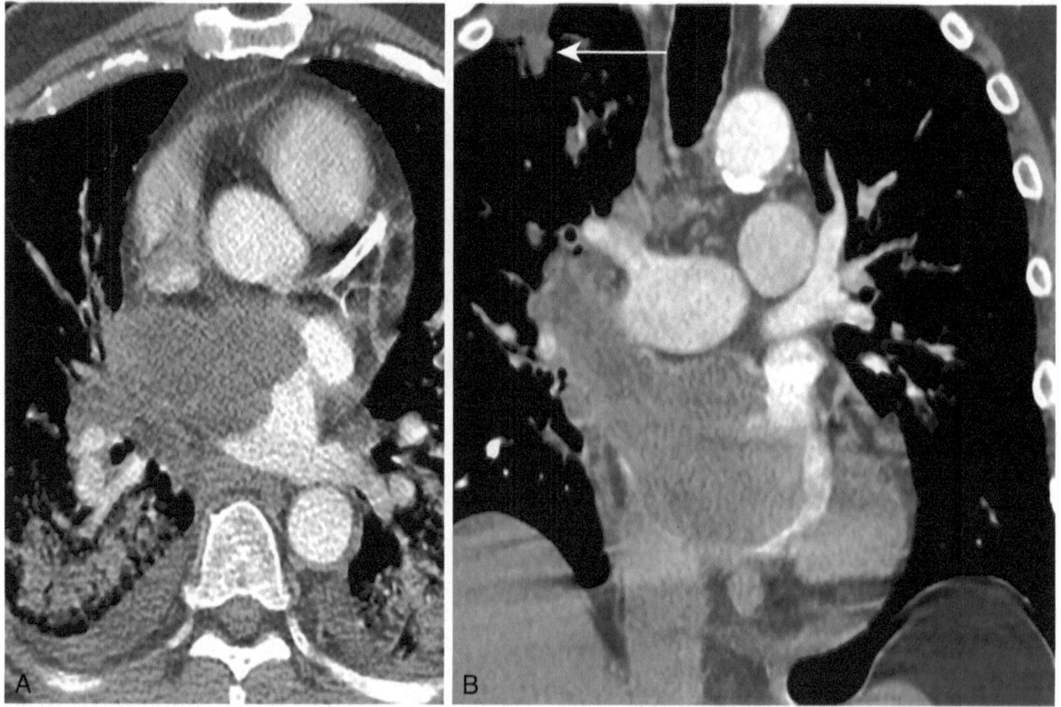

FIGURE 24.10 Non–small cell lung cancer (NSCLC) with invasion of the left atrium. Axial **(A)** and coronal **(B)** chest computed tomography images demonstrate direct right superior pulmonary vein and left atrial invasion by right upper lobe NSCLC *(arrow)*. Note the small bilateral pleural effusions and lower lobe parenchymal opacities related to pulmonary edema.

sequences with and without gadolinium are valuable in these cases.

Nodal Involvement

There are four N categories in the current TNM staging classification. The presence and location of affected regional lymph nodes determine different categories: none (N0), ipsilateral peribronchial and hilar (N1) (Fig. 24.11), ipsilateral mediastinal (N2), and contralateral mediastinal and supraclavicular (N3) (Fig. 24.12). A nodal involvement is presumed if primary cancer extends into a neighboring node. Despite its high value in preoperative staging, CT has its limitation in accurately detecting involved regional

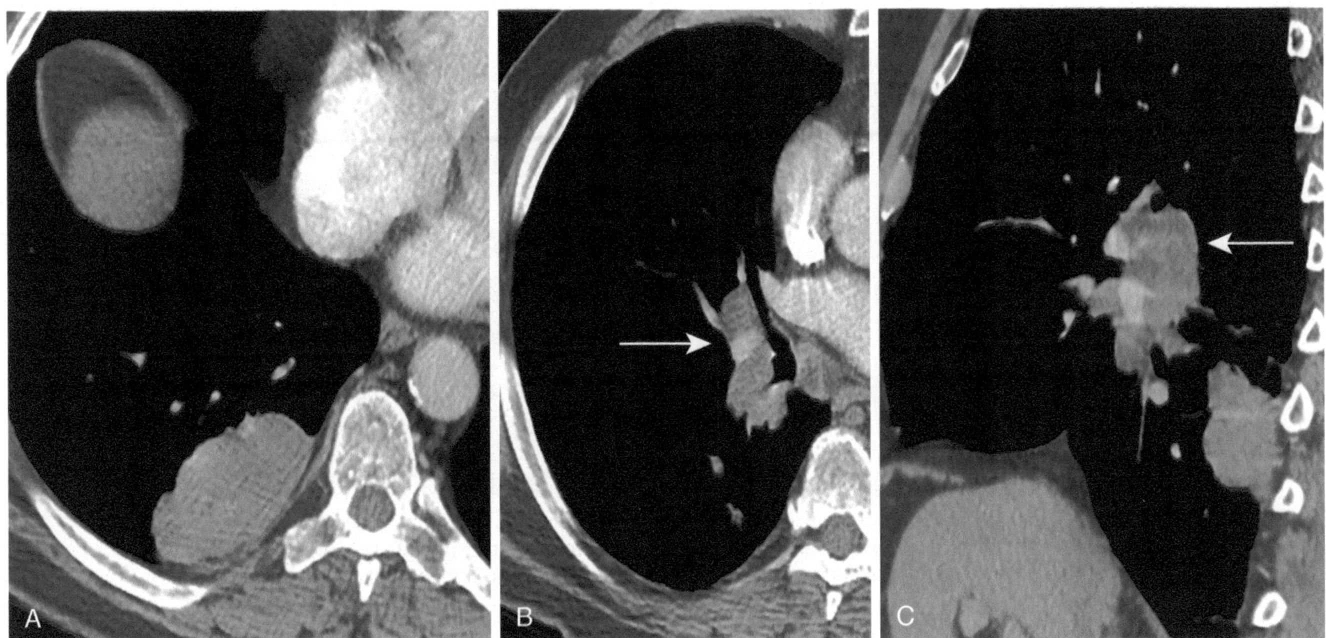

FIGURE 24.11 Non–small cell lung cancer with ipsilateral hilar lymph nodes (N1). Axial (**A** and **B**) and sagittal (**C**) chest computed tomography images demonstrate a mass in the posterior basal segment of the right lower lobe with enlarged metastatic right hilar lymph nodes *(arrows)*.

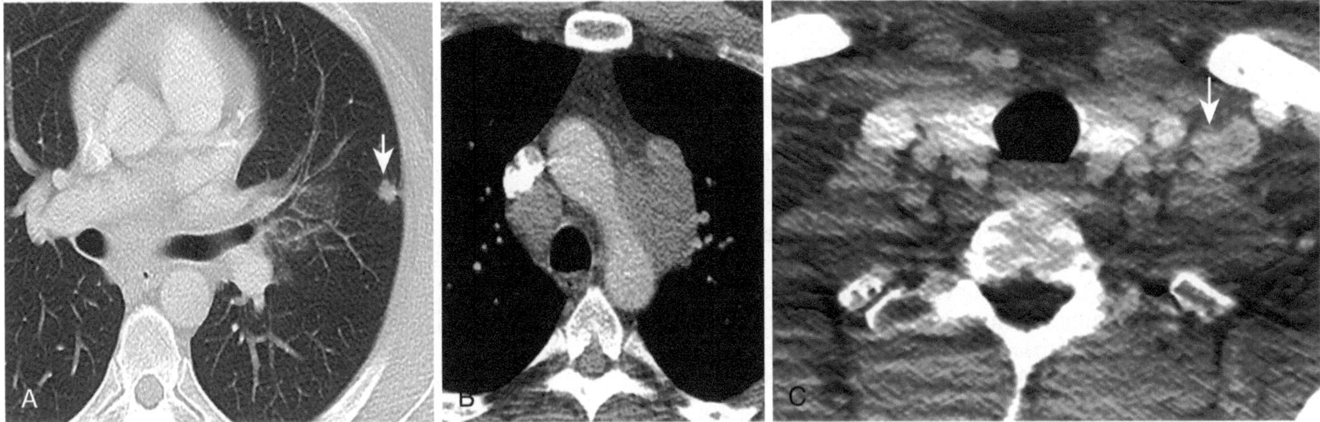

FIGURE 24.12 Non–small cell lung cancer (NSCLC) with bilateral mediastinal and supraclavicular lymph nodes. **A** to **C**, Axial chest computed tomography images demonstrate 9-mm peripheral spiculated NSCLC in the left upper lobe *(arrow)* and enlarged metastatic lymph nodes in the anteroposterior window, lower right paratracheal, and left supraclavicular lymph node stations *(arrow)*.

lymph nodes in the case of lung cancer. This is mostly because CT predominantly uses size criteria for detection of nodal involvement. Indeed, in many cases, a lymph node may be involved and of normal size; alternatively, a lymph node may be enlarged but without neoplastic involvement. As mentioned previously, combined PET/CT has higher sensitivity and specificity than CT alone in determining nodal involvement; nevertheless, correlation with tissue sampling is usually required. Current recommendations include resection of at least three nodes from N1 and N2 stations during surgery for accurate staging. When available, minimally invasive procedures are preferred for nodal sampling and biopsy before definitive surgery. Although each has limitations, a combination of two techniques can allow access to the sampling of almost all hilar and mediastinal lymph nodes (see Table 24.3).

Metastasis

There are two M categories: M0 (no metastasis) and M1 (metastasis). Metastatic pleural or pericardial effusion or nodules classify the tumor into an M1 (Fig. 24.13). This category also includes tumor with associated nodules in the contralateral lung. A solitary metastasis in an extrathoracic organ is M1b and multiple extrathoracic metastases is M1c. Currently, it is controversial if patients with T1 tumors should undergo extensive preoperative imaging for detection of metastasis, given the rarity of metastasis in these cases. CT and total-body PET/CT are currently primary imaging modalities in the assessment of distant metastasis. All cases of small cell lung cancer (SCLC) require screening imaging of the brain. For non-small cell lung cancers (NSCLCs), CT and MRI of the head are performed in cases of advanced

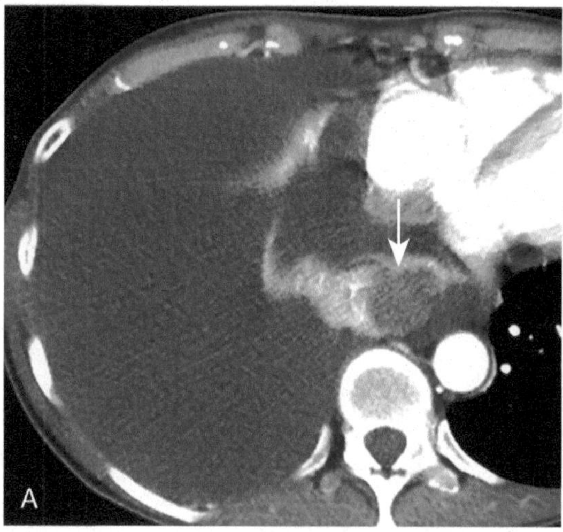

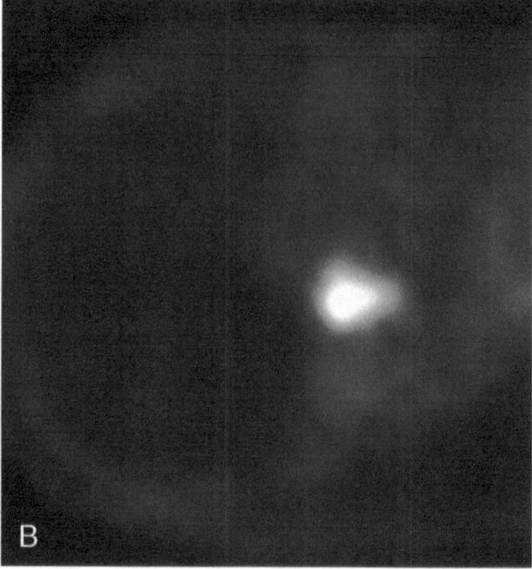

FIGURE 24.13 Lung adenocarcinoma with malignant pleural effusion. **A,** Axial computed tomography image demonstrates a mass in the collapsed right lower lobe *(arrow)* and a large malignant right pleural effusion. **B,** Positron emission tomography scan demonstrates corresponding increased fludeoxyglucose uptake in the mass.

tumor stage or if neurologic symptoms are present. Adrenal glands are one of the most common organs affected by lung cancer metastasis. When adrenal gland adenoma, the most common adrenal mass, cannot be differentiated from metastasis on CT scan (if the mass is of >10 HU in density and does not show delayed washout after intravenous contrast), a further assessment with either PET/CT or MRI usually is sufficient for diagnosis.

Changes From the Last TNM Staging Edition

The current eighth TNM staging edition includes several changes from the prior edition, predominantly regarding T factor. Central tumors extending into the main bronchus are now classified as T2 independently of their proximity to the carina. These tumors remain as T2 even if associated with complete lung collapse. The tumors that invade the diaphragm, previously classified as T3, are now moved up into the T4 category. Finally, tumors larger than 7 cm are now classified as T4, and those larger than 5 cm but smaller than 7 cm are in T3. A minor change in the M category is made for distinguishing cancers with single distant solid organ metastasis from those with multiple metastases.

GROUP STAGES AND TREATMENT

Based on T, N, and M factors, four staging groups, I through IV, are determined. Each stage has subdivisions (Table 24.4). The stage I group includes T1 and T2a N0M0 cancers, stage II includes T1 and T2 N1 M0 and T2b and T3 N0M0 cancers, and stage IV includes any cancer with distant metastases (M1). All other cancers are part of stage III group and include all T4, T3 N>0 cancers, and all N2 and N3. This staging classification applies to NSCLC, SCLC, and bronchopulmonary carcinoid tumors. The Veterans Administration Lung Study Group (VALSG) staging system for SCLC is still in use and consists of two categories: limited stage and advanced stage. According to the TNM classification, limited-stage SCLC corresponds to any tumor without distant metastasis (M0) and multiple pulmonary nodules extending outside of a single radiation field (some T3 and T4 tumors). In the context of NSCLC, stages I to IIIA are considered resectable, and IIIB is potentially resectable in select cases. Stage IV patients are considered inoperable and are treated with only chemotherapy. Some stage III cancers usually require neoadjuvant chemotherapy and preoperative radiotherapy. Definitive radiation therapy is the treatment for patients not considered for surgery. Adjuvant chemotherapy has improved survival in patients with stage II cancers. It is possible to predict prognosis and survival rate in patients who received standard therapy based on staging (Table 24.5).

TABLE 24.4 Stage Groupings

T/M	Category	N0	N1	N2	N3
T1	T1a	IA1	IIB	IIIA	IIIB
	T1b	IA2	IIB	IIIA	IIIB
	T1c	IA3	IIB	IIIA	IIIB
T2	T2a	IB	IIB	IIIA	IIIB
	T2b	IIA	IIB	IIIA	IIIB
T3	T3	IIB	IIIA	IIIB	IIIC
T4	T4	IIIA	IIIA	IIIB	IIIC
M1	M1a	IVA	IVA	IVA	IVA
	M1b	IVA	IVA	IVA	IVA
	M1c	IVB	IVB	IVB	IVB

M, Metastasis; *N,* node; *T,* tumor.
Modified from Detterbeck FC, Boffa DJ, Kim AW, Tanoue LT. The eighth edition lung cancer stage classification. Chest 2017;151:193-203.

It is important to understand that the staging system just described is not the only factor used in determining management strategy and prognosis itself. In fact, many other clinical and environmental factors are considered, including but not limited to the patient's general medical condition, tumor histologic subtype, treatment availability and accessibility, and response to treatment.

MULTIPLE CANCERS

If there are two lung cancers of different histopathologic characteristics diagnosed at the same time by imaging

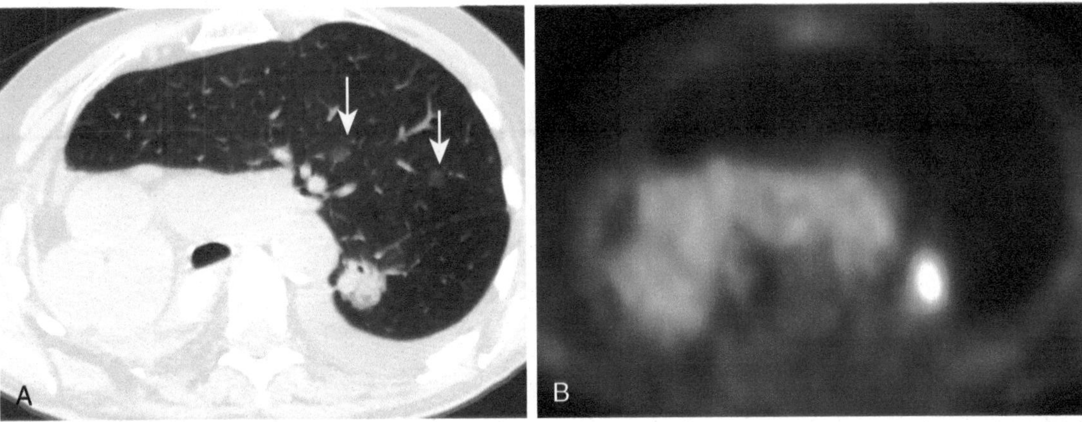

FIGURE 24.14 Multifocal lung cancers. **A,** Multiple ground-glass nodules in the left upper lobe *(arrows)* and a solid nodule in the left lower lobe. The tumor, node, metastasis (TNM) staging is based on the larger left lower lobe nodule. The patient also underwent remote right pneumonectomy for adenocarcinoma of the lung. **B,** Positron emission tomography scan shows fludeoxyglucose avidity of only the left lower lobe nodule.

TABLE 24.5 **Overall 2- and 5-Year Survival Rates According to Clinical Stage**

Stage	2-Year Survival Rate (%)	5-Year Survival Rate (%)
IA1	97	92
IA2	94	83
IA3	90	77
IB	87	68
IIA	79	60
IIB	72	53
IIIA	55	36
IIIB	44	26
IIIC	24	13
IVA	23	10
IVB	10	0

Modified from Detterbeck FC, Boffa DJ, Kim AW, Tanoue LT. The eighth edition lung cancer stage classification. Chest 2017;151:193-203.

modalities, each tumor should receive its own separate TNM classification. On the other hand, if two lung cancers have the same histology, these should be considered as "one primary lung cancer with satellite nodule" and be classified into TNM stage depending on the location of the satellite nodule with relation to the primary tumor. Finally, adenocarcinoma of the lung with a predominantly lepidic growth pattern occasionally presents with multiple scattered ground-glass and part solid nodules. In this context, the tumor is classified as one TNM stage according to the nodule or mass with the highest T category (Fig. 24.14).

SUGGESTED READINGS

Adams K, Shah PL, Edmonds L, et al. Test performance of endobronchial ultrasound and transbronchial needle aspiration biopsy for mediastinal staging in patients with lung cancer: systematic review and meta-analysis. *Thorax*. 2009;64:757-762.

AJCC. *AJCC Cancer Staging Manual*. 8th ed. New York, NY: Springer; 2016.

Cerfolio RJ, Ojha B, Bryant AS, et al. The accuracy of integrated PET-CT compared with dedicated PET alone for the staging of patients with nonsmall cell lung cancer. *Ann Thorac Surg*. 2004;78:1017-1023.

De Leyn P, Dooms C, Kuzdzal J, et al. Revised ESTS guidelines for preoperative mediastinal lymph node staging for non-small-cell lung cancer. *Eur J Cardiothorac Surg*. 2014;45(5):787-798.

Detterbeck F, Arenberg D, Asamura H, et al. The IASLC Lung Cancer Staging Project: background data and proposals for the application of TNM staging rules to lung cancer presenting as multiple nodules with ground glass or lepidic features or a pneumonic-type of involvement in the forthcoming eighth edition of the TNM classification. *J Thorac Oncol*. 2016;11:666-680.

Detterbeck F, Arenberg D, Asamura H, et al. The IASLC Lung Cancer Staging Project: background data and proposed criteria to distinguish separate primary lung cancers from metastatic foci in patients with two lung tumors in the forthcoming eighth edition of the TNM Classification for Lung Cancer. *J Thorac Oncol*. 2016;11:651-665.

Detterbeck FC, Boffa DJ, Kim AW, et al. The eighth edition lung cancer stage classification. *Chest*. 2017;151:193-203.

Eberhardt W, Mitchell J, Crowley J, et al. The IASLC Lung Cancer Staging Project: proposals for the revision of the M descriptors in the forthcoming (8th) edition of the TNM Classification of Lung Cancer. *J Thorac Oncol*. 2015;10:1515-1522.

Fischer B, Lassen U, Mortensen J, et al. Preoperative staging of lung cancer with combined PET-CT. *N Engl J Med*. 2009;361:32-39.

Goldstraw P, Chancky K, Crowley J, et al. The IASLC Lung Cancer Staging Project: proposals for Revision of the TNM Stage Groupings in the Forthcoming (Eighth) Edition of the TNM Classification for Lung Cancer. *J Thoracic Oncol*. 2015;1:39-51.

Haggar AM, Perlberg JL, Froelich JW, et al. Chest wall invasion by carcinoma of the lung: detection by MR imaging. *AJR Am J Roentgenol*. 1987;148:1075-1078.

Kinsey CM, Arenberg DA. Endobronchial ultrasound-guided transbronchial needle aspiration for non-small cell lung cancer. *Am J Respir Crit Care Med*. 2014;189:640-649.

Kligerman S, Digumarthy S. Staging of non-small cell lung cancer using integrated PET/CT. *AJR Am J Roentgenol*. 2009;193:1203-1211.

Lanuti M. Mediastinoscopy and other thoracic staging procedures. In: Kaiser LR, Kron IL, Spray TL, eds. *Mastery of Cardiothoracic Surgery*. Philadelphia: Lippincott Williams & Wilkins; 2014:14-27.

Libshitz HI, McKenna RJ. Mediastinal lymph node size in lung cancer. *AJR Am J Roentgenol*. 1984;143:715-718.

McLoud TC, Filion RB, Edelman RR, et al. MR imaging of superior sulcus carcinoma. *J Comput Assist Tomogr*. 1989;13:233-239.

Pennes DR, Glazer GM, Wimbish KJ, et al. Chest wall invasion by lung cancer: limitations by CT evaluation. *AJR Am J Roentgenol*. 1985;144:507-511.

Rami-Porta R, Bolejack V, Crowley J, et al. The IASLC Lung Cancer Staging Project. Proposals for the revisions of the T descriptors in the forthcoming eighth edition of the TNM Classification for Lung Cancer. *J Thorac Oncol*. 2015;10:990-1003.

Roberts PF, Follette DM, von Haag D, et al. Factors associated with false-positive staging of lung cancer by positron emission tomography. *Ann Thorac Surg*. 2000;70:1154-1160.

Staples CA, Müller NL, Miller RR, et al. Mediastinal nodes in bronchogenic carcinoma comparison between CT and mediastinoscopy. *Radiology*. 1988;167:367-372.

Teran MD, Brock MV. Staging lymph node metastases from lung cancer in the mediastinum. *J Thorac Dis*. 2014;6:230-236.

Travis D, Asamura H, Bankier AA, et al. The IASLC Lung Cancer Staging Project: proposals for coding T categories for subsolid nodules and assessment of tumor size in part solid tumors in the forthcoming eighth edition of the TNM Classification of Lung Cancer. *J Thorac Oncol*. 2016;11:1204-1223.

UyBico SF, Wu CC, Suh RD, et al. Lung cancer staging essentials: the new TNM staging system and potential imaging pitfalls. *Radiographics*. 2010;30:1163-1181.

Chapter 25

Interventional Techniques

Florian J. Fintelmann, Jo-Anne O. Shepard, and Amita Sharma

INTRODUCTION

The most common interventional procedures in thoracic radiology are drainage of air or fluid collections followed by percutaneous transthoracic needle biopsy (PTNB) of lung and mediastinal lesions. Other procedures are placement of localization markers in lung parenchyma to facilitate resection or radiation and thermal ablation to treat primary and secondary neoplasms.

BIOPSY OF LUNG AND MEDIASTINUM

Indications and Contraindications

Percutaneous transthoracic needle biopsy is commonly performed to diagnose persistent or growing pulmonary nodule(s). Feasibility of PTNB depends on nodule size, location, and consistency. As a general rule, lesions measuring at least 1 cm in diameter can be biopsied. The solid component of part solid lesions should be targeted. Overall, sensitivity and specificity of 93% to 98% and 98% to 100%, respectively, have been reported for the diagnosis of malignancy. Many surgeons value preoperative PTNB of suspicious nodules because PTNB allows them to plan a definitive curative procedure rather than rely on intraoperative frozen-section analysis. Advanced lung cancers are also commonly biopsied for molecular profiling and identification of mutations amenable to targeted therapy. PTNB is also used to confirm malignancy in nonsurgical candidates before radiotherapy, thermal ablation, or chemotherapy. Other indications for PTNB include the workup of mediastinal masses; hilar masses when bronchoscopy results are negative; single or multiple pulmonary nodules in a patient with a known extrathoracic malignancy; and suspected infectious lesions manifesting as nodules, masses, or focal consolidation, particularly in immunocompromised patients.

There are several alternatives to PTNB. Bronchoscopy is preferred for airspace opacities, central lesions adjacent to or involving the airways, and hilar masses. Navigational bronchoscopy may be able to sample peripheral lesions. Transbronchial needle aspiration combined with endobronchial ultrasound (EBUS) can establish neoplastic involvement of mediastinal nodes for the purposes of staging lung cancer. Video-assisted thoracoscopic surgery (VATS) enables the resection and diagnosis of peripheral subpleural pulmonary lesions. However, both EBUS and VATS require general anesthesia and are more expensive than bronchoscopy or PTNB.

Most contraindications to TNB are relative rather than absolute (Box 25.1). However, patients need to be cooperative and be able to maintain a certain position. Consensus guidelines suggest that bleeding risk is moderate and that coagulopathy should be evaluated and managed accordingly (Table 25.1). Although a minimum of 50,000/mL platelets is recommended, we prefer to biopsy patients with a platelet count above 100,000/mL. Although severe pulmonary hypertension is a relative contraindication, PTNB of peripheral lesions can be safely attempted in patients with moderate pulmonary hypertension (<50 mm Hg). Other relative contraindications include bullae or severe emphysema in the path of the lesion to be biopsied; severe chronic obstructive pulmonary disease (COPD), defined by a forced expiratory volume in 1 second (FEV_1) of less than 1 L or 35% predicted; and intractable cough. Diagnosis of diffuse lung disease is established with VATS wedge resection because tissue from PTNB is usually inadequate.

BOX 25.1 Relative Contraindications for Biopsy of the Lung and Mediastinum and Thermal Ablation of Lung Lesions

- Uncorrectable coagulopathy
- Severe pulmonary hypertension (right ventricular systolic pressure >50 mm Hg)
- Forced expiratory volume in 1 second <1 L or 35% predicted
- Emphysema along the projected needle path
- Pneumonectomy
- Uncooperative patient
- Risk of injury caused by proximity of target to critical structures (vessel, nerve, airway)

Sedation Plan

Lung and mediastinal biopsies can be performed with local anesthesia in cooperative patients. Local anesthesia supplemented with conscious sedation minimizes respiratory motion and maximizes patient comfort and immobility while obviating the need for breath-holding. Intravenous (IV) conscious sedation consists of a short-acting anxiolytic such as midazolam and an opioid such as fentanyl. Oversedation can cause significant atelectasis that obscures nodules in the dependent lung. General anesthesia may be necessary if conscious sedation is contraindicated because of cardiorespiratory comorbidities. In these cases, low-volume ventilation is preferable because positive pressure increases the risk for a large pneumothorax.

Tools and Technical Principles

Computed tomography (CT) is most often used for image guidance. Ultrasound may be better suited for chest wall lesions or small peripheral nodules abutting the pleura. Fluoroscopy was historically the choice for large masses. However, CT allows more precise visualization.

TABLE 25.1 Adapted Society of Interventional Radiology 2012 Consensus Guidelines for Periprocedural Management of Coagulation Status and Hemostasis Risk in Image-guided Interventions

		Bleeding Risk		
		Low	**Moderate**	**Significant**
Preprocedure laboratory testing	INR	Recommended for patients receiving warfarin or known or suspected liver disease	Recommended	Recommended
	aPTT	Recommended for patients receiving IV UFH	Recommended for patients receiving IV UFH	Recommended for patients receiving IV UFH
	Platelet count	Not routinely recommended	Not routinely recommended	Recommended
	Hematocrit	Not routinely recommended	Not routinely recommended	Recommended
Management	INR	Correct to <2.0	Correct to <1.5	Correct to <1.5
	aPTT	No consensus	No consensus	Stop or reverse heparin for values >1.5× control
	Platelets	Transfusion recommended for counts <50,000/mL	Transfusion recommended for counts <50,000/microL	Transfusion recommended for counts <50,000/microL
	Hematocrit	No recommended threshold for transfusion	No recommended threshold for transfusion	No recommended threshold for transfusion
	Clopidogrel	Withhold for 5 days before procedure	Withhold for 5 days before procedure	Withhold for 5 days before procedure
	Aspirin	Do not withhold	Do not withhold	Withhold for 5 days before procedure
	LMWH (therapeutic dose)	Withhold one dose before procedure	Withhold one dose before procedure	Withhold for 24 hr or up to two doses

aPTT, Activated partial thromboplastin time; *INR,* international normalized ratio; *IV,* intravenous; *LMWH,* low-molecular-weight heparin; *UFH,* unfractionated heparin.

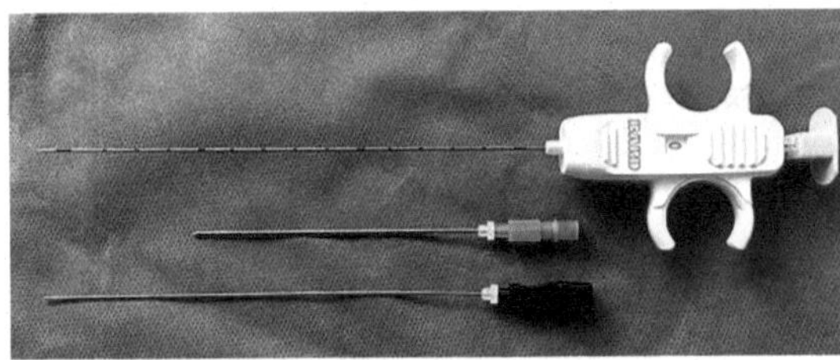

FIGURE 25.1 Lung biopsy tools. Photograph shows a 16-cm, 20-gauge spring-loaded biopsy device; a 10-cm, 19-gauge Chiba Ultrathin introducer needle; and a 15-cm, 22-gauge Chiba needle (*top* to *bottom*). With the stylet removed from the 19-gauge Chiba needle, the 22-gauge needle or a 20-gauge spring-loaded biopsy device can be advanced through the introducer needle.

CT fluoroscopy combines the advantages of standard fluoroscopy with CT guidance.

Percutaneous transthoracic needle biopsy is best performed with a coaxial technique because this allows several specimens to be obtained with only one pleural puncture. To this end, the stylet of a 19-gauge introducer needle can be exchanged for a 22-gauge Chiba needle or a 20-gauge spring-loaded core biopsy device (Fig. 25.1), both of which need to be 5 cm longer than the introducer needle. The length of the introducer needle itself should exceed the depth of the lesion from the skin by 3 to 5 cm to allow for sufficient purchase outside the patient. Extrapleural lesions in the mediastinum and chest wall should be biopsied with a 17-gauge introducer needle in combination with an 18-gauge core biopsy device.

Procedure

Patient positioning is a critical first part of the procedure. It is key to make every effort to ensure the patient is comfortably immobilized in a position that allows access to the target and prevents motion during the procedure. The prone position is preferred because it minimizes chest wall movement, and the patient cannot see the needle. Biopsies are also performed with patients in the supine position, depending on how the target can be accessed without having to traverse a fissure. When planning the needle path, interlobar fissures, pulmonary vessels, bullae, and areas of severe emphysema should be avoided to minimize complications. Review of preprocedure contrast-enhanced CT examinations is helpful to identify vessels, and if a nodule represents an aneurysm or arterial venous malformation, it should not be biopsied. The periphery of consolidations should be targeted to avoid larger vessels. Central lesions are best approached with the needle parallel to major pulmonary arteries and veins. Whereas anterior mediastinal masses are best sampled using a parasternal approach (Fig. 25.2), a paravertebral approach is used for posterior mediastinal lesions (Fig. 25.3). Large masses may contain areas of necrosis that are best visualized with IV contrast (see Fig. 25.2). Such areas should be avoided because they often produce nondiagnostic samples. If a lesion is cystic or cavitary, a tangential approach should be used to sample the wall (Fig. 25.4). Review of a recent positron emission tomography (PET) examination can identify the viable portion of large masses, which should be targeted for maximum yield (see Fig. 25.4).

After the patient has been positioned, conscious sedation should be started. CT slices are then obtained through the lesion with a localizing grid on the overlying skin. In the prone position, internally rotating the shoulders can move the scapula laterally. Ribs, fissures, and large vessels can be moved out of the needle path by tilting the CT gantry (Fig. 25.5). The skin overlying the target is marked, and a sterile field is set up. After the injection of local anesthesia, a small incision is made. The introducer

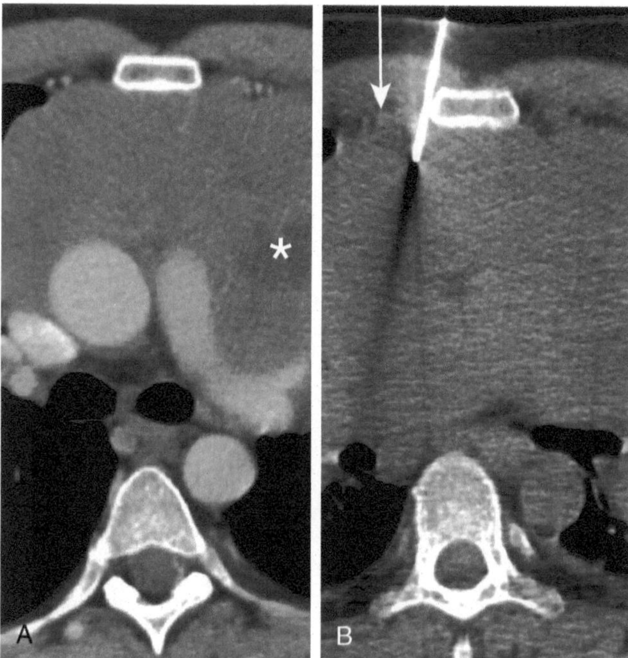

FIGURE 25.2 Parasternal approach. **A,** Diagnostic contrast-enhanced axial computed tomography (CT) image demonstrates a large anterior mediastinal mass with focal hypoattenuation representing necrosis *(asterisk)*. Note the contrast in the internal thoracic arteries. **B,** Intraprocedural CT image with the patient in the supine position demonstrates sampling using a right parasternal approach to avoid the right internal thoracic artery *(arrow)* and sample the solid part of the mass.

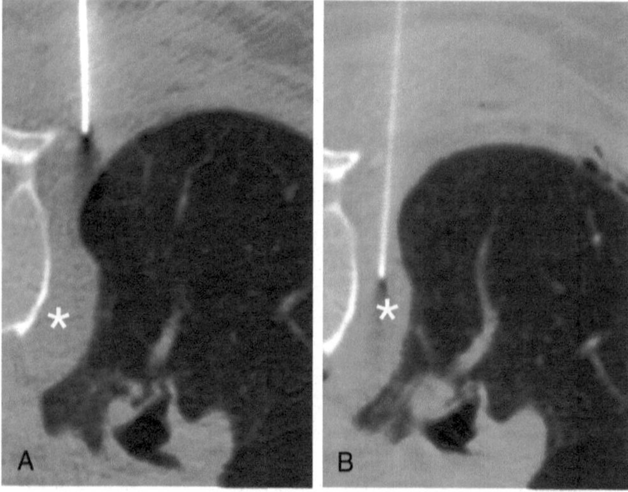

FIGURE 25.3 Hydrodissection. **A,** Axial intraprocedural computed tomography image with the patient in a prone position demonstrates a right paraspinal mass *(asterisk)* and an introducer needle in soft tissues superficial to the pleura. **B,** After hydrodissection to displace the lung laterally, air bubbles are noted in the right extrapleural space, and the introducer needle has been advanced into the right paraspinal mass *(asterisk)* using an extrapleural approach.

needle is advanced through the chest wall in parallel to the CT gantry (Fig. 25.6, *A*). Repeat imaging is performed to check for alignment of the needle with the target and to measure the residual distance from the needle tip to the pleura (Fig. 25.6, *B*). The goal is to perfectly align the introducer needle with the target before puncturing

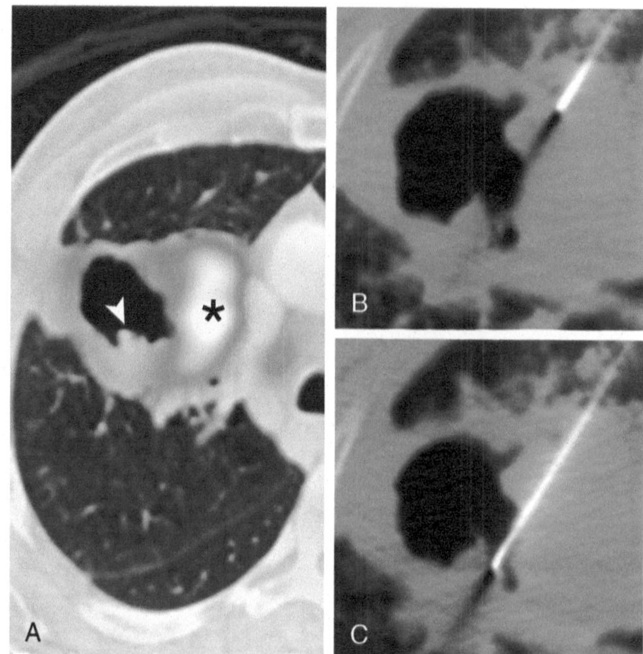

FIGURE 25.4 Cavitary lesion biopsy. **A,** Fused axial contrast-enhanced positron emission tomography/computed tomography (CT) image demonstrates a thick-walled right upper lobe cavitary mass with focal fludeoxyglucose (FDG) uptake in the medial wall *(asterisk)* and debris dependently *(arrowhead)*. **B,** Intraprocedural CT image demonstrates the tangential approach to obtain tissue cores from the FDG-avid solid wall found to be carcinoma. **C,** The needle is redirected to obtain fine-needle aspirates of intracavitary debris, which was superinfection with *Aspergillus*.

the pleura because it is difficult to reposition the needle after the lung is entered, and attempting to do so often produces a pleural tear. The parietal pleura is sensitive to pain, and numbing with lidocaine is advised, especially if the procedure is performed without conscious sedation. The pleura is then punctured by advancing the introducer needle quickly and decisively by about 2 cm. When in the lung, the introducer needle tip is incrementally advanced into the lesion (Fig. 25.6, *C*). The stylet is then exchanged for a 22-gauge aspiration needle a small amount of saline is placed in the introducer needle hub to reduce the risk of air embolism. Through the saline meniscus, a 22-gauge Chiba needle connected to a syringe is advanced into the target. An aspirate is obtained via a series of up-and-down motions and gentle suction to draw cells into the needle (Fig. 25.7). It is important not to move the tip of the introducer needle out of the nodule and not to advance the Chiba needle through the posterior wall of the nodule because this increases the risk of pulmonary hemorrhage. The specimen is expelled on glass slides and immediately handed to a cytopathology technologist. Preliminary rapid onsite evaluation of the fine-needle aspirate may suggest repositioning of the introducer needle and determine what additional samples are required. Additional aspirates can be obtained in saline solution for subsequent preparation of a cellblock or flow cytometry. If onsite cytologic evaluation for malignancy is negative, aspirates should be sent to the microbiology laboratory. Tissue cores increase the chances of establishing the diagnosis of a specific neoplasm and benign lesions. Molecular profiling of lung cancer can

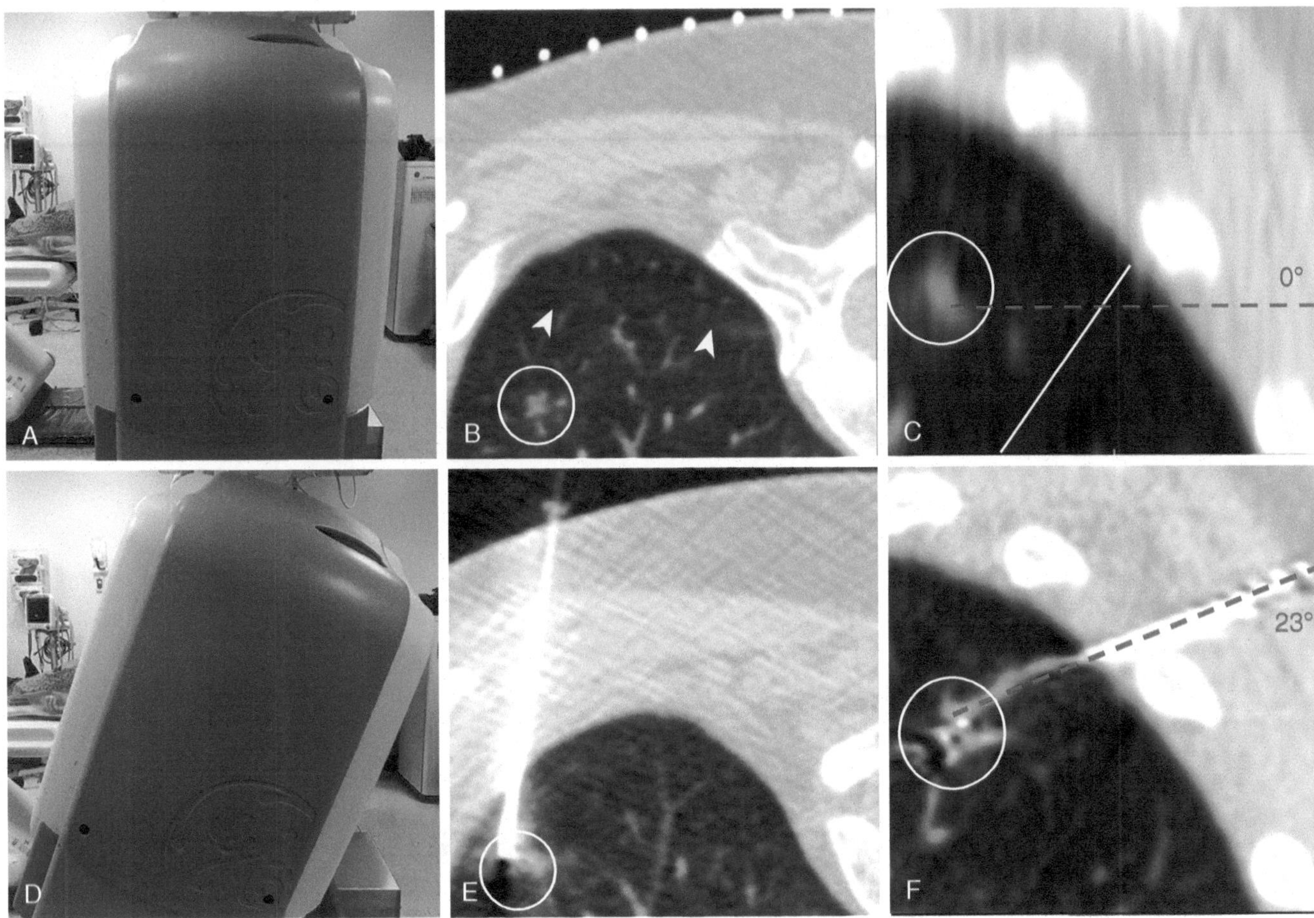

FIGURE 25.5 Computed tomography (CT) gantry angulation. **A,** Photograph shows the CT gantry at 0 degrees. **B,** Axial intraprocedural CT image with the patient in a prone position shows that with the angle at 0 degrees, the major fissure *(arrowheads)* is between the grid overlying the skin and the biopsy target, a right upper lobe ground-glass nodule *(circle)*. **C,** Sagittal reformat confirms that the major fissure (line) is between the skin and the target *(circle)*, along the needle path *(dashed line)*. **D,** Photograph shows the CT gantry angled toward the head of the patient by 23 degrees. **E,** Axial intraprocedural CT image with the patient in a prone position shows that with the CT gantry at 23 degrees, the needle reaches the biopsy target *(circle)* while avoiding the major fissure. **F,** Sagittal reformat confirms that the major fissure *(line)* is no longer in the needle path *(dashed line)* to the target *(circle)*.

be performed with 20-gauge tissue cores or cellblock of fine-needle aspirates. As a general principle, tissue cores should be obtained whenever it is safe, especially in the absence of rapid onsite evaluation during the procedure, and if a benign entity is suspected, such as a hamartoma or granuloma.

Computed tomography images are obtained at the end of the procedure before the introducer needle is removed. If a small pneumothorax is present, air can be aspirated from the pleural space through the introducer needle as it is removed. If a large pneumothorax is present, a chest tube can be placed at this time.

Postprocedure Care

After the needle is removed, patients are immediately rolled over from the CT table onto a stretcher to place the puncture side dependent. The patient remains in this position for 3 hours after the procedure without moving or talking. This position increases atelectasis, decreases lung excursion, and thus maximizes apposition of the pleural surfaces. Oxygen is administered per nasal cannula to accelerate the absorption of intrapleural air. Reducing the partial pressure of nitrogen in the alveoli compared with the pleural space increases the diffusion gradient for nitrogen. Chest radiographs are obtained at 1 hour and 3 hours after the procedure to evaluate for a delayed pneumothorax. If a small pneumothorax is present, it is followed for an additional 2 hours, and if there is no change in size, the patient can be discharged. However, symptomatic or enlarging pneumothoraces require chest tube insertion. There is controversy about whether patients with small-bore chest tubes require admission or are best managed as outpatients. We prefer to admit patients who require a chest tube because many have air leaks that require suction. However, most chest tubes can be removed within 24 to 48 hours. Patients who recover without complications are discharged home accompanied by an escort. They are instructed to immediately seek hospital attention at the nearest emergency department in case of severe chest pain, shortness of breath, or increasing hemoptysis. Continuous positive airway pressure ventilation or bilevel positive airway

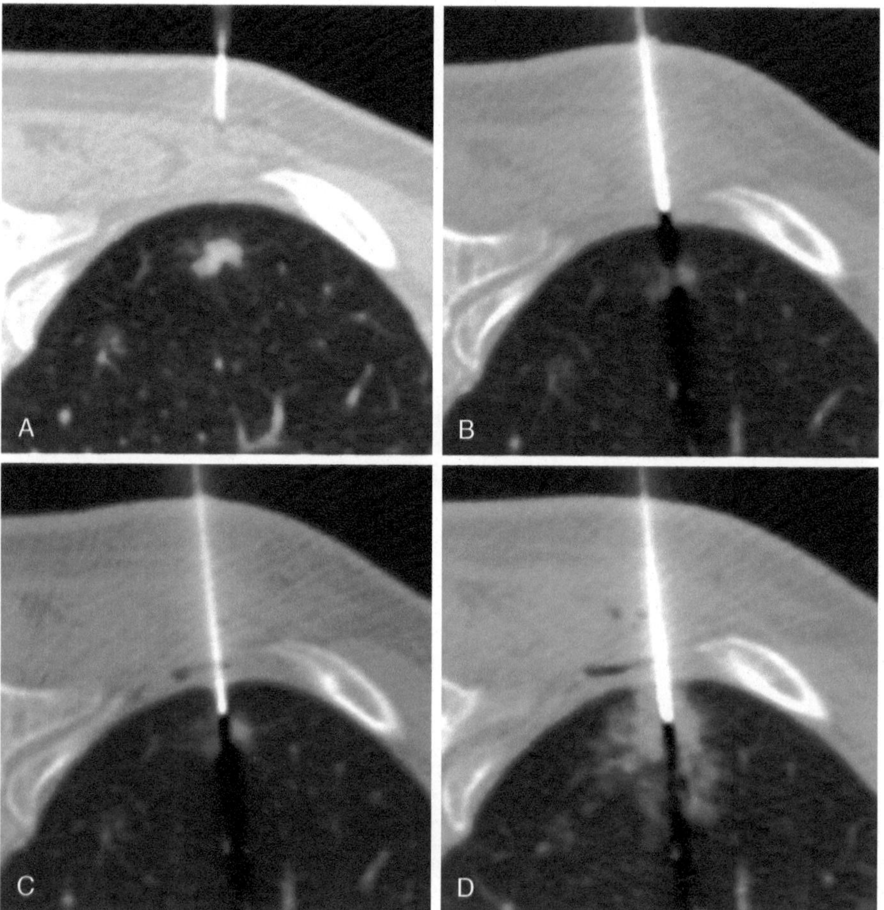

FIGURE 25.6 Introducer needle positioning. **A,** Axial intraprocedural computed tomography image with the patient in a prone position demonstrates a lidocaine needle marking the skin entry site. **B,** The introducer needle is advanced to the pleura. **C,** The pleura is punctured with the introducer needle in perfect alignment with the target. **D,** Blood products around the target may occur after tissue sampling.

BOX 25.2 Summary of Post–Lung Biopsy Care

Roll patient from computed tomography table onto stretcher with the needle entry side in a dependent position immediately upon withdrawing the introducer needle.

Lie on needle entry site for 3 hours without moving or talking.

Continue oxygen per nasal cannula at 2 L/min.

Obtain chest radiographs 1 hour and 3 hours post procedure to exclude delayed pneumothorax.

Discharge with escort with instructions to refrain from strenuous activity for 48 hours.

Resume blood thinners after 24 hours. Continue all other medications immediately.

pressure ventilation should be discontinued for at least 24 hours after PTNB to prevent a delayed pneumothorax. Postprocedure care is summarized in Box 25.2.

Complications

The most common complications of PTNB are pneumothorax and hemoptysis (Table 25.2). Pneumothorax has been reported in 0% to 60% of patients, with an average of approximately 20%. Risk factors for the development of pneumothorax include the size and depth of the lesion, the presence of emphysema and COPD, the number of pleural punctures, and the transgression of a fissure. Whereas most small pneumothoraces resolve without intervention, larger pneumothoraces require aspiration or chest tube insertion. The percentage of pneumothoraces requiring chest tube insertion ranges from about 2% to 15%. The risk of pneumothorax decreases when lesions are sampled without traversing aerated lung. For this reason, an extrapleural approach should be chosen whenever possible. The injection of saline (hydrodissection) can create or widen an extrapleural path by displacing the lung (see Fig. 25.3).

A small amount of pulmonary hemorrhage surrounding the biopsy target is common (Fig. 25.6, *D*). Hemoptysis occurs in 1% to 10% of cases and is usually mild and self-limited. Because blood is a strong irritant of the airways, even a small amount of hemorrhage can lead to coughing. Airway obstruction can lead to cardiorespiratory arrest. The procedure should be aborted if the cough cannot be controlled with small doses of fentanyl IV. Patients with significant hemorrhage should be placed biopsy side down to prevent transbronchial aspiration of blood into the contralateral lung. Encouraging coughing and suctioning the mouth will help clear the airway. The patient may need bronchoscopy to help clear the airways. As a last resort, lobe-selective bronchial blockade can be attempted

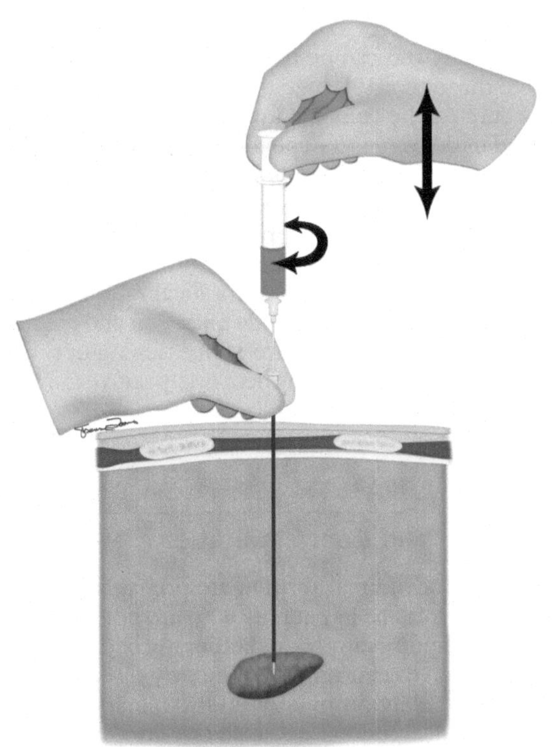

FIGURE 25.7 Fine-needle aspiration technique. Illustration shows how the fine needle is advanced into the target through the introducer needle. Note that the introducer needle tip is just within the lesion. Aspirate is obtained by moving the fine needle into the nodule while performing a combination of up–down and rotatory motions and applying gentle suction with the syringe. Note how the other hand stabilizes the introducer needle hub to prevent inadvertent dislodgment. The introducer needle hub had been filled with saline before removal of the stylet to prevent air embolism.

TABLE 25.2 **Complications of Lung Biopsy by Likelihood**

Complication	Average Likelihood (%)
Pneumothorax	20
Pneumothorax requiring chest tube insertion	5
Hemoptysis	5
Hemothorax	1.5
Tract seeding	0.6
Death	0.15
Air embolism	0.06–0.4

Sources: Manhire A, Charig M, Clelland C, et al. Guidelines for radiologically guided lung biopsy. Thorax 2003;58(11):920-936; AJR Am J Roentgenol 2011;196(6); Wiener RS, Wiener DC, Gould MK. Risks of transthoracic needle biopsy: how high? Clin Pulm Med 2013;20(1):29-35.

by combining a double-lumen endotracheal tube with a bronchial blocker. Hemothorax is rare unless the patient has a bleeding diathesis.

Malignant seeding of the biopsy track is rare and has been reported in malignant pleural tumors such as mesothelioma. The use of an introducer needle with a coaxial technique provides protection from seeding.

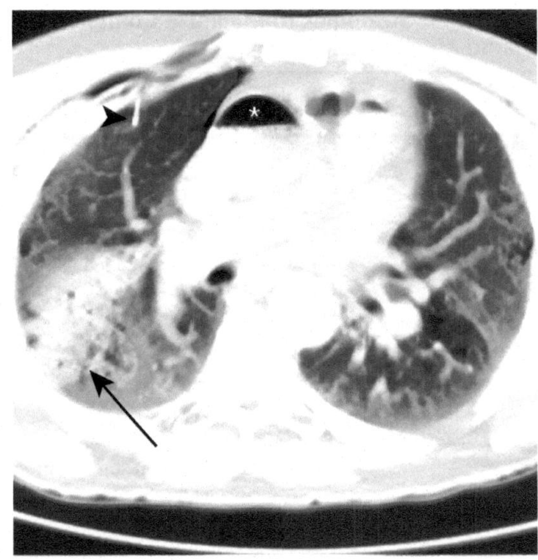

FIGURE 25.8 Air embolism. Axial computed tomography image obtained during lung biopsy at an outside hospital with the patient in a supine position demonstrates an air–blood level in the ascending aorta *(asterisk)*. Part of the biopsy needle is seen in the right upper lobe *(arrowhead)*, and hemorrhage is noted dependently *(arrow)*. Small pneumothorax is present.

Systemic arterial air embolism is another rare complication that may result in myocardial infarction, stroke, and death (Fig. 25.8). The mechanism is presumed to be air entry from the needle, cavity, or airway into a pulmonary vein, precipitated by coughing and positive-pressure ventilation. Keeping saline in the introducer needle during fine-needle aspiration and core needle biopsy likely lessens the danger of air embolism. If a patient becomes unresponsive during the procedure or air is seen in vessels, the patient should be placed in the left lateral decubitus position with the head down, and 100% oxygen should be administered. Strategies to minimize complications are summarized in Table 25.3.

PERCUTANEOUS LOCALIZATION TECHNIQUES

Minimally invasive surgical techniques such as VATS can access the lung through several small incisions between the ribs. Avoidance of a thoracotomy is associated with decreased morbidity and mortality. VATS does not allow the surgeon to palpate the whole lung, and lesion identification may be difficult, particularly for small, deep, or ground-glass attenuation nodules. It has been reported that up to 40% of VATS resections require conversion to open procedures. Image-guided placement of markers can aid in the localization of small tumors for minimally invasive surgical resection or radiation therapy.

Markers used for percutaneous CT-guided preoperative localization include wires, liquids, radioisotopes, and fiducials. The methods of wire localization include hook wires, which are traditionally used in breast localization, and micro-coils, originally developed for vascular embolization. A coaxial needle is used to place the marker in or adjacent to the nodule; the hook wire comes out onto the patient's skin, and the micro-coil end sits coiled in the pleural space. The patient is transferred to the operating room (OR), and the surgeon uses the position of the wire as a map from

TABLE 25.3 Strategies to Minimize Complications From Lung and Mediastinal Biopsy

Complication	Strategies to Decrease Risk
Pneumothorax	• Single pleural puncture • Patient immobilization • Constant respirations (no breath-holding maneuvers) • No talking or coughing during procedure • If possible, choose extrapleural approach • If bilateral lesions, select side of prior surgery • Consider blood patch or pleural plug • Drain pleural effusion prior to biopsy • Recover lying on the pleural puncture site without talking or coughing
Hemorrhage	• Optimize coagulation profile • Avoid proximal segmental vessels >4 mm; vessels are best seen on preprocedure contrast-enhanced CT • Position needle tip within lesion
Air embolus	• Use saline seal during needle exchange • Avoid pulmonary veins • Patient immobilization • Constant respirations (no breath-holding maneuvers) • No talking or coughing during procedure
Nondiagnostic sample	• Target solid part and avoid areas of necrosis • Send aspirate to microbiology if rapid onsite cytology evaluation is negative for malignancy • Obtain tissue cores of solid lesions, especially if benign etiology is suspected • Follow-up imaging of patients with discordant result

CT, Computed tomography.

the pleura through the lung to the nodule. The wire may be associated with patient discomfort, and the route of entry is determined by the surgical approach, rather than a radiologist's preference, which may lead to difficulties in placement.

Liquid markers that have been used for localization include methylene blue dye, barium, and lipiodol. These are injected into or adjacent to the nodule. The methylene blue is also injected along the coaxial needle path as it is removed to mark an entry point in the pleura that the surgeon can follow toward the nodule. Methylene blue quickly diffuses through the parenchyma, and immediate transfer to the OR is necessary. Barium and lipiodol are identified by fluoroscopy in the operating room. They do not diffuse through the lung parenchyma, so a temporal delay in removal is not such a problem, but they can induce an intense inflammatory reaction that can affect histologic evaluation. Anaphylactic reactions have also been reported with use of these liquid markers.

The most common radioisotope marker used for preoperative localization is technetium-99M (Tc-99M) labeled macroaggregated albumin (traditionally used in perfusion studies). The radioisotope is mixed with nonionic iodinated contrast to allow CT confirmation of its position after injection. The radioisotope, and therefore the nodule, is located in the OR with a handheld Geiger counter. There is reported difficulty in identifying deep lesions, and the 6-hour half-life of Tc-99M necessitates surgical excision of the nodule within 6 to 12 hours.

Fiducial markers consist of 3- and 5-mm gold seeds that are inert and can be deposited into or adjacent to the nodule through a 19-gauge coaxial needle (Fig. 25.9). The procedure can be combined with a biopsy if requested. The method of delivery is independent of the surgical approach, and because the gold seeds are inert, they can remain in the lung for many days before surgery. In the OR, they are easily identified at fluoroscopy, and an image of the wedge resection specimen can confirm complete excision. An identical technique is used for localization planning for radiation. Complications include migration and embolization into airways and vessels. Careful positioning of the coaxial needle before fiducial deployment is imperative in preventing these complications.

THERMAL ABLATION

Indications and Contraindications

Indications for thermal ablation are primary and secondary thoracic neoplasms in patients who are not candidates for surgery, chemotherapy, or radiotherapy because of comorbidities or have recurrent or refractory disease after these treatments. Selection by a multidisciplinary tumor board is advised. Ideal lesions are small (<3 cm), but microwave ablation can successfully treat larger lesions (Table 25.4). Pain palliation due to chest wall invasion is another indication. Chest wall lesions are best treated with cryoablation.

Contraindications are similar to those for lung and mediastinal biopsy (see Box 25.1). Consensus guidelines suggest that the bleeding risk is moderate or significant, depending on the complexity of the case. Coagulopathy should be evaluated and managed accordingly (see Table 25.1).

Tools and Technical Principles

Thermal ablation can be performed using heat (radiofrequency and microwave) or cold (cryoablation). Radiofrequency and microwave ablation convert the energy of electromagnetic waves into heat. Temperatures above 60°C cause cell death by irreversible protein denaturation and coagulation necrosis. Cryoablation relies on the rapid release of argon gas to create temperatures as low as −140°C, while subsequent release of helium thaws the tissue. A cycle of freezing and thawing causes destruction of tissue.

Sedation Plan

Conscious sedation or general anesthesia is required in addition to local anesthesia to guarantee patient immobility and analgesia. An adequate effect can be achieved with a combination of IV fentanyl and midazolam administered in small doses during probe placement, with the addition of IV meperidine during treatment. Cryoablation requires less pain medication because of the inherent analgesia induced by freezing. General anesthesia is reserved for patients who have airway abnormalities, require continuous oxygen therapy, and cannot be positioned comfortably otherwise.

Procedure

Planning the treatment area and type and number of probes required to ablate the tumor plus a safety margin is the first

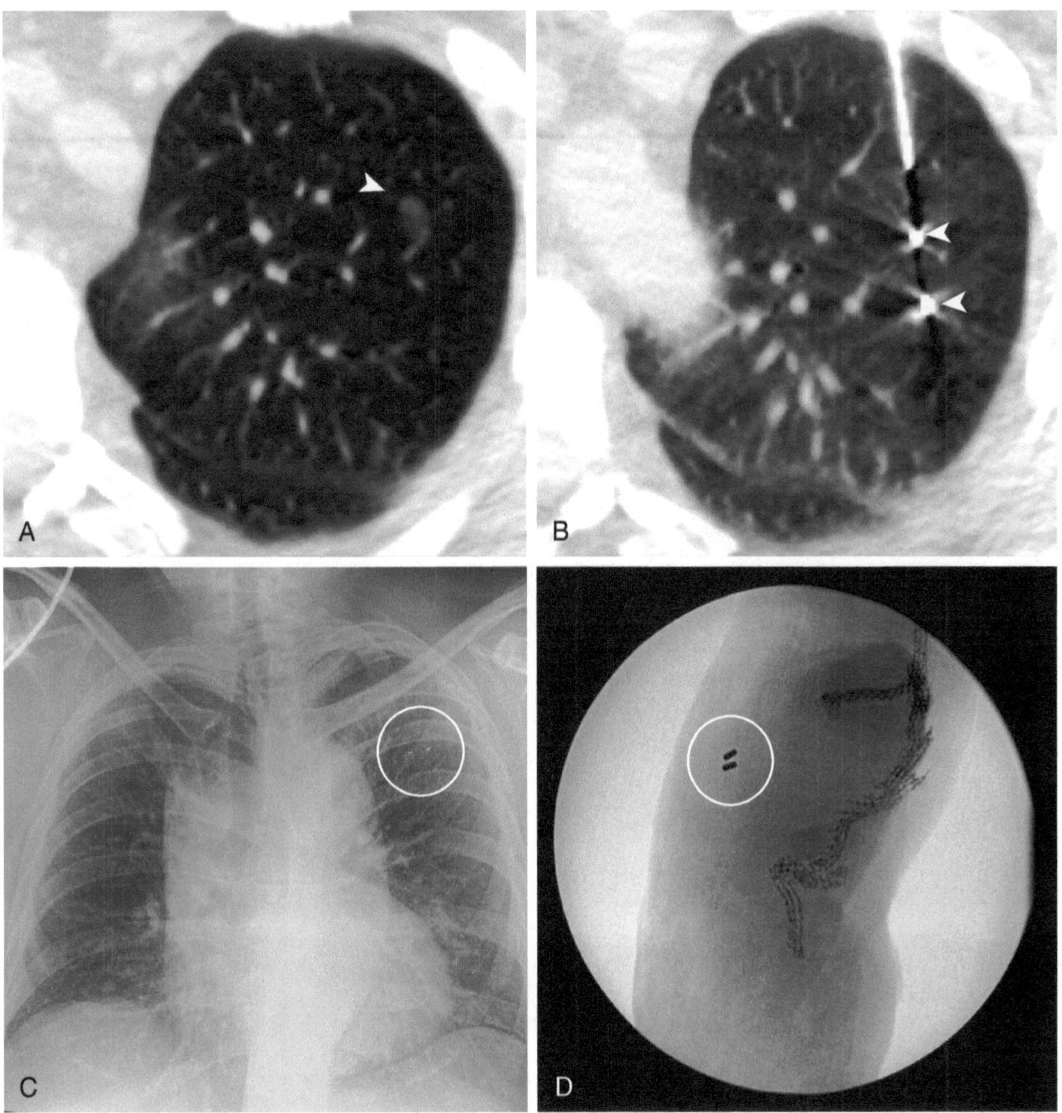

FIGURE 25.9 Fiducial placement. **A,** Axial intraprocedural computed tomography image with the patient in a supine position shows an enlarging 8-mm left upper lobe ground-glass nodule *(arrowhead)*. **B,** Two gold fiducial markers *(arrowheads)* are placed on either side of the nodule using a coaxial needle. **C,** Preoperative chest radiograph confirms two markers unchanged in position *(circle)*. **D,** Radiograph of wedge resection specimen shows two fiducial markers in the specimen *(circle)*, during excision of the adjacent adenocarcinoma.

TABLE 25.4 **Comparison of Perceived Advantages and Disadvantages of Thermal Ablation Techniques**

	Radiofrequency	Microwave	Cryoablation
Coverage of lesions ≤3 cm	++	+++	+++
Coverage of lesions >3 cm	+	+++	++
Lung lesions ≤1.5 cm from pleura	+ (pain)	+ (air leak)	+++
Chest wall lesions	+	++	+++
Mediastinal lesions	+	+	++
Predictability of treatment zone	++(+)	+	++(+)
Compatibility with pacer or AICD and surgical clips	No	Some issues	No issues

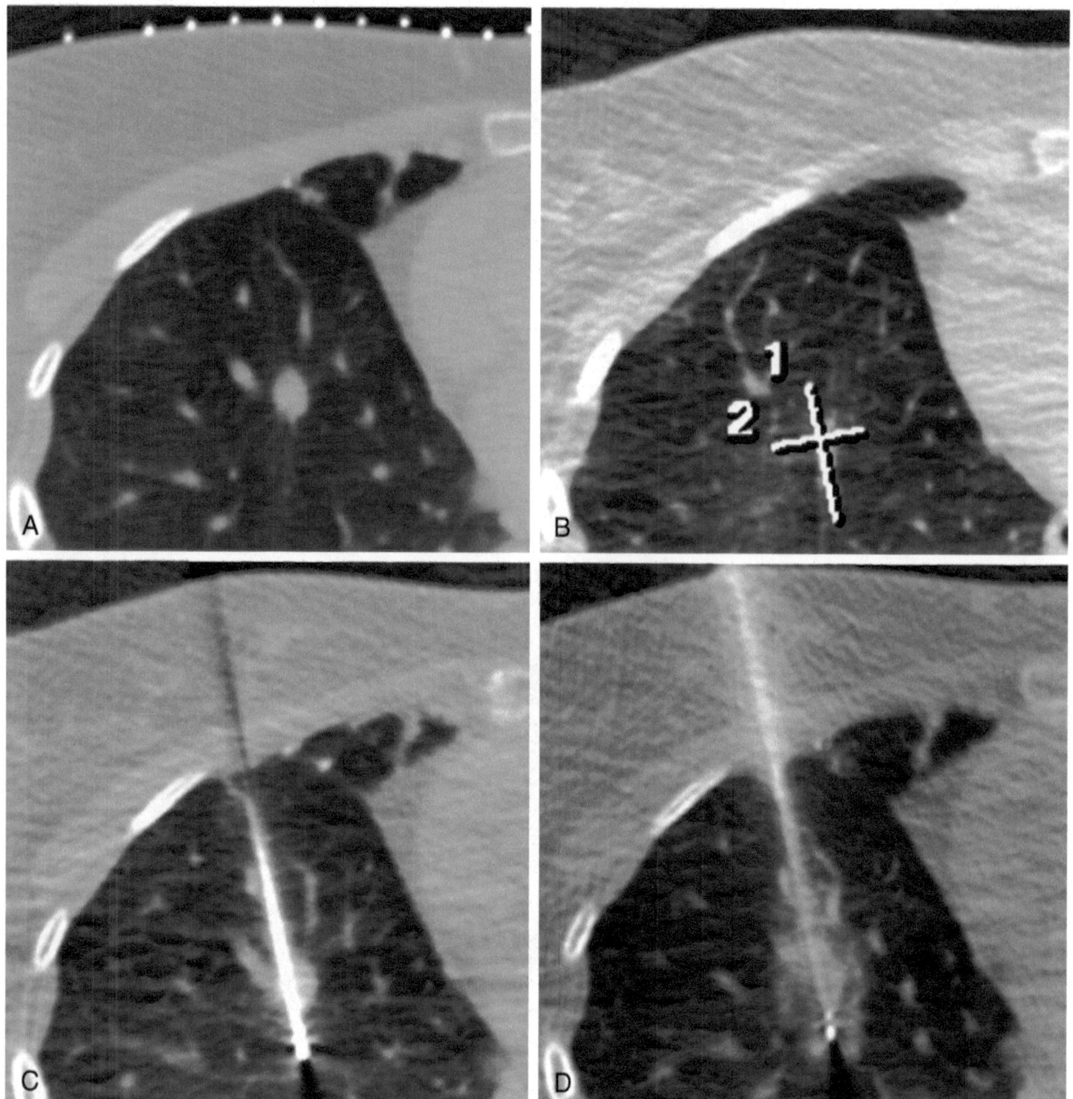

FIGURE 25.10 Thermal ablation of a middle lobe 10 mm adeno carcinoma. **A,** Axial intraprocedural computed tomography image with the patient in a supine position demonstrates a grid on the skin overlying a right lower lobe 1.2-cm lung cancer. **B,** Calipers indicate the dimension of the desired ablation zone. **C,** A radiofrequency ablation electrode is placed through the center of the nodule with the tip beyond the nodule. **D,** Ground-glass opacities around the nodule after completion of the treatment indicate an adequate treatment zone, which encompasses the target.

crucial step. Details depend on the particular modality and design of the ablation probe(s) used. The steps involved in placement of ablation probes are the same as those for introducer needle placement for biopsy. After treatment is started, it is important to frequently monitor the size of the treatment zone. A halo of ground-glass opacity is seen around treated parenchymal tumors (Fig. 25.10).

Postprocedure Care

In addition to care that would be rendered after a biopsy, ablation patients are usually admitted for overnight observation to control pain and monitor for complications. Imaging follow up includes contrast-enhanced CT with or without fludeoxyglucose PET to detect complications and recurrence. Successfully treated lesions are expected to gradually decrease in size (Fig. 25.11). Irregular nodular peripheral enhancement measuring more than 10 mm, growth of the ablation zone after 3 months, and enlargement of regional or distant lymph nodes after 6 months may indicate residual or recurrent disease (Fig. 25.12).

Complications

Structures such as chest wall, nerves, bones, esophagus, pericardium, and bronchi can be damaged during thermal ablation. Blood flow in vessels close to the tumor creates a "thermal sync" by taking heat (or cold) away from the tumor, which can result in inadequate treatment. Pneumothorax, pulmonary hemorrhage, hemoptysis, pleural effusion, persistent air leak, and infection are possible. Pacemakers and intracardiac defibrillators can malfunction because of interference with electromagnetic waves. The likelihood of complications varies by treatment modality (Table 25.5). In addition, the patient may experience a

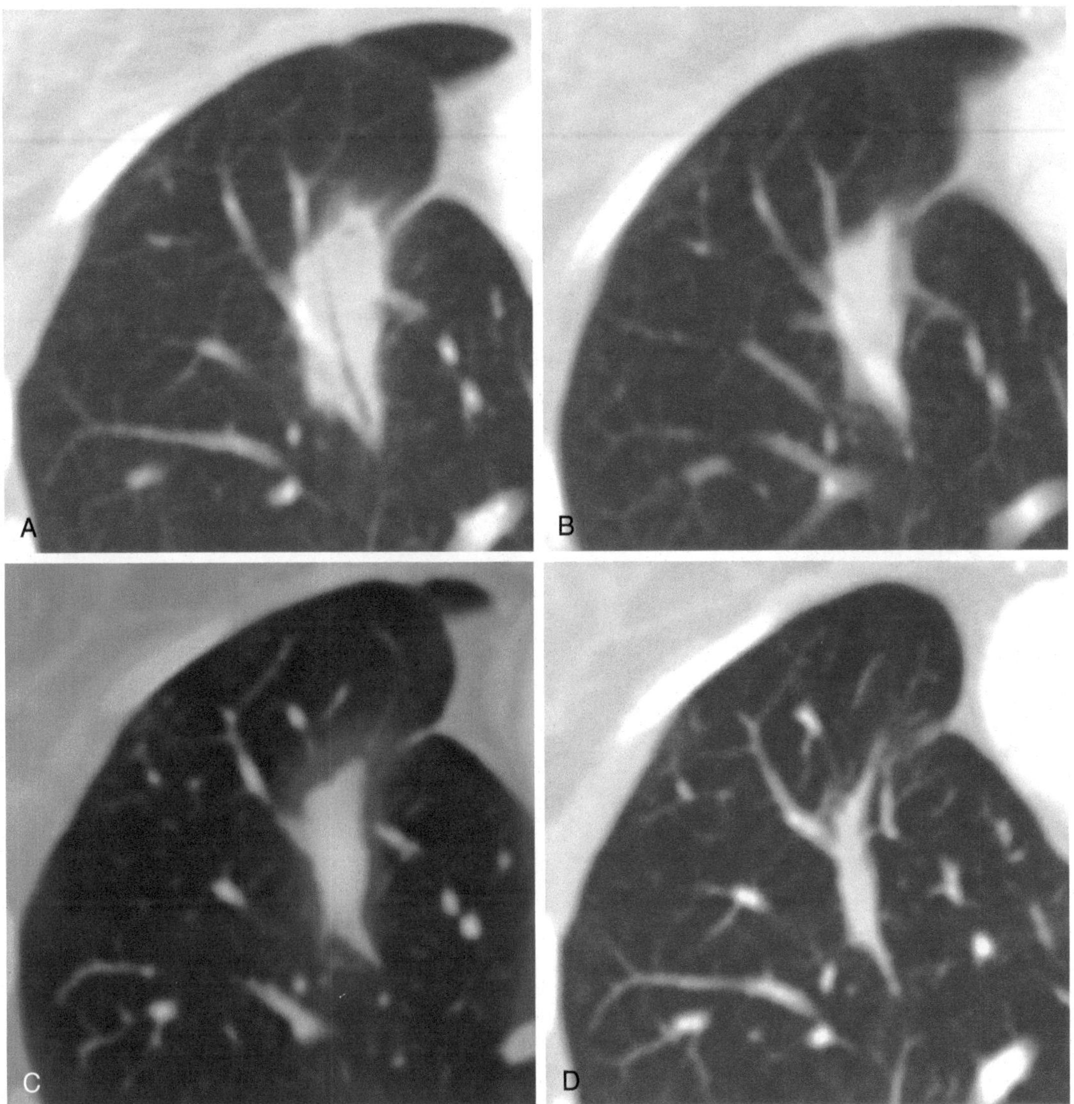

FIGURE 25.11 Expected findings after radiofrequency ablation (RFA) of a right lower lobe lung cancer in the same patient. **A,** Axial computed tomography (CT) image at 1 month after RFA demonstrates the postablation zone. **B,** At 3 months, the postablation zone has decreased in size. **C,** At 6 months, axial fused positron emission tomography/CT image shows uniform fludeoxyglucose uptake and further decrease of the postablation zone. **D,** At 15 months, the postablation zone continues to decrease in size.

TABLE 25.5 **Likelihood of Complications Associated With Thermal Ablation Techniques**

	Radiofrequency	Microwave	Cryoablation
Thermal sink	+++	+	++
Pain	+++	++	+
Bleeding	++	+	+++
Bronchopleural fistula	+++	+++	+

postablation syndrome with flulike symptoms the first week after the procedure. Skin burns can occur if the radiofrequency grounding pads are placed incorrectly. Hemothorax, acute respiratory distress syndrome, cardiac arrhythmias, air embolus, transient mediastinal nerve injury, and death are rare.

THORACENTESIS AND PLEURAL DRAINAGE

Indications and Contraindications

Diagnostic thoracentesis is indicated to determine the cause of pleural fluid. Therapeutic thoracentesis provides symptomatic relief for patients with large pleural effusions.

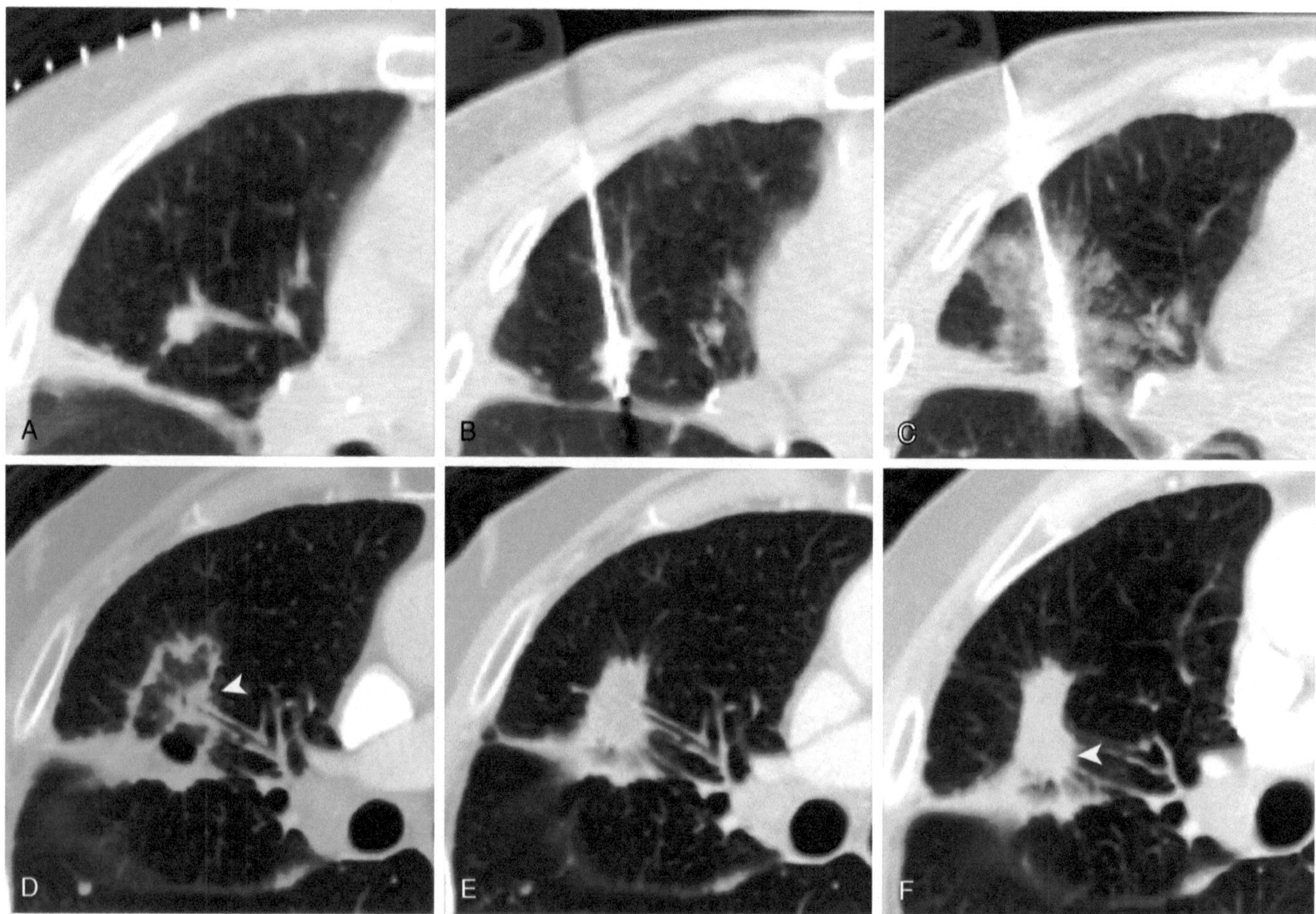

FIGURE 25.12 Recurrent disease after radiofrequency ablation (RFA). **A,** Axial intraprocedural computed tomography image with the patient in a supine position shows a 10-mm right upper lobe nodule. **B,** Placement of an 18-gauge RFA electrode through the lesion. **C,** Ground-glass opacity surrounding the lesion immediately after the procedure indicates an adequate ablation zone. **D,** At 1 month after ablation, there is an expected reverse halo sign. The treated nodule is visible in the medial edge of the postablation zone *(arrowhead)*. An adjacent vessel is likely to have reduced the treatment zone around the nodule because of heat sink effect. **E,** At 6 months post ablation, there is expected contraction of the treatment zone laterally. **F,** At 12 months post ablation, there is eccentric growth in the medial edge of the postablation zone, indicating a recurrent tumor *(arrowhead)*, confirmed to represent a 1-cm adenocarcinoma at right upper lobectomy.

Drainage (chest tube thoracostomy or insertion) is indicated to evacuate pneumothorax, loculated pleural effusion, and blood products, especially when infection is suspected.

Contraindications include an uncooperative patient and uncorrectable coagulopathy. Consensus guidelines suggest that bleeding risk is low for thoracentesis and moderate for chest tube insertion. Coagulopathy should be evaluated and managed accordingly (see Table 25.1).

Tools and Technical Principles

Diagnostic thoracentesis can be performed with a 20-gauge needle. A 7-French catheter works well for therapeutic thoracentesis. The diameter and number of catheters required for drainage vary by indication: Whereas a single 12-French catheter is sufficient to evacuate a pneumothorax, at least one 16-French catheter is required to drain a hemothorax or empyema (Fig. 25.13) because fluid is more viscous.

Sampling of large layering pleural effusions may not require image guidance. Ultrasound guidance increases the likelihood of obtaining a diagnostic sample if the pleural effusion is small while decreasing the risk of pneumothorax. CT is reserved for drainage of loculated pleural effusions to minimize the risk of bleeding and bronchopleural fistula.

Sedation Plan

Local anesthesia is sufficient for thoracentesis. Conscious sedation should be considered for insertion of drainage catheters.

Procedure

If possible, the patient should sit on the side of the bed and lean over a side table to open up the intercostal spaces. If the patient cannot sit upright, the procedure can be performed in the lateral decubitus position with the fluid-filled side down. Imaging is used to visualize the largest fluid pocket, and the entry point is marked on the overlying skin. The trajectory should be above the rib to avoid injury of the intercostal neurovascular bundle. After sterilizing the field, local anesthesia is provided to skin and parietal pleura using 15 cc of 1% lidocaine. The catheter is then inserted either over a wire (Seldinger technique) or mounted on a trocar. The catheter is secured by hand, and samples are obtained for analysis. Pleural fluid should be sent to the laboratory to evaluate Light's criteria (cholesterol, lactate dehydrogenase, and protein), and a sample should be sent to the microbiology laboratory with a request for Gram stain and cultures with sensitivities. A third sample should be sent for cytology and cell count in patients older than 35 years of age with large pleural effusions of unknown etiology. Fluid can be removed for therapeutic purposes by connecting the catheter to vacuum bottles. Chest tubes are secured to the skin with silk sutures and connected to a chest drainage system. Cloth tape is used to secure all connections of the catheter to the chest drainage system. The chest drainage system is initially set to water seal and kept below the patient to facilitate evacuation of fluid.

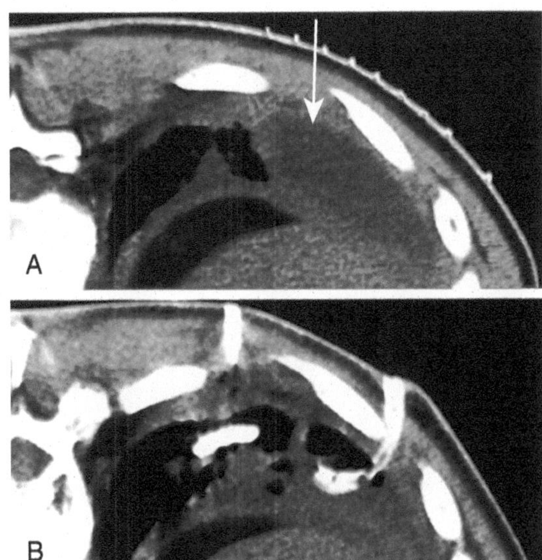

FIGURE 25.13 Empyema drainage. **A,** Axial intraprocedural computed tomography image with the patient in a prone position demonstrates a grid on the skin over right pleural thickening *(arrow)* surrounding loculated pleural fluid consistent with an empyema. **B,** Empyema was evacuated with two chest tubes.

Postprocedure Care

A chest radiograph should be obtained to evaluate for residual fluid, reexpansion pulmonary edema, and pneumothorax, as well as to document the position of any drainage catheters. Chest drainage systems should be connected to wall suction at 20 cm H_2O and tubing should be flushed with 20 cc of sterile saline every 8 hours to prevent clogging. Daily chest radiographs should be obtained to assess for tube migration and residual fluid or air. Instillation of tissue plasminogen activator or DNase through indwelling chest tube(s) helps to break up internal septations and facilitates complete drainage. Refractory fluid pockets can be addressed by placing additional catheters under CT guidance. The decision to remove a chest tube is based on the reason that the tube was placed, imaging findings, and current output (Fig. 25.14). Chest tubes can be removed at the bedside while the patient is exhaling or humming.

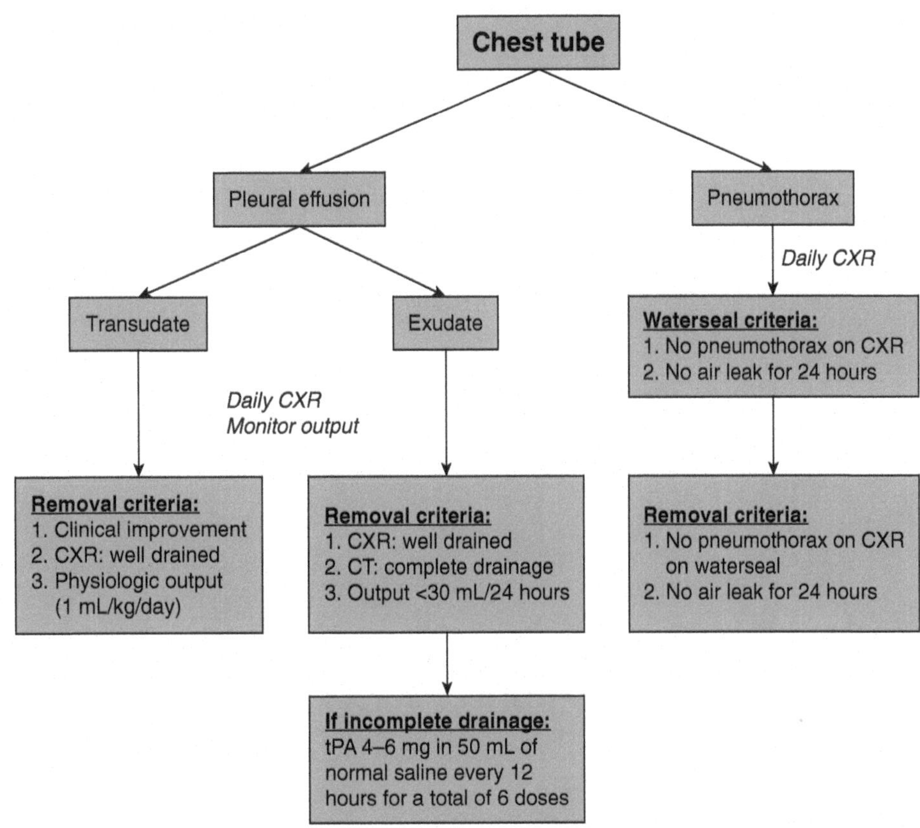

FIGURE 25.14 Criteria for chest tube removal. *CT,* Computed tomography; *CXR,* chest radiography; *tPA,* tissue plasminogen activator. (Adapted from McDermott S, Levis DA, Arellano RS. Chest drainage. Semin Intervent Radiol 2012;29(4):247-255. Thieme Medical Publishers Inc. www.thieme.com; reprinted by permission.)

The site should be covered with a dry airtight dressing. It is prudent to obtain a chest radiograph after drain removal to document the absence of a pneumothorax.

Complications

Risks of thoracentesis include pain, bleeding, and infection, as well as pneumothorax. Patients are likely to experience the urge to cough after about 500 cc of fluid has been removed and the lung starts to reexpand. Rapid removal of large fluid volumes (>1 L) may result in unilateral reexpansion pulmonary edema. Chest tube insertion can result in airway injury if the tube enters the lung parenchyma, manifested as an air leak despite tight tubing connections. Consent for chest tube insertion should include the fact that the dwell time of the tube is unknown.

SUGGESTED READINGS

Dupuy DE. Image-guided thermal ablation of lung malignancies. *Radiology*. 2011;260:633-655.

Klein JS, Zarka MA. Transthoracic needle biopsy. *Radiol Clin North Am*. 2000;38:235-266, vii.

McDermott S, Levis DA, Arellano RS. Chest drainage. *Semin Intervent Radiol*. 2012;29:247-255.

O'Neill AC, et al. Rapid needle-out patient-rollover time after percutaneous CT-guided transthoracic biopsy of lung nodules: effect on pneumothorax rate. *Radiology*. 2012;262:314-319.

Patel IJ, Davidson JC, Nikolic B, et al. Consensus guidelines for periprocedural management of coagulation status and hemostasis risk in percutaneous image-guided interventions. *J Vasc Interv Radiol*. 2012;23(6):727-736.

Sharma A, Abtin F, Shepard J-AO. Image-guided ablative therapies for lung cancer. *Radiol Clin North Am*. 2012;50:975-999.

Sharma A, et al. Increase in fluorodeoxyglucose positron emission tomography activity following complete radiofrequency ablation of lung tumors. *J Comput Assist Tomogr*. 2013;37:9-14.

Wilcox ME, et al. Does this patient have an exudative pleural effusion? *JAMA*. 2014;311:2422.

Wu CC, Maher MM, Shepard J-AO. CT-guided percutaneous needle biopsy of the chest: preprocedural evaluation and technique. *AJR Am J Roentgenol*. 2011;196:W511-W514.

Wu CC, Maher MM, Shepard J-AO. Complications of CT-guided percutaneous needle biopsy of the chest: prevention and management. *AJR Am J Roentgenol*. 2011;196:W678-W682.

Index

Page numbers followed by "*b*" indicate boxes, "*f*" indicate figures and "*t*" indicate tables.

C

D

E

F

G

H

M

N

T